坎贝尔骨科手术学
手外科

Campbell's Operative Orthopaedics

第 14 版
（影印版）

Frederick M. Azar, MD

James H. Beaty, MD

人民卫生出版社
·北京·

图书在版编目（CIP）数据

坎贝尔骨科手术学 . 手外科 : 英文 /（美）弗雷德
里克·M.阿扎尔（Frederick M. Azar），（美）詹姆斯·
H. 比蒂（James H. Beaty）主编 . —影印本 . —北京：
人民卫生出版社，2021.12

ISBN 978-7-117-32518-9

Ⅰ. ①坎⋯　Ⅱ. ①弗⋯　②詹⋯　Ⅲ. ①骨科学 – 外科
手术 – 英文②手 – 外科手术 – 英文　Ⅳ. ①R68

中国版本图书馆 CIP 数据核字（2021）第 241279 号

人卫智网	www.ipmph.com	医学教育、学术、考试、健康，
		购书智慧智能综合服务平台
人卫官网	www.pmph.com	人卫官方资讯发布平台

图字：01–2021–6747 号

坎贝尔骨科手术学
手　外　科

Kanbeier Guke Shoushuxue
Shou Waike

主　　编：Frederick M. Azar　James H. Beaty
出版发行：人民卫生出版社（中继线 010-59780011）
地　　址：北京市朝阳区潘家园南里 19 号
邮　　编：100021
E - mail：pmph @ pmph.com
购书热线：010-59787592　010-59787584　010-65264830
印　　刷：三河市宏达印刷有限公司（胜利）
经　　销：新华书店
开　　本：889×1194　1/16　　印张：40.5
字　　数：1928 千字
版　　次：2021 年 12 月第 1 版
印　　次：2022 年 1 月第 1 次印刷
标准书号：ISBN 978-7-117-32518-9
定　　价：516.00 元

打击盗版举报电话：**010-59787491**　**E-mail：WQ @ pmph.com**
质量问题联系电话：**010-59787234**　**E-mail：zhiliang @ pmph.com**

坎贝尔骨科手术学
手外科

Campbell's Operative Orthopaedics

第 14 版
（影印版）

Frederick M. Azar, MD

Professor

Department of Orthopaedic Surgery and Biomedical Engineering University of Tennessee–Campbell Clinic

Chief of Staff, Campbell Clinic

Memphis, Tennessee

James H. Beaty, MD

Harold B. Boyd Professor and Chair

Department of Orthopaedic Surgery and Biomedical Engineering University of Tennessee–Campbell Clinic

Memphis, Tennessee

Editorial Assistance

Kay Daugherty *and* **Linda Jones**

人民卫生出版社
·北 京·

Elsevier (Singapore) Pte Ltd.
3 Killiney Road,
#08–01 Winsland House I,
Singapore 239519
ELSEVIER Tel:（65）6349–0200; Fax:（65）6733–1817

This English Reprint of Part ⅩⅧ from Campbell's Operative Orthopaedics, 14E by Frederick M. Azar and James H. Beaty was undertaken by People's Medical Publishing House and is published by arrangement with Elsevier (Singapore) Pte Ltd.

Part ⅩⅧ from Campbell's Operative Orthopaedics, 14E by Frederick M. Azar and James H. Beaty由人民卫生出版社进行影印，并根据人民卫生出版社与爱思唯尔（新加坡）私人有限公司的协议约定出版。

Notice

Practitioners and researchers must always rely on their own experience and knowledge in evaluating and using any information, methods, compounds or experiments described herein. Because of rapid advances in the medical sciences, in particular, independent verification of diagnoses and drug dosages should be made. To the fullest extent of the law, no responsibility is assumed by Elsevier, authors, editors or contributors in relation to the adaptation or for any injury and/or damage to persons or property as a matter of products liability, negligence or otherwise, or from any use or operation of any methods, products, instructions, or ideas contained in the material herein.

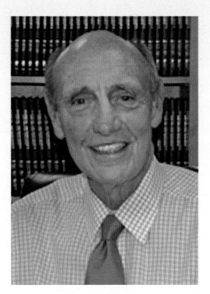

S. Terry Canale, MD

It is with humble appreciation and admiration that we dedicate this edition of *Campbell's Operative Orthopaedics* to Dr. S. Terry Canale, who served as editor or co-editor of five editions. He took great pride in this position and worked tirelessly to continue to improve "The Book." As noted by one of his co-editors, "Terry is probably the only person in the world who has read every word of multiple editions of *Campbell's Operative Orthopaedics*." He considered *Campbell's Operative Orthopaedics* an opportunity for worldwide orthopaedic education and made it a priority to ensure that each edition provided valuable and up-to-date information. His commitment to and enthusiasm for this work will continue to influence and inspire every future edition.

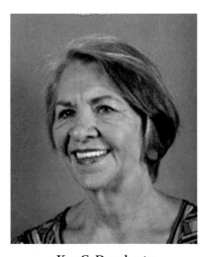

Kay C. Daugherty

It is with equal appreciation and regard that we dedicate this edition to Kay C. Daugherty, the managing editor of the last nine editions *Campbell's Operative Orthopaedics*. Over the last 40 years, she has faithfully and tirelessly edited, reshaped, and overseen all aspects of publication from manuscript preparation to proofing. She has a profound talent to put ideas and disjointed words into comprehensible text, ensuring that each revision maintains the gold standard in readability. Each edition is a testament to her dedication to excellence in writing and education. A favorite quote of Mrs. Daugherty to one of our late authors was, "I'll make a deal. I won't operate if you won't punctuate." We are grateful for her many years of continual service to the Campbell Foundation and for the publications yet to come.

CONTRIBUTORS

FREDERICK M. AZAR, MD
Professor
Director, Sports Medicine Fellowship
University of Tennessee–Campbell Clinic
Department of Orthopaedic Surgery and
  Biomedical Engineering
Chief-of-Staff, Campbell Clinic
Memphis, Tennessee

JAMES H. BEATY, MD
Harold B. Boyd Professor and Chair
University of Tennessee–Campbell Clinic
Department of Orthopaedic Surgery and
  Biomedical Engineering
Memphis, Tennessee

MICHAEL J. BEEBE, MD
Instructor
University of Tennessee–Campbell Clinic
Department of Orthopaedic Surgery and
  Biomedical Engineering
Memphis, Tennessee

CLAYTON C. BETTIN, MD
Assistant Professor
Director, Foot and Ankle Fellowship
Associate Residency Program Director
University of Tennessee–Campbell Clinic
Department of Orthopaedic Surgery and
  Biomedical Engineering
Memphis, Tennessee

TYLER J. BROLIN, MD
Assistant Professor
University of Tennessee–Campbell Clinic
Department of Orthopaedic Surgery and
  Biomedical Engineering
Memphis, Tennessee

JAMES H. CALANDRUCCIO, MD
Associate Professor
Director, Hand Fellowship
University of Tennessee–Campbell Clinic
Department of Orthopaedic Surgery and
  Biomedical Engineering
Memphis, Tennessee

DAVID L. CANNON, MD
Associate Professor
University of Tennessee–Campbell Clinic
Department of Orthopaedic Surgery and
  Biomedical Engineering
Memphis, Tennessee

KEVIN B. CLEVELAND, MD
Instructor
University of Tennessee–Campbell Clinic
Department of Orthopaedic Surgery and
  Biomedical Engineering
Memphis, Tennessee

ANDREW H. CRENSHAW JR., MD
Professor Emeritus
University of Tennessee–Campbell Clinic
Department of Orthopaedic Surgery and
  Biomedical Engineering
Memphis, Tennessee

JOHN R. CROCKARELL, MD
Professor
University of Tennessee–Campbell Clinic
Department of Orthopaedic Surgery and
  Biomedical Engineering
Memphis, Tennessee

GREGORY D. DABOV, MD
Assistant Professor
University of Tennessee–Campbell Clinic
Department of Orthopaedic Surgery and
  Biomedical Engineering
Memphis, Tennessee

MARCUS C. FORD, MD
Instructor
University of Tennessee–Campbell Clinic
Department of Orthopaedic Surgery and
  Biomedical Engineering
Memphis, Tennessee

RAYMOND J. GARDOCKI, MD
Assistant Professor
University of Tennessee–Campbell Clinic
Department of Orthopaedic Surgery and
  Biomedical Engineering
Memphis, Tennessee

BENJAMIN J. GREAR, MD
Instructor
University of Tennessee–Campbell Clinic
Department of Orthopaedic Surgery and
  Biomedical Engineering
Memphis, Tennessee

JAMES L. GUYTON, MD
Associate Professor
University of Tennessee–Campbell Clinic
Department of Orthopaedic Surgery and
  Biomedical Engineering
Memphis, Tennessee

JAMES W. HARKESS, MD
Associate Professor
University of Tennessee–Campbell Clinic
Department of Orthopaedic Surgery and
  Biomedical Engineering
Memphis, Tennessee

ROBERT K. HECK JR., MD
Associate Professor
University of Tennessee–Campbell Clinic
Department of Orthopaedic Surgery and
  Biomedical Engineering
Memphis, Tennessee

MARK T. JOBE, MD
Associate Professor
University of Tennessee–Campbell Clinic
Department of Orthopaedic Surgery and
  Biomedical Engineering
Memphis, Tennessee

DEREK M. KELLY, MD
Professor
Director, Pediatric Orthopaedic Fellowship
Director, Resident Education
University of Tennessee–Campbell Clinic
Department of Orthopaedic Surgery and
  Biomedical Engineering
Memphis, Tennessee

SANTOS F. MARTINEZ, MD
Assistant Professor
University of Tennessee–Campbell Clinic
Department of Orthopaedic Surgery and
  Biomedical Engineering
Memphis, Tennessee

ANTHONY A. MASCIOLI, MD
Assistant Professor
University of Tennessee–Campbell Clinic
Department of Orthopaedic Surgery and
  Biomedical Engineering
Memphis, Tennessee

BENJAMIN M. MAUCK, MD
Assistant Professor
Director, Hand Fellowship
University of Tennessee–Campbell Clinic
Department of Orthopaedic Surgery and
  Biomedical Engineering
Memphis, Tennessee

MARC J. MIHALKO, MD
Assistant Professor
University of Tennessee–Campbell Clinic
Department of Orthopaedic Surgery and
  Biomedical Engineering
Memphis, Tennessee

WILLIAM M. MIHALKO, MD PhD
Professor, H.R. Hyde Chair of Excellence in
  Rehabilitation Engineering
Director, Biomedical Engineering
University of Tennessee–Campbell Clinic
Department of Orthopaedic Surgery and
  Biomedical Engineering
Memphis, Tennessee

ROBERT H. MILLER III, MD
Associate Professor
University of Tennessee–Campbell Clinic
Department of Orthopaedic Surgery and
 Biomedical Engineering
Memphis, Tennessee

G. ANDREW MURPHY, MD
Associate Professor
University of Tennessee–Campbell Clinic
Department of Orthopaedic Surgery and
 Biomedical Engineering
Memphis, Tennessee

ASHLEY L. PARK, MD
Clinical Assistant Professor
University of Tennessee–Campbell Clinic
Department of Orthopaedic Surgery and
 Biomedical Engineering
Memphis, Tennessee

EDWARD A. PEREZ, MD
Associate Professor
University of Tennessee–Campbell Clinic
Department of Orthopaedic Surgery and
 Biomedical Engineering
Memphis, Tennessee

BARRY B. PHILLIPS, MD
Professor
University of Tennessee–Campbell Clinic
Department of Orthopaedic Surgery and
 Biomedical Engineering
Memphis, Tennessee

DAVID R. RICHARDSON, MD
Associate Professor
University of Tennessee–Campbell Clinic
Department of Orthopaedic Surgery and
 Biomedical Engineering
Memphis, Tennessee

MATTHEW I. RUDLOFF, MD
Assistant Professor
Co-Director, Trauma Fellowship
University of Tennessee–Campbell Clinic
Department of Orthopaedic Surgery and
 Biomedical Engineering
Memphis, Tennessee

JEFFREY R. SAWYER, MD
Professor
Co-Director, Pediatric Orthopaedic
 Fellowship
University of Tennessee–Campbell Clinic
Department of Orthopaedic Surgery and
 Biomedical Engineering
Memphis, Tennessee

BENJAMIN W. SHEFFER, MD
Assistant Professor
University of Tennessee–Campbell Clinic
Department of Orthopaedic Surgery and
 Biomedical Engineering
Memphis, Tennessee

DAVID D. SPENCE, MD
Assistant Professor
University of Tennessee–Campbell Clinic
Department of Orthopaedic Surgery and
 Biomedical Engineering
Memphis, Tennessee

NORFLEET B. THOMPSON, MD
Instructor
University of Tennessee–Campbell Clinic
Department of Orthopaedic Surgery and
 Biomedical Engineering
Memphis, Tennessee

THOMAS W. THROCKMORTON, MD
Professor
Co-Director, Sports Medicine Fellowship
University of Tennessee–Campbell Clinic
Department of Orthopaedic Surgery and
 Biomedical Engineering
Memphis, Tennessee

PATRICK C. TOY, MD
Associate Professor
University of Tennessee–Campbell Clinic
Department of Orthopaedic Surgery and
 Biomedical Engineering
Memphis, Tennessee

WILLIAM C. WARNER JR., MD
Professor
University of Tennessee–Campbell Clinic
Department of Orthopaedic Surgery and
 Biomedical Engineering
Memphis, Tennessee

JOHN C. WEINLEIN, MD
Assistant Professor
Director, Trauma Fellowship
University of Tennessee–Campbell Clinic
Department of Orthopaedic Surgery and
 Biomedical Engineering
Memphis, Tennessee

WILLIAM J. WELLER, MD
Instructor
University of Tennessee–Campbell Clinic
Department of Orthopaedic Surgery and
 Biomedical Engineering
Memphis, Tennessee

A. PAIGE WHITTLE, MD
Associate Professor
University of Tennessee–Campbell Clinic
Department of Orthopaedic Surgery and
 Biomedical Engineering
Memphis, Tennessee

KEITH D. WILLIAMS, MD
Associate Professor
University of Tennessee–Campbell Clinic
Department of Orthopaedic Surgery and
 Biomedical Engineering
Memphis, Tennessee

DEXTER H. WITTE III, MD
Clinical Assistant Professor in
 Radiology
University of Tennessee–Campbell Clinic
Department of Orthopaedic Surgery and
 Biomedical Engineering
Memphis, Tennessee

PREFACE

When Dr. Willis Campbell published the first edition of *Campbell's Operative Orthopaedics* in 1939, he could not have envisioned that over 80 years later it would have evolved into a four-volume text and earned the accolade of the "bible of orthopaedics" as a mainstay in orthopaedic practices and educational institutions all over the world. This expansion from some 400 pages in the first edition to over 4,500 pages in this 14th edition has not changed Dr. Campbell's original intent: "to present to the student, the general practitioner, and the surgeon the subject of orthopaedic surgery in a simple and comprehensive manner." In each edition since the first, authors and editors have worked diligently to fulfill these objectives. This would have not been possible without the hard work of our contributors who always strive to present the most up-to-date information while retaining "tried and true" techniques and tips. The scope of this text continues to expand in the hope that the information will be relevant to physicians no matter their location or resources.

As always, this edition also is the result of the collaboration of a group of "behind the scenes" individuals who are involved in the actual production process. The Campbell Foundation staff—Kay Daugherty, Linda Jones, and Tonya Priggel—contributed their considerable talents to editing often confusing and complex author contributions, searching the literature for obscure references, and, in general, "herding the cats." Special thanks to Kay and Linda who have worked on multiple editions of *Campbell's Operative Orthopaedics* (nine editions for Kay and six for Linda). They probably know more about orthopaedics than most of us, and they certainly know how to make it more understandable. Thanks, too, to the Elsevier personnel who provided guidance and assistance throughout the publication process: John Casey, Senior Project Manager; Jennifer Ehlers, Senior Content Development Specialist; and Belinda Kuhn, Senior Content Strategist.

We are especially appreciative of our spouses, Julie Azar and Terry Beaty, and our families for their patience and support as we worked through this project.

The preparation and publication of this 14th edition was fraught with difficulties because of the worldwide pandemic and social unrest, but our contributors and other personnel worked tirelessly, often in creative and innovative ways, to bring it to fruition. It is our hope that these efforts have provided a text that is informative and valuable to all orthopaedists as they continue to refine and improve methods that will ensure the best outcomes for their patients.

Frederick M. Azar, MD
James H. Beaty, MD

CONTENTS

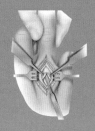

CHAPTER 1

BASIC SURGICAL TECHNIQUE AND POSTOPERATIVE CARE

David L. Cannon

The hand is the most complex and versatile structure in the human body. Formed of 27 bones, the hand and wrist require more than 30 muscles and a vast web of ligaments and tendons to move them into the myriad postures required for the countless tasks the hand performs every day. The complexity of hand function is reflected by the large amount of brain space dedicated to it. Injury to or dysfunction of any element of hand function can cause significant disability. Because of the importance of the hand to every aspect of life, it is essential for the surgeon to make the correct diagnosis and perform the appropriate and needed procedures, avoiding both undertreatment and overtreatment.

PREOPERATIVE PLANNING AND PREPARATION

A carefully taken history and detailed physical examination of the involved part are frequently sufficient to determine the appropriate diagnosis. Routine anteroposterior, lateral, and oblique radiographic hand and wrist views may be supplemented with additional special views of the wrist, thumb base, and fifth carpometacarpal joint. MRI and CT can provide sufficient additional information to clarify some bone and soft-tissue problems in the hand and wrist. Radionuclide bone scanning may show areas of bone involvement before they can be seen on plain radiographs. Electrodiagnostic studies (electromyography and nerve conduction velocities) may localize areas of nerve compression and reveal other conditions (e.g., peripheral neuropathy). In patients with suspected but undiagnosed systemic illnesses, such as the inflammatory arthritides, assessment by appropriate medical specialists is helpful in determining appropriate nonoperative management. Patients who are taking warfarin, corticosteroids or other antiinflammatory medications, immunosuppressive drugs, aspirin, herbal and complementary preparations, and medications for diabetes may require modification of dosage or discontinuation of the medications during the immediate preoperative and intraoperative periods.

Most important is that the patient and surgeon have realistic expectations regarding the operative outcome before the procedure is performed. The patient should understand the options; the alternatives to surgery; the expected outcome with and without surgical treatment; the potential risks, hazards, and benefits of the surgery; the nature and location of the incisions; the potential need for incisions to be made on other parts of the body for the harvesting of grafts; and the possible use of internal fixation, drains, and other types of implants. The patient should understand the nature of immobilization after surgery, including the use of splints and casts, and he or she should understand that recovery and rehabilitation might be prolonged, especially after major reconstructive procedures.

As part of the preoperative preparation, patients are instructed to keep their hands clean for several days before surgery and to avoid skin injury to minimize the potential for infection. From currently available information, an infection rate of 0.5% to 3.0% might be expected. If the patient has evidence of cuts or skin or remote infections, the operation may best be delayed. If the fingernails are long or dirty, they should be trimmed and cleaned to remove potential sources of bacterial contamination, and excessive hair in the incision area should be removed before scrubbing the operative extremity.

PERIOPERATIVE ANTIBIOTICS

Although surgical site infections are uncommon after hand surgery, postoperative infection can occur, causing impairment of hand function, delaying rehabilitation and return to work. Severe infection may require multiple surgical procedures and result in permanent damage to the hand. The routine use of perioperative antibiotics for many orthopaedic procedures in the hand remains questionable. In three large series (one retrospective study involving 8850 patients, one prospective, randomized study involving 1340 patients, and one retrospective analysis of 516,986 patients gathered from a multistate commercial insurance claims database) there was no significant difference in the frequency of infection in patients who received perioperative antibiotics and those who did not. The prospective study also found no difference between elective and emergency surgery, between operations lasting 2 hours and those lasting longer, or between "clean" and "crush/dirty" wounds. Even in "high-risk" patients (smokers, those with diabetes mellitus, and those with longer operative procedure times) in the retrospective study, pro-phylactic antibiotics did not reduce the frequency of surgical site infection. Another study that evaluated the use of anti-biotics for carpal tunnel release in patients with a prosthetic joint also found that antibiotics were not indicated. Although numerous studies have concluded that antibiotic prophylaxis should not be routinely administered for surgery of the hand, the rate of antibiotic use has steadily increased, with antibiot-ics being used in one of five clean soft-tissue hand surgeries.

ARRANGEMENT AND ROUTINE IN THE OPERATING ROOM

Because surgical results depend considerably on the skill, judg-ment, and precise work of the surgeon, intraoperative distrac-tions should be kept to a minimum. It is important for the surgeon to establish a standard routine that is followed regularly. Each assistant can then depend on this routine. The activities of the assistants in following this routine should not be disrupted by the surgeon with irregular, unexpected, or inconsistent demands. A standard routine makes it possible for assistants to know what is expected of them at each step in the operation and allows them to perform without hesitation, delay, or wasted motion.

The operating room should always be pleasant. If a local anesthetic is being used and the patient is awake, loud or inappropriate noises or bursts of conversation may alarm the patient and should be avoided. Sometimes music of the patient's choosing is comforting.

If the surgical procedure is being arranged with the oper-ating room staff, it is helpful to make requests regarding spe-cial needs for the case under consideration. Making advance arrangements for instruments, sutures, operating micro-scope, special implants, additional assistants, and other items enhances the efficiency of the operating team on the day of the procedure. Radiology support, including the use of C-arm fluoroscopy, should be arranged beforehand as well.

Five "be" attitudes on the part of the surgeon can increase efficiency in the operating room: (1) be punctual—if possible, be early; (2) be available—being present signifies to the surgical team that you are a member of the team; (3) be predictable—the less variation in the operating room routine, the more efficient it becomes; (4) be progressive—go from simple to complex; and (5) be gracious—it costs nothing, but buys a lot of goodwill.

The operating surgeon usually sits on a firm, comfortable, and stable stool and occasionally stands for some procedures. When sitting, the surgeon's knees are almost level with the hips and the feet rest flat on the floor without strain. The working surface of the operating hand table should be at elbow height to provide a comfortable support for the forearms. When the light is directed perpendicular to the surgeon's view, it shines directly on the operative field, and shadows are avoided.

Seated opposite the surgeon, the assistant should view the operative field from 8 to 10 cm higher than the surgeon to allow a clear line of vision without having to bend forward and obstruct the surgeon's view. Although mechanical hand holders are available, they are not as good as a motivated and well-trained assistant (Fig. 1.1). It is especially helpful for the assistant to be familiar with each procedure. Usually, the pri-mary duty of the assistant is to hold the patient's hand stable, secure, and motionless, retracting the fingers to provide the surgeon with the best access to the operative field (Fig. 1.2A and B). Using a mechanical holder such as a lead hand is bet-ter with untrained assistants.

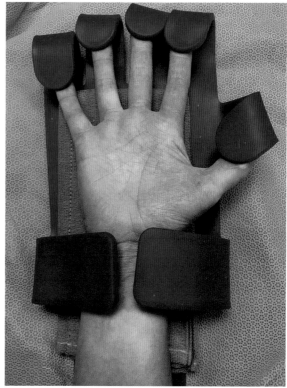

FIGURE 1.1 Mechanical hand positioner/holder.

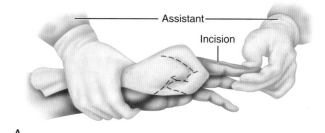

A

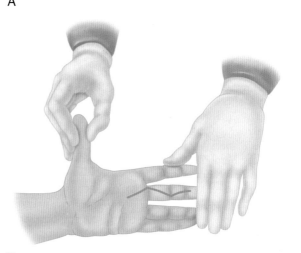

B

FIGURE 1.2 **A,** Assistant holds patient's hand firm and motionless and exposes operative field for midlateral digital inci-sion. **B,** Ideal position for assistant to stabilize patient's hand as surgeon makes zigzag incision.

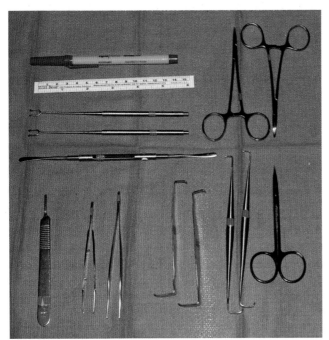

TABLE 1.1

Maximal Doses of Local Anesthetics for Brachial Plexus Blocks

ANESTHETIC	MAXIMAL RECOMMENDED DOSE
Bupivacaine	2.5 mg/kg
Bupivacaine with epinephrine	3.0 mg/kg
Levobupivacaine	2.0 mg/kg
Levobupivacaine with epinephrine	3.0 mg/kg
Ropivacaine	2.0 mg/kg
Ropivacaine with epinephrine	3.0 mg/kg

These amounts should be used as a guideline only; practitioners should use their clinical judgment when administering local anesthetics.
Modified from Bruce BG, Green A, Blaine TA, Wesner LV: Brachial plexus blocks for upper extremity orthopaedic surgery, *J AAOS* 20:38, 2012.

FIGURE 1.3   Basic instruments for any surgical procedure on hand. Octagonal knife handle is preferable to flat handle because knife is more commonly held by precision pinch in hand surgery. Instruments shown are knife handle, small rat-tooth forceps, dissecting scissors, small hemostats, ruler, marking pencil, double-hook Lovejoy retractors, and probe.

The hand operating table should be stable and immobile. Space should be sufficient for the patient's hand and for resting the elbows and forearms of the surgeon and assistant, minimizing muscle fatigue. For most procedures, the surgeon should sit on the axillary side of the involved extremity, allowing the anatomy of either hand to be seen in the same relative position. Some procedures on the dorsum of the hand and wrist may be performed more easily from the cephalic side. If the surgeon changes sides, keep in mind the change in routine to avoid anatomic disorientation.

The tray holding the basic instruments is often placed on a shelf extending from the operating table, level with the working surface. The instruments always should be arranged in the same order (Fig. 1.3). This arrangement allows the surgeon to save time by routinely reaching for instruments from the basic tray. With practice, this can be done without the surgeon looking at the instruments.

Using an instrument pan or designated "hands-free" zone, the surgeon discards an instrument after using it, and the surgery technician returns it to its place on the tray. The discarded knife, tissue forceps, and dissecting scissors that are used constantly are not retrieved by the surgery technician unless requested by the surgeon. Special instruments should be readily available on another large table so that they can be handed quickly to the surgeon on request. Additional knife blades and special sutures and needles also should be immediately available.

Numerous hand conditions, such as infection, foreign bodies, and fractures, may now be effectively treated in procedure rooms with local anesthesia as opposed to formal operating rooms when appropriate. Studies have shown a significant reduction in the cost of these procedures without a significant difference in risk of complications.

CHOICE OF ANESTHESIA

Drugs used for local and regional anesthesia should become effective within a few minutes after injection, should cause minimal local irritation, and should have low systemic toxicity. Lidocaine seems to fulfill these requirements. Mepivacaine (Carbocaine) is longer acting but may be slower in onset. Many surgeons prefer bupivacaine (Marcaine) because it is effective for 8 hours or longer. It can be used for axillary brachial block to avoid the use of a general anesthetic. Each of these agents has a toxicity level based on milligrams per kilogram of body weight, and this should be calculated before administration (Table 1.1).

Unsatisfactory anesthesia for hand and upper extremity operations prevents the surgeon from accomplishing his or her goals and is likely to compromise the surgical result. For accurate and precise work, the part must be motionless, the procedure should be completely painless, and the patient should be comfortable. All anesthetic techniques carry some risks, and the selection of the technique depends on the needs of the patient and the preferences of the surgeon and anesthesiologist. The selection should be part of the preoperative planning.

At times, general anesthesia is preferred. Factors that favor the use of this type of anesthesia include extensive and prolonged hand and upper extremity operations, performance of procedures on other parts of the body (chest or abdomen or harvesting of various tissue grafts), extensive operations in young children, the presence of infection in a region that would preclude injecting a local anesthetic agent, and the preference of a particularly uneasy or anxious patient.

Regional anesthesia has many advantages in hand and upper extremity surgery. Satisfactory regional anesthesia can be achieved for emergency procedures performed on patients with a full stomach; in these situations and in elective operations, a regional anesthetic blocks vasoconstrictive afferent impulses from the surgical wound and avoids some of the unpleasant postoperative complications of general anesthesia. Outpatient surgery can be performed safely using regional anesthetic blocks, which reduce the need for postoperative nursing care. A regional anesthetic may allow operations to be done on the hand and upper extremity in patients with unstable cardiac or severe pulmonary or renal problems that would create an increased risk with general anesthesia. In a recent study of 27,041 patients who had hand surgery, local and regional anesthesia, with and without sedation, resulted in fewer postoperative complications than general anesthesia. In addition, avoiding sedation entirely was shown to decrease the risk of complications after surgery in patients over the age of 65 years.

Regional anesthesia is less satisfactory in children or extremely nervous, anxious, or uncooperative adults. It should be avoided in patients with documented, true allergies to local anesthetic agents and in patients taking anticoagulants. A regional anesthetic agent may be difficult to administer in patients with contractures or involvement of joints that limit positioning of the limb for satisfactory blocks and in patients whose veins or blood pressure elevation do not allow the use of the intravenous technique. Care should be taken when administering regional anesthetic agents to avoid complications such as overdosage, intravascular injection (when doing nerve blocks), pneumothorax (when doing supraclavicular brachial plexus blocks), and the dissemination of infection.

For operations on the hand and upper extremity, four methods of regional anesthesia are in widespread use: (1)

brachial plexus blocks using the interscalene, axillary, or supraclavicular approach; (2) intravenous regional blocks; (3) peripheral nerve blocks distal to the axilla, including blocks of the median, radial, ulnar, and digital nerves; and (4) local infiltration of anesthetic agents, including the wide-awake, local anesthesia, no tourniquet (WALANT) technique. It is helpful to have the patient satisfactorily sedated before surgery. In many situations, especially in elective surgery, simple nerve blocks at the wrist or fingers require little premedication. The use of regional anesthesia requires that sufficient time be allowed in the immediate period before surgery for preparation of the patient, for the administration of the regional anesthetic agents, and for the anesthetic to become effective before the skin incision is made.

BRACHIAL PLEXUS BLOCKS

The traditional approaches for administering anesthesia to the major components of the brachial plexus include the axillary, interscalene, and supraclavicular and infraclavicular routes (Fig. 1.4). The axillary and interscalene approaches we use most commonly probably are safer than the supraclavicular route,

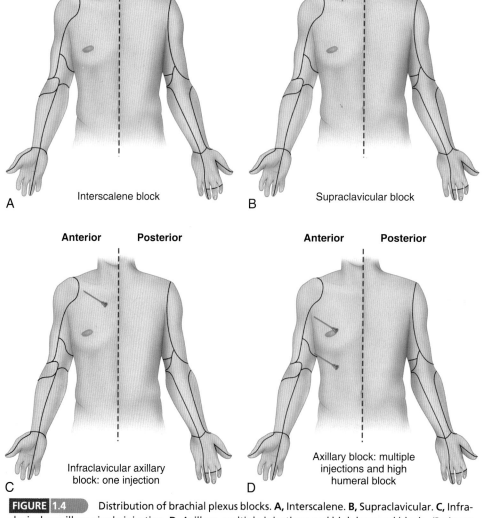

FIGURE 1.4   Distribution of brachial plexus blocks. **A,** Interscalene. **B,** Supraclavicular. **C,** Infraclavicular axillary, single injection. **D,** Axillary, multiple injections and high humeral block. (Redrawn from Chelly JE, editor: *Peripheral nerve block*, ed 3, Philadelphia, 2008, Lippincott Williams & Wilkins.)

which carries the risk of a low incidence (1% to 5%) of pneumothorax. Infraclavicular and supraclavicular blocks are more commonly done now with ultrasound guidance. The interscalene block covers the supraclavicular nerves emanating from the third and fourth cervical roots and is ideal for shoulder surgery. Interscalene blocks can also be used for elbow surgery. Supraclavicular blocks are useful for surgery in the upper arm distal to the shoulder, whereas infraclavicular blocks can provide regional anesthesia for surgery of the elbow, forearm, wrist, and hand. An axillary block provides anesthesia similar to that of an infraclavicular block. Access to the axillary space requires the patient to abduct the arm 90 degrees, which may be difficult for those with trauma or contractures. Needle placement for brachial plexus blocks was traditionally based on anatomic landmarks and nerve localization with a nerve stimulator, but more recent approaches use an ultrasound approach. A meta-analysis of 13 studies comparing neurostimulation with ultrasound-guided blocks found that ultrasound-guided blocks were more likely to be successful, took less time, had a faster onset, and decreased the risk of vascular puncture. A study of the multiple-injection technique for axillary block showed that ultrasound guidance resulted in fewer needle passes, a shorter time to onset of anesthesia, and less procedure-related pain than nerve stimulation techniques. Limitations of ultrasound include availability, a limited plane of view, and highly operator-dependent image quality.

Short- and long-acting local anesthetic agents can be used for brachial plexus blocks. The dose depends on the agent used, the technique used, and the preference of the administering physician. Although the amount of anesthetic used is not standardized, maximal amounts have been recommended (Table 1.1). Evidence exists that multiple-injection block is more effective than single or double-injection block in obtaining and maintaining anesthesia; no statistically significant differences have been noted regarding secondary analgesia failure, complications, or patient discomfort.

Complications of brachial plexus blocks are few (<1%). Reported systemic complications include cardiac arrest, respiratory failure, and seizures. Peripheral nerve injury can be caused by mechanical trauma from needles or catheters, drug neurotoxicity, ischemia, compression, or stretch, but permanent neurologic sequelae occur in less than 1% of patients. Pneumothorax is most common with supraclavicular blocks (as high as 6%) but has been reported with interscalene and infraclavicular blocks. Ultrasound-guided technique has been suggested to reduce the risk of pneumothorax: a prospective study found no clinically apparent pneumothoraces in 510 patients who had ultrasound-guided supraclavicular blocks.

Contraindications to axillary brachial plexus block include infection in the axilla, axillary lymphadenopathy, and malignancy.

Dysesthesias and "brachialgia" may persist after brachial plexus blocks, and the patient should understand this before the block. It also might create difficulty in patients who require fine manipulation of the hands in their occupation.

INTRAVENOUS REGIONAL ANESTHESIA

The intravenous regional anesthesia technique using a double tourniquet (Bier) is useful, especially for procedures of relatively short duration (60 to 90 minutes). A specially designed double tourniquet is used. The patient should be satisfactorily premedicated, and intravenous infusion should be in place in

the contralateral arm. The usual anesthetic agent is lidocaine. In most situations, 30 to 60 mL of 0.5% lidocaine provides sufficient and safe anesthesia. Adjuncts to lidocaine also have shown some benefit in analgesia and tourniquet pain. The dosage used should take the patient's age and body weight into consideration. Satisfactory anesthesia can be obtained in a short time. The tourniquet is left inflated for a minimum of 30 minutes after injection of the anesthetic agent into the extremity. In the usual situation, the limb is exsanguinated; the proximal tourniquet is inflated to a level 100 mm Hg greater than the systolic pressure (usually 250 to 300 mm Hg); and, using sterile technique, the anesthesiologist intravenously introduces the previously determined volume of anesthetic agent (Fig. 1.5). As the more proximal tourniquet becomes uncomfortable, the distal

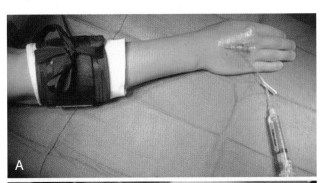

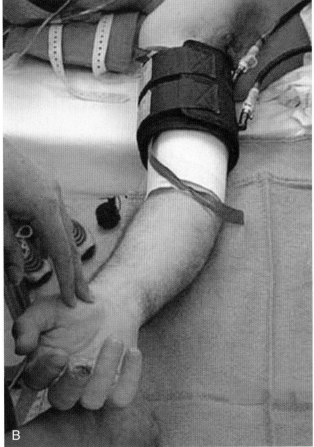

FIGURE 1.5 Continuous intravenous regional anesthesia with forearm **(A)** and upper arm **(B)** tourniquet (see text). (A from anesthesiologynews.com; B from University of Pittsburgh Nurse Anesthesia Program.)

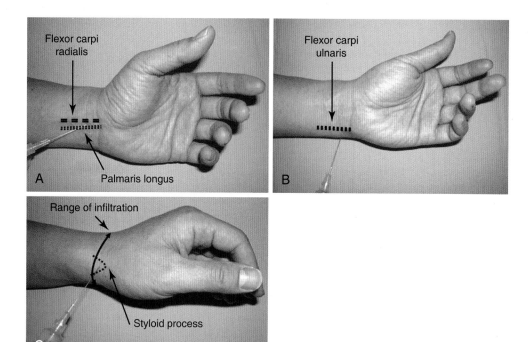

FIGURE 1.6 Technique of peripheral nerve blocks. **A,** Ulnar nerve, superficial branch. **B,** Median nerve. **C,** Superficial radial nerve.

tourniquet is inflated and the proximal tourniquet is deflated. Reported reactions during intravenous regional anesthesia include anesthetic toxicity, cardiac arrhythmias (bradycardia and cardiac arrest), unconsciousness, seizures, vertigo, nystagmus, and compartment syndrome.

The use of a forearm tourniquet for intravenous regional anesthesia has been suggested, with reported advantages of safety, preservation of hand motor function, lower anesthetic dose, and reduced risk of complications. One study of 430 patients demonstrated no major complications when tourniquet time was less than 20 minutes.

PERIPHERAL NERVE BLOCKS

The median, radial, and ulnar nerves can be blocked at the wrist. In terms of surgical time, tourniquet time, and postoperative pain, no difference has been noted between forearm blocks and brachial plexus blocks; however, forearm blocks are extremely helpful for brief procedures (Fig. 1.6), and a tourniquet may not be required or may be used only for a short period (usually ≤30 minutes). Blocks at the wrist can be especially useful for procedures such as tenolysis and capsulotomy because motion of the fingers can be observed during surgery. The patient can be kept comfortable, and a tourniquet can be used longer than 30 minutes if the patient is adequately sedated. Kocheta and Agrawal described adding posterior interosseous and anterior interosseous nerve blocks to a wrist block for more effective carpal surgery. Regardless of the surgical location, it is essential to know the location of the respective nerves before attempting regional blocks. Ultrasound may be useful in this regard. One study found that nonultrasound-guided median nerve blocks at the wrist were unreliable in effectiveness and took up to 40 minutes for maximal numbness to occur and up to 100 minutes for maximal anesthesia. Contraindications to peripheral nerve blocks include infection in the proposed area of injection, history of

allergy to the anesthetic, or a patient who is unable to communicate pain.

DIGITAL NERVE BLOCKS

Digital nerve blocks provide excellent anesthesia for procedures on the fingers (Fig. 1.7). Usually, perineural injection around the digital nerves proximal to the finger web spaces is a safer technique than injection of the nerves at the base of the fingers. Because ischemia may develop after injection of an anesthetic agent in a circle around the base of the finger, this technique should be avoided. Digital blocks using a transthecal (flexor sheath) approach have shown no advantage compared with the traditional digital block technique (Fig. 1.8), but may be tolerated better because it is a single injection rather than two separate injections. We rarely use epinephrine in the local anesthetic agent in the digits, although it can be used safely.

If hemostasis is required, traditionally a Penrose drain or a French rubber catheter applied around the finger has provided satisfactory and safe ischemia. Commercially available finger tourniquets and the finger of a rubber glove cut to allow it to be rolled onto the finger as a tourniquet also are effective tools (Fig. 1.9). Pressures achieved beneath these tourniquets cannot be determined accurately; caution is advised. At times, especially in the elderly and patients with vascular disorders in the fingers (e.g., Raynaud disease, atherosclerosis, diabetes), vascular insufficiency may develop in the digit, and care should be taken when using digital tourniquets in these patients (Fig. 1.10). If a rubber glove is used, special attention is essential to ensure it is removed at the end of the procedure: there are reports of catastrophic consequences after such a tourniquet was left on a digit.

LOCAL INFILTRATION

Local infiltration of an anesthetic agent may be used for more proximal conditions that do not require deep, extensive

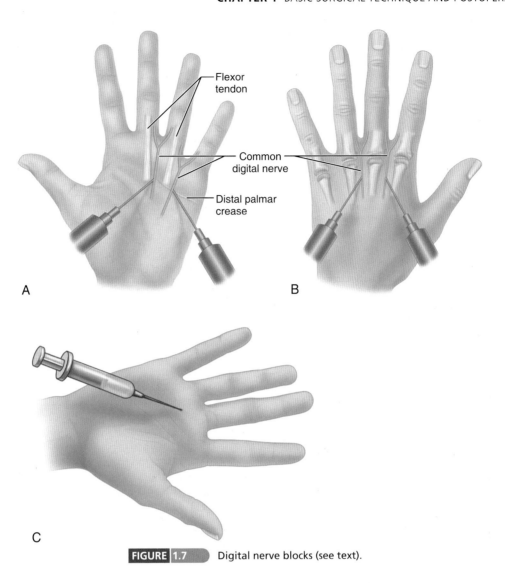

Flexor tendon

Common digital nerve

Distal palmar crease

A

B

C

FIGURE 1.7 Digital nerve blocks (see text).

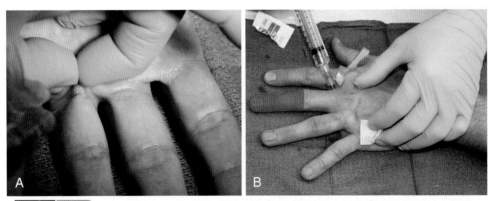

FIGURE 1.8 For procedures that require anesthesia from midmiddle phalanx distally (e.g., nail bed regions and distal interphalangeal joint distributions and fusions) digital anesthesia can be easily achieved by single volar injection technique. **A,** Just proximal to palmar digital crease, through pinched skin 3 to 5 mL of local anesthetic is injected superficial to flexor sheath. **B,** Anesthesia achieved *(colored area)* from block of proper and dorsal sensory digital nerve branches. Note, if more proximal anesthesia is needed, additional block can be given at metacarpophalangeal joint dorsally as shown.

dissection. This method is satisfactory for trigger digit release, small scar revision, and excision of benign masses from the skin and subcutaneous tissues of the forearm, hand, and fingers.

■ WALANT APPROACH

There has been a move away from the traditional tourniquet and sedation protocol to the WALANT approach for outpatient hand and wrist surgery. Suggested benefits of the

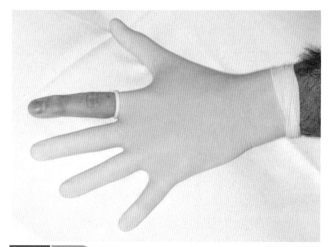

FIGURE 1.9 Rubber glove tourniquet (see text). (From Henley J, Brewer JD: Newer hemostatic agents used in the practice of dermatologic surgery, *Dermatol Res Pract.* 2013:270289, 2013. Epub August 7, 2013.)

WALANT approach include (1) increased patient comfort and convenience, (2) decreased operative time for minor procedures such as carpal tunnel and trigger finger releases, (3) significant cost reductions, and (4) ability to see sutured tendons, and bones and joints with fracture fixation, during a full range of active movement, which can improve functional outcomes. The WALANT approach can be used for a variety of outpatient hand and wrist procedures, with the location of injection and the volume of anesthetic agent differing between them (Table 1.2). Although the technique is not appropriate for all patients, it can be used in most patients who can, for instance, have dental procedures without sedation. Specific procedures for which WALANT is effective include flexor tendon repair, tendon transfer, and soft-tissue releases. It has also been used for phalangeal and metacarpal fracture treatment. The primary advantage of this procedure is that it avoids the use of a tourniquet, reducing patient pain and the risk of injury to the nerves or skin. Patient satisfaction is high with this method because there are no sedation side effects, and faster recovery has been noted. Also postoperative narcotic use has been reported to be less than with other forms of anesthesia.

WALANT uses a combination of lidocaine or bupivacaine and epinephrine to obtain hemostasis and anesthetize the area of the surgical procedure. As with any local anesthetic use, adverse reactions are possible but rare. Nevertheless, patients require monitoring for hypotension, seizures, cardiac dysrhythmias, and other complications. In the past the use of epinephrine in the hand or foot was believed to cause necrosis and gangrene, but this has been refuted by several studies.

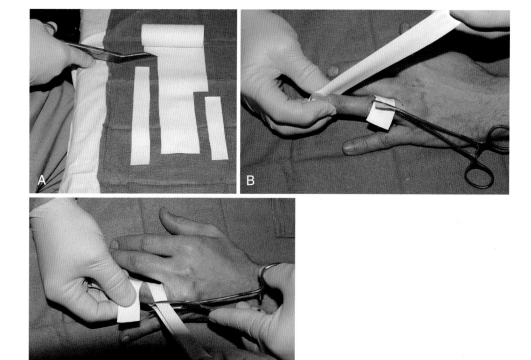

FIGURE 1.10 Broad-based finger tourniquet can be cut from Esmarch wrap, which usually accompanies upper extremity packages. **A,** Long and short strips 2.5 cm wide are cut from opposite sides of Esmarch bandage. **B,** Short strip is loosely applied across finger base and is held in place with curved hemostat. Longer strip is used to exsanguinate finger. **C,** Tension is applied to short section, and hemostat is applied close to dorsal skin with the two limbs of short Esmarch section fully opposed.

TABLE 1.2

Typical Volumes Used for Common Operations

OPERATION	TYPICAL VOLUME OF 1% LIDOCAINE WITH 1:100,000 EPINEPHRINE AND 8.4% BICARBONATE (MIXED 10 mL:1 mL)	LOCATION OF INJECTION
Carpal tunnel	20 mL	10 mL between ulnar and median nerves (5 mm proximal to wrist crease and 5 mm ulnar to median nerve); another 10 mL under incision
Trigger finger	4 mL	Subcutaneously beneath the center of the incision
Finger sensory block (SIMPLE)	2 mL	Volar middle of proximal phalanx just past palmar-finger crease
Finger soft-tissue lesions or other surgery when finger base tourniquet is not desirable and finger epinephrine is used for hemostasis	5 mL volar distributed among 5 phalanges, 4 mL dorsal split between 2 phalanges	2 mL volar and 2 mL dorsal subcutaneous midline fat, in both proximal and middle phalanges. Distal phalanx gets only 1 mL midline volar, just past the DIP crease
PIP arthrodesis	8 mL total, 4 mL volar (2 in each phalanx) and 4 mL dorsal (2 in each phalanx)	2 mL midvolar and another 2 mL middorsal of both proximal and middle phalanges
Thumb MCP arthrodesis and collateral ligament tears of the MCP joint	15 mL	2 mL on each of volar and dorsal aspects of proximal phalanx and the rest all around the metacarpal head
Dupuytren contracture or zone II flexor tendon repair	15 mL/ray	10 mL (or more) in the palm; 2 mL in the proximal and middle phalanges and 1 mL in the distal phalanx (if required)
Trapeziectomy or Bennett fracture	40 mL	Radial side of the hand under the skin and all around the joint, including the median nerve. If LRTI is performed, decrease concentration to 0.5% lidocaine with 1:200,000 epinephrine, and also inject all around where FCR or APL will be dissected
Metacarpal fractures	40 mL	All around the metacarpal where dissection or K-wires will occur

APL, Abductor pollicis longus; *DIP*, distal interphalangeal joint; *FCR*, flexor carpi radialis; *LRTI*, ligament reconstruction and tendon interposition; *MCP*, metacarpophalangeal joint; *PIP*, proximal interphalangeal joint; *SIMPLE*, single subcutaneous injection in the middle of the proximal phalanx with lidocaine and epinephrine.
Modified from Lalonde DH, Wong A: Dosage of local anesthesia in wide awake hand surgery, *J Hand Surg* 38:2025, 2013.

In a multicenter, prospective study of 3110 patients who had hand or finger epinephrine injections, none developed skin necrosis or digital tissue loss. If a local adverse reaction occurs from the use of epinephrine in the finger, phentolamine, a vasodilator, can be used for reversal of epinephrine-induced vasoconstriction.

▌WALANT ADMINISTRATION (BOX 1.1)

Two mL of 1% lidocaine with epinephrine (1:100,000) is injected into the palmar and dorsal subcutaneous tissues (Fig. 1.11). If only a sensory block is required, a single subcutaneous dose of lidocaine and epinephrine is injected in the midline of the proximal phalanx (SIMPLE technique) (Fig. 1.11A). Lalonde and Wong recommend no more than 1 mL for distal phalangeal procedures. Although some studies support the safe use of up to 35 mg/kg of lidocaine with epinephrine, the accepted maximal dose is 7 mg/kg (50 mL for 150 lb patient).

Some surgeons prefer bupivacaine to lidocaine because of its longer action, but intravascular bupivacaine has been associated with cardiotoxicity, and the pain block provided by bupivacaine lasts only half the time as the return to normal sensation. Pain while the area is still numb is a common complaint in patients. Adding epinephrine will prolong the pain relief but only for about 1.5 hours; patients should be informed that pain sensation will return before the numbness resolves. Using lidocaine, pain and sensation return at the same time, and most surgeries in the hand can be done within the anesthesia time provided by lidocaine with epinephrine (5 hours in the wrist, 10 hours in the finger). Bupivacaine can be used for procedures expected to last 3 hours, although pain may be severe thereafter.

Maximal vasoconstriction after injection of lidocaine with epinephrine can be expected at 25 minutes, after which time optimal visibility of the operative field is obtained. McKee et al. recommend waiting 30 minutes after injection before incision.

PREPARATION AND DRAPING FOR ELECTIVE SURGERY

Regardless of the procedure, the method of preparing and draping the upper extremity and hand should be the same. This helps to standardize the routine and allows movement

BOX 1.1

Tips for Administering WALANT (Lalonde & Wong 2013)

- Pain during administration can be reduced by several methods:
  - Buffering the solution: a solution of lidocaine 1% with 1:100,000 epinephrine has a pH of 4.2, which likely contributes to the pain with injection. A 1:20 ratio of 8.4% sodium bicarbonate to lidocaine 1% with 1:100,000 epinephrine has a more physiologic pH of 7.4. A Cochrane review concluded that patients much preferred buffered lidocaine to unbuffered lidocaine; the difference was even more pronounced when the solution contained epinephrine.
  - Warming the solution.
  - Using a smaller needle (27- or 30-gauge or smaller).
  - Choosing the correct angle for needle insertion: A randomized, controlled crossover trial of 65 patients showed that injections with needles oriented at 90 degrees were significantly less painful than those with needles oriented at 45 degrees.
  - Injecting the solution under the dermis: In their double-blind, prospective trial, Arndt et al. found that subdermal injections produced less pain than intradermal injections. Strazar et al. suggested that this occurred because the space-occupying effect of the solution stretches the tissue, producing more pain in the densely innervated dermal tissue.

From: Steiner MM, Calandruccio JH: Use of wide-awake local anesthesia no tourniquet in hand and wrist surgery, *Orthop Clin North Am* 49(1):63, 2018.

about the operative field while minimizing the risk of bacterial contamination. The preparation of other areas for graft donor sites varies depending on the requirements of the procedure. If skin, tendon, bone, nerve, or other grafts are required, the patient should be positioned to allow easy access to the specific areas. Care should be taken to pad and protect neurovascular structures. The electrocautery grounding pads should be attached in a safe and secure manner. Usually, the hand and forearm are scrubbed before the time of the surgery. The hair is removed with electric clippers from the areas where skin incisions will be made on the hand, forearm, and elsewhere as needed; this often is done before the patient is transported to the operating room. A well-padded tourniquet is applied to the arm or the forearm, depending on the surgeon's preference; however, it is not inflated until all preparations have been completed (unless a Bier block is being used). After the patient has been satisfactorily anesthetized, the hand and forearm are scrubbed by an assistant with an antiseptic solution of choice. Iodophor soaps and skin preparation solutions and combinations of chlorhexidine and alcohol have been found to be effective (Table 1.3). A waterproof sheet is placed on the well-padded hand surgery table, followed by a sterile drape-sheet. Combinations of sterile towels and sheets are applied, leaving exposed the upper extremity and hand and other areas that may require access during the operation. The gloves used in preparation of the surgical field are removed, and the surgeon dons a gown and gloves and sits down, usually on the axillary side of the forearm. The operating lights are adjusted, and the skin incisions are outlined.

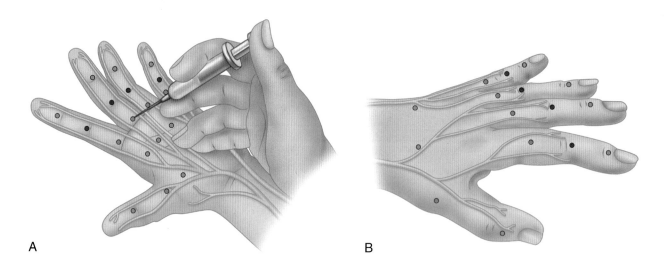

A   B

FIGURE 1.11 Sites of injection of local anesthesia in finger and hand surgery. **A,** Volar injections. When only a sensory block of finger is required (SIMPLE technique), 2 mL are injected into the areas designated by the blue dots. To obtain hemostasis and local anesthesia for palmar finger surgery, 1% lidocaine with epinephrine 1:100,000 is injected into midline subcutaneous fat between digital nerve in each area designated by dot. **B,** Dorsal injections. For hemostasis and local anesthesia, injection is into midline subcutaneous fat in each area designated by dot. In both volar and dorsal injections, 2 mL are injected at site of blue and red dots, 1 mL at site of green dots, and 5 mL at site of the orange dots. (From Lalonde D, Martin A. Epinephrine in local anesthesia in finger and hand surgery: the case for wide-awake anesthesia, *J Am Acad Orthop Surg* 21:443–447, 2013.)

TABLE 1.3

Antiseptic Solutions

Alcohol	Good immediate skin disinfectant, but dries quickly and has less long-term effect
	95% alcohol better than 75% because of dilution by moist skin
Hexachlorophene (pHisoHex)	Forms a film that retains bacteriostatic properties
	Easily washed off
	Requires multiple applications to be effective
	May be toxic in infants
	Effective against gram-positive organisms; less effective against gram-negative organisms
Iodine	Side effects
Alcoholic (tincture)	Frequent skin irritation (can be lessened by adding iodine)
Aqueous (Lugol's solution)	True allergic reactions
Iodophors (povidone-iodine [Betadine])	Advantages over iodine
Iodine and polyvinyl pyrrolidine or povidone	Slower release of iodine
	Fewer skin reactions
	Effective against gram-negative and gram-positive organisms
Chlorhexidine (Hibiclens) 70% alcoholic solution	Some studies have shown it superior to Betadine and pHisoHex
	Repeated washings may have a cumulative effect

Adapted from Green DP: General principles. In Wolfe SW, Hotchkiss RN, Pederson WC, Kozin SH, editors: *Green's operative hand surgery*, ed 6, Philadelphia, 2011, Elsevier.

TOURNIQUET

A bloodless field is essential for accurate dissection to avoid damaging small vital structures. The inherent dangers of tourniquet use are ischemia and its complications, including muscle contracture and nerve paralysis. Because the pressure can be monitored and controlled more reliably with a pneumatic tourniquet, complications are believed to be less likely with this type than with an elastic or rubber bandage tourniquet. Regardless of the tourniquet used, temporary or permanent disproportionate or prolonged edema, stiffness, diminished sensibility, and weakness or paralysis may result. Based on animal studies, Pedowitz et al. emphasized that biochemical, biomechanical, microvascular, and cellular mechanisms combine to produce significant neuromuscular injury from the use of tourniquets even at clinically allowable pressures and durations.

When operations are performed with the patient under local anesthesia and last less than 30 minutes, an elastic (Martin) bandage provides sufficient hemostasis and may be used safely. Wrapping of the bandage is begun at the fingertips and proceeds proximally on the forearm. It is applied in layers that overlap less than 5 to 6 mm. When the midforearm is reached, four or five layers of the elastic are overlapped. Wrinkles are avoided. The pressure is increased with each layer so that only moderate stretching is needed. The bandage is unwrapped, beginning distally, from the hand up to the midforearm. The overlapped layers in the midforearm are left in place until the operation is finished. For some procedures done with local infiltration or wrist block anesthesia, a pneumatic tourniquet can be used rather than an elastic wrap tourniquet. The tourniquet can be applied above or just below the elbow and left inflated 30 minutes without extreme discomfort.

Although the tourniquet is generally applied to the upper arm, several reports have indicated that forearm tourniquets are safe and reliable. The use of a forearm tourniquet with regional blocks has been reported to allow the dosage of local anesthetic to be decreased to almost half of that required with an upper arm tourniquet, and the frequency and severity of tourniquet pain have been reported to be less with a forearm tourniquet (procedures of 25 minutes or less or distal to the wrist with regional block). Both a longer duration of sensory block and prolonged postoperative analgesia have been described with the use of a forearm tourniquet.

The usual procedure for tourniquet application involves first the application of several layers of Webril wrapped smoothly around the middle of the upper arm near the axilla. The tourniquet is usually applied by the surgeon, an experienced assistant, or the anesthesiologist. Wrinkles are avoided because their presence may cause blisters, pinching of the skin, and necrosis. The limb is exsanguinated by elevation for 2 to 5 minutes or by wrapping with an elastic bandage about 10 cm wide beginning at the fingertips and proceeding to just distal to the tourniquet. With automatic tourniquets, inflation is usually rapid enough to avoid trapping excessive blood in the arm during inflation. Wrapping of the limb should be avoided in patients with infections in the limb or in whom malignant tumors are suspected. Instead, to allow venous drainage, the limb is elevated for 5 to 10 minutes. The tourniquet inflation pressure generally should not exceed 100 mm Hg systolic blood pressure for adults and children. The wider cuffs minimize focal compression of nerves beneath the cuff; however, smaller cuffs are required for children. When the tourniquet has been released, it and the underlying cotton wrapping should be removed to avoid venous congestion.

Improvements in design have resulted in the development of "automatic" pneumatic tourniquets that allow the setting of pressures within a safe range and for specific periods of time. Alarms notify the surgeon and anesthesiologist when the preset time has passed. Pneumatic tourniquets are available in several widths with Velcro strap fasteners. There is no absolute rule as to how long a tourniquet can remain safely inflated on the arm. The reports of most authors suggest that the "recovery time" or revascularization time between periods of tourniquet inflation is related to the length of time the tourniquet has been inflated (Table 1.4). In practice, the usual limit is considered to be 2 hours. If this limit is exceeded, the risk of paralysis may be increased. Usually, if the operation lasts longer than 2 hours, the tourniquet is released for at least 15 minutes and the limb is elevated with minimal compression applied to the incisions with sterile dressings. The limb is again exsanguinated with an elastic wrap, and the tourniquet is reinflated.

INSTRUMENTS

For the accurate work required in hand surgery, instruments with small points are necessary; the handles, however, should

TABLE 1.4

Tourniquet Time and Revascularization

TOURNIQUET TIME	NO. PATIENTS	PH		PO_2 (mm Hg)		PCO_2 (mm Hg)	
		RANGE	MEAN	RANGE	MEAN	RANGE	MEAN
Preinflation		7.38–7.42	7.4	40–50	45	35–40	38
0.5 h	50	7.29–7.35	7.31	22–27	24	45–53	50
1 h	40	7.15–7.22	7.19	19–22	20	60–66	62
1.5 h	26	7.02–7.10	7.04	6–16	10	80–88	85
2 h	12	6.88–6.96	6.9	0–6	4	92–110	104

From Wilgis EFS: Observations on the effect of tourniquet ischemia, *J Bone Joint Surg* 53A:1343, 1971.

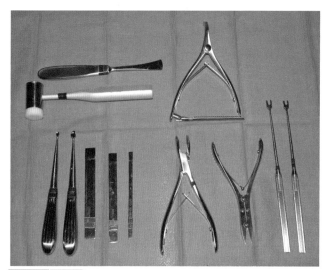

FIGURE 1.12 Instruments for small bone surgery include osteotomes, bone cutter, rongeur, awl, small curet, and small hammer.

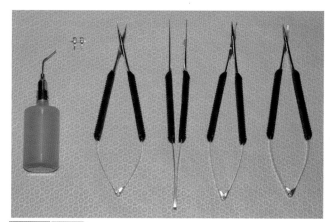

FIGURE 1.13 Instruments useful in microvascular and digital nerve surgery include small irrigation bulb, microvascular clamp, microneedle holder, pickups, and scissors of assorted lengths.

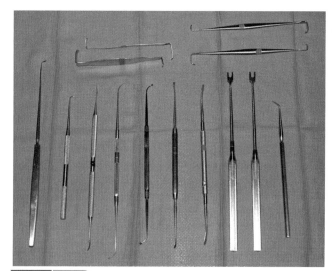

FIGURE 1.14 Certain dental instruments are often useful for dissection of ligaments and bone. Retractors of numerous designs have been used in hand surgery, but modified tonsil prong *(left)* has proved to be most useful.

be large enough to allow a firm, secure grip. The four basic instruments are the knife, the small forceps, the dissecting scissors, and the mosquito hemostat (Fig. 1.3). The knife blade should be firmly attached to the handle and changed when necessary. The knife should be used for most dissection, to avoid tearing through the tissues with a blunt instrument. The forceps should be carefully checked before surgery for cleanliness and precision of closure. The scissors should have sharp double points, preferably curved, to dissect neurovascular bundles. Instruments used for fine surgery on soft tissues are shown in Figs. 1.12 to 1.15.

A mosquito hemostat or small forceps is preferred for clamping vessels because they cause minimal tissue damage. Vessels should be clamped as seen, even when a tourniquet is used. An electric cautery, especially of the bipolar type, is helpful. Retractors should be of the small single-hook or double-hook type and should have handles long enough to keep the assistant's hands out of the surgeon's working area. Small self-retaining retractors are also useful in certain situations.

For drilling holes in bone, small steel twist drill points provided in most surgical drill sets are satisfactory. Drill bits and small, sharp-pointed Kirschner wires may be required. Air-powered or battery-powered drills allow precise placement of drill holes and wires. Needle holders with narrow noses and smooth jaws are used for tying fine suture material. Numerous varieties of braided and nonbraided sutures are available to meet the procedure's requirements. Most sutures are available with swaged, straight, or curved needles.

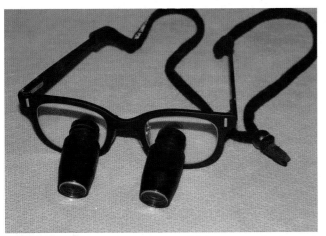

FIGURE 1.15 Magnifying glasses for fine surgery on soft tissues. It is possible to achieve magnification of 6× with magnification lens on glasses frame. The magnification lens becomes too heavy for mounting, however, if more than 6× magnification is needed.

BASIC SKIN TECHNIQUE
INCISIONS

As long as certain principles are observed, skin incisions can be made anywhere on the hand (Figs. 1.16 and 1.17). Incisions within deep creases should be avoided. Here subcutaneous fat is sparse, and moisture tends to accumulate, macerating the skin edges. An incision should be long enough to expose the deep structures without excessive stretching of the skin edges; greater exposure is possible if the skin and subcutaneous fat are dissected from the underlying fascia. Incision placement applies only to the skin surface; entries into deeper structures are made according to their anatomy and may be opposite in direction to those made in the skin. For example, the skin incision over the radial surface of the wrist for de Quervain stenosing tenosynovitis may be transverse, yet the underlying incision in the stenosed sheath is longitudinal.

Generally, shorter incisions may suffice on the dorsum of the hand because here the skin is more mobile. A straight or lazy-S longitudinal incision on the middorsum of the wrist allows structures to be exposed from the extreme radial side to the extreme ulnar side of the wrist.

Parallel or nearly parallel incisions that are too close together or too long should be avoided because healing may be slow or skin necrosis may occur caused by impairment of

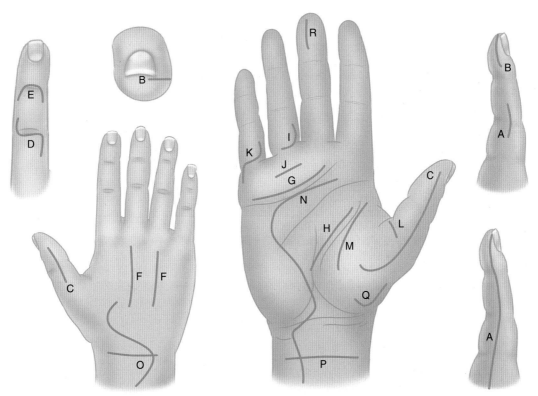

FIGURE 1.16 Correct skin incisions in hand: *A,* Midlateral incision in finger. *B,* Incision for draining felon. *C,* Midlateral incision in thumb. *D,* Incision to expose central slip of extensor tendon. *E,* Inverted-V incision for arthrodesis of distal interphalangeal joint. *F,* Incision to expose metacarpal shaft. *G,* Incision to expose palmar fascia distally. *H,* Incision to expose structures in middle of palm. *I,* L-shaped incision of base of finger. *J,* Short transverse incision to expose flexor tendon sheath. *K,* S-shaped incision in base of finger. *L,* Incision to expose proximal end of flexor tendon sheath of thumb. *M,* Incision to expose structures in thenar eminence. *N,* Extensive palmar and wrist incision. *O,* Incisions in dorsum of wrist. *P,* Transverse incision in volar surface of wrist. *Q,* Incision in base of thumb. *R,* Alternative incision to drain a felon.

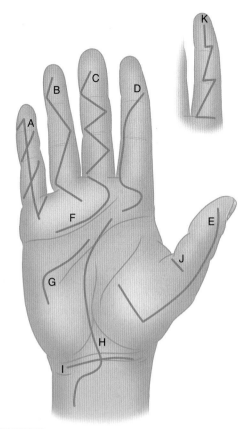

FIGURE 1.17   Additional correct skin incisions in hand: *A,* Z-plasty incision often used in Dupuytren contracture (McGregor). *B* and *C,* Zigzag incisions for Dupuytren contracture or exposure of flexor tendon sheath. *D,* Volar flap incision. *E,* Incision to expose structures in volar side of thumb and thenar area. *F,* Incision in distal palm for trigger finger or other affections of proximal tendon sheath. *G,* Incision to form flap over hypothenar area. *H,* Incision to expose structures in middle of palm; it may be extended proximally into wrist. *I,* Short transverse incision in volar surface of wrist. *J,* Short transverse incision to release trigger thumb. *K,* Digital palmar oblique incision.

the blood supply. Scars that adhere to the underlying structures, especially bone, should be avoided if possible. The offset incision is helpful: the first incision is carried through the skin and subcutaneous fat, and after a flap is undermined on one side, the deep approach is made through the fascia and muscle parallel with but offset from the skin incision.

Joint motions are approximately perpendicular to the long axis of skin creases, and incisions should not cross a crease at or near a right angle because the resulting scar contracture may limit motion. Although true elsewhere in the body, this principle is more important when dealing with the hand, especially the fingers, because the development of contractures results in significant impairment of function.

FINGER INCISIONS

The midlateral finger incision allows the neurovascular bundle to be carried volarward with the volar flap of the incision, or the dissection can be carried superficial to the neurovascular bundle. If the dissection is taken superficial to the neurovascular bundle, care must be taken to avoid making the skin flaps too thin.

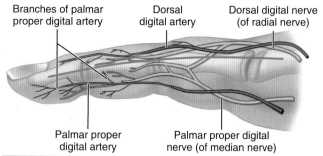

Branches of palmar proper digital artery   Dorsal digital artery   Dorsal digital nerve (of radial nerve)

Palmar proper digital artery   Palmar proper digital nerve (of median nerve)

FIGURE 1.18   Midlateral skin incision in finger extending from metacarpophalangeal joint to lateral edge of nail. To avoid flexor skin creases, it is placed slightly posterolateral. **SEE TECHNIQUE 1.1.**

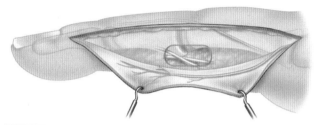

FIGURE 1.19   Midlateral approach especially to expose flexor tendon sheath. On radial sides of index and middle fingers and on ulnar side of little finger is dorsal branch of digital nerve that should be preserved if possible. Volar flap containing neurovascular bundle has been developed and reflected. Window has been cut in sheath to show relationships of flexor tendons. **SEE TECHNIQUE 1.1.**

MIDLATERAL FINGER INCISION

TECHNIQUE 1.1

- To carry the neurovascular bundle volarward, begin the incision on the midlateral aspect of the finger at the level of the proximal finger crease and carry it distally to the proximal interphalangeal joint just dorsal to the flexor skin crease; continue it distally along the middle phalanx, dorsal to the distal flexor skin crease, and proceed toward the lateral edge of the fingernail (Fig. 1.18). Because flexor skin creases extend slightly over halfway around the finger, the incision is slightly posterolateral.
- Develop the dorsal flap a little to aid in closure of the incision.
- The radial sides of the index and middle fingers and the ulnar side of the little finger should be preserved when possible, especially dorsal branches of the digital nerves (Fig. 1.19).
- Develop the volar flap by continuing into the subcutaneous fat over the proximal and middle phalanges, but, because fat is scanty over the proximal interphalangeal joint, be careful not to enter it by mistake.
- Immediately after incising the fat, carry the dissection volarward deep to the neurovascular bundle and expose the tendon sheath. The sheath can be incised, or the neurovascular bundle can be exposed by further dissection

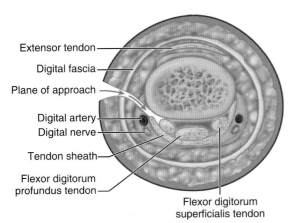

Extensor tendon
Digital fascia
Plane of approach
Digital artery
Digital nerve
Tendon sheath
Flexor digitorum
profundus tendon
Flexor digitorum
superficialis tendon

FIGURE 1.20 Cross section of finger to show midlateral approach when used to expose flexor tendons. **SEE TECHNIQUE 1.1.**

(Fig. 1.20). The opposite neurovascular bundle also can be exposed because of its anterolateral position.

- For the second basic midlateral incision, the skin flap is developed superficial to the neurovascular bundle.
- Make the same midlateral skin incision, but just distal to the distal flexor skin crease, and carry the incision obliquely into the pulp of the finger.
- As the volar skin flap is developed through the subcutaneous fat, carefully isolate the neurovascular bundle; it can best be found at the middle of the middle phalanx.
- Expose the bundle by dissecting the fat from its volar surface, and expose the flexor tendon sheath.
- If necessary, the skin flap can be developed further by dissecting into the depths of the pulp distally, being careful not to disturb the nerves and arteries, and by extending the incision into the palm proximally.

Using the principles just outlined and illustrated, many other extensile exposures of the finger are possible. The popular volar zigzag finger incision (Fig. 1.17B and C) does not require mobilizing either neurovascular bundle and directly exposes the volar surface of the flexor tendon sheath. When used on a contracted skin surface, however, it tends to straighten out and result in a more linear scar than is desirable; here multiple Z-plasty incisions are more satisfactory. In either type of incision, the neurovascular bundles must be protected.

The volar midline oblique incision (Fig. 1.17K) is useful for a variety of procedures and often can be used instead of a volar zigzag incision. It generally is safe and easily closed. In the approach to the flexor sheath, the incision crosses the flexion creases obliquely in the midline of the finger between the neurovascular bundles.

■ THUMB INCISIONS

Midlateral incisions described for the fingers also are suitable for the thumb; the radial side is more accessible, and an incision here can be extended by curving its proximal end at the midmetacarpal area and creating a flap on the palmar surface of the thumb (Fig. 1.16C). Care should be taken to avoid the dorsal branch of the superficial radial nerve to the radial side of the thumb. This incision can be used for tendon grafts without an additional palmar incision because the flap can be developed sufficiently to expose most of the flexor surface of

the thumb. Fat is scanty on the lateral aspects of the thumb interphalangeal joint, and the volar plate may be opened by mistake when seeking the flexor tendon sheath. When a transverse incision for trigger thumb is made at the level of the metacarpophalangeal joint, the two digital nerves of the thumb, located to either side of the flexor tendon as in the fingers, must be carefully avoided (Fig. 1.16L).

■ PALMAR INCISIONS

As a rule, distal palmar incisions are transverse; in the proximal palm, they tend to be more longitudinal, with the distal end curving radially and paralleling the closest major skin crease. An incision of any desired length can be made across the palm, provided that the underlying digital nerves and other vital structures are protected. After the skin and underlying fat have been incised, the latter is dissected from the palmar fascia and is carried with the skin flaps. It may be desirable, although tedious, to preserve small vessels perforating the palmar fascia if wide undermining of the skin flaps is necessary; otherwise, most of the vital structures are deep to the palmar fascia. In the distal palm, structures lying between the metacarpal heads are not protected by the palmar fascia. After the skin flaps have been retracted, the fascia can be incised in any direction necessary for ample exposure; excision of the fascia may be desirable. The tendons and, parallel to them, the neurovascular bundles can then be seen. The superficial volar vascular arch should be protected when deeper exposure is required. Incisions in the more proximal palm should parallel the thenar crease; however, when extended proximal to the wrist, they should not cross the flexor wrist creases at a right angle. The most important structure in the thenar area is the recurrent branch (motor) of the median nerve, which should be exposed and protected if its exact location is in doubt. In addition, care should be taken to avoid injury to the palmar cutaneous branches of the median and ulnar nerves. Anatomic studies have shown that there is no single longitudinal incision in the proximal palm that completely avoids the palmar cutaneous branches of the median and ulnar nerves (Figs. 1.21 and 1.22).

BASIC SKIN CLOSURE TECHNIQUES

Early closure of hand wounds may lessen the chance of infection and excessive scarring, which may destroy the gliding mechanism essential to hand movements. Immediate coverage is imperative when bone, cartilage, or tendon is exposed because of desiccation of these underlying structures. Whenever possible, direct skin suture without tension is the best method of closure. On the dorsum of the hand or wrist, this is sometimes possible even after considerable loss of the mobile skin by extending the wrist to relieve tension; care should be taken, however, to not hyperextend the metacarpophalangeal joints (Fig. 1.23). When a large defect here is closed in this manner, flexion of the wrist and fingers is limited, and replacement of skin by grafting may be necessary later. The advantages of primary closure by direct suture are jeopardized unless each suture is accurately and patiently placed because not only the epidermis but also each plane of tissue should meet its corresponding plane. In the digits, palm, and dorsum of the hand, subcutaneous sutures are almost never necessary. Placing too few sutures or placing them too close to the skin edges jeopardizes satisfactory wound closure: the underlying tissues heal poorly, the skin edges tend to separate

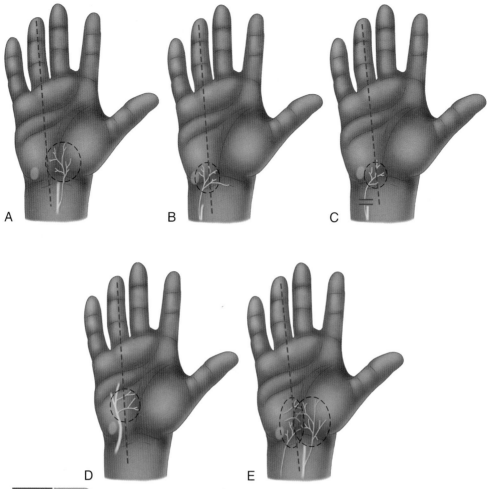

FIGURE 1.21 Cutaneous innervation of palm. **A,** Palmar cutaneous branch of median nerve, present in 100% of specimens. **B,** Palmar cutaneous branch of ulnar nerve, present in 16% of specimens. **C,** Nerve of Henle, present in 40%. **D,** Transverse palmar cutaneous branches of ulnar nerve, present in 96%. **E,** Cutaneous nerves at risk for being transected by traditional incision used for carpal tunnel surgery.

between the sutures, and necrosis occurs around the sutures (Fig. 1.24). The apical stitch is extremely useful for suturing a sharp angle in a laceration or in an elective flap because it holds effectively without embarrassing the circulation at the apex (Fig. 1.25). Sometimes a "dog ear" of redundant tissue is left after closure of a wound with uneven edges. This "dog ear" can be excised one side at a time after splitting it down the middle to create two triangles; each triangle is then excised at its base. The line of excision of one side is used to mark the line of excision of the other. Another method of excising a "dog ear" is shown in Fig. 1.26.

When closure without excessive tension by direct suture is impossible, some type of skin graft may be chosen without prolonged delay, usually within about 5 days. The types of skin grafts most frequently used are described in chapter 2. Sometimes leaving palmar wounds open is advantageous, such as in Dupuytren disease or other long-standing contractures. Transverse wounds, even gaps as large as 2 to 3 cm, appear to heal uneventfully in 6 to 8 weeks. This open palmar technique allows egress of fluid, perhaps reducing swelling

and infection rates. In similar fashion, even palmar digital and proximal interphalangeal skin gaps can heal by secondary intention.

Z-PLASTY

Z-plasty is an application of the transposition type of local flap whereby suitably constructed skin flaps are brought from adjacent areas to release a contracture. Typically, Z-plasty produces a gain in length along the central limb, which undergoes a change in orientation. Its primary use is in the release of a long, narrow contracture surrounded by tissue mobile enough to allow some shifting and manipulation without the danger of necrosis from impaired blood supply. Z-plasty should not be used in attempting to close a wide fusiform defect, nor should it be used in the primary closure of a wound, unless the wound consists only of a laceration similar to a surgical incision.

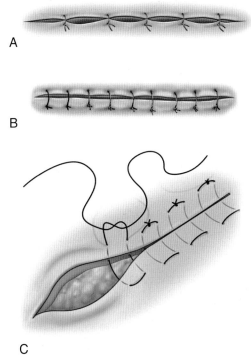

A

B

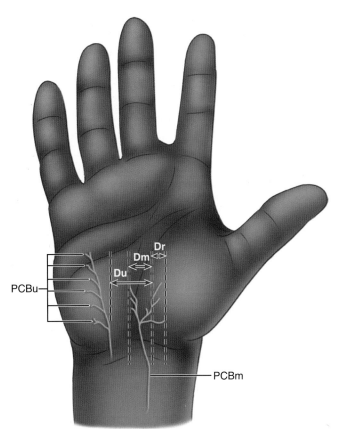

FIGURE 1.22　Distribution of subbranches of palmar cutaneous branches of median *(PCBm)* and ulnar *(PCBu)* nerves. *Du,* Distance from origin of palmar cutaneous branch of ulnar nerve to thenar crease (mean 23 mm); *Dm,* distance from terminal end of most ulnar subbranch of palmar cutaneous branch of median nerve to thenar crease (mean 12 mm); *Dr,* distance from terminal end of most radial subbranch of palmar cutaneous branch of median nerve to thenar crease (mean 5 mm).

C

FIGURE 1.24　**A,** Skin closed by insufficient number of sutures placed too superficially and too close to skin edges. **B,** Skin closed by sufficient number of sutures placed more deeply and well away from skin edges. **C,** Horizontal mattress suturing spreads tension along the wound edge.

FIGURE 1.25　Apical stitch is useful for suturing a sharp angle in laceration or in elective flap.

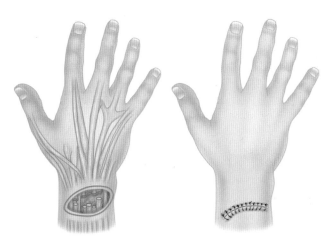

FIGURE 1.23　Small defects of skin and subcutaneous tissue on dorsum of hand or wrist can be closed after wrist has been extended to relieve tension. This closure may require grafting later to permit wrist flexion while making a fist.

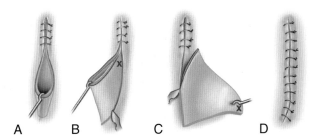

A　　B　　C　　D

FIGURE 1.26　Method of excising "dog ear." **A,** Fold of skin is caught at its apex by hook. **B,** Fold is retracted to one side, and skin is incised along base of fold on opposite side; point *X* forms apex of flap. **C,** Skin is unfolded, and resulting flap is excised. **D,** Skin closure has been completed.

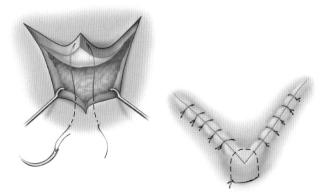

Figure 1.27

- Make the central limb of the Z along the line of the contracture to be released (Fig. 1.28).
- Make the other two limbs of the Z equal in length to that of the central limb; the angle between each limb and the central limb must be equal to each other and should be about 60 degrees or less. An increase in this angle would not allow transposition of the flap without severe tension; a decrease makes the Z less effective in releasing tension and impairs the blood supply to each flap.
- Handle the points of the flaps with care because they are most likely to undergo necrosis; suture each point with an apical stitch.
- Multiple Z-plasties (Figs. 1.29 and 1.30) can be used when a scar is too long to allow correction with one Z-plasty and when the scars resulting from the flap rotation would be in more desirable positions.

McGregor modified the standard multiple Z-plasty for use in the fixed palmar skin of the hand and fingers (Fig. 1.17A). The length of its limbs may vary, making adjoining flaps larger or smaller as desired; however, the length of the

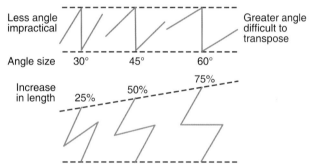

FIGURE 1.27 Angles permissible in performing Z-plasties. Angle that central limb of Z makes with each of the other two limbs should be 45 to 60 degrees. When angle is less than 45 degrees, blood supply to flap is impaired; when angle is more than 60 degrees, flaps cannot be transposed without severe tension. **SEE TECHNIQUE 1.2.**

limbs of each individual Z must be equal. The oblique limbs are curved to broaden the tips of the flaps, increasing their blood supply. A three-flap arrangement of skin can be useful for relieving web contractures in the second, third, or fourth webs (Fig. 1.31).

CARE AFTER SURGERY

Care after surgery must be managed so that tissues are allowed to heal and functions of the affected part are restored as rapidly as possible. Care begins with the application of the dressing. The routine dressing is applied as follows. A closely woven patch of nonadherent gauze (Xeroform or Adaptic) is placed over each incision. Granulation tissue cannot grow through this material and cause it to adhere; the gauze also prevents the wound from becoming macerated. After the hand has been positioned properly, sponges that have been moistened in saline or glycerin solution can be placed carefully around it. Moist sponges conform to the contours of the hand more accurately and distribute pressure more evenly than do dry ones. They also promote absorption of blood. A roll of cotton or synthetic sheet padding is wrapped around the hand and forearm. Finally, an appropriate splint, of plaster or fiberglass, is applied and is held in position with a roll of 2-inch or 3-inch gauze bandage. Immediately before the tourniquet is removed, the hand is kept constantly elevated to prevent edema and hemorrhage after surgery. Splints and bandages on children tend to slip distally but can be controlled effectively by applying a long-arm splint or cast and a tube of stockinette that encloses the entire extremity. Adults responsible for children's postoperative care should be competent in evaluating the vascular status of the fingers and hand.

Elevation should be maintained for at least 48 hours; this can be done by positioning the hand on a pillow resting on the chest, with a sling that positions the hand higher than the elbow (Fig. 1.32A), by light overhead suspension that elevates the hand and forearm while the elbow rests on the bed, or by using a preformed rubber sponge block (Fig. 1.32B). A simple solution is to use two pillows pinned together over two rolled towels (Fig. 1.33).

Body activity increases edema of the hand, and merely supporting it in a sling while the patient is ambulatory is not effective. Fingers not splinted should be exercised. The shoulder is

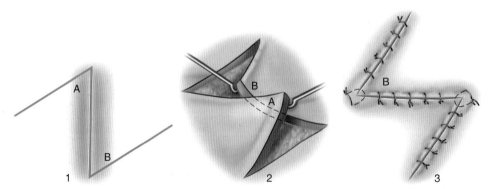

FIGURE 1.28 Simple Z-plasty to release long, narrow contracture. *1,* Central limb of Z is made along line of contracture, and other two limbs are to be made where shown. *2,* Incisions are made, and flaps are shifted. *3,* Flaps are sutured in their new positions. Note apical stitches at *A* and *B.* **SEE TECHNIQUE 1.2.**

likely to become stiff, especially in older patients, and should be abducted and elevated toward the head several times daily.

Although sutures usually are removed 10 to 14 days after surgery, they may not require removal until the splint is discarded, sometimes even at 3 or 4 weeks. Complete redressing of wounds may be unnecessary unless hematoma or infection is suspected. In these instances, the dressing should be opened as needed and the splint should be reapplied. Even when no complications are suspected, wound inspection at about 7 days may allow timely management of unexpected infection or skin necrosis.

Active use of the hand is the most effective way to reestablish motion after surgery. Physical therapy and occupational therapy techniques, protocols, and modalities are helpful in educating the patient to reintegrate the hand and upper extremity into vocational, recreational, and other activities of daily living. Hand therapy has been of immeasurable importance in assisting patients in their recovery. Often the best therapy is the patient's usual work; if possible, patients should be offered the opportunity to return to work as part of the treatment, even if on a limited basis. The return to the activities of daily living and work also seems to have a beneficial psychologic effect.

Applying excessive heat to the hand and forced passive manipulation of joints by the patient, therapist, or surgeon usually are contraindicated. The patient, therapist, and surgeon should function as a well-integrated team, planning and organizing the patient's course of treatment, with scheduled progress evaluations. In most settings, the surgeon should take the lead in planning, prescribing, and monitoring the therapy program. The patient should not be forced into therapeutic interventions that are markedly painful. Causes of pain should be determined, internal splinting should be incorporated when indicated, and timelines and therapeutic endpoints should be outlined.

Insufficient postoperative pain management can negatively affect patient satisfaction and outcomes. However, with

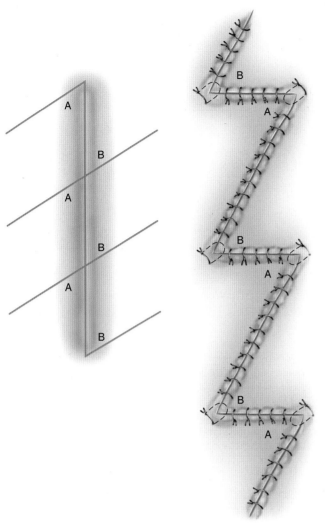

FIGURE 1.29 Multiple Z-plasties to release scar too long to be released by single Z-plasty. **SEE TECHNIQUE 1.2.**

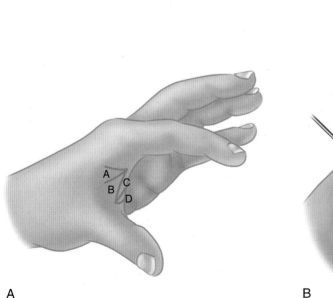

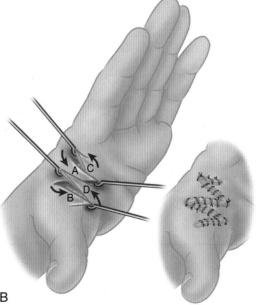

A   B

FIGURE 1.30 Four-flap Z-plasties are useful in reducing first web contractures secondary to narrow linear scar and with normal elastic surrounding tissue. **A,** Outline of flaps. **B,** Flaps are rotated. *Inset,* Flaps are sutured in place. **SEE TECHNIQUE 1.2.**

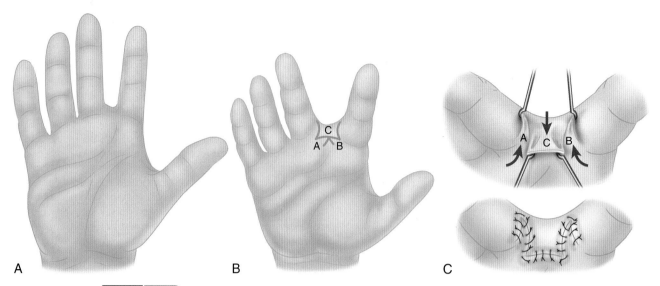

FIGURE 1.31 To correct linear contracture of second, third, or fourth web caused only by narrow scar, dorsal flap may be fashioned using technique shown. **A,** Web contracture. **B,** Flaps are outlined. **C,** Flaps are rotated in place. *Inset,* Flaps are sutured.

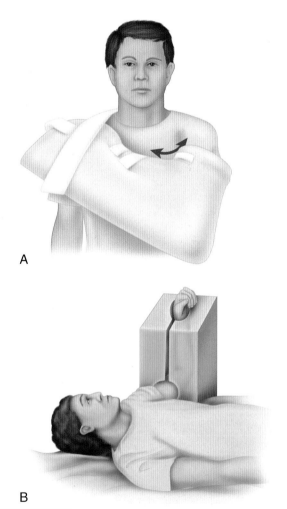

FIGURE 1.32 Postoperative elevation can be maintained with a sling that keeps hand higher than elbow **(A)** or with preformed rubber sponge block **(B)**.

the ever-increasing abuse of prescription opioids, obtaining adequate pain control after surgery can be challenging. Most studies agree on the use multi-modal pain management strategies to decrease narcotic use. Depending on the type and scope of procedure, Ilyas et al. and Stepan et al. advocate prescribing no more than four to 10 narcotic pills after surgery. Kelley et al. developed a helpful algorithm for acute postoperative pain management in patients undergoing hand surgery (Fig. 1.34).

SPLINTING

Splinting serves several purposes: (1) to immobilize all or part of the hand in a position that promotes healing and prevents deformity; (2) to correct an existing deformity and promote function in that part; and (3) to supply power to compensate for weakness, especially in muscles affected by peripheral nerve palsy. Splints may function to prevent motion (static splints) or to assist motion (dynamic splints).

Immobilizing splints are used most frequently after an operation for a limited time only or intermittently to ensure correct position of joints and to relax muscles; they also are used to prevent further deformity, as in an arthritic hand. The splint should permit unaffected parts to function as normally as possible. They should be comfortable and light. Care should be taken so that the splint does not cause excessive skin pressure, especially over joints, because pressure sores may develop and interfere with the therapy program, delaying the patient's progress. An orthotist or therapist should be available for making technical adjustments requiring special skills, but the patient should be able to apply the splint, remove it, and make minor adjustments. Useful splints are illustrated in Figs. 1.35 to 1.42. The patient should thoroughly understand the reason for splint wear and should be educated about its value. As treatment progresses, faithful use can be determined by observing the patient's skill in applying and removing the splint.

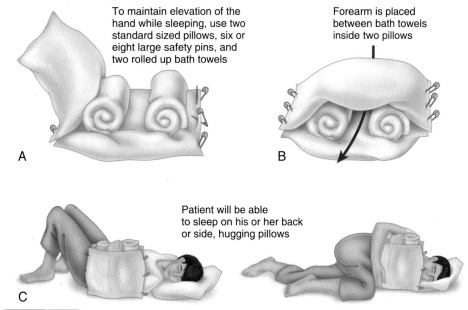

To maintain elevation of the hand while sleeping, use two standard sized pillows, six or eight large safety pins, and two rolled up bath towels

Forearm is placed between bath towels inside two pillows

Patient will be able to sleep on his or her back or side, hugging pillows

A

B

C

FIGURE 1.33 A simple method of hand elevation uses two pillows, two rolled towels, and several safety pins. (Redrawn from Green DP: General principles. In Wolfe SW, Hotchkiss RN, Pederson WC, Kozin SH, editors: *Green's operative hand surgery,* ed 6, Philadelphia, 2011, Elsevier.)

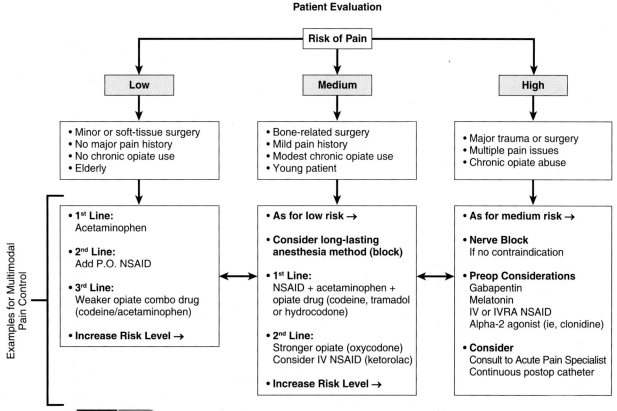

Patient Evaluation

Risk of Pain

Low

Medium

High

- Minor or soft-tissue surgery
- No major pain history
- No chronic opiate use
- Elderly

- Bone-related surgery
- Mild pain history
- Modest chronic opiate use
- Young patient

- Major trauma or surgery
- Multiple pain issues
- Chronic opiate abuse

Examples for Multimodal Pain Control

- **1st Line:** Acetaminophen

- **2nd Line:** Add P.O. NSAID

- **3rd Line:** Weaker opiate combo drug (codeine/acetaminophen)

- **Increase Risk Level →**

- **As for low risk →**

- **Consider long-lasting anesthesia method (block)**

- **1st Line:** NSAID + acetaminophen + opiate drug (codeine, tramadol or hydrocodone)

- **2nd Line:** Stronger opiate (oxycodone) Consider IV NSAID (ketorolac)

- **Increase Risk Level →**

- **As for medium risk →**

- **Nerve Block** If no contraindication

- **Preop Considerations** Gabapentin Melatonin IV or IVRA NSAID Alpha-2 agonist (ie, clonidine)

- **Consider** Consult to Acute Pain Specialist Continuous postop catheter

FIGURE 1.34 Algorithm for pain control in patients after hand surgery. *P.O.*, Oral; *IV*, intravenous; *combo*, combination. (From: Kelley BP, Shauver MJ, Chung KC: Management of acute postoperative pain in hand surgery: a systematic review, *J Hand Surg Am* 40(8):1610, 2015.)

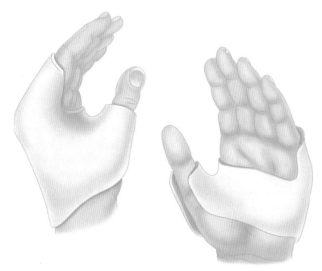

FIGURE 1.35   Splint is comfortable and has very low profile, which encourages wearing while recovery is progressing in median-ulnar nerve palsies. It permits pinch and some grasping while maintaining metacarpophalangeal joints in slight flexion. It blocks metacarpophalangeal joint extension and prevents clawing.

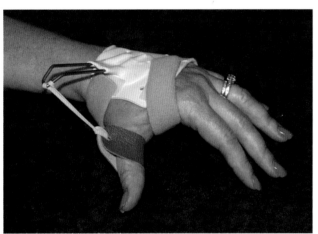

FIGURE 1.36   Splint for low median nerve palsy dynamically holds thumb in abduction, extension, and opposition, preventing adduction contracture of thumb. Splint is light and compact.

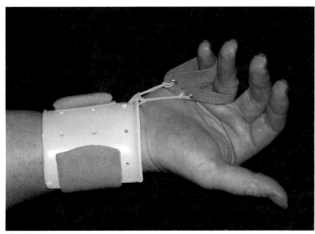

FIGURE 1.37   Splint for ulnar nerve palsy dynamically forces metacarpophalangeal joints of ring and little fingers into flexion. Part of palm is covered by rubber bands, which is a disadvantage.

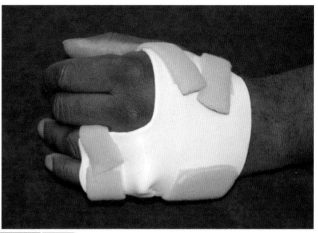

FIGURE 1.38   Splint for ulnar nerve palsy prevents hyperextension deformity of metacarpophalangeal joints of ring and little fingers. It also conforms to shape of transverse metacarpal arch and has no attachments that hinder function of hand.

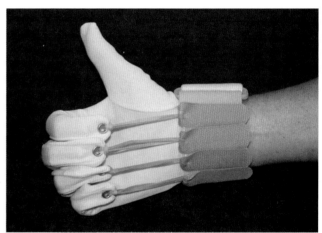

FIGURE 1.39   Flexor glove dynamically forces fingers into flexion, exerting continuous force on proximal interphalangeal and metacarpophalangeal joints. Sometimes it also flexes wrist when proximal eyelets are too far proximal, and, when desirable, it may be applied over volar wrist splint.

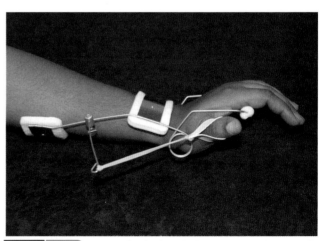

FIGURE 1.40   Splint for high radial nerve palsy dynamically splints digits in extension.

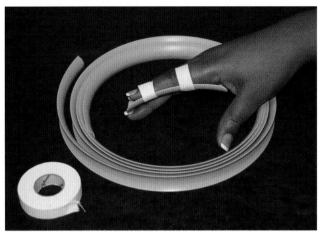

FIGURE 1.41 Preformed plastic gutter splints for digits are easily adjustable in length and support soft tissue or fracture healing.

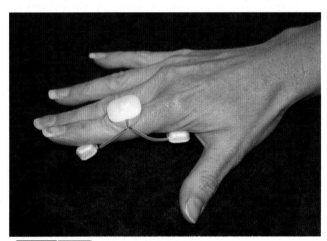

FIGURE 1.42 Proximal interphalangeal extension splint.

REFERENCES

GENERAL/ANATOMY

Aydun N, Uraloglu M, Yilmaz Burhanoglu AD, Sensöz O: A prospective trial on the use of antibiotics in hand surgery, *Plast Reconstr Surg* 126:1617, 2010.

Bykowski MR, Sivak WN, Cray J, et al.: Assessing the impact of antibiotic prophylaxis in outpatient elective hand surgery: a single-center, retrospective review of 8,850 cases, *J Hand Surg [Am]* 36A:1741, 2011.

Dunn JC, Fares AB, Kusnezov N, et al.: Current evidence regarding routine antibiotic prophylaxis in hand surgery, *Hand (N Y)*, 2017, Mar 1:1558944717701241.

Edmunds I, Avakian Z: Hand surgery on anticoagulated patients: a prospective study of 121 operations, *Hand Surg* 15:109, 2010.

Gurses IA, Coskun O, Gayretyli O, et al.: The relationship of the superficial radial nerve and its branch to the thumb to the first extensor compartment, *J Hand Surg [Am]* 39:480, 2014.

Garon MT, Massey P, Chen A, et al.: Cost and complications of percutaneous fixation of hand fractures in a procedure room versus the operating room, *Hand (N Y)* 13(4):428, 2018.

Hyatt BT, Saucedo JM: Beside procedures in hand surgery, *J Hand Surg Am*, 2018.

Johnson SP Zhong L, Chung KC, Waljee JF: Perioperative antibiotics for clean hand surgery: a national study, *J Hand Surg Am* 43(5):407, 2018.

Kazmers NH, Presson AP, Xu Y, Howenstein A: Cost implications of varying the surgical technique, surgical setting, and anesthesia type for carpal tunnel release surgery, *J Hand Surg Am*, 2018.

Tyser AR, Kocheta A, Agrawal Y: Landmark technique for a wrist block, *JBJS Essent Surg Tech* 8(1):37, 2018.

Li K, Sambare TD, Jiang SY, et al.: Effectiveness of preoperative antibiotics in preventing surgical site infection after common soft tissue procedures of the hand, *Clin Orthop Relat Res* 476(40):664, 2018.

Sandrowski K, Edelman D, Rivlin M, et al.: A prospective evaluation of adverse reactions to single-dose intravenous antibiotic prophylaxis during outpatient hand surgery, *Hand (N Y)*, 2018, Jul 1:1558944718787264.

Tosti R, Fowler J, Dwyer J, et al.: Is antibiotic prophylaxis necessary in elective soft tissue hand surgery? *Orthopedics* 35:e829, 2012.

Vallera C, LaPorte DM: Preoperative evaluation for hand surgery in adults, *J Hand Surg Am* 36A:1394, 2011.

Zeng W, Paul D, Kemp T, Elfar J: Prosthetic joint infections in patients undergoing carpal tunnel release, *J Am Acad Orthop Surg* 25(3):225, 2017.

ANESTHESIA

Albino FP, Fleury C, Higgins JP: Putting it all together: recommendations for improving pain management in plastic surgical procedures: hand surgery, *Plast Reconstr Surg* 134:1265, 2014.

Al Youha S, Lalonde DH: Update/review: changing of use of local anesthesia in the hand, *Plast Reconstr Surg Glob Open* 2:e150, 2014.

Arslanian B, Mehrzad R, Kramer T, Kim DC: Forearm Bier block: a new regional anesthetic technique for upper extremity surgery, *Ann Plast Surg* 23:156, 2014.

Badiger SV, Desai SN: Comparison of nerve stimulation-guided axillary brachial plexus block, single injection versus four infections: a prospective randomized double-blind study, *Anesth Essays Res* 11(1):140, 2017.

Bashir MM, Oayyum R, Saleem MH, et al.: Effect of time interval between tumescent local anesthesia infiltration and start of surgery on operative field visibility in hand surgery without tourniquet, *J Hand Surg Am* 40:1606, 2015.

Bismil MSK, Bismil OMK, Harding D, et al. Transition to total one-stop wide-awake hand surgery service-audit: a retrospective review. *J R Soc Med Sh Rep* 3:23, 2013.

Blackburn EW, Shafritz AB: Why do Bier blocks work for hand surgery … most of the time? *J Hand Surg Am* 35A:1022, 2010.

Bruce BG, Green A, Blaine TA, Wesner LV: Brachial plexus blocks for upper extremity orthopaedic surgery, *J Am Acad Orthop Surg* 20:38, 2010.

Caggiano NM, Avery 3rd DM, Matullo KS: The effect of anesthesia type on nonsurgical operating room time, *J Hand Surg Am* 40:1202, 2015.

Calder K, Chung B, O'Brien C, et al.: Bupivacaine digital blocks: how long is the pain relief and temperature elevation? *Plast Reconstr Surg* 131:1098, 2013.

Cantlon MB, Yang SS: Wide awake hand surgery. *Bull Hosp Jt Dis* 75:47-51, 2017.

Chin KJ, Alakkad H, Cubillos JE: Single, double or multiple-injection techniques for non-ultrasound guided axillary brachial plexus block in adults undergoing surgery of the lower arm, *Cochrane Database Syst Rev* 8:CD003842, 2013.

Chin KJ, Handoll HH: Single, double or multiple-injection techniques for axillary brachial plexus block for hand, wrist or forearm surgery in adults, *Cochrane Database Syst Rev* 7:CD003842, 2011.

Chowdhry S, Seidenstricker L, Cooney DS, et al.: Do not use epinephrine in digital blocks: myth or truth? part II. a retrospective review of 1111 cases, *Plast Reconstr Surg* 126:2031, 2010.

Davison PG, Cobb T, Lalonde DH: The patient's perspective on carpal tunnel surgery related to the type of anesthesia: a prospective cohort study, *Hand (NY)* 8:47, 2013.

Dufeu N, Marchand-Maillet F, Atchabahian A, et al.: Efficacy and safety of ultrasound-guided distal blocks for analgesia without motor blockade after ambulatory hand surgery, *J Hand Surg Am* 39:737, 2014.

Fletcher SJ, Hulgur MD, Varma S, et al.: Use of a temporary forearm tourniquet for intravenous regional anaesthesia: a randomised controlled trial, *Eur J Anaesthesiol* 28:133, 2011.

Gianesello L, Pavoni V, Coppini R, et al.: Comfort and satisfaction during axillary brachial plexus block in trauma patients: comparison of techniques, *J Clin Anesth* 22:7, 2010.

Gregory S, Lalonde DH, Leung LTF: Minimally invasive finger fracture management. wide-awake closed reduction, K-wire fixation, and early protected movement, *Hand Clin* 30:7, 2014.

Gupta B, Verma RK, Kumar S, Chaudhary G: Comparison of analgesic efficacy of dexmedetomidine and midazolam as adjuncts to lidocaine for intravenous regional anesthesia, *Anesth Essays Res* 11(1):62, 2017.

Gurich Jr RW, Langan JW, Teasdall RJ, et al.: Tourniquet deflation prior to 20 minutes in upper extremity intravenous regional anesthesia, *Hand (N Y)* 13(2):223, 2018.

Hagert E, Lalonde DH: Wide-awake wrist arthroscopy and open TFCC repair, *J Wrist Surg* 1:55, 2012.

Hogan ME, vanderVaart S, Perampaladas K, et al.: Systematic review and meta-analysis of the effect of warming local anesthetics on injection pain, *Ann Emerg Med* 58:86, 2011.

Hustedt JW, Chung A, Bohl DD, et al.: Comparison of postoperative complications associated with anesthetic choice for surgery of the hand, *J Hand Surg Am* 42:1, 2017.

Iqbal HJ, Doorgakant A, Rehmatullah NNT, et al.: Pain and outcomes of carpal tunnel release under local anaesthetic with or without a tourniquet: a randomized controlled trial, *J Hand Surg Eur* 43(8):808, 2018.

Kang RA, Chung YH, Ko JS, et al.: Reduced hemidiaphragmatic paresis with a "corner pocket" technique for supraclavicular brachial plexus block single-center, observer-blinded, randomized controlled trial, *Reg Anesth Pain Med* 43(7):720, 2018.

Kocheta A, Agrawal Y: Landmark technique for a wrist block, *JBJS Essent Surg Tech* 8:E7, 2018.

Lalonde D: Minimally invasive anesthesia in wide awake hand surgery, *Hand Clin* 30:1, 2014.

Lalonde DH: Wide-awake extensor indicis proprius to extensor pollicis longus tendon transfer, *J Hand Surg Am* 39:2297, 2014.

Lalonde D, Eaton C, Amadio PC, Jupiter JB: Wide-awake hand and wrist surgery: a new horizon in outpatient surgery, *Instr Course Lect* 64:249, 2015.

Lalonde D, Martin A: Epinephrine in local anesthesia in finger and hand surgery: the case for wide-awake anesthesia, *J Am Acad Orthop Surg* 21:443, 2013.

Lalonde D, Martin A: Tumescent local anesthesia for hand surgery: improved results, cost effectiveness, and wide-awake patient satisfaction, *Arch Plast Surg* 41:312, 2014.

Lalonde DH, Martin AL: Wide-awake flexor tendon repair and early tendon mobilization in zones 1 and 2, *Hand Clin* 29:207, 2013.

Lalonde D, Martin A: Tumescent local anesthesia for hand surgery: improved results, cost effectiveness, and wide-awake patient satisfaction, *Arch Plast Surg* 41:312, 2014.

Lalonde DH, Wong A: Dosage of local anesthesia in wide awake hand surgery, *J Hand Surg* 38A:2025, 2013.

Lam NC, Charles M, Mercer D, et al.: A triple-masked, randomized, controlled trial comparing ultrasound-guided brachial plexus and distal peripheral nerve block anesthesia for outpatient hand surgery, *Anesthesiol Res Pract* 2014:324083, 2014.

Lee HJ, Cho YJ, Gong HS, et al.: The effect of buffered lidocaine in local anesthesia: a prospective, randomized double-blind study, *J Hand Surg Am* 38:971, 2013.

Lin E, Choi J, Hadzic A: Peripheral nerve blocks for outpatient surgery: evidence-based indications, *Curr Opin Anaesthesiol* 26:467, 2013.

Lovely LM, Chishti YZ, Woodland JL, Lalonde DH: How much volume of local anesthesia and how long should you wait after injection for an effective wrist median nerve block? *Hand (N Y)* 13(3):281, 2018.

Martires KJ, Malbasa CL, Bordeaux JS: A randomized controlled crossover trial: lidocaine injected at a 90-degree angle causes less pain than lidocaine injected at a 45-degree angle, *J Am Acad Dermatol* 65:1231, 2011.

McKee DE, Lalonde DH, Thoma A, et al.: Optimal time delay between epinephrine injection and incision to minimize bleeding, *Plast Reconstr Surg* 131:811, 2013.

Middleton SD, Jenkins PJ, Muir AY, et al.: Variability in local pressures under digital tourniquets, *J Hand Surg Eur* 39:637, 2014.

Miller A, Kim N, Ilyas AM: Prospective evaluation of opioid consumption following hand surgery performed wide awake versus with sedation, *Hand (N Y)* 12(6):606, 2017.

Nelson R, Higgins A, Conrad J, et al.: The wide-awake approach to Dupuytren's disease: fasciectomy under local anesthetic with epinephrine, *Hand (NY)* 5:117, 2010.

Perretta DJ, Gotlin M, Brock K, et al.: Brachial plexus blockade causes subclinical neuroapathy: a prospective observational study, *Hand (N Y)* 12(1):50, 2017.

Rozanski M, Neuhaus V, Reddy R, et al.: An open-label comparison of local anesthesia with or without sedation for minor hand surgery, *Hand (N Y)* 9:399, 2014.

Sasor SE, Cook JA, Duquette SP, et al.: Tourniquet use in wide-awake carpal tunnel release, *Hand (N Y)*, 2018, Jul 1 1558944718787853.

Soberén Jr JR, Crookshank 3rd JW, Nossaman BD, et al.: Distal peripheral nerve blocks in the forearm as an alternative to proximal brachial plexus blockade in patients undergoing hand surgery: a prospective and randomized pilot study, *J Hand Surg Am* 41(10), 2016.

Sørensen AM, Dalsgaard J, Hansen TB: Local anaesthesia versus intravenous regional anaesthesia in endoscopic carpal tunnel release: a randomized controlled trial, *J Hand Surg Eur* 38:481, 2013.

Srikumaran U, Stein BE, Tan EW, et al.: Upper-extremity peripheral nerve blocks in the perioperative pain management of orthopaedic patients: AAOS exhibit selection, *J Bone Joint Surg* 95A:e197, 2013.

Steiner MM, Calandruccio JH: Use of wide-awake local anesthesia no tourniquet in hand and wrist surgery, *Orthop Clin North Am* 49(1):63, 2018.

Strazar AR, Leynes PG, Lalonde DH: Minimizing the pain of local anesthesia injection, *Plast Reconstr Surg* 132:675, 2013.

Tang JB: Wide-awake primary flexor tendon repair, tenolysis, and tendon transfer, *Clin Orthop Surg* 7:275, 2015.

Van Demark RE, Becker HA, Anderson MC, Smith VJS: Wide-awake anesthesia in the in-office procedure room: lessons learned, *Hand (N Y)* 13(4):481, 2018.

Vinycomb TI, Sahhar LJ: Comparison of local anesthetics for digital nerve blocks: a systematic review, *J Hand Surg Am* 39:744, 2014.

Warrender WJ, Lucasti CJ, Ilyas AM: Wide-awake hand surgery: principles and techniques, *J Bone Joint Surg Rev* 6(5):e8, 2018.

Wong KH, Huq NS, Nakhooda A: Hand surgery using local anesthesia, *Clin Plast Surg* 40:567, 2013.

Xing SG, Tang JB: Surgical treatment, hardware removal, and the wide-awake approach for metacarpal fractures, *Clin Plast Surg* 41:463, 2014.

Zencirci B: Comparison of nerve stimulator and ultrasonography as the techniques applied for brachial plexus anesthesia, *Int Arch Med* 4:4, 2011.

Zhu AF, Hood BR, Morris MS, Ozer K: Delayed-onset digital ischemia after local anesthetic with epinephrine injection requiring phenolamine reversal, *J Hand Surg Am* 42(6):e1, 2017.

INCISIONS

Catalano LW, Zlotolow DA, Purcelli Lafer M, et al.: Surgical exposures of the wrist and hand, *J Am Acad Orthop Surg* 20:48, 2010.

Xu X, Lao J, Zhao X: How to prevent injury to the palmar cutaneous branch of median nerve and ulnar nerve in a palmar incision in carpal tunnel release, a cadaveric study, *Acta Neurochir (Wien)* 155:1751, 2013.

SKIN CLOSURE

Dosani A, Khan SK, Gray S, et al.: Clinical outcome and cost comparison of carpal tunnel wound closure with monocryl and ethilon: a prospective study, *Hand Surg* 18:189, 2013.

Hundeshagen G, Zapata-Sirvent R, Goverman J, Branski LK: Tissue rearrangements: the power of the Z-plasty, *Clin Plast Surg* 44(4):2017.

Kundra RK, Newman S, Saithna A, et al.: Absorbable or non-absorbable sutures? A prospective, randomised evaluation of aesthetic outcomes in patients undergoing elective day-case hand and wrist surgery, *Ann R Coll Surg Engl* 92:665, 2010.

POSTOPERATIVE MANAGEMENT

Ahsan ZS, Carvalho B, Yao J: Incidence of failure of continuous peripheral nerve catheters for postoperative analgesia in upper extremity surgery, *J Hand Surg Am* 39:324, 2014.

Albino FP, Fleury C, Higgins JP: Putting it all together: recommendations for improving pain management in plastic surgical procedures: hand surgery, *Plast Reconstr Surg* 134(4 Suppl 2):126S, 2014.

Gauger EM, Gauger EJ, Desai MJ, Lee DH: Opioid use after upper extremity surgery, *J Hand Surg Am* 43(5):470, 2018.

Haddock NT, Weinstein AL, Sinno S, Chiu DT: Thrombin and topical local anesthetic for postoperative pain management, *Ann Plast Surg* 73:30, 2014.

Harrison RK, DiMeo T, Klinefelter RD, et al.: Multi-modal pain control in ambulatory hand surgery, *Am J Orthop (Belle Mead NJ)* 47(6), 2018.

Ilyas AM, Miller AJ, Graham JG, Matzon JL: Pain management after carpal tunnel release surgery: a prospective randomized double-blinded trial comparing acetaminophen, ibuprofen, and oxycodone, *J Hand Surg Am* 43(10):913, 2018.

Kelley BP, Shauver MJ, Chung KC: Management of acute postoperative pain in hand surgery: a systematic review, *J Hand Surg Am* 40(8):1610, 2015.

Labrum 4th JT, Ilyas AM: Perioperative pain control in upper extremity surgery: prescribing patterns, recent developments, and opioid-sparing treatment strategies, *hand (N Y)*, 2018, Jul 1:1558944718787262.

Stepan JG, London DA, Osei DA, et al.: Perioperative celecoxib and postoperative opioid use in hand surgery: a prospective cohort study, *J Hand Surg Am* 43(4):346, 2018.

Yang G, McClinn EP, Chung KC: Management of the stiff finger: evidence and outcomes, *Clin Plast Surg* 41:501, 2014.

TOURNIQUET

Brewster MB, Upadhyay PK, Hill CE: Finger tourniquets: a review of national patient safety agency recommendations, available devices and current practice, *J Hand Surg Eur* 40:214, 2015.

Chiao FB, Chen J, Lesser JB, et al.: Single-cuff forearm tourniquet in intravenous regional anaesthesia results in less pain and fewer sedation requirements than upper arm tourniquet, *Br J Anaesth* 111:271, 2013.

Drolet BC, Okhah Z, Phillips BZ, et al.: Evidence for safe tourniquet use in 500 consecutive upper extremity procedures, *Hand (N Y)* 9:494, 2014.

Lim E, Shukla L, Barker A, Trotter DJ: Randomized blinded control trial into tourniquet tolerance in awake volunteers, *ANZ J Surg* 85:636, 2015.

Martin-Smith JD, van der Rijt R, Kelly J: Finger tourniquets: two safe and cost effective techniques and a discussion of the literature, *Hand Surg* 18:2283, 2013.

Middleton SD, Jenkins PJ, Muir AY, et al.: Variability in local pressures under digital tourniquets, *J Hand Surg Eur* 39:637, 2013.

Oragui E, Parsons A, White T, et al.: Tourniquet use in upper limb surgery, *Hand (N Y)* 6(2):165, 2011.

SPLINTING

MacLean SB, Dhillon S, Dias R: Safe and re-usable splinting for hand surgery, *Ann R Coll Surg Engl* 92:169, 2010.

Rocchi I, Merolli A, Morini A, et al.: A modified spica-splint in postoperative early-motion management of skier's thumb lesion: a randomized clinical trial, *Eur J Phys Rehabil Med* 50:49, 2014.

The complete list of references is available online at Expert Consult.com.

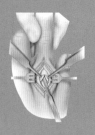

CHAPTER 2

ACUTE HAND INJURIES

David L. Cannon

The hand and fingers are the body parts most often injured in the workplace. In the United States, annually, more than 1 million emergency department visits are caused by work-related hand trauma. For an acutely injured hand, restoration of function is the goal of treatment. It is necessary to prevent infection, salvage injured parts, and promote primary healing. Although nerves and tendons may be repaired in the primary phase of care, their management is secondary in importance to thorough cleansing and debridement, correct stabilization of fractures and dislocations, and wound closure or coverage with skin grafts or skin flaps. Through patient history taking and careful physical examination, the surgeon must personally appraise the injury to decide which primary procedures can be done safely and which secondary procedures may be necessary later. Determining the best treatment in a timely manner for each individual patient must take into account not only the type and severity of injury but also the type of employment, hobby, or sport of the patient. Long-term impairment is a risk if patients are not returned to work or activities expeditiously. Level of pain, reduced hand function, psychosocial issues, education, compensation, and legal factors have all been found to be associated with resumption of activities.

HISTORY

The history should provide the following information accurately and concisely: (1) the exact time of injury (to determine the interval before treatment), (2) the first aid measures given and by whom and where, (3) the nature, amount, and time of receiving any medication, (4) the exact mechanism of injury (to determine the amount of crushing, contamination, and blood loss), (5) the nature, time, and amount of food and liquid taken by the patient (information necessary

for selection of the anesthetic), and (6) the patient's age, occupation, place of employment, handedness, and general health status. The time since injury is important to determine because immediate, urgent surgery is required for severely contaminated wounds, wounds in which infection of a deep space is suspected, wounds with vascular injuries that cause hemorrhage or compromise perfusion, high-pressure injuries, and wounds for which amputation or replantation may be needed.

EXAMINATION

The evaluations to be performed before wound inspection are (1) radiographs of the hand to check for injuries to bone and for foreign objects, (2) vascular and neurologic function, and (3) motor function of the hand, including examination of possible tendon injury (see chapter 3). These examinations can provide 90% of the information needed to determine appropriate treatment. In addition, it reduces anxiety in the patient if the wound can be covered most of the time. Once that has been accomplished, the wound is examined for size, depth, and location; zone of additional injury; sepsis or contamination; and what procedures will be necessary Techniques for detailed evaluation of tendon and nerve injuries are described in chapter 3 and 5, respectively, and evaluation of fractures and dislocations is described in chapter 4.

Antibiotics, sedation, blood transfusions, tetanus prophylaxis, and other measures are provided as indicated (Table 2.1). Before sedatives or narcotics are given, the patient should be advised as to the extent of the injuries, the general plan of treatment, and the prognosis, especially with regard to any possible amputation. The patient also should be forewarned when skin grafts or distant skin flaps are anticipated (Fig. 2.1).

TABLE 2.1

Antibiotic Prophylaxis for Hand Injuries

CLINICAL SITUATION	ANTIBIOTIC PROPHYLAXIS
Low-risk, traumatic injuries (clean wounds with easily demarcated borders, no devitalized tissue)	None
Injuries in immunocompromised patients (e.g., patient with human immunodeficiency virus infection, diabetes)	Gram-positive cocci coverage
Wounds with devitalized tissue	Gram-positive cocci coverage if wound, tendon, or joint space is contaminated*
Animal and human bites (other than superficial abrasions)	First-generation cephalosporin. In patients with bites that may contain *Pasteurella multocida* or *Eikenella corrodens*, consider penicillin or amoxicillin-clavulanate potassium (Augmentin). In immunocompromised patients, consider erythromycin or amoxicillin-clavulanate. In patients with sepsis and petechial rash, consider intravenous ciprofloxacin (Cipro) and clindamycin (Cleocin).†
Puncture wounds	Case-by-case decision

*If the wound is contaminated, debridement is required.
†Patients with sepsis or petechial rash should be hospitalized.
Adapted from Daniels JM II, Zook EG, Lynch JM: Hand and wrist injuries, part II: emergent evaluation, *Am Fam Physician* 69:1949–1956, 2004.

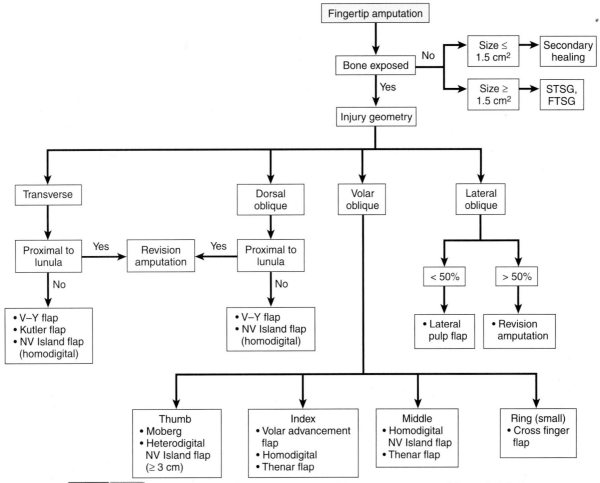

FIGURE 2.1   Algorithm to help guide decision-making in management of fingertip injuries based on digit, geometry, location, and size. *STSG*, Split-thickness skin graft; *FTSG*, full-thickness skin graft. (From Christoforou D, Alaia M, Craig-Scott S: Microsurgical management of acute traumatic injuries of the hand and fingers, *Bull Hosp Jt Dis* 71:6–16, 2013.)

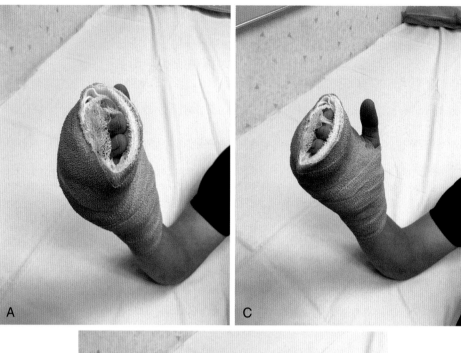

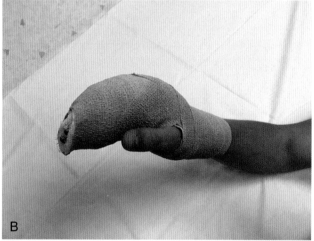

FIGURE 2.2   A-C, Splints.

In the mangled hand or in patients with multiple trauma, evaluation begins by identifying life-threatening injuries, followed by identification of the injured structures. Damage-control orthopaedics may be required when definitive treatment cannot be accomplished in the emergency department. Urgent temporary measures, such as minimizing ischemia time, debriding the wound, splinting the hand, administering antibiotics, and preparing the injury site for secondary repair at a later date, offer the best chance for optimizing hand function.

SPLINTING

When splinting is necessary, it is important to remember that improper technique should be avoided, as it can lead to joint stiffness, skin breakdown, or worsening deformity. A splint should be used to relax muscles, maintain correct position, and immobilize the hand in a position that will prevent further injury. Immobilization should be above and below the injury or deformity but not farther, allowing function to the unaffected parts (Fig. 2.2) (see chapter 1).

ANESTHESIA

A digital block, regional block, or general anesthetic may be selected, depending on the patient's age and general condition, the severity of the injury, other injuries, the interval since the last ingestion of food or drink, and whether or not a distant flap will be necessary (see chapter 1 for more details). Some surgeons have expanded the indications for the wide-awake local anesthesia with no tourniquet (WALANT) technique to acute surgery of the hand (see chapter 1).

TOURNIQUET

A tourniquet is necessary while the wound is being cleansed and inspected and while the deep structures are being repaired. When the viability of an area of skin is questionable because of a crushing or avulsing injury, a tourniquet should be used as briefly as possible. For a large wound with fractures, elevation of the hand for 2 minutes is better than wrapping it with an elastic (Martin) bandage before inflation of the tourniquet. This prevents further crushing and displacement of fracture fragments (for more information on the tourniquet, see chapter 1).

CLEANSING AND DRAPING OF HAND

After the patient or the part is anesthetized and the tourniquet is applied, the first aid dressing is removed and the wound is thoroughly irrigated with normal saline solution, generally through a pulsating lavage apparatus to provide a stream with enough force to loosen small foreign particles and to remove large hematomas. Antiseptics generally are not used in the wound because of potential tissue toxicity. Small bleeding vessels, which sometimes are more easily seen under saline solution, are clamped with mosquito hemostats and cauterized. Small flaps and tags of devitalized fat and fascia seen floating in the solution can be removed at their bases. Nerve ends are not debrided. Ragged skin edges may be trimmed, but complete excision of the edges of the wound usually is unnecessary in the hand.

As the deeper parts of the wound are cleaned, they are carefully searched for foreign materials, especially if there is suspicion that they contain broken glass, wood, or pieces of glove or when the wound has been caused by a gunshot. Cleaning should not be hurried; it must be thorough to help prevent infection. Primary healing without infection is necessary to limit the scar and to allow additional early reconstruction, if needed. When cleaning is complete, all instruments, gloves, and drapes used during this process are discarded and the hand is redraped (see chapter 1 for the details of draping and of the routine in the operating room).

After a diligent effort has been made to convert the contaminated wound into a clean one in the operating room, the wound is reexamined. The circulatory status of the skin is assessed with the usual observations of color and capillary refill in the digit and bleeding of the skin after needle or scalpel puncture and with a Doppler probe for the larger vessels in the hand and upper extremity.

The tissues in the depths of the wound, including exposed bones, tendons, vessels, and nerves, are assessed in an orderly, anatomic manner to avoid error; the skin also is examined carefully. Only after an accurate assessment of the damage can correct decisions be made as to which structures can be repaired primarily. Bones and joints are inspected to assess bone loss, the extent of periosteal stripping, and fracture stability. This evaluation allows estimation of potential bone healing and the advisability of early joint motion after internal fixation of fractures. Conclusions drawn from the first examination may be wrong, so suspected tendon and nerve injury should be confirmed by direct inspection. Usually, the damage has been underestimated.

Evaluating the skin damage is most important because primary wound closure depends on skin viability. Frequently, some skin appears to be lost when actually it has only retracted; this is especially true of L-shaped wounds on the dorsum of the hand. When skin is crushed or flaps of skin are avulsed, the possibility of necrosis must be seriously considered. Releasing the tourniquet may be necessary for accurate evaluation. A valuable sign that skin is viable is a prompt pink blush (about 6 seconds) after release of the tourniquet. The extent of bleeding from the skin edges, the color of the skin immediately after compression, and the amount of undermining of the skin edges must be observed. Necrosis, infection, and scarring can occur if flaps of doubtful viability are retained. The extent of skin loss from the injury itself and after surgical excision of nonviable flaps must be evaluated, and plans must be made for complete coverage. Passive finger motion often delivers severed tendons into the wound. Small hematomas seen within synovial sheaths may be indications of further tendon injury.

CONSIDERATIONS FOR AMPUTATION

Considerations for amputation are discussed in other chapter.

ORDER OF TISSUE REPAIR

Setting priorities for repair of injured structures is important. After the wound is cleaned, the bony architecture must be reestablished immediately if possible (see chapter 4) or within a few days after the wound becomes clean; otherwise, the soft tissues contract, making bone repair difficult or impossible without soft-tissue grafting. Although definitive closure may not be possible, the bony architecture should be reestablished. Stabilize the thumb for opposition, the index and long fingers for pinch and manipulation, and the ring and small fingers for grasp. It is preferable to close the wound within the first 5 days. If the injury and wound conditions permit, tendons and nerves should be repaired at the time of primary or secondary skin closure. While awaiting repair, nerves contract, especially in the fingers and palm. Consideration should be given to tagging the nerve ends with a small suture to the soft tissues of the palm. If repairs of nerves and tendons are delayed, repair or reconstructions may be done later. (See chapter 3 and 5 for additional discussions of nerve and tendon repair and reconstruction.)

ARTERIAL INJURIES

Generally, the best treatment of major upper extremity arterial injury (subclavian, axillary, brachial) includes immediate diagnosis, emergent angiography, and surgical exploration and repair. The best management of injuries to the radial or ulnar arteries in the forearm and wrist is controversial. If the palmar arterial arches are complete, hand survival and function are possible if one or both arteries are transected. Problems with pain, cold intolerance, and weakness may occur later. Unrepaired single artery injuries generally cause insignificant changes in hand circulation, but combined arterial and nerve injury can result in disabling symptoms of pain and cold intolerance. At 10-year follow-up, cold sensitivity that limited activity was reported by 78% of 97 people with various hand injuries, although most reported a low degree of disability. In about 20% of patients, either the radial artery or the ulnar artery does not have a connection with the superficial palmar arterial arch. Pulse volume measurements and digital oximetry are helpful in assessing adequacy of circulation to the hand and digits.

Several options are available for treatment of radial and ulnar arterial injuries, alone or in combination. If an injury involves only one artery in a young person without nerve injury and with the intact artery providing adequate circulation, ligation remains a satisfactory option. In younger and older patients with inadequate circulation through the intact artery, especially if a nerve injury is present, repair of the injured artery is preferable. If both arteries are transected, repair of both arteries should be performed, especially in older patients and in patients with concomitant nerve injury. In a series of 28 patients with upper extremity arterial injuries treated at an urban trauma center, most (22) were treated with primary repair or ligation; six required saphenous vein bypasses, and two required endovascular procedures. The overall limb salvage rate was 96% (successful repair in 27 of 28 patients).

BOX 2.1

Basic Principles of Soft-Tissue Reconstruction

- Further injury to the upper extremity must be prevented.
- Aggressive debridement of all necrotic and nonviable tissue, including bone, is essential.
- Bone stability must be achieved.
- Acute coverage should begin with the simplest technique needed to cover the wound.
- Secondary reconstructions that will be needed should be considered at the time of soft-tissue coverage and primary reconstruction.
- Composite soft-tissue reconstruction should be considered when there is soft-tissue loss.
- Amputation may be better than limb salvage.

Modified from Wolf JM, Athwal GS, Shin AY, Dennison DG: Acute trauma to the upper extremity: what to do and when to do it, *J Am Acad Orthop Surg* 91:1240, 2009.

Injuries to the palmar arterial arch and the digital arteries require exploration and repair if circulatory impairment threatens digital viability. Microvascular techniques usually are required for these injuries. (See chapter 14 for a discussion of ulnar tunnel syndrome.)

A 15-year study of upper extremity arterial injuries that involved 167 patients with 189 arterial injuries identified the brachial artery as the most frequently injured vessel (55%). Risk factors for limb loss were early graft failure, compartment syndrome, associated skeletal and brachial plexus damage, and a military mechanism of injury. Some studies also have reported worse functional outcomes in arterial injuries caused by blunt trauma than by penetrating trauma.

CONSIDERATIONS FOR SKIN CLOSURE

Soft-tissue coverage may be the most important step in the treatment of acute hand injuries because it plays such a large part in determining how all other repaired and reconstructed structures heal and ultimately function. Although early definitive closure is desirable, this is not always possible, especially with severe crush injuries and contaminated wounds. Because swelling causes wounds to enlarge and skin to contract, closure becomes progressively more difficult. The use of rubber bands or surgical "vessel loops" can help bring the wound edges closer together without creating ischemia or increasing the risk of compartment syndrome. The use of negative pressure therapy, such as with a vacuum-assisted closure device, may allow the wound to granulate so that a simpler coverage method can be used. Negative pressure therapy should not be used for long periods, however, because it may compromise the gliding motion of muscles and tendons. In some patients, viability of the skin is unknown at the time of surgical evaluation, which is an indication for use of negative pressure wound therapy. Stabilizing the wound by immobilization in a functional position and applying negative pressure wound therapy has been shown to promote early healing in these patients.

The traditional "reconstructive ladder" generally follows a progression from simple (primary closure, healing by secondary intention) to more complex coverage methods (skin grafting, flap coverage). Wolf et al. outlined several basic principles of soft-tissue reconstruction in acute hand injuries (Box 2.1).

Primary skin closure is desirable and usually can be done in all sharply incised, clean wounds. The purpose of primary skin closure is to obtain early healing and to prevent infection, granulation tissue, edema, and excessive scar production. Misjudgment may lead to delayed healing as a result of hematoma, swelling, and infection, any of which may require reopening the wound for drainage or additional debridement. Certain wounds should never be closed primarily, including severely contaminated or crush wounds caused by farm machinery, human bites, tornado missiles, and augers. High-velocity missile wounds, other combat wounds, and wounds contaminated with animal or human feces or fertilizer also should not be closed primarily.

When in doubt, the wound should be left open after careful debridement using an anesthetic. Within 24 to 48 hours, the wound should be reinspected, and if it is sufficiently clean, it can be closed by direct suture or by skin graft. If possible, a wound should be closed within about 5 days of injury. Generally, a wound should not be left open to granulate and heal by secondary intention, unless it cannot be made sufficiently clean to allow skin grafting or closure. Closure of some wounds may be facilitated with the use a vacuum-assisted closure system to reduce the size of the wound and close dead space. An experienced microsurgical team is essential to the success of this method of managing severe hand injuries. The ability to take a "second look" at the wound, additional assessment of limb viability, more precise operative planning, and better control over scheduling of the procedure have been cited as advantages to a delayed approach.

METHODS AND INDICATIONS FOR SKIN CLOSURE
DIRECT SUTURE

Unless the wound is severely contaminated or crushed, consideration should be given to primary closure of every wound of the hand (except those mentioned previously) because healing by primary intention is the desired result. Treatment of some lacerations without suturing may be satisfactory in certain patients. Most clean lacerations without tendon or nerve involvement can be closed by simple direct suture of the skin and splinted. Usually the subcutaneous tissue is not sutured separately, but care should be taken to avoid inversion of the skin edges. Careful hemostasis is necessary. Closure is easier when all viable skin edges have been preserved during the initial cleansing. A skin defect on the dorsal surface of the hand can be converted to a transverse elliptical one and closed in a transverse line. Because of the mobility of the dorsal hand skin, this type of closure is possible here and is made easier when the wrist is extended.

Because sutures are by definition "foreign bodies," they may generate an inflammatory response, interfere with wound healing, and increase the risk of infection; the number and diameter of sutures used for wound closure should be kept to the minimum necessary.

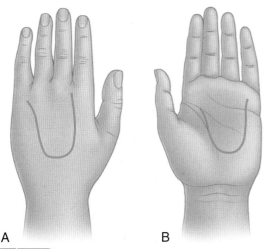

FIGURE 2.3 Flap attached distally on dorsum of hand **(A)** is less likely to survive than is similar one on palm **(B)**.

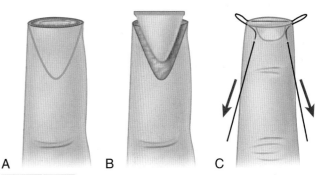

FIGURE 2.4 Purse-string suture attachment of flap for finger amputation. **A,** Design and dissection of flap. **B,** Advancement of flap to cover defect without tension. **C,** Two ends of continuous V-string suture are pulled until desired curve of fingertip is achieved. (Redrawn from Hassanpour SE, Hosseini SN, Abdolzadeh M: Purse-string suture as a complementary technique with conventional flaps in repairing fingertip amputation, *Tech Hand Up Extrem Surg* 15:94–98, 2011.)

SKIN GRAFTS

Skin grafts obtained from the patient (autografts) are either split thickness or full thickness. Wounds with distally attached flaps may have enough skin for primary closure but not enough venous drainage for the skin to survive. This deficient drainage causes engorgement and venous distention and finally thrombosis and necrosis; the color of the flap changes from a deep blue to purple and then to black. The retrograde flap is often the result of a crushing or tearing injury, and the nature of this injury jeopardizes the survival of the flap further. Such a flap on the dorsal surface of the hand or forearm is less likely to survive than one on the palm (Fig. 2.3). If doubt exists, the skin should be excised and replaced with a split graft (see Technique 2.1).

If skin is lost and no deep structures (nerves, tendons, joints, or cortical bone) have been exposed, it should be replaced immediately with a split-thickness graft or occasionally with a full-thickness graft. Other types of skin grafts that may have applications in the injured hand include allografts from other human donors and xenografts from other species (e.g., porcine skin). Both are used for temporary coverage while a capillary bed develops. Although an allograft may revascularize, rejection occurs, and it is replaced with an autograft.

SKIN FLAPS

When a skin defect leaves deep structures exposed, a split-thickness or full-thickness skin graft is insufficient coverage for nerves, tendons, and cortical bone. These structures do not readily support a skin graft and require good blood supply to survive. A skin flap is necessary to provide subcutaneous tissue for coverage and for sufficient vascularity. The nomenclature of flaps depends on the location, blood supply, and technique of transfer. By location, a flap may be termed *local* or *distant*. The blood supply determines whether the flap is *random* or *axial*. Random flaps receive their circulation through the subdermal or subcutaneous plexus of vessels and do not have a named artery supplying them. Axial pattern flaps receive their circulation from a named artery. Axial flaps also are subdivided by the major tissue of the flap into *cutaneous, musculocutaneous,* and *fasciocutaneous* flaps. The technique of transfer of a flap determines whether it is a *pedicled flap* to be transferred in two stages or a *free flap,* which is transferred in a single step, with vascular anastomoses.

COVERAGE OF SPECIFIC AREAS WITH FLAPS

Fingertip injuries with only skin loss less than 1 cm square usually can be treated satisfactorily with healing by secondary intention. If the defect is larger without exposed bone, a full-thickness skin graft provides good coverage and the potential for return of some sensation. Hassanpour et al. described the use of a purse-string suture in conjunction with conventional flap coverage of 41 fingertip amputations to restore nail and finger contour and improve the aesthetic and functional results (Fig. 2.4). They reported only one poor functional result; cosmetic results were excellent or good in all nine female patients and in 26 of the 32 male patients. The use of local, rotational, advancement, and neurovascular island flaps for amputations and injuries of the fingertip and thumb is discussed in other chapter.

A large skin defect on the dorsum of a finger that exposes tendons not covered with paratenon should be covered with a flap. Frequently, a double local flap can be constructed by rotating a proximally based local flap on one side and a distally based local flap on the other side of the defect to cover the exposed tendon. The donor defects are covered with split grafts. For more proximal dorsal injuries, local rotational flaps from the same finger are insufficient and a reverse cross finger flap from the dorsum of an adjacent finger may be used. A "flag" flap, which is an axial flap, may be used for proximal palmar and dorsal digital defects (see Fig. 2.22). If multiple fingers are involved, or if a larger area needs to be covered, a subpectoral flap may be appropriate. Thick subcutaneous fat, as is found on the lower abdomen, is not preferred on a flap, especially on the finger.

Skin defects on the volar surface of a finger that expose tendons may be covered with a cross finger flap. The flap is raised from the dorsal surface of an adjacent finger and extends from the midline of one of its lateral surfaces to that of the other; the flap is a little wider than the defect it is to cover. Although such a flap from the dorsal surface of one finger can be used to cover a defect on the volar surface of another, the reverse is never indicated. Skin defects on the palm or dorsum of the hand that expose vital structures can be covered with a local flap, a flap from an adjacent unsalvageable finger, a flap from the opposite forearm or upper

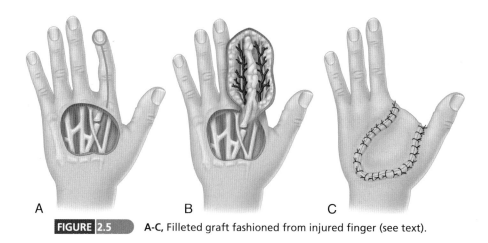

FIGURE 2.5   **A-C,** Filleted graft fashioned from injured finger (see text).

arm, an axial pattern flap from the same forearm or hand, a flap from the abdomen, or a free flap, depending on the size of the defect and the presence and location of any associated injuries. Although cross arm and cross forearm flaps provide good skin, immobilizing both upper extremities is a disadvantage. In suitable situations, an arterialized axial flap from the same forearm allows comfortable positioning of the upper limb. An abdominal flap from the same side also permits comfortable positioning of the arm. To ensure survival of the random pattern flap (because it must be applied immediately), its base should be as wide as its length. The length-to-width ratio may exceed 3 : 1 with axial pattern flaps such as the groin pedicle flap. The donor area and the raw part of the flap that does not make contact with the defect should be covered with split-thickness skin grafts. A local rotation flap is unlikely to survive, however, if undermining of the skin is extensive, especially if the skin is already crushed or contused from the injury. A filleted injured finger makes an excellent pedicle graft when this technique is applicable (Fig. 2.5). In some situations, free tissue transfer by microvascular technique provides the best coverage.

More recently, the use of "artificial skin" or skin substitutes has been reported for initial coverage of severe hand wounds, burns, and contracture release procedures. Although these products are not substitutes for adequate surgical debridement and standard coverage strategies such as grafts and flaps, they may be useful in selected patients. The product most frequently reported in the hand literature is a bilayer dermal regeneration template (Integra; Integra LifeSciences Corp., Plainsboro, NJ). The dermal layer is made of bovine type I collagen, and the epidermal layer is made of silicone. Weigert et al. reported the use of Integra for management of 15 severe traumatic hand wounds with bone, joint, or tendon exposure; split-thickness grafting was done at an average of 26 days after injury. In 13 of the 15 hands, a durable, functional, and aesthetic coverage was obtained with this technique. Advantages of the skin substitutes include potentially less need for local rotational or free-flap coverage, ease of use, and immediate availability in large quantities and different sizes. Disadvantages include its high cost, the learning curve for use, and a higher risk of seroma or hematoma formation.

MANAGEMENT OF DONOR AREA

Several acceptable methods are used for treating the donor area. In one, the donor area is dressed with one layer of finely woven nylon or silk gauze. If the dressing prevents drying, the donor area tends to become macerated and secondary infection and necrosis may occur; this area itself may require skin grafting later. Otherwise the part is left uncovered, and drying of the area is encouraged. In another technique, a synthetic adhesive film is placed over the donor site. Serum and blood accumulate daily for 1 to 2 days, and the film is changed. After 7 to 10 days, this can be removed and the area is left open, usually with satisfactory healing. Bed sheets should be kept off the donor site with a bed cradle support.

GRAFTS AND FLAPS
FREE GRAFTS

When free skin grafts are to be obtained, remember that "the thinner the graft, the better the take"; however, when the graft is expected to be permanent, "the thicker the graft, the better the function." A thick graft is better able to withstand friction and constant use than a thin one and contracts only about 10%; a thin graft may contract 50% to 75%. The sooner the graft can be applied, the better. As long as there is no sepsis, it is not necessary to wait for granulation to begin before skin grafting. Sepsis can be identified with swabs for culture or with wound biopsy for a quantitative colony count. For the graft to survive, it must reestablish its nutrition before death of its entire thickness occurs; great care is needed in operative technique and in aftercare to ensure that it remains undisturbed and in direct contact with the recipient area during healing. This takes careful planning, especially in children. The graft cannot survive if a hematoma separates it from the underlying vascular bed; rarely, it may survive a gross infection. For primary coverage of acute wounds, free skin grafts usually are of thin or medium thickness. They usually do not survive on bare cortical bone, bare tendon, or bare cartilage. Except for fingertip injuries, full-thickness free skin grafts are used infrequently on the hand. Such grafts or thick split grafts can be used, however, for the palmar surface because it contains elastic tissue, and in growing children these contract less and tend to accommodate growth. Because the survival of a full-thickness graft is so uncertain, it is best used only in elective surgery for skin coverage in the palm; it should be used rarely in acute injuries, with the possible exception of the fingertips.

SPLIT-THICKNESS SKIN GRAFTS

Frequently, only a small or postage stamp graft is needed, and it can be obtained within the same operative field from the forearm;

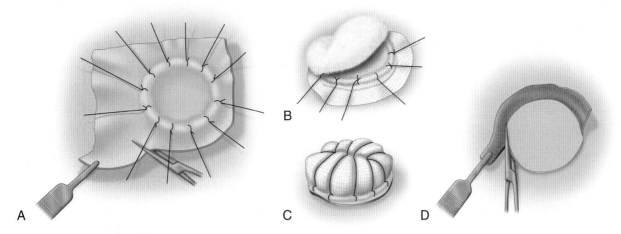

FIGURE 2.6 Technique of applying split-thickness graft. **A,** Graft has been sutured over defect, and redundant edges of graft are being trimmed. **B,** Sheet of finely meshed gauze and pack of moist cotton or gauze have been placed over graft. **C,** Sutures have been tied over pack. **D,** Necrotic edges of graft are being trimmed away after graft has healed. **SEE TECHNIQUE 2.1.**

however, taking a graft from this area can be undesirable because it leaves a slight scar. The hypothenar area of the palm can be used to obtain satisfactory split-thickness skin grafts, especially for skin loss on the fingertips. More suitable donor areas for these and larger grafts are the anterior and lateral aspects of the thigh and the medial aspect of the arm just inferior to the axilla. In some older women, skin is available inferior to a pendulous breast without leaving a readily visible scar. Split-thickness skin grafts vary in thickness from 0.008 inch in infants to 0.015 inch in adults. In elderly individuals and children, the lower abdominal wall or buttock skin is used if the graft is more than 0.010 inch.

▮ OBTAINING SKIN GRAFTS WITH A DERMATOME

Electrically powered dermatomes are not difficult to assemble and use; even an inexperienced operator can cut consistently good grafts 7.5 cm wide. Skin glue is not required, but light lubrication of the skin with mineral oil or petrolatum is helpful. Bony prominences are not satisfactory donor sites with these dermatomes. The Reese drum dermatome does require skin glue and must be operated with precision, but it is excellent for cutting grafts more than 7.5 cm wide. Usually it controls the thickness of the grafts more accurately. The following suggestions are offered about this dermatome: (1) stretch the rubber tape tightly on the drum, (2) wait at least 3 minutes for the glue to dry before applying the dermatome to the skin, (3) rotate the drum slowly, and lift up gently while cutting the graft, and (4) keep the blade from slipping around the drum to avoid being struck on the palmar side of the wrist. When using a dermatome, cut the graft larger than the recipient area.

APPLYING SPLIT-THICKNESS GRAFTS

The recipient area for a split-thickness graft must have a vascular bed and be free of active bleeding and gross infection. If the recipient area is unsuitable, preparation may require several days of enzymatic debridement, multiple dressing changes, and surgical debridement to remove dead and infected material. Applying mesh to the graft is helpful if a large area is to be covered. It also allows the free drainage of serum and blood from beneath the graft (see Fig. 2.6B).

TECHNIQUE 2.1

- Place the graft on the recipient area without trimming or excessive handling.
- The graft border may be attached with sutures or skin staples to secure it in its new position.
- Trim the redundant edge (Fig. 2.6A).
- When suturing the graft in place, it is much easier to insert a small curved needle first through the graft and then through the skin around the recipient area than to do the reverse.
- Apply a stent dressing, or a finely meshed nonadherent gauze (Xeroform or Adaptic), and hold in place with a bulky dressing secured by circumferential conforming gauze (Fig. 2.6B and C). If necessary, cover with a thin layer of plaster for splinting.

POSTOPERATIVE CARE The dressing usually is changed after 5 to 7 days; any necrotic graft is removed, and a fresh dressing is applied (Fig. 2.6D). When an area of necrosis is large, regrafting may be necessary. When necrosis is anticipated, or when another procedure is planned in which a split-thickness graft is to be used, a graft larger than needed initially may be cut and refrigerated at 0°C to 5°C in lactated Ringer solution or in a saline solution to which penicillin has been added; then it can be used at any time up to 21 days.

FREE FULL-THICKNESS GRAFTS

When a full-thickness graft is used, the recipient area must be free of infection and hemostasis must be complete. Preferred donor areas include the groin or the medial aspect of the arm, where the skin is thin and where the defect created by

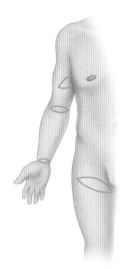

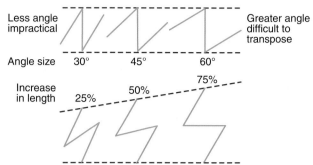

Less angle impractical   Greater angle difficult to transpose

Angle size   30°   45°   60°

Increase in length   25%   50%   75%

FIGURE 2.9 Angles permissible in performing Z-plasties. Angles that central limb of Z make with each of other two limbs should be between 45 and 60 degrees. When angles are less than 45 degrees, blood supply to flap is impaired; when they are more than 60 degrees, flaps cannot be transposed without severe tension.

FIGURE 2.7 Sites from which to obtain full-thickness skin grafts. Groin or medial aspect of arm is preferable (see text).

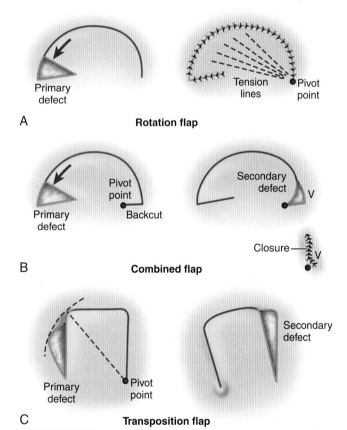

A   **Rotation flap**

B   **Combined flap**

C   **Transposition flap**

FIGURE 2.8 A-C, Principles of three types of local flaps. In each type, defect to be covered is converted into triangular one. Flap may be rotated **(A)** or transposed **(C)** or both **(B)**. **B,** Back-cut in combined flap decreases tension on flap but also decreases blood supply to flap; defect created by this back-cut is closed as shown. **C,** Defect created by transposing flap must be covered with split-thickness graft.

APPLYING FULL-THICKNESS GRAFTS

TECHNIQUE 2.2

- Make a pattern on sterile tape or gauze of the area to be covered. Using this pattern, outline the anticipated graft on the donor area with methylene blue or a skin marker. It should be slightly larger than the pattern to allow for the necessary margin in suturing and for shrinkage.
- Remove the graft with a sharp knife by dissection between the fat and the skin; do not take any fat with the graft.
- Suture it in place and excise the redundant edges.
- Apply a stent dressing and support the hand with a plaster splint for at least 7 to 10 days before redressing. At that time, dark blisters of the superficial layer of the graft may be seen, but this usually does not indicate deep necrosis.

SKIN FLAPS

Skin grafts usually do not "take" on exposed bone, cartilage, or tendon. The scarring beneath a skin graft interferes with function in areas where a flexible and mobile bed is needed for tendon and joint motion. Skin flaps are used in such areas where a layer of subcutaneous tissue is required. Flap coverage can be used in the primary closure of a hand wound or in a secondary procedure to replace scars, skin of poor quality, or necrotic skin. It can be obtained locally or from a distant part. If the area to be covered is small, a local flap may be indicated (Fig. 2.8) or a Z-plasty may suffice (Figs. 2.9 to 2.11).

LOCAL FLAPS

Local flaps may be designated as advancement, rotation, translation, and transposition types. Use of an advancement flap involves mobilizing a small flap of skin to cover an adjacent defect without using a skin graft for the donor defect. These are used to cover fingertip amputations. Rotation flaps are raised on a curved radius with undermining of the flap and closed under modest tension without a skin-grafted donor defect (see Fig. 2.8A). Translation flaps usually are rectangular and are used to close an adjacent defect. The flap

removing the graft can be closed by undermining and suturing the skin edges (Fig. 2.7). Sometimes an associated injury makes a detached piece of skin and underlying fat available; in this instance, the skin can be stabilized on a dermatome drum and a full-thickness graft can be excised from the fat.

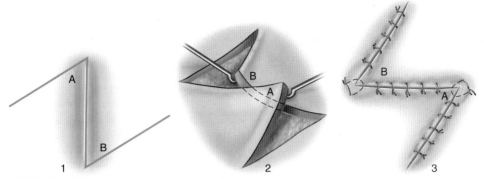

FIGURE 2.10 Simple Z-plasty to release a long, narrow contracture. *1,* Central limb of Z is to be made along line of contracture, and other two limbs are to be made where shown. *2,* Incisions have been made, and flaps are being shifted. *3,* Flaps have been sutured in their new positions. Note special stitches at *A* and *B.*

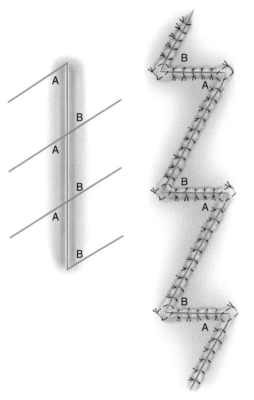

FIGURE 2.11 Multiple Z-plasties to release scar too long to be released by single Z-plasty.

is moved around a pedicle base and is closed without tension. Translation flaps require a skin graft for the donor site (Fig. 2.12). Transposition flaps usually are moved across an adjacent area of normal skin to close an adjacent defect without tension. Skin grafting at the donor site is necessary (Fig. 2.13). Based on cadaver dissections and injection studies, skin flaps based on the anastomoses between the palmar digital artery and the dorsal metacarpal artery have been used to cover the volar surface of an adjacent finger (Fig. 2.14), a reverse adipofascial flap has been successful for finger amputations at the level of the nail fold (lunula to proximal nail matrix) (Fig. 2.15), and "excellent" results were reported in 40 patients with a more proximally based adipofascial "turnover flap" for

coverage of the dorsum of the distal and middle phalanges (Fig. 2.16). This flap is based on dorsal branches of the digital arteries, providing pedicle lengths of 10 mm proximal or distal to the proximal interphalangeal joint. The advantages of a local flap over one from a distant part are that the involved hand is not tied to the distant donor and in many instances finger motions may continue. If the defect is too large to be covered with a local flap, an axial arterialized pedicle flap from the forearm, a distant flap from the abdomen, or a free tissue transfer is indicated.

■ LOCAL FLAPS IN FINGERS

Figure 2.8 illustrates the principles of three types of local flaps. In the fingers, either they are random pedicle flaps, receiving their circulation through the base of a skin pedicle, or they can be designed with circulation through the proper digital artery or one of its branches (Fig. 2.17). Local flaps used in the fingers usually are of the simple transposition type. This type covers vital structures but leaves a defect that must be covered with a split-thickness graft (see Fig. 2.13). A common error in designing a local flap is to make it too short. The fixed point of pivot from which the advancement is made is at the border of the base that is opposite the defect. If the corresponding border of the flap is not long enough, tension occurs when the flap is sutured in its new bed.

Skin to be used for a local flap should not be damaged because necrosis may occur. Developing a local skin flap requires undermining and minimal tension on the flap.

■ LOCAL FLAPS FROM THE DORSUM OF THE HAND

Local flaps used over the dorsum of the hand may be of any of the types previously listed. The inclusion of the fascia in a random fasciocutaneous flap is helpful in this area, and various vascularized flaps can be developed on the basis of the first dorsal metacarpal artery (Fig. 2.18). In addition, the abductor digiti quinti and the palmaris brevis can be mobilized as pedicled muscle flaps to cover adjacent areas.

A variety of local flaps can be used in the hand and fingers. They include local rotation flaps from the dorsum of the hand to fill defects in the web spaces (Fig. 2.19), cross finger flaps (Figs. 2.20 and 2.21), thenar flaps, and other transposition flaps, such as the "flag" flap (Fig. 2.22). A better understanding of the circulation to the dorsoulnar side of the hand

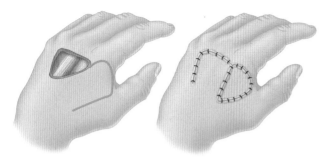

and thumb has led to the development of a dorsoulnar thumb flap (Figs. 2.23 and 2.24).

FIGURE 2.12 Translation flap raised from skin in continuity with area of skin loss. Donor area is covered by graft. (Redrawn from Tubiana R, editor: *The hand*, vol 2, Philadelphia, 1985, Saunders.)

■ CROSS FINGER FLAPS

Cross finger flaps (see Fig. 2.20) are useful for covering a defect of the skin and other soft tissues on the volar surface of the finger when tendons and neurovascular structures are exposed and a small amount of subcutaneous fat is needed. They also are useful for some amputations of the thumb. These grafts are best avoided in patients older than 50 years, in patients with hands with arthritic changes or a tendency to finger stiffness for some other reason, and in patients with local infection.

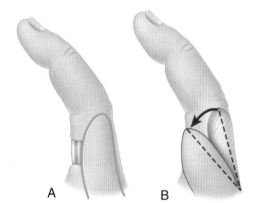

FIGURE 2.13 Simple transposition type of local flap. **A,** Deep structures on anterolateral aspect of finger are exposed and must be covered by local flap; flap has been outlined. **B,** Flap has been transposed, and defect created on posterolateral aspect of finger has been covered by split-thickness graft. Note radius *(broken lines)* of arc *(arrow)* of transposition.

APPLYING CROSS FINGER FLAPS

TECHNIQUE 2.3

- Excise the edges of the defect so that it is rectangular, with its longer sides parallel to the long axis of the finger but not crossing skin creases.
- Measure its dimensions, placing the injured finger against the donor finger to determine where to locate the base of the proposed flap.
- Cut the flap from the donor finger through the skin and subcutaneous tissues, leaving its base attached to the side adjacent to the recipient finger (Fig. 2.25).
- Make the flap 4 to 6 mm wider than the defect and long enough to cover the defect (allowing for normal skin contraction) and to provide a bridge between the fingers.
- If necessary, the flap may be raised from one midlateral line of the donor finger to the other, but be careful to avoid incising the volar surface of the donor finger.

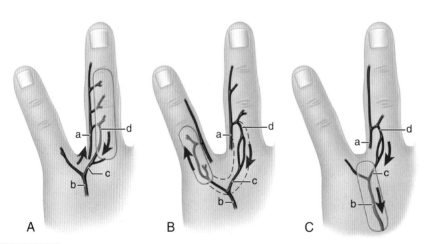

FIGURE 2.14 Vascular basis of dorsal digital and metacarpal skin flaps. **A,** Extended dorsal phalangeal island skin flap on dorsal aspect of proximal and middle phalanges. **B,** Boomerang flap on dorsal aspect of proximal phalanx (subcutaneous vascular pedicle of flap indicated by *dashed lines*). **C,** Reverse dorsal metacarpal artery island flap based on vascular anastomoses between dorsal cutaneous branches of palmar digital artery and dorsal digital branches of dorsal metacarpal artery. *Arrows* show direction of blood flow. Palmar digital artery *(a)*; dorsal perforating branch of palmar metacarpal arteries from deep palmar arch *(b)*; dorsal digital artery *(c)*; dorsal cutaneous branches of palmar digital artery *(d)*.

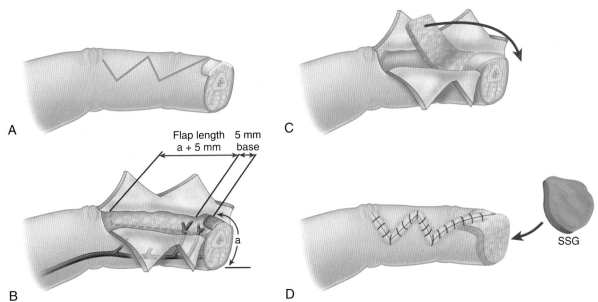

FIGURE 2.15   Reverse adipofascial flap. **A,** Z incision. **B,** Instead of Z incision, quadrangular incision is marked on dorsum of finger as alternative, leaving 5 mm as basis of flap just proximal to germinal matrix. a = defect + germinal matrix; flap length = a + 5 mm to cover the basis. **C,** Skin flaps are raised, leaving paratenon intact, and adipofascial flap is raised from proximal to distal until marked basis is reached. **D,** Adipofascial flap is turned over to defect, and skin flaps are sutured to remain open above base of flap. Split-thickness skin graft (*SSG*) is ready to be applied. (Redrawn from Laoulakos DH, Tsetsonis CH, Michail AA, et al: The dorsal reverse adipofascial flap for fingertip reconstruction, *Plast Reconstr Surg* 112:121–125, 2003.)

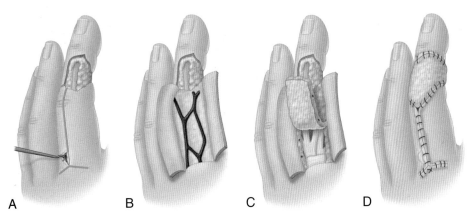

FIGURE 2.16   Turnover flap. **A,** Arterial flap: H-shaped incision of donor site. **B,** Skin deepidermization. **C,** Adipofascial flap transposed over defect. **D,** Final aspect. Skin graft in place. (Redrawn from Braga-Silva J, Kuyven CR, Albertoni W, et al: The adipofascial turn-over flap for coverage of the dorsum of the finger: a modified surgical technique, *J Hand Surg* 29A:1038–1043, 2004.)

- When raising the flap, make the incisions through the subcutaneous tissue but not through the peritenon of the extensor expansion (Fig. 2.26).
- If possible, avoid using skin distal to the distal interphalangeal joint so as not to injure the nail bed. The skin over the dorsal surface of the proximal interphalangeal joint also should be avoided unless needed for width. If necessary, the base of the flap can be freed further by cutting the oblique fibers of the deep tissue that attaches the skin to the extensor tendon and periosteum along the side of the finger. Handle the flap with small hooks to prevent crushing and necrosis.

- Release the tourniquet and obtain absolute hemostasis.
- Reinflate the tourniquet.
- Cut a thick split graft (0.018 inch) from the forearm or thigh and suture it to the donor area and to the undersurface of the bridge.
- Apply the flap to the recipient area and suture it in place with the finest suture (5-0 or 6-0 nylon); the entire recipient area should be in contact with the flap.
- Leave the sutures long at the edges of the free split graft and fashion a stent dressing.
- Avoid excessive tension on sutures transverse to the long axis of the finger to avoid vascular compromise.

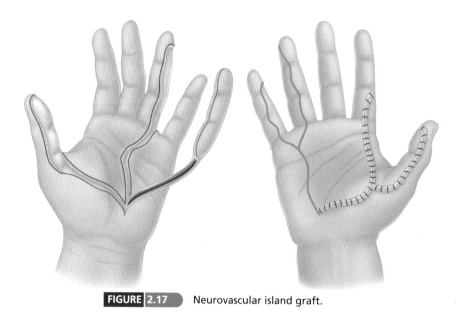

FIGURE 2.17 Neurovascular island graft.

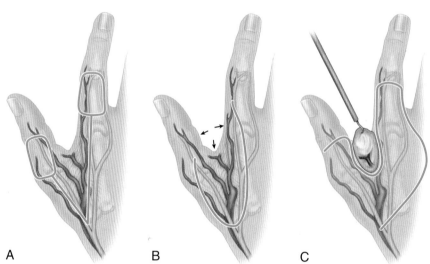

A   B   C

FIGURE 2.18 Design of various flaps in first web space. **A,** Proximally based flaps: based on first dorsal metacarpal artery and branches. Island flap pedicle includes first dorsal metacarpal artery and its branches, first dorsal interosseous fascia, subcutaneous tissue and veins, and radial nerve branches and accompanying artery. **B,** Distally based flap: based on one of distal perforators *(arrows)*. **C,** Double flap from web space: fascial flap based on first dorsal metacarpal artery *(marked in drawing by hook)* and cutaneous flap based on artery accompanying radial nerve *(green line)*.

- Cover the suture line with nonadhering gauze, place moist cotton pledgets around the graft, and apply gauze wrapping.
- To ensure immobility of the recipient finger, place an oblique Kirschner wire through the interphalangeal joint.
- A volar splint of plaster or fiberglass also can be used if additional support is needed.

POSTOPERATIVE CARE The flap can be detached after 12 to 14 days. The skin margins of the recipient finger should be trimmed so that the junction of the normal skin with the graft is at a midlateral position on the finger. Motion of both fingers can be started the day after the flap is detached.

This technique can be altered so that the base of the flap is proximal rather than lateral; such a flap is useful for covering a defect near the tip of an adjacent finger or thumb (see Fig. 2.21). Rotation of the flap is necessary, and care should be taken to prevent strangulation at the base and necrosis. Rotated flaps that are based proximally can be used to cover defects on the same finger (see Fig. 2.13).

FOREARM FLAPS FOR HAND COVERAGE

Two arterialized pedicle flaps from the forearm (the radial forearm flap and the posterior interosseous flap) have been found useful for covering defects in the hand. Each has a consistently reliable arterial supply. However, variations in forearm vascular anatomy, especially in the posterior interosseous artery, may preclude use of these flaps.

▨ RADIAL FOREARM FLAP

The radial artery supplies blood to the distal, palmar, and lateral forearm skin (an area approximately 16 × 8 cm). The flap territory is supplied through a branch of the radial artery arising about 7 cm from the radial styloid (Fig. 2.27). The radial forearm flap, which is innervated by branches of the musculocutaneous nerve, is thin and can be used as an osteocutaneous flap with a portion of the radius, a

fasciocutaneous flap on the pedicle, or a free tissue transfer. As a pedicle flap, it can be mobilized to cover many parts of the hand (Fig. 2.28). Some surgeons find the donor defect and the sacrifice of the radial artery objectionable. If the flap is used as a fascial flap, the skin can be closed with minimal scarring and the flap can be covered with a skin graft. A preoperative Allen test is required to assess the adequacy of ulnar arterial flow. If the status of the ulnar artery cannot be determined, arteriography should give a definitive picture of hand circulation. The general technique by Foucher et al. is described; however, every detail of dissection and application is not provided, so a review of the vascular and neural anatomy is recommended (Fig. 2.29).

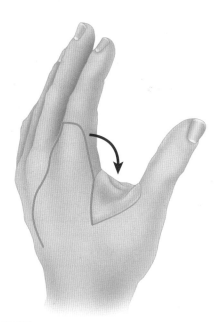

FIGURE 2.19 Transposition flap. Dorsal flap to cover thumb web space. (Redrawn from Tubiana R, editor: *The hand*, vol 2, Philadelphia, 1985, Saunders.)

APPLYING A RADIAL FOREARM GRAFT

TECHNIQUE 2.4

(FOUCHER ET AL.)
- After preparation of the wound to be covered, if it is suitable to receive the flap, proceed with flap design.
- Design a flap centered over the radial artery. The largest flaps obtained by Foucher et al. were 16 cm long × 9 cm wide.
- Expose the radial artery at the proximal and distal borders of the flap.
- Ligate the radial artery proximal to the flap.
- At the proximal border of the flap, identify, dissect, and preserve the musculocutaneous nerve.

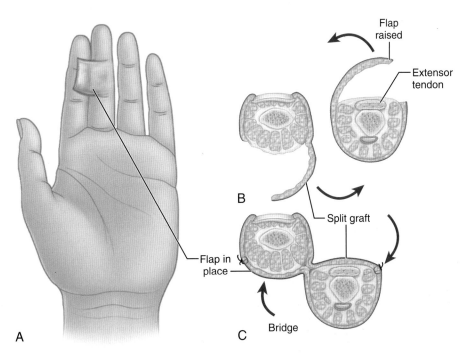

FIGURE 2.20 Cross finger flap. **A,** Laterally based pedicle flap has been raised from middle finger and has been applied to distal pad of index. **B and C,** Cross sections of two fingers show how cross finger flap has been applied and how raw surfaces of donor finger and of bridge between two fingers have been covered with split-thickness skin graft (see text).

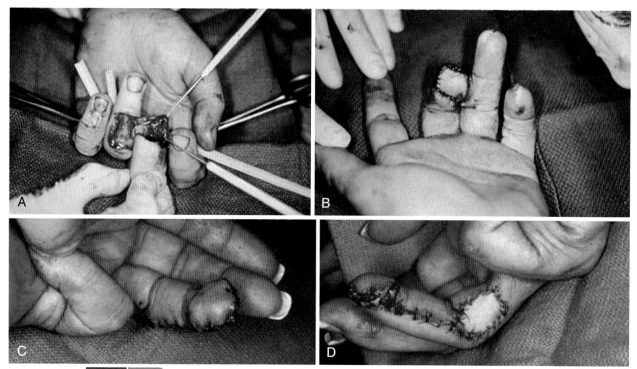

FIGURE 2.21 **A** and **B,** Volar angulated fingertip injury with loss of pulp pad and bone exposed treated with cross finger flap from dorsum of adjacent finger. **C** and **D,** Results. (From Netscher D, Murphy K, Fiore N: Hand surgery. In Townsend CM, Beauchamp RD, Evers BM, Mattox KL, editors: *Sabiston textbook of surgery*, ed 19. Philadelphia, 2012, Elsevier.)

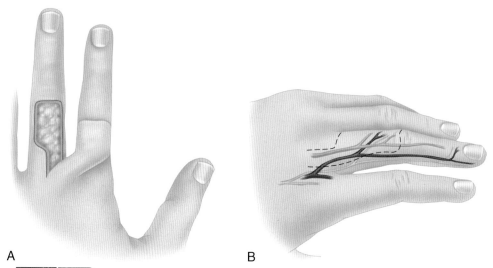

FIGURE 2.22 "Flag flap." **A,** Skin can be moved over distance to palmar surface or to neighboring digit. **B,** "Flag staff" contains pedicle consisting of dorsal vein, dorsal branch of digital artery, and dorsal branch of digital nerve.

- Incise the anterior (medial) border, extending beyond the forearm midline if needed.
- Progressively raise the medial two thirds of the flap (medial to the radial artery), leaving the perimysium intact. Ensure that the radial artery and veins are taken as a single block from the radial groove.
- On reaching the distal end of the pedicle, dissect the lateral border of the flap laterally and medially.

- Leave the cephalic vein and the superficial radial nerve intact.
- Dissect from proximal to distal to mobilize the flap; avoid damage to the venae comitantes. If necessary, lengthen the pedicle by dissecting to the angle between the first and second metacarpals.
- Delicately dissect the vessels from the abductor pollicis longus, extensor pollicis brevis, and extensor pollicis

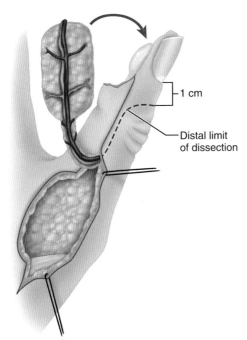

FIGURE 2.23 Dorsoulnar flap harvested from inner side of thumb metacarpophalangeal area reaches distal area of thumb. (Redrawn from Brunelli F, Vigasio A, Valenti P: Arterial anatomy and clinical application of the dorsoulnar flap of the thumb, *J Hand Surg* 24A:803–811, 1999.)

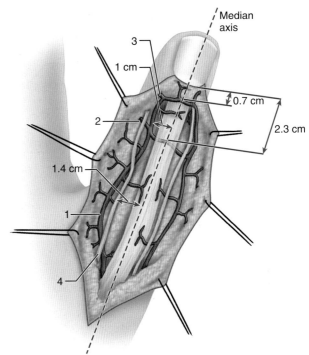

FIGURE 2.24 Dorsal arterial supply to thumb showing ulnar dorsal collateral artery (*1*) and its anastomosis with ulnar palmar digital artery at neck of first phalanx (*2*) and with arcade at proximal nail fold (*3*). Topographic position of essential structures: distance between dorsal arcade of proximal nail fold and cuticle of nail is 0.7 cm, distance between palmar anastomosis and cuticle of nail is 2.3 cm, distance between median axis of thumb and ulnar dorsal collateral artery (*1*) at level of neck of first phalanx is 1 cm, and distance between median axis of thumb and ulnar dorsal collateral nerve (*4*) at level of head of first metacarpal bone is 1.4 cm. (Redrawn from Brunelli F, Vigasio A, Valenti P: Arterial anatomy and clinical application of the dorsoulnar flap of the thumb, *J Hand Surg* 24A:803–811, 1999.)

longus, opening the retinacular sheaths to allow passage of the flap beneath the tendons.
- Obtain hemostasis with bipolar electrocoagulation of the numerous small vessels. On completion, a pedicle of about 8 cm is obtained, which allows rotation to many parts of the hand.
- Proceed with other requirements of the specific injury.

POSTOPERATIVE CARE Flap circulation should be monitored for at least 24 h. If flap viability is uncertain, the flap should be monitored until it is safe to allow the patient to return home. Sutures that appear too tight are removed. Causes of vasospasm (smoking, cold drinks, an excessively cold environment, and emotional upsets) should be avoided. Skin sutures are removed in 10 to 14 days, and rehabilitation appropriate for the specific injury is begun.

■ POSTERIOR INTEROSSEOUS FLAP

The posterior interosseous artery, usually a branch of the common interosseous artery, supplies a skin flap territory on the dorsal surface of the forearm. In the distal forearm, the posterior interosseous artery joins the anterior interosseous artery at the distal part of the interosseous space. Over its course, the posterior artery gives four to six cutaneous branches, passing through the septum between the extensor digiti minimi and extensor carpi ulnaris muscles, supplying an area of skin in about the middle third of the dorsum of the forearm (Fig. 2.30). Flap islands 1.5 × 4 cm to 9 × 11 cm were obtained by Büchler and Frey. Using the "retrograde" flap, an arc of

rotation up to 19 cm centered over the distal radioulnar joint allowed coverage of sites as far distal as the dorsum of the proximal interphalangeal joint. Anatomic variation may preclude development of the flap as planned. If anatomic variation interferes with the pedicle, three options have been suggested to improve reliability of the flap: (1) performing additional venous anastomosis if venous congestion is encountered after insetting the flap, (2) changing the flap to a free flap if anatomic variation prevents the elevation of a distally based flap owing to compromise of the nerve branches, and (3) raising the flap with a wide base, incorporating branches of the anterior and posterior interosseous arteries in patients with possible peripheral vascular disease. Preoperative evaluation should include consideration of injury at the wrist, location of the defect on the distal finger, the need for sensation, the presence of peripheral arterial disease, and the presence of injury on the volar forearm with damage to the anterior interosseous artery. The technique of Zancolli and Angrigiani, with recommendations by Chen et al., is described next. Because every detail of dissection and application is not provided, review of the vascular anatomy with an alternative plan in mind is recommended.

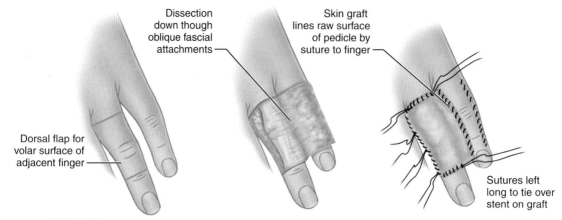

FIGURE 2.25   Technique of applying cross finger flap, using skin from dorsum of two phalanges. **SEE TECHNIQUE 2.3.**

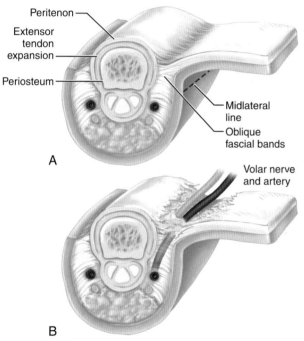

FIGURE 2.26   Details of raising cross finger flap. **A,** Incision has been carried to, but not through, peritenon of extensor expansion; note oblique fascial bands. **B,** Incision has been continued to sever oblique fascial bands but avoids damage to volar digital artery and nerve. **SEE TECHNIQUE 2.3.**

APPLYING A POSTERIOR INTEROSSEOUS FLAP

In dissecting the posterior interosseous flap, observe the following recommendations of Chen et al.: (1) dissect a cutaneous vein proximal for venous anastomosis; (2) note variations in size, location, and relationship to nerves of the posterior interosseous artery; and (3) observe for venous congestion after flap inset.

TECHNIQUE 2.5

(ZANCOLLI AND ANGRIGIANI; CHEN ET AL.)

■ After the wound to be covered has been prepared and is suitable to receive the flap, proceed with flap design. On the dorsal (posterior) surface of the forearm, draw a line between the lateral epicondyle and the distal radioulnar joint along the course of the posterior interosseous artery (Fig. 2.31). Design a flap that is centered on this line and preserve the cutaneous branches.

■ Mark point A 2 cm proximal to the ulnar styloid that represents the distal anastomosis between the anterior and posterior interosseous arteries and the rotation point of the flap pedicle. From point A, measure to the most distal point to be covered on the hand, point B. Transfer this length back proximally along the longitudinal line to a new point, C. Measure the length of the cutaneous defect to be covered, and transfer that length along the line X-X1 from the proximal point distally to a new point. Distance C-D is the flap length, and distance A-B is the length of the vascular pedicle. The width of the flap is determined by measuring the width of the defect to be covered and transferring that shape along the X-X1 line between points C and D.

■ Begin the skin incision at the distal point of anastomosis between the interosseous arteries. Incise only the skin proximally along the radial (lateral) side of the flap; do not include the fascia in the flap.

■ Dissect the flap medially toward line X-X1, observing the cutaneous branches, dissecting and protecting them. Open the fascia longitudinally over the extensor digiti minimi and the extensor carpi ulnaris muscles.

■ Use gentle blunt dissection between these two muscles to expose the posterior interosseous artery with its venae comitantes.

■ Preserve the posterior interosseous nerve.

■ Electrocauterize the muscular branches of the artery.

■ Section the posterior interosseous artery proximally near its origin near the distal edge of the supinator muscle.

■ Open the ulnar (medial) side of the flap with a skin incision along the ulnar border of the flap.

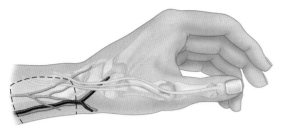

FIGURE 2.27 Outline of radial forearm flap centered on radial artery.

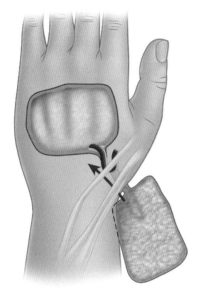

FIGURE 2.28 Flap can be used to cover dorsum of hand.

- Gently elevate the flap distally to the distal anastomosis with the anterior interosseous artery.
- Gently dissect the vascular pedicle as far distally as possible to gain more length.
- Arrange the flap appropriately to cover the recipient wound.
- Proceed with the other requirements of the specific injury.
- If the donor skin defect does not exceed 3 to 4 cm in width, close it primarily; otherwise, cover it with skin graft.

POSTOPERATIVE CARE Flap circulation should be monitored closely for at least 24 hours. If flap viability is uncertain, the flap should be monitored until it is safe to allow the patient to return home. Sutures that appear to be too tight and that may compromise flap circulation are removed. Potential causes of vasospasm (smoking, cold drinks, excessively cold room, emotional upsets) should be avoided. Skin sutures are removed in about 10 days. Rehabilitation appropriate for the specific injury is then begun.

ABDOMINAL FLAPS

In addition to the flaps previously discussed, the size of the defect and the thickness of the flap required may make it necessary to use a remote pedicle flap from the abdominal

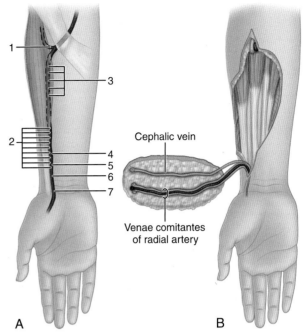

FIGURE 2.29 **A,** Schematic representation of cutaneous branches of radial artery (*1* = anterior recurrent radial artery, *2* = cutaneous branch of superficial radial artery, *3* = cutaneous branch of deep radial artery, *4* = dorsal branch to the wrist, *5* = palmar branch to the wrist, *6* = branch to the scaphoid, *7* = distal radial artery). **B,** Reversed forearm flap showing venae comitantes and cephalic vein.

region. Traditionally, flaps from the abdomen have been used as tubed pedicle flaps or as direct flaps. The tubed pedicle technique requires the formation of a bipedicle tube and 6 weeks of maturation followed by detachment of one end of the tube to be applied to the hand, followed by another 3 to 6 weeks before the flap is completely detached and "inset" into the defect. The direct abdominal flaps typically are limited in their length-to-width ratio because of the random circulation. It rarely is safe to use such a flap with a length-to-width ratio that varies significantly from 1 : 1. A better understanding of the skin circulation has led to the development and use of axial pattern flaps that have a defined arteriovenous supply. Axial pattern flaps allow a safe length-to-width ratio of at least 3 : 1, the possibility of covering either the dorsal or palmar surface, and a sufficiently long pedicle to allow arm and hand movement. Because such flaps usually do not require a delay in detachment of one end, they are useful for coverage of acute hand injuries. Microvascular surgical coverage options using free flaps are discussed in other chapter.

■ RANDOM PATTERN ABDOMINAL PEDICLE FLAPS

A random pattern abdominal flap to be applied to the hand should have its base either distal, toward the superficial epigastric vessels, usually on the same side as the affected hand, or proximal, above the umbilicus toward the thoracoepigastric vessels, usually on the opposite side (Fig. 2.32). The flaps above the umbilicus should not be used in a patient with a "barrel chest" associated with chronic lung disease. Abdominal

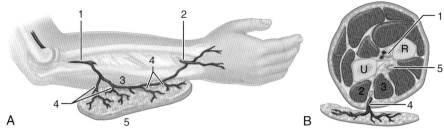

FIGURE 2.30   **A,** Anatomy of interosseous arteries. Common interosseous artery (*1*) divides into anterior interosseous artery (*2*), running volar to interosseous membrane, and posterior interosseous artery (*3*). Distally, anterior interosseous artery approaches posterior compartment of forearm (*2*) and gives branches to dorsal aspect of wrist and forearm that anastomose with cutaneous branches of posterior interosseous artery (*4*). Area of skin on dorsal aspect of forearm irrigated by posterior interosseous artery (*5*). **B,** Transverse section at middle third of forearm where posterior interosseous artery runs immediately beneath superficial fascia of dorsal aspect of forearm. *1,* Anterior interosseous artery; *2,* extensor carpi ulnaris muscle; *3,* extensor digiti minimi muscle; *4,* posterior interosseous artery between muscles *2* and *3,* with some branches perforating superficial fascia to reach skin; *5,* posterior interosseous nerve. *R,* Radius; *U,* ulna.

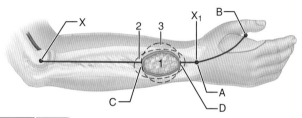

FIGURE 2.31   Technique to correct contracture of first web space. Four points (*A,B,C,* and *D*) marked on skin. Width of flap depends on defect in first web space. Different shapes (*2* and *3*) can be used (see text). (Redrawn from Zancolli EA, Angrigiani C: Posterior interosseous island forearm flap, *J Hand Surg* 13B:130–135, 1988.)

flaps obtained from areas above the umbilicus usually avoid the fat "storage areas." If the flap is obtained from the infraumbilical area, the recipient grafted area usually increases in bulk because the infraumbilical area skin adds fat.

APPLYING A RANDOM PATTERN ABDOMINAL PEDICLE FLAP

TECHNIQUE 2.6

- On sterile paper, make a pattern of the defect and outline it on the abdomen; outline the flap, making it sufficiently larger than the pattern to allow for normal skin contraction and for the pedicle "bridge" between the abdomen and the defect. As a rule, the flap should be rectangular to avoid a circular outline when the flap is attached to the hand. Avoid making the flap too thick. If possible, follow the principles of appropriate hand incisions (see chapter 1) to avoid tension lines and excessive scarring.
- Using sharp dissection, raise the skin flap of the desired size and thickness (Figs. 2.33 and 2.34).
- Maintain hemostasis and handle the fat carefully to avoid necrosis.

- To close the donor site defect, widely undermine the skin margins and suture them together or apply a split-thickness skin graft, or both.
- With a split skin graft, cover the part of the raw, exposed undersurface of the flap pedicle that does not cover the hand defect. Slightly undermine the edges of the defect on the hand and apply the flap over the entire defect. Suture the edges of the flap to the edges of the defect and suture the free edge of the split graft to the edge of the defect nearest to the base of the pedicle, covering all raw surfaces.
- Place strips of nonadhering gauze (Xeroform or Adaptic) over the suture line and a dry dressing on the flap; be careful to prevent kinking, tension, and rotation at its base.
- Using flannel cloth reinforced with plaster or wide adhesive tape, apply a bandage around the trunk and shoulder supporting the hand. The flap should be easily accessible for inspection through the dressing.
- When marked pronation or supination of the forearm is necessary to prevent tension on the flap, a heavy transverse Steinmann pin through the radius and ulna just proximal to the wrist is helpful in maintaining this position.

POSTOPERATIVE CARE The flap should be inspected almost hourly during the first 48 hours for circulatory compromise produced by tension or torsion or for the development of a hematoma. Sutures that appear to be too tight should be removed because the pressure they apply on the flap may be sufficient to produce ischemia.

If an area becomes necrotic, it should be excised and covered with a split skin graft. Gross infection from necrosis or hematoma usually results in failure. The area should be redressed frequently to avoid offensive odor and reduce the chance of infection. Usually the flap can be detached safely after 3 weeks. In children, the flap usually can be detached after 2 weeks.

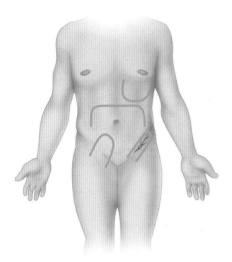

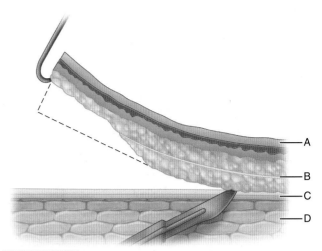

FIGURE 2.32   Example of abdominal flaps (see text for details regarding length and width of flaps). Lower abdominal flap may be made narrower in relation to its length if it contains superficial circumflex iliac artery and vein *(lower right)* or superficial epigastric artery and vein.

FIGURE 2.34   Cross-section of abdominal pedicle flap being raised. *A,* Epidermis and dermis; *B,* superficial fascia of abdomen; *C,* deep fascia of abdomen; *D,* muscularis. *Dotted line* indicates extent of defatting of portion of pedicle to be applied to hand. Base or stem should retain sufficient fat to retain its shape to prevent kinking. (From Kelleher JC, Sullivan JG, Baibak GJ, et al: Use of a tailored abdominal pedicle flap for surgical reconstruction of the hand, *J Bone Joint Surg* 52A:1552–1562, 1970.) **SEE TECHNIQUE 2.6.**

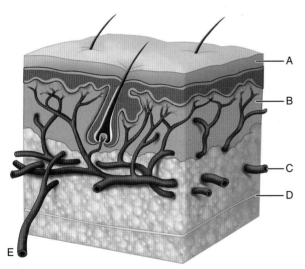

FIGURE 2.33   Dissection of skin and subcutaneous fat. *A,* Epidermis; *B,* dermis; *C,* subdermal plexus of vessels; *D,* superficial fascia; *E,* arteries perforating muscularis and deep fascia to join subdermal plexus of vessels. (From Kelleher JC, Sullivan JG, Baibak GJ, et al: Use of a tailored abdominal pedicle flap for surgical reconstruction of the hand, *J Bone Joint Surg* 52A:1552–1562, 1970.) **SEE TECHNIQUE 2.6.**

GROIN PEDICLE FLAP

Before the 1973 description by Daniel and Taylor of its successful use as a free flap, the iliofemoral (groin) flap, popularized by McGregor, was widely used in reparative and reconstructive surgery of the upper extremity. Advantages of the groin flap include (1) its location in an area sparse in hair, (2) minimal donor site morbidity, (3) multiple arteriovenous supply, (4) potential for incorporating bone with the overlying skin flap even when used as a pedicle flap, and (5) potentially large size. Disadvantages include (1) problems with color matching, (2) possibility of damage to vessels from previous inguinal surgery, and (3) thickness of the flap in obese patients.

The groin pedicle flap usually receives its arterial supply from the superficial circumflex iliac branch of the femoral artery. Its venous drainage is through the superficial inferior epigastric and superficial circumflex iliac veins. For a discussion of variations in the vasculature, especially as they pertain to the use of a free flap, see other chapter.

TECHNIQUE 2.7

- Position the patient supine or turned slightly away from the affected side with sandbags or bolsters beneath the scapula and pelvis on the side of the flap to allow free access to the flank if a large flap is required.
- To help determine the central axis of the flap, identify and locate the course of the superficial circumflex iliac artery using a Doppler probe, usually about 2.5 cm distal and parallel to the inguinal ligament.
- After skin preparation and draping, use a suitable material, such as sterile paper or plastic sheeting, to outline

■ AXIAL PATTERN FLAPS

Of the three axial pattern pedicle flaps that have been used often for hand coverage (deltopectoral, groin, and hypogastric), the groin and hypogastric flaps have been found to be the most useful. Other axial pattern flaps that have been transferred as vascularized free flaps are discussed in other chapter.

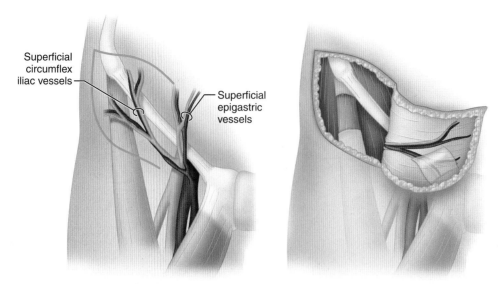

Superficial circumflex iliac vessels

Superficial epigastric vessels

FIGURE 2.35   Groin pedicle flap. **SEE TECHNIQUE 2.7.**

the recipient defect with allowances for skin contraction. Place the pattern in the inguinal region, parallel with the inguinal ligament, along the course of the superficial circumflex iliac artery (Fig. 2.35).

- Although unusual, a groin flap 20 × 30 cm has been elevated in some situations. The usual dimensions fall within a width of about 10 cm and a length extending about 5 cm posterolateral to the anterior superior iliac spine. Landmarks to remember and refer to include the (1) pubic tubercle, (2) anterior superior iliac spine, (3) inguinal ligament, and (4) pulsation of the femoral artery.
- Incise the skin along the outline of the pattern, tapering the margins of the flap to a narrower pedicle of skin overlying the vessels that lie about 2.5 cm distal to the inguinal ligament near the medial border of the sartorius.
- Incise the skin and subcutaneous tissue down to the deep fascia and continue to elevate the flap in this plane.
- While dissecting along the superior margin of the flap, identify, ligate, or cauterize and divide the superficial epigastric vessels to ensure that the superficial circumflex iliac vessels are kept within the flap.
- Approach the lateral border of the sartorius with care because these vessels penetrate the sartorius fascia near this point.
- At the lateral margin of the sartorius, incise the fascia and carefully elevate it to the medial border.
- At the medial border of the sartorius, the superficial circumflex iliac artery usually has a deep branch. Dissection of the flap medial to the medial border of the sartorius requires division of this branch and might place the trunk of the artery at risk. Usually a sufficient skin flap can be elevated without extending the dissection medial to the sartorius.
- Dissect and handle the flap gently, maintaining hemostasis throughout the procedure.
- When elevation of the flap is complete, determine the best hand and forearm position for attachment of the flap. Determine also the amount of the flap required to cover the hand defect and manage the intervening pedicle bridge of skin by forming a tube in the pedicle or by applying a split skin graft to the raw, exposed area on the

pedicle. If forming a tube causes excessive pressure on the pedicle vessels, a split skin graft provides safer coverage of this exposed tissue.

- While preparing the recipient area on the hand or forearm, cover the raw deep surface of the flap with moist gauze to prevent drying. Usually, groin flaps have a pale appearance after elevation. If there is any doubt regarding the axial arterial integrity after flap elevation, it may be necessary to replace the flap in its donor area, allowing a delay of 10 to 14 days.
- After the recipient area has been prepared, elevate the skin at the margin of the defect to allow easier insetting of the flap.
- After elevation of small to medium-sized flaps, close the donor site by mobilizing the skin margins, flexing the hip, and closing the subcutaneous and skin layers.
- Close the donor site before attaching the flap to the hand defect.
- Securely attach the flap skin to the skin margins of the recipient hand defect with a nonstrangulating suture technique.
- Apply a nonadherent gauze (e.g., Adaptic, Xeroform) to the suture lines and pad the axilla with absorbent padding to avoid maceration of the axillary skin.
- With the help of assistants, elevate the patient's torso using a board or similar device to support the back while the shoulder, arm, and forearm are included in a circumferential flannel wrapping, incorporating the torso and affected extremity.
- Secure the cloth wrap by wrapping over it with adhesive tape.
- Create a small window in the bandage to allow inspection of the flap. Take care at all times while moving or assisting the patient not to pull the arm away from the body.

POSTOPERATIVE CARE The flap is protected by avoiding pulling on the affected arm. The flap is inspected and its circulatory status is evaluated hourly for the first 48 hours. If excessive tension, pedicle torsion, or hematoma becomes evident, the limb is repositioned, the bandage is changed, or sutures are removed to relieve ischemia. Any necrotic areas are promptly excised, and hematomas are evacuated. Bandages are changed, and the wound is cleaned

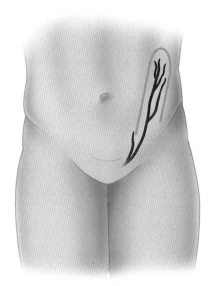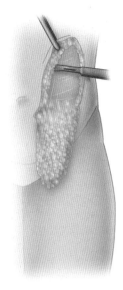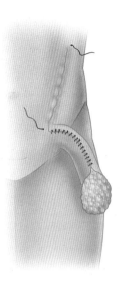

FIGURE 2.36   Hypogastric (superficial epigastric) flap. **SEE TECHNIQUE 2.8.**

frequently to decrease any unpleasant odor. Usually the flap can be detached at 3 to 4 weeks. If there is any doubt concerning the axial artery or vascularity of the flap, or if the pedicle bridge is to be used to cover the defect, the remainder of the flap is not detached for another 1 to 2 weeks. This helps minimize the risk of necrosis of portions of the flap.

HYPOGASTRIC (SUPERFICIAL EPIGASTRIC) FLAP

Since its initial description by Shaw and Payne, wide application has been found for the hypogastric flap, and it has proven extremely useful for coverage of the hand and forearm. Its arteriovenous pedicle consists of the superficial epigastric artery and vein (Fig. 2.36). The axis of the flap usually is oriented in a superolateral direction, with the base near the inguinal ligament centered at about the midpoint of the ligament. Flaps measuring 18 cm long × 7 cm wide have been used. Its advantages and disadvantages are similar to those described for the groin pedicle flap (see earlier). Usually a bone graft cannot be incorporated into the skin flap. During preoperative planning, it is important to examine the abdomen on the affected side for the presence of previous surgical or traumatic scars that might have damaged the arterial supply.

TECHNIQUE 2.8

- Position the patient and elevate the affected side with a sandbag as needed. After skin preparation and draping, use a suitable material, such as sterile paper, to outline the recipient defect, making allowances for skin contraction.
- Place the pattern over the distribution of the superficial epigastric artery, arranging the base of the flap along the inguinal ligament. Arrange the axis of the flap so that it extends superiorly and slightly laterally from the ingui-

nal ligament and is centered at about the midpoint of the ligament. Avoid exceeding a length-to-width ratio of more than 3 : 1.
- Make the skin incisions along the skin markings of the pattern outline, with two parallel incisions extending superiorly and tapering toward the superiormost extreme of the flap. The distal extent of the dissection should not extend inferior to the inguinal ligament.
- Extend the skin incision through the subcutaneous tissue so that the plane of dissection is at the level of the Scarpa fascia.
- Elevate the flap inferiorly to the level of the inguinal ligament and cover the deep subcutaneous tissues with moistened gauze.
- Prepare the recipient site on the hand and mobilize and elevate the skin at the margins of the defect on the hand to allow ease of attachment of the flap to the hand.
- Close or skin graft the donor site before attaching the flap to the hand defect.
- After the elevation of small to medium-sized flaps, the donor site usually can be closed by mobilizing the skin margins and closing the subcutaneous and skin layers.
- Attach the flap skin to the skin margins of the recipient hand defect with a nonstrangulating suture technique.
- Apply a nonadherent gauze (e.g., Adaptic, Xeroform) to the suture lines.
- With the help of an assistant, lift the patient's torso and support it with a board or similar device while the shoulder, arm, and forearm are incorporated in a circumferential flannel wrap around the torso and affected extremity.
- Wrap over the cloth wrap with wide adhesive tape to secure the dressing.
- Arrange the bandage so that the flap can be inspected.
- Take care while moving the patient so that the flap is not disrupted by pulling on the arm.

POSTOPERATIVE CARE Postoperative care is similar to that for the groin pedicle flap procedure. Pulling on the affected arm or shoulder should be avoided to prevent disruption of the suture line. The flap should be inspected hourly for the first 48 hours to evaluate its appearance and circulatory status. If there are any signs of excessive tension, pedicle kinking, or hematoma formation, the limb should be repositioned, the bandage changed, sutures removed, and other necessary corrections made to avoid or correct ischemic changes. Necrotic tissue is excised promptly, and hematomas are evacuated. The wound is cleaned and the bandage is changed frequently to minimize drainage and odor. The flap can be detached safely at 3 to 4 weeks. If the vascular status of the flap is doubtful, or if the pedicle bridge is required to cover more of the hand defect, the axial artery is divided, or the pedicle is partially divided, and the remainder of the flap is inset into the defect 1 to 2 weeks later.

- Suture the flap in place so that it lies flat; avoid strangulating its base, and trim only slightly any "dog ears" that may be produced at the margins of the base to preserve the blood supply of the flap.

POSTOPERATIVE CARE Flap circulation should be monitored closely for at least 24 h. If flap viability is uncertain, the flap should be monitored until it is safe for the patient to return home. The hand should be elevated to avoid excessive edema. Potential causes of vasospasm (smoking, cold drinks, excessively cold room, emotional upsets) should be avoided. Skin sutures are removed in 10 to 14 days. When flap healing is progressing satisfactorily, rehabilitation appropriate for the specific injury is begun.

FILLETED GRAFTS

A filleted graft is a flap of tissue fashioned from a nearby part, usually a finger, from which the bone has been removed but in which one or more neurovascular bundles have been retained. In the hand, such a graft is indicated only when deep tissues, such as tendons, nerves, and joints, are exposed and when a nearby damaged finger is to be sacrificed because it is not salvageable. A filleted graft is never used at the expense of a salvageable, useful part.

A filleted graft is especially convenient when other injuries more proximal in the same extremity would interfere with positioning the hand to receive a flap from a distant part. The advantages of this graft are that (1) it can be applied in a one-stage procedure at the time of injury and is obtained from within the same surgical field as the injured part; (2) its survival is almost ensured because one or more of its neurovascular bundles are preserved; (3) its skin is similar to that which is to be replaced; (4) it is not attached to a distant part, and consequently after surgery the hand can be splinted in the position of function and elevated; and (5) it provides an adequate thumb web when the index finger is the donor.

APPLYING A FILLETED GRAFT

TECHNIQUE 2.9

- Because the main vessels course anterolaterally through the digit, it is easier to fashion a flap with its base anterior and cover a defect on the dorsum of the hand than vice versa (see Fig. 2.5).
- Make a midline dorsal incision along the full length of the finger and skirt it around the nail distally. Deepen the dissection to the extensor tendon.
- Remove this tendon, the underlying bone, and the flexor tendons and their sheath, but preserve the fat in which the neurovascular bundles are located; take care to avoid damaging these bundles.
- Spread the flap created and place it on the donor area. If it is too wide, trim its edges, or if it is too long, excise its end; in the latter instance, ligate the digital vessels and resect the digital nerves far enough proximally to prevent their being caught in the scar.

SKIN COVERAGE
GRANULATING AREAS

A granulating area on the hand rarely should be left to heal with a scar. If a hand has not been covered completely with skin during the treatment of an acute injury, a split-thickness graft should be applied as soon as the surface is clean enough to support it. Even if the entire granulating surface is not clean, any portion that is clean enough should be covered. Exposed tendons, joints, or cortical bone should be covered with flap grafts (see previously).

SCARS

A scar is a poor substitute for skin; it is nonelastic, and its sensation is abnormal. The absence of elasticity restricts the motion of otherwise unobstructed underlying joints and interferes with the nutrition of adjacent parts. Often the scar adheres to joints, tendons, and ligaments, further limiting motion. A scar contracts during healing and does not stretch later. Attempts to stretch a scar may be beneficial only in that normal surrounding skin is stretched. When a linear scar is left spanning a joint, the intermittent stretching from active motion causes it to hypertrophy. Forced passive stretching causes any scar to rupture and fissure, only to heal and become thicker. A scar not only lacks normal sensation but also may become painful when it adheres to nerve endings.

Scars cannot be entirely eliminated because the process of healing depends on the production of scar tissue. A scar can be replaced partially, however, by tissue of better quality, and the direction or location of its lines can be changed so that they interfere less with function. A scar can be treated surgically (1) to eliminate deformity, (2) to restore joint motion, (3) to provide better skin coverage for vulnerable parts or to permit operation on deeper structures such as tendons or nerves, (4) to relieve pain, and (5) occasionally to improve the appearance of the hand. Sometimes the excision of normal skin is necessary in moving the lines of the scar to a more desirable location.

If possible, a scar should not be replaced until it has matured, usually after a minimum of 3 months. It should be treated earlier, however, when it severely limits joint motion. When a metacarpophalangeal joint is held in extension or a proximal interphalangeal joint is held in flexion, a severe secondary contracture develops in the joint unless the offending scar is treated as soon as possible without awaiting its maturation. For the purposes of treatment, scars may be classified as linear scars and area scars; either type may be volar or dorsal and may or may not involve the deep structures.

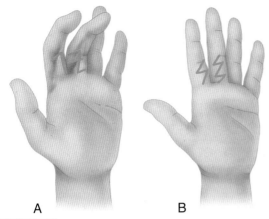

FIGURE 2.37 Flexion contractures caused by linear scars **(A)** can be released by Z-plasties **(B)**.

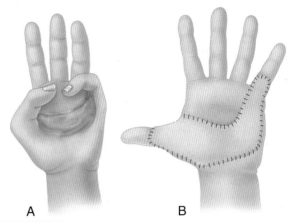

FIGURE 2.39 Area scar on palm **(A)** has been replaced by graft **(B)** with margins that follow rules that guide location and direction of hand incisions.

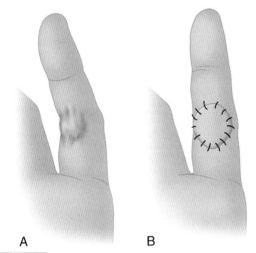

FIGURE 2.38 Area scar **(A)** has been replaced by full-thickness skin graft **(B)** that is larger than scar.

■ METHODS OF CORRECTING LINEAR SCARS

Disabling linear scars usually result from surgical incisions or traumatic lacerations that cross flexor creases. When such a scar on a finger is narrow and is surrounded by normal tissue (Fig. 2.37), it can be released by a Z-plasty (see chapter 1), but a scar more than 2 mm wide on the volar surface is difficult to correct in this way because the skin here is less mobile than that on the dorsal surface. In some instances, the scar must be replaced by a full-thickness free graft (see Technique 2.2), a cross finger flap (see Technique 2.3), or a local flap (see Fig. 2.8). On the palm, a linear scar may represent loss of skin substance, and, in this instance, a free, split-thickness graft or a full-thickness graft is indicated; correcting a scar contracture here by Z-plasty is difficult. On the dorsum of the hand, most disabling linear scars may be corrected by Z-plasty.

■ METHODS OF CORRECTING AREA SCARS

An area scar represents an initial skin loss greater than the area of the final scar because it has contracted during healing; it always must be replaced by a graft that is larger than the scar (see Fig. 2.38). Because the skin for any graft should be as similar to the lost skin as possible, a local flap (see Fig.

2.8) or cross finger flap (see Technique 2.3) is preferable only if a small area is lost. If the area is large, if bare bone or tendon is left after excision of the scar, or if a reconstructive procedure is planned, a distant ("remote") flap, or vascularized free flap, containing skin and subcutaneous fat is necessary. Deeper parts of the scar may be excised when the flap is applied, but tendons or nerves must not be repaired until later. The tendons or nerves are exposed through an incision along the edge of the flap and not through it.

An area scar on the dorsum of the hand involving only the skin can be replaced by a medium or thick split graft of carefully planned size. The normal adult hand has about 5 cm of extra skin longitudinally on the dorsum to allow flexion of the wrist and fingers and about 2.5 cm of extra skin transversely to allow development of the metacarpal arch when making a fist. A graft here must allow for some of this extra skin and for previous shrinkage of the scar and later shrinkage of the graft and must be placed while the hand is in the position of function; otherwise, it would be much too tight. Burm et al. found that the greatest amount of skin could be grafted to the dorsum of the hand with the hand in the "fist" position and that the anatomic position allowed for more skin than the "safe" position. In most clinical situations, however, interphalangeal flexion contracture is possible if the fingers are held flexed too long.

For an area scar on the palm, similar skin cannot be used because it is found only on the sole of the foot (palmar skin withstands friction and shock and is more sensitive than dorsal skin). If the scar is superficial, a split-thickness graft can be used. If deep vulnerable structures are involved, a full-thickness graft is preferable, although it is harder to handle, is less likely to survive, and must be limited in size by the fact that it leaves a defect in the donor area that must be closed by suture after its edges are undermined.

For an insensitive large area scar on the radial side of an otherwise normal index finger or on the area of pinch of the thumb, a neurovascular island graft may be indicated. When a graft is applied to the hand, the rules that guide the location and direction of hand incisions (see chapter 1) must be followed carefully because the graft heals to the normal skin with a linear scar (Fig. 2.39).

REFERENCES

Aydin HU, Savvidou, Ozyurekoglu T: Comparison of homodigital dorsolateral flap and cross-finger flap for the reconstruction of pulp defects, *J Hand Surg Am*, 2018 Oct 23, [Epub ahead of print].

Azzena B, Amabile A, Tiengo C: Use of acellular dermal regeneration template in a complete finger degloving injury: case report, *J Hand Surg* 35A:2057, 2010.

Balbo R, Avonto I, Marenchino D, et al.: Platelet gel for the treatment of traumatic loss of finger substance, *Blood Transfus* 8:255, 2010.

Berger MJ, Regan WR, Seal A, Briston SG: Reliability of the "Ten Test" for assessment of discriminative sensation in hand trauma, *J Plast Reconstr Aesthet Surg* 69(10):1411, 2016.

Bush K, Meredith S, Demsey D: Acute hand and wrist injuries sustained during recreational mountain biking: a prospective study, *Hand* 8:397, 2013.

Cannon TA: High-pressure injection injuries of the hand, *Orthop Clin North Am* 47(3):617, 2016.

Carty MJ, Blazar PE: Complex flexor and extensor tendon injuries, *Hand Clin* 29:283, 2013.

Chang JH, Shieh SJ, Kuo LC, Lee YL: The initial anatomical severity in patients with hand injuries predicts future health-related quality of life, *J Trauma* 71:1352, 2011.

Christoforou D, Alaia M, Craig-Scott S: Microsurgical management of acute traumatic injuries of the hands and fingers, *Bull Hosp Jt Dis* 71(6), 2013.

DeGeorge Jr BR, Rodeheaver GT, Drake DB: Operative technique for human composite flexor tendon allograft procurement and engraftment, *Ann Plast Surg* 72:S191, 2014.

DePutter CE, Selles RW, Polinder S, et al.: Economic impact of hand and wrist injuries: health-care costs and productivity costs in a population-based study, *J Bone Joint Surg* 94A:e56, 2012.

Dorf E, Blue C, Smith BP, Koman LA: Therapy after injury to the hand, *J Am Acad Orthop Surg* 18:464, 2010.

Dunn JC, Fares AB, Kusnezov N, et al.: Current evidence regarding routine antibiotic prophylaxis in hand surgery, *Hand (N Y)*, 2017, Mar 1 [Epub ahead of print].

Dunn JC, Means Jr KR, Desale S, Giladi AM: Antibiotic use in hand surgery: surgeon decision making and adherence to available evidence, *Hand*, 2018, Nov 22. [E-pub ahead of print].

Eisele A, Dereskewitz C, Kus S, et al.: Factors affecting time off work in patients with traumatic hand injuries: a bio-psycho-social perspective, *Injury* 49(10):1822, 2018.

Ellis CV, Kulber DA: Acellular dermal matrices in hand reconstruction, *Plast Reconstr Surg* 130(5 Suppl 2):256S, 2012.

Frech A, Pellegrini L, Fraedrich G, et al.: Long-term clinical outcome and functional status after arterial reconstruction in upper extremity injury, *Eur J Vasc Endovasc Surg* 52(1):119, 2016.

Fritz J, Efron DT, Fishman EK: Multidetector CT and three-dimensional CT angiography of upper extremity arterial injury, *Emerg Radiol* 22:269, 2015.

Ghareeb PA, Daly C, Liao A, Payne D: Current trends in the management of ballistic fractures of the hand and wrist: experiences of a high-volume level I trauma center, *Hand (NY)* 13(2):176, 2018.

Guo E, Xie Q, Zhu Z, et al.: Laparoscopy-assisted chimeric peritoneal-deep inferior epigastric perforator flap for reconstruction of hand and foot, *Wounds* 30(2):36, 2018.

Gustafsson M, Hagberg L, Holmefur M: Ten years follow-up of health and disability in people with acute traumatic hand injury: pain and cold sensitivity are long-standing problems, *J Hand Surg Eur* 36:590, 2011.

Haddock NT, Ehrlich DA, Levine JP, Saadeh PB: The crossover composite filet of hand flap and heterotopic thumb replantation: a unique indication, *Plast Reconstr Surg* 130:634e, 2012.

Hassanpour SE, Hosseini SN, Abdolzadeh M: Purse-string suture as a complementary technique with conventional flaps in repairing fingertip amputation, *Tech Hand Up Extrem Surg* 15:94, 2011.

Hile D, Hile L: The emergent evaluation and treatment of hand injuries, *Emerg Med Clin North Am* 33:397, 2015.

Kandamany N, Naasan A: The composite Moberg flap for reconstruction of complex thumb tip injuries, *Plast Reconstr Surg* 133:235, 2014.

Lee MC, Jany YJ, Yun IS, et al.: Comparative skin evaluation after split-thickness skin grafts using 2 different acellular dermal matrices to cover composite forearm defects, *J Hand Surg Am* 42(4):297, 2017.

Lesiak AC, Shafritz AB: Negative-pressure wound therapy, *J Hand Surg Am* 38:1828, 2013.

Machol 4th JA, Fang RC, Matloub HS: The free fillet flap after traumatic amputation: a review of literature and case report, *Hand* 8:487, 2013.

Marom BS, Ratzon NZ, Carel RS, Sharabi M: Return to work barriers among manual workers after hand injuries: 1-year follow-up cohort study, *Arch Phys Med Rehabil* 100(3):422, 2019.

McKee DM: Acute management of burn injuries to the hand and upper extremity, *J Hand Surg* 35A:1542, 2010.

Murphy GR, Gardiner MD, Glass GE, et al.: Meta-analysis of antibiotics for simple hand injuries requiring surgery, *Br J Surg* 103(5):487, 2016.

Netscher DT: Regarding "fingertip reconstruction with simultaneous flaps and nail bed grafts following amputation, *J Hand Surg Am* 39:171, 2014.

Neutel N, Houpt P, Schuurman AH: Prognostic factors for return to work and resumption of other daily activities after traumatic hand injury, *J Hand Surg Eur* 44(2):203, 2019.

Panattoni JB, De Ona IR, Ahmed MM: Reconstruction of fingertip injuries: surgical tips and avoiding complications, *J Hand Surg Am* 40:1016, 2015.

Pannell WC, Heckmann N, Alluri RK, et al.: Predictors of nerve injury after gunshot wounds to the upper extremity, *Hand (N Y)* 12(5):501, 2017.

Patterson JM, Boyer MI, Ricci WM, Goldfard CA: Hand trauma: a prospective evaluation of patients transferred to a level I trauma center, *Am J Orthop (Belle Mead NJ)* 39:196, 2010.

Schmitt T, Talley J, Chang J: New concepts and technologies in reconstructive hand surgery, *Clin Plast Surg* 39:445, 2012.

Rabarin F: Saint Cast Y, Jeudy J, et al: cross finger flap for reconstruction of fingertip amputations: long-term results, *Orthop Traumatol Surg Res* 102(4 Suppl):S225, 2016.

Richards T, Clement R, Russell I, Newington D: Acute hand injury splinting – the good, the bad and the ugly, *Ann R Coll Surg Engl* 100(2):92, 2018.

Senarath-Yapa K, Bell DR: "Front and back" flaps for multiple dorsal and planar digital skin loss, *J Hand Surg Eur* 35:721, 2010.

Shichinohe R, Yamamoto Y, Kawashima K, et al.: Factors that affected functional outcome after a delayed excision and split-thickness skin graft on the dorsal side of burned hands, *J Burn Care Res* 38(5):e851, 2017.

Shim HS, Choi JS, Kim SW: A role for postoperative negative pressure wound therapy in multi-tissue hand injuries, *Biomed Res Int* 2018:3629643, 2018.

Sivak WN, Ruane EJ, Hausman SJ, et al.: Decellularized matrix and supplemental fat grafting leads to regeneration following traumatic fingertip amputation, *Plast Reconstr Surg Glob Open* 4(1):e1094, 2016.

Smith Jr DJ: Techniques and outcomes for hand surgery: summary of recent literature, *Clin Plast Surg* 41:615, 2014.

Soni A, Pham TN, Ko JH: Acute management of hand burns, *Hand Clin* 33(2):229, 2017.

Tang L, Pafitanis G, Yang P, et al.: Combined multi-lobed flaps: a series of 39 extensive hand and multi-digit injuries one-staged reconstructions using modified designs of ALT, DPA and chimeric linking flaps, *Injury* 48(7):1527, 2017.

Thomson CH, Shah AK, Köhler G, et al.: Mid-palm hand amputation: reconstruction of the superficial palmar arch, *J Plast Reconstr Aesthet Surg* 66:1155, 2013.

To P, Atkinson CT, Lee DH, Pappas ND: The most cited articles in hand surgery over the past 20-plus years: a modern-day reading list, *J Hand Surg Am* 38:983, 2013.

Tosti R, Eberlin KR: "Damage control" hand surgery: evaluation and emergency management of the mangled hand, *Hand Clin* 34(1):17, 2018.

Turker T, Capdarest-Arest N: Management of gunshot wounds to the hand: a literature review, *J Hand Surg Am* 38:1641, 2013.

Vigouroux F, Choufani C, Grosset A, et al.: Application of damage control orthopedics to combat-related hand injuries, *Hand Surg Rehabil* 37(6):342, 2018.

Weigert R, Choughri H, Casoli V: Management of severe hand wounds with Integra dermal regeneration template, *J Hand Surg Eur* 36E:185, 2011.

Werdin F, Tenenhaus M, Becker M, Rennekampff HO: Healing time correlates with the quality of scarring: results from a prospective randomized control donor site trial, *Dermatol Surg* 44(4):521, 2018.

Xing SG, Tang JB: Extending applications of local anesthesia without tourniquet to flap harvest and transfer in the hand, *Hand Clin* 35(1):97, 2019.

The complete list of references is available online at ExpertConsult.com.

CHAPTER 3

FLEXOR AND EXTENSOR TENDON INJURIES

David L. Cannon

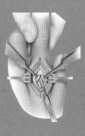

FLEXOR TENDONS

A basic knowledge of the anatomy of the flexor tendons, especially in the forearm, wrist, and hand, is assumed, as is an understanding of the essential biomechanical aspects of flexor digitorum profundus and sublimis function in the fingers. Tendon nutrition is believed to derive from two basic sources: (1) the synovial fluid produced within the tenosynovial sheath and (2) the blood supply provided through longitudinal vessels in the paratenon, intraosseous vessels at the tendon insertion, and vincular circulation (Fig. 3.1). An ischemic area is present in the flexor digitorum superficialis beneath the A2 pulley at the proximal phalanx. Two zones of ischemia are present in the flexor digitorum profundus—beneath the A2 pulley and beneath the A4 pulley. Tendon healing is believed to occur through the activity of extrinsic and intrinsic mechanisms, occurring in three phases: inflammatory (48 to 72 hours), fibroblastic (5 days to 4 weeks), and remodeling (4 weeks to about 3.5 months). The extrinsic mechanism occurs through the activity of peripheral fibroblasts and seems to be the dominant mechanism contributing to the formation of scar and adhesions. Intrinsic healing seems to occur through the activity of the fibroblasts derived from the tendon.

Although tendon adhesions occur and are associated with tendon injury and healing, they are not believed to be essential to the tendon repair process itself. Experimentally, it has been shown that tendon injury alone is insufficient to produce adhesions, whereas tendon injury with injury to the synovial sheath combined with immobilization leads to extensive adhesions. Techniques to prevent adhesion formation include the use of physical barriers and chemical agents. None has proved reliable in the clinical setting. Cytokine manipulation, gene therapy, and mesenchymal stem cell therapies are other areas of promising research into methods of controlling the formation of adhesions. Experiments suggest that cyclic tension applied to healing tendons stimulates the intrinsic healing response more than does the lack of tension. Findings such as these have led to the development of postoperative mobilization techniques to diminish the formation of adhesions and enhance the end result. To provide tendon repairs of sufficient strength to permit passive and active motion rehabilitation, researchers have produced a considerable amount of information regarding suture material, size, and core and peripheral suturing techniques, described subsequently in this chapter.

EXAMINATION

Evaluation of a patient with an injured hand involves the usual assessments of the patient's general condition and the possibility of other injuries, including the use of radiographs to exclude fractures. Careful examination of the neurovascular status of the hand precedes the evaluation of tendon function. Even when gross deformity is absent, the posture of the hand often provides clues as to which flexor tendons are severed

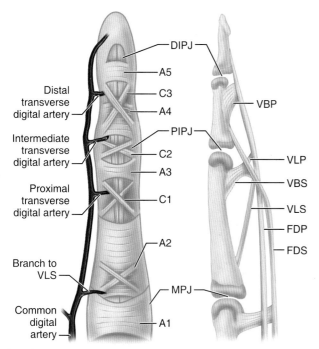

FIGURE 3.1   Vascular supply to flexor tendons is by four transverse communicating branches of digital arteries. *DIPJ,* Distal interphalangeal joint; *FDP,* flexor digitorum profundus; *FDS,* flexor digitorum sublimis; *MPJ,* metacarpophalangeal joint; *PIPJ,* proximal interphalangeal joint; *VBP,* vinculum breve profundus; *VBS,* vinculum breve superficialis; *VLP,* vinculum longum profundus; *VLS,* vinculum longum superficialis.

(Fig. 3.2). Traditionally, the "finger points the way" toward the injured structures. Errors are always possible when examining for flexor tendon injuries. Movements of the injured hand by the patient or the examiner can cause sufficient pain to limit motion and cause confusion. This is seen also when examining the hand after nerve injuries.

When both flexor tendons of a finger are severed, the finger lies in an unnatural position of hyperextension, especially compared with uninjured fingers. Flexor tendon injuries can be tentatively confirmed by several passive maneuvers. Passive extension of the wrist does not produce the normal "tenodesis" flexion of the fingers. If the wrist is flexed, even greater unopposed extension of the affected finger is produced. Gentle compression of the forearm muscle mass at times shows concomitant flexion of the joints of the uninvolved fingers, whereas the injured finger does not show this flexion, indicating separation of the tendon ends. Gently pressing the fingertip of each digit reveals loss of normal tension in the injured finger.

Tendon function is evaluated with voluntary active movements of the finger, usually directed by the examiner. This examination is unreliable and probably worthless, however, when evaluating an excited, uncooperative child or an anxious, uncooperative, or intoxicated adult. Demonstrating the maneuvers requested using the examiner's hand or the patient's uninjured hand before evaluating the injured hand can be helpful. If the wound is distal to the wrist, the injured finger should be stabilized to obtain specific joint movements. With the proximal interphalangeal joint stabilized, the flexor digitorum profundus is presumed severed if the distal interphalangeal joint cannot be actively flexed (Fig. 3.3). If neither the proximal nor the distal interphalangeal joint can be actively flexed with the metacarpophalangeal joint stabilized, both flexor tendons probably are severed.

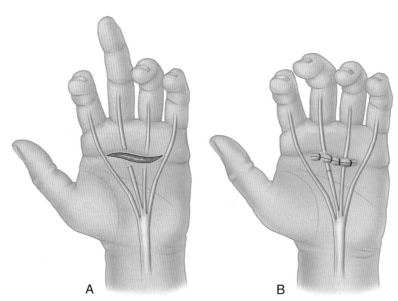

FIGURE 3.2   **A,** If long finger remains extended when hand is at rest, flexor tendons have been severed. **B,** This finger becomes normally flexed after profundus tendon or profundus tendon and sublimis tendons have been repaired.

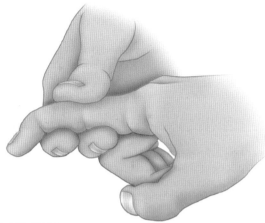

FIGURE 3.3   If distal interphalangeal joint can be actively flexed while proximal interphalangeal joint is stabilized, profundus tendon has not been severed.

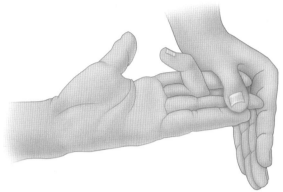

FIGURE 3.4   If proximal interphalangeal joint can be actively flexed while adjacent fingers are held completely extended, sublimis tendon has not been severed (see text).

The method used to show the transection of a flexor digitorum superficialis tendon with an intact flexor profundus tendon involves maintaining the adjacent fingers in complete extension, anchoring the profundus tendon in the extended position, and removing its influence from the proximal interphalangeal joint. When a flexor superficialis tendon has been severed, and the two adjacent fingers are held in maximal extension, flexion of the interphalangeal joint usually is impossible (Fig. 3.4). The exception to this evaluation is the result of the independent function of the index finger flexor digitorum profundus; a technique advocated by Lister is helpful in evaluating an isolated injury to this tendon. In this examination, the patient is requested to pinch and pull a sheet of paper with each hand, using the index fingers and thumbs. In the intact finger, this function is accomplished by the flexor superficialis with the flexor digitorum profundus relaxed, allowing hyperextension of the distal interphalangeal joint so that maximal pulp contact occurs with the paper. If the flexor superficialis is injured, the distal interphalangeal joint hyperflexes and the proximal interphalangeal joint assume an extended position.

In the thumb, to check the integrity of the flexor pollicis longus tendon, the metacarpophalangeal joint of the thumb is stabilized. If the flexor pollicis longus tendon is divided, flexion at the interphalangeal joint is absent.

If a wound is located at the level of the wrist, the joints of a finger can be actively flexed even though the tendons to that finger are severed. This is the result of intercommunication of the flexor profundus tendons at the wrist, particularly in the little and ring fingers.

Sometimes a definitive diagnosis of flexor tendon transection may be impossible. These maneuvers do not detect a partially divided tendon. A partially divided tendon usually is functional; however, finger motion can be limited by pain, and the examination indicates tendon injury without allowing a definite diagnosis of tendon transection. Ultrasound and MRI may be helpful but are not always needed. When a definite diagnosis of tendon injury cannot be made, surgical exploration usually is indicated.

BASIC TENDON TECHNIQUES

The purpose of tendon suture is to approximate the ends of a tendon or to fasten one end of a tendon to adjoining tendons or to bone and to hold this position during healing. When tendons are being sutured, handling should be gentle and delicate, causing as little reaction and scarring as possible. Pinching and grasping of the uninjured surfaces should be avoided because this can contribute to the formation of adhesions. Strickland stressed six characteristics of an ideal tendon repair: (1) easy placement of sutures in the tendon, (2) secure suture knots, (3) smooth juncture of tendon ends, (4) minimal gapping at the repair site, (5) minimal interference with tendon vascularity, and (6) sufficient strength throughout healing to permit application of early motion stress to the tendon. In general, studies have shown that four, six, and eight core sutures with epitendinous repair best accomplish the objectives of achieving a predictable clinical outcome of near ideal functional restoration.

■ SUTURE MATERIAL

A variety of satisfactory suture materials are available for tendon repair. Although monofilament stainless steel has the highest tensile strength, it is difficult to handle, tends to pull through the tendon, and makes a large knot. Although it can be used satisfactorily in the distal forearm, its disadvantages limit its use in the fingers. Most absorbable sutures, including catgut and the polyglycolic acid group (Dexon, Vicryl), become weak too early after surgery to be effective in tendon repair. Synthetic sutures of the caprolactam family (Supramid) and nylon maintain their resistance to disrupting forces longer than polypropylene (Prolene) and polyester suture. Polydioxanone (PDS) has been shown to be as strong as polypropylene. A comparison of polyglycolide-trimethylene carbonate (Maxon) and polydioxanone found that the polydioxanone repairs maintained better strength over 28 days. Monofilament nylon permitted earlier gap formation and failure of the repair compared with braided polyester. In a biomechanical study, braided polyethylene and braided stainless steel wire were most suitable mechanically. Braided polyester was intermediate, and monofilament sutures of nylon and polypropylene were least satisfactory. In clinical situations, most surgeons find that the braided polyester sutures (Ticron, FiberWire, Mersilene) provide sufficient resistance to disrupting forces and gap formation, handle easily, and have satisfactory knot characteristics; consequently, these sutures are widely used.

A 4-0 suture is estimated to be 66% stronger than a 5-0 suture, and a 3-0 suture 52% stronger than a 4-0 suture. Based on cadaver experiments, the use of a 3-0 suture results in a twofold to threefold increase in fatigue strength and a 3-0 suture in a two-strand or four-strand configuration is recommended if an early active motion program is used. In most situations, a 3-0 suture may be useful to repair tendons in the forearm, palm, and larger digits, whereas a 4-0 suture may handle better in smaller digits. Epitendinous repair usually is done with 5-0 or 6-0 monofilament suture (Prolene).

Several newer devices and technologies appear promising. In a cadaver biomechanical analysis, an intratendinous, crimped, single-strand, multifilament stainless steel device (Teno Fix; Ortheon Medical, Winter Park, FL) compared favorably with four-strand cruciate repairs. A multicenter, randomized, and blinded clinical trial compared the stainless steel tendon repair device with a control group of four-strand cruciate suture repairs. The intratendinous device group had a lower rupture rate (0 vs. 18% in the controls) and compared favorably in other outcome measures, such as grip and pinch strength and DASH (disability, arm, shoulder, hand) scores. More clinical reports are needed using this device, the motion-stable wire suture of Towfigh, and the shape memory alloy suture to determine their place in the management of flexor tendon injuries. The use of the neodymium: yttrium-aluminum-garnet laser does not seem to weld tendons, according to a study in chickens. A knotless barbed suture has been described in the literature. One study found it to be as strong as a four-strand configuration for epitendinous repair, while one cadaver study found the barbed suture technique to be inferior to the conventional 4-0 suture with cyclic loading.

■ SUTURE CONFIGURATIONS

In the process of seeking the strongest intratendinous suture arrangement to allow early passive and active motion, numerous suture configurations at the repair site have been developed and studied (Fig. 3.5).

An abundance of research has shown that four-strand, six-strand, and eight-strand core sutures create stronger repairs, reduce the possibility of gap formation, and permit greater active forces to be applied to the repaired tendons, allowing earlier active motion than the traditional two-strand core sutures (Fig. 3.6). A global survey of clinical practices by Tang et al. confirms the efficacy of multistrand (four to eight) 3-0 or 4-0 core sutures with 6-0 epitendinous sutures. A human cadaver comparison of the Kessler, modified Kessler, Savage, Lee, augmented Becker, and Tsuge core suture methods by Zobitz et al. found no difference in maximal failure force or force to produce a 1.5-mm gap. Continuing the interest in multiple-strand modifications, such as those of Savage (six strands) (Fig. 3.7) and Lee (four strands) (Fig. 3.8), the grasp of a "cross-stitch" (Fig. 3.9) of 6-0 braided

polyester was found to be 117% stronger than a modified Kessler core suture with a conventional epitendinous repair.

The locked cruciate, the modified double Tsuge, and the modified Becker repairs have been shown to provide sufficient strength to support an early active motion rehabilitation program. The Tang and cruciate repairs (Fig. 3.10) have shown better tensile strength and elastic properties compared with the Silfverskiöld, Robertson, and modified Kessler repairs.

A cadaver study found that the cruciate four-strand suture technique provided stronger resistance to gap formation and had greater ultimate tensile strength than the Kessler, Strickland, or Savage techniques. When Kessler, Strickland, and modified Becker techniques were compared, only the Becker repair was strong enough to tolerate forces estimated for an active motion rehabilitation plan. The Strickland repair had less tendency to gap. In a group of canine tendons, the Becker repair was associated with greater friction between the tendon and sheath than the modified Kessler repair. A four-strand adaptation of the Kessler repair was found to be significantly stronger than the modified Kessler technique (Fig. 3.11). It is a straightforward modification that might be done with more ease in areas of the flexor sheath where access to the tendon is limited. Such techniques allow satisfactory purchase on the tendon so that satisfactory tensile strength is maintained during the early healing phase. Early active motion rehabilitation programs may have a beneficial effect on tendon healing and may reduce adhesion formation significantly.

Intratendinous crisscross suture techniques (Bunnell, Kleinert modification of Bunnell) tend to jeopardize the intratendinous circulation (Fig. 3.12). Although placement of sutures in the volar half of the tendon has been recommended to avoid injury to the circulation, experimental work showed that the mean strength of repairs sutured in the dorsal half of the tendon was 58.3% greater than that in the volar half. Locking the sutures as they pass through the tendons traps bundles of the tendon fibers, preventing the suture from pulling out of the tendon and increasing the resistance to gap formation. These techniques have been shown to be dependable in the fingers. No suture material or technique can be relied on to maintain tendon repairs with unlimited active movement in the early postoperative period. Most investigators report that the strength of the tendon repair diminishes considerably in the first 10 days. Thereafter, the strength of the repair gradually increases, so that by the end of 10 to 12 weeks considerable active forces can be applied in the rehabilitation program.

Continuous epitendinous sutures, placed circumferentially around the repair site, decrease the bulk of the repair site, minimizing the risk of triggering. This addition also enhances the strength of the core suture repair, supports 50% of the load to failure, and resists gap formation. In biomechanical tests of human cadaver tendons, the epitenon-first technique (Fig. 3.13) was found to be 22% stronger than the modified Kessler technique. A comparison of four circumferential techniques without core sutures in sheep tendons found that the interlocking horizontal mattress suture had the highest load to failure, greatest resistance to gap formation,

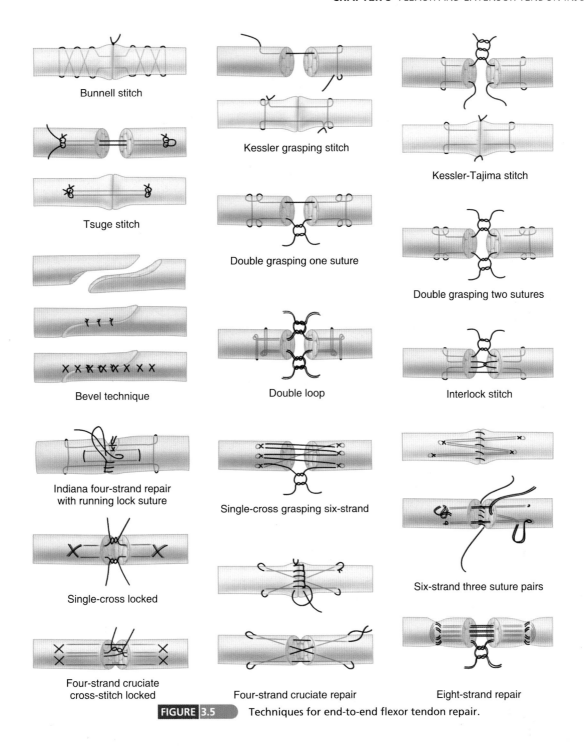

FIGURE 3.5 Techniques for end-to-end flexor tendon repair.

Bunnell stitch

Tsuge stitch

Bevel technique

Indiana four-strand repair with running lock suture

Single-cross locked

Four-strand cruciate cross-stitch locked

Kessler grasping stitch

Double grasping one suture

Double loop

Single-cross grasping six-strand

Four-strand cruciate repair

Kessler-Tajima stitch

Double grasping two sutures

Interlock stitch

Six-strand three suture pairs

Eight-strand repair

and highest stiffness and was believed to be best overall (Fig. 3.14). Peripheral sutures placed 2 mm from the repair site provide a stronger repair than placement of the sutures 1 mm from the repair site.

To minimize compression and bulking of the repair site, most techniques advocate the placement of temporary or permanent partial epitendinous sutures to secure the tendon ends before placement of core sutures. The partial epitendinous repair can then be completed or removed if a cross-stitch type of epitendinous repair is preferred. Alternatively, a tendon approximator or hypodermic needles can be used to stabilize the tendon ends in apposition so that the core suture is not used to approximate the ends.

END-TO-END SUTURE TECHNIQUES

MODIFIED KESSLER-TAJIMA SUTURE

A modification of the Kessler and Tajima techniques incorporates several advantages of each. Separate pieces of suture are used so that the tendon ends can be passed

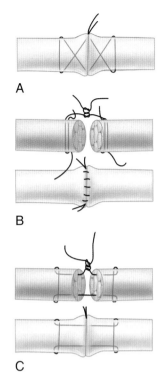

A

B

C

FIGURE 3.6 **A,** Crisscross stitch. **B,** Mason-Allen (Chicago) stitch. **C,** Modified Kessler stitch with single knot at repair.

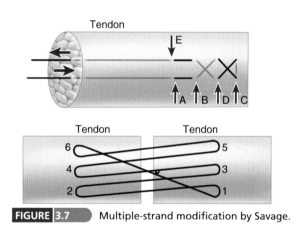

FIGURE 3.7 Multiple-strand modification by Savage.

within the flexor sheath, using the free ends of the suture as traction sutures. The knots are tied within the tendon. The sutures are locked with each exit from the tendon.

TECHNIQUE 3.1

(STRICKLAND, 1995)

- Use separate sutures introduced into each tendon end.
- Introduce a suture into one cut surface of the tendon, staying along the volar portion of the tendon, and exit 5 to 10 mm from the cut edge.
- Grasp approximately 25% of the diameter of the tendon with passage of the needle and lock the suture on the side of the tendon with a knot.

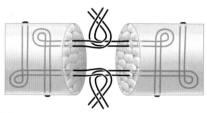

FIGURE 3.8 Four-strand technique (Lee). Two knots are made within repair site.

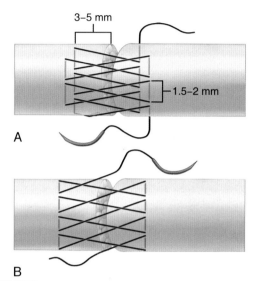

A

B

FIGURE 3.9 Two basic versions of cross-stitch. **A,** Suturing starts on far side of repair and proceeds toward operator. Simple overlap of each preceding grasp by approximately 50% automatically produces weave pattern without need for special needle passages. Symmetric placement of grasps (used here for clarity) is unnecessary in actual practice. Grasp size, overlap, and distance to tendon edge can be adapted to needs as suturing progresses. **B,** Suturing starts on near side of repair; overlapping is unnecessary.

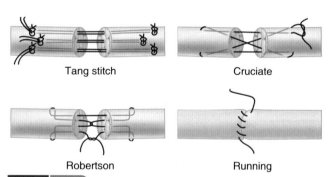

Tang stitch   Cruciate

Robertson   Running

FIGURE 3.10 Tendon suture techniques. (See text.) (Redrawn from Tang JB, Gu YT, Rice K, et al: Evaluation of four methods of flexor tendon repair for postoperative active mobilization, *Plast Reconstr Surg* 107:742–749, 2001.)

- Pass the suture transversely behind this locked knot across the tendon and onto the tendon surface and lock the suture again.
- Pass the suture into the tendon behind the second knot and exit on the cut surface.

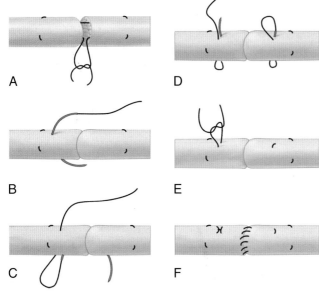

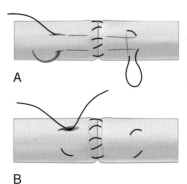

FIGURE 3.11 **A,** Standard Kessler core stitch is inserted using a round-bodied needle. Suture is tied with knot between cut ends. **B,** Second suture is inserted at right angles to first, again using round-bodied needle. **C,** Needle is passed along tendon, across junction, and out of tendon. If needle is too short, it can be brought out at junction and then passed in again. **D,** Rest of suture is inserted. **E,** Suture is tied under carefully judged tension to match first, with knot on outside of tendon. **F,** Repair is completed with epitendinous suture.

FIGURE 3.13 **A,** Epitenon-first technique. After placement of running epitendinous suture, core suture is placed within tendon. **B,** Completion of epitenon-first suture. Final knot is buried within tendon.

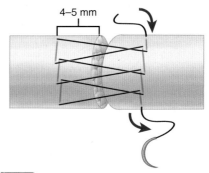

FIGURE 3.14 Interlocking horizontal mattress suture.

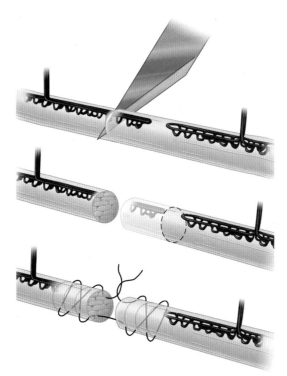

FIGURE 3.12 Flexor tendon with segmental vascular system, each segment supplied by one dorsal vinculum vessel. Tendon is cut within one segmentally vascularized portion *(top).* Shadowed area *(middle)* indicates area devascularized by transection of tendon. Intratendinous sutures contribute further to impaired microcirculation in tendon ends *(bottom).*

- Repeat this process on the opposite side of the cut tendon, locking the suture with each exit and maintaining the suture repair on the volar third of the cut surface of the tendon.
- Tie the knots within the tendon.
- Add a running-lock dorsal epitendinous suture of 5-0 or 6-0 nylon.
- On completion of the back wall suture, add a horizontal mattress suture of 4-0 braided polyester to the core suture configuration.
- Tie all knots of the core sutures.
- Complete the palmar (volar) running-lock peripheral epitendinous suture (Fig. 3.15).

FLEXOR TENDON REPAIR USING SIX-STRAND REPAIR (ADELAIDE TECHNIQUE)

TECHNIQUE 3.2

(SAVAGE AND RISITANO)
- The tendon repair comprises three grasping stitches in each tendon end and six strands of 4-0 Ethibond suture.

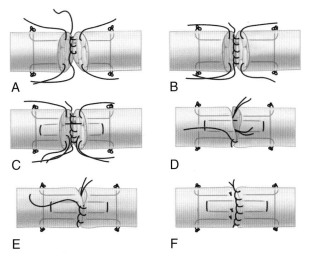

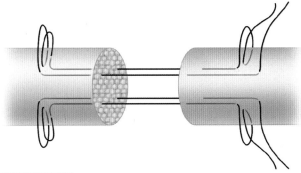

FIGURE 3.16   Modified Tsuge suture technique. **SEE TECHNIQUE 3.3.**

FIGURE 3.15   Simplified four-strand repair in which basic two-strand core suture is supplemented by horizontal mattress suture and running-lock stitch. **A,** Tajima core sutures in place. Back wall (dorsal) running-lock peripheral epitendinous stitch in progress. **B,** Back wall suturing completed. **C,** Mattress core suture added in palmar tendon gap. **D,** All core sutures tied. **E,** Completion of running-lock peripheral epitendinous suture. **F,** Repair completed. **SEE TECHNIQUE 3.1.**

- To make the grasping stitch (see Fig. 3.7), insert the needle into the tendon end and bring it out at A, reinsert at B, bring it opposite D, reinsert at C, bring it out opposite of C, reinsert at D, bring it out at B, reinsert at E, and finally bring out of the tendon end.
- As a practical point, grip the tendon end with a toothed forceps while inserting the suture, putting a small bundle of tendon fibers in tension where the grasping stitch is made. The number of grasping stitches is based on the size of the tendons.
- Insert six such grasping stitches, each about 1 to 1.5 mm in diameter and about 5 to 10 mm from the tendon end, sequentially around the tendon, avoiding the vincular area (see Fig. 3.7B).

FOUR- OR SIX-STRAND REPAIR

TECHNIQUE 3.3

(CHUNG, MODIFIED TSUGE)
- Insert the needle laterally into the proximal tendon end on the volar surface within 1 cm from the intended repair site.
- Run the strand longitudinally across the repair site and take it out 1 cm past the repair site at the distal tendon end.
- Pass the needle transversely in the distal part, taking the strand across the loop, and reinsert it into the distal tendon end; cross the repair site at the dorsal surface and exit

at the proximal end dorsally. Then reintroduce the suture transversely to make a loop.
- Tie a knot at this site.
- Perform the same suture passage as just described but on the opposite side of the tendon (Fig. 3.16).
- To complete the repair use a peripheral 6-0 monofilament running polypropylene suture (see Fig. 3.13).

MULTIPLE LOOPED SUTURE TENDON REPAIR

TECHNIQUE 3.4

(TANG ET AL.)
- Place one thread of 4-0 or 5-0 looped nylon in the center of the palmar half of the tendon. Pass it farther through to avoid placing knots at the same level on the tendon surface.
- Place one thread in each of the two respective sides of the dorsal half of the tendon.
- Place these suture threads to form the tips of a triangle in cross section of the tendon. The knots on the tendon surface are arranged in a triangular fashion (see Fig. 3.10).
- Make the knots as described for the modified Tsuge technique.
- Place epitendinous stitches with 6-0 nylon at the four cardinal points to smooth the ends of the tendon.

SIX-STRAND DOUBLE-LOOP SUTURE REPAIR

TECHNIQUE 3.5

(LIM AND TSAI)
- Place core sutures as shown in Figure 3.17 to minimize tendon constriction.

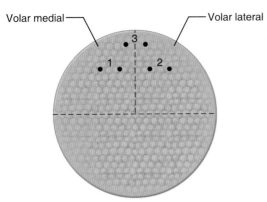

FIGURE 3.17   Cross section of a flexor tendon of right digit with placement of core sutures (double-loop 6-strand repair): *(1)* placement of first loop suture from proximal to distal in medial volar quadrant; *(2)* second loop suture from distal to proximal in lateral volar quadrant; *(3)* rerouting of both loop sutures to meet at repair site in midportion of tendon. (Redrawn from Gill RS, Lim BH, Shatford RA, et al: A comparative analysis of the six-strand double-loop flexor tendon repair and three other techniques: a human cadaveric study, *J Hand Surg* 24:1315–1322, 1999.) **SEE TECHNIQUE 3.5.**

- Holding the tendon parts slightly overlapped, superficially stitch the tendon 1.25 cm from the proximal end and transverse to the length of the tendon fibers.
- Lock the stitch by passing the needle through the loop suture and tighten with firm pressure to remove slack and increase resistance to gapping.
- Insert the needle close to the locked suture, taking a deeper, longitudinal bite of the medial volar quadrant tendon, running parallel to the tendon fibers and exiting the cut end.
- Reinsert the needle into the facing cut end of the distal tendon and exit 1 cm from the tendon end.
- Place a similar locking suture 1.25 cm from the distal cut end of the lateral volar quadrant of the tendon into the proximal cut end, and surface 1 cm from the end. Avoid inserting the needle too far from the locking suture because this leads to tendon bunching.
- Approximate the posterior wall of the tendon with 6-0 Prolene running epitenon sutures. Posterior running epitenon sutures help to correct the position of the tendon ends and control tension.
- Lock the ends of the two core sutures by taking a transverse bite and passing the needle through the loop.
- Insert the needles close to the second set of locked sutures, and surface through the tendon ends.
- Divide the loop suture, leaving the proximal loop ends longer than the distal loop ends, to make the four suture ends easier to identify.
- Tie the suture ends intratendinously. Four square throws provide a sturdy knot. Take care that all six strands are under the same tension, otherwise the benefit of using multiple strands is reduced (Fig. 3.5).
- Smooth the anterior walls of the tendon ends with a simple running epitenon suture (see Fig. 3.13).

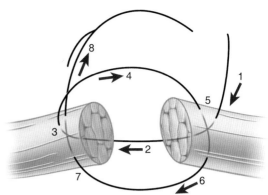

FIGURE 3.18   Double right-angle suture with single monofilament or multifilament wire suture threaded on curved needle.

EIGHT-STRAND REPAIR

TECHNIQUE 3.6

(WINTERS AND GELBERMAN)
- Insert the needle into the tendon at the repair site and extend it through the posterolateral quadrant, exiting 1 cm from the cut tendon edge.
- Working counterclockwise, insert the needle just distal to its previous exit point to anchor the tendon transversely.
- Complete the first posterolateral rectangle by paralleling the first suture pass with the tendon edge.
- Carry out the procedure in the same way in the opposite tendon stump, completing a dorsal rectangle.
- Advance the needle into the palmar half of the tendon and duplicate the previous steps, with the needle finally exiting the repair site opposite and palmar to the initial entry site.
- Place tension on the double-stranded suture to allow apposition of the tendon.
- Tie a four-throw surgeon's knot at the repair site (see Fig. 3.5).
- Use a 6-0 nylon epitendinous running suture to invaginate the free ends of the tendon (see Fig. 3.13).

DOUBLE RIGHT-ANGLED SUTURE

To suture the severed ends of a tendon together without shortening, a double right-angled stitch can be used. This suture technique is useful proximal to the palm. Although the apposition of the tendon ends is not as neat as after the other end-to-end suture techniques described, the method is easier and is used more often when several tendons have been severed in the distal forearm and proximal palm (Fig. 3.18).

FISH-MOUTH END-TO-END SUTURE (PULVERTAFT)

A tendon of small diameter can be sutured to one of large diameter by the method shown in Figure 3.19. This method commonly is used to suture tendons of unequal size.

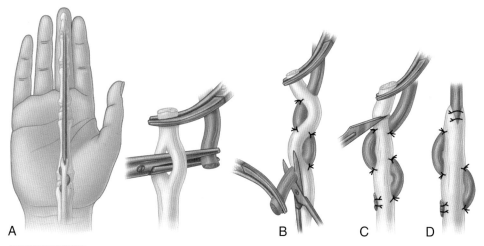

FIGURE 3.19 Pulvertaft technique of suturing tendon of small diameter to one of larger diameter. **A,** Smaller tendon is brought through larger tendon and anchored with one or two sutures after tension is adjusted. **B,** Tendon is brought through more proximal hole and is anchored again with one or two sutures after tension is adjusted. **C,** After excess is cut flush with larger tendon, exit hole can be closed with one or two sutures. **D,** Excess of larger tendon is trimmed as shown to permit central location of smaller tendon. This so-called fish mouth is closed with sutures.

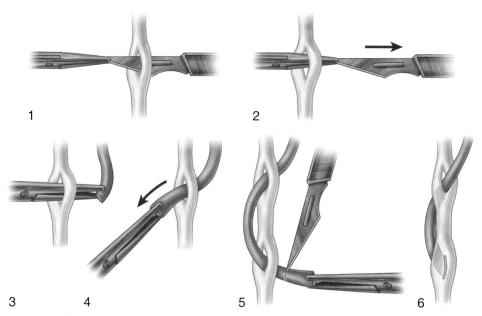

FIGURE 3.20 Steps in technique of end-to-side anastomosis. End of tendon has been buried (6). Sutures are appropriately placed to fasten tendons together. **SEE TECHNIQUE 3.7.**

END-TO-SIDE REPAIR

End-to-side repair frequently is used in tendon transfers when one motor must activate several tendons.

TECHNIQUE 3.7

- Pierce the recipient tendon through the center with a No. 11 Bard-Parker knife blade and grasp the blade on the opposite side with a straight hemostat (Fig. 3.20).
- Withdraw the blade, carrying the hemostat with it; with the latter, gently grasp the end of the tendon to be transferred and bring it through the slit.
- Repeat this technique with any adjacent tendons, placing the slits so that the transferred tendon approaches the recipient tendon at an acute angle to its line of pull.
- Suture the tendon at each passage with a vertical mattress stitch.
- Bury the end of the transferred tendon in the last tendon pierced.

ROLL STITCH

The roll stitch is especially useful for suturing extensor tendons over or near the metacarpophalangeal joints.

TECHNIQUE 3.8

- Use a 4-0 monofilament wire or 4-0 monofilament nylon threaded on a small, curved needle (Fig. 3.21).
- Pass the suture through the skin just medial or lateral to the divided tendon and through the proximal segment of the tendon near its margin from superficial to deep and then through the deep surface of the distal segment, to emerge on its superficial surface.
- Pass it proximally and through the opposite margin of the proximal segment and bring it out through the skin on the opposite side of the tendon from which it was introduced.

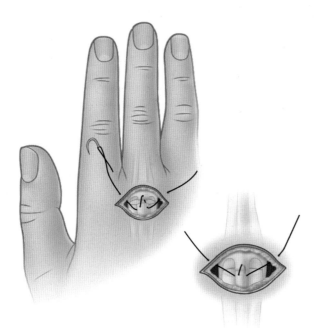

FIGURE 3.21   Roll stitch using 4-0 wire or 4-0 monofilament nylon is especially useful in suturing lacerated extensor tendon over or near head of metacarpal. **SEE TECHNIQUE 3.8.**

- Ensure that the suture slides easily in the skin and tendon. At about 4 weeks, the suture can be removed by pulling on one of its ends.

TENDON-TO-BONE ATTACHMENT

The attachment of tendon to bone (usually distal phalanx) for repair or grafting frequently requires a pull-out technique. Several methods have been described (Figs. 3.22 and 3.23). Tendon-to-tendon repair of grafts may be preferable in children to avoid physeal injury (Fig. 3.24). For tendon-to-bone repairs, the core suture techniques used most often have included the Kessler and a modification of the Bunnell crisscross suture (Fig. 3.25) in which the pull-out wire is looped over a straight needle that is passed transversely through the tendon approximately 10 mm from the cut end. This leaves the pull-out wire attached to a loop of the suture proximally in the tendon to be passed into the bone distally (Fig. 3.26).

PULL-OUT TECHNIQUE FOR TENDON ATTACHMENT

TECHNIQUE 3.9

- The modified Bunnell crisscross suture is accomplished with at least one crossing of the sutures within the tendon.

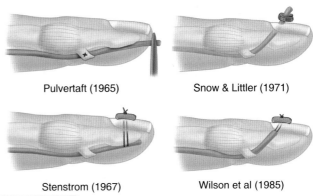

Pulvertaft (1965)   Snow & Littler (1971)

Stenstrom (1967)   Wilson et al (1985)

FIGURE 3.22   Tendon attachment through finger flap.

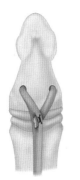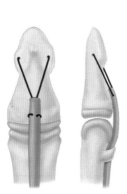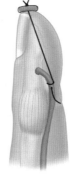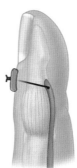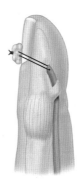

Koch (1944) & Pulvertaft (1965)   Sood & Elliot (1999)   Bunnell (1940)   Eyre–Brook (1954)   Tubiana (1969)

FIGURE 3.23   Tendon-to-bone attachment.

- Bring the needle out through the cut end of the tendon and pass it through the tunnel in the bone and out the opposite side of the bone and the skin.
- Pass the needle through felt and a button and tie it over the button.
- Pass the pull-out wire retrograde out through the skin with a needle.
- At 3 to 4 weeks, to remove the wire, cut the button from the wire suture and pull the pull-out wire retrograde

(proximally) to remove it. The crisscross intratendinous suture may bind and is sometimes difficult to remove; another disadvantage is the retrograde traction on the tendon, which has been attached to bone. This can increase the risk of separation of the tendon from the bone.

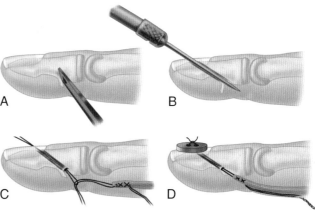

FIGURE 3.26   One method of attaching tendon to bone. **A,** Small area of cortex is raised with osteotome. **B,** Hole is drilled through bone with Kirschner wire in drill. **C,** Bunnell crisscross stitch is placed in end of tendon, and wire suture is drawn through hole in bone. **D,** End of tendon is drawn against bone.

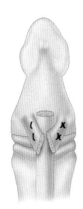

FIGURE 3.24   Tendon-to-tendon suture.

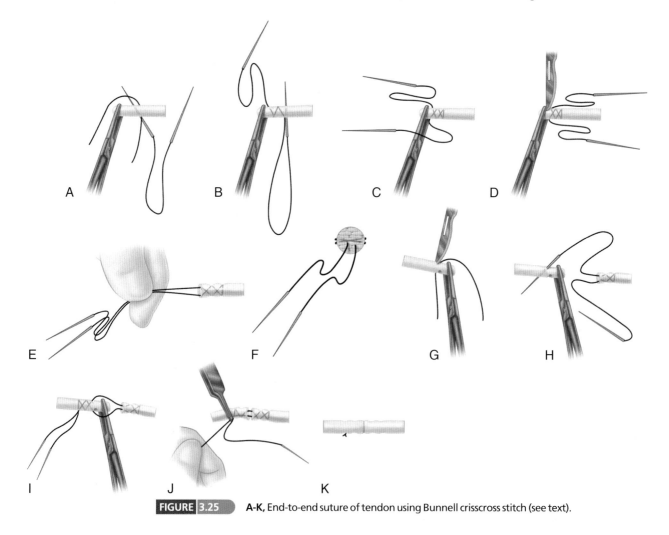

FIGURE 3.25   **A-K,** End-to-end suture of tendon using Bunnell crisscross stitch (see text).

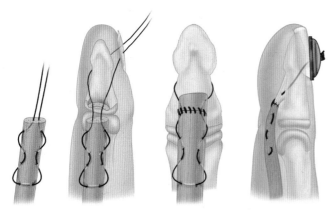

FIGURE 3.27   Zone I injury. Profundus tendon is advanced and reinserted into distal phalanx using pull-out wire suture and tie-over button. **SEE TECHNIQUE 3.9.**

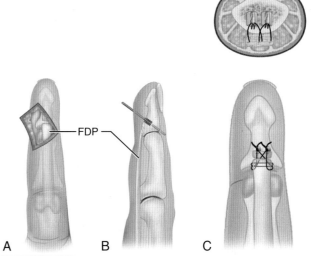

FIGURE 3.28   Suture anchor tendon attachment. Volar **(A)** and lateral **(B)** views showing avulsed flexor digitorum profundus tendon and surgical exposure. **C,** Volar and cross-sectional views showing suture anchor placement in the distal phalanx and suture technique. *FDP,* Flexor digitorum profundus.

- Using another technique, place the suture in a single loop within the tendon by passing the needle from the cut surface into the tendon and out of the tendon, across the surface of the tendon, and back through the tendon to the cut surface (Fig. 3.27).
- Pass the loop of suture into the tunnel in the bone and secure it over a piece of felt and a button in the fashion previously described. At the time of suture removal, cut one side of the suture and remove in an antegrade fashion, minimizing the risk of disrupting the bony attachment. As an alternative to passing the tendon through bone, the suture can be brought around small bones, such as the distal phalanx.
- To attach a tendon to bone, use a small osteotome or dental chisel to roughen the site of insertion or to raise a small area of cortex to accept the tendon (see Fig. 3.26). If several tendon ends are to be fixed to bone, they are best inserted into a large hole drilled in the bone.
- After an area of cortex has been elevated or a large hole made, perforate the bone with a small Kirschner wire in a power drill.
- Using the first needle as described for the end-to-end suture, run the suture diagonally two or three times through the end of the tendon.
- Loop a pull-out wire over the second needle and complete the crisscross diagonal suture.
- Using the needles, pass the two ends of the suture through the bone and snug the tendon against it. If the bone is large enough, and if space is available, suture anchors may be used to attach the distal end of the tendon to bone.
- To avoid injuring the nail bed, which may occur if a pull-out suture is passed through drill holes in the nail bed, pass the suture closely along the palmar surface of the distal phalanx and out the distal end of the digit, just palmar to the tip of the fingernail, and then through the felt and button, as for the usual pull-out technique. Injury to the nail bed also may be avoided if the suture passage is made distal to the lunula of the nail bed.

SUTURE ANCHOR TENDON ATTACHMENT

The use of a suture anchor has been shown to be as effective as a pull-out wire or suture but without the potential complications with the fingernail that can occur with the pull-out technique. Two suture anchors are placed in the distal phalanx from distal-volar to proximal-dorsal so that they gain purchase in the thickest portion of the distal phalanx to provide the greatest pull-out strength (Fig. 3.28).

TIMING OF FLEXOR TENDON REPAIR

If a wound is caused by a sharp object such as a knife and is reasonably clean, some tendons of the hand can be repaired at the time of primary wound closure. Usually, a primary tendon repair is done within the first 12 hours of injury. This can be extended to within 24 hours of injury in rare situations. A so-called *delayed primary repair* is one that is done within 24 hours to approximately 10 days. After 10 to 14 days, the repair is considered to be secondary; and after about 4 weeks, the secondary repair is a "late" secondary repair.

Primary repair can be performed in patients who have a clean wound with either a tendon injury or a tendon injury combined with a neurovascular bundle injury or a fracture if it can be fixed and stabilized satisfactorily. If this is impossible, a secondary repair should be considered. A secondary repair is indicated if the tendon injury is associated with complicating factors that could compromise the end result. These factors include extensive crushing with bony comminution near the level of tendon injury, severe neurovascular injury, severe joint injury, and skin loss requiring a coverage procedure, such as skin grafting or flap coverage.

PARTIAL FLEXOR TENDON LACERATIONS

After partial tendon lacerations, complications reported by many authors include rupture, triggering, and tendon entrapment. Experimental work suggests that a partially lacerated tendon retains varying amounts of its strength. A tendon with a 60% laceration can retain 50% or more of its strength and a tendon with a 90% laceration can retain only slightly more than 25% of its strength. Studies in human cadaver tendons found that the loads required to rupture 50% and 75% tendon lacerations were higher than the physiologic loads measured during normal active motion. In canine flexor tendons with lacerations of 30% and 70% of the cross-sectional area, with and without repair, no significant differences were seen in the structural properties of the repaired versus the unrepaired tendons, suggesting that partial lacerations of 70% of the cross-sectional area could be treated without repair. Excellent results were reported in 14 of 15 patients treated conservatively with "greater than half the width" partial lacerations of flexor tendons in zone II. Considering these findings, a reasonable clinical approach to managing the major problems related to partial tendon lacerations would be as follows.

If a tendon is lacerated 60% or more it is treated the same as a complete transection. A core suture is placed in the tendon, and the surface of the tendon is sutured with a continuous 6-0 nylon suture. The flexor sheath is repaired when possible. Postoperative management of a 60% or greater tendon laceration is the same as for a complete transection, with immobilization, early controlled passive motion, and restoration of forceful activities at 10 to 12 weeks.

If the laceration is less than 60%, the injury is evaluated for the risk of triggering. If triggering is seen, the flap of tendon is smoothly debrided and the flexor sheath is repaired to help avoid entrapment or triggering of the flap in the defect in the flexor sheath. Postoperatively, the part is protected with dorsal block splinting for 6 to 8 weeks and more forceful activities are resumed gradually after approximately 8 weeks.

PRIMARY FLEXOR TENDON REPAIR

Certain anatomic differences in the flexor surface of the hand influence the method and outcome of tendon repair. These differences allow the division of the flexor surface into five zones (Fig. 3.29). Zone I extends from just distal to the insertion of the sublimis tendon to the site of insertion of the profundus tendon. Zone II is in the critical area of pulleys (Bunnell's "no man's land") between the distal palmar crease and the insertion of the sublimis tendon. Zone III comprises the area of the lumbrical origin between the distal margin of the transverse carpal ligament and the beginning of the critical area of pulleys or first anulus. Zone IV is the zone covered by the transverse carpal ligament. Zone V is the zone proximal to the transverse carpal ligament and includes the forearm.

As a rule, all flexor tendons should be repaired at whatever level they are severed. Because of the vincular system of the profundus tendon, when both have been severed, some surgeons believe the results are better when both are repaired than when the profundus tendon alone is repaired. If possible, especially with sharp injuries, it is better to stabilize fractures and suture digital nerves and tendons initially than to delay and perform a secondary procedure for tendon repair. If performed later, it may be necessary to do a tendon graft. Repairing the flexor sheath over the tendon repair is controversial. If the area of tendon repair appears to catch on the sheath, and if the sheath can be repaired easily, repair is appropriate. If the sheath cannot be repaired, a circumferential epitendinous suture with a "funnel" opening of the sheath along one side is helpful. Historically, it has been taught that at least the A2 and A4 annular pulley areas of the flexor

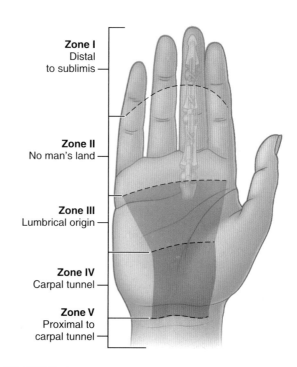

FIGURE 3.29 Flexor zones of hand. Designated zones on flexor surface of hand are helpful because treatment of tendon injuries may vary according to level of severance.

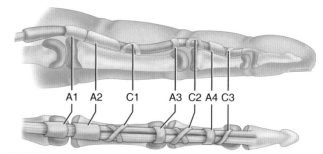

FIGURE 3.30 This anatomic diagram of various parts of flexor sheath is helpful in understanding gliding of tendon. Maintenance of second anulus (A2) and fourth anulus (A4) is essential to retain appropriate angle of approach and prevent "bowstringing" of flexor tendons or tendon graft.

sheath be preserved to prevent tendon bowstringing and flexion deformity of the finger (Figs. 3.30 and 3.31); however, several authors have shown it not to be clinically relevant.

◼ ZONE I

The flexor digitorum profundus tendon can be repaired primarily by direct suture to its distal stump or by advancement and direct insertion into the distal phalanx when the distance is 1 cm or less. Extreme care should be exercised when advancing a flexor profundus tendon. The 1-cm rule regarding advancement includes the amount of tendon that is excised, the "kinking" or bunching up that may occur, and the length of tendon inserted into bone. Excessive trimming and advancement of the tendon can result in a finger that is held in a flexed position compared with other fingers (the finger "cascade"). Although the finger may function reasonably well, uneven tension can be applied to the common muscle belly of the flexor profundus tendons and can lead to limited flexion of the remaining

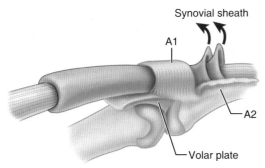

FIGURE 3.31 Diagram of relationship of synovial layers (there are two) and anulus.

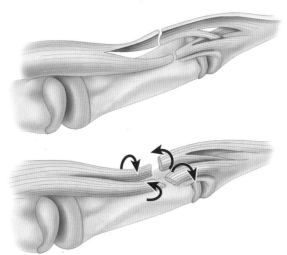

FIGURE 3.32 Flexor digitorum sublimis spiral. Flexor digitorum sublimis separates just distal to level of metacarpophalangeal joint with finger in extension. It winds around profundus tendon to chiasma of Camper, where it decussates to insert in middle phalanx. Superficial portion of proximal sublimis tendon becomes deep at level of chiasma of Camper. If laceration is sustained in sublimis at midpoint of this spiral arrangement of both slips, proximal and distal ends rotate through 90 degrees, but in different directions. An unwary surgeon would be presented with two ends that do match, that appear to lie in good relationship, and that can be so sutured. If this is done, channel for profundus tendon is obliterated. If error is not noted and corrected, effect would be to block excursion of tendon and eliminate satisfactory motion.

profundus tendons (the "quadriga effect" described by Verdan). In such a situation, lengthening of the tendon at the wrist should be considered or, if excessive shortening has occurred, tendon grafting may be considered.

A pull-out wire technique can be used to attach the proximal tendon end to its distal stump (see Fig. 3.27) or directly to the bone after advancement (see Fig. 3.26). When the diagnosis of interruption of this tendon is delayed, and the tendon has retracted into the palm, its vinculum has been disrupted and a decision must be made regarding repair. Three types of flexor tendon ruptures have been described, depending on the level to which the tendon has retracted. In type 1, the tendon is found retracted into the palm. If it is within 7 to 10 days of the injury, the tendon should be threaded back into the finger and reattached with a pull-out wire into the distal phalanx. In type 2 ruptures, the tendon has retracted to the level of the proximal interphalangeal joint. At times, despite the passage of a few months, these tendons can be reattached as well. In type 3, the tendon has retracted only to the level of the distal interphalangeal joint and usually has a bony fragment attached to it. These also usually can be treated by reattachment. Although satisfactory function can be achieved, limitation of distal interphalangeal joint motion is to be expected, regardless of the level of rupture.

Old, untreated injuries to the flexor profundus in zone I can be treated by tendon grafting, tenodesis, or arthrodesis of the distal joint, depending on the finger involved and the age and needs of the patient. Flexor tendon grafting in such situations in the presence of an intact and functioning sublimis tendon has been recommended for the index and long fingers in specific situations.

All authors recommend careful patient selection: highly motivated patients between 10 and 21 years old may be considered candidates for grafting. The flexor profundus of the ring finger can be grafted after tendon injuries in zone I for specific needs (e.g., skilled technicians, musicians). Because of the risk of damaging the intact flexor sublimis and the additional potential complications of flexor tendon grafting, patients who are older, who have joint stiffness, who are noncompliant, or who do not understand the difficulty in achieving a successful result should not be considered for flexor tendon grafting. Some authors pass the tendon graft around the sublimis tendon. Two-stage tendon grafting also has been advocated.

◼ ZONE II

Primary repair of flexor tendons in the fibroosseous sheath (Bunnell's "no man's land"), which was controversial until the

major contributions of Verdan and of Kleinert, is now widely accepted. If repair is done under satisfactory conditions by an experienced surgeon, satisfactory function can be expected in 80% or more of patients. Generally, the results of flexor tendon repair are better in younger patients than in patients older than 40 years of age. The results of primary flexor tendon repair also are better than secondary repair or staged reconstruction with a graft. Here especially, the primary surgeon has the greatest influence on the final result. To make the decision and perform a primary repair, a surgeon should be sufficiently skilled to perform a tendon graft or tenolysis later if the primary repair fails.

Primary repairs at this level frequently fail because of adhesions in the area of the pulleys. Exacting wound care is crucial. If the timing of tendon repair is in doubt, the wound should be cleaned and the repair made later by an experienced surgeon.

Technical concerns during the repair procedure include the management of lacerations of the profundus and sublimis tendons, the appropriate orientation of the profundus with the sublimis slips, the attachment of the sublimis slips in the thin flat area, the management of the flexor sheath, including the annular thickening (pulleys), the postoperative management, and the timing and technique for tenolysis. Most surgeons recommend repair of the flexor profundus and sublimis tendons in zone II. Care should be taken when the flexor sublimis has been injured in the area just proximal to the proximal interphalangeal joint and distally where the orientation of the proximal and distal portions of the tendon can be misinterpreted and repairs may be incorrectly done with the sublimis slips malrotated (Fig. 3.32). A report in the

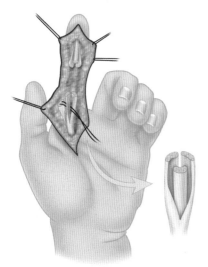

FIGURE 3.33 Separated position of two tendon ends in distal palm after flexor tendon interruption and proximal retraction. Profundus must be correctly positioned in sublimis hiatus before passing tendons distally into digit. Anatomic relationship of profundus and sublimis tendon stumps must be reestablished so that they can be correctly repaired to corresponding distal tendon stumps. In some cases, profundus must be passed back through hiatus created by sublimis slips to lie palmar to Camper chiasma and to recreate position of tendons at level of tendon laceration.

literature noted that a portion of the A2 pulley can be incised to improve tendon gliding, and all of A2 can be incised if the remainder of the sheath and pulleys is intact. Care also should be taken to deliver the flexor profundus tendon through the split portion of the flexor sublimis when the profundus tendon has retracted proximally (Fig. 3.33).

As indicated previously, many suture configurations have been advocated. In zone II, a core suture with four or more strands, locking components, and buried knots is usually preferred. The educational and clinical experience of the surgeon and the particular demands of each case may allow the use of other appropriate techniques. Traditionally, it has been recommended that the intratendinous configuration of the core sutures should remain in the volar third of the tendon to avoid impairment of the intratendinous circulation. Placing sutures in the dorsal half of the tendon was found to provide a mean strength to the repair that was 58% greater than for sutures placed in the volar half of the tendon. A running, circumferential 5-0 or 6-0 nylon is used by most surgeons to complete a smooth repair and to minimize adhesion formation to the sheath and "triggering" on the sheath. A peripheral suture increases the strength of the repair, and a four-strand core suture combined with a peripheral suture allows a postoperative routine of light active flexion with the wrist extended, leading to better function and fewer complications. The choice of suture material depends on the experience and preference of the individual surgeon; however, most authors prefer a synthetic braided suture, usually of polyester material (Mersilene, Ticron, Tevdek, FiberWire), whereas others have had success with monofilament nylon and wire suture. Usually 3-0 or 4-0 sutures are required. Generally, a pull-out suture technique is unnecessary in zone II. The postoperative management is paramount, as discussed subsequently (see "Primary Suture of Flexor Tendons").

Tenolysis may be required in an estimated 18% to 25% of patients after flexor tendon repair. Usually, tenolysis is considered when the patient has reached a plateau in postoperative rehabilitation and when all wounds are supple and flexible and the skin is soft with minimal or no induration around the scars. Fracture and joint injuries should be healed, and there should be no or minimal residual joint contractures. A near-normal passive range of motion is preferred. Normal sensation is preferred; however, if digital nerves have been repaired, progress toward return of sensation should be observed. For these criteria to be met usually requires 5 to 6 months after the tendon repair. Three months is considered to be the earliest time for flexor tenolysis, assuming no improvement in motion in the previous 1 to 2 months. Flexor tenolysis is a technically demanding procedure and should be undertaken by someone who has training and experience in this type of surgery. Function in the finger can be improved by 50% by tenolysis (see also "Flexor Tendon Injuries in Children").

■ ZONE III

At zone III, the muscle bellies of the lumbricals and the tendons frequently are interrupted. Additional incisions often are needed to expose this area further. All tendons can be repaired primarily if wound conditions are satisfactory or if repair is delayed only a few days. If conditions permit, primary repair of sharply severed nerves is crucial because delaying the repair even a few weeks results in significant gaps between the nerve ends. If wound conditions preclude tendon and nerve repair, the ends of the tendons and nerves are sutured to adjacent fascia to prevent undue retraction. Lumbrical muscle bellies usually are not sutured because this can increase the tension of these muscles and result in a "lumbrical plus" finger (paradoxic proximal interphalangeal extension on attempted active finger flexion).

■ ZONE IV

All tendons and nerves in zone IV can be repaired primarily when wound conditions are satisfactory; however, for exposure it may be necessary to release partially or completely the transverse carpal ligament. Should complete release be necessary, the wrist should not be placed in flexion past neutral position, but the fingers should be brought into slightly more flexion than usual to permit relaxation of the musculotendinous units. Flexion of the wrist beyond neutral may permit subluxation of the repaired tendons out of their normal bed and then bowstringing them just under the sutured skin. When it is technically possible to accomplish tendon repair and retain part of the transverse carpal ligament, this problem is eliminated. Alternatively, the transverse carpal ligament can be released in a Z-lengthening configuration, allowing its repair after tendon repair and providing a pulley for the tendons. The flexor digitorum profundus tendons at this level may not be distinctly separated, and frequent interdigitations may be present.

■ ZONE V

Because zone V is proximal to the transverse carpal ligament, tendon gliding after repair usually is better here than in more distal zones. All tendons and nerves lacerated in this area should be repaired primarily when wound conditions are satisfactory, as advised earlier. The chief difficulty of repair here usually is one of exposure, which requires a proximal extension and possibly a distal extension of the typical transverse laceration. Blood clots within the tenosynovium usually serve as clues to locating severed tendons. At this level, the profundus tendons are not completely separated into individual tendon units. The sublimis tendons usually are distinctly separated, their muscle bellies extend more distally, and the severed ends usually are more easily matched. If the necessary expertise is unavailable, primary repair can be delayed and the wound cleaned. Results are not likely to be compromised by a brief delay of several days. At this level, excision of some of the tenosynovial covering is necessary to identify and remove the hematoma; however, a total synovectomy usually is not indicated. An isolated laceration of the palmaris longus tendon does not absolutely require repair.

■ DELAYED REPAIR OF ACUTE INJURIES

Delayed repair in any zone may be necessary in the presence of severe wound contamination, crushing or avulsing injuries, soft-tissue loss, multiple comminuted fractures, or lack of available surgical skill. Delayed repairs of tendons are reasonable also if other injuries require immediate surgery. In such circumstances, a patient's condition might not permit definitive management of tendons and nerves, and it is appropriate to clean the limb as well as possible and loosely close the wound or leave it open but covered with a sterile bandage and splint. Plans should be made for definitive management of the wound and injured structures. Undue complications usually are not encountered if the repair of tendons is delayed for 2 to 3 days as long as the wound has been thoroughly cleaned. Prolonged delay may permit unacceptable retraction of tendons and nerves, especially in zones III, IV, and V. If it seems that definitive management of the tendons and nerves may be delayed, an attempt should be made to secure the ends of the tendons and nerves to the adjacent soft tissues to prevent retraction before achieving satisfactory wound closure.

■ PRIMARY SUTURE OF FLEXOR TENDONS

The preparations and techniques for primary and delayed primary suture of flexor tendons vary from zone to zone. The techniques are discussed according to the requirements of each zone. Generally, further exposure of the tendon to be sutured may be necessary. Additional incisions (Fig. 3.34) should be made without crossing flexion creases at a right angle. Usually, less exposure is needed distally than proximally because the distal segment of the tendon may be delivered into the wound by flexing the distal joints. Also, the distal segment is not subject to retraction by muscle, as are the proximal segments. Regardless of the zone in which the tendon is injured, careful attention should be given to the anatomic location of the respective tendons and their relationships to each other and other structures. Meticulous, gentle, and atraumatic technique should be used in the handling of the tendons. Each tendon is delivered by grasping it with a small-tipped forceps with teeth. Crushing of the cut surface of the tendon with instruments such as Allis forceps, Kocher clamps, and hemostats should be avoided. Although the tip of the tendon can be held with a small hemostat, the crushed portion should be excised before the suture is tied. Sometimes this can shorten the tendon needlessly. Suturing techniques should be exact so that the tendon ends are held together accurately and distraction, gap formation, and exposure of raw surfaces at the junction are avoided.

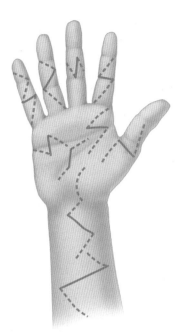

FIGURE **3.34**   Exposures for primary suture of tendons. *Solid lines* indicate examples of skin lacerations, and *broken lines* show direction in which they can be enlarged to obtain additional exposure (see text).

REPAIR IN ZONES I AND II

TECHNIQUE 3.10

ZONE I

- When the flexor profundus tendon has been injured in zone I at or near its insertion, approach the distal end of the finger by extending the laceration with an oblique incision into the central portion of the pulp or through a midradial or midulnar incision.
- Avoid injury to the terminal branches of the digital nerve, and avoid devascularizing any skin flaps that are elevated. Usually the insertion of the flexor profundus is easily seen. At times, the proximal stump of the tendon will have retracted very minimally.
- Extend the incision proximally, using a volar zigzag (Bruner), midradial, midulnar, or midline oblique incision (Fig. 3.35A). Avoid injury to the neurovascular bundles.
- Elevate the skin flap by going either dorsal or volar to the neurovascular bundle.
- Expose the fibroosseous flexor sheath (Fig. 3.35B). If the proximal end of the tendon can be seen, attempt to deliver it into the wound by grasping it with a small forceps, such as an Adson or a finer tissue forceps. If the tendon has retracted more proximally, extend the incision as needed, in a midradial or a midulnar incision or by extending the skin incision in a volar zigzag or midline oblique incision, avoiding injury to the neurovascular bundle.
- Open the thin cruciform portion of the sheath to assist in delivering the tendon. Open the sheath by an L-shaped incision or with a trapdoor with a Z-plasty arrangement to allow easier closure if needed.

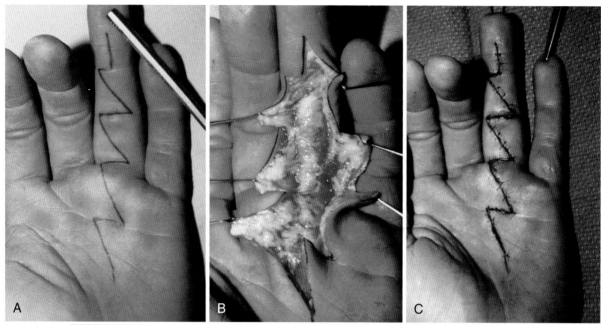

FIGURE 3.35 **A,** Incision outlined on digit and palm. **B,** Exposure of flexor tendon sheath after flap elevation. **C,** Closed incision. **SEE TECHNIQUE 3.10.**

- If the tendon has retracted, place a grasping suture in its end, using one of the techniques previously described. When opening the flexor sheath over the middle phalanx, it is important to preserve the A4 pulley. If the flexor tendon cannot be maintained in such a way that it can be repaired easily, insert a small-gauge (25-gauge or 26-gauge) hypodermic needle, Keith needle, or Bunnell needle through the skin, through the tendon, and out the skin on the opposite side of the finger as a temporary tendon retention device. These needles are removed when the tendon repair has been accomplished.
- Although a pull-out wire of the Bunnell type can be attached in such an arrangement, it is not always necessary, especially if the antegrade pull-out wire technique is used as opposed to the Bunnell retrograde pull-out technique (see Figs. 3.26 and 3.27).
- Using straight needles, pass the suture out through the distal pulp of the finger, usually exiting just palmar to the hyponychium.
- As an alternative, the proximal end of the tendon can be attached distally, using a pull-out technique in which a tunnel is drilled in bone and the needles are passed through the tunnel and out through the fingernail or around the distal phalanx. Regardless of the suture material selected, 4-0 suture is usually used.
- After ascertaining satisfactory rotation and attachment of the tendon, close the wound with fine 4-0 or 5-0 monofilament nylon sutures (Fig. 3.35C).

ZONE II

- In zone II, the wound usually must be extended with proximal and distal incisions (Fig. 3.36). Regardless of which approach is used, carefully reflect the skin flaps and avoid injury to neurovascular structures during the dissection.

- If digital nerves have been transected, gently dissect them and delay their repair until after the tendons are repaired to avoid disruption.
- Expose the flexor sheath in the area of injury and sufficiently proximal and distal to allow location of the tendon ends. As indicated previously, the distal tendon end usually can be identified easily with passive flexion of the distal interphalangeal joint. Avoid injury to the sheath, particularly the A2 and A4 pulleys.
- If opening of the flexor sheath is required, this is best done in the filamentous cruciate areas of the sheath. Small openings in the sheath can be made in the distal tendon insertion, C2 and C3, and C1 areas where the sheath is filamentous (see Fig. 3.30). These openings can be made in several configurations. An L-shaped opening allows ease of closure and facilitates passage of the tendon through the sheath (Lister). If several days have passed, and the tendon sheaths are contracting, opening the sheath with a Z-lengthening configuration helps to allow partial closure of the sheath in difficult situations.
- Deliver the flexor tendon into the finger by milking the forearm, hand, and wrist and flexing the wrist and fingers to allow the proximal end to be delivered if possible. If it cannot be delivered easily, a transverse incision at the distal palmar crease may be necessary to locate the tendon in the palm.
- When the proximal end of the tendon has been identified, place a core suture using the definitive suture material in a locking fashion so that the suture material can be used for traction in passing the suture through the sheath.
- In a fresh, acute injury, passage of the tendon usually is not difficult. After several days, tendon edema and sheath contracture may require additional techniques. The proximal end of the tendon can be passed easily through the sheath and between the slips of the sublimis using a piece

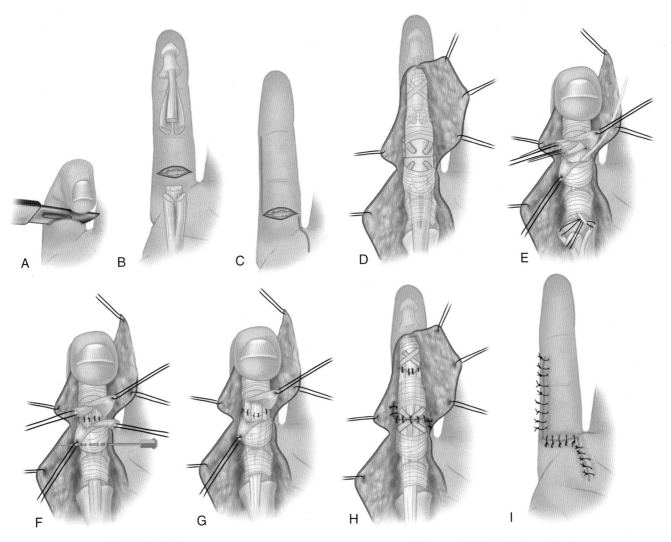

FIGURE 3.36 Strickland technique of flexor tendon repair in zone II. **A,** Knife laceration through zone II with digit in full flexion. **B,** Level of flexor tendon retraction of same finger after digital extension. **C,** *Green lines* depict radial and ulnar incisions to allow wide exposure of flexor tendon system. **D,** Flexor tendon system of involved finger after reflection of skin flaps. In this case, laceration has occurred through C1 cruciate pulley area. Note proximal and distal position of severed flexor tendon stumps resulting from flexed attitude of finger at time of injury. *Green lines* indicate lateral incisions in cruciate-synovial portions of sheath, which are used to provide exposure for tendon repair. **E,** Reflection of small triangular flaps at cruciate-synovial sheath allows distal flexor tendon stumps to be delivered into wound by passive flexion of distal interphalangeal joint. Profundus and sublimis stumps are retrieved proximal to A1 pulley, using small catheter or infant feeding gastrostomy tube. **F,** Proximal flexor tendon stumps are maintained at repair site by means of transversely placed small-gauge hypodermic needle, followed by repair of flexor digitorum sublimis slips. **G,** Completed repair of both tendons with distal interphalangeal joint in full flexion. **H,** Extension of distal interphalangeal joint delivers repair under intact distal flexor tendon sheath. Repair of cruciate (C1)-synovial pulley has been completed. **I,** Wound repair at conclusion of procedure.

of pediatric feeding tubing or plastic intravenous connecting tubing, as recommended by Lister.
■ Deliver the tubing into the flexor sheath between the slips of the sublimis.
■ Pass the suture into the tubing. Clamp the tubing with the suture within it and "lead" the flexor tendon through the sheath following the plastic tubing and suture.

■ As an alternative method, fashion a 20- or 22-gauge wire into a loop, and pass it proximally in the sheath to use as a snare for the suture, which is delivered through the sheath followed by the tendon. The tendon also can be sutured to tubing of various types and delivered following the tubing through the sheath as well.

- When the proximal end of the tendon has been delivered to the area of repair, secure it in the sheath using a transverse 25- or 26-gauge hypodermic needle for temporary fixation with little or no long-term harmful effects. This is used as a temporary stabilizing device.
- Stabilize the distal end of the tendon in a similar way.
- Introduce the core suture, using a four-strand to eight-strand method. Care should be taken at this point to ensure that the profundus tendon is not malrotated. Reference to the vincular attachment and the relationship to the sublimis is helpful in this regard.
- Tie the knots and complete the tendon repair with circumferential 5-0 or 6-0 nylon inverting suture or cross-stitch (see Fig. 3.14) to minimize exposure of the cut surface of the tendon.
- If the flexor sublimis has been transected just proximal to the proximal interphalangeal joint, take care regarding the arrangement of its slips of the sublimis and the so-called flexor digitorum sublimis "spiral" (see Fig. 3.32). The flexor digitorum sublimis winds around the profundus tendon after it divides at the metacarpophalangeal joint. It inserts into the volar surface of the middle phalanx after decussating. This allows the superficial portion of the sublimis tendon to become deep in the chiasma of Camper. A laceration in this area allows the proximal and distal ends of the sublimis tendons to rotate 90 degrees in opposite directions. The tendon lies in *apparently* satisfactory alignment; however, if it is sutured in this alignment, it causes binding of the flexor profundus tendon.
- An additional technical problem can be encountered if the flexor sublimis tendon has been transected more distally, near the proximal interphalangeal joint or its insertion. Here the tendon is quite thin, and it is difficult to achieve satisfactory placement of core sutures. Try to place a locked core suture in the tendon because a simple repair with 5-0 or 6-0 nylon would be insufficient to prevent rupture. Use small suture anchors to repair the sublimis if the bone and working space permit secure insertion.
- Sometimes it can be extremely difficult technically to accomplish a flexor sublimis repair. Although most surgeons recommend against sublimis excision, if in the surgeon's judgment sublimis repair cannot be satisfactorily accomplished, or such repair would compromise profundus function, excise the sublimis tendon in the area.
- Usually the sublimis tendon is repaired before the profundus tendon. Tie the knots; use the circumferential 6-0 nylon sutures as needed; and repair the sheath, conditions permitting, with 5-0 or 6-0 nylon.
- Close the wound with interrupted 5-0 nylon and remove the temporary retaining needle.
- Avoid hyperextension of the finger and immobilize the hand in a padded compression dressing with the fingers and the thumb immobilized with a dorsal splint.
- Splint the wrist in 45 to 50 degrees of flexion; splint the fingers in flexion at the metacarpophalangeal joints to 50 to 60 degrees, with the proximal and distal interphalangeal joints extended.
- If one or more pulleys are damaged and cannot be repaired, they should be reconstructed at the time of primary tendon repair to avoid bowstringing and restriction of motion.

- The flexor sheath/pulley reconstruction can be protected with orthotic thermoplastic rings during postoperative rehabilitation of the flexor tendon and while the patient is regaining motion (see discussion of staged tendon reconstruction later).

REPAIR IN ZONES III, IV, AND V

TECHNIQUE 3.11

ZONE III

- In zone III, the area between the distal edge of the transverse carpal ligament and the proximal portion of the A1 pulley, perform flexor tendon repair in a manner similar to zone II repair. Incisions that extend the wound proximally and distally may be required. Avoid crossing flexion creases at right angles. Also avoid injuring neurovascular structures and devascularizing the skin flaps.
- Achieve proper orientation of the tendon before repair. At times, if tendons have retracted into the carpal tunnel or more proximally, partial release of the transverse carpal ligament may be required to deliver them distally into the palm.
- Although the flexor sheath is not involved in the palm, use careful technique in the placement of sutures; it probably is best to use an intratendinous core suture in the palm to avoid exposure of the suture material to adjacent structures. Satisfactory healing and functional results can be expected after repair of the tendons in the palm.
- Apply a compressive, bulky dressing and immobilize the thumb, fingers, and wrist. Immobilize the wrist at about 45 degrees of flexion, with the fingers at about 50 to 60 degrees of flexion and the interphalangeal joints extended.

ZONE IV

- In zone IV, the area of the carpal tunnel, an injury directly to the base of the palm usually also involves the median nerve. If a laceration occurs just proximal to the wrist flexion crease, flexor tendon injury, especially with the fingers flexed, in zone IV should be suspected.
- Extend the laceration distally into the palm and proximally into the forearm, taking care to cross flexion creases obliquely. If the laceration occurs beneath the transverse carpal ligament, partial or complete release of the transverse carpal ligament may be required.
- Preserve, if possible, a portion of the transverse carpal ligament to avoid bowstringing postoperatively.
- If it cannot be preserved, release it in a Z-lengthening configuration so that it can be repaired and help minimize the risk of postoperative bowstringing.
- Repair the flexor profundus and sublimis tendons in the carpal tunnel; probably the best suture configuration is an intratendinous one with a locking core suture to hold the tendons with minimal exposure of cut surface and suture material.
- In the carpal tunnel, ensure proper orientation and location of the individual tendons. The usual arrangement of

the flexor sublimis tendons in the carpal tunnel, with the middle and ring finger tendons superficial to the index and small finger tendons, is helpful to recall in this situation. Partial tenosynovectomy may be required to diminish the bulky and edematous tissue that may follow the repair.

- Close the skin with 4-0 nylon and apply the bandage and dorsal splint to maintain the wrist in approximately 45 degrees of flexion.
- If the transverse carpal ligament has been completely released and repair is impossible, bring the wrist nearly to neutral and flex the fingers more acutely to diminish pressure on the volar skin and to minimize bowstringing.
- If the transverse carpal ligament is partially intact or has been repaired, immobilize the wrist in about 45 degrees of flexion, with the fingers in 50 to 60 degrees of flexion at the metacarpophalangeal joints and the interphalangeal joints in full extension.

ZONE V

- In zone V, the volar forearm proximal to the transverse carpal ligament, multiple tendons, nerves, and vessels frequently are injured by major lacerations, often from broken glass or in violent altercations with knives. In this area, it is important to identify the tendons accurately.
- Because of their common muscle origin, when the sublimis and profundus tendons are divided, particularly at the wrist, they can be delivered into the wound as a group by finding and pulling distally on one tendon.
- Properly match the tendon ends by careful attention to their location and level in the wound, their relation to neighboring structures, their diameters, the shape of their cross sections, and the angle of the cuts through each tendon. Although it is not a disgrace to open an anatomy book in the operating room to be certain of anatomic relationships, it is inexcusable to sew the median nerve to the flexor pollicis longus, the palmaris longus, or some other tendon.
- The proximal and distal ends of the median nerve usually can be identified easily in their appropriate anatomic location and from their more yellowish color and the presence of a volar midline vessel and the nerve fascicles, which usually can be identified in the median nerve's severed ends.
- Although 4-0 sutures usually are used in the palm and more distally, 3-0 nylon may be sufficient for suturing tendons in the distal forearm. Repairs done in the distal forearm do not absolutely require an intratendinous repair. A double right-angled or mattress suture may be satisfactory in the forearm.
- Repair nerves and vessels if needed after the tendon repairs in the forearm, working from the repair of deep structures to more superficial structures.
- Close the wounds with 4-0 nylon and immobilize the limb with the wrist flexed approximately 45 degrees and the metacarpophalangeal joints flexed 50 to 60 degrees with the interphalangeal joints in full extension.

POSTOPERATIVE CARE Excellent results can be achieved using either of two postoperative mobilization techniques. In one (Kleinert), active finger extension is used with passive flexion achieved using a rubber band attached to the fingernail and at the wrist (Fig. 3.37). This subsequently has been modified with a roller in the palm to alter the line of force of the rubber band. The second technique (Duran) involves a controlled passive motion technique with dorsal blocking of the fingers (Fig. 3.38). The margin of safety with early passive motion rehabilitation is increased if the tendon repairs have been done with the stronger multistrand techniques (four or more). Multistrand repairs are used if an early active motion program is considered. Children younger than approximately 10 years old and noncompliant patients cannot be entrusted with understanding and following the complexities of either of these techniques, and a more conservative postoperative management routine should be selected, depending on the judgment of the surgeon and the therapist.

Although some patients may be allowed to remove a splint in the first week after surgery, we have found it safer to leave the nonremovable postoperative dorsal splint in place. Passive flexion and extension of the proximal and distal interphalangeal joints are demonstrated in the first postoperative day. The wrist usually is positioned in 20 to 45 degrees of flexion with the metacarpophalangeal joints in 50 to 70 degrees of flexion and interphalangeal joints left in the neutral position. Before closure of the wound, the amount of passive movement of the fingertip required to create a 3- to 5-mm excursion of the tendon is determined (Fig. 3.39). This amount of movement is started the day after surgery. A removable splint can be used 3 days after surgery in some compliant patients (Fig. 3.40). The patient is instructed in an exercise program, including eight repetitions of proximal and distal interphalangeal and composite passive flexion and extension of the joints twice daily. A "place and hold" exercise can be added for compliant patients if a strong multistrand repair has been done. This is continued for at least 3 to 4 weeks, at which time a removable splint can be applied.

The controlled active motion program requires the attachment of a suture through the tip of the fingernail or a garment hook glued to the nail allowing the attachment of an elastic band (see Fig. 3.37A). A dorsal splint holds the wrist in 20 to 30 degrees of flexion and the metacarpophalangeal joints at 40 to 60 degrees. The interphalangeal joints are splinted in extension. The rubber band is passed beneath a roller or a safety pin in the palm and is secured to another safety pin at the level of the distal forearm (see Fig. 3.37B). The safety pin maintains the finger in flexion of 40 to 60 degrees at the proximal interphalangeal joint with no tension on the rubber band. The rubber band should allow full extension of the proximal interphalangeal joint against the traction of the rubber band. With this form of controlled mobilization, it is believed that the flexor tendon repair is not stretched and the movement that is allowed can enhance healing. Beginning on the first day after surgery, active extension exercises within the limitations of the splint are encouraged. If the patient does not seem able to understand and cooperate with this technique, it should be abandoned in the first week.

After 3 weeks, the dorsal splint is removed and a wrist band with a hook for the rubber band is used for an additional 3 weeks. The patient actively extends the digit against the resistance of the rubber band. No passive extension or

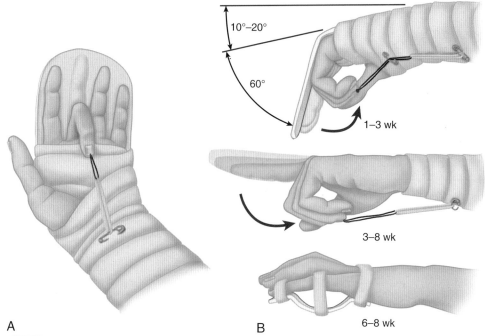

FIGURE 3.37 **A,** After primary flexor tendon repair or flexor tendon graft, wrist and hand are held in posterior plaster splint. Additionally, involved finger is held in flexion by elastic band attached at wrist level and at fingernail by wire through nail or glued-on garment hook. This permits active finger extension and protected passive flexion. **B,** Immediate controlled mobilization of repaired flexor tendon is achieved with extension block splint and proper rubber band traction, allowing proximal interphalangeal joint extension against traction and flexion of 40 to 60 degrees. At 3 to 8 weeks, rubber band is attached to elastic bandage cuff at wrist. After removal of rubber band traction, night splinting can be used at 6 to 8 weeks if necessary. **SEE TECHNIQUE 3.11.**

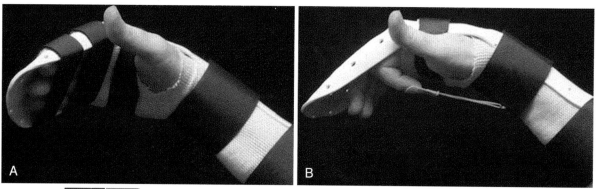

FIGURE 3.38 **A,** Splint with dynamic flexion for Kleinert protocol. Note minimal distal interphalangeal joint flexion and relatively severe proximal interphalangeal joint flexion in resting position. **B,** Dorsal protective splint for modified Duran protocol. Note that fingers are held in interphalangeal joint extension when at rest. (From Pettengill KM: The evolution of early mobilization of the repaired flexor tendon, *J Hand Ther* 18:157–168, 2005.) **SEE TECHNIQUE 3.11.**

active flexion is permitted. The wrist band splint is discontinued at 6 to 8 weeks, and dynamic extension splinting is used to prevent contractures of the proximal interphalangeal joint. At 8 to 10 weeks, strengthening exercises are permitted, and the patient progresses to using the hand normally at 10 to 12 weeks after the repair.

FLEXOR TENDON INJURIES IN CHILDREN
Management of injured flexor tendons in children younger than 10 years old is difficult and demanding. The same

principles previously outlined apply to the management of flexor tendon injuries in a young patient.

The diagnosis of tendon and associated injuries may be more difficult in children because examination is less reliable as a result of their anxiety. Because of the extremely small tolerances between the flexor sheath and flexor tendons, even more attention to the use of meticulous technique is required. Finer sutures, such as 5-0, may be required for repair of the tendons because of their small size; 6-0 and 7-0 sutures may be required for the circumferential repair of the surface of

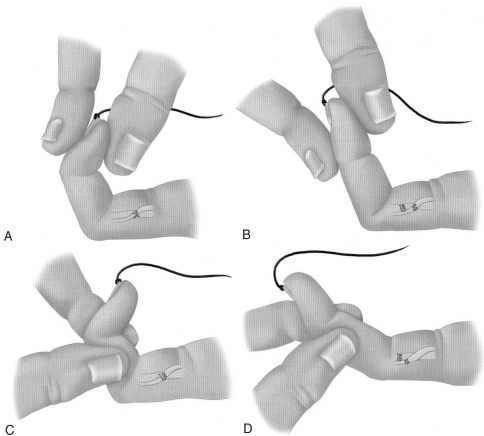

FIGURE 3.39 **A,** Diagram of controlled passive motion exercise. Metacarpophalangeal joint should remain in normal balanced position. Extension of distal interphalangeal joint is sufficient to move anastomosis 3 to 5 mm. Only distal interphalangeal joint moves during this exercise. **B,** Note distal migration of anastomosis of flexor digitorum profundus tendon away from that of flexor digitorum sublimis tendon. **C,** When middle phalanx is extended, both anastomoses glide distally. Only proximal interphalangeal joint moves during this exercise. **D,** Anastomoses are moved away from fixed structures that may have been injured. Elastic traction returns finger to original position.

the tendon. Because of the inability of very young children to cooperate with a postoperative rehabilitation program, their immobilization after surgery usually is more extensive and prolonged, frequently requiring the use of long arm casts until 28 days from repair. Several studies have found that the postoperative regimen has little effect on the outcome of tendon repair in children. Total active motion appears to correlate best with age at the time of injury, with children older than 10 years at the time of injury regaining the most motion (82%) compared with children 4 to 10 years of age (77%) and children younger than age 4 years (54%). In a report by Sikora et al., 40 of 47 patients with an average age of 8 years achieved 100% motion of their fingers after 4 weeks of immobilization postoperatively. The retraining and rehabilitation of very young children are unpredictable, leading some surgeons to delay flexor tendon surgery in infants to a later age of 3 to 4 years to allow for better technical repair and to increase the chances of postoperative cooperation. The results after flexor tenolysis tend to be better the older the child. Should tendon grafting be required in tendon reconstruction, the sources of tendon grafts also are limited.

FLEXOR TENDON RUPTURES

Although rupture of flexor tendons is not as common as that of extensor tendons, it does occur and often is not diagnosed. The most common tendon to be avulsed in athletes is the flexor digitorum profundus at its insertion in the ring finger. It can produce a small bony avulsion or articular fracture seen on a radiograph. MRI can help to define tendon rupture. Traumatic rupture usually occurs at the insertion of the tendon. Frequently, a patient's initial complaint is that of a mass in the palm without awareness of any loss of finger function. The flexor tendons most frequently ruptured are the profundus tendons and more rarely the sublimis tendons or the flexor pollicis longus. These ruptures occur most often in men in their twenties and thirties, and about 20% may be associated with synovitis. Intratendinous rupture of the flexor profundus can occur in individuals involved in activities requiring forceful flexion against resistance.

■ TREATMENT

Direct repair, tendon grafting, or tendon transfer has been recommended for the treatment of these injuries. Factors found

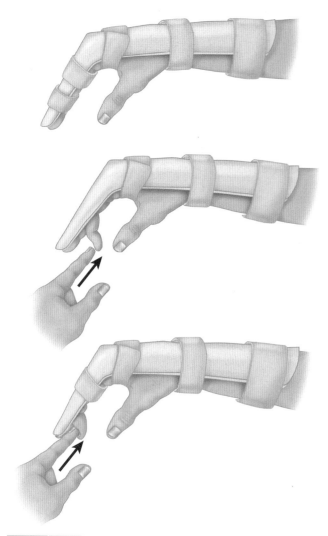

Passive flexion of interphalangeal joints, which is done several times each day for 4 to 5 weeks. Duran and Houser popularized early passive motion after tendon repair.

to influence the treatment and outcome are (1) the length of time between injury and treatment, (2) the extent to which the tendon retracts, (3) the blood supply to the avulsed tendon, and (4) the presence of bony fragments seen on a radiograph. These factors allow the classification of these injuries into three types. In type 1, the tendon retracts completely into the palm and is held there by the lumbrical origin. In type 2, the tendon retracts to the level of the proximal interphalangeal joint with a long vinculum intact, presumably maintaining blood supply. In type 3, usually a bony fragment is involved. The fragment may be comminuted or noncomminuted and may be nonarticular or intraarticular.

For type 1 injuries, reinsertion into the distal phalanx is recommended if the injury is detected within 7 to 10 days. After this period, the distal end of the tendon likely has become kinked and softened, prohibiting delivery into the finger and attachment to the distal phalanx. A midlateral or volar oblique incision usually is used. The sheath is opened through a transverse incision distal to the A2 pulley. Absence of the tendon end in this area indicates retraction into the palm. A transverse incision near the distal palmar crease exposes the flexor sheath proximal to the A1 pulley and allows location of the

tendon end, which can be delivered by a variety of techniques using sutures, the retrograde passage of pediatric feeding tubing or intravenous tubing, or wire loops to allow antegrade passage of the tendon without additional injury to the tendon sheath. The tendon is attached to the distal phalanx with a pull-out wire, preferably of the antegrade type rather than the traditional retrograde Bunnell pull-out wire (see Fig. 3.27). This is left in place for 3 to 4 weeks, during which time the limb is immobilized in a dorsal splint with the wrist in flexion, the metacarpophalangeal joint in 70 to 80 degrees of flexion, and the interphalangeal joints in extension. The pull-out wire is removed at 3 to 4 weeks. If a type 1 injury is seen late, consideration should be given to flexor tendon grafting in a young, cooperative patient for the index, long, or ring finger, or, as alternatives, tenodesis or arthrodesis should be considered, depending on the needs and activities of the patient.

Type 2 injuries with the tendon retracted to the level of the proximal interphalangeal joint can be repaired at a later time than injuries in which the tendon is retracted into the palm, because the circulation is thought to be maintained. Some of these avulsions have been satisfactorily repaired several months after injury.

Type 3 injuries with an avulsion fracture close to the level of the distal interphalangeal joint also can be treated by fracture fixation at a later time because of the preservation of the circulation. Early passive motion is encouraged with the finger immobilized, and if a pull-out wire technique is used, the aforementioned postoperative treatment is followed. A word of caution with types 2 and 3 injuries, however: the tendon can be avulsed from the bony fragments and are then treated as type 1 injuries.

In many patients seen late, regardless of the level of retraction, if satisfactory reattachment is impossible, consideration should be given to arthrodesis or tenodesis. A select group of motivated patients in the 10- to 20-year age range may achieve satisfactory function after flexor tendon grafts through the intact sublimis tendon in the index and long (middle) fingers.

■ POSTREPAIR RUPTURE

If flexor tendon rupture after a primary repair is detected promptly, satisfactory results can be achieved if the finger is explored and the ruptured tendon is located and repaired. If detection of the rupture is delayed, end-to-end repair rarely is possible and tendon graft reconstruction may be required. The flexor tendon can rupture after tenolysis. In these situations, judgment is required in making the decision regarding exploration and repair versus tendon grafting. If the tendon has ruptured in a densely scarred area, satisfactory function after reexploration and repair is unlikely and consideration should be given to delayed tendon grafting. When a rupture of the flexor pollicis longus tendon is seen early, the tendon can be reattached to the distal phalanx; when seen late, a tendon graft may be necessary because of muscle shortening and tendon degeneration (see Technique 3.16).

REPAIR OF FLEXOR TENDON OF THUMB

The thumb also can be arbitrarily divided into zones according to the specific anatomic structures in the zone that influence the type of repair that is chosen for the flexor pollicis longus. Zone I includes the area at the interphalangeal joint and the insertion of the flexor pollicis longus. Zone II includes the

TABLE 3.1

Methods of Repairing the Flexor Pollicis Longus Based on the Zone of Injury and Timing of Repair

ZONE	SHARP CUT	TENDON LOSS	MINIMAL SCAR	SEVERE SCAR
I	Direct	Advancement	Advancement (or direct)	Advancement
II	Direct	Advancement and lengthening	Advancement and lengthening	Advancement and lengthening
III	Direct	Advancement and lengthening	Advancement and lengthening	Advancement and lengthening
IV	Direct	Free tendon graft	Free tendon graft	Two-stage free tendon graft
V	Direct	Tendon transfer (or bridge graft)	Direct	Tendon transfer

From Urbaniak JR: Repair of the flexor pollicis longus, *Hand Clin* 1:69–76, 1985.

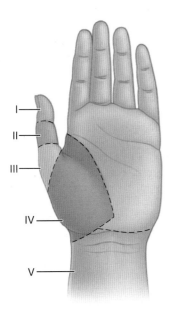

FIGURE 3.41 Anatomic zones of flexor pollicis longus that influence type of repair.

fibroosseous sheath extending just proximal to the metacarpal head and the metacarpophalangeal joint. Zone III includes the area of the metacarpal beneath the thenar muscles. Zone IV corresponds to the carpal tunnel, and zone V corresponds to the distal forearm just proximal to the wrist (Fig. 3.41).

Urbaniak proposed an organized system of selecting repair methods for the flexor pollicis longus depending on the location of the injury and the timing of repair (Table 3.1). Supporting the recommendations for direct repair of zone II injuries, the results after end-to-end repair within the flexor digital sheath have been reported to be as good as those after delayed tendon reconstruction.

To locate the flexor pollicis longus, volar zigzag incisions over the thumb and linear incisions in the region of the thenar eminence and at the wrist may be required (see Fig. 3.34). An early mobilization routine can be used after flexor pollicis longus repair similar to routines used for finger flexors. Postoperative immobilization includes splinting with the wrist flexed 30 to 45 degrees and the metacarpophalangeal and interphalangeal joints slightly extended. The splint is left intact for about 3 weeks, and a removable splint is applied for an additional 3 weeks to protect the wrist and finger against excessive hyperextension. Active flexion is begun at about 3

weeks, and passive extension and more vigorous activities can begin at 8 to 12 weeks.

■ ZONE I

When the long flexor tendon of the thumb is divided in zone I within 1 cm of its insertion, it can be sutured primarily to the distal stump or advanced and sutured directly into the bone. Some of the flexor sheath may require division. When this tendon is transected more proximally than 1 cm from its insertion, further advancement becomes necessary and lengthening of the tendon by Z-plasty just proximal to the wrist should be done. This tendon is unique in that it can be advanced without disturbing its blood supply because it does not have a vinculum. Tendon advancement rather than tendon grafting has been recommended because paratendinous adhesions are not as likely to form after advancement.

■ ZONE II

In zone II, the critical pulley area at the thumb metacarpophalangeal joint, a portion of the pulley can be excised to lessen the possibility of adherence to the pulley of the site of the tendon suture. Primary repair is unpredictable, however, and a later graft might be the better choice, unless the surgeon is experienced in tendon repair. Advancement of the tendon distally to be sutured to a stump that is shortened to lie distal to the metacarpophalangeal pulley has the advantage of moving the repair site from beneath the area of a pulley. Lengthening of the tendon at the wrist by Z-plasty also may be required for this procedure. Urbaniak recommended an end-weave repair at the site of lengthening just proximal to the wrist.

■ ZONE III

In zone III, with a laceration of the flexor pollicis longus tendon, the proximal end frequently retracts to near the wrist level. Usually the proximal end can be retrieved easily with atraumatic grasping of the tendon end in the sheath. If the tendon end cannot be retrieved easily, persistent grasping and probing should be avoided, and the tendon can be located through a separate incision at the wrist, between the radial artery and the flexor carpi radialis. Primary repairs in this zone can be performed when the two ends are retrieved and apposed by flexing the wrist and the distal joint of the thumb. When retrieval of the proximal tendon requires an additional incision at the wrist, the tendon should be carefully rethreaded through its normal route. This can be done by inserting a 22-gauge wire loop, a suture passer, or a tendon carrier through the sheath from the distal end, delivering a suture attached to the tendon, and threading it through from proximal to distal.

ZONE IV

In zone IV, the tendon rarely is cut because it is protected in part by a shelf of the radiocarpal bones. There is no contraindication to repair at this level as long as the repair technique is atraumatic and the two ends are recoverable. The creation of a lump of suture material sufficient to cause median nerve compression within the closed space of the carpal tunnel should be avoided.

ZONE V

In zone V, primary repair of the flexor pollicis longus tendon is indicated. Usually the location of the tendon ends and end-to-end repair are not difficult.

SECONDARY REPAIR AND RECONSTRUCTION OF FLEXOR TENDONS

If flexor tendons cannot be repaired within the first 10 to 14 days (delayed primary repair), the repair is considered to be secondary. After 1 month, delivery of the flexor tendon through the fibroosseous sheath and the pulleys is extremely difficult, and in those circumstances, in the absence of extensive scarring and destruction of the tendon sheath, traditional single-stage flexor tendon grafting can be done. In the presence of extensive disturbance of the flexor sheath and pulleys, joint contractures, and nerve injury, two-stage tendon grafting should be considered.

Generally, tendons can be repaired secondarily by direct suture at the site of division, by tendon graft, or by tendon transfer. Before tendons are secondarily repaired, certain requirements must be met, which are as follows: (1) wound erythema and swelling should be minimal; (2) skin coverage must be adequate; (3) the tissues through which the tendon is expected to glide must be relatively free of scar; (4) the alignment of bones must be satisfactory, and any fractures must be healed or fixed securely; (5) joints must have a useful range of passive motion; and (6) sensation in the involved digit must be undamaged or restored, or it should be possible to repair damaged nerves directly or with nerve grafts at the time of tendon repair. Secondary repair of tendons also may be delayed for reconstruction of the flexor pulleys, especially the critical A2 and A4 pulleys. During these reconstructions, a silicone rubber temporary prosthesis (Hunter and Salisbury) is useful to maintain the lumen of the tendon sheath while the grafted pulleys are healing. This is followed later by the insertion of the flexor tendon graft.

FLEXOR TENDONS OF FINGERS
ZONE I (DISTAL HALF OF FINGER)

If the profundus tendon has been lacerated or avulsed, it is best reattached within a few days, before it retracts into the palm and before avulsion of the vinculum occurs. If treated early, an avulsed or lacerated profundus tendon can be advanced *no more than* 1 cm and reattached as discussed under primary repair (see discussion of flexor tendon rupture). After a few days, the tendon end swells, and it becomes difficult or impossible to thread the tendon through the bifurcation of the sublimis. Rethreading the swollen profundus also can jeopardize proximal interphalangeal joint movement. Profundus function can be restored by a tendon graft, but only when indicated. Flexor tendon grafting through the intact sublimis tendons is unpredictable, and preoperative discussions should allow the patient to have a clear understanding of the uncertainties. Occupational requirements, such as those found in the playing of stringed musical instruments and work done by technicians, artisans, and artists, are also important when considering the need for flexor tendon grafting through an intact flexor sublimis.

As noted previously, flexor tendon grafting through an intact sublimis has been recommended for the index and long fingers for children and young adults, and rarely in the ring and little fingers.

ZONE II (CRITICAL AREA OF PULLEYS)

When the sublimis tendon alone has been divided in the critical area of pulleys, secondary repair is unnecessary because the profundus tendon provides satisfactory function, and profundus function can be jeopardized by attempts at repair of the flexor sublimis. Hyperextension deformities of the proximal interphalangeal joint occasionally occur after the laceration of a sublimis tendon in a very flexible hand. This can be treated with techniques such as tenodesis.

When the profundus tendon alone has been divided in zone II, the sublimis tendon provides ample flexion of the proximal interphalangeal joint. In the "delayed primary" period (10 to 14 days), meticulous repair of the flexor profundus can result in satisfactory function. During the "late secondary" period (4 weeks), it is doubtful that a direct repair would be successful. Under these circumstances, consideration should be given to distal tenodesis or distal joint arthrodesis, depending on the needs of the patient. Unless the distal joint is extremely hyperextensible and "flail," rarely is extensive surgical treatment for this problem necessary. Tenodesis or arthrodesis may be necessary in the index or long finger but rarely in other digits. When both tendons have been divided, and if conditions do not permit primary or delayed primary repair of the tendons, flexor function can be restored with a single-stage tendon graft when all prerequisites are met in the fingers (healed and stable wound, flexible joints, and good or improving sensibility).

ZONES III, IV, AND V (FOREARM AND PALM)

Flexor tendons in the forearm and palm can be repaired 3 or 4 weeks after injury by direct suture because flexing the wrist usually accommodates the gap sufficiently to overcome muscle retraction. After 4 or 5 weeks, the muscles become tightly contracted and a graft is necessary at times to bring the tendon ends together. This may be in the form of a short segmental graft between the tendon ends (Fig. 3.42). When tendons have been destroyed, profundus tendons take priority, and attaching available proximal sublimis tendons to distal profundus tendons may provide satisfactory function. The tendons can be attached with a mattress suture or with a strong multiple-strand technique, using 4-0 nonabsorbable suture or monofilament wire, especially in the distal forearm.

PROFUNDUS ADVANCEMENT

TECHNIQUE 3.12

(WAGNER)

- Make a volar oblique, zigzag, or midlateral incision over the profundus insertion. Incise the tendon sheath at the C4 pulley area and retract it, preserving the annular pul-

split profundus stump and tie the suture at the end of the finger through a button.

- Do not disturb the capsular attachment of the profundus stump because it protects the volar plate and helps to ensure a gliding surface and mobile joint.
- Repair any divided digital nerves at this time.
- Close the wound and apply a dorsal splint with the wrist in 45 degrees of flexion, the metacarpophalangeal joints in 60 to 70 degrees of flexion, and the interphalangeal joints in full extension.

POSTOPERATIVE CARE Refer to the discussion of postoperative care for primary repair. Remove the pull-out suture approximately 28 days postoperatively.

RECONSTRUCTION OF FINGER FLEXORS: SINGLE-STAGE TENDON GRAFT

When the sublimis and profundus tendons have been divided in the critical area of the pulleys, flexor tendon grafting may be indicated if a delay in treatment has occurred, if there is segmental loss of tendon, if a gap cannot be closed because of myocontracture, or if other conditions exist that may lead the surgeon to select tendon grafting. The following requirements should be met before a tendon graft is done: (1) the skin is pliable; (2) any wounds are well healed; (3) edema has subsided; (4) the joints allow a full passive range of motion; and (5) sensation in the finger is normal or at least one digital nerve is intact (one divided digital nerve can be sutured at the time of grafting if the other nerve is intact). The A2 and A4 pulley systems also should be intact; otherwise, these should be reconstructed in a separate staged procedure before tendon grafting (see later discussion of technique for pulley reconstruction). Age is a strong prognostic factor. Results are best in patients 10 to 30 years old, and the worst results occur in the very young and in patients older than 50 years.

TECHNIQUE 3.13

- Make a zigzag or volar oblique incision on the volar aspect of the finger to expose the underlying flexor sheath up to the proximal finger crease, or make a volar oblique or midlateral incision (see Fig. 3.34); carefully avoid entering the proximal interphalangeal joint, which has thin subcutaneous fat laterally. Avoid injuring the neurovascular bundles, and make the flaps wide and thick enough to prevent necrosis.
- Expose the flexor sheath and preserve as much of the unscarred sheath as possible.
- Excise no more than absolutely necessary of the A2 and A4 pulley systems; complete excision of either may result in limited excursion of the grafted tendon.
- Free the scarred sublimis and profundus tendons and carefully preserve all of the volar plate of the proximal and distal interphalangeal joints. In the patient with hyperextensible

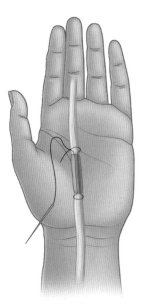

FIGURE 3.42 Long-standing flexor tendon interruptions in palm may require short segmental graft or "minigraft" to avoid excessive tension.

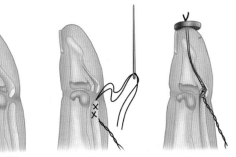

FIGURE 3.43 Wagner technique of profundus advancement. **SEE TECHNIQUE 3.12.**

leys. Usually the proximal end of the profundus has retracted into the palm. This can be determined by making another opening in the sheath distal to the A2 pulley. If the tendon cannot be seen, it probably is in the palm.

- Make a transverse incision near the distal palmar crease to recover it.
- Carefully thread the tendon through the bifurcation of the sublimis and into the distal end of the finger; if this cannot be done accurately and with assurance that the relation of the sublimis to the profundus is normal, the following two choices are available: (1) abandon the procedure because profundus and sublimis function may be impaired, or (2) make a volar oblique incision over the proximal phalanx, open a portion of the A2 pulley, and deliver the profundus tendon under direct vision.
- Resect the distal segment of the profundus at a level just proximal to the distal interphalangeal joint, and split its distal stump in a transverse plane (Fig. 3.43). Take no more than 1 cm of tendon.
- With a Bunnell retrograde pull-out wire suture or an antegrade pull-out wire (see Figs. 3.26 and 3.27), fix the distal end of the proximal segment of tendon into the

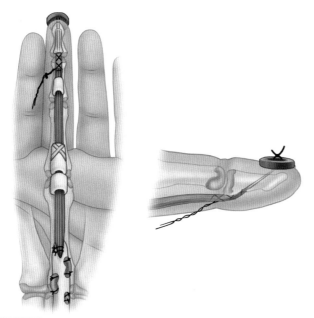

FIGURE 3.44 Repair of finger flexor tendons by tendon graft. Graft has been sutured in place. Proximal and distal pulleys have been narrowed. **SEE TECHNIQUE 3.13.**

joints, tenodesis of the sublimis helps prevent a swan-neck deformity.

- Divide both tendons at their insertions and bring them out through a transverse palmar incision made over the midbelly of the lumbrical muscles.
- Use a small chisel to raise a flap of bone just distal to the distal interphalangeal joint on the volar surface of the distal phalanx for later insertion of the profundus tendon graft (see Fig. 3.26).
- Under this bone flap, drill a small hole with a Kirschner wire large enough to accommodate two 4-0 monofilament wire sutures.
- Pass the sutures in the graft out through the nail (Fig. 3.44), or if there is concern about nail deformity, pass the sutures out through the distal end of the distal phalanx or through the distal tendon insertion and out the tip of the finger in the hyponychium.
- As an alternative to using a pull-out suture for distal insertion, suture the proximal end of the tendon into a split in the remaining distal tendon stump (see Fig. 3.43) if the stump is large enough to receive and hold a suture. With children, this method avoids the need for later removal of the pull-out suture.
- Through the proximal palmar incision, divide the sublimis tendon as far proximally as possible and discard it; retain the profundus tendon for attachment to the graft.
- In 10% to 15% of individuals, the palmaris longus tendon is absent, but when present, it can be taken from the same forearm and used as the graft.
- Expose the palmaris longus tendon through a transverse incision just proximal to its insertion at the wrist and through another in the upper forearm.

- Dissect the tendon at its musculotendinous junction proximally and detach it distally after dissecting out the various portions of its insertion; draw the tendon out through the proximal forearm incision.
- Place a monofilament 4-0 pull-out wire suture in the distal end of the palmaris longus tendon before dividing it proximally. As an alternative, use a 4-0 or 3-0 nylon suture. Arrange the pull-out wire in the retrograde Bunnell technique or use a single-loop antegrade pull-out wire. This suture is much more easily placed when the proximal end of the tendon has been stabilized.
- Thread the pull-out wire through the hole in the distal phalanx. Pass the needles in the suture through sterile felt and tie the distal ends of the suture. The distal attachment can be reinforced with an absorbable mattress suture.
- Bring the palmaris longus tendon proximally through the intact tendon sheath and into the palm by wetting the tendon and passing it with a suture passer, or use a 22-gauge wire loop to pass the tendon proximally.
- A careful attempt must be made to attach the tendon to the graft under appropriate tension.
- Place the wrist in neutral and the finger in full extension and place tension on the musculotendinous junction proximally and on the graft attached to the finger distally.
- At the point where the tendon and graft are to be joined, mark the junction with a methylene blue pen.
- Adjust the tension so that when the wrist is in extension, the finger is automatically brought into about the same amount or slightly more flexion as the adjoining digits. The amount of flexion should increase in the ulnar digits.
- The best method used to suture the proximal junction is the fish-mouth "weave" insertion described by Pulvertaft (see Fig. 3.19), which makes it easier to adjust the tension. Do not suture the lumbrical muscle to the tendon junction because this tends to increase tension in the lumbrical muscle, contributing to the "lumbrical plus" finger.
- Attach the tendon ends and close the palmar and digital wounds without subcutaneous sutures.
- Insert a drain in the proximal palmar wound if needed, especially if the tourniquet is to be deflated after a splint has been applied.
- Place the wrist in 40 to 45 degrees of flexion with the metacarpophalangeal joints in 60 degrees of flexion and the interphalangeal joint in full extension. The wrist should not be placed in forced flexion because this can increase postoperative pain and put pressure on the median nerve.
- Cover the wounds with a layer of nonadhesive material and a moist, molded dressing.
- Apply a posterior short arm splint to hold the wrist in flexion. In children, a long arm cast is applied to keep the dressing from shifting distally.
- It is crucial to prevent a postoperative hematoma. Release the tourniquet before wound closure and keep manual pressure on the wound for 5 minutes. Ascertain hemostasis using electrocautery.
- As an alternative, ascertain hemostasis, close the wound, and apply a moist, conforming dressing to the volar aspect of the finger with the wrist held in flexion by a posterior splint; elevate the hand, deflate the tourniquet, and maintain pressure on the palmar surface of the hand while the patient is awakening from anesthesia.

POSTOPERATIVE CARE The hand is elevated for the first 24 to 48 hours. Drains are removed after about 24 hours or when drainage subsides. Postoperative management and rehabilitation depend on the philosophy, experience, and preferences of the surgeon and therapist. Satisfactory results have been reported with the use of an early postoperative mobilization technique. Other surgeons are more conservative, basing their rehabilitation program on the concept that the avascular tendon graft must revascularize and go through a weakened phase before beginning any significant motion. If a controlled passive motion rehabilitation program is pursued, the patient should be evaluated carefully for his or her ability to comply and should be closely supervised several times weekly for at least 4 weeks. No active flexion, overextension, or passive hyperextension should be permitted. The pull-out suture is removed approximately 28 days after surgery. Protected motion is continued for at least 4 more weeks (total of 8 weeks). Strengthening is begun at 8 weeks after the tendon graft; however, normal forceful activity is not permitted before 12 to 14 weeks (see discussion of postoperative care for primary repair).

■ DONOR TENDONS FOR GRAFTING

Donor tendons for grafting, in order of preference, are the palmaris longus, the plantaris, and the long extensors of the toes. In rare cases, the index extensor digitorum communis, the extensor indicis proprius, and the flexor digitorum sublimis are used.

▌PALMARIS LONGUS

The palmaris longus is the tendon of choice because it fulfills the requirements of length, diameter, and availability without producing a deformity. The presence of this tendon should be determined before any grafting procedure; its presence can be exhibited by having the patient appose the tips of the thumb and little finger while flexing the wrist (Fig. 3.45). The tendon is reported to be present in one arm in 85% of individuals and in both arms in 70%. The tendon is flat, is surrounded by paratenon, and is long enough for a graft about 15 cm long. The tendon is excised as follows. A short transverse incision is made directly over the tendon just proximal to the flexion crease of the wrist. The tendon is grasped at its end with a hemostat, and traction is applied so that it can be palpated easily in a proximal direction. A second transverse incision is made over the tendon at the junction of the middle and proximal thirds of the forearm. The tendon is identified and divided, and the segment to be used as a graft is withdrawn. Should paratenon be desired, a long curved incision over the forearm is necessary; this method is much more disabling, and, as an alternative, a tendon stripper similar to that devised for the plantaris tendon (Fig. 3.46) can be used. Occasionally, there is a double palmaris longus tendon, or it can have multiple insertions or an associated aberrant muscle. Any of these would make it difficult to withdraw it from only two transverse incisions.

▌PLANTARIS TENDON

The plantaris tendon is equally satisfactory for a graft as the palmaris tendon, has the advantage of being almost twice as long (enough to provide two grafts), but is not as accessible (Figs. 3.47 and 3.48). It reportedly is present in 93% of individuals. The tendon is anteromedial to the Achilles tendon proximal to the heel and can be obtained for grafting as follows. A small, medial, longitudinal incision is made just anterior to the insertion of the Achilles tendon. The tendon is identified as a slip distinctly separate from the Achilles tendon (Fig. 3.46). The tendon is divided near its insertion and

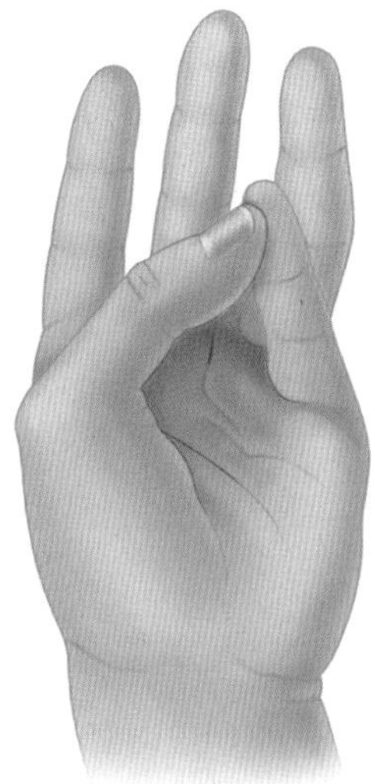

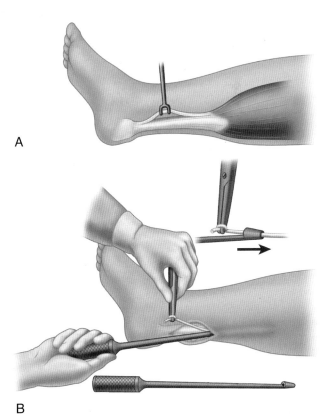

A

B

FIGURE 3.46   Method of removing plantaris tendon for grafting (see text). **A,** Plantaris tendon is separated from Achilles tendon. **B,** Brand tendon stripper.

FIGURE 3.45   Method of showing presence of palmaris longus tendon (see text).

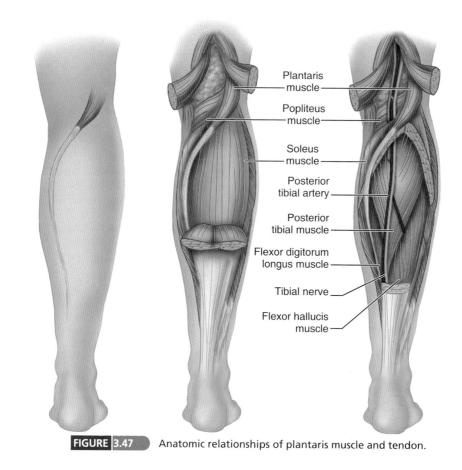

FIGURE 3.47　Anatomic relationships of plantaris muscle and tendon.

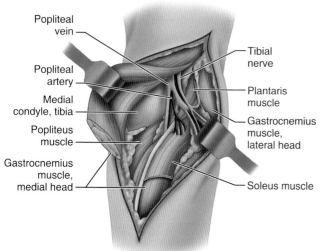

FIGURE 3.48　Anatomic relationships of plantaris muscle and tendon.

threaded through the loop of a tendon stripper made for this purpose. The knee is kept in full extension. The distal end of the tendon is clamped with a hemostat and held taut while the stripper is passed up the leg until the resistance of the gastrocsoleus fascia is encountered; this resistance is overcome with additional force on the stripper. The stripper is advanced proximally for about 25 cm, where resistance is again met as the loop of the stripper meets the belly of the muscle. The loop of the stripper is palpated through the skin, and a longitudinal incision 5 cm long is made over it. The gastrocnemius

muscle belly is freed from around the plantaris tendon, and the tendon is divided under direct vision and withdrawn. If a tendon stripper is unavailable, the tendon is removed through multiple short transverse incisions.

LONG EXTENSORS OF TOES

Tendons of the long extensors of the toes are not as desirable as the palmaris longus or the plantaris tendons because there are many attachments between them, especially as the cruciate ligament is approached proximally. Every toe except the little toe has an extensor brevis tendon to dorsiflex it after excision of the long extensor tendon. The extensor hallucis longus is much larger than the other extensors, and the extensor of the second toe is much more intimately related to the dorsalis pedis artery. The extensor of the third toe is probably easiest to remove and use. Multiple short transverse incisions are made over the tendon, and the tendon is removed by elevating the skin proximal to each incision and dissecting to a more proximal level. Another incision is made at this point, and the procedure is repeated. The divided end of the tendon is extracted through each successive incision and removed through the proximal incision (Fig. 3.49A). A tendon can be removed much more easily through a long curved incision along the course of the tendon (Fig. 3.49B), but such an incision temporarily prevents weight bearing and results in an unsightly scar.

EXTENSOR INDICIS PROPRIUS, EXTENSOR DIGITORUM COMMUNIS OF INDEX

The extensor tendons to the fingers rarely are used as tendon grafts. The extensor indicis proprius tendon usually is long enough for a single flexor tendon graft but rarely is used. It is divided distally at its insertion into the ulnar side of the extensor hood through a small transverse incision and proximally just proximal to the extensor retinaculum through a short longitudinal incision. The distal end of the proximal segment of tendon is sutured to the extensor digitorum communis to help maintain independent extension of the index finger. If the extensor digitorum communis to the index finger is selected, it is divided in a similar fashion through a small transverse incision over the proximal portion of the extensor hood, repairing the distal remnant to the extensor indicis proprius tendon. It is released as well through a short longitudinal incision over the extensor retinaculum proximal to the wrist.

FLEXOR DIGITORUM SUBLIMIS

A flexor digitorum sublimis tendon should not be excised simply as a graft, but at times one is available when removed in conjunction with an amputation or flexor tendon grafting. The tendon usually is too thick, so its central part can

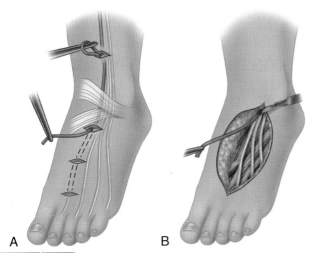

FIGURE 3.49 Methods of obtaining long extensor tendon of toe for grafting (see text). **A,** Long extensor tendon of second toe is removed through four short transverse incisions. **B,** Same tendon is removed through one long longitudinal incision.

undergo necrosis when it is used as a graft, producing a local reaction that causes adhesions. The tendon can be split longitudinally to make it thinner, but this leaves a raw surface where adhesions are even more likely to develop.

■ COMPLICATIONS
▌"LUMBRICAL PLUS" FINGER

The "lumbrical plus" finger develops when the pull of the profundus musculotendinous unit is applied through the lumbrical muscle, rather than through a flexor tendon graft distal to the lumbrical muscle origin. The pull of the profundus muscle, applied through the lumbrical muscle, creates extension of the proximal and distal interphalangeal joints. This usually occurs if the tension on a tendon graft is not appropriately set and the graft is relatively too "long" (Figs. 3.50 and 3.51). The condition also may be seen when amputations have occurred through the middle phalanx after avulsion of the insertion of the flexor digitorum profundus or division of the flexor profundus tendon. The long finger seems to be most commonly involved. Usually, with gentle flexion effort, the patient can nearly make a fist with the grafted finger; however, when forceful flexion is attempted, the interphalangeal joints extend with "paradoxic extension." According to Parkes, the test for the "lumbrical plus" finger is to show first that the patient has full passive flexion of all joints of the finger. In strong gripping or active flexion of all fingers, flexion is incomplete and partial extension of the interphalangeal joints occurs. The treatment of this condition consists of transection of the involved lumbrical tendon through a longitudinal incision in the web space to the radial side of the involved finger, usually after use of a local anesthetic. If the tendon otherwise functions satisfactorily, this should cure the problem.

▌"QUADRIGA" EFFECT

If the tension on the tendon graft is set too tightly, when the patient attempts to flex the fingers, the grafted finger flexes and reaches the palm before the remaining fingers. This blocks full excursion of the proximal flexor musculotendinous units and reduces the ability to flex the uninjured digits, usually occurring in the long, ring, and little fingers. This limitation of excursion also can occur if the flexor digitorum sublimis spiral is not corrected in the repair of any injury to

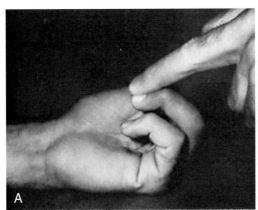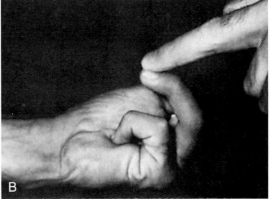

FIGURE 3.50 "Lumbrical plus" finger. In this patient, tendon graft that is too long has been inserted. **A,** Gentle flexion results in coordinated flexion of grafted ring finger and adjacent small finger. **B,** Powerful flexion of hand results in good flexion of small digit but paradoxic extension of interphalangeal joints of grafted ring finger against examiner's digit.

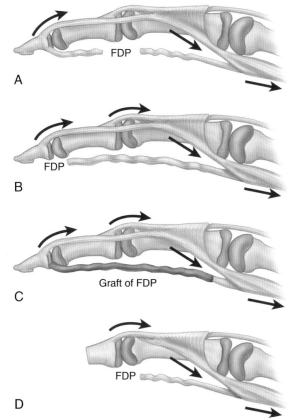

A

B

C   Graft of FDP

D

FDP (appears in A, B, D)

FIGURE 3.51   Conditions that cause "lumbrical plus" finger. **A,** Severance of flexor digitorum profundus *(FDP)* (produces paradoxic extension). **B,** Avulsion of FDP. **C,** Overly long flexor tendon graft. **D,** Amputation through middle phalanx.

the flexor profundus and sublimis, with improper repair of an oblique laceration allowing triggering or blocking of motion to occur and blocking of tendon motion because of eversion of the tendon repair. This has been emphasized by Verdan and elucidated further by Lister.

■ RECONSTRUCTION OF FLEXOR TENDON PULLEYS

Injury to the important annular thickenings of the fibroosseous sheath (especially the A2 and A4 pulleys) may have occurred at the time of tendon injury, or they may have been destroyed during previous surgical procedures, either at the time of a primary repair or subsequently during tenolysis. When reconstructive procedures, including tenolyses and single-stage and two-stage graft reconstructions, are attempted without reconstruction of the pulleys, the result usually is unsatisfactory. Without pulleys, the angle of approach of the tendon to its insertion is altered, retinacular restraints are damaged, a flexion contracture frequently develops at the proximal interphalangeal joint, bowstringing of palmar skin occurs, and tendon excursion is lost. If the finger is left without the function of the A2 and A4 pulleys, it cannot function satisfactorily after tenolysis, and tendon graft reconstruction fails. Reconstruction of the A2 and A4 pulley systems is indicated when insufficient pulley remnants are left after tenolysis and as part of a single-stage or two-stage tendon graft reconstruction. In the involved digit, all fractures and joint injuries should be healed, neurovascular defects should be minimal

or improving, and there should be good soft-tissue coverage with minimal scarring.

In two situations, flexor tenolysis and single-stage flexor tendon grafting, the pulley reconstruction can be jeopardized at the time that motion is begun. Usually this problem can be overcome in the postoperative period using rings, taped bands, or thermoplastic rings, as recommended by Strickland et al., to protect the pulley reconstruction.

Use of the pulley reconstruction in the two-stage tendon graft reconstruction allows the grafted material to heal satisfactorily so that by the time of the second stage of the tendon grafting procedure the pulley reconstruction has sufficiently healed. The results usually are better in young adults and adolescents because younger individuals are less likely to develop joint stiffness. Donor grafts for pulley reconstruction include a flexor sublimis tendon that is sacrificed and split longitudinally; portions of the extensor retinaculum at the wrist or ankle, as advocated by Lister; sublimis tendon; fascia lata in rare situations; and the palmaris longus if it is not needed for flexor tendon grafting (see earlier section "Donor Tendons for Grafting").

RECONSTRUCTION OF FLEXOR TENDON PULLEYS

TECHNIQUE 3.14

- Make a zigzag (see Fig. 1.17, lines *B* and *C*), midlateral (see Fig. 1.18), or volar oblique (see Fig. 1.17, line *D*) incision exposing the area of the flexor tendons. Make the exposure wide enough to show all of the flexor pulley system.
- Excise the scarred tendons and surrounding scar tissue. Retain any part of the sheath that is not scarred, however, especially in the area of the distal joint and the A1 pulley system in the palm.
- Bring the tendons out through an additional palmar incision and complete their excision.
- If a two-stage tendon reconstruction is planned, insert a Silastic rod (Hunter) of appropriate size and attach it distally either to the remaining profundus tendon stump or to the bone by a small screw (Fig. 3.52), as described for the two-stage Hunter rod technique.
- Place the rod proximally at the forearm or palmar level in a scar-free area away from the profundus tendon.
- Leave the profundus tendon attached to the lumbrical muscle to maintain its length.
- Several techniques are available for pulley reconstruction. If a tendon graft is to be used for a pulley substitute, use a thin strip measuring at least 6 cm in length and 0.25 cm in width. If the original fibroosseous rim of the flexor sheath is satisfactory, weave the tendon through this rim and secure it with mattress sutures. Weave the strip over the silicone rod beginning at about the A2 pulley level (Fig. 3.53).
- The A2 and A4 pulleys can be reconstructed individually in this method. If the fibroosseous rim is insufficient, pass

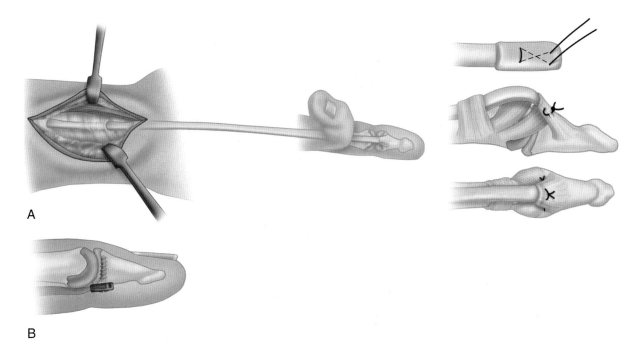

A

B

FIGURE 3.52 **A,** Stage 1. Distal implant juncture; suture to profundus stump. **B,** Distal implant juncture; metal endplate implant model with screw fixation to distal phalanx. **SEE TECHNIQUE 3.14.**

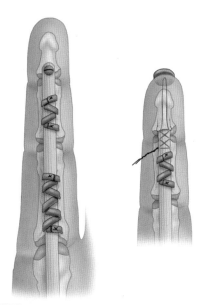

FIGURE 3.53 Reconstruction of flexor tendon pulleys. **SEE TECHNIQUE 3.14.**

the tendon graft around the phalanx and suture it to itself with several mattress sutures.
- Over the proximal phalanx (A2 pulley reconstruction), pass the tendon over the silicone rod and around the proximal phalanx deep to the extensor tendon. Over the middle phalanx (A4 pulley reconstruction), pass the tendon around the middle phalanx superficial to the extensor tendon and suture it to itself. In each case, the circling pulley reconstruction is rotated so that the suture portion is to the side of the finger.

- In another technique, advocated by Lister, extensor retinaculum from the wrist can be harvested and used as an encircling pulley reconstruction as well (Fig. 3.54). Pass a piece of thread around the finger to estimate the amount of length of the tendon graft material that would be required for the pulley reconstruction.
- Avoid reconstructing the pulley over the proximal interphalangeal joint because this can restrict motion.
- When pulley reconstruction is done concomitant with flexor tenolysis, plan to incorporate an orthotic protection (ring) in the rehabilitation period.
- Close the wound loosely and support the hand with a dorsal splint.

POSTOPERATIVE CARE If pulley reconstruction is part of the first stage of a two-stage tendon reconstruction, passive motion of the finger joints usually is started at 7 to 10 days. The patient is instructed in passive finger exercises. Strapping to adjacent fingers can be helpful. For tenolysis, active motion is begun in the first 72 hours and the therapy program progresses gradually. For staged tendon reconstruction, 3 months may be required to allow for healing and restoration of flexibility and sheath reconstitution before the second stage.

RECONSTRUCTION OF FINGER FLEXORS BY TWO-STAGE TENDON GRAFT

For patients with excessive scarring, joint stiffness, and possible nerve injury, a two-stage procedure for tendon repair may be indicated. A patient who has a severely contracted, scarred digit, especially if neurovascular insufficiency is significant, may be a candidate for an arthrodesis or even amputation as reasonable alternatives to staged tendon reconstruction. The

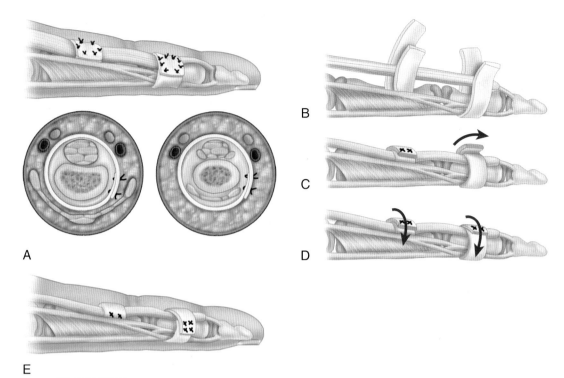

FIGURE 3.54 **A,** Reconstructive tissue is passed around phalanx and tendon deep to extensor tendon over proximal phalanx and superficial to it over middle. **B** and **C,** Graft is sutured securely because suture represents only weak point in this reconstruction. Overlapped repair is rotated around to side of digit, creating strong pulley with synovial gliding surface on its inner aspect. **D** and **E,** Intervening windows should be reconstructed with synovial tissue from dorsum of foot adjacent to retinaculum. **SEE TECHNIQUE 3.14.**

patient should understand the extensive rehabilitation and effort involved in recovery after a minimum of at least two operations that would be required for such a tendon reconstruction. The first stage consists of excising the tendon and scar from the flexor tendon bed and preserving or reconstructing the flexor pulley system. A Dacron-impregnated silicone rod is inserted to maintain the tunnel in the area of the excised tendons until passive motion and sensitivity have been restored to the digit. The rod is attached distally to bone or a tendon stump. It is passed proximally into the distal forearm to a level about 5 cm proximal to the wrist crease to allow proximal extension of the sheath into the forearm. The second stage consists of removal of the rod and insertion of a tendon graft (Fig. 3.55).

STAGE 1: EXCISION OF TENDON AND SCAR AND RECONSTRUCTION OF FLEXOR PULLEY

TECHNIQUE 3.15

- Make a zigzag (see Fig. 1.17, lines *B* and *C*) or midlateral (see Fig. 1.18) incision to expose the entire flexor sheath area. If scars are present, it is best to follow them with the incision to avoid ischemia in skin flaps.

- Expose the palm either by a continuation of the zigzag incision or through an additional incision at the level of the A1 pulley.
- Excise the profundus and sublimis tendons, but retain a stump of the profundus tendon 1 cm long at the distal phalanx.
- If pulley reconstruction is planned, preserve the insertion of the sublimis to reinforce the pulleys. Save excised tendon as graft material for pulley reconstruction. Retain only the unscarred portions of the flexor pulley system, but some portions of the A2 and A4 pulleys are the minimum required.
- Extend the dissection into the palm; if the lumbrical muscle is scarred and contracted, excise it.
- Transect the profundus tendon at the level of the lumbrical.
- Select a Dacron silicone rod of appropriate size and rinse it in saline to remove lint. Usually a smaller rod is selected to provide a snug fit in the sheath.
- Insert the rod into the palm and continue blunt dissection proximally so that the rod extends above the wrist level. Excision of the entire sublimis tendon may be necessary to make room for the rod at the wrist.
- Attach the rod distally beneath the stump of the profundus with 3-0 monofilament steel wire or nylon reinforced with two 4-0 nonabsorbable sutures through the Dacron portion of the rod.
- As an alternative, secure the rod to the distal phalanx with a screw.

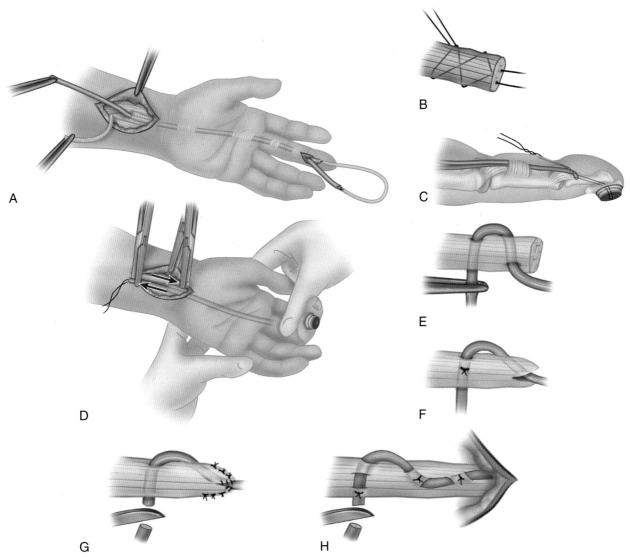

FIGURE 3.55 Passive gliding technique using Hunter tendon prosthesis. Stage 2: Removal of prosthesis and insertion of tendon graft. **A,** Graft has been sutured to proximal end of prosthesis and pulled distally through new tendon bed. Note mesentery-like attachment of new sheath visible in forearm. **B,** Distal anastomosis. Bunnell pull-out suture in distal end of tendon graft. **C,** Distal anastomosis. Complete Bunnell suture with button over fingernail. Reinforcing sutures are usually placed through stump of profundus tendon. **D,** Proximal anastomosis. Measuring excursion of tendon graft and selecting motor. If procedure is done with local anesthesia (see text), true amplitude of active muscle contraction can be measured. **E,** Proximal anastomosis graft is threaded through tendon motor muscle two or three times for added strength. **F,** Proximal anastomosis. Stump is "fish-mouthed" after method of Pulvertaft, tension is adjusted, and one suture is inserted as shown. Further adjustment of tension can be accomplished simply by removing and shortening or lengthening as necessary. **G,** Proximal anastomosis. After appropriate tension has been selected, anastomosis is completed. **H,** Proximal anastomosis. Technique when graft is anastomosed to common profundus tendon. **SEE TECHNIQUE 3.16.**

- After seating the prosthesis, passively flex the fingers to observe any tendency toward buckling. Traction on the prosthesis determines the need for possible further modification of the pulley system, either by excising more scar tissue or by reconstructing a defective area in the system, especially at the A2 and A4 levels.

- Repair digital nerves as needed and close the wound after obtaining satisfactory hemostasis.
- Apply a bulky compressive dressing and a dorsal splint with the wrist at about 35 degrees of flexion, the metacarpophalangeal joints at 60 to 70 degrees of flexion, and the interphalangeal joints extended.

POSTOPERATIVE CARE After closing the wound, the hand is supported by a splint and gentle passive motion of the finger joints is started at 7 to 10 days. The hand should be examined regularly for synovitis or buckling of the rod. If buckling is seen, external rings are worn on the fingers to support the implant. If synovitis develops, prompt and complete immobilization usually is sufficient for resolution. The second stage is done when the finger is soft, supple, and well healed with mobile joints. The earliest time for the second stage is about 8 weeks, but 3 months usually is required, depending on the patient's needs and the surgeon's judgment.

STAGE 2: ROD REMOVAL AND TENDON GRAFT INSERTION

TECHNIQUE 3.16

- Using appropriate anesthesia, open the previous incision to expose the flexor sheath over the distal portion of the middle phalanx near the distal joint and make another incision proximally in the palm or the forearm.
- Select a donor tendon, depending on the planned proximal attachment. A palmaris longus probably would suffice for a single tendon with a proximal attachment in the palm. Longer tendons would be required for attachments from the forearm to the finger. The plantaris or the extensor digitorum longus tendon to the three central toes makes a sufficiently long tendon graft. Motor tendons usually selected include the profundus mass for the long, ring, and little fingers. If suitable, the profundus to the index is used for the index finger. The sublimis muscles also can be used for motors for the tendon grafts. For thumb flexor tendon reconstruction, the flexor pollicis longus or the sublimis muscles can be used. In certain selected situations, the sublimis to the ring finger can be used as motor and tendon without the need for a free tendon graft.
- While the tendon grafts are being harvested, deflate the tourniquet and cover the wounds with sterile bandages and compress.
- After the tendon grafts have been harvested, exsanguinate the limb and reinflate the tourniquet.
- Suture the flexor graft to the proximal end of the implant and pull the implant distally through the sheath, trailing the tendon graft with it (Fig. 3.55A).
- Separate the implant from the tendon graft and discard the implant.
- Use a pull-out technique to secure the distal attachment of the tendon graft to the distal phalanx (Fig. 3.55B and C) or the distal end of the flexor tendon, as previously described (see Fig. 3.43).
- If the palm is not involved with scarring, a short graft can be used and the proximal attachment is made to the profundus tendon at the lumbrical origin with a Pulvertaft fish-mouth weave (Fig. 3.55F and G). If the profundus is unsatisfactory, an adjacent sublimis can be used as a motor in the palm.

- If the profundus tendons of the long, ring, and little fingers are chosen for common motors, use an interweaving technique for the proximal attachment.
- In some circumstances, the proximal attachment is in the forearm.
- In the forearm, select the appropriate motor muscle and obtain the length of the flexor tendon graft by allowing the dorsum of the hand and wrist to lie flat on the operating table.
- Inspect the "cascade of the fingers" (Schneider) with each finger more flexed than the finger to its radial side.
- Pass the tendon graft in an interweave method without being sutured and apply traction to the graft until the finger shows its proper position relative to its adjacent fingers (Fig. 3.55D); place a mattress suture through the motor tendon and the tendon graft.
- After testing passive movement with wrist flexion and extension, place the hand on the table and observe the finger as it assumes its position in relation to the adjacent fingers. If the position is satisfactory, complete the attachment of the graft with a Pulvertaft weave with mattress sutures (Fig. 3.55E to H).
- Deflate the tourniquet, obtain satisfactory hemostasis, and close the wound using drains as needed.
- Apply a bulky compression dressing with a short arm dorsal splint and maintain the wrist in about 35 degrees of flexion, the metacarpophalangeal joints in 70 degrees of flexion, and the interphalangeal joints in full extension.

POSTOPERATIVE CARE An early protected motion program generally is recommended. A more conservative approach can be used if there is concern about rupture and disruption at the tendon attachments. If an early protected motion program is initiated, it usually begins 3 days after the operation. If a rubber band attachment to the fingernail is used as a part of the passive component of the protected motion routine, the therapist and the surgeon should closely supervise the program to avoid proximal and distal interphalangeal joint contractures. The pull-out suture is removed at 4 weeks. In a compliant patient, the dorsal splint is removed at 4 weeks also and the rubber band is attached to a wrist cuff to provide additional protection for 1 to 2 more weeks. Blocking exercises are begun at 4 to 5 weeks. Static splints are used to help avoid recurrence of flexion contractures present before stage 1. Dynamic and static splints are added as needed, possibly by 4 to 5 weeks in patients with poor pull-through. In patients with satisfactory motion, dynamic and static splints can be added at 6 to 8 weeks. Heavy resistance should be avoided early in the program.

For patients who cannot be closely supervised by the surgeon or therapist, a safer routine would involve splinting of the hand without the rubber band traction for approximately 3 weeks after surgery and initiation of finger mobilization after that time. At about 3 weeks, an active and passive range-of-motion exercise routine can be started, with blocking and more active exercises begun at 4 weeks. Protection against hyperextension should be maintained for 6 to 7 weeks after surgery, and heavy resistance should not be forced for 9 to 12 weeks.

■ LONG FLEXOR OF THUMB

The flexor pollicis longus tendon can be repaired secondarily by direct suture at any level within the thumb if the two ends can be approximated without excessive tension. Within the first few weeks after injury, tension of the muscle from contracture can be overcome by flexing the wrist. Avoid repair of the flexor pollicis longus at the proximal pulley, opposite the metacarpophalangeal joint, because the suture line is likely to adhere to the pulley. This repair can be accomplished by tendon advancement or tendon advancement with lengthening at the wrist, as described earlier (see "Primary Flexor Tendon Repair"). Another alternative in difficult situations is tendon transfer of the ring finger flexor sublimis to substitute for flexor pollicis longus function. Urbaniak recommended that this tendon transfer be reserved for patients who have lost function of the flexor pollicis longus muscle belly because of anterior interosseous nerve injury, loss of blood supply, or muscle damage. As a last resort, the thumb interphalangeal joint can be stabilized by arthrodesis (see chapter 10) or tenodesis (see Technique 3.22).

FLEXOR TENDON GRAFT

TECHNIQUE 3.17

- Make an incision on the radial side of the thumb from a point near the base of the nail to near the middle of the metacarpal and angle it toward the palm to end near the middle of the thenar eminence.
- Elevate the skin and subcutaneous tissue as a flap with its base toward the palm; carefully dissect the branch of the radial nerve and its corresponding vessel, and retract them with this flap.
- Dissect the digital neurovascular bundle, which lies well toward the anterior aspect of the thumb.
- Identify the pulley and open the tendon sheath and the pulley sufficiently to insert the tendon graft, but leave a segment of the pulley at least 1 cm wide intact over the metacarpophalangeal joint to prevent bowstringing of the tendon.
- Also leave intact the oblique pulley at the proximal and middle thirds of the proximal phalanx.
- Free the flexor tendon, but do not enter the interphalangeal joint or damage its volar plate.
- Make a transverse incision 2.5 cm long proximal to the flexor crease of the wrist and identify the flexor pollicis longus tendon and withdraw it; if possible, tag the distal end of the tendon with a suture before withdrawing it, and use this suture as a guide in threading the graft into the thumb.
- Obtain a tendon graft from an appropriate site, usually the palmaris longus or toe extensor digitorum longus tendons.
- Anchor the graft at the point of insertion of the original tendon as described for a flexor tendon graft of a finger.
- Use the end-weave technique to suture the proximal end of the graft to the distal end of the flexor pollicis longus tendon at a level proximal to the wrist so that the junc-ture does not enter the carpal tunnel or encroach on the median nerve when the thumb and wrist are extended.
- The graft should be under enough tension to flex slightly the interphalangeal joint of the thumb when the wrist is in the neutral position. Test the tension on the graft by placing one mattress suture through the end weave.
- With the wrist in maximal extension, full flexion of the thumb is produced. With the wrist in maximal passive flexion, full extension of the thumb should be produced.
- When the tension is satisfactory, the additional mattress sutures are placed to secure the juncture.
- As an alternative method, the proximal end of the graft can be sutured to the tendon opposite the middle of the thumb metacarpal; this requires only one incision and helps avoid potential median nerve complications.
- Close the wound with 5-0 nylon or a similar suture without subcutaneous sutures. Apply a dorsal splint to the wrist, hand, and thumb with the wrist in 45 degrees of flexion and the interphalangeal joint of the thumb in extension.

POSTOPERATIVE CARE At 4 weeks, the pull-out suture is removed, and active motion is begun. Splint protection against hyperextension is continued for 7 to 8 weeks. At 7 weeks, active flexion can be increased to approach heavy resistance by 9 to 10 weeks.

TWO-STAGE FLEXOR TENDON GRAFT FOR FLEXOR POLLICIS LONGUS

In the unusual situation in which there is extensive disruption of the flexor pollicis longus in its course from the carpal tunnel distally in its passage beneath the thenar muscles to the thumb and the tendon insertion and, especially if there are associated joint contractures and pulley reconstruction is required, staged tendon grafting using the silicone rod technique (Hunter) is appropriate.

TECHNIQUE 3.18

(HUNTER)
- The incision and approach to the thumb are similar to those described for the single-stage flexor tendon graft. After the pulley has been reconstructed, and the silicone rod has been placed beneath the pulley reconstruction and secured distally in a manner similar to that described for the silicone rod technique in the finger, suture the distal end of the silicone rod to the stump of flexor tendon with wire and nonabsorbable sutures.
- Pass the rod proximally through the course of the flexor pollicis longus beneath the thenar muscles and further proximally through the carpal tunnel into the distal forearm adjacent to the flexor pollicis longus tendon.
- After wound closure, apply a dorsal splint to maintain the wrist in slight flexion and to provide an increased length for the sheath of the flexor pollicis longus.
- Passive motion is begun, and after satisfactory wound healing and motion have been achieved, the second stage is done, usually 2 to 3 months after the first stage.

- Harvest a free tendon graft of sufficient length, usually the plantaris or extensor digitorum longus from a toe.
- Make limited incisions in the distal attachment of the thumb and proximally at the wrist for passing the tendon graft attached to the rod.
- Attach the graft to the proximal end of the rod and pull it distally through the sheath.
- Remove the rod and discard. Complete the distal attachment with a pull-out technique similar to a single-stage tendon graft. The proximal attachment is accomplished with an end weave (Pulvertaft) using mattress sutures, and the tension is set in a manner similar to that described in the single-stage graft technique for the flexor pollicis longus (see Technique 3.17).

POSTOPERATIVE CARE Postoperative care after two-stage tendon grafting is similar to that for the single-stage grafting technique.

TRANSFER OF RING FINGER FLEXOR SUBLIMIS TO FLEXOR POLLICIS LONGUS

TECHNIQUE 3.19

- Expose the flexor pollicis longus insertion through a mid-lateral or volar zigzag incision. Avoid injury to neurovascular structures and the annular thickenings of the flexor sheath of the thumb. Open only enough of the sheath to identify the flexor pollicis longus tendon insertion, and leave it attached to its insertion.
- Make a transverse palmar incision at the level of the proximal flexion crease of the ring finger.
- Acutely flex the metacarpophalangeal and proximal interphalangeal joints of the ring finger to allow harvesting the greatest length of the tendon.
- Transect the flexor sublimis tendon and close the palmar incision with continuous 4-0 nylon sutures.
- Make a longitudinal incision at the wrist to the radial side of the distal forearm. Identify the transected flexor sublimis tendon to the ring finger and deliver it into the proximal wrist incision.
- Identify the proximal end of the transected flexor pollicis longus tendon, either at the wrist incision or by using a palmar incision over the thenar eminence (see chapter 1).
- If the flexor pollicis longus tendon is mobile in its sheath, the distal end of the sublimis tendon can be attached to the flexor pollicis longus, and then the tendon can be delivered by applying traction to the distal end of the flexor pollicis longus tendon from its insertion. If this is the case, detach the flexor pollicis longus from its insertion, deliver the sublimis tendon distally, and attach it with a pull-out technique using the retrograde Bunnell technique or the antegrade pull-out technique.
- If the flexor pollicis longus cannot be moved easily in its sheath, dissect and mobilize the tendon and excise it as

required by the scarred conditions in the palm and thumb; use a 22-gauge wire loop to pass retrograde down the course of the flexor pollicis longus to deliver the sublimis tendon distally through the palm and into the thumb for its insertion.

- Obtain adequate hemostasis and close the wound in a routine manner using 4-0 or 5-0 monofilament nylon sutures.
- Apply a compressive dressing and a dorsal short arm splint that immobilizes the wrist in 25 to 30 degrees of flexion, allowing the thumb metacarpophalangeal and interphalangeal joints to be in extension or only slight flexion. Drains usually are unnecessary.

POSTOPERATIVE CARE Any drains are removed at approximately 24 hours or when drainage has ceased. Although an early postoperative mobilization program can be undertaken, it is usually unnecessary. The sutures are removed at 10 to 14 days. The pull-out suture is removed at 4 weeks. The initial splint is left in place for approximately 4 weeks, and then gentle active motion is begun. The thumb is protected with an additional removable dorsal splint for another 3 to 4 weeks, and motion exercises are increased. Forceful resistance activities are not undertaken for 10 to 12 weeks.

■ FLEXOR TENOLYSIS AFTER REPAIR AND GRAFTING

In addition to the complications that can occur after any surgical procedure, tendon repair and grafting can be complicated by the adherence of the tendon to the sheath and its lack of gliding and consequent loss of motion. Tenolysis should not be considered until it can be documented that the patient has not made significant progress over several months while cooperating with an organized progressive therapy program. Usually at least 3 months should have passed since the initial surgical procedure, and in some situations 4 to 6 months may be required to make an accurate assessment of the patient's progress. In addition to documenting a lack of progression in the physical therapy program and motion at the distal and proximal interphalangeal joints, the following requirements should have been met: (1) all soft tissue and skin scars should be soft, pliable, and flexible and should be healed; (2) fractures and joint injuries should have healed; (3) the passive range of motion in the digital joints should be as near normal as possible; (4) the sensibility, under ideal circumstances, should be normal or there should be demonstrable recovery of nerve function after nerve repair; and (5) the patient should be showing progression with strengthening exercises and should realistically understand the expectations after such a procedure; the patient also should understand that at the time of the procedure, if the extent of scar and adhesion is excessive, the first stage of a two-stage flexor tendon graft procedure would be a likely option. The patient also should understand that if tenolysis is successful, the risk of tendon rupture after tenolysis can be 10% or greater. After a failed graft, a fresh tendon graft should be used instead of a tenolysis.

FLEXOR TENOLYSIS AFTER REPAIR AND GRAFTING

TECHNIQUE 3.20

- Make the incision through the existing skin scar. When elevating the skin flaps, avoid injury to neurovascular structures and the annular portions of the fibroosseous sheath.
- Using great care, dissect the scar tissue from the tendon. Sometimes the tendon and fibroosseous sheath are indistinguishable. Similarly, the tendon sometimes adheres to the phalanx, particularly in areas of healed fracture callus.
- Use sharp dissection and periosteal elevators to free the flexor tendon from the adherent periosteum and fibroosseous sheath.
- After determining that the tendon has been completely released in the digit, make an incision in the distal forearm, identify the appropriate flexor tendon, and show with traction on the proximal tendon that the finger can be moved through a nearly normal full range of motion.
- If a regional or local block anesthetic is used for the tenolysis, the patient can voluntarily show the amount of motion in the finger. If it can be shown that the annular pulleys are not present, or if the remaining pulleys are insufficient for proper finger function, perform pulley reconstruction at the time of tenolysis.
- If the flexor tendon cannot be salvaged because of extensive injury, insert a silicone rod (Hunter) beneath any pulley reconstruction as the first stage of a two-stage flexor tendon graft reconstruction.
- If the flexor tendon graft has ruptured or cannot be salvaged, insert a silicone rod as the first stage of a two-stage flexor tendon graft.
- If flexion contractures are present at the proximal and distal interphalangeal joints, release these by capsulotomy, usually by release of the proximal extensions of the palmar plate.
- Usually corticosteroids are not instilled.
- Sometimes, especially with comminuted fractures in which irregular bony surfaces are exposed, silicone sheeting has been interposed between the tendon and the bone and removed later after satisfactory motion has been established.

POSTOPERATIVE CARE A compression dressing is applied, usually with the fingers in mild flexion. Postoperative rehabilitation is begun with active motion on the first day after surgery. Indwelling catheters for pain control with local anesthetics rarely are used, although they can be helpful in controlling immediate postoperative pain.

■ ADHERENCE OF TENDONS

When a tendon completely adheres to bone, specific active movements of one or more joints distal to the area of adherence are lost. Specific passive movements also are limited because the adherent tendon acts as a checkrein. When a profundus tendon is stuck to the shaft of the proximal phalanx, the two distal finger joints cannot be flexed actively by this tendon; however, the proximal interphalangeal joint can be actively flexed by the sublimis tendon. The metacarpophalangeal joint also can be actively flexed by the profundus and sublimis tendons, along with the intrinsics. Adherence of the profundus tendon to the shaft of the proximal phalanx also checks full passive or active extension of the two distal finger joints. Active extension of the distal interphalangeal joint can be increased by passive flexion of the proximal interphalangeal joint; likewise, active extension of the proximal interphalangeal joint can be increased by passive flexion of the distal interphalangeal joint. Extension of the wrist can initiate flexion of the metacarpophalangeal joint through the adherent tendon.

▌ADHERENCE OF A TENDON TO A FRACTURE SITE

The adherence of a tendon to a fracture site usually is associated with (1) volar angulation of a phalangeal fracture after poor reduction, (2) external pressure against the tendon, forcing it against the fracture during healing, (3) crush injuries, or (4) laceration of the tendon sheath. A sublimis tendon usually adheres to the proximal phalanx, causing a flexion contracture of the proximal interphalangeal joint; a profundus tendon usually adheres to the middle phalanx, causing a flexion contracture of the distal interphalangeal joint. An extensor tendon usually adheres to the metacarpal shaft or proximal phalanx. Surgery may be indicated when the tendon fails to loosen by active exercise, as determined by measurements of motion of adjacent joints.

FREEING OF ADHERENT TENDON

TECHNIQUE 3.21

(HOWARD)
- Make a longitudinal incision parallel to the lateral margin of the involved metacarpal and away from any previous scar.
- Free the tendon from the bone and smooth the bone with a rasp or osteotome.
- Remove all scar tissue from the tendon.
- Place a Silastic sheet over the bone and anchor it with sutures at its corners (Fig. 3.56).

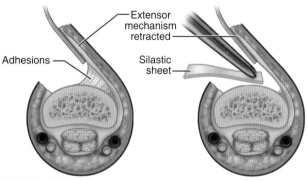

FIGURE 3.56 Howard technique to free adherent extensor tendon. **SEE TECHNIQUE 3.21.**

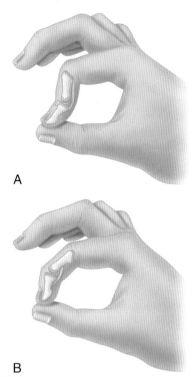

A

B

FIGURE 3.57   Tenodesis for irreparable damage to profundus tendon. **A,** Before tenodesis, distal interphalangeal joint is unstable and hyperextends during pinch. **B,** After tenodesis, joint is stable and remains partially flexed during pinch.

- Immobilize the part for 5 days and then begin voluntary motion. Improvement can be expected up to 1 year postoperatively.

TENODESIS

Tenodesis is useful when the profundus has been damaged, flexor tendon grafting is impossible, and the fingertip is more useful functionally when partially flexed and stabilized than when extended; this usually is true of the index finger (Fig. 3.57) and for other fingers in certain occupations as well. The operation is possible only when the distal stump of the profundus tendon is long enough to anchor proximal to the distal interphalangeal joint.

TECHNIQUE 3.22

- Make a midlateral incision (see Fig. 1.18) or volar oblique incision and identify the stump of the tendon.
- Flex the distal interphalangeal joint 30 degrees and note the length of profundus tendon required for tenodesis.
- Insert a Bunnell pull-out wire suture in the tendon and excise any redundant tendon (Fig. 3.58).
- With the joint in the desired position, insert a Kirschner wire obliquely across it and cut off the wire beneath the skin.

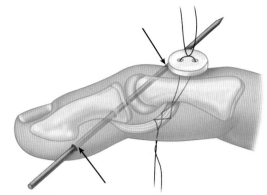

FIGURE 3.58   Technique of tenodesis (see text). Kirschner wire is cut off beneath skin at points indicated by arrows. **SEE TECHNIQUE 3.22.**

- At the level of intended tenodesis, roughen the bone of the middle phalanx with a dental chisel and then drill two small holes through it from anterior to posterior.
- On the palmar cortex, connect the holes and make a small cortical window with a small curet.
- With straight needles, thread the ends of the wires through the holes, leading the tendon into the cortical opening and through the dorsum of the finger, and tie them through a button over the middle phalanx. A pullout technique using the Bunnell retrograde or the antegrade technique usually is required.
- Bring the Bunnell pull-out wire through the volar surface of the finger.
- Close the wound with 5-0 nylon.
- Apply a bandage. Although external splinting usually is unnecessary, a small splint is good protection from postoperative bumping and pain.

POSTOPERATIVE CARE   The splint and sutures are removed at 10 to 14 days. The pull-out wire suture is removed at 4 weeks, and the Kirschner wire is removed at 5 or 6 weeks. Active motion of uninvolved fingers is encouraged. Heavy resistance activities are not begun for 6 to 8 weeks.

EXTENSOR TENDONS
ANATOMY

As traditionally described, the extensor tendons pass from the forearm onto the dorsum of the hand through the six compartments beneath the extensor retinaculum. From the radial (lateral) side to the ulnar (medial) side of the retinaculum, the compartments contain the following numbers of tendons: two, two, one, five, one, and one. The first compartment contains the extensor pollicis brevis and the abductor pollicis longus; the second, the extensors carpi radialis longus and brevis; the third, the extensor pollicis longus; the fourth, the four tendons of the extensor digitorum communis plus the extensor indicis proprius; the fifth, the extensor digiti quinti; and the sixth, the extensor carpi ulnaris. In a cadaver study, the anatomic patterns of the extensors to the fingers were further defined (Fig. 3.59). The most common patterns included

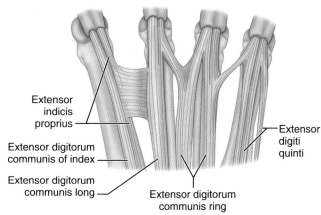

Extensor indicis proprius

Extensor digitorum communis of index

Extensor digitorum communis long

Extensor digitorum communis ring

Extensor digiti quinti

FIGURE 3.59 Most common pattern of extensor tendons on dorsum of hand: single extensor indicis proprius tendon, which inserts ulnar to extensor digitorum communis of index; single extensor digitorum communis of index; single extensor digitorum communis long; double extensor digitorum communis ring; absent extensor digitorum communis small; and double extensor digiti quinti with double insertion.

a single extensor indicis proprius inserting to the ulnar side of the index extensor digitorum communis, a single extensor digitorum communis to the index finger, a single extensor digitorum communis to the long finger, a double extensor digitorum communis to the ring finger, an absent extensor digitorum communis to the small finger, and a double extensor digiti quinti with double insertions.

Anatomic variations in the extensor tendons are common. In the first dorsal compartment, septation occurs in 20% to 60% of specimens. The abductor pollicis longus may have multiple slips in 56% to 98% of dissections. Common variations in the extensors to the fingers include a double extensor indicis proprius, double or triple extensor digitorum communis to the long finger, single or triple extensor digitorum communis to the ring finger, and single or double extensor digitorum communis to the small finger. Variations in the juncturae tendinum have been classified into three major types (Fig. 3.60).

EXAMINATION

An extensor tendon (Fig. 3.61) is presumed to be divided between the proximal and distal interphalangeal joints when active extension of the distal interphalangeal joint is lost. Initially, a gross mallet finger deformity may be absent because the surrounding capsule and other soft tissues have not yet been stretched by the strong flexor digitorum profundus. The division of the central slip of an extensor tendon between the metacarpophalangeal and proximal interphalangeal joints results in loss of extension of the proximal interphalangeal joint only after the lateral bands subluxate anteriorly. Because the metacarpophalangeal and distal interphalangeal joints may be actively extended, this lesion is easily overlooked during the initial examination. When the entire extensor expansion, including the lateral bands, is divided at this level, extension of the joints distal to the wound is lost; such a lesion is unlikely, however, because the expansion covers a convex surface of bone, which usually blocks the injuring object before the division is complete. When the extensor tendon is divided just proximal to the metacarpophalangeal joint, the

two distal finger joints can be extended by the lateral bands and their connecting transverse fibers, but extension of the metacarpophalangeal joint is incomplete. Partial or complete extension of the finger may be possible when a single extensor tendon is divided at the wrist because of the presence of accessory communicating tendons (juncturae tendinum), as shown in Figure 3.60.

When checking the long extensor tendon of the thumb, the examiner must stabilize the metacarpophalangeal joint and must test carefully for active extension of the interphalangeal joint and active retropulsion of the thumb toward the dorsum of the hand. Division of this tendon often is overlooked because an intact short thumb extensor can actively extend the thumb as a unit. Although the short thumb extensor cannot extend the interphalangeal joint alone, the thumb intrinsic muscles assist with interphalangeal extension in some patients.

EXTENSOR TENDON REPAIR

To emphasize the different anatomic relationships of the extensor tendons and their attachments, the extensor surface of the hand has been divided into eight zones (Fig. 3.62). Even-numbered zones are over bones; odd-numbered zones are over joints; the forearm area of extensor muscle bellies is considered as a ninth zone. The acute (primary) and chronic (delayed, secondary) management of the extensor tendon injuries within each zone are discussed together. Similarly, extensor tendon ruptures, excluding ruptures in rheumatoid arthritis, are discussed within their individual zones. For additional discussion of extensor tendon ruptures, see chapter 10.

■ ZONE I

Zone I is at the level of the distal interphalangeal joint. Mallet finger deformities usually result from closed avulsion of the insertion of the tendon, sometimes with a small bone fragment, and can be treated by splinting alone (see the subsequent discussion of mallet finger). An open transection of the central slip insertion at the distal phalanx usually is repaired with a roll stitch (see Fig. 3.21), or a dermotenodermal suture, and protected with a small transarticular Kirschner wire.

▍ EXTENSOR TENDON RUPTURE

For a closed extensor tendon rupture from its insertion into the distal phalanx, the treatment usually is nonsurgical. The distal interphalangeal joint is constantly held in hyperextension on a splint (Fig. 3.63) for 6 to 8 weeks and at night only for 2 to 4 additional weeks; this allows the tendon to heal, prevents stretching when the splint is removed, and usually provides a satisfactory result. The last degrees of extreme flexion of the distal joint may be lost; however, the flexion posture of the joint usually is corrected. Splint treatment within 2 weeks of injury has been found to be as effective as splinting more than 4 weeks after injury. This treatment can be successful in some patients 3 months after injury (see discussion of treatment of chronic mallet finger subsequently). High patient satisfaction was reported at an average of 5 years after splint treatment of mallet deformities, with and without fracture. Osteoarthritic changes, seen in 48%, were usually associated with fractures. For a discussion of mallet finger deformities caused by fractures of the distal phalanx, see chapter 4.

Mallet finger deformities in children may be caused by traumatic separation of the epiphysis (Fig. 3.64). These deformities can be readily recognized with radiographs. Early

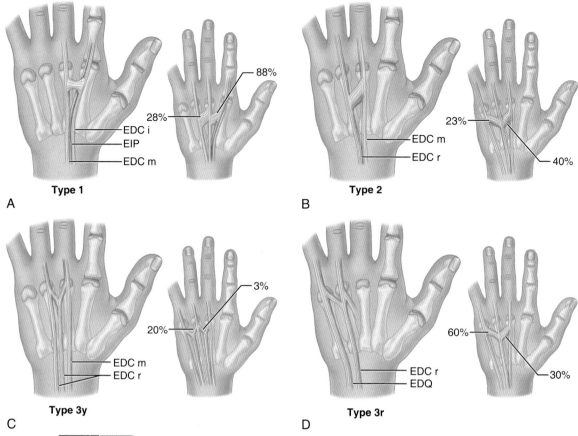

FIGURE 3.60 Juncturae tendinum. **A,** Type 1 (thin filamentous type) between extensor digitorum communis *(EDC)* tendons of long *(EDC m)* and index *(EDC i)* fingers; juncturae did not connect to extensor indicis proprius *(EIP)* tendon. Numbers on right indicate incidence of type 1 juncturae in second and third intermetacarpal spaces. There were no type 1 juncturae present in any other spaces. **B,** Type 2 (thicker) juncturae between EDC tendons of ring *(EDC r)* and *(EDC m)* fingers. Incidences of type 2 juncturae in third and fourth intermetacarpal spaces are shown on right; they were not present in any other spaces. **C,** Type 3 (subtype y), in which Y-shaped tendon and juncturae appear as split tendon inserting into two adjacent digits, between EDC r and EDC m fingers. Incidences of type 3y juncturae in third and fourth intermetacarpal spaces are shown on right; they were not present in any other spaces. **D,** Type 3 (subtype r), more oblique R-shaped juncturae between EDC to EDC r and most radial of three extensor digitorum quinti *(EDQ)* tendons to small finger. Most frequent orientation and incidences of type 3r juncturae in third and fourth intermetacarpal spaces are shown on right; they were not present in any other spaces.

detection usually allows straightforward reduction with hyperextension of the distal interphalangeal joint. The finger is splinted for 3 to 4 weeks, and healing is rapid compared with injury of the extensor tendon itself. Growth disturbance is possible but rare.

ACUTE TRANSECTION OF EXTENSOR TENDON

Treatment of an open injury of the extensor tendon insertion requires repair of the tendon. Extension of the skin laceration proximally may be required to grasp the tendon and mobilize it to its insertion, where a roll suture (see Fig. 3.21) or dermotenodermal suture usually is sufficient to hold the insertion for healing. The repair can be protected with a transarticular Kirschner wire. The wound is closed, and the finger is temporarily splinted for comfort and to avoid additional trauma. The suture is removed after approximately 3 weeks,

the Kirschner wire is removed at approximately 4 weeks, and the finger is splinted for an additional 4 weeks to protect the repair. Progressive motion exercises are begun and continued until maximal function has been achieved.

CHRONIC MALLET FINGER (SECONDARY REPAIR)

A mallet finger caused by avulsion of the extensor tendon from the distal phalanx can be satisfactorily treated by splinting 12 weeks after injury, as described for an acute injury. Prolonged splinting and splinting longer than 12 weeks may be successful; the duration of splinting may be limited by the patient's tolerance of the splinting. After 12 weeks, if

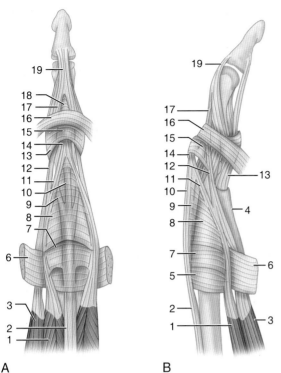

FIGURE 3.61 Anatomy of extensor apparatus of fingers. **A,** Dorsal. **B,** Lateral. *1,* interosseous muscle; *2,* extensor digitorum communis tendon; *3,* lumbrical muscle; *4,* flexor tendon sheath; *5,* sagittal bands; *6,* transverse metacarpal ligament; *7,* interosseous hood; *8,* interosseous hood, oblique fibers; *9,* extensor lateral band; *10,* extensor middle band; *11,* interosseous middle band; *12,* interosseous lateral band; *13,* oblique retinacular ligament; *14,* central extensor tendon; *15,* spiral fibers; *16,* transverse retinacular ligament; *17,* lateral extensor tendon; *18,* triangular lamina; *19,* terminal extensor tendon.

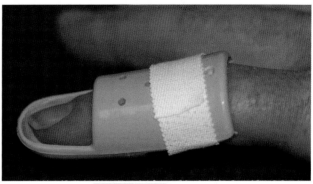

FIGURE 3.63 Stack splint.

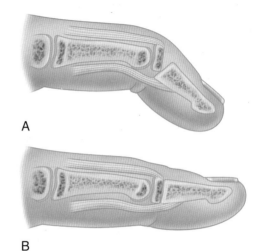

FIGURE 3.64 **A,** Displacement of epiphysis of distal phalanx can cause digit to assume mallet finger posture. **B,** Hyperextension of phalanx usually affords satisfactory reduction of displaced epiphysis.

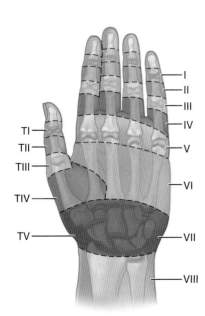

FIGURE 3.62 Indications for surgery of extensor tendon lacerations vary according to level of pathologic condition; various zones have been designated.

the distal phalanx droops severely, but passive extension in the distal interphalangeal joint still is satisfactory, surgery may be indicated, depending on the patient's needs.

TECHNIQUE 3.23

- Make a small V-shaped or U-shaped incision, convex distally, with the tip no closer than 5 mm proximal to the nail base on the dorsum of the finger. Avoid injury to the germinal matrix of the nail.
- Develop the flap gently in the plane between the tendon and the subcutaneous fat. Elevate the flap proximally to expose the extensor tendon with its intervening scar.
- Attempt to identify the junction of the normal tendon with the scar and sever the tendon transversely proximal to the joint, leaving the insertion of the tendon into bone.
- Resect sufficient scar or tendon to allow closure of the gap with the finger in maximal extension.
- To support and protect the repair, immobilize the joint with a transarticular 0.045-inch Kirschner wire.
- Repair the extensor tendon with 4-0 monofilament nylon or 4-0 monofilament wire as a pull-out roll stitch (see Fig. 3.21). No additional sutures are required.

- Close the skin with interrupted 5-0 nylon. As an alternative, use 4-0 nylon as a dermotenodermal suture.
- Maintain the finger in extension and apply a compressive dressing. Support the finger with a volar splint for postoperative comfort and to avoid reinjury in the recovery period.

POSTOPERATIVE CARE The sutures are removed at 10 to 14 days, and the distal joint is maintained in extension, with the Kirschner wire protected by a small metal splint, for 4 weeks. The Kirschner wire is removed after 4 to 6 weeks, and the repair is protected with a splint for 8 weeks. Normal activities are progressively resumed.

CHRONIC MALLET FINGER (SECONDARY REPAIR)

TECHNIQUE 3.24

(FOWLER)
- Make a midlateral finger incision (see Fig. 1.17) from just distal to the proximal interphalangeal joint to a point level with the middle of the proximal phalanx.
- Open the deep tissues until the edge of the lateral band of the extensor hood is located.
- Elevate this edge with a small hook and, with the finger in extension, continue elevating the expansion until the deep surface of the central slip is exposed at the proximal interphalangeal joint.
- Elevate the entire extensor hood from the proximal phalanx.
- Using the point of a No. 11 Bard-Parker knife blade and beginning on the deep surface of the central slip, free the insertion of the central slip from the proximal edge of the middle phalanx (Fig. 3.65). Releasing this central slip allows the entire extensor mechanism to displace proximally; the tension increases on the distal end and is transmitted to the avulsed tendon where the tendon has become too long after healing to the distal phalanx by scar.
- Close the wound with interrupted 5-0 nylon suture, apply a compressive dressing, and protect the finger with a splint for postoperative comfort.

POSTOPERATIVE CARE The sutures are removed at 10 to 14 days, and the splint is maintained with the proximal interphalangeal joint in no more than 30 degrees of flexion and the distal joint in extension. Prevention of acute flexion of the proximal interphalangeal joint prevents the capsule of the joint from being torn after release of the central slip. The splint is removed at 3 weeks, and another splint is applied to immobilize the distal interphalangeal joint. The distal interphalangeal joint is held in extension for 4 additional weeks on a small metal splint, allowing full motion of the proximal interphalangeal and metacarpophalangeal joints.

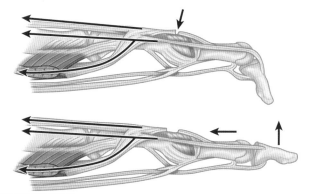

FIGURE 3.65   Tenotomy of central slip (Fowler procedure) to correct mallet finger; this results in proximal retraction of extensor apparatus. **SEE TECHNIQUE 3.24.**

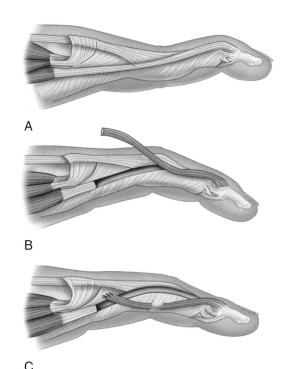

A

B

C

FIGURE 3.66   Technique of correcting recurrent hyperextension and locking of proximal interphalangeal joint. **A,** Lateral view of extensor hood and flexor tendon sheath. **B,** One lateral band of hood has been detached proximally. **C,** Detached band has been threaded through small pulley made in flexor tendon sheath opposite proximal interphalangeal joint and has been sutured to hood under enough tension to create slight flexion contracture of joint. **SEE TECHNIQUE 3.25.**

CORRECTION OF AN OLD MALLET FINGER DEFORMITY BY TENDON TRANSFER OR TENDON GRAFT

The technique used to correct hyperextension locking deformity in the proximal interphalangeal joint by transferring a lateral band of the extensor mechanism also can be used to correct an old mallet finger deformity when passive motion is satisfactory and any arthritic changes in the distal joint are no worse than moderate (Fig. 3.66). Successful treatment of posttraumatic mallet deformities has been reported with reconstruction of the oblique retinacular ligament with a palmaris tendon graft passed from the distal phalanx proximally along the path of the oblique retinacular ligament, spiraling volar to the flexor tendon sheath between the neurovascular bundle and the flexor sheath, across to the opposite side of the proximal phalanx volar to the proximal interphalangeal joint and secured to the base of the proximal phalanx through a drill hole using a pull-out technique (the spiral oblique retinacular ligament).

TENDON TRANSFER FOR CORRECTION OF OLD MALLET FINGER DEFORMITY

TECHNIQUE 3.25

(MILFORD)
- Make a lateral incision on the least scarred side of the digit and expose the extensor mechanism and the flexor sheath (Fig. 3.66A).
- Detach one lateral band just beyond the metacarpophalangeal joint of the finger and dissect it loose entirely to its insertion distally (Fig. 3.66B).
- Make a small pulley by opening the flexor tendon sheath with two parallel incisions opposite the proximal interphalangeal joint.
- Pass the lateral band of tendon slip from distal to proximal through the pulley, bringing the end to be sutured to the extensor hood a bit dorsal to its original position on the lateral side of the extensor mechanism (Fig. 3.66C).
- Correct tension on this transfer is essential and holds the proximal interphalangeal joint slightly flexed while the distal joint is fully extended.
- Protect this repair with a transarticular 0.045-inch Kirschner wire obliquely placed across the proximal interphalangeal joint.
- Close the wound with interrupted 5-0 nylon suture and apply a conforming, compressing dressing, supporting the finger, hand, and wrist with a volar plaster splint over adequate padding for postoperative comfort and protection.

POSTOPERATIVE CARE The sutures are removed at 10 to 14 days. At 4 weeks, the transarticular Kirschner wire is removed. Between exercise periods the finger is protected with a volar removable splint, which should be worn at night and during the day except for exercise periods. Wearing of this splint can be discontinued after about 8 weeks, and gradual improvement in motion may progress.

TENDON GRAFT FOR CORRECTION OF OLD MALLET FINGER DEFORMITY

TECHNIQUE 3.26

- Make a dorsal angular incision exposing the distal phalanx and short midradial and midulnar incisions to approach

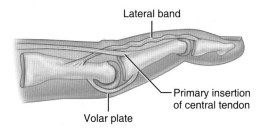
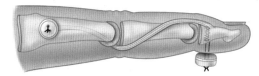
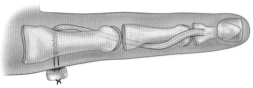

FIGURE 3.67 Palmaris longus tenodesis for oblique retinacular ligament reconstruction for swan-neck deformity, called the spiral oblique retinacular ligament. Pathologic condition of swan-neck deformity involves hyperextension of proximal interphalangeal joint with extensor lag at distal joint, combined with laxity of volar plate. Palmaris longus can be used to provide tenodesis to correct imbalance at both joints. **SEE TECHNIQUE 3.26.**

the radial side of the proximal interphalangeal joint and the ulnar aspect of the proximal phalanx (Fig. 3.67).
- Make a vertical hole in the distal phalanx between the extensor tendon insertion and the nail germinal matrix using a small, sharp gouge.
- Use a hemostat for gentle blunt dissection proximally along the radial side of the middle phalanx following the lateral band, passing dorsal to the Cleland ligament to the proximal interphalangeal joint, and create a tunnel that spirals to the palmar surface between the neurovascular bundles and the volar surface of the flexor sheath, exiting through the ulnar incision at the base of the proximal phalanx.
- Make a transverse hole through the base of the proximal phalanx volar to the lateral band, passing from the ulnar side to the radial side.
- Harvest a palmaris or plantaris tendon graft (Fig. 3.46).
- Use a 22-gauge or smaller stainless steel wire placed through the holes in the bone and along the tunnel that spirals from the distal phalanx along the radial side and volar to the flexor sheath to guide the tendon graft into its appropriate position.
- Apply longitudinal tension to the proximal end of the graft and demonstrate that the distal and the proximal interphalangeal joints will be extended.
- Secure the distal bony attachment of the tendon to the distal phalanx using an antegrade pull-out wire technique over a felt-and-button gently applied to the pulp of the distal phalanx. Set the tension on the graft by adjusting it with the proximal and the distal interphalangeal joints at neutral extension, and secure the proximal free ends

of the tendon graft with a button-over-felt applied to the radial side over the base of the proximal phalanx. With these attachments, passive extension of the proximal interphalangeal joint should show full passive extension of the distal interphalangeal joint with a tenodesis effect.

- Take care in adjusting the tension on the tendon graft to avoid excessive pull, which can cause proximal interphalangeal joint flexion and distal interphalangeal joint extension, or a boutonniere posture. If necessary, transfix the proximal interphalangeal joint in extension with a 0.045-inch Kirschner wire to protect the tenodesis.
- Immobilize the hand with the wrist slightly extended, the metacarpophalangeal joint flexed, and the proximal and distal interphalangeal joints fully extended.
- Apply a well-padded volar plaster splint for postoperative comfort and protection.

POSTOPERATIVE CARE The sutures are removed at 10 to 14 days. At about 4 weeks, Kirschner wires are removed, and the affected digit is protected with a dorsal splint that holds the proximal interphalangeal joint in 20 degrees of flexion and the distal interphalangeal joint at neutral. The pull-out wires are removed at approximately 3 weeks. Active-assisted flexion exercises are begun after removal of the Kirschner wires (approximately 4 weeks), and hyperextension is avoided beyond a position of about 20 degrees of flexion. From 6 to 10 weeks after surgery, the protective splint gradually is extended 5 to 10 degrees. Stretching of the proximal interphalangeal joint beyond 5 to 10 degrees of flexion should be avoided.

■ ZONE II

Zone II is the area over the middle phalanx. The flat tendon in this area may limit the suture configuration. Lateral tendons lacerated proximal to the insertion can be sutured with a figure-of-eight mattress stitch or a roll stitch (see Fig. 3.21). The Kleinert modification of the Bunnell suture (Fig. 3.68) and the modified Kessler sutures are stronger than a figure-of-eight or mattress suture for repair of extensor tendons in zone II. A continuous suture reinforced with a Silfverskiöld cross-stitch (see Fig. 3.9) provides a strong repair as well.

■ ZONE III

Zone III is the area of the proximal interphalangeal joint.

▌RUPTURE OR ACUTE TRANSECTION OF THE CENTRAL SLIP OF THE EXTENSOR EXPANSION (BOUTONNIERE DEFORMITY)

Rupture or laceration of the central slip of the extensor expansion at or near its insertion results in loss of active extension of the proximal interphalangeal joint and consequently

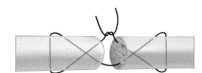

FIGURE 3.68   Kleinert modification of Bunnell crisscross suture technique.

persistent flexion of the joint. If left untreated, the collateral ligaments and volar plate of the proximal interphalangeal joint become contracted. The lateral bands of the extensor expansion subluxate volarward and are held there by the transverse retinacular ligaments, which also become contracted. This results in an established boutonniere deformity. The lateral bands, because they lie volar to the transverse axis of rotation of the proximal interphalangeal joint, act as flexors of the joint. The contracted oblique retinacular ligaments and the lateral bands force the distal interphalangeal joint into hyperextension, which may be increased by any attempt to extend the proximal interphalangeal joint passively.

Buttonholing also can be caused by traumatic rotation of a digit at the proximal interphalangeal joint while partially flexed. Rotation can cause a condyle of the proximal phalanx to protrude through the capsule and disrupt the triangular ligament area between the lateral band and the central tendon. This condylar herniation can cause a volar subluxation of the lateral band. A rupture of the extensor mechanism occurs, but the central tendon may not separate completely. The collateral ligament may be partially disrupted, and there may be an accompanying dislocation of the proximal interphalangeal joint. After such an injury, the proximal interphalangeal joint cannot be fully extended because of hemorrhage and swelling. The joint remains in its flexed position, and the subluxated lateral band contracts, allowing the transverse retinacular ligament also to contract, securely holding the subluxated lateral band. With anterior dislocation of the proximal interphalangeal joint, complete rupture of the central slip and lateral ligament may occur (Fig. 3.69).

Boutonniere deformities that are diagnosed early in closed wounds before fixed contractures occur can be treated conservatively. If the patient can show some active extension of the proximal interphalangeal joint, this suggests that an incompletely ruptured central slip may be present. Conservative treatment consists of splinting the proximal interphalangeal joint in full extension while permitting the distal interphalangeal joint to be actively flexed. Excessive pressure leading to skin necrosis over the proximal interphalangeal joint area should be avoided. Extension should be maintained around the clock for 4 to 6 weeks and continued nightly for several more weeks. When a boutonniere deformity is traumatic, and the diagnosis of complete rupture, transection, or laceration of the central slip can be made, it should be exposed surgically and repaired.

REPAIR OF CENTRAL SLIP OF THE EXTENSOR EXPANSION CAUSING BOUTONNIERE DEFORMITY

TECHNIQUE 3.27

- Expose the extensor mechanism dorsally with a lazy-S or bayonet incision.
- Place the proximal interphalangeal joint in full extension and hold it in this position with a 0.045-inch Kirschner wire inserted obliquely across the joint.
- Repair the disruption of the central slip with a roll stitch of 4-0 monofilament nylon or wire. If there is sufficient ten-

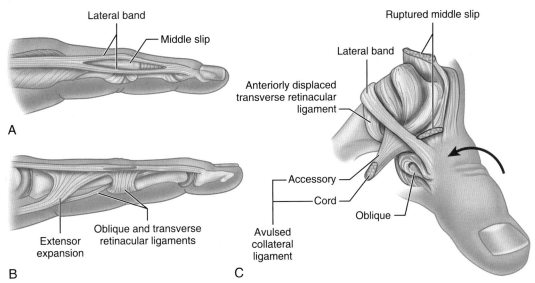

FIGURE 3.69 **A** and **B**, Dorsolateral and lateral views of extensor mechanism. **C**, Anterior dislocation of proximal interphalangeal joint with rupture of middle slip, avulsed collateral ligament, and partial tear of distal fibers of transverse retinacular ligament. Lateral band is displaced anteriorly.

don, use a core suture, supplemented with a Silfverskiöld cross-stitch (see Fig. 3.9). If there is an insufficient insertion, a suture anchor may provide satisfactory attachment of the central slip to the middle phalanx.

- Close the wound and apply a volar splint over a gently compressing dressing.

POSTOPERATIVE CARE The sutures are removed at 10 to 14 days, the transarticular wire is removed at 3 to 4 weeks, and gradual protected flexion is allowed. A volar splint is worn to protect the repair for an additional 4 weeks except for exercise. Evans reported better results in patients who began a program of early "short arc" exercises 2 to 11 days after central slip repair compared with patients who had 3 to 6 weeks of continuous postoperative immobilization. This technique may be considered in patients who do not require transarticular wire stabilization and whose injuries and compliance permit.

CHRONIC BOUTONNIERE DEFORMITY (SECONDARY REPAIR AND RECONSTRUCTION)

In neglected, undiagnosed, or chronic boutonniere deformity, the central slip of extensor expansion has retracted and the lateral bands loosen and subluxate volarward after their dorsal transverse retaining fibers have stretched additionally. This subluxation allows the proximal interphalangeal joint to flex, the lateral bands become contracted, and a fixed flexion contracture of the proximal interphalangeal joint with hyperextension of the distal interphalangeal joint occurs (Fig. 3.70A). Before any surgical procedure, splinting and stretching should be done to relieve contractures of the proximal and distal interphalangeal joints. Reconstruction after rupture or laceration of the central slip of the extensor expansion is difficult and requires a precise and extensive procedure to restore the function of the damaged central slip and to release the associated

contractures. For the boutonniere deformity with a flexible proximal interphalangeal joint, the Fowler/Dolphin tenotomy of lateral bands distal to the central slip insertion may restore proximal interphalangeal joint extension and allow distal interphalangeal joint flexion (Fig. 3.71). A variety of techniques have been described for reconstructing the extensor mechanism, including the central slip flap of Snow (Fig. 3.72), the lateral band flaps of Aiache (Fig. 3.73), the lateral band relocation of Matev, and the dorsal shift of the lateral bands of Littler, described here. Tendon grafts may be necessary if there is a significant segmental defect in the extensor mechanism. If the joint has significant arthrosis, proximal interphalangeal joint arthrodesis or arthroplasty may be considered.

RECONSTRUCTION OF THE EXTENSOR MECHANISM FOR CHRONIC BOUTONNIERE DEFORMITY

TECHNIQUE 3.28

(LITTLER, MODIFIED)
- Make a dorsal curved incision centered over the proximal interphalangeal joint (Fig. 3.70B), exposing the lateral bands.
- Using the point of a probe, dissect deep to each transverse retinacular ligament from its origin near the volar plate to its insertion on the border of the lateral band.
- Using small scissors, divide each transverse retinacular ligament near its midportion.
- Free the insertions of the lateral band so that they can be replaced dorsally.
- On the radial side, separate with sharp dissection, leaving intact the radial fibers of the lateral band representing

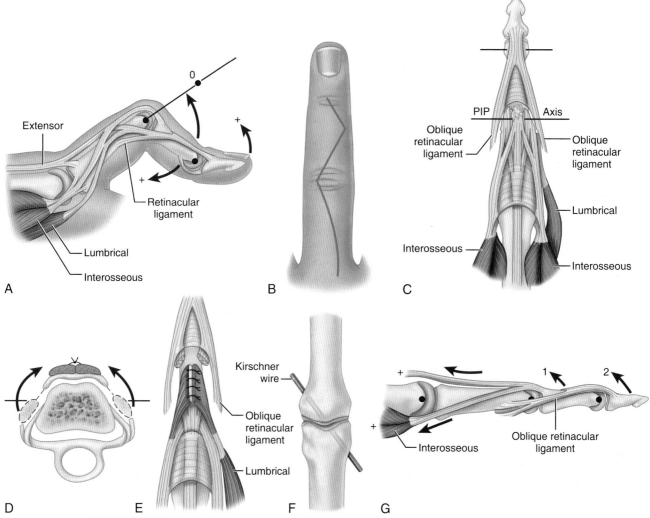

FIGURE 3.70 Littler technique for repair of old boutonniere deformity. **A,** Typical deformity with flexion of proximal interphalangeal joint and extension of distal interphalangeal joint. Lateral bands have subluxated volarward. **B,** Dorsal curved longitudinal incision is made. **C,** Insertions of lateral bands are completely freed except for radialmost fibers of radial lateral band. **D** and **E,** Lateral bands are shifted dorsally and proximally and are sutured together and to soft tissues over proximal third of middle phalanx and to central tendon. **F,** Proximal interphalangeal joint (PIP) is fixed in full extension by Kirschner wire. **G,** After repair, proximal interphalangeal joint is extended by extensor hood and distal interphalangeal joint by preserved lumbrical muscle and oblique retinacular ligament. **SEE TECHNIQUE 3.28.**

the contribution of the lumbrical muscles and the oblique retinacular ligament.
- This should preserve active extension of the distal interphalangeal joint.
- At this point, the insertions of the lateral band should be completely free except for the radialmost fibers of the radial lateral band (Fig. 3.70C).
- Shift the bands dorsally and proximally and suture them to the soft tissue and periosteum over the proximal third of the middle phalanx (Fig. 3.70D and E).
- Suture them to the attenuated central tendon with the proximal interphalangeal joint held in full extension.
- Support the repair with a transarticular 0.045-inch Kirschner wire obliquely placed across the joint (Fig. 3.70F).

- Leave the divided transverse retinacular ligaments unsutured.
- Close the wound with 5-0 interrupted monofilament nylon suture.
- Use a volar splint for immediate postoperative protection and comfort.

POSTOPERATIVE CARE The sutures are removed at 10 to 14 days. At 3 to 4 weeks, the transarticular Kirschner wire is removed, and protected motion is allowed. A volar splint is used on the finger to protect the proximal interphalangeal joint, allowing distal interphalangeal flexion for another 4 weeks. This splint is worn during the day and night and is removed for exercise three to four times daily.

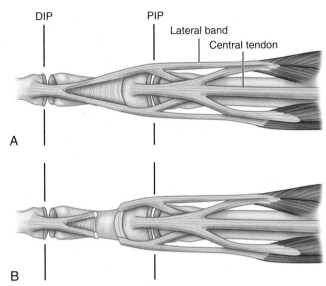

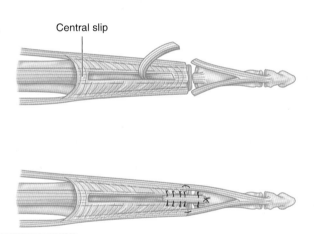

FIGURE 3.71 Extensor tenotomy for supple boutonniere deformity. **A** and **B,** Lateral bands are released distal to insertion of central slips. The resulting lateral proximal migration of extensor mechanism reduces tension at distal interphalangeal joint *(DIP)* and increases extensor tension at proximal interphalangeal joint *(PIP).*

FIGURE 3.72 Severed extensor mechanism over proximal interphalangeal joint *(above)*; retrograde flap of central slip has been elevated. After suture of severed central slip and lateral bands, retrograde flap is brought over juncture as batten.

■ ZONE IV

Zone IV includes the area over the proximal phalanx. Lacerations over the proximal phalanx may cause an incomplete injury to the tendon because of the broad tendon covering the phalanx. If full active proximal interphalangeal joint extension is present, closed treatment with splinting may suffice. If proximal interphalangeal joint extension is limited, exploration of the wound is needed to determine the extent of injury. A core stitch of the modified Bunnell configuration of Kleinert or the modified Kessler stitch, reinforced with a cross-stitch (see Fig. 3.9), provides a strong repair and does not shorten the tendon, according to Newport et al. Postoperative extension splinting is maintained for 6 to 8 weeks, and a "short arc" range-of-motion rehabilitation program may be started.

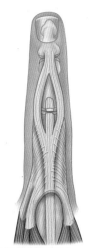
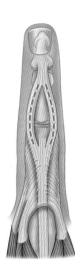
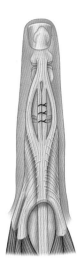

FIGURE 3.73 Injury to middle slip. Lateral bands are freed, and oblique and transverse retinacular ligaments are elevated from middle phalanx *(left)*. Each lateral band is slit longitudinally into two parts *(center)*. Medial halves of lateral bands are sutured together and to capsule in midline *(right)*.

■ ZONE V

Zone V includes the area at the metacarpophalangeal joint. For a clean laceration, repair of the tendon with a core suture reinforced with a cross-stitch is indicated. If the tendon injury occurs as the result of a tooth injury, repair of the tendon is delayed until it is clear that there are no septic complications, or until the infection is controlled.

▮ TRAUMATIC DISLOCATION OF THE EXTENSOR TENDON AT THE METACARPOPHALANGEAL JOINT

Traumatic dislocation of the extensor tendon toward the ulnar aspect of the metacarpophalangeal joint occurs most commonly in the long finger. The dislocation usually occurs as a result of a tear in the proximal radial portion of the shroud ligament (sagittal bands) and the more proximal fascia as the finger is suddenly extended against a force, as in a flicking or thumping motion. Ulnar side disruption with radial displacement of the tendon is rare. More violent mechanisms may cause collateral ligament and joint surface injury. If seen within the first few days, this dislocation can be treated effectively with splinting of the metacarpophalangeal joint and wrist in extension for 3 to 4 weeks, followed by 3 to 4 weeks of removable splinting or buddy taping to the adjacent finger on the radial side in the case of ulnar displacement. A relative-motion splint technique, which allows immediate controlled active motion, can be used in select patients. Merritt also reported its use after sagittal band injuries and after repair of closed extensor tendon ruptures in patients with rheumatoid arthritis (Fig. 3.74). If the condition goes undetected and becomes chronic, a repair using a section of the central fibers of the extensor mechanism at the metacarpophalangeal joint can be successful. Rayan and Murray described three clinical types of sagittal band injuries (Fig. 3.75): type I injuries show no extensor instability, type II injuries are injuries with extensor tendon subluxation, and type III injuries have extensor tendon dislocation. In their series of 28 nonrheumatoid patients, those treated within 3 weeks of injury achieved satisfactory results with nonoperative splinting. Patients with more severe or chronic involvement frequently required operative treatment.

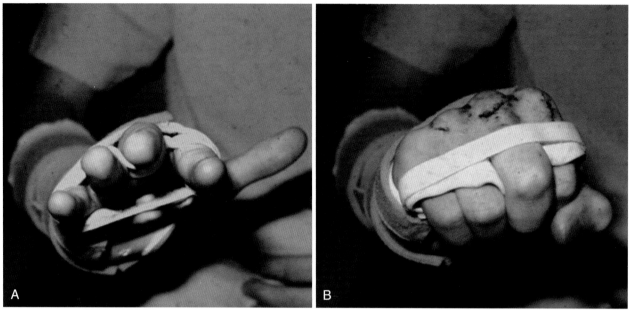

FIGURE 3.74   Immediate active motion after long finger extensor repair. **A,** Wrist is splinted for 3 weeks. **B,** Finger is splinted for 6 weeks.

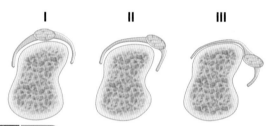

FIGURE 3.75   Three types of sagittal band injury. Type I, mild injury with no instability; type II, moderate injury with extensor tendon subluxation; type III, severe injury with tendon dislocation.

REPAIR OF TRAUMATIC DISLOCATION OF THE EXTENSOR TENDON

TECHNIQUE 3.29

- Use of an intravenous regional block or local infiltration anesthetic allows the patient to attempt active extension of the finger before wound closure to ensure that the extensor tendon remains centralized.
- Make a curved incision on the radial side of the metacarpophalangeal joint to expose the joint and the subluxating extensor tendon.
- Release the ulnar sagittal band if it is contracted.
- Direct repair of the radial sagittal band may be possible, although it may require reinforcement.
- Several methods can be used to recentralize the extensor tendon. In one method, create a loop by removing a 5-cm lateral margin of the central tendon at this level, leaving the distal insertion of this segment attached.
- Pass the proximal segment through a small window made with vertical incisions in the capsule and through the

superficial portion of the joint capsule, and suture the proximal end to the extensor tendon. In some patients, the extensor tendon can be found "shucked" from the dorsum of the sagittal band. In these patients, the tendon can be reattached to its bed with three or four 4-0 nonabsorbable sutures.

- Otherwise, fashion a narrow slip (3- to 4-mm) of the sagittal band vertical fibers by making vertical parallel incisions from dorsal to palmar on the radial side to create a strip about 8 mm long, based dorsally.
- Pass this slip dorsally through a narrow slit in the extensor tendon and suture the slip back on itself with two or three 4-0 nonabsorbable sutures.
- The technique of Carroll et al. includes release of the ulnar sagittal band and elevation of a distally based tendon strip from the ulnar side of the extensor digitorum communis.
- Make the strip long enough to pass beneath the radial side of the extensor digitorum communis, dorsal to the joint, deep to the radial collateral ligament, and dorsally again to suture it to the extensor digitorum communis tendon dorsally (Fig. 3.76).
- Adjustment of the tension is essential to maintain the central alignment of the subluxating extensor tendon and to allow flexion of the metacarpophalangeal joint.
- Close the wound and apply a splint to maintain the finger in radial deviation to prevent ulnar deviation and to prevent metacarpophalangeal joint flexion.

POSTOPERATIVE CARE The sutures are removed after 10 to 14 days, and the splint is maintained with the metacarpophalangeal joint extended for 4 weeks. A removable splint is applied to block metacarpophalangeal joint flexion, leaving the proximal interphalangeal free to move. Gradual improvement of motion is allowed, and the finger is taped to the adjacent radial-side finger to protect the repair. Protected motion and splinting are maintained for

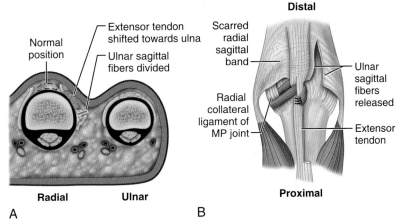

FIGURE 3.76 **A,** Cross section of metacarpal head in which ulnar subluxation of extensor tendon is shown. **B,** Ulnar-based loop formed from extensor tendon passed in distal-to-proximal direction around radial collateral ligament and sutured to extensor tendon. *MP,* Metacarpophalangeal. **SEE TECHNIQUE 3.29.**

about 8 weeks, and a gradual increase in activities is allowed thereafter. Casting may be required for 4 weeks to maintain extension of the metacarpophalangeal joint in uncooperative or noncompliant patients or patients with limited ability to understand or in a poor social situation. The relative-motion splint has been shown to work well from the postoperative period to 8 weeks in select patients (see Fig. 3.74).

■ ZONE VI

Zone VI is the area of the metacarpals of the fingers. Wounds should be explored in patients who cannot hyperextend the metacarpophalangeal joint even though weak active extension may be present. Intact adjacent tendons pulling through the juncturae tendinum and the presence of intact proprius tendons to the index and small fingers may conceal a complete transection of extensor tendons in zone VI. Adequate exposure is required to retrieve tendons that may retract proximally. The size and diameter of the tendons over the metacarpals permits the use of a 3-0 or 4-0 core suture with an epitendinous suture. Considering the studies of extensor tendon repair techniques, either the Becker repair or the Kleinert modification of the Bunnell repair should provide sufficient resistance to gap formation, while permitting metacarpophalangeal and proximal interphalangeal joint motion. Postoperatively, continuous dynamic splinting or static followed by dynamic splinting is used for 6 to 8 weeks.

■ ZONE VII

Zone VII is the area of the wrist under the dorsal carpal ligament (extensor retinaculum). At this level, the tendons have mesotenon. They are retained by the dorsal carpal ligament, which acts as a pulley, and are ensheathed in fibroosseous canals similar to the digital flexor sheath. More extensive incisions and dissection may be required to retrieve lacerated tendons because they tend to retract proximally into the forearm. Primary repair of extensor tendons here can be done with a 3-0 or 4-0 core suture, supplemented with a circumferential epitendinous suture. Access to the tendons may require

elevation of the extensor retinaculum. A straightforward removal of the proximal or distal portion of the retinaculum may allow sufficient exposure of the tendons for repair, while preserving sufficient retinaculum to avoid bowstringing of the tendons. Using another method, the extensor retinaculum is opened with a Z-lengthening incision, which allows repair of the retinaculum over the tendon repairs. Splinting the wrist after repair in a position of moderate extension instead of full extension helps limit the bowstring effect. Tendons repaired in this zone may become stuck in their canals as they heal.

The relative-motion splint, with or without immobilization of the wrist, has been reported to facilitate normal extensor tendon function and reduce the risk of morbidity to the adjacent digits after repairs in zones IV through VII. The splint places the repaired tendon(s) in 15 to 20 degrees greater metacarpophalangeal joint extension than adjacent digits for a continuous 6-week period. The wrist is placed in a separate splint at approximately 20 to 25 degrees of extension for 3 weeks to avoid tension on the suture (see Fig. 3.74). The goal is to recover full flexion and extension of the interphalangeal and metacarpophalangeal joints as soon as possible after repair.

■ ZONE VIII

Zone VIII is the area of the distal forearm, proximal to the extensor retinaculum (dorsal carpal ligament). In this zone, many extensor tendons are covered by their respective muscles. Careful dissection is required to identify the proximal portion of the muscle belly, which is appropriate for attachment of the tendon. The tendinous portion of the musculotendinous unit can be sutured to the muscle belly with a carefully placed 3-0 mattress or figure-of-eight suture to minimize the tendency of sutures to cut out or pull through the muscle. A volar splint is applied from the elbow to the proximal interphalangeal joints to maintain the wrist in full extension postoperatively. This permits maximal relaxation of the musculotendinous unit because it is difficult to maintain muscle-to-muscle repair by any suture technique.

■ ZONE IX

Lacerations of the extensor muscle bellies in the proximal forearm (zone IX of Doyle) may have associated vessel and nerve injuries. If treated early, the muscle bellies usually require several mattress or figure-of-eight sutures to hold the muscle together. If difficulty is encountered with suturing techniques, tendon grafts can be used in a weaving technique through the muscle belly from one side of the laceration to the other. The wrist is held in appropriate extension and the metacarpophalangeal joints in about 30 degrees of flexion with the proximal interphalangeal joints left free. This splint or some similar protection is needed for about 6 weeks.

SECONDARY REPAIR OF EXTENSOR TENDONS

An extensor tendon usually can be repaired secondarily by direct suture at the level of the metacarpophalangeal joint or on the dorsum of the hand. After 4 to 6 weeks, when the proximal segment has retracted or when a segment of tendon has been destroyed, the options for treatment include transfer of the extensor indicis proprius tendon to the distal segment, side-to-side suture of the distal segment to an intact adjoining extensor tendon, or segmental tendon graft. For severe injuries in which whole segments of tendon have been lost, tendon grafting may be necessary. If multiple tendons have been abraded, or avulsed, or if the muscle has been denervated and has become fibrotic and scarred, transferring a suitable muscle, such as the flexor carpi ulnaris or flexor carpi radialis, with attachment to the distal segment can provide satisfactory function. An interposition graft may be required in such situations as well (see section on technique of tendon transfers).

EXTENSORS OF THE THUMB
◼ ZONES TI AND TII

Zone TI includes the thumb interphalangeal joint; zone TII includes the proximal phalanx. Closed injuries to the extensor pollicis longus in these zones can be treated with prolonged splinting for 8 or more weeks, as for mallet finger injuries in the fingers. Associated fractures of the distal phalanx involving 50% or more of the joint or fractures with distal fragment subluxation usually require reduction and internal fixation.

When an extensor pollicis longus tendon has been divided at the interphalangeal joint, its proximal segment does not retract appreciably because the adductor pollicis, abductor pollicis brevis, and extensor pollicis brevis insert into the extensor expansion; consequently, the tendon can be repaired primarily or secondarily without grafting or tendon transfer. A 4-0 core suture, supplemented with an epitendinous cross-stitch, usually is sufficient. Transarticular pinning of the interphalangeal joint for 4 weeks permits active motion of the metacarpophalangeal joint. Splinting is maintained for another 4 weeks after pin removal. Active motion is begun after the total period of splinting.

◼ ZONES TIII AND TIV

Zone TIII is at the metacarpophalangeal joint; zone TIV is over the thumb metacarpal. Injuries to the extensor pollicis brevis in these zones usually are repaired. When the tendon has been divided at the metacarpophalangeal joint or more proximally, its proximal segment retracts rapidly. By 1 month after injury, a fixed contracture of the muscle usually has developed. The contracture often can be overcome by rerouting the tendon from around the Lister tubercle and placing it in a straight line; when this maneuver does not provide enough length, the extensor indicis proprius tendon can be

transferred, and in this instance only one suture line is necessary instead of the two a graft would require.

◼ ZONE TV

Zone TV includes the third extensor compartment and the area of the first dorsal compartment. The extensor pollicis longus, extensor pollicis brevis, and abductor pollicis longus tendons may be injured in this zone. The superficial radial nerve also is at risk for injury. Tendons injured in the first dorsal compartment usually are mobilized from that compartment to minimize adhesion formation. Repairs to all injured tendons are done with 3-0 or 4-0 core sutures supplemented with a circumferential epitendinous suture.

When the tendon is divided at a level far enough proximal for the distal end of the palmaris longus tendon to reach the end of its distal segment, this tendon can be transferred instead of the extensor indicis proprius. A graft is necessary to bridge a long defect when a tendon transfer is either impossible or undesirable. If a graft is selected, it should be rerouted from around the Lister tubercle to avoid adhesion and abrasion of the graft.

A splint is applied with the wrist in near full extension and the thumb extended and abducted. The splint should begin distal to the elbow but extend to the thumb tip and to the distal palmar crease. This immobilizes the thumb but releases the movement of the fingers. The splint should be maintained for 4 weeks, and then the thumb is gradually permitted to move, with the wrist splinted in extension for another 4 weeks. Due to noncompliance or an inability to understand, some patients may require casting for 4 weeks postoperatively.

REFERENCES

TENDON HEALING

De Jong JP, Nguyen JT, Sonnema AJ, et al.: The incidence of acute traumatic tendon injuries in the hand and wrist: a 10-year population-based study, *Clin Orthop Surg* 6:196, 2014.

Henn 3rd RF, Kuo CE, Kessler MW, et al.: Augmentation of zone II flexor tendon repair using growth differentiation factor 5 in a rabbit model, *J Hand Surg* 35A:1825, 2010.

Peltz TS, Haddad R, Scougall PJ, et al.: Structural failure mechanisms of common flexor tendon repairs, *Hand Surg* 20:369, 2015.

Tan V, Nourbakhsh A, Capo J, et al.: Effects of nonsteroidal anti-inflammatory drugs on flexor tendon adhesion, *J Hand Surg* 35A:941, 2010.

Thomopoulos S, Kim HM, Das R, et al.: The effects of exogenous basic fibroblast growth factor on intrasynovial flexor tendon healing in a canine model, *J Bone Joint Surg* 92A:2285, 2010.

Yao J, Korotkova T, Smith RL: Viability and proliferation of pluripotential cells delivered to tendon repair sites using bioactive sutures-an in vitro study, *J Hand Surg* 36A:252, 2011.

Zhao C, Sun YL, Kirk RL, et al.: Effects of a lubricin-containing compound on the results of flexor tendon repair in a canine model in vivo, *J Bone Joint Surg* 92A:1453, 2010.

POSTOPERATIVE CARE

Bal S, Oz B, Gurgan A, et al.: Anatomic and functional improvements achieved by rehabilitation in Zone II and Zone V flexor tendon injuries, *Am J Phys Med Rehabil* 90:17, 2011.

Burns MC, Derby B, Neumeister MW: Wyndell Merritt immediate controlled active motion (ICAM) protocol following extensor tendon repairs in zone IV-VII: review of literature, orthosis design, and case study – a multimedia article, *Hand* 8:17, 2013.

Canham CD, Hammert WC: Rehabilitation following extensor tendon repair, *J Hand Surg Am* 38:1615, 2013.

Chesney A, Chauhan A, Kattan A, et al.: Systematic review of flexor tendon rehabilitation protocols in zone II of the hand, *Plast Reconstr Surg* 127:1583, 2011.

Chinchalkar SJ, Larocerie-Salgado J, Suh N: Pathomechanics and management of secondary complications associated with tendon adhesions following flexor tendon repair in zone II, *J Hand Microsurg* 8(2):70, 2016.

Chung B, Chiu DTW, Thanik V: Relative motion flexion splinting for flexor tendon lacerations: proof of concept, *Hand* 14(2):193, 2019.

Collocott SJF, Kelly E, Foster M, et al.: A randomized clinical trial comparing early active motion programs: earlier hand function, TAM, and orthotic satisfaction with a relative motion extension program for zones V and VI extensor tendon repairs, *J Hand Ther* Pii:S0894-1130(18)30082–30086, 2019.

De Spirito D, Giunchi D: The pull-out K-wire anchorage: the "shepherd's crook" technique, *Tech Hand Up Extrem Surg* 21(3):85, 2017.

Hammond K, Starr H, Katz D, Seiler J: Effect of aftercare regimen with extensor tendon repair: a systematic review of the literature, *J Surg Orthop Adv* 21:246, 2012.

Howell JW, Peck F: Rehabilitation of flexor and extensor tendon injuries in the hand: current updates, *Injury* 44:397, 2013.

Merritt WH: Relative motion splint: active motion after extensor tendon injury and repair, *J Hand Surg Am* 39(6):1187, 2014.

Neuhaus V, Wong G, Russo KE, Mudgal CS: Dynamic splinting with early motion following zone IV/V and TI to TIII extensor tendon repairs, *J Hand Surg Am* 37:933, 2012.

Ng CY, Chalmer J, Macdonald DJ, et al.: Rehabilitation regimens following surgical repair of extensor tendon injuries of the hand – a systematic review of controlled trials, *J Hand Microsurg* 4:65, 2012.

Rigo IZ, Rokkum M: Predictors of outcome after primary flexor tendon repair in zone 1, 2, and 3, *J Hand Surg Eur* 41(8):793, 2016.

Sameem M, Wood T, Ignacy T, et al.: A systematic review of rehabilitation protocols after surgical repair of the extensor tendons in zones V-VIII of the hand, *J Hand Ther* 24:365, 2011.

Starr HM, Snoddy M, Hammond KE, Seiler 3rd JG: Flexor tendon repair rehabilitation protocols: a systematic review, *J Hand Surg Am* 38:1712, 2013.

Trumble TE, Vedder NB, Seiler 3rd JG, et al.: Zone-II flexor tendon repair: a randomized prospective trial of active place-and-hold therapy compared with passive motion therapy, *J Bone Joint Surg* 92A:1381, 2010.

Wong AL, Wilson M, Girnary S, et al.: The optimal orthosis and motion protocol for extensor tendon injury in zones IV-VII: a systematic review, *J Hand Ther* 30(4):447, 2017.

FLEXOR TENDON REPAIR

Al-Qattan MM: Flexor tendon repair in zone III, *J Hand Surg Eur* 36:48, 2011.

Al-Qattan MM, Al-Rakan MA, Al-Hassan TS: A biomechanical study of flexor tendon repair in zone II: comparing a combined grasping and locking core suture technique to its grasping and locking components, *Injury* 42:1300, 2011.

Bommier A, McGuire D, Boyer P, et al.: Results of heterodigital flexor digitorum profundus hemi-tendon transfer for 23 flexor tendon injuries in zones 1 or 2, *J Hand Surg Eur* 43(5):487, 2018.

Bunata RE, Simmons S, Roso M, Kosmopoulos V: Gliding resistance and triggering after venting or A1 pulley enlargement: a study of intact and repaired flexor tendons in a cadaver model, *J Hand Surg* 36A:1316, 2011.

Chen J, Wang K, Katirai F, Chen Z: A new modified Tsuge suture for flexor tendon repairs: the biomechanical analysis and clinical application, *J Orthop Surg Res* 9:136, 2014.

Corradi M, Bellan M, Frattini M, et al.: The four-strand staggered suture for flexor tendon repair: in vitro biomechanical study, *J Hand Surg* 35A:948, 2010.

De Kraker M, Selles RW, Zuidam JM, et al.: Outcome of flexor digitorum superficialis oppenensplasty for type II and IIIA thumb hypoplasia, *J Hand Surg Eur* 41(3):258, 2016.

Dy CJ, Daluiski A: Update on zone II flexor tendon injuries, *J Am Acad Orthop Surg* 22:791, 2014.

Elliot D, Giesen T: Primary flexor tendon surgery: the search for a perfect result, *Hand Clin* 29:191, 2013.

Farzad M, Layeghi F, Asgari A, et al.: A prospective randomized controlled trial of controlled passive mobilization vs. place and active hold exercises after zone 2 flexor tendon repair, *Hand Surg* 19:53, 2014.

Firestone DE, Lauder AJ: Chemistry and mechanics of commonly used sutures and needles, *J Hand Surg* 35A:486, 2010.

Foo TL, Mak DS: Wire loop technique to retrieve flexor tendon, *J Hand Surg* 36A:1115, 2011.

Gan AW, Neo PY, He M, et al.: A biomechanical comparison of 3 loop suture materials in a 6-strand flexor tendon repair technique, *J Hand Surg Am* 37:1830, 2012.

Gibson PD, Sobol GL, Ahmed IH: Zone II flexor tendon repairs in the United States: trends in current management, *J Hand Surg* 42(2):e99, 2017.

Gil JA, Skjong C, Katarincic JA: Flexor tendon repair with looped suture: 1 versus 2 knots, *J Hand Surg Am* 41(3):422, 2016.

Giesen T, Reissner L, Besmens I, et al. Flexor tendon repair in the hand with the M-Tang technque (without peripheral sutures), pulley division, and early active motion, *J Hand Surg (European Volume)* 43(5):474, 2018.

Gordon L, Matsui J, McDonald E, et al.: Analysis of a knotless flexor tendon repair using a multifilament stainless steel cable-crimp system, *J Hand Surg Am* 38:677, 2013.

Griffin M, Hindocha S, Jordan D, et al.: An overview of the management of flexor tendon injuries, *Open Orthop J* 6:28, 2012.

Hirpara KM, Sullivan PJ, O'Sullivan ME: A new barbed device for repair of flexor tendons, *J Bone Joint Surg* 92B:1165, 2010.

Jordan MC, Schmitt V, Jansen H, et al.: Biomechanical analysis of the modified Kessler, Lahey, Adelaide, and Becker sutures for flexor tendon repair, *J Hand Surg Am* 40:1812, 2015.

Kannas S, Jeardeau TA, Bishop AT: Rehabilitation following zone II flexor tendon repairs, *Techn Hand Up Extrem Surg* 19:2, 2015.

Karjalainen T, He M, Chong AK, et al.: Nickel-titanium wire in circumferential suture of a flexor tendon repair: a comparison to polypropylene, *J Hand Surg* 35A:1160, 2010.

Kim YJ, Baek JH, Park JS, Lee JH: Interposition tendon graft and tension in the repair of closed rupture of the flexor digitorum profundus in zone III or IV, *Ann Plast Surg* 80(3):238, 2018.

Kim HM, Nelson G, Thomopoulos S, et al.: Technical and biological modifications for enhanced flexor tendon repair, *J Hand Surg* 35A:1031, 2010.

Kollitz KM, Parsons EM, Weaver MS, Huang JI: Platelet-rich plasma for zone II flexor tendon repair, *Hand* 9:217, 2014.

Kucukguven A, Uzun H, Menku FD, et al. Endoscopic retrieval of retracted flexor tendons: an atraumatic technique, *J Plast Reconstr Aesthet Surg* 72(4):622, 2019.

Lalonde DH: An evidence-based approach to flexor tendon laceration repair, *Plast Reconstr Surg* 127:885, 2011.

Lee SK, Goldstein RY, Zingman A, et al.: The effects of core suture purchase on the biomechanical characteristics of a multistrand locking flexor tendon repair: a cadaveric study, *J Hand Surg* 35A:1165, 2010.

Low TH, Ahmad TS, Ng ES: Simplifying four-strand flexor tendon repair using double-stranded suture: a comparative ex vivo study on tensile strength and bulking, *J Hand Surg Eur* 37:101, 2012.

Maddox GE, Ludwig J, Craig ER, et al.: Flexor tendon repair with a knotless, bidirectional barbed suture: an in vivo biomechanical analysis, *J Hand Surg Am* 40:963, 2015.

Marrero-Amadeo IC, Chauhan A, Warden SJ, Merrell GA: Flexor tendon repair with a knotless barbed suture: a comparative biomechanical study, *J Hand Surg* 36A:1204, 2011.

McDonald E, Gordon JA, Buckley JM, Gordon L: Comparison of a new multifilament stainless steel suture with frequently used sutures for flexor tendon repair, *J Hand Surg* 36A:1028, 2011.

Momeni A, Grauel E, Chang J: Complications after flexor tendon injuries, *Hand Clin* 26:179, 2010.

Moriya K, Yoshizu T, Maki Y, et al.: Clinical outcomes of early active mobilization following flexor tendon repair using the six-strand technique: short-and long-term evaluations, *J hand Surg Eur* 40:250, 2015.

Moriya K, Yoshizu T, Tsubokawa N, et al.: Clinical results of releasing the entire A2 pulley after flexor tendon repair in zone 2C, *J Hand Surg (European Volume)* 41E(8):822, 2016.

Moriya K, Yoshizu T, Tsubokawa N, et al.: Outcomes of release of the entire A4 pulley after flexor tendon repairs in zone 2A followed by early active mobilization, *J Hand Surg (European Volume)* 41E(4):400, 2016.

Moriya T, Zhao C, An KN, Amadio PC: The effect of epitendinous suture technique on gliding resistance during cyclic motion after flexor tendon repair: a cadaveric study, *J Hand Surg* 35A:552, 2010.

Myer C, Fowler JR: Flexor tendon repair: healing, biomechanics, and suture configurations, *Orthop Clin North Am* 47(1):219, 2016.

Netscher DT, Badal JJ: Closed flexor tendon ruptures, *J Hand Surg Am* 39:2315, 2014.

Neumann JA, Leversedge FJ: Flexor tendon injuries in athletes, *Sports Med Arthrosc* 22:56, 2014.

O'Brien 3rd FP, Parks BG, Tsai MA, Means KR: A knotless bidirectional-barbed tendon repair is inferior to conventional 4-strand repairs in cyclic loading, *J Hand Surg Eur* 41(8):809, 2016.

Okcesiz IE, Ege A, Turhan E, et al.: The longer pull-out suture as a transmission suture for early active motion of repaired flexor tendon at the proximal zone-2, *Arch Orthop Trauma Surg* 131:573, 2011.

Orkar KS, Watts C, Iwuagwu FC: A comparative analysis of the outcome of flexor tendon repair in the index and little fingers: does the little finger fare worse? *J Hand Surg Eur* 37:20, 2012.

Osei DA, Stephan JG, Calfee RP, et al.: The effect of suture caliber and number of core suture strands on zone II flexor tendon repair: a study in human cadavers, *J Hand Surg Am* 39:262, 2014.

Pan ZJ, Qin J, Zhou X, Chen J: Robust thumb flexor tendon repairs with six-strand M-Tang method, pulley venting, and early active motion, *J Hand Surg Eur* 42E(9):909, 2017.

Peltz TS, Haddad R, Scougall PJ, et al.: Influence of locking stitch size in a four-strand cross-locked cruciate flexor tendon repair, *J Hand Surg* 36A:450, 2011.

Piper SL, Wheeler LC, Mills JK, et al. Outcomes after primary repair and staged reconstruction of one I and II flexor tendon injuries in children, *J Pediatr Orthop* 2016. [Epub ahead of print].

Poggetti A, Novi M, Rosati M, et al.: Treatment of flexor tendon reconstruction failures: multicentric experience with Brunelli active tendon implant, *Eur J Orthop Surg Traumatol* 28(5):877, 2018.

Polfer EM, Sabino JM, Katz RD: Zone I flexor digitorum profundus repair: a surgical technique, *J Hand Surg Am* 44(2):164, 2019.

Saito K, Kihara H: A randomized controlled trial of the effect of 2-step orthosis treatment for a mallet finger of tendinous origin, *J Hand Ther* 29(4):433, 2016.

Sandow MJ, McMahon M: Active mobilisation following single cross grasp four-strand flexor tenorrhaphy (Adelaide repair), *J Hand Surg Eur* 36:467, 2011.

Savvidou C, Tsai TM: Clinical results of flexor tendon repair in zone II using a six strand double loop technique, *J Hand Microsurg* 7:25, 2015.

Schaller P, Baer W: Motion-stable flexor tendon repair with the Mantero technique in the distal part of the fingers, *J Hand Surg Eur* 35:51, 2010.

Scherman P, Haddad R, Scougall P, Walsh WR: Cross-sectional area and strength differences of fiberwire, prolene, and ticron sutures, *J Hand Surg* 35A:780, 2010.

Schreck MJ, Holbrook HS, Koman LA: Technique of dynamic flexor digitorum superficialis transfer to lateral bands for proximal interphalangeal joint deformity correction in severe Dupuytren disease, *J Hand Surg Am* 43(2):192, 2018.

Starnes T, Saunders RJ, Means Jr KR: Clinical outcomes of zone flexor tendon repair depending on mechanism of injury, *J Hand Surg Am* 37:2532, 2012.

Takeuchi N, Mitsuyasu H, Hotokezaka S, et al.: Strength enhancement of the interlocking mechanism in cross-stitch peripheral sutures for flexor tendon repair: biomechanical comparisons by cyclic loading, *J Hand Surg Eur* 35:46, 2010.

Takeuchi N, Mitsuyasu H, Kikuchi K, et al.: The biomechanical assessment of gap formation after flexor tendon repair using partial interlocking cross-stitch peripheral sutures, *J Hand Surg Eur* 36:584, 2011.

Tang JB: Clinical outcomes associated with flexor tendon repair, *Hand Clin* 21:199, 2005.

Tang JB: New developments are improving flexor tendon repair, *Plast Reconstr Surg* 141(6):1427, 2018.

Tang JB: Recent evolutions in flexor tendon repairs and rehabilitation, *J Hand Surg Eur* 43(5):469, 2018.

Tang JB: Wide-awake primary flexor tendon repair, tenolysis, and tendon transfer, *Clin Orthop Surg* 793:275, 2015.

Yaseen Z, English C, Stanbury SJ, et al.: The effect of the epitendinous suture on gliding in a cadaveric model of zone II flexor tendon repair, *J Hand Surg Am* 40:1363, 2015.

Zeplin PH, Zahn RK, Meffert RH, Schmidt K: Biomechanical evaluation of flexor tendon repair using barbed suture material: a comparative ex vivo study, *J Hand Surg* 36A:446, 2011.

SECONDARY REPAIR, RECONSTRUCTION, AND TENDON GRAFTS

Angelidis IK, Thorfinn J, Connolly ID, et al.: Tissue engineering of flexor tendons: the effect of a tissue bioreactor on adipoderived stem cell–seeded and fibroblast-seeded tendon constructs, *J Hand Surg* 35A:1466, 2010.

Clark TA, Skeete K, Amadio PC: Flexor tendon pulley reconstruction, *J Hand Surg* 35A:1685, 2010.

Dy CJ, Daluiski A, Do HT, et al.: The epidemiology of reoperation after flexor tendon repair, *J Hand Surg Am* 37:919, 2012.

Dy CJ, Lyman S, Schreiber JJ, et al.: The epidemiology of reoperation after flexor pulley reconstruction, *J Hand Surg Am* 38:1705, 2013.

Ikeda J, Zhao C, Sun YL, et al.: Carbodiimide-derivatized hyaluronic acid surface modification of lyophilized flexor tendon: a biomechanical study in a canine in vitro model, *J Bone Joint Surg* 92A:388, 2010.

Jakubietz MG, Jakubietz DF, Gruenert JG, et al.: Adequacy of palmaris longus and plantaris tendons for tendon grafting, *J Hand Surg* 36A:695, 2011.

Moore T, Anderson B, Seiler 3rd JG: Flexor tendon reconstruction, *J Hand Surg* 35A:1025, 2010.

Pulos N, Bozentka DJ: Management of complications of flexor tendon injuries, *Hand Clin* 31:293, 2015.

Sun S, Ding Y, Ma B, Zhou Y: Two-stage flexor tendon reconstruction in zone II using Hunter's technique, *Orthopedics* 33:880, 2010.

Zhao C, Sun YL, Ikeda J, et al.: Improvement of flexor tendon reconstruction with carbodiimide-deerivatized hyaluronic acid and gelatin-modified intrasynovial allografts: study of a primary repair failure model, *J Bone Joint Surg* 92A:2817, 2010.

FLEXOR TENDON INJURIES IN CHILDREN

Al-Qattan MM: A six-strand technique for zone II flexor-tendon repair in children younger than 2 years of age, *Injury* 42:1262, 2011.

Al-Qattan MM: Finger zone II flexor tendon repair in children (5-10 years of age) using three "figure of eight" sutures followed by immediate active mobilization, *J Hand Surg* 36:291, 2011.

Sikora S, Lai M, Arneja JS: Pediatric flexor tendon injuries: a 10-year outcome analysis, *Can J Plast Surg* 21:181, 2013.

Singer G, Zwetti T, Amann R, et al.: Long-term outcome of paediatric flexor tendon injuries of the hand, *J Plast Reconstr Aesthet Surg* 70(7):908, 2017.

Von der Heyde R: Flexor tendon injuries in children: rehailitative options and confounding factors, *J Hand Ther* 28:195, 2015.

FLEXOR TENDONS

Lied L, Lydersen S, Finsen V: Cold intolerance after flexor tendon injury: disposing factors and long term prognosis, *Scand J Surg* 99:187, 2010.

Lifchez SD: Flexor tendon injuries, *Orthopedics* 34:710, 2011.

Sügün TS, Krabay N, Toros T, et al.: Validity of ultrasonography in surgically treated zone 2 flexor tendon injuries, *Acta Orthop Traumatol Turc* 44:452, 2010.

EXTENSOR TENDON REPAIR

Afifi AM, Richards A, Medoro A, et al.: The extensor tendon splitting approach to the proximal interphalangeal joint: do we need to reinsert the central slip? *J Hand Surg Eur* 35:188, 2010.

Altobelli GG, Connelly S, Haufler C, et al.: Outcomes of digital zone IV and V and thumb zone TI to TIV extensor tendon repairs using a running interlocking horizontal mattress technique, *J Hand Surg Am* 38:1079, 2013.

Carty MJ, Blazar PE: Complex flexor and extensor tendon injuries, *Hand Clin* 29:283, 2013.

Chauhan A, Jacobs B, Andoga A, Baratz ME: Extensor tendon injuries in athletes, *Sports Med Arthrosc* 22:45, 2014.

Chung KC, Jun BJ, McGarry MH, Lee TQ: The effect of the number of cross-stitches on the biomechanical properties of the modified Becker extensor tendon repair, *J Hand Surg Am* 37:231, 2012.

Colantoni Woodside J, Bindra RR: Rerouting extensor pollicis longus tendon transfer, *J Hand Surg Am* 40:822, 2015.

Dwyer CL, Ramirez RN, Lubahn JD: A brief review of extensor tendon injuries specific to the pediatric patient, *Hand* 10:23, 2015.

Fischer LH, Abzug JM, Osterman AL, et al.: Complications of common hand and wrist surgery procedures: flexor and extensor tendon surgery, *Instr Course Lect* 63:97, 2014.

Hall B, Lee H, Page R, et al.: Comparing three postoperative treatment protocols for extensor tendon repair in zones V and VI of the hand, *Am J Occup Ther* 64:682, 2010.

Henderson J, Sutcliffe M, Gillespie P: Epitendinous suture techniques in extensor tendon repairs: an experimental evaluation, *J Hand Surg Am* 36:1968, 2011.

Henderson J, Sutcliffe M, Gillespie P: The tension band principle and angular testing of extensor tendon injuries, *J Hand Surg Eur* 36:297, 2011.

Iwamoto T, Sakuma Y, Momohara S, et al.: Modified extensor pollicis longus rerouting technique for Boutonniere deformity of the thumb in rheumatoid arthritis, *J Hand Surg Am* 41(6):e129, 2016.

Kang L, Carlson MG: Extensor tendon centralization at the metacarpophalangeal joint: surgical technique, *J Hand Surg Am* 35:1194, 2010.

Lee SK, Dubey A, Kim BH, et al.: A biomechanical study of extensor tendon repair methods: introduction to the running-interlocking horizontal mattress extensor tendon repair technique, *J Hand Surg* 35A:19, 2010.

Lutz K, Pipicelli J, Grewal R: Management of complications of extensor tendon injuries, *Hand Clin* 31:301, 2015.

Matzon JL, Bozentka DJ: Extensor tendon injuries, *J Hand Surg* 35A:854, 2010.

McMurtry JT, Isaacs J: Extensor tendon injuries, *Clin Sports Med* 34:167, 2015.

Merritt WH: Relative motion splint: active motion after extensor tendon injury and repair, *J Hand Surg Am* 39:1187, 2014.

Patillo D, Rayan GM: Open extensor tendon injuries: an epidemiologic study, *Hand Surg* 17:37, 2012.

Posner MA, Green SM: Diagnosis and treatment of finger deformities following injuries to the extensor tendon mechanism, *Hand Clin* 29:269, 2013.

Savvidou C, Thirkannad S: Hemilateral band technique for reconstructing gap defects in the terminal slip of the extensor tendon, *Tech Hand Up Extrem Surg* 15:177, 2011.

Türker T, Hassan K, Capdarest-Arest N: Extensor tendon gap reconstruction: a review, *J Plast Surg Hand Surg* 23:1, 2015.

The complete list of references is available online at Expert Consult.com.

CHAPTER 4

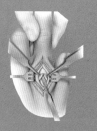

FRACTURES, DISLOCATIONS, AND LIGAMENTOUS INJURIES OF THE HAND AND WRIST

James H. Calandruccio

Although general management principles apply to the hand, functional impairment may follow seemingly minor trauma from resultant secondary sensory loss, motion restriction, and weakness. When treating fractures, anatomic and radiographic perfection does not always lead to normal function and early and accurate detection of soft-tissue injuries may require more specialized and urgent treatment. Often, it is better to accept a less than anatomic fracture position and strive to obtain good function through proper splinting and early motion. In general, a closed approach to the management of hand fractures and dislocations is preferred to operation; when surgery is required, the least complicated procedure to accomplish the desired functional result should be chosen. With few exceptions, prolonged immobilization (>3 weeks) is not indicated in treating hand injuries. Because clinical fracture union often precedes radiographic evidence of union by many weeks, early motion can be encouraged when clinical stability is ensured.

Angulation and lack of fracture apposition frequently are much more obvious on radiographs than on clinical examination. Fracture rotation may become clinically obvious only after a composite fist is attempted and demonstrates finger override or deviation (Fig. 4.1). Observing the plane of the fingernails (Fig. 4.2) at the time of reduction or fixation helps to determine rotation; passively flexing all fingers fully at the metacarpophalangeal, proximal interphalangeal (PIP), and distal interphalangeal joints at one time also helps to verify the appropriate fracture rotation after fracture reduction or internal fixation. When closed reduction methods are used for rotationally unstable fractures, taping the injured finger to an uninjured finger may help correct or prevent rotational

change. In this instance, we prefer not to use gauze or cast padding between the fingers and sometimes use the tape as a derotation device (Fig. 4.3).

The small finger has a normal tendency to overlap the ring finger. This becomes most apparent when the small finger can be only partially flexed while the ring finger is fully flexed. This "normal" overlap is permitted by the rotation allowable at the fifth carpometacarpal joint and the fact that each fingertip when flexed individually points to the scaphoid tuberosity. Only when full composite small finger flexion is possible in conjunction with the ring finger can proper rotational alignment be ascertained. When small finger fracture healing has been achieved, passive external rotation seldom is possible and further internal rotation is accentuated. Anteroposterior, lateral, and oblique radiographs are necessary to determine the fragment positions before and after reduction. Splay lateral views of the digits in varying amounts of flexion to prevent phalangeal overlap may show only one digit in a true lateral projection. Oblique views often are helpful in assessing reduction of articular fractures. True lateral views of the ring and small finger metacarpals can be obtained with the hand in 10 degrees of supination and the index and middle fingers in 10 degrees of pronation. Lateral tomograms or CT scans in the sagittal plane occasionally are necessary to evaluate displacement when a splint is applied. Even when the fracture is being reduced under direct vision, radiographs can prevent errors in alignment and can reveal small fragments of bone not seen before reduction. Shaft fractures are best evaluated by multiple images with the bone parallel to the film or image source, and articular fractures may require views projecting the joint surfaces perpendicular to the radiation beam.

PRINCIPLES OF TREATMENT

For most metacarpal and phalangeal fractures, closed manipulation, proper splinting, and protected motion generally produce good functional results. There are exceptions, however, when operative treatment, usually open reduction and internal fixation or closed manipulation and percutaneous pinning, may provide superior results. Percutaneous pinning should be attempted before edema obliterates external landmarks. If necessary, the extremity can be elevated for 24 to 48 hours before reduction and pinning. Fracture fixation, especially by open means, is preferably performed when the soft-tissue envelope is not markedly swollen; sometimes a delay in fixation of 7 to 10 days is warranted. Some form of fixation is most often indicated in the following instances: (1) when a displaced fracture involves a significant portion of the articular surface; (2) when a fracture is part of a major ligamentous or tendinous avulsion; (3) when a fracture is so severely displaced that interposition of tendons or other soft tissue prevents realignment by manipulation; (4) when multiple

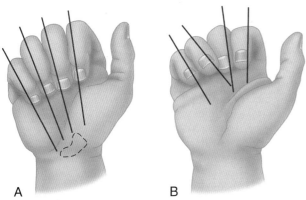

FIGURE 4.1   Malrotation of metacarpal or phalangeal fractures must be corrected. **A,** Normally, all fingers point toward the scaphoid tuberosity when a fist is made. **B,** Malrotated fracture causes affected finger to typically deviate into supinated posture.

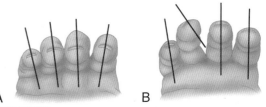

FIGURE 4.2   Observing plane of fingernails helps in detecting malrotation of fractures; comparison with opposite hand may be helpful. **A,** Normal alignment of fingernails. **B,** Alignment of fingernails with malrotation of ring finger.

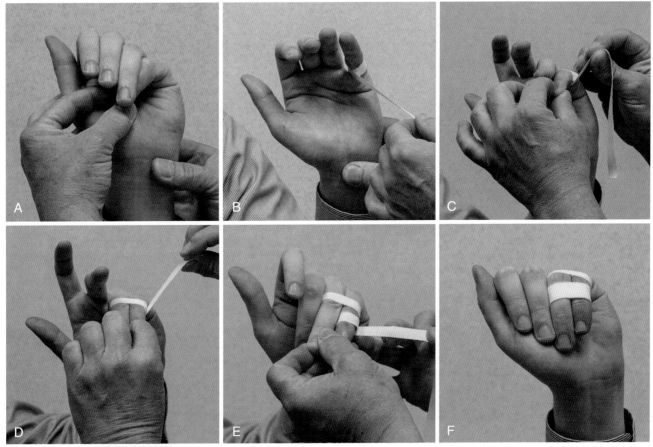

FIGURE 4.3   **A,** Simulation of typical rotational deformity caused by fracture of fifth digit. **B to D,** External rotation reduction maneuver combined with a buddy finger taping technique to hold reduction. **E and F,** Second strip of tape placed distal to proximal interphalangeal joint in similar fashion.

fractures are involved, and the hand cannot be held in the position of function without internal fixation; and (5) when a fracture is open (internal fixation allows wound care after surgery without loss of reduction).

Severely comminuted closed fractures usually should not be opened because internal fixation of multiple fragments may be impossible. Limited percutaneous pinning occasionally is indicated.

Dislocations can be managed by manipulation and early function. Many are self-reduced, and functional motion through "buddy taping" to an adjacent finger generally provides a good result. It is important, however, to examine for associated ligamentous injury or tendon avulsion. Surgery is required most often for the following conditions:

- Unstable thumb or finger carpometacarpal joint dislocations
- Thumb metacarpophalangeal joint injuries with complete ulnar collateral ligament rupture
- Dislocations in which a tendon is trapped, preventing manipulative reduction
- Chronic undiagnosed dislocations
- "Buttonhole" dislocations

OPEN FRACTURES AND DISLOCATIONS

Open fractures and dislocations require wound debridement and irrigation and then reduction. If an open dislocation is self-reduced and a contaminant is suspected, redislocation and wound cleansing should be done. Finger motion should begin as soon as soft-tissue healing and fracture and joint stability permit. Fixation should permit wound inspection or dressing changes without loss of fracture alignment.

Severely traumatized hands commonly are accompanied by soft-tissue defects, and additional incisions are usually unnecessary to access the fracture. Fractures should be fixed under direct vision or percutaneously, and segmental defects of tubular bones may be held to length by wire spacers or rods to prevent collapse while the wound is healing (Fig. 4.4). Massive trauma to the hand may require extensive reconstructive efforts to restore bony integrity (Fig. 4.5).

Judgment is required to determine whether the wound is sufficiently clean to permit primary closure or whether it should be left open for repeat debridement and irrigation. Loose skin-edge approximation is recommended because soft-tissue edema over the next 48 hours will further increase tension on the traumatized tissues and possibly compromise otherwise viable flaps. At 48 hours, the wound can be reevaluated in the operating room and plans made at that time for closure. The goal is to close the wound within the first 4 to 5 days before granulation tissues form and contractures develop. Exposed tendons without their paratenon or sheath soon necrose without appropriate coverage (see chapter 2 for a discussion of methods of and indications for skin closure). We no longer routinely culture acute open hand injuries in the emergency department. Thorough irrigation and debridement usually are adequate for primary fracture treatment. Routine use of antibiotics for fresh injuries probably is not necessary; however, when essential tissue has borderline viability and contamination remains after irrigation and debridement, antibiotic use is justified.

BASIC FRACTURE TECHNIQUES

Physician judgment is required to form logical treatment plans including, when applicable, suitable internal and external fracture fixation implants. Plating of small tubular bones, especially of the phalanges, can cause skin sloughs, tendon adherence or ruptures, joint contractures, and other complications. External fixation pins can impinge on tendons or ligaments and interfere with motion. Percutaneously placed pins may damage nerves, and tendons or ligaments may be tethered as well.

Rarely is more fixation needed than that afforded by external splinting, Kirschner wires, and minifragment screws. Unstable, long, oblique, or spiral fractures may be best treated with interfragmentary screw fixation alone, although a variety of fixation techniques may be indicated (Fig. 4.6).

The same instruments used in handling the soft tissues can be used to manipulate the bones; a straight Kocher clamp, hemostat, or towel clip is usually sufficient to reduce provisionally metacarpal or phalangeal shaft fractures before fracture fixation. Kirschner wires sharpened on both ends permit antegrade and retrograde drilling when necessary. A small hand-held power Kirschner-wire driver or drill without a cumbersome air supply line aids in accurate in-plane placement. A trocar-pointed wire has greater initial holding power than either a diamond or diagonally cut wire; in addition, initial bone engagement and placement at an acute angle are easier with a trocar-pointed wire. The Kirschner wire should project as short a distance as possible to prevent pin bending during insertion. After insertion, the wires may be cut off flat and the ends left protruding or left beneath the skin. Kirschner wires usually can be removed under local anesthesia, using a pointed extractor with grooved, corrugated, and parallel jaws. A diamond or carbide-tipped needle holder likewise is useful for gripping and removing small Kirschner wires.

Regardless of the method chosen for fracture fixation, the fractured bone ends should be in close approximation or apposition to promote healing. Sometimes a second wire is needed, however, to control rotation. When possible, the fractured finger should be flexed fully at the metacarpophalangeal, proximal and distal interphalangeal joints and compared with the adjacent uninjured finger or fingers before definitive rotational control is achieved, especially if there are doubts regarding correct fracture rotational alignment.

Outpatient surgery center services are usually selected when wounds are grossly contaminated or when fractures require implants other than Kirschner wires. In addition, young children and patients with medical conditions requiring cardiovascular monitoring should be treated at a surgical center. Wide-awake local anesthesia with no tourniquet (WALANT) can be incorporated in the office setting for less complex fractures that can be treated with Kirschner wires. Patients with Raynaud or Berger disease and patients with other epinephrine-intolerant conditions are not candidates for WALANT procedures. The WALANT technique uses a 30-gauge needle to liberally infiltrate in a tumescent fashion the region to be operated, including the subperiosteal regions of the fractures to be treated (Fig. 4.7). A 10 mL syringe is filled with 10 mL of 1% lidocaine with 1:100,000 epinephrine, after which an additional 1 mL of 8.4% sodium bicarbonate is drawn into the same syringe (a typical 10 mL syringe can hold 11 mL of solution). The addition of 8.4% sodium bicarbonate to the 1% lidocaine with 1:100,000 epinephrine in a 1:10 ratio normalizes the lidocaine pH of 4.2, thus reducing the burning sensation associated with local anesthetic infiltration. Simple procedures may require 10 to 20 mL of this solution; however,

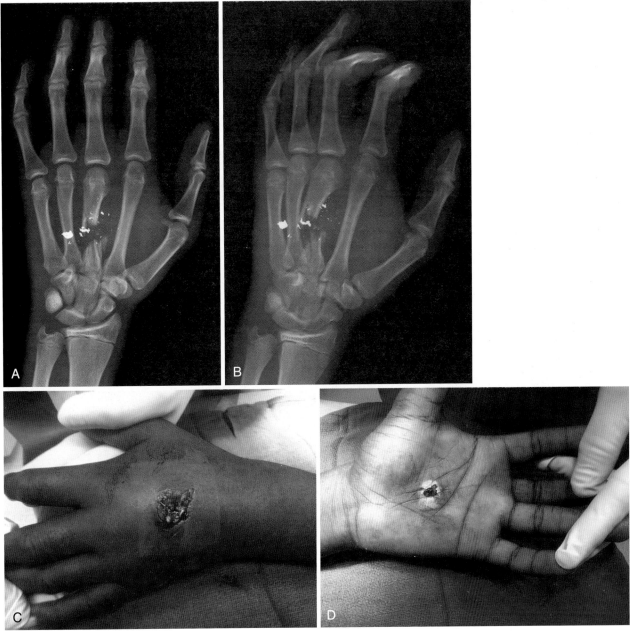

FIGURE 4.4   **A** and **B,** Comminuted middle finger metacarpal shaft fracture with intercalary bone loss from self-inflicted handgun injury in 17-year-old boy. **C** and **D,** Clinical appearance of hand before debridement.

50 mL of this mixture is permissible in an average 70 kg (155 lb) man, assuming 7 mg/kg maximum dosage of lidocaine.

THUMB

Thumb stability is essential for most hand functions. Offset intraarticular fractures or persistent subluxation or dislocation can cause limitation of motion, pain, and weakness of pinch and of grip. Secondary metacarpophalangeal hyperextension deformities can follow thumb basal joint dorsal displacement and severely weaken pinch and grip strength. Thus, reestablishing stability and congruency to the thumb trapeziometacarpal joint is critical to thumb and hand function.

BENNETT FRACTURE

In 1882, Bennett, an Irish surgeon, described an intraarticular fracture through the base of the first metacarpal in which the shaft is laterally dislocated by the unopposed pull of the abductor pollicis longus (Fig. 4.8). The medial projection of the thumb metacarpal base on which the volar oblique ligament attaches remains in place. Reduction by traction is easy but is difficult to maintain. The use of a cast that maintains reduction by pressure on the base of the metacarpal also often is unsatisfactory because immobilization is incomplete and verification of alignment by radiographs through the overlying cast is difficult. Too much pressure may cause skin necrosis, and too little allows loss

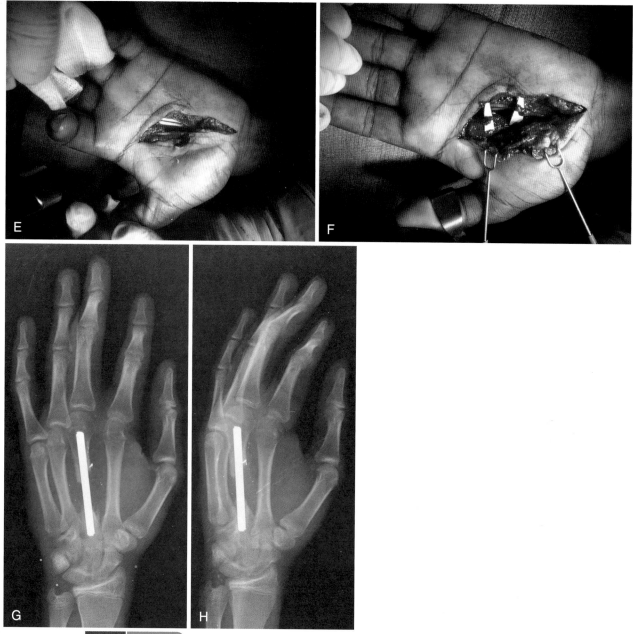

FIGURE 4.4, Cont'd E and F, Surgical debridement of devitalized second and third dorsal interossei and incidental deficit of second web space common digital nerve. G and H, Intramedullary fixation with large Kirschner wire.

of reduction. Some controversy surrounds the acceptable limits of displacement. Articular incongruity of 1 to 3 mm seems to be well tolerated, provided that union and joint stability are achieved. The technique of closed pinning described by Wagner (Figs. 4.9 and 4.10) is preferred, but should reduction be unsatisfactory, open reduction is indicated (Fig. 4.11). Long-term patient-reported outcomes following displaced Bennett fractures treated by closed reduction and Kirschner wire fixation show excellent functional results according to Middleton et al. At a mean follow-up of 11.5 years the 62 patients in this study had a high

level of patient satisfaction and none required a revision or salvage procedure.

Open reduction and direct exposure of the thumb basal joint may be required when adequate reduction cannot be achieved by closed or percutaneous fragment manipulation techniques. We have found that thumb metacarpal base fractures and the trapeziometacarpal joint are best seen through a Wagner type approach (Fig. 4.11). The volar capsule (between the abductor pollicis longus tendon and beak ligament) is structurally unimportant and can be reflected off the metacarpal base for joint exposure.

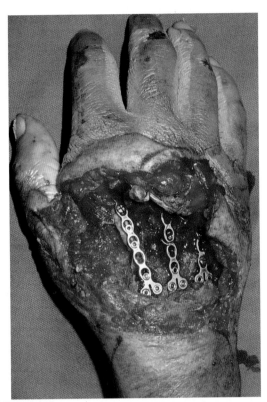

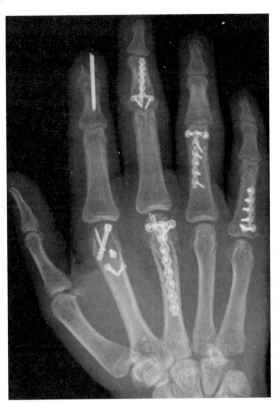

FIGURE 4.5 Intraoperative photo showing open second, third, and fourth metacarpals after plate fixation and before soft-tissue flap coverage. (From Cheah AE, Yao J: Hand fractures: indications, the tried and true and new innovations, *J Hand Surg Am* 41[6]:712-722, 2016.)

FIGURE 4.6 Multiple fractures in hand treated with a variety of methods ranging from pinning of distal phalanx to plate and screw fixation of proximal and middle phalanges and metacarpals. Note cannulated headless screw fixation of index metacarpal head fracture. (From Cheah AE, Yao J: Hand fractures: indications, the tried and true and new innovations, *J Hand Surg Am* 41[6]:712-722, 2016.)

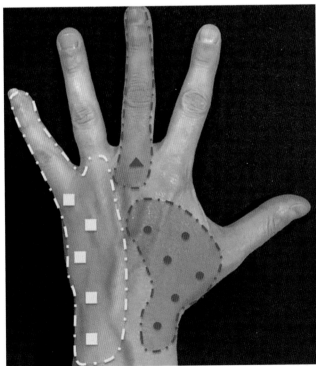

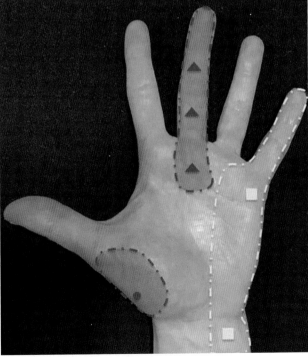

FIGURE 4.7 Sites of local anesthetic injection for various hand fractures. Local anesthetic should first be delivered proximally to perform regional block of sensory nerves that innervate entire region of surgical trauma Injection sites and region of anesthesia are illustrated for phalangeal fractures *(red triangles)*, first metacarpal base fractures *(blue circles)*, and fifth metacarpal fractures *(yellow squares)*. (From Hyatt BT, Rhee PC: Wide-awake surgical management of hand fractures: technical pearls and advanced rehabilitation, *Plast Reconstr Surg* 143:800-810, 2019.)

CLOSED PINNING

TECHNIQUE 4.1   *Figures 4.8 to 4.10*

(WAGNER)
- Maintaining fracture reduction by manual traction and pressure, drill an appropriate-gauge Kirschner wire into the base of the metacarpal across the joint and into the trapezium.

- Check the reduction by radiographs; if it is accurate, cut the wire near the skin.
- Apply a forearm cast, holding the wrist in extension and the thumb in abduction; leave the thumb interphalangeal joint free.
- Sometimes more than one Kirschner wire is required, and the wire may engage carpal bones other than the trapezium for adequate fixation. Fixation merely to the volar oblique fragment may be insufficient to prevent loss of fracture reduction.

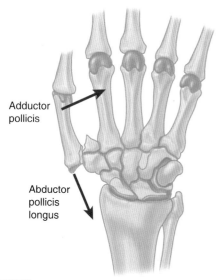

Adductor pollicis

Abductor pollicis longus

FIGURE 4.8   In Bennett fracture first metacarpal shaft is displaced by divergent pull of the adductor pollicis and abductor pollicis longus muscles.

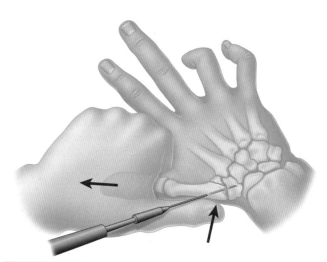

FIGURE 4.9   Wagner technique of closed pinning of Bennett fracture (see text).

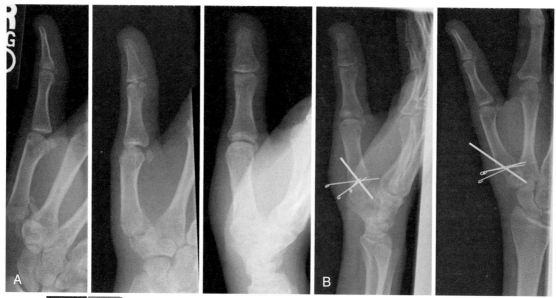

FIGURE 4.10   Bennett fracture. **A,** Young man with 6-week-old Bennett fracture and accompanying dorsal trapezial rim fracture. **B,** Results of fixation after callus excision and fracture fragment reduction.

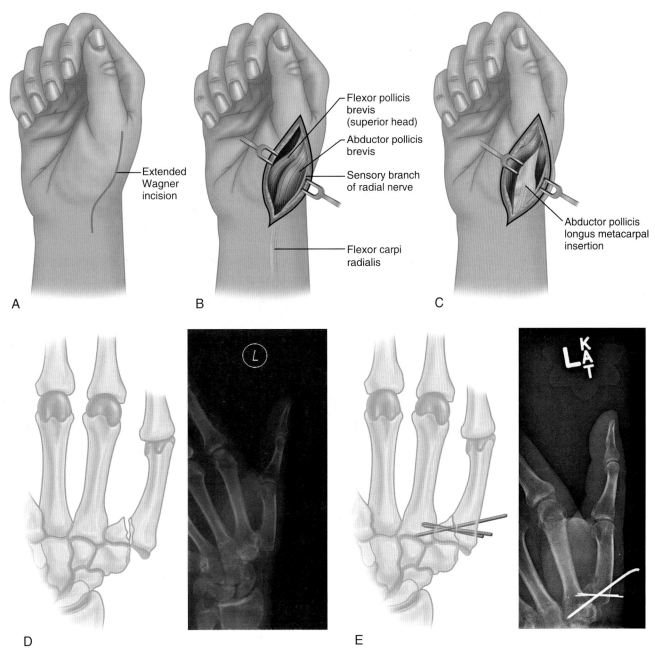

FIGURE 4.11 **A,** Extended Wagner incision. Thenar incision between glabrous and nonglabrous skin, extended ulnarly across wrist crease to radial side of flexor carpi radialis tendon. **B,** Thenar musculature. Note: protect all crossing sensory branches before exposing abductor pollicis brevis and flexor pollicis brevis muscle fascia. **C,** Reflection of thenar muscles from abductor pollicis longus insertion. The volar capsule is sharply elevated away from trapeziometacarpal joint, leaving intact ligamentous attachments to metacarpal beak. **D,** Malunited Bennett fracture. **E,** After fixation of fracture malunion.

OPEN REDUCTION

TECHNIQUE 4.2

(WAGNER; FIG. 4.11)
- Begin a curved incision on the dorsoradial aspect of the first metacarpal, and curve it volarward at the wrist flexion crease. Carefully protect the sensory branches crossing this area.
- To expose the fracture, partially strip the soft tissue from the proximal end of the metacarpal shaft and open the carpometacarpal joint.
- Align the articular surface of the larger fragment with that of the smaller fragment and under direct vision drill a wire across the joint fracture site to maintain the reduction.

- Often additional Kirschner wires are added to the provisional, smaller-caliber wires (Fig. 4.12).
- As an alternative, fixation can be achieved with a 2.0- or 2.7-mm screw (Fig. 4.13).
- After closing the wound, apply a forearm-based thumb spica splint.

POSTOPERATIVE CARE The cast is removed for wound inspection at 2 to 3 weeks but is replaced and worn until 4 weeks after surgery. Wires can be removed, but immobi-

lization may be necessary for 2 to 4 more weeks. If screw fixation is used, active range of motion and intermittent splinting can be initiated at 10 to 14 days in a compliant patient with secure fixation.

■ COMPLICATIONS

Malunion with persistent subluxation may progress to painful carpometacarpal joint arthritis. Reduction should not be attempted after 6 weeks. For a malunion that is recognized before degenerative changes are noted, an intraarticular osteotomy through an extended Wagner approach may be warranted (Fig. 4.11). When degenerative arthritis has developed, arthrodesis or arthroplasty is advised.

CORRECTIVE OSTEOTOMY

TECHNIQUE 4.3

- Make a 2- to 3-cm curved incision along the subcutaneous border of the thumb metacarpal base between the glabrous and nonglabrous skin. Protect all cutaneous nerves in the area (Fig. 4.11).
- Sharply elevate the thenar muscles, and reflect them anteriorly and distally without detaching the abductor pollicis longus metacarpal base tendon insertion. A capsulotomy between the abductor pollicis longus and metacarpal beak is made to assess the malunion and the degree of arthrosis (Fig. 4.11C).
- Assess the articular surface gap, and offset and determine the segment of bone to be removed to restore articular

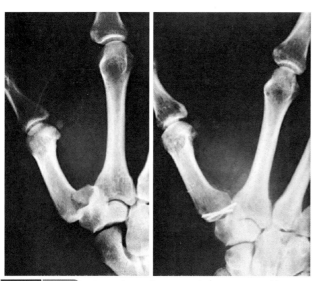

FIGURE 4.12 Comminuted Bennett fracture treated by open reduction. Two Kirschner wires were necessary to keep articular fragments reduced. **SEE TECHNIQUE 4.2.**

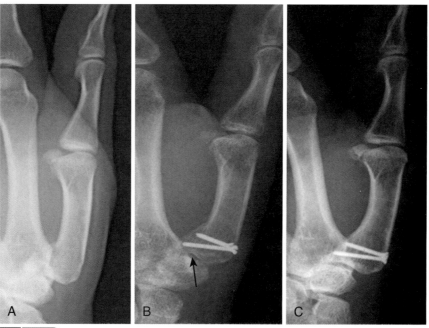

FIGURE 4.13 Gedda type II fracture: preoperative (**A**), 4 months (**B**), and 71 months (**C**) after operation. Step presented in **B** *(black arrow)* has completely remodeled with time. (From Leclere FMP, Jenzer A, Hüsler R, et al: 7-year follow-up after open reduction and internal screw fixation in Bennett fractures. *Arch Orthop Trauma Surg* 132:1045-1051, 2012.)

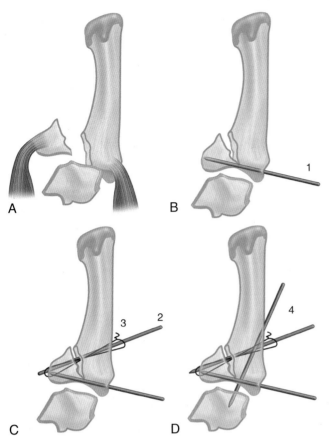

FIGURE 4.14   **A,** Bennett fracture malunion. **B,** Reduction of the fracture with temporary Kirschner wire fixation *(1)*. **C,** Second Kirschner wire *(2)*, wire loop *(3)*, and bone graft to fill defect. **D,** Temporary Kirschner wire crossing trapeziometacarpal joint to prevent subluxation *(4)*. (Redrawn from Mahmoud M, El Shafie S, Menorca RMG, Elfar JC: Management of neglected Bennett fracture in manual laborers by tension fixation, *J Hand Surg Am* 39:1728-1733, 2014.) **SEE TECHNIQUE 4.3.**

congruity. Curets, dental picks, and fine osteotomes are most suitable for disengaging the fragments. Working from distal to proximal, the periosteum and the excess callus can be stripped off of the bone. Gentle supination of the thumb allows careful separation of the volar lip with the callus attached as one piece and preservation of the capsular attachment to the volar fragment.

■ Within the malunion site, freshen the opposing bone surfaces, excising fibrous tissue, callus, and joint debris. The articular components can then be repositioned and fixed temporarily with small-caliber Kirschner wires. Definitive fixation can be achieved with larger-caliber wires to supplement the provisional fixation, interfragmentary screw(s), or tension band fixation (Fig. 4.14).

ROLANDO FRACTURE (COMMINUTED FIRST METACARPAL BASE) AND OTHER FRACTURES INVOLVING THE FIRST CARPOMETACARPAL JOINT

In 1910, Rolando described a Y-shaped fracture involving the thumb metacarpal base that usually does not result in diaphyseal

displacement as in a Bennett fracture. We have found that in most Rolando-type fractures the joint surface fragments can be reasonably well fixed with the use of small wires placed directly under the subchondral bone and supplemented with a larger transarticular and occasionally transmetacarpal pinning (Fig. 4.15). Because of the likelihood of posttraumatic arthritis after these fractures or after intraarticular trapezial fractures, accurate reduction is important. Many fractures can be reduced by traction and held by open or closed pinning. Open reduction and fixation with a minifragment T-plate may be plausible if the articular fragments are of sufficient size (Technique 4.4).

The combination of tension band wiring and an external fixator can result in an acceptable reduction. The external fixator is used to align the comminuted fragments and to restore length, and tension band wiring provides stability (Fig. 4.16). If the fracture is stable, the external fixator can be removed; if not, the fixator should remain in place for 8 weeks.

Severely comminuted fractures may require a combination of external fixation, limited internal fixation, and bone grafting. This technique showed good results despite persistent joint irregularities. Although the quality of reduction does not correlate with the late occurrence of symptoms and osteoarthritic changes, it is recommended that the joint articulation be restored to as close to normal as possible.

OPEN REDUCTION AND INTERNAL FIXATION

TECHNIQUE 4.4

(FOSTER AND HASTINGS)

■ Make a palmar radial incision similar to the approach to Bennett fracture (see Technique 4.2). Extend the radial end of the incision distally along the diaphyseal portion of the thumb metacarpal. Protect sensory branches of the radial nerve to prevent the development of a painful neuroma.

■ Reduce the two large basilar fragments (Fig. 4.17A and B), and provisionally fix them with a Kirschner wire (Fig. 4.17C).

■ Use a small T-plate or L-plate that accepts 2.7-mm screws on the thumb metacarpal.

■ Place the transverse portion of the T-plate on the basilar fragments of the metacarpal (Fig. 4.17D).

■ The previously placed Kirschner wire should slide through one of the two holes in the transverse portion of the plate. If it does not, place a second Kirschner wire in line with one of the two holes in the transverse portion of the plate and remove the first wire.

■ With a 2-mm drill bit, drill through the free hole in the transverse portion of the plate and through the dorsal and palmar fragments (Fig. 4.17E).

■ Tap the hole with a 2.7-mm tap.

■ Overdrill the hole in the dorsal fragment using a 2.7-mm drill bit for a lag screw effect.

■ Insert a 2.7-mm cortical screw of appropriate length to compress the palmar articular fragment against the dorsal articular fragment (Fig. 4.17F).

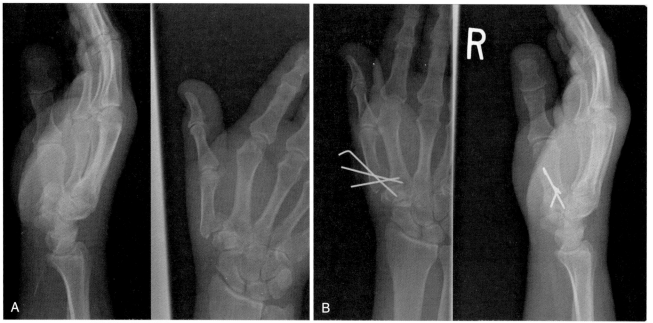

FIGURE 4.15   Rolando fracture. **A,** Male construction worker with comminuted fracture of base of thumb. **B,** Reduction required open approach with initial articular segment reduction with multiple 0.035-inch Kirschner wires, followed by metacarpal-trapezial pinning with 0.062-inch Kirschner wire.

- Repeat the same technique with the second proximal plate hole.
- The exact fracture pattern may vary and require use of a lag screw separate from the plate holes or two screws placed off center through the two proximal plate holes to compress the articular fragments together.
- Reduce the metacarpal to the stabilized intraarticular fragments and attach to the long portion of the T-plate or L-plate with 2.7-mm screws (Fig. 4.17G).
- Close the incision appropriately and apply a soft compressive dressing and thumb spica splint.

POSTOPERATIVE CARE Active range-of-motion exercises are begun within 5 to 7 days.

- Loosen the external fixation and adjust to a position where the flexion deformity of the thumb metacarpal distal to the fracture is eliminated. Usually this creates a larger defect of bone substance on the volar aspect of the proximal metaphyseal-diaphyseal junction that may require bone grafting to minimize subsequent settling of the fracture.

POSTOPERATIVE CARE External fixation is left in place for an average of 6 weeks (range, 5 to 12 weeks) until fracture stability is adequate. Interval radiographs should be obtained to assess the healing process. After the fixator has been removed, active and passive range-of-motion exercises are begun. A removable thumb spica splint is worn for an additional 6 to 12 weeks.

TECHNIQUE 4.5

(BUCHLER ET AL.)

- Place the AO mini external fixator between the thumb and index metacarpals in a quadrilateral frame configuration.
- Perform open reduction through a radial palmar approach, elevating the thenar musculature from its carpal origin for exposure of the thumb carpometacarpal joint (Fig. 4.18A).
- With the external fixator in slight distraction, gently elevate and align the displaced, depressed osteochondral joint fragments, using the opposite joint surface as a template for reduction (Fig. 4.18B).
- Depending on the fracture configuration, fix with an interfragmentary screw, Kirschner wires, or a combination of both.

THUMB CARPOMETACARPAL JOINT DISLOCATION

Dislocation of the thumb carpometacarpal joint is a rare injury, and all those reported have been dorsal dislocations. Based on cadaver studies, the dorsoradial ligament and the volar oblique ligament are the most important ligaments in preventing dislocation. When this injury occurs without fracture and is recognized early, the dislocation should be reduced and the joint immobilized for 4 to 6 weeks to prevent recurrence. Careful assessment of joint stability immediately after reduction is advised. Dislocations reduced on the day of injury may be stable immediately after reduction, and cast immobilization can be sufficient to maintain reduction and prevent long-term instability. Open reduction and pinning with repair of the dorsoradial ligament is necessary to ensure better joint stability if the joint is unstable after reduction.

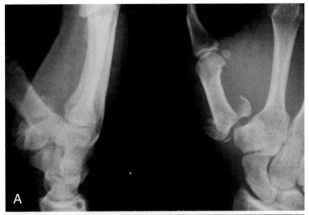

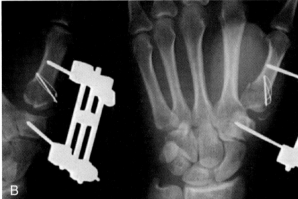

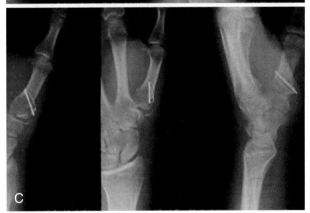

FIGURE 4.16 Rolando fracture (**A**) treated by external fixation distractor (**B**) and tension band wiring (**C**). Distractor was left in place for 8 weeks because fracture was unstable; excellent carpometacarpal and metacarpophalangeal function was obtained. (Courtesy of Robert Belsole, MD, and Thomas Greene, MD.)

LIGAMENT RECONSTRUCTION FOR RECURRENT DISLOCATION

TECHNIQUE 4.6

(EATON AND LITTLER)
- Make a dorsoradial incision along the proximal half of the first metacarpal and curve its proximal end ulnarward around the base of the thenar eminence parallel with the distal flexor crease of the wrist.
- Expose the carpometacarpal joint of the thumb subperiosteally and the volar aspect of the trapezium extraperiosteally. Isolate the distal part of the flexor carpi radialis tendon from its position on the ulnar aspect of the trapezial crest.
- In the distal forearm, expose the same tendon through a longitudinal incision, and split from its radial side a strip of tendon 6 cm long; free the strip proximally, continue the split distally, and leave the strip attached to the base of the second metacarpal (Fig. 4.19).
- Before proceeding further, reduce the first metacarpal on the trapezium and pass a Kirschner wire through this joint while holding it in appropriate orientation. Care should be taken in placing the wire so as not to interfere with the site where the transverse hole will be drilled through the first metacarpal and through which the tendon transfer eventually will pass.
- Reroute the tendon strip previously raised from behind the ridge of the trapezium, and pass it directly from the base of the second metacarpal to that of the first metacarpal.
- Drill a hole transversely through the base of the first metacarpal ulnar to the extensor pollicis brevis tendon and emerging extraarticularly from the volar beak region of the thumb metacarpal base.
- Pass the strip of tendon through this hole, loop it back deep to the abductor pollicis longus tendon, draw it tight, and suture it to the periosteum near its exit or the abductor pollicis longus bony insertion, which serves as an excellent suture site.
- Loop the tendon strip around the flexor carpi radialis near its insertion and suture it to the base of the first metacarpal.

POSTOPERATIVE CARE The thumb is immobilized for 4 to 6 weeks in extension and abduction. A home exercise program is initiated with interval splint wear for 4 to 6 weeks. A formalized therapy program is sometimes required to regain unprotected use 3 to 6 months after surgery.

Immobilization for 6 weeks is indicated after the repair. If reduction is delayed beyond 3 weeks, ligament reconstruction is advised.

In idiopathic or traumatic recurrent thumb carpometacarpal joint dislocation or subluxation, intermetacarpal ligament reconstruction may be indicated. The operation is most helpful when the joint is unstable and painful and when degeneration of its articular surfaces is minimal. This procedure should not be done solely to relieve symptoms or subluxations of this joint from osteoarthritis.

THUMB METACARPOPHALANGEAL FRACTURES AND DISLOCATIONS

Fractures around the thumb metacarpophalangeal joint usually involve the ulnar margins of the proximal phalanx from ulnar collateral ligament avulsion injuries. When the fragment is small and displaced less than 2 to 3 mm, the injury does not require surgery. Biplanar films should always be taken before evaluating joint stability. Displaced fractures of this sort are treated similarly to ulnar collateral ligament injuries. Impaction fractures with less than 20

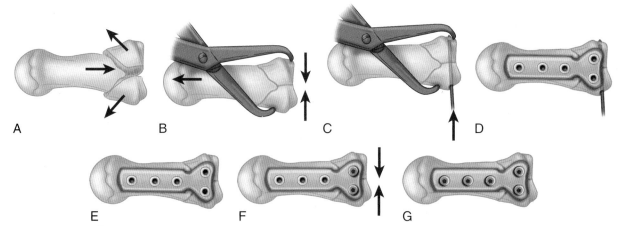

FIGURE **4.17**   Technique of open reduction and internal fixation of T-type Rolando fracture with miniplate and screws. **A,** Fracture. **B,** Reduction and traction. **C,** Provisional fixation with Kirschner wire. **D,** Positioning of plate. **E,** Offset drilling of two proximal holes. **F,** Tightening of two proximal screws compresses proximal fragments. **G,** Fixing rest of metacarpal to proximal fragments. **SEE TECHNIQUE 4.4.**

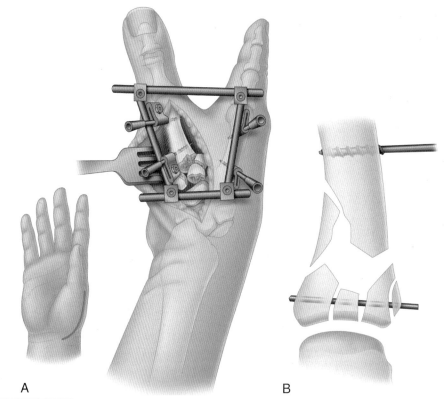

FIGURE **4.18**   Buchler technique. **A,** Palmar radial approach to carpometacarpal joint of thumb. **B,** Use of articular surface of trapezium as template and bone grafting technique. **SEE TECHNIQUE 4.5.**

degrees of dorsal angulation or joint separation less than 2 mm often can be treated nonoperatively. Angulated and displaced fractures probably are best treated operatively (Fig. 4.20).

Dislocation of any of the metacarpophalangeal joints is possible from hyperextension injuries, but dorsal dislocation of the thumb metacarpophalangeal joint is the most common type of metacarpophalangeal dislocation injury (Fig. 4.21).

These injuries are classified as *simple* (reducible using closed technique) or *complex* (irreducible with closed technique). Simple dislocations manifest with hyperextension deformity at the metacarpophalangeal joint, whereas complex dislocations show more parallelism between the proximal phalanx and the metacarpal. The volar plate, sesamoids, or flexor tendon may become entrapped, preventing reduction. Early closed reduction may be easy, provided that the thumb is maintained in adduction to relax its intrinsic muscles. In one method, minimal if any tension is used, the metacarpophalangeal joint is hyperextended, and the examiner uses his or her thumb to push forward the proximal end of the proximal phalanx over the end of the metacarpal head. This tends to

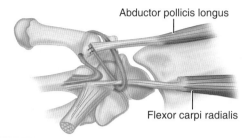

FIGURE 4.19 Volar and radial ligament reconstruction with strip from tendon of flexor carpi radialis, which is left attached at its insertion at base of second metacarpal. Course of tendon strip creates reinforcement of volar, dorsal, and radial aspects of joint. **SEE TECHNIQUE 4.6.**

diminish the buttonhole effect on the metacarpal neck that traction accentuates. Flexing the thumb interphalangeal joint also can help to relax the flexor pollicis longus. After reduction, the collateral ligaments should be checked for stability. Rarely is collateral instability found with pure dorsal dislocations. The thumb should be immobilized in 20 degrees of flexion for 4 weeks. If this method is unsuccessful, repeated attempts are contraindicated; open reduction should be done to disengage the metacarpal head from a buttonhole slit in the volar capsule and the flexor pollicis brevis muscle. A volar-radial or a dorsal approach can be used. In 1876, Farabeuf recommended a dorsal surgical approach for irreducible dislocations of the thumb metacarpophalangeal joint. The dorsal approach provides access to the dorsally displaced volar plate, which is the main obstacle to reduction and is tethered tightly over the metacarpal head and neck. The volar plate, a fibrocartilaginous structure similar in appearance to articular cartilage, is divided longitudinally so that it slips around the metacarpal head and permits reduction of the proximal phalangeal base. Motion is started within a few days of surgery.

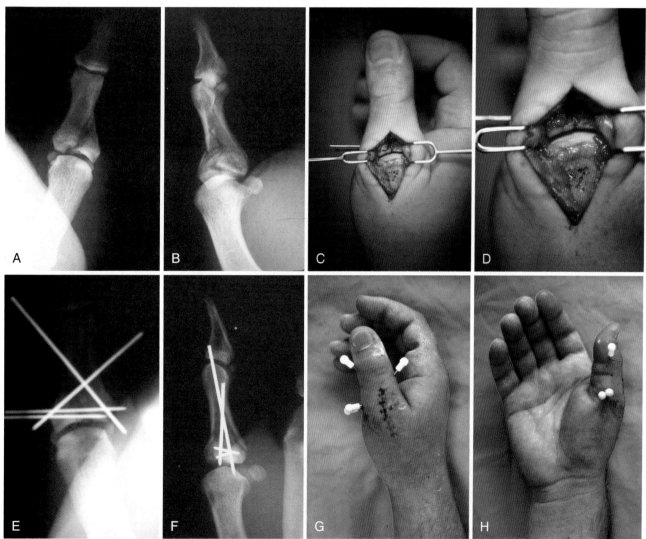

FIGURE 4.20 **A** and **B,** Comminuted displaced fracture of base of thumb proximal phalanx in young man. **C,** Exposure of dorsal joint through by splitting the extensor pollicis brevis longitudinally. **D,** Direct joint inspection permits anatomic reduction. **E** and **F,** Fracture fixation with simple Kirschner wires. **G** and **H,** Wires capped outside skin for easy removal 4 weeks after surgery.

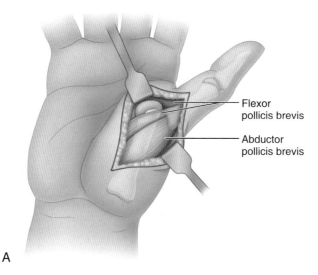

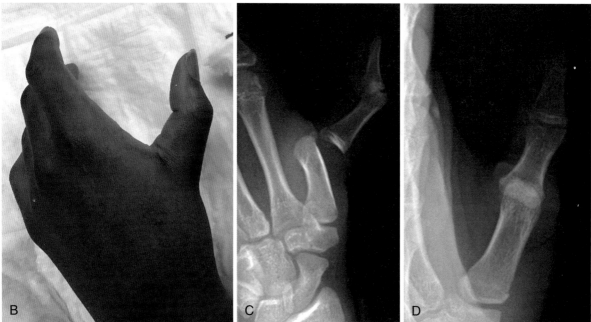

FIGURE 4.21 **A,** Dislocation of metacarpophalangeal (MCP) joint of thumb. Metacarpal head has penetrated joint capsule; if traction were applied to thumb, metacarpal neck would be caught by capsule and reduction would be impossible. Traction should not be applied; rather, metacarpal should be adducted and dislocated joint should be hyperextended, while proximal end of proximal phalanx is pushed against and over metacarpal head with interphalangeal joint flexed to reduce tension on flexor pollicis longus. **B,** Clinical appearance of sports-related complex dorsal thumb MCP joint dislocation in a 15-year-old boy. **C** and **D,** Lateral and posteroanterior images of thumb prior to open reduction.

OPEN REDUCTION—VOLAR APPROACH

TECHNIQUE 4.7

- Make an incision to expose the volar aspects of the metacarpophalangeal joint, exposing the metacarpal head articular surface.

- The proximal phalangeal base lies on the dorsal aspect of the metacarpal head and neck, and the metacarpal head protrudes through the anterior capsule.
- Disengage the flexor pollicis brevis muscle, releasing the metacarpal head.
- Flex the thumb, and push the head through the capsular rent to complete the reduction.
- With the joint in 20 degrees of flexion, secure it with a Kirschner wire.

■ In the rare event that the volar plate is found to be detached from the proximal phalanx, surgical repair is justified.

POSTOPERATIVE CARE The thumb is held in 20 degrees of flexion by a plaster splint. After 4 weeks, the splint and Kirschner wire are removed and active motion is begun.

Palmar dislocation of the thumb proximal phalanx is rare, but sometimes it can be irreducible if the metacarpal head is trapped between the extensor pollicis longus and extensor pollicis brevis tendons. Reduction is achieved by opening the dorsal aponeurosis and relocating the extensor tendon.

THUMB METACARPOPHALANGEAL JOINT ULNAR COLLATERAL LIGAMENT RUPTURE

Injury to the thumb metacarpophalangeal joint ulnar collateral ligament is commonly referred to as *gamekeeper thumb* or *skier's thumb*, although the original "gamekeeper" description (Campbell, 1955) referred to an attritional ulnar collateral ligament injury. Snow skiing accidents and falls on an outstretched hand with forceful radial and palmar abduction of the thumb are the usual causes. Changes in ski pole design have not been shown to reduce the incidence of this injury. Patients commonly report pain, swelling, and ecchymosis around the metacarpophalangeal joint. Tenderness is greatest over the ulnar aspect of the joint but often is not localized. Differentiating between an incomplete and complete ulnar collateral ligament rupture is necessary because incomplete ruptures are treated nonoperatively and complete ruptures usually require surgery. Stener described the anatomic pathology found in 39 complete ruptures of the ulnar collateral ligament of the thumb. In 25 of the 39 patients, he found the adductor aponeurosis interposed between the ruptured ulnar collateral ligament and its site of insertion on the base of the proximal phalanx. On clinical examination, a prominent lump can be palpated that represents the ulnar collateral ligament being proximally and superficially displaced by the adductor aponeurosis. Pathologic rotation of the thumb also may be evident. If left uncorrected, this lesion prevents proper healing and leads to chronic instability and subsequent arthrosis. Other injuries associated with tears of the ulnar collateral ligament include avulsion fractures, dorsal capsular tears, and volar plate tears. The following protocol is recommended to differentiate between complete and incomplete tears.

Plain radiographs should be obtained prior to any stress examinations. A minimally displaced (<2 mm) avulsion fracture signifies a complete avulsion without a Stener lesion. This fracture usually heals with casting. To prevent the development of a Stener lesion, the joint should not be stressed. If a Salter-Harris type I or type II fracture is present in a child, stress films are contraindicated.

After plain radiographs have been reviewed, anteroposterior stress radiographs can be obtained of both thumbs for comparison purposes. A local anesthetic may be necessary. The surgeon can stress the joint while obtaining the radiographs, but this may be awkward, especially when the surgeon wears lead gloves. It may be easier to tape the tips of both thumbs together and have the patient actively abduct both thumbs over a roll of tape placed as a fulcrum between the thumb metacarpophalangeal joints while the anteroposterior radiograph is taken. As an alternative, both thumbs can be held together at the interphalangeal joint level with a rubber band, and an image can be obtained while the patient tries to separate the hands (Fig. 4.22). An injured thumb that shows more than 30 degrees of instability compared with the uninjured side indicates a complete rupture. Ultrasonography, arthrography, and MRI also have been used successfully to distinguish complete from incomplete tears; moreover, ulnar collateral ligament retraction more than 3 mm and interposed soft tissue are reasonable guides to surgical intervention (Figs. 4.23 to 4.26). Incomplete ruptures of the ulnar collateral ligament of the thumb are common and require only proper protection for restoration of function, although pain and swelling may persist for several months. A thumb spica cast or functional brace is recommended for 4 to 6 weeks.

Acute complete rupture of the ulnar collateral ligament should be surgically repaired (Fig. 4.27). If the diagnosis is delayed for 1 month or longer, fibrosis makes ligament identification and repair more difficult, although repair can be done by dissecting out the ligament from within the fibrotic mass and reattaching it appropriately (Fig. 4.28). The detached tendinous insertion of the adductor muscle can be advanced and reattached to furnish a dynamic reinforcement. If the repair is done several months after the injury, a graft can be used to

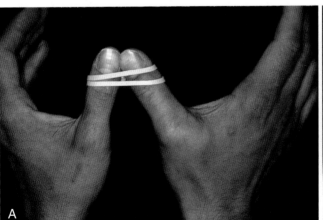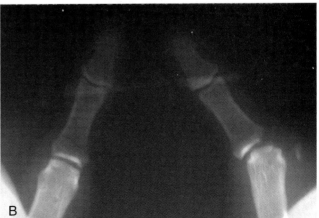

FIGURE 4.22 **A,** Rubber band is used to oppose interphalangeal joints while patient actively tries to separate hands. **B,** Image showing significant differential laxity.

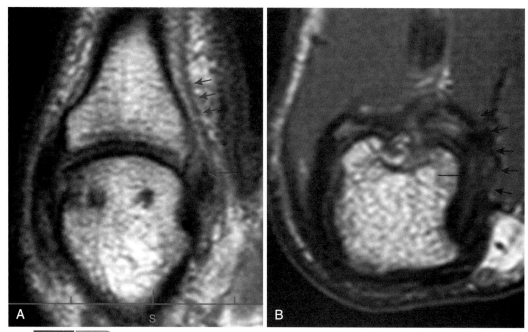

FIGURE 4.23 T2-weighted MRI appearance of a group 1 ulnar collateral ligament injury, demonstrating sprain or partial tear injury of ligament. **A,** Sagittal view. **B,** Axial view demonstrating increased signal associated with partial tear in the ulnar collateral ligament *(large arrow)* lying beneath adductor aponeurosis *(small arrows).* (From Milner CS, Manon-Matos Y, Thirkannad SM: Gamekeeper's thumb—a treatment-oriented magnetic resonance imaging classification, J Hand Surg Am 40[1]:90-95, 2015.)

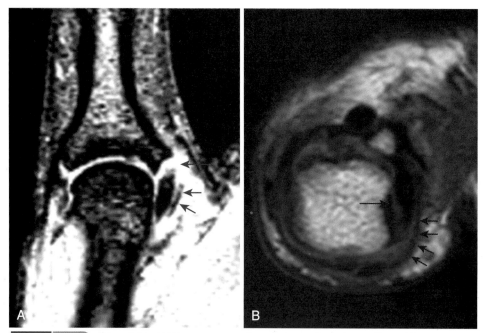

FIGURE 4.24 T2-weighted MRI appearance of group 2 complete ulnar collateral ligament tear less than 3 mm. Sagittal **(A)** and axial **(B)** views demonstrating complete tear *(large arrow)* with proximally attached end remaining beneath adductor aponeurosis *(small arrows).* (From Milner CS, Manon-Matos Y, Thirkannad SM: Gamekeeper's thumb—a treatment-oriented magnetic resonance imaging classification, J Hand Surg Am 40[1]:90-95, 2015.)

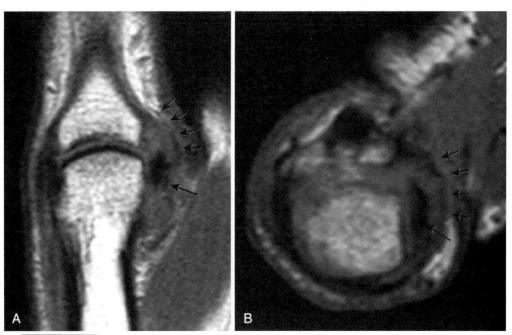

FIGURE 4.25 Sagittal (**A**) and axial (**B**) T2-weighted MRI images of group 3 complete tear in ulnar collateral ligament with more than 3 mm separation. In this example, free end of ligament has become reflected proximally (*large arrow,* sagittal image) while remaining beneath adductor aponeurosis *(small arrows)* as quasi-Stener lesion. (From Milner CS, Manon-Matos Y, Thirkannad SM: Gamekeeper's thumb—a treatment-oriented magnetic resonance imaging classification, J Hand Surg Am 40[1]:90-95, 2015.)

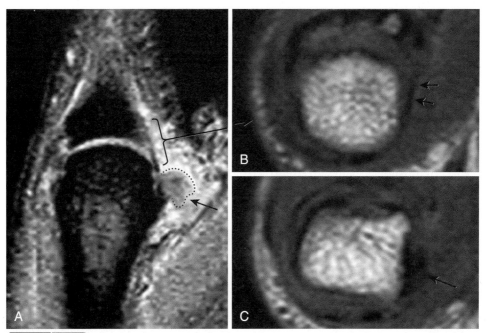

FIGURE 4.26 Sagittal (**A**) and twin-level (**B**) axial T2-weighted MRI images of group 4 thumb ulnar collateral ligament Stener lesion. **B,** Direct approximation of adductor aponeurosis against joint capsule *(small arrows).* **C,** More proximal axial view of joint where rolled-up free end of ulnar collateral ligament (outlined in *red* in **A,** *large arrows*) lies proximal to free edge of adductor aponeurosis. (From Milner CS, Manon-Matos Y, Thirkannad SM: Gamekeeper's thumb—a treatment-oriented magnetic resonance imaging classification, *J Hand Surg Am* 40[1]:90-95, 2015.)

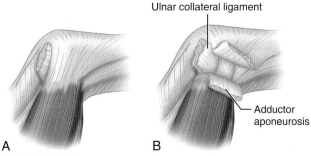

FIGURE 4.27 Complete rupture of ulnar collateral ligament of metacarpophalangeal joint of thumb. **A,** Ligament is ruptured distally and is folded back so that its distal end points proximally. **B,** Adductor aponeurosis has been divided, exposing the remainder of the ligament and MP joint.

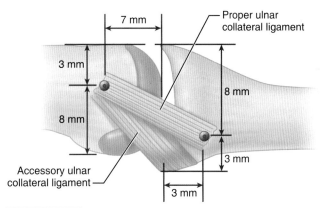

FIGURE 4.28 Mean locations of origin and insertion of proper ulnar collateral ligament of thumb metacarpophalangeal joint. (Redrawn from Bean CHG, Tencer AF, Trumble TE: The effect of thumb metacarpophalangeal ulnar collateral ligament attachment site on joint range of motion: an in vitro study, *J Hand Surg* 24A:283-287, 1999.)

replace the ligament. The graft can be box-like with a strip of fascia or palmaris longus tendon passed through the proximal and distal attachments of the ligament, or the extensor pollicis brevis tendon, either split or in total, can be threaded through bone and attached by pull-out sutures to reconstruct the ligament. Arthrodesis of the metacarpophalangeal joint may be indicated when arthritic changes within the joint or global joint instability is present.

REPAIR BY SUTURE

TECHNIQUE 4.8

- Make a slightly curved dorsoulnar longitudinal incision based radially or a bayonet-shaped incision with the transverse segment at the joint level over the metacarpophalangeal joint.
- Protect the superficial radial nerve terminal branches, which innervate the lateral margins of the thumb pulp.

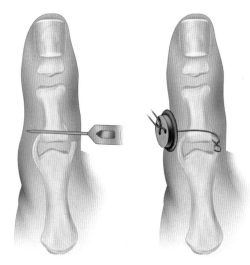

FIGURE 4.29 Repair of acute rupture of ulnar collateral ligament of metacarpophalangeal joint of thumb. *Note:* Button often is replaced by direct suture or suture anchor fixation to proximal phalangeal base. **SEE TECHNIQUE 4.8.**

Identify them as they pass distally on each side at the dorsolateral aspect of the metacarpophalangeal joint deep to the subcutaneous fat. The nerve branches usually are retracted dorsally but can be retracted volarly as well, depending on the nerve branch location.

- If a Stener lesion is present, the ulnar collateral ligament can be seen with its distal hemorrhagic end flipped up in the subcutaneous tissue just proximal to the adductor aponeurosis.
- Incise the adductor aponeurosis expansion longitudinally, and separate the thin tendinous sheet from the underlying capsule.
- Identify the ulnar collateral ligament, and establish its failure site, often an avulsion from the volar ulnar proximal phalanx base. If the ulnar collateral ligament has been detached from the proximal phalanx, it can be reinserted with a suture, suture anchor, or pull-out wire. When the ligament disruption is associated with a significant avulsion bone fragment, fixation with a small-caliber Kirschner wire or even a minifragment screw is possible. In most cases, before the repair, a Kirschner wire is placed across the metacarpophalangeal joint to hold it in approximately 20 degrees of flexion.
- To insert a pull-out wire, use a Kirschner wire and drill through the proximal end of the proximal phalanx (Fig. 4.29).
- Place a Bunnell pull-out suture through the avulsed end of the ligament, pass the ends of the suture through the phalanx, and, while holding the joint in slight flexion, tie them over a padded button on the radial side.
- Pass the twisted pull-out wire loop through the skin near the incision before closure.
- The same technique is used when a small bone fragment is avulsed by the ligament if the tear is complete and the bone fragment is displaced. If the operating surgeon prefers not to use a Bunnell pull-out wire or if one is unavailable, the following technique is recommended.

- After identifying the site of avulsion, drill two holes beginning on the ulnar base and exiting on the radial base of the proximal phalanx using a 0.035-inch Kirschner wire.
- Place a 3-0 Mersilene grasping suture into the ligament and pass it through the drill holes.
- With adequate dorsal exposure, tie this suture directly over the radial aspect of the proximal phalanx for permanent placement.
- With either technique, the metacarpophalangeal joint should be transfixed with a Kirschner wire in slight flexion and neutral adduction.
- Repair the dorsal capsule and volar plate to strengthen the repair further.
- Repair the dorsal aponeurosis.
- Splint the thumb, maintaining the first web space.

POSTOPERATIVE CARE A removable thumb spica brace or splint is worn for 3 to 4 weeks for comfort between range-of-motion and strengthening exercises. The pull-out wire and Kirschner wire are removed at 4 to 6 weeks. Tension band wiring, although technically demanding and not part of our routine management, may preclude the use of a pull-out wire.

■ CHRONIC ULNAR COLLATERAL LIGAMENT RECONSTRUCTION

Procedures designed to restore range of motion and stability for chronic ulnar collateral ligament injuries are numerous. Stability at long-term follow-up has been associated with "anatomic repairs" in which the graft is directed to reconstruct both proper and accessory ulnar collateral ligament limbs. We favor more anatomic type repairs such as those described by Glickel et al., Jobe, and others. Tendon anchor systems such as suture anchors and tenodesis screws are preferred by some for early construct stability; however, the adjunct provisional metacarpophalangeal joint stabilization in 20 degrees of flexion with Kirschner wires probably is sufficient during the graft incorporation period. A palmaris longus graft is preferred; if the palmaris longus is absent, common alternative autogenous sources include a portion of the flexor carpi radialis or a toe extensor tendon.

ANATOMIC GRAFT RECONSTRUCTIONS

TECHNIQUE 4.9

(GLICKEL)
- Expose the thumb metacarpophalangeal joint through a mid-axial or lazy-S incision centered over the joint line, taking care to isolate and protect the radial nerve dorsal sensory branch (Fig. 4.30A).
- Save the extensor mechanism sagittal band fibers. Release the extensor mechanism oblique fibers from the extensor pollicis longus longitudinally and vertically from the sagittal band proximally. This leaves a triangular section of the extensor mechanism to reflect palmarward.

- Retract the sagittal band proximally, exposing the proximal phalanx base and metacarpophalangeal joint. Excise the fibrotic ulnar collateral ligament stumps. Evaluate the joint, and note if significant degenerative changes preclude reconstruction.
- Make gouge holes in the proximal phalanx, first in the palmar aspect (7-o'clock position) and a second more dorsally (11-o'clock position) just distal to the joint surface (Fig. 4.30B). Connect these, preserving the bone bridge.
- Make a hole in the metacarpal head ligament fossa ulnarly, and direct this hole across the metacarpal head radially and more proximally. Make a 5-mm incision over this site for tendon passage.
- Harvest a tendon graft, and pass this through the proximal phalangeal base holes with either a stainless steel wire or small curved needle. Place a Kirschner wire through the metacarpal head so as not to obstruct the metacarpal head tunnel. Pass the two tendon graft limbs under the sagittal band and through the metacarpal neck to exit radially (Fig. 4.30C). Take tension off the graft by slightly overcorrecting the reduction, and reduce the palmar subluxation if present.
- Once the correct tension has been established, secure the graft either over a button or a catheter tip (Fig. 4.30D and E). Alternately, the graft can be secured with either a screw or anchor or sutured to bone. Carefully drive the Kirschner wire across the joint, redirecting it if there is any question of graft engagement. Close the triangular oblique extensor expansion flap and skin in routine fashion.

POSTOPERATIVE CARE The reconstruction is protected for 5 weeks in a thumb spica cast after which the Kirschner wire is removed and therapy is begun.

JOBE FOUR-LIMB RECONSTRUCTION

TECHNIQUE 4.10

- Expose the ulnar side of the thumb metacarpophalangeal joint as described in Technique 4.9, with the usual superficial sensory nerve protection.
- Separate the capsular tissue, and excise the old ulnar collateral ligament from its origin and insertion attachments.
- Identify the planned sites of the two pairs of holes according to normal anatomic positions (Fig. 4.31A) for normal metacarpophalangeal joint anatomy. The distal holes correspond to the proper and accessory ulnar collateral ligament phalangeal attachments. Make these two phalangeal holes 2.75 mm in diameter, and leave a bone bridge of 3 to 4 mm between them (Fig. 4.31B). Carefully channel these together with a small curved curet or other appropriate instrument.
- Make two 3-mm holes in the metacarpal head, the most distal hole in the ulnar collateral ligament fossa and another approximately 5 mm more proximally (Fig. 4.31A and B). Communicate these, protecting the bone bridge. Pass the tendon graft (palmaris longus or equivalent)

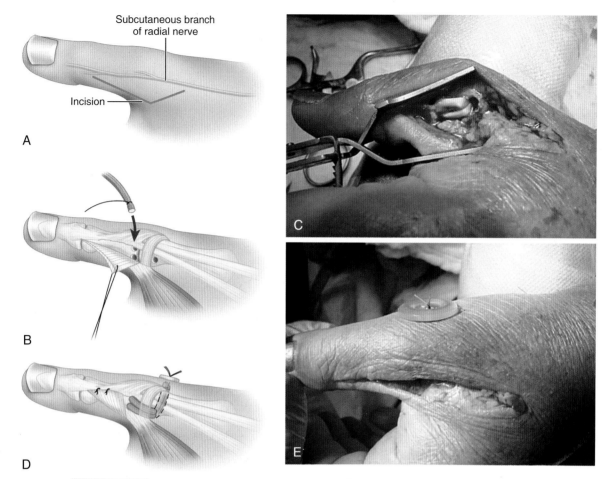

Subcutaneous branch
of radial nerve

Incision

A

B

D

C

E

FIGURE 4.30 Ulnar collateral ligament reconstruction described by Glickel et al. **A,** Incision. **B,** Two gouge holes made on ulnar side of proximal phalangeal base and one across metacarpal neck. **C to E,** Passage and fixation of tendon graft. (Redrawn from Glickel SZ, Malerich M, Pearce SM, Littler JW: Ligament replacement for chronic instability of the ulnar collateral ligament of the metacarpophalangeal joint of the thumb, *J Hand Surg* 18A:930-941, 1993.) **SEE TECHNIQUE 4.9.**

through the phalangeal holes, and pass the two limbs through the ulnar collateral ligament fossa hole and subsequently out the more proximal hole (Fig. 4.31C).
- Assess joint reduction, and adjust tension on the two free limbs. Fold the limbs distally, and use nonabsorbable sutures to secure the construct (Fig. 4.31D and E).
- A biotenodesis screw also can be used to secure the two limbs in the ulnar collateral ligament fossa (Fig. 4.32). For screw fixation, make only one hole in the fossa and continue it across the metacarpal head. Grasp the two limbs of the free graft, and pass them through the hole in the metacarpal head that has been reamed for the appropriate tenodesis screw. Adjust tension on the free suture ends; once appropriate joint reduction and tension are achieved, advance the tenodesis screw into the metacarpal head. Excise the tendon ends and/or suture emerging from the radial side of the metacarpal head. If necessary, protect the construct with a Kirschner wire transfixing the joint in 20 degrees of flexion.

- Close the extensor expansion and wound in routine fashion, and apply a thumb spica splint.

POSTOPERATIVE CARE The reconstruction is protected for 4 to 6 weeks, after which the Kirschner wire and splint are removed and joint motion exercises are initiated.

RADIAL COLLATERAL LIGAMENT INJURIES

Although radial collateral ligament injuries occur less frequently than ulnar collateral ligament injuries, improper treatment can lead to chronic painful instabilities, especially during activities requiring "push off." No lesions comparable to that described by Stener exist; if proper protection is provided, adequate healing of the ligament should occur. Incomplete tears and tears not associated with volar or rotational subluxation can be treated in a cast for 4 to 6 weeks. Complete tears, particularly if rotational and with volar

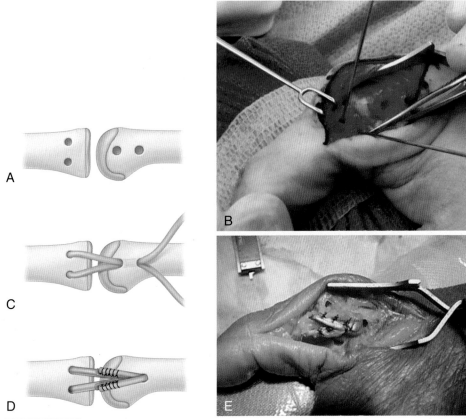

FIGURE 4.31 Jobe four-limb reconstruction of ulnar collateral ligament. **A** and **B**, Position of metacarpal and phalangeal holes for passage of tendon graft. **C**, Passage of graft. **D** and **E**, Final position of graft fixed with sutures. **SEE TECHNIQUE 4.10.**

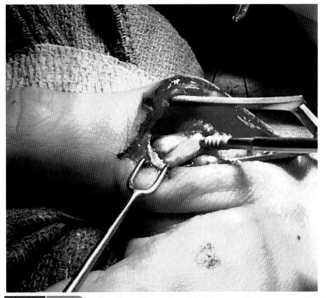

FIGURE 4.32 Fixation of graft with biotenodesis screw. **SEE TECHNIQUE 4.10.**

subluxation after casting, should be treated with direct ligament repair. Chronic instability should be treated with open repair, radial collateral ligament reefing, supplemental palmaris longus tendon graft, or advancement of the abductor pollicis brevis.

FINGER METACARPALS

CARPOMETACARPAL FRACTURE-DISLOCATIONS

Fracture-dislocation of the metacarpal bases often is not recognized because of swelling and metacarpal overlap on lateral plain films. The fifth metacarpal base is most commonly dorsally displaced, and concomitant fourth metacarpal base involvement is frequent; however, all four metacarpals may be dislocated dorsally or volarly. A true lateral radiograph is needed for accurate diagnosis because swelling can obscure the deformity (Fig. 4.33). The loss of parallel joint surfaces at the carpometacarpal articulations in a posteroanterior radiograph is indicative of this injury (Fig. 4.34). Sometimes a CT scan is beneficial to determine the extent of joint surface involvement and to guide appropriate intervention. When the injury is seen early, manual reduction is easy, but Kirschner wire fixation usually is necessary to prevent redislocation. Open reduction and pinning are useful in patients in whom closed reduction is unsuccessful. Excellent

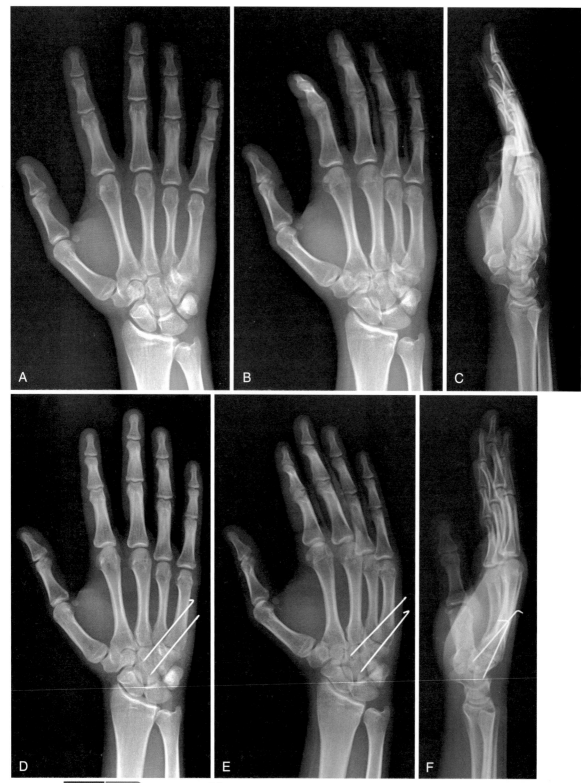

FIGURE 4.33   A to C, Small finger carpometacarpal fracture-subluxation in 34-year-old man. D to F, Ring and small finger carpometacarpal joints were reduced closed and stabilized with two 0.045-inch Kirschner wires.

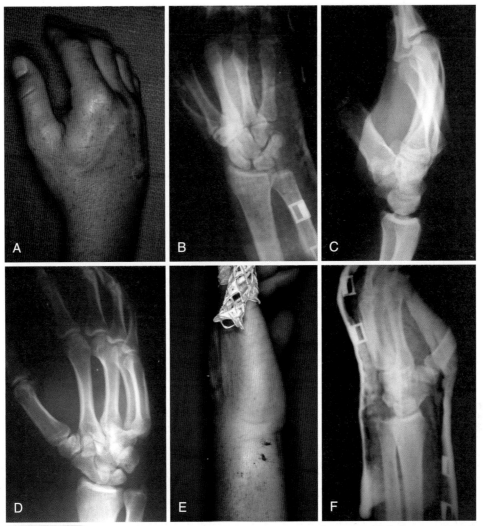

FIGURE 4.34 Dislocation of fourth and fifth carpometacarpal joints. **A,** Clinical appearance of hand before reduction. Note dorsoulnar hand swelling consistent with injury. **B,** Posteroanterior view. **C,** Lateral view. **D,** Oblique view. **E** and **F,** Traction was adequate to reduce, and splint was satisfactory to maintain reductions.

long-term results can be achieved with open reduction and internal fixation because better reduction can be obtained and transfixing of the tendons and nerves avoided. When seen late, the injury requires open reduction, and sometimes the proximal end of the metacarpal must be resected and the carpometacarpal joint treated by either fusion or interposition arthroplasty.

INTRAARTICULAR FRACTURE OF THE FIFTH METACARPAL BASE

Bora and Didizian called attention to a potentially disabling intraarticular fracture at the base of the fifth metacarpal (Fig. 4.35). If the injury is not reduced properly, a malunion may result in weakness of grip and a painful joint. The joint consists of the fifth metacarpal base articulating with the hamate and the adjoining fourth metacarpal. The extensor carpi ulnaris tendon attaches proximally to the fifth metacarpal dorsal base. The joint permits approximately 30 degrees of normal flexion and extension and the rotation necessary in grasp and palmar cupping. This displaced intraarticular fracture might

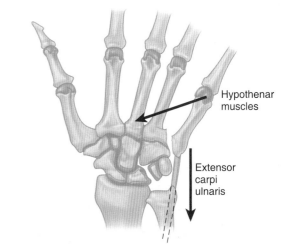

Hypothenar muscles

Extensor carpi ulnaris

FIGURE 4.35 Unstable fracture of base of fifth metacarpal may permit proximal displacement of shaft similar to Bennett fracture (see text).

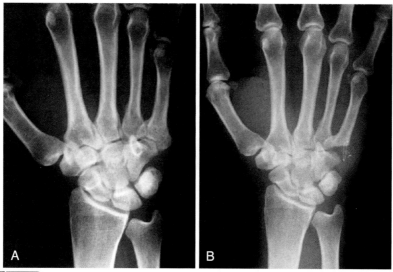

FIGURE 4.36   **A,** This malunited fracture of base of fifth metacarpal was painful. **B,** Resection arthroplasty is preferred over osteotomy. Tendon of extensor carpi ulnaris must be reattached.

be compared with a Bennett fracture because the pull of the extensor carpi ulnaris has a great tendency to displace the metacarpal shaft proximally, similar to the thumb metacarpal displacement in a Bennett fracture by the abductor pollicis longus. In addition to the routine anteroposterior and lateral views, a radiograph should be made with 30 degrees of pronation to give a better view of the articular surface for accurate diagnosis. This fracture often can be reduced by traction and percutaneous pinning and is then protected by a cast. Fractures that are not recognized early and are healing in a displaced position may benefit from correction osteotomy of the malunion or resection arthroplasty (Fig. 4.36) or fusion.

FINGER METACARPOPHALANGEAL DISLOCATIONS

Metacarpophalangeal dislocations are less common than interphalangeal dislocations. They occur most often in the index finger, and Kaplan's original description clearly indicates the pathoanatomy (Fig. 4.37). The fibrocartilaginous plate avulses from its weakest attachment, the volar aspect of the second metacarpal neck. The flexor tendons and the pretendinous band are displaced ulnarly and the lumbrical radially to the metacarpal head. The fibrocartilaginous plate is displaced dorsally over the metacarpal head, where it becomes wedged between the base of the proximal phalanx and the metacarpal head. The lateral collateral ligaments, which are now abnormally displaced, lock the phalanx in the abnormal dorsal position. Distally, the natatory ligament is situated dorsal to the metacarpal head with the volar plate; proximally, the superficial transverse ligament extends across the metacarpal neck volarly. The dislocated metacarpal head lies between the natatory ligament and the superficial transverse ligament of the palmar fascia. The flexor tendons and pretendinous bands are on one side, and the lumbrical muscle is on the other. Contrary to the noose concept, Afifi et al. showed in a cadaveric model that the volar plate was the sole anatomic structure requiring release for reduction of the metacarpophalangeal joint.

When the dislocation is incomplete, reduction by manipulation is easy. When complete, with the head of the metacarpal displaced volarward and the base of the phalanx dorsalward,

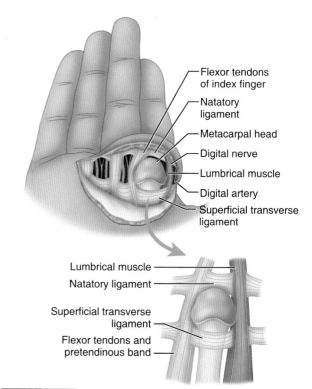

FIGURE 4.37   Kaplan open reduction of dislocation of second metacarpophalangeal joint. *Inset,* Diagram of four structures that surround the metacarpal head. **SEE TECHNIQUE 4.11.**

open reduction often is required. The major obstruction preventing reduction of the metacarpophalangeal joint is the displaced volar fibrocartilaginous plate lying dorsal to the metacarpal head. Sometimes, however, manipulation alone can be successful; 50% can be reduced by closed means. The joint is hyperextended, the proximal phalangeal articular surface is forced firmly against the metacarpal neck, and while this force is maintained the joint is flexed. Sometimes this maneuver traps the displaced fibrocartilaginous plate and carries it to its normal position anterior to the metacarpal head.

OPEN REDUCTION

TECHNIQUE 4.11

(KAPLAN)
- Begin an incision in the thenar crease at the radial base of the index finger, continue it into the proximal palmar crease, and divide all the constricting bands.
- Make the first incision to free the constriction of the cartilaginous plate (Fig. 4.37).
- Incise the free edge of the torn ligament to the junction of the periosteum with the proximal phalanx. The incision must penetrate the entire thickness of the plate. Division of the plate alone is insufficient, however.
- Divide completely the transverse fibers of the taut natatory ligament, and make another longitudinal incision through the transverse fibers of the superficial transverse metacarpal ligament.
- This third incision, which should extend to the ulnar side of the first lumbrical muscle, releases the constriction below the metacarpal head.
- The proximal phalangeal base should return to its normal place over the metacarpal head. This permits the immediate replacement of the second metacarpal head in line with the other metacarpal heads, following which the flexor tendons, the volar plate, and the nerves and vessels are restored to their normal positions.
- Close the wound in a routine manner, and immobilize the finger in functional position for about 1 week.

OPEN REDUCTION—DORSAL APPROACH

Becton et al. suggested that the dorsal approach has several advantages over the volar approach. The dorsal approach provides full exposure of the fibrocartilaginous volar plate, which is the structure blocking reduction. The digital nerves are not as likely to be cut, and should there be an occult fracture of the metacarpal head, this can be reduced and fixed more easily.

TECHNIQUE 4.12

(BECTON ET AL.)
- Over the metacarpophalangeal joint, make a 4-cm midline incision, splitting longitudinally the underlying extensor tendon and joint capsule as well. The fibrocartilaginous plate may be difficult to distinguish from the metacarpal head because its torn margin may not be visible and has the same color and similar compliance as the metacarpal head articular cartilage.
- Make a small incision to ensure that the tissue is the volar plate; complete the longitudinal incision (Fig. 4.38).
- Flex the wrist volarward to release the tension on the flexor tendons; place traction on the finger and flex the metacarpophalangeal joint, reducing the dislocation.

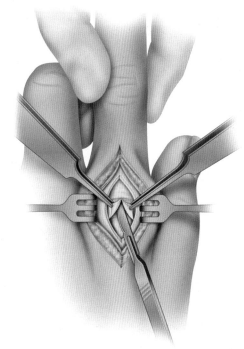

FIGURE **4.38**   Dorsal surgical approach to dislocated metacarpophalangeal joint. Volar plate caught over dorsal area of metacarpal head is incised longitudinally, and reduction is easily achieved. (Redrawn from Becton JL, Christian JD Jr, Goodwin HN, Jackson JG: A simplified technique for treating the complex dislocation of the index metacarpophalangeal joint, *J Bone Joint Surg* 57A:698-700, 1975.) **SEE TECHNIQUE 4.12.**

- Observe to see if any free cartilage is missing from the metacarpal head; this may be lodged in the joint.
- Suture the extensor tendon and skin.

POSTOPERATIVE CARE Begin early metacarpophalangeal joint flexion exercises, and protect the metacarpophalangeal joint from hyperextension with a splint for 3 weeks.

METACARPAL SHAFT OR NECK FRACTURES

Isolated metacarpal shaft fractures can be treated by closed methods if there is no excessive shortening, angulation, or rotational malalignment. The intervolar plate or intermetacarpal ligaments usually sufficiently suspend the middle and ring metacarpal shafts so that loss of length (which may occur in oblique or comminuted fractures) is usually functionally insignificant. When several metacarpals are fractured and there is open soft-tissue trauma, internal fixation is indicated. Correct rotational alignment is the most important factor in reduction (Figs. 4.39 and 4.40). Transverse midshaft fractures with significant apex dorsal angulation can be fixed with intramedullary wires, and certain oblique fractures can be fixed with interfragmentary screws. Intramedullary screws have been designed and used for a variety of tubular long bone hand fractures (Fig. 4.41). Using cannulated headless screws for various fractures was retrospectively reviewed by del Piñal et al., and the authors concluded that a single screw was sufficient for fixation of unstable metacarpal and phalangeal shaft fractures.

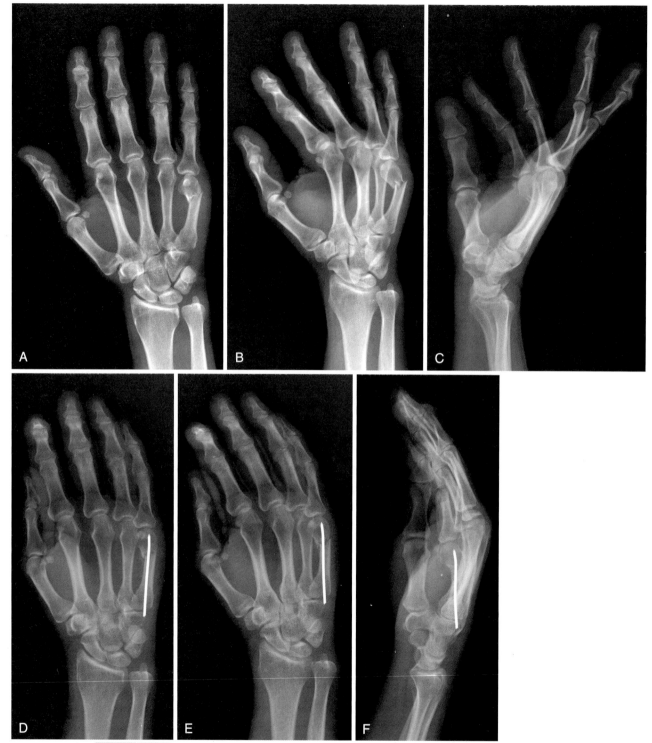

FIGURE 4.39   **A** to **C**, Fifth metacarpal neck fracture with 80-degree apex dorsal angulation and rotational deformity. **D** to **F**, After reduction to acceptable angulation, single pin was used to allow buddy taping to ring finger to ensure correct rotational alignment.

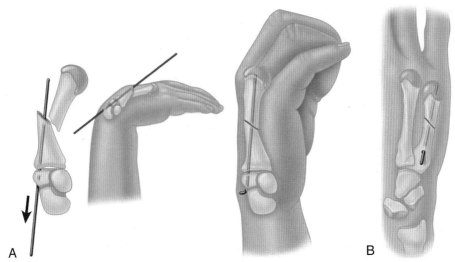

FIGURE 4.40   **A** and **B,** Open reduction and medullary fixation of fracture of metacarpal shaft and neck. **SEE TECHNIQUE 4.13.**

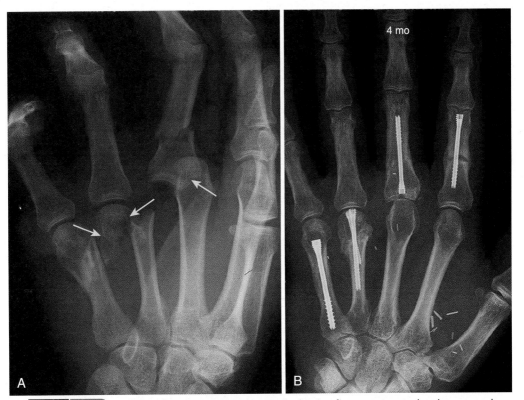

FIGURE 4.41   **A,** Severe subcapital comminution in the ring finger metacarpal and compound dislocation on base of middle finger (*arrows* point to area of comminution). **B,** Radiographs at 4 months. There is primary bone healing of little finger metacarpal and some callus on others, suggesting secondary wound healing. (From del Piñal F, Moraleda E, Rúas JS, et al: Minimally invasive fixation of fractures of the phalanges and metacarpals with intramedullary cannulated headless compression screws, *J Hand Surg Am 40[4]:692-700, 2015.*)

OPEN REDUCTION AND FIXATION OF METACARPAL SHAFT FRACTURE

TECHNIQUE 4.13

- Introduce a Kirschner wire at the fracture site, and drill it out through the skin at the metacarpal base; while drilling, force a bow in the wire convex toward the palm and hold the wrist in flexion so that the wire emerges on the dorsum of the wrist.
- Reduce the fracture, and drill the wire in the opposite direction into the distal fragment, stopping just proximal to the metacarpophalangeal joint.
- Cut off the proximal end under the skin (Fig. 4.40).
- Apply a splint holding the wrist in extension.
- A fracture of the metacarpal neck can be treated similarly if open reduction is necessary.

PERCUTANEOUS PINNING OF METACARPAL SHAFT FRACTURE

TECHNIQUE 4.14

- With the metacarpophalangeal joint acutely flexed, introduce a 0.062-inch Kirschner wire into the metacarpal head, and drill it to the level of the fracture. By manual pressure and manipulation of the wire and with the aid of an image intensifier, reduce the fracture and drill the wire out the dorsum of the wrist as described in Technique 4.13.
- Withdraw the wire until the distal tip is just proximal to the metacarpophalangeal joint.

Oblique metacarpal shaft fractures that are twice the length of the shaft diameter can be treated with interfragmentary screw fixation. The advantages of such fixation include less periosteal stripping and reduced implant prominence. Fracture site protection is advised for 6 weeks. Radiographic evidence of healing usually is lacking because of the anatomic fracture reduction.

Short oblique or transverse fractures with unacceptable angulation or displacement can be stabilized with plate-and-screw fixation or aligned by intramedullary fixation using a 0.062-inch Kirschner wire (Fig. 4.42). Image intensification is required for correctly establishing the entry portal in the middle of the metacarpal base and for ensuring that the wire crosses the fracture and enters the distal canal.

PERCUTANEOUS PINNING OF A METACARPAL SHAFT FRACTURE

TECHNIQUE 4.15

- Use general or regional block anesthesia.

- Use a fluoroscopic image to find the middle of the metacarpal base proximally and dorsally, and mark the area with a skin pen (Fig. 4.42A).
- Make a 0.5-cm longitudinal incision beginning 1.0 to 1.5 cm proximal to this mark.
- Spread bluntly down through the soft tissues to the base of the fractured metacarpal.
- Use as a trocar a pair of iris scissors to make an entry portal in the proximal metacarpal base in line with the long metacarpal axis (Fig. 4.42B).
- Cut the pointed end from a 0.062-inch Kirschner wire, and gently curve the end of the wire to assist in gaining entry into the medullary canal.
- Use fluoroscopy to ensure intramedullary containment of the wire, especially across the fracture site (Fig. 4.42C).
- If the wire is not easily passed across the fracture site, make a limited open incision to reduce the fracture.
- After the fracture is reduced, tamp the curved portion of the Kirschner wire into the metacarpal head, cut the wire squarely, and bury it below the skin away from sensory nerves and extensor tendons (Fig. 4.42D).

POSTOPERATIVE CARE A hand-based splint is applied, and buddy taping is used for fracture rotational control if needed. The sutures are removed at 10 to 14 days, and a removable hand-based splint is applied. The Kirschner wire is removed at 6 to 8 weeks, depending on clinical and radiographic healing (Fig. 4.42E and F).

METACARPAL HEAD FRACTURES

Intraarticular metacarpal head fractures, especially of the fourth and fifth metacarpals, often are caused by the patient striking an opponent's teeth in a fistfight. Compound injuries are almost always caused by human bites (see section on human bite treatment in chapter 16 for wound care and appropriate antibiotics). Many intraarticular metacarpal head fractures require open reduction and internal fixation, particularly if the articular surface is incongruous. These can be fixed with Kirschner wires. Occasionally, these fractures result in osteonecrosis of the displaced fragment (Fig. 4.43).

Although screws and plates have limited application in acute metacarpal fractures, the surgeon should be familiar with the techniques and equipment available to make a proper judgment in treatment of the individual patient. Complications of this method of treatment have been reported in 42% of patients.

OPEN REDUCTION AND PLATE FIXATION

The indications for plate fixation of the metacarpals are (1) multiple fractures with gross displacement or additional soft-tissue injury, (2) displaced diaphyseal transverse, short oblique, or short spiral fractures, (3) comminuted intraarticular and periarticular fractures, (4) comminuted fractures with shortening or malrotation or both, and (5) fractures with substance loss or segmental defects.

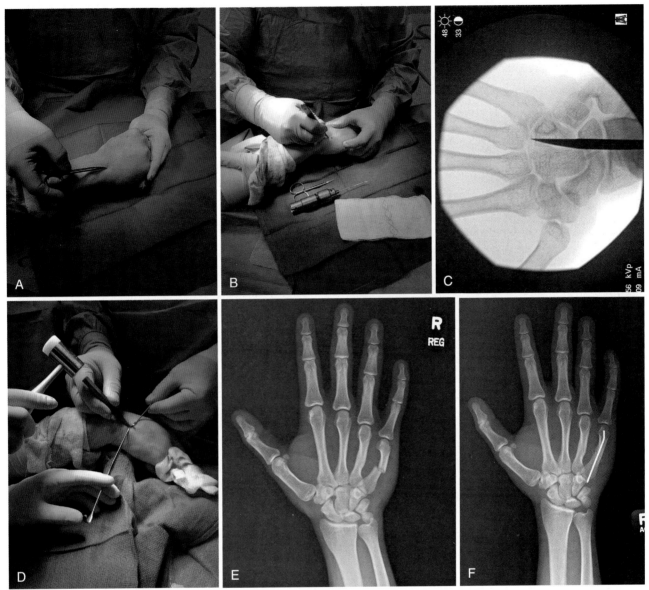

FIGURE 4.42   Percutaneous pinning of metacarpal shaft fracture. **A,** Skin marking to indicate middle of metacarpal base as determined by fluoroscopy. **B,** Incision proximal to metacarpal base. **C,** Fluoroscopic view shows correct entry position of intramedullary wire. **D,** Curved portion of Kirschner wire is tamped into metacarpal head. **E** and **F,** Anteroposterior preoperative and postoperative radiographs of patient with metacarpal shaft fracture treated with percutaneous pinning. **SEE TECHNIQUE 4.15.**

TECHNIQUE 4.16

- Plate fixation requires reduction, provisional stabilization by Kirschner wires or reduction clamps, and plate application.
- Expose the fracture surfaces sufficiently to allow anatomic reduction.
- Provisional fixation with reduction forceps is more difficult in the central metacarpals than the more accessible border index and small metacarpals. Because, in most instances, reduction forceps currently available are inadequate for clamping the plate to bone proximally and distally for provisional fixation, have an assistant hold the reduction and contour chosen plate to the metacarpal dorsum.
- For transverse fractures when an adequate palmar cortical buttress is restored, apply the plate as a dorsal tension band plate.
- Use a 2.7-mm dynamic compression plate across the fracture. In stable fractures, use a less bulky one fourth tubular plate and eccentric placement of the screws for compression. Tighten both screws terminally using the force of three digits on the screwdriver.
- To function as a tension band, contour the plate exactly to or slightly beyond the dorsal metacarpal bow to restore the anterior cortical buttress. Without anterior but-

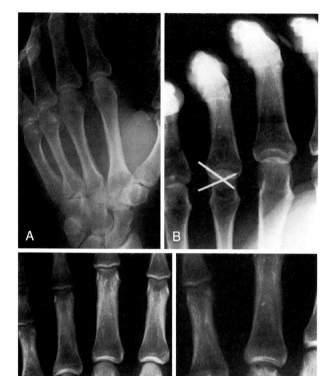

FIGURE 4.43   **A,** Radiograph of hand of 20-year-old man who sustained horizontally directed fracture of fourth metacarpal head with palmar fragment displaced proximally. **B,** Fracture was reduced and held in place with Kirschner wires. **C,** At 4 months, radiographs showed early osteonecrosis of metacarpal head. **D,** At 2½ years, radiographs showed some remodeling but definite incongruities of metacarpal head. (From McElfresh EC, Dobyns JH: Intra-articular metacarpal head fractures, *J Hand Surg* 8A:383-393, 1983.)

tressing, the plate bends and fatigues. When an anterior buttress is properly restored, the plate is protected from bending stress and is subjected mainly to tensile stress.
- Stabilize short oblique and spiral fractures by an interfragmentary screw followed by a dorsal plate to neutralize rotational stresses.
- When a T-shaped plate or oblique L-plate is used, apply the side arm or arms first because a rotational deformity can occur as the screws in the side arm or arms draw the underlying bone fragment up to the plate.
- For intraarticular fractures, lag the two articular fragments together with a screw separate from the plate and placed perpendicular to the fracture site.
- Alternatively, eccentrically place the two screws in the T or L portion of the plate away from the fracture to compress the two fragments on terminal screw tightening.
- With distal metaphyseal metacarpal fractures, dorsal plating may interfere with the extensor mechanism. To avoid

the interference, use a 2-mm condylar plate, applied dorsoradially and dorsoulnarly through the dorsal tubercle of origin of the collateral ligament.
- Plate fixation for metacarpal fractures should include screw purchase in at least four cortices distal and proximal to the fracture. The choice of plates must be tailored to the individual situation. Stabilize short oblique or spiral fractures requiring neutralization plating with a one fourth tubular plate and 2.7-mm dynamic compression plate or a one third tubular plate. Such a strut plate requires protection from loading and early bone grafting.

OPEN REDUCTION AND SCREW FIXATION

Screw fixation alone may be indicated in long oblique or spiral fractures and displaced intraarticular fractures (Fig. 4.44). The screw size and number will vary according to the fracture pattern. Not all metacarpal fractures shafts can accept even 2-mm screws; thus, smaller screws may adequately suit some fracture needs.

TECHNIQUE 4.17

- Fracture reduction follows local debridement of hematoma and soft tissue.
- Limit periosteal stripping to 1 or 2 mm, only enough to ensure anatomic reduction.
- Use reduction forceps or Kirschner wires for temporary fixation.
- Plan screw placement according to the fracture anatomy.
- For compressive forces, which act to deform and shorten the metacarpals, place a screw at 90 degrees to the bone's long axis. For torsional stress, place screws at 90 degrees to the fracture. The best compromise for resistance against axial and torsional loading is a screw that bisects the angle between a line 90 degrees to the fracture and 90 degrees to the bone's long axis.
- Check that screw placement near the fracture spikes is accurate to ensure bicortical purchase.
- The 2-mm screws are useful for shaft fractures, and the 2.7-mm screws are better for metaphyseal fractures.
- Countersink the screw head to allow for better load distribution and reduce screw head prominence.
- Interfragment gliding hole screws compress fracture surfaces together and convert the screws' torsional load to an axial load. Some metacarpal head fractures can be fixed with a single screw; fractures of the metaphysis and diaphysis require a minimum of two screws. Stable fixation by screws alone is possible for fractures with a length twice the bone diameter and fixed with two or more screws.

■ MINICONDYLAR PLATE FIXATION
Minicondylar plates sometimes are useful for metacarpal and phalangeal periarticular injuries. Indications may include (1)

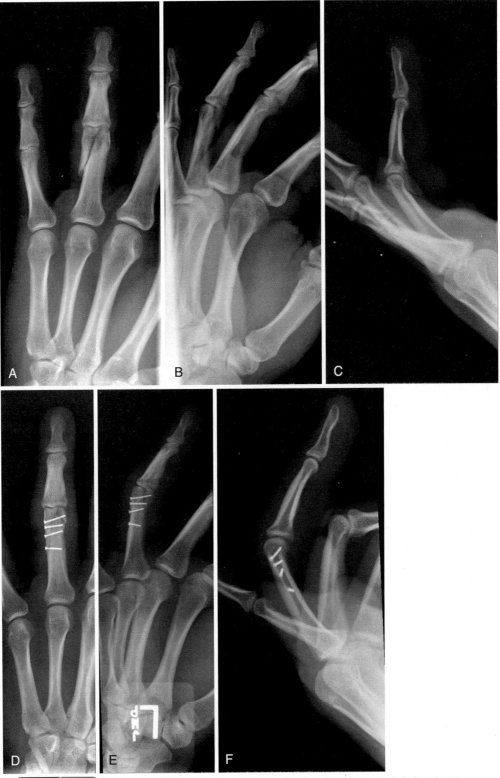

FIGURE 4.44   **A** to **C,** Three-part displaced intraarticular fracture of proximal phalanx in 27-year-old man. **D** to **F,** After open reduction and fixation with minifragment screws. Note that small screw heads do not interfere with collateral ligament function. **SEE TECHNIQUE 4.17.**

acute fractures associated with partial or complete flexor tendon disruption treated with primary tenorrhaphy and early motion, partial or complete extensor tendon injuries that are functionally competent or repaired so as to withstand early tensile loading, and periarticular injuries in which the risk

of joint stiffness is great because of the severity and location of associated soft-tissue injury, (2) replantation of digits, (3) metaphyseal osteotomies of phalanges or metacarpals, especially in conjunction with capsulotomy or tenolysis, (4) digit reconstruction (osteoplastic, pedicle graft, free composite tissue transfer) with need for stable skeletal fixation, and (5) arthrodesis. The three contraindications are: (1) use in the vicinity of open physes, (2) joint fragments narrower than 6 mm for the 2-mm plate or 5 mm for the 1.5-mm plate, and (3) condylar blade and screw intraarticular insertion, with the exception of the dorsal recess of the metacarpal head.

■ WIRING TECHNIQUES

Various wire configurations including tension band, 90-90, and cerclage can be used as sole methods of or supplements to fracture fixation. Although cerclage techniques may theoretically result in osteonecrosis, we have found this adjunct to be useful on occasion (Fig. 4.45).

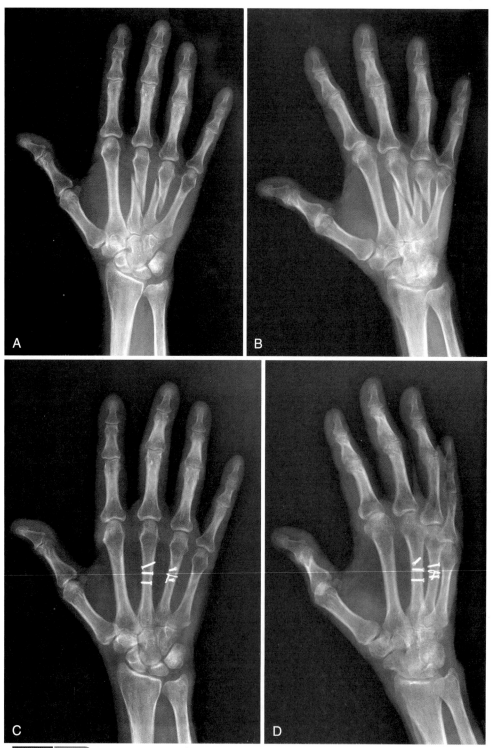

FIGURE 4.45   **A** and **B,** Middle and ring metacarpal shaft fractures in 75-year-old woman with shortening and obliquity suitable for interfragmentary fixation. **C** and **D,** Postoperative radiographs show anatomic reduction. Note that sagittal bending moment of ring metacarpal shaft fracture was offset by supplemental 24-gauge cerclage wire fixation.

PHALANGES
FRACTURE OF THE MIDDLE OR PROXIMAL PHALANX

A direct blow on the dorsum of the fingers often is the cause of middle and proximal phalangeal fractures. Angulation is toward the palm, and the fingers may assume a claw position (Fig. 4.46). When multiple or open, these fractures should be stabilized surgically. They can be approached through a longitudinal dorsolateral incision or, for a proximal phalangeal fracture, through one placed dorsally over the phalanx. The latter incision extends from the metacarpophalangeal to the PIP joint in an S curve.

OPEN REDUCTION

TECHNIQUE 4.18

(PRATT)
- Expose the extensor tendon, and incise it longitudinally in its center; retract it to each side to expose the fracture site (Fig. 4.47A and B).
- Drill a Kirschner wire into the distal fragment under direct vision; after reducing the fracture, drill it retrograde (Fig. 4.47C and D).

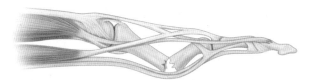

FIGURE 4.46   Full flexion of metacarpophalangeal joint is required to relax proximal phalangeal deforming forces and maintain reduction.

- Correct any rotational deformity, although some shortening may be acceptable.
- Repair the extensor tendon.
- Support the finger in the position of function and the wrist in extension.
- Sometimes an unstable oblique fracture of a middle or proximal phalanx can be treated by closed reduction and percutaneous pinning with a Kirschner wire inserted across the fracture. The Kirschner wire should be inserted midlaterally to avoid injury to the extensor hood and the flexor tendon (Fig. 4.48).

POSTOPERATIVE CARE The finger is splinted for 2 to 3 weeks, allowing protected early range of motion. The wire is removed in 3 to 4 weeks.

Belsky and Eaton described a useful technique for pinning multiple proximal phalangeal fractures. The fractured phalanx is held reduced with the metacarpophalangeal joint flexed to 90 degrees, while a single Kirschner wire is drilled from the dorsal aspect of the metacarpal head across the metacarpophalangeal joint and along the medullary canal to cross the fracture (Fig. 4.49). The wire should not cross the PIP joint and should be left exposed proximally to allow removal at 3 to 4 weeks. Some proximal phalangeal base intraarticular fractures may require open reduction and internal fixation. When restoration of near-anatomic joint surface articulation is necessary and early motion desirable, screw fixation may be preferable (Fig. 4.50).

Open or severely comminuted phalangeal fractures, especially of the proximal phalanx, may be unsuitable for internal fixation using traditional methods. In such cases, external fixation using a mini external fixator may be appropriate.

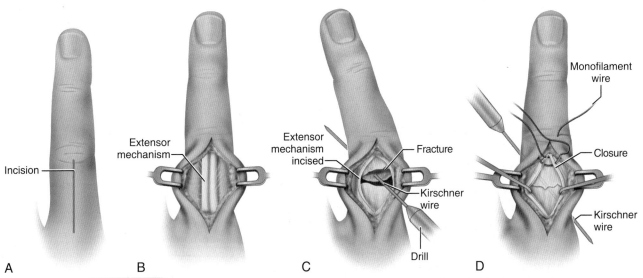

FIGURE 4.47   A through **D,** Some phalangeal shaft fractures may be suitable for crossed Kirschner wire fixation. Double-ended Kirschner wires can be used in an antegrade and retrograde fashion to preposition the Kirschner wires in the desired alignment. **SEE TECHNIQUE 4.18.**

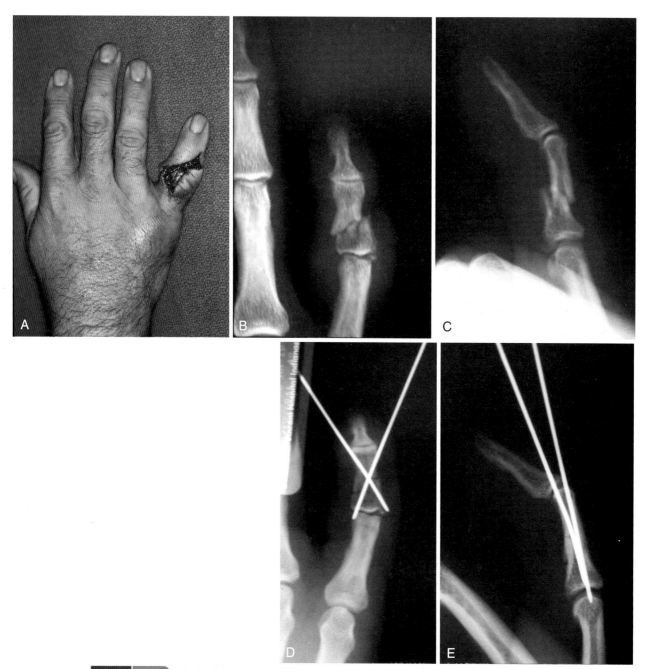

FIGURE 4.48   **A,** Crush injury to small finger resulting in middle phalangeal fracture. **B** and **C,** Fracture was inherently unstable and required stabilization. **D** and **E,** Pratt technique of crossed Kirschner wire fixation provided good alignment and stability.

PROXIMAL INTERPHALANGEAL JOINT FRACTURE-DISLOCATION

A PIP joint fracture-dislocation as a rule results in an unstable dorsal displacement of the middle phalanx caused by disruption of the attachment of the volar fibrocartilaginous plate. If a large, single volar fragment involving more than 50% of the joint surface is present, open reduction and internal fixation can be done with one or more Kirschner wires, minifragment screws, minifragment volar plate, or a wire loop pull-out. If the fragment or fragments include less than 40% of the articular surface, active motion of the PIP joint while maintaining the finger in an extension block splint may give satisfactory results, especially in cases without gross displacement. In PIP fracture-dislocations that have a comminuted surface of the middle phalanx of greater than 40%, instability usually persists because the collateral ligaments are attached to the volar fragment. Surgical intervention usually is required such cases, which may involve closed reduction and transarticular Kirschner wire placement, percutaneous fragment reduction and dorsal block pinning, static or dynamic external fixation, volar plate arthroplasty, and hemi-hamate osteoarticular autografts.

Extension block pinning is a simple technique for managing dorsal PIP joint fracture-subluxations and appears to be an attractive alternative to more complex techniques. A series of 12 patients with up to 75% articular involvement of the middle phalangeal base were treated by Bear et al., who

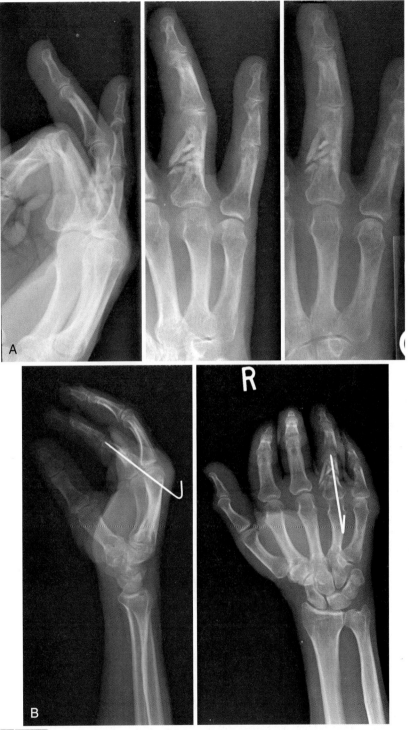

FIGURE 4.49 Belsky-Eaton pinning. **A,** Markedly unstable proximal phalangeal fracture treated by percutaneous pinning **(B)** across metacarpophalangeal joint. Metacarpophalangeal joint should be flexed at least 60 to 70 degrees, and proximal interphalangeal joint is not crossed.

reported an average 84 degrees motion and low pain scores at 3-year follow-up (Fig. 4.51). Similar range of PIP motion was found by Maalla et al. in 22 patients, 16 patients of whom had normal joint contours. In a smaller series of patients, Vitale et al. reported favorable outcomes when a percutaneous wire was used for fracture reduction in conjunction with a dorsal block pin.

Preservation of the proximal phalanx articular surface is necessary for most joint preservation or reconstructive procedures. Even in old, healed, displaced fractures cases treated up to 2 years after injury, Eaton and Malerich reported volar plate arthroplasty being successfully employed (Fig. 4.52).

An alternative treatment involves reconstruction of the middle phalanx volar lip by autogenous osteoarticular graft.

When dorsal subluxation of the PIP joint persists with 30 degrees of PIP joint flexion, an autogenous hemi-hamate osteoarticular graft has been recommended. A size-matched segment of the distal hamate articular surface is carefully shaped to match the contour of the middle phalanx (Fig. 4.53). We have found this technique useful, and in selected patients the need to protect the repair with provisional

pinning appears unnecessary because intraoperatively dramatic stability is achieved. Successful outcomes are dependent on accurate graft fashioning to "cup" to the proximal phalangeal head. Suboptimal results will be obtained when the graft is placed flatly and recurrent dorsal subluxation ensues. Some indications for this procedure include delayed presentations of PIP joint dorsal fracture subluxations with middle phalanx volar lip fractures exceeding 50% of the articular surface, failed volar plate arthroplasty, and failed dynamic traction or extension block splinting.

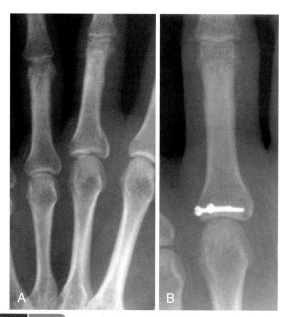

FIGURE 4.50   **A** and **B,** Comminuted intraarticular fracture in middle finger proximal phalanx base of avid tennis player treated by screw fixation.

HEMI-HAMATE AUTOGRAFT

TECHNIQUE 4.19

(WILLIAMS ET AL.)

- Expose the PIP joint through a volar V-shaped incision (apex radial or ulnar) from the palmar digital crease to the distal interphalangeal joint flexion crease.
- Protect the neurovascular bundles, and open the flexor sheath between the A2 and A4 pulleys. Retract the flexor tendons to the side by releasing them from the accessory collateral ligaments.
- Excise any bone fragments from the volar plate, and retract the volar plate proximally. This exposes the middle phalangeal fracture site and the proximal phalangeal head.
- Release the collateral ligaments, leaving a small portion attached to the middle phalangeal base to facilitate volar plate reattachment during closure. "Shotgun" the PIP

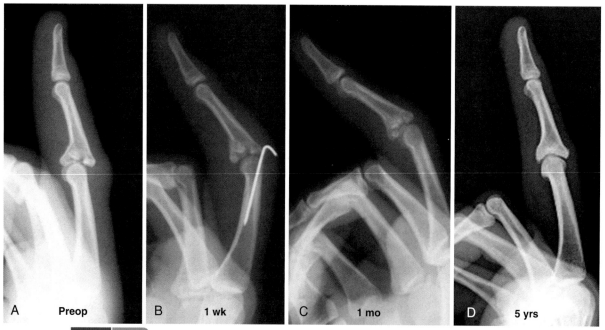

FIGURE 4.51   **A,** Preoperative and **(B-D)** follow-up lateral radiographs of patient treated with extension-block pinning. Initial images show V sign, indicative of instability. Remodeling of proximal interphalangeal joint surface was consistently noted, as can be seen here **(D)** at 5-year follow-up. (From Bear DM, Weichbrodt MT, Huang C, et al: Unstable dorsal proximal interphalangeal fracture-dislocations treated with extension-block pinning, *Am J Orthop (Belle Mead NJ)* 44:122-126, 2015.)

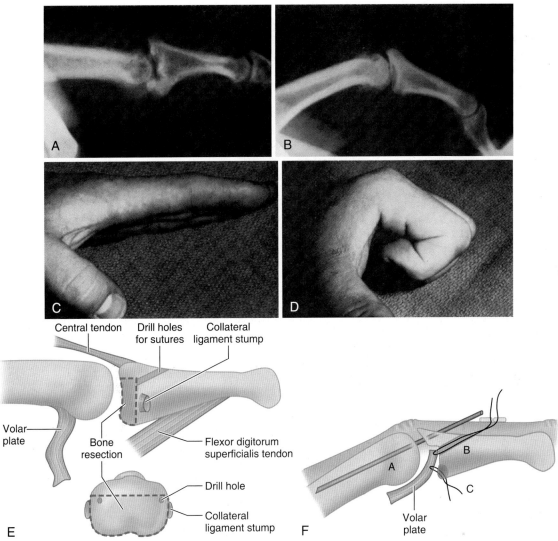

FIGURE 4.52 **A,** Radiograph 1 year after fracture-dislocation. Patient had pain and only 20 degrees of motion. **B,** Radiograph 14 months after arthroplasty. Note smooth, congruous articular arc. **C,** Active extension 14 months after arthroplasty of proximal interphalangeal joint. **D,** Active flexion 14 months after arthroplasty of proximal interphalangeal joint. **E** and **F,** Schema of volar plate advancement. (**A** to **D** from Eaton RG, Malerich MM: Volar plate arthroplasty for the proximal interphalangeal joint: a ten-year review, *J Hand Surg* 5A:260-268, 1980.)

joint by hyperextension and remove remaining bone fragments (Fig. 4.54A).
- Prepare the middle phalangeal base with a rongeur and oscillating saw, taking care to remove bone necessary for the graft. Take special care not to remove much dorsal bone to prevent fracture. Measure the defect with calipers.
- Under fluoroscopic guidance, make a 3-cm incision transversely at the ring and small finger carpometacarpal bases.
- Make a capsulotomy, and locate the distal surface of the hamate. Mark the desired graft centered on the distal hamate articular ridge. The graft should be slightly larger than the defect to allow further contouring.
- Make the axial hamate cut (Fig. 4.54B, *line A*) and sagittal hamate cut (Fig. 4.54B, *lines B and C*) with an osteotome or sagittal saw.

- The coronal cut can be made with a curved osteotome and is facilitated by removing a small notch of bone proximal to the axial cut (Fig. 4.54B, *line A*). Make sure not to make the cut too oblique because the graft must be contoured to cup the proximal phalangeal head.
- Contour the graft, place it into the defect, and, if necessary, place bone graft under the distal end of the graft to make it cup shaped.
- Provisionally fix the graft with a 0.9-mm Kirchner wire in the graft center, and fix the graft in place with 1.0- to 1.5-mm volar to dorsal screws. A third screw can be used if the graft is large enough in the provisional pin fixation site.
- Reduce the joint, and assess the reduction fluoroscopically. Note that the hamate articular cartilage is thicker than that of the proximal phalangeal base and an apparent

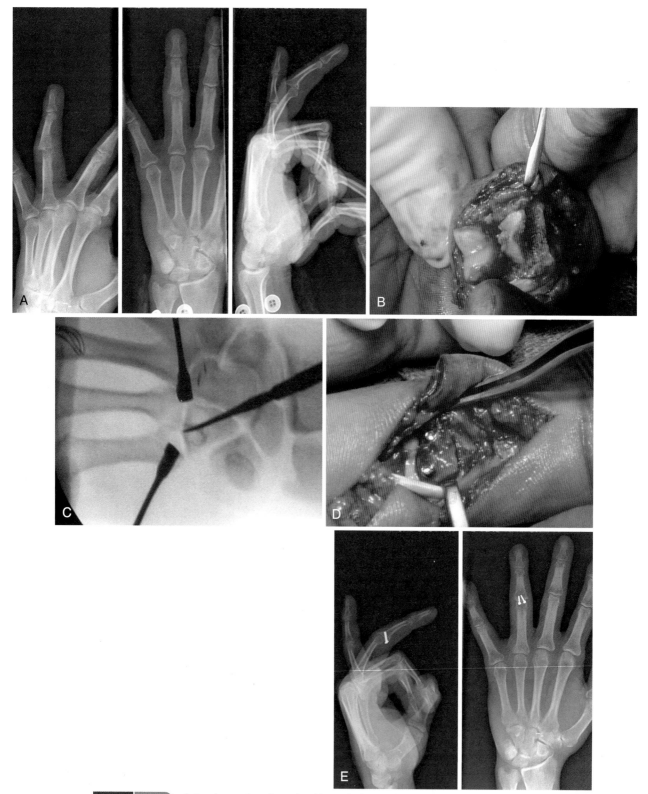

FIGURE 4.53 **A,** Persistent dorsal proximal interphalangeal joint subluxation with nonreconstructible middle phalangeal volar lip fracture. **B,** Volar exposure of middle phalangeal base and geometrical preparation of defect for graft. **C,** Fluoroscopic view of distal hamate donor site. **D,** Fixation of graft with two minifragment screws to replicate middle phalangeal base concavity. **E,** Concentric joint without collapse or dorsal subluxation at 2 years after surgery. **SEE TECHNIQUE 4.20.**

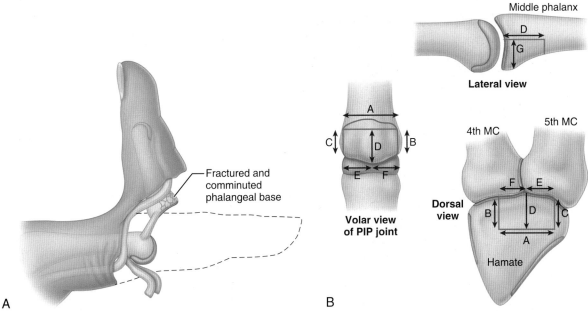

FIGURE 4.54 Hemi-hamate autograft for unstable proximal interphalangeal fracture-dislocation. **A,** "Shotgunned" proximal interphalangeal joint showing exposure of fracture and intact articular cartilage at base of middle phalanx. **B,** Prepared base of middle phalanx and corresponding donor site on hamate. *PIP,* Proximal interphalangeal. **SEE TECHNIQUE 4.19.**

radiographic step-off should not be worrisome as long as the visual reduction is satisfactory.

- Contour the graft distally to contour with the middle phalangeal cortex. Reattach the volar plate to the collateral ligament stumps. The reflected flexor sheath may be interposed between the flexor tendons and the volar plate.
- Deflate the tourniquet, obtain hemostasis, and apply a dorsal splint to block the PIP joint in 20 degrees of flexion.

POSTOPERATIVE CARE One week after surgery, range-of-motion exercises are begun, edema control measures are instituted, and a figure-of-eight splint is applied with a 15-degree extension block to provide lateral stability.

Some fractures around the PIP joint result in poor outcomes despite achievement of a concentric reduction (Fig. 4.55). Persistent swelling, limited motion, and intrinsic imbalance commonly accompany comminuted fractures of the middle phalangeal base regardless of the method of open reduction.

◼ CLOSED REDUCTION AND EXTENSION BLOCK SPLINTING

Marked comminution of the middle phalangeal shaft may be treated better by traction than by internal devices. These more complex injuries are not suited to open reduction techniques, and maintaining the undisturbed soft tissues around the fracture fragments seems to allow faster healing (Fig. 4.56). Numerous commercially available devices can be used to support the fracture, but few allow early motion at the PIP and distal interphalangeal joints.

After closed reduction, a malleable metal dorsal splint can be incorporated in a forearm gauntlet plaster cast so that the involved finger is maintained in flexion at the PIP joint and the metacarpophalangeal joint (Fig. 4.57). Because instability occurs when the PIP joint is extended, the angle at which it occurs can be determined before application of the plaster. The PIP joint is blocked in flexion 15 degrees short of this demonstrated position of instability. The proximal phalanx should be held securely against the dorsal splint to avoid extension at the PIP joint caused by further flexion of the metacarpophalangeal joint. Immediate flexion motion of the PIP joint is permitted. Full extension is not permitted for 6 to 12 weeks; however, an increased amount of extension may be permitted each week, and the patient is encouraged to increase flexion (Fig. 4.58).

OPEN REDUCTION

TECHNIQUE 4.20

(EATON AND MALERICH)

- Make a volar incision using an elongated V with the flap based radially.
- Excise the flexor tendon sheath from the proximal phalanx sufficiently to allow the tendons to be retracted to one side to view the entire joint.
- Hyperextend the joint to identify the fracture in fresh injuries.
- The volar plate is still attached to the bone fragments of the middle phalanx. Detach the accessory collateral ligament from both sides, freeing the volar plate.
- Detach the bone fragments by sharp dissection at the distal margin of the volar plate. In acute injuries, the collateral ligaments and joint capsule need not be incised.

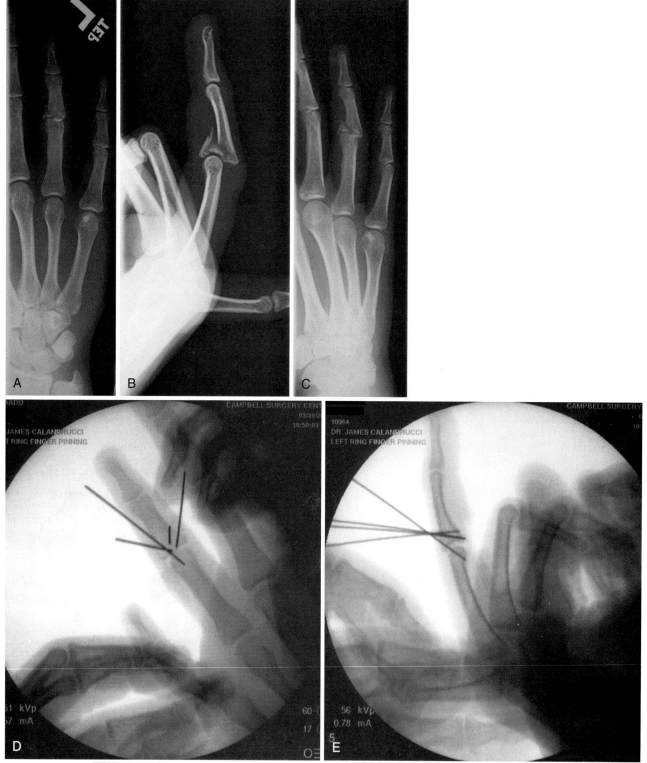

FIGURE 4.55   Proximal interphalangeal joint fracture-dislocation in 15-year-old softball player. Anterior **(A)**, lateral **(B)**, and oblique **(C)** views of markedly comminuted and unstable proximal interphalangeal joint fracture-dislocation. **D** and **E,** Reduction was obtained through volar approach. Persistent joint enlargement and limited motion resulted despite dorsal capsulectomy and aggressive physical therapy.

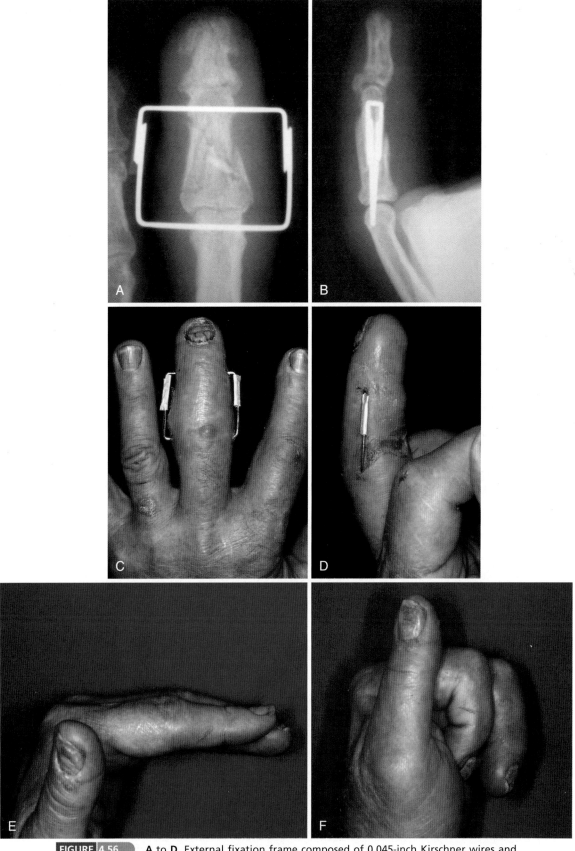

FIGURE 4.56 **A** to **D,** External fixation frame composed of 0.045-inch Kirschner wires and portions of disposable neurotip tube. Early motion is possible because axis pin passes through proximal head center. **E** and **F,** Clinical result 10 weeks after surgery.

- Drill two small holes at the extreme margin of a trough created at the middle phalanx by the bone deficit.
- Place the pull-out wire through each corner of the volar plate and through the drill holes to emerge dorsally.
- Place traction on these wires to snug the volar plate into the articular defect, effectively resurfacing the joint.
- Maintain reduction by flexing the joint no more than 35 degrees (Fig. 4.52E).
- Check congruity of reduction with a radiograph, and insert a Kirschner wire across the joint to maintain reduction.
- Place the hand and finger in a splint.

MALUNITED FRACTURES

- In old injuries in which the fractures have malunited, divide the volar plate as far distally as possible. It may be necessary to excise both collateral ligaments.
- Create a transverse trough at the proximal edge of the middle phalanx, and extend it completely across the bone to avoid an angular deformity when attaching the volar plate.
- The passive PIP joint motion should be 110 degrees, so as to easily touch the distal palmar crease with the fingertip. If passive motion is not 110 degrees, perform a dorsal capsular release and then attach the volar plate as described earlier.

POSTOPERATIVE CARE The splint is worn for 2 weeks, after which the Kirschner wire is removed and active guarded flexion is started with a dorsal block splint. At 5 weeks, full extension should be accomplished; and if not, a dynamic splint should be used. The pull-out wires can be removed at 3 weeks.

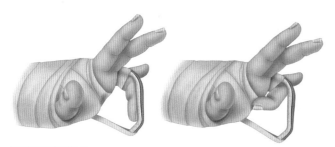

FIGURE 4.57   Extension-block splinting. (Redrawn from McElfresh EC, Dobyns JH, O'Brien ET: Management of fracture-dislocation of the proximal interphalangeal joints by extension-block splinting, *J Bone Joint Surg* 54A:1705-1711, 1972.)

■ DYNAMIC EXTERNAL SPLINT REDUCTION

Several methods are commonly used to reduce PIP joint fracture-subluxations. These techniques rely on coupling distraction and volarly directed forces across the joint. Common to most of these devices is achieving distraction force through pins placed through the rotation axes of the proximal and distal interphalangeal joints. The method by which the volarly

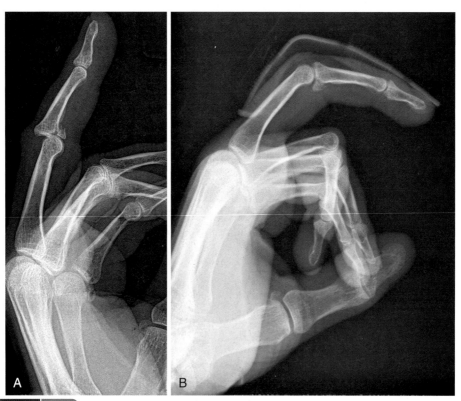

FIGURE 4.58   Dorsal fracture-dislocation of proximal interphalangeal joint in 54-year-old male patient. Before (**A**) and after reduction (**B**) lateral views showing treatment with dorsal block splint.

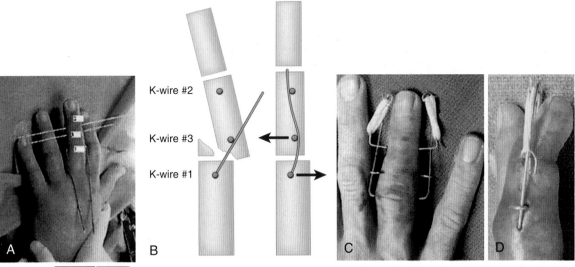

K-wire #2

K-wire #3

K-wire #1

A B C D

FIGURE 4.59 Dynamic distraction external fixation. **A,** Application of Kirschner wires. **B,** Lever-assisted reduction of fracture-dislocation. **C** and **D,** Assembled fixator. (From Ruland RT, Hogan CJ, Cannon DL, Slade JF: Use of dynamic distraction external fixation for unstable fracture-dislocations of the proximal interphalangeal joint, *J Hand Surg* 33A:19-25, 2008.) **SEE TECHNIQUE 4.21.**

directed forces are achieved differs according to the chosen technique.

DYNAMIC DISTRACTION EXTERNAL FIXATION

TECHNIQUE 4.21

(RULAND ET AL.)
- Under fluoroscopic guidance, attempt a closed reduction; make limited open incisions to achieve concentric reduction when necessary.
- Place a 0.045-inch Kirschner wire through the proximal phalangeal head rotational axis center. Bend the ends of this wire along the longitudinal axis of the digit, and rotate it dorsally for placement of the second pin.
- Place the second pin at the distal metadiaphyseal junction of the middle phalanx parallel to the distal interphalangeal joint. Place the third wire in the middle third of the middle phalanx, distal to the fracture site along the axis created by the first two wires (Fig. 4.59A).
- Rotate the first wire over the third wire (fulcrum) and under the second wire, thus providing a dorsally directed force on the proximal phalangeal head and a palmarly directed force on the middle phalangeal base (Fig. 4.59B).
- Fashion the free ends of the first wire into upward hooks and those of the second wire into downward hooks (Fig. 4.59C and D). Apply dental rubber bands (two usually are sufficient) between the hooks to serve as in-line traction across the PIP joint.
- Intraoperatively have the patient flex and extend the finger under fluoroscopic guidance. If concentric reduction is not present, apply a third rubber band.

- *Note:* If a pilon fracture is present, the use of a fulcrum wire is not necessary and may cause fracture angulation. In these cases the third wire is merely used for frame control.

POSTOPERATIVE CARE Immediate supervised range-of-motion exercises are begun, and weekly radiographs are made to evaluate the reduction and maintenance of the joint space. If the joint space exceeds that of the adjacent fingers, the rubber bands are reduced in number. At 6 weeks or when there is sign of radiographic union, the fixator is removed. Use of antibiotics is recommended when pin sites are of concern.

DYNAMIC INTRADIGITAL EXTERNAL FIXATION

TECHNIQUE 4.22

- Drive two parallel 0.045-inch Kirschner wires through the centers of the proximal and middle phalangeal heads.
- Bend the proximal phalangeal wire at 90 degrees on either side of the finger toward the distal pin. Then bend it again backward beginning about 1.0 cm distal to the distal pin and then again forward to engage the distal pin.
- Adjust the traction force by merely altering the angle of the wire engagement distally (Fig. 4.60).

When necessary, make midlateral incisions to assist in fracture reduction. Kapur et al. described another method to apply fixed distraction across an interphalangeal joint, incorporating Jurgan Pin Balls (Jurgan Development, Madison, WI) and Kirschner wires (Fig. 4.61). They used this

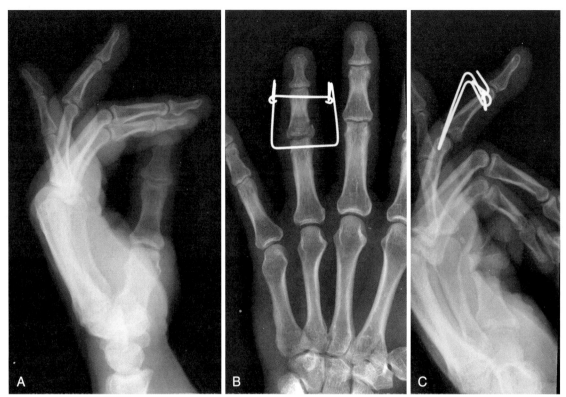

FIGURE 4.60 **A,** Proximal interphalangeal joint fracture-subluxation. **B** and **C,** Dynamic external fixation. **SEE TECHNIQUE 4.22.**

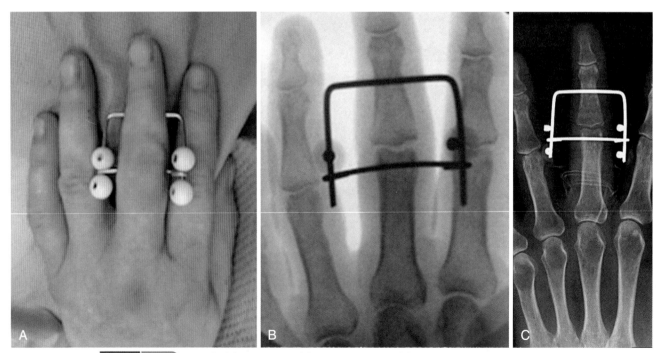

FIGURE 4.61 External fixator in situ (**A**), intraoperatively (**B**), and postoperatively (**C**). (From Kapur B, Paniker J, Casaletto J: An alternative technique for external fixation of traumatic intra-articular fractures of proximal and middle phalanx, *Tech Hand Surg* 19:163-167, 2015.)

technique in 20 patients for a variety of fractures involving the proximal and middle phalanges, including oblique, spiral, and volar plate injuries, and reported near-normal motion, no rotational deformity, normal grip strength, and no functional deficit of the involved finger as reported by the patients.

INTERPHALANGEAL DISLOCATIONS

Most interphalangeal dislocations are dorsal and usually are reduced immediately by the patient or a bystander. The collateral ligaments usually are not ruptured and provide adequate stability for early protected range of motion after closed reduction. If one or both of the collateral ligaments are completely ruptured in a young adult, and the joint is unstable, the ligaments should be repaired, especially if the rupture is on the radial side of the index finger. If the joint remains unstable with persistent dorsal subluxation, the joint may be pinned in 20 degrees of flexion for 2 to 3 weeks. Alternatively, a pin can be used merely as a dorsal block, permitting flexion exercises of the joint early.

In contrast to dorsal dislocations, volar PIP joint dislocations often cannot be reduced with closed techniques. Entrapment of the lateral band around the head of the proximal phalanx may block reduction, and open reduction may be necessary. Nonconcentric reduction after a closed reduction, usually caused by soft tissue or bony interposition, also requires open reduction (Figs. 4.62 and 4.63).

Unstable joints that are the result of acute trauma or reconstructive efforts can be managed with numerous small dynamic external fixators. These devices allow early motion while maintaining reduction of the joint.

■ UNSTABLE PROXIMAL INTERPHALANGEAL JOINT SECONDARY TO CHRONIC COLLATERAL LIGAMENT RUPTURE

In rare instances, the PIP joint may be grossly unstable laterally. A tendon graft can be used to replace the collateral ligament (Fig. 4.64).

TENDON GRAFT TO REPLACE RUPTURED COLLATERAL LIGAMENT

TECHNIQUE 4.23

- Make a midlateral incision over the PIP joint on the side of the collateral ligament insufficiency.
- Incise the transverse retinacular ligament, and reflect the extensor mechanism dorsally.
- Excise any scar tissue from around the origin and insertion of the cord fibers.
- Drill a hole completely through the bone on each side of the joint (Fig. 4.65).
- Obtain the necessary graft material, such as the palmaris longus tendon.
- Tie a 4-0 suture or 34-gauge wire loop around each end of the graft, and bring one end out through one of the holes on the side opposite the injury.
- Pass the other end of the graft across the joint and through the hole in the other bone in the appropriate direction.
- Pass each wire loop on the ends of the graft through a piece of felt and then through separate holes in a single button.

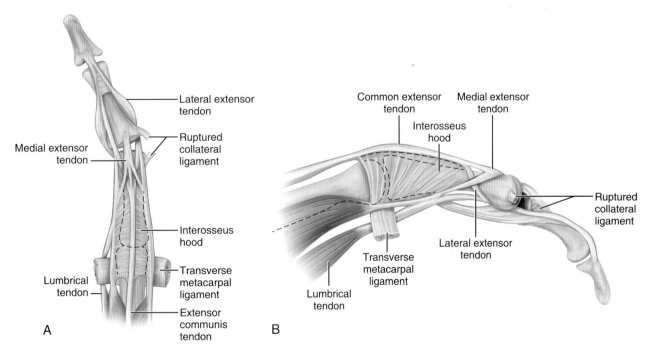

FIGURE 4.62 Irreducible dislocation of proximal interphalangeal joint. Collateral ligament has been torn, and lateral band of extensor hood has been trapped within joint. **A,** Dorsal view. **B,** Lateral view.

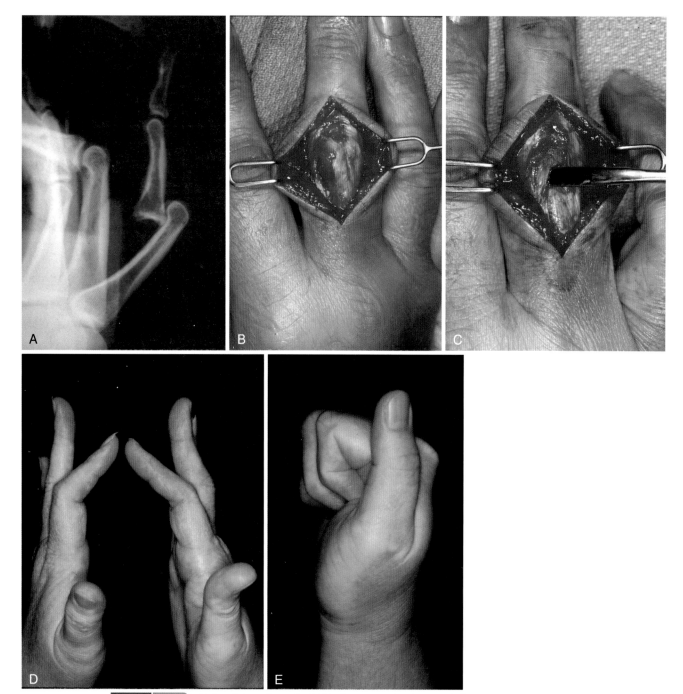

FIGURE 4.63 Volar dislocation of middle finger proximal interphalangeal joint. **A,** Injury suggestive of central slip injury. **B,** Proximal phalangeal radial condyle buttonholed through extensor mechanism with lateral band trapped volarly. **C,** Lateral band reduced. **D** and **E,** Despite acute anatomic repair and good flexion, extensor lag of 20 degrees persisted.

- Pull the graft snug, and tie the two wires together over the button.
- Additionally, an accessory collateral ligament can be created if necessary. Section a portion of the tendon sheath on the side opposite the defect; maintain its insertion into the bone on the side of the involved collateral ligament, and fold this fascia-like sheath over the grafted tendon. Suture it to the graft with the finger in extension. Transfix the joint with an oblique Kirschner wire.

POSTOPERATIVE CARE At 3 weeks, the Kirschner wire is removed and motion is begun. The button and wire loop are removed at 4 to 6 weeks.

▣ UNDIAGNOSED INTERPHALANGEAL DISLOCATIONS

Failure to diagnose interphalangeal dislocations is rare but does occur because swelling soon obscures the landmarks

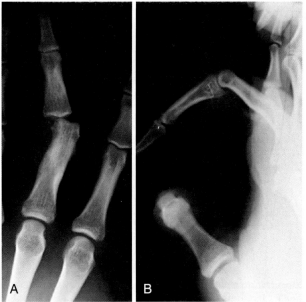

FIGURE 4.64 **A,** Chronically unstable proximal interphalangeal joint permitted tilting and produced pain on pinch. **B,** Alignment by segmental graft from palmaris longus tendon attached through bone.

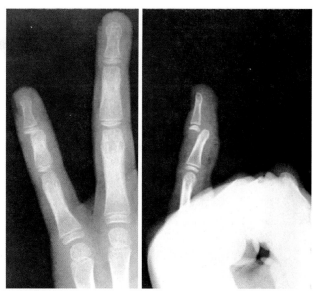

FIGURE 4.66 Radiographs of interphalangeal dislocation in child. Injury had gone undiagnosed for 1 month because deformity appeared slight externally. After open reduction, flexion of 30 degrees was eventually possible.

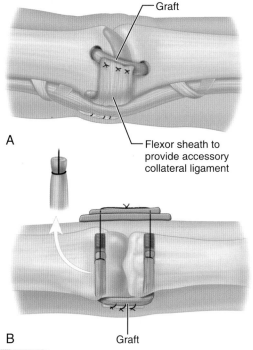

Graft

Flexor sheath to provide accessory collateral ligament

Graft

FIGURE 4.65 **A** and **B,** Reconstruction of collateral ligament of proximal interphalangeal joint with tendon graft. **SEE TECHNIQUE 4.23.**

OPEN REDUCTION AND FIXATION WITH A KIRSCHNER WIRE

TECHNIQUE 4.24

- Make a midlateral incision at the level of the affected interphalangeal joint.
- Expose the joint, remove the granulation tissue and the remaining hematoma, and reduce the joint under direct vision.
- Often, the volar plate lies between the joint surfaces and both collateral ligaments must be excised.
- Hold the joint with an oblique Kirschner wire, and place the finger in a splint.
- If at surgery the joint is found to be completely destroyed, it should be arthrodesed.

POSTOPERATIVE CARE In 2 weeks, the wire can be removed, and active motion is begun.

■ DISTAL PHALANGEAL FRACTURES

Distal phalangeal fractures caused by crushing injuries usually are comminuted and require only splinting. Treatment is primarily directed at managing the associated soft-tissue injuries, such as nail bed lacerations. When a circular wound is present that nearly amputates the fingertip, a Kirschner wire or a 22-gauge hypodermic needle is valuable in supporting the bone while the soft tissues heal (Fig. 4.68). Prolonged tenderness and hypoesthesia of the fingertip after the fracture are common for many months.

that make early diagnosis easy. If the dislocation is not diagnosed within the first week, joint cartilage may be eroded by pressure from the articular edge of the dislocated phalanx; open reduction is then usually necessary (Figs. 4.66 and 4.67).

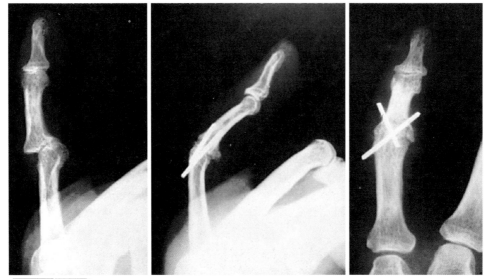

FIGURE 4.67 Undiagnosed interphalangeal dislocation in adult complicated by infected wound. Bone has been eroded. At 6 weeks after injury, infection had been controlled, and joint was arthrodesed.

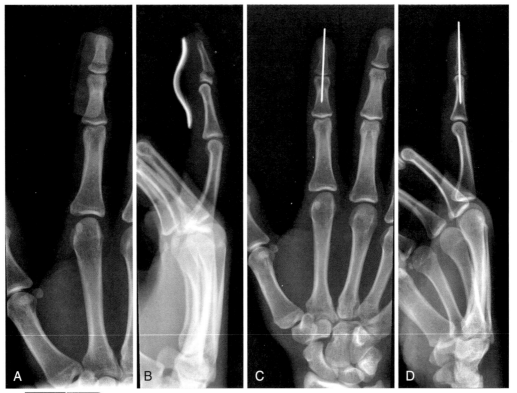

FIGURE 4.68 **A** and **B,** Displaced and angulated distal phalangeal fracture associated with nail bed laceration in 22-year-old college student. **C** and **D,** After bone fixation, which permitted subsequent realignment and repair of nail bed.

■ MALLET FINGER

Disruption of the terminal extensor tendon frequently results in a distal interphalangeal joint extension lag and is commonly referred to as a *baseball* or *mallet finger deformity.* Full passive distal interphalangeal joint extension usually remains, and PIP joint hyperextension may develop because of secondary volar plate laxity from proximal migration of the extensor apparatus resulting in a swan neck deformity. The usual cause is a forceful blow to the tip of the finger causing sudden flexion; however, a hyperextension injury with fracture of the dorsal lip of the distal phalanx also may manifest as mallet deformity. Although closed injuries are more common, open injuries caused by lacerations and crush abrasions also occur. Approximately 40% of mallet fingers result from minor

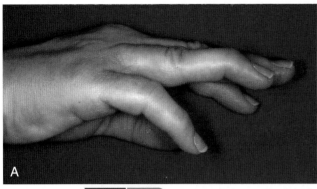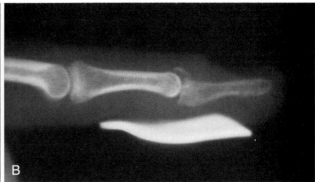

FIGURE 4.69 **A,** Acute type 1 mallet finger with secondary "swanning" of proximal interphalangeal joint. **B,** Aluminum splint achieving full extension of distal interphalangeal joint.

injuries. Mallet fingers are classified into four types according to associated soft-tissue injuries and the fracture pattern:

Type 1: Closed or blunt trauma with loss of tendon continuity with or without a small avulsion fracture.

Type 2: Laceration at or proximal to the distal interphalangeal joint with loss of tendon continuity.

Type 3: Deep abrasion with loss of skin, subcutaneous cover, and tendon substance.

Type 4: *4A,* transphyseal fracture in children; *4B,* hyperflexion injury with fracture of articular surface of 20% to 50%; *4C,* hyperextension injury with fracture of the articular surface usually greater than 50% with early or late volar subluxation of the distal phalanx.

Type 1 mallet fingers are the most common. Differentiating small avulsion type 1 fractures from the larger type 4 fractures is important because the subluxation or dislocation present in type 4 fractures determines treatment.

Treatment for type 1 mallet fingers usually consists of continuous distal interphalangeal joint extension splinting with a molded polythene (Stack) or aluminum splint for 6 to 8 weeks (Fig. 4.69). Night splinting usually is recommended for an additional 2 to 6 weeks. Volar or dorsal splints can be used, but care must be taken when applying them to prevent skin maceration and ulceration. Hyperextension of the distal interphalangeal joint should be avoided because it causes skin blanching, which possibly contributes to skin breakdown. Although open type 2 injuries can be treated with closed reduction after appropriate wound care, splint management can be difficult. Direct repair of the extensor tendon can be done by tendon suture repair and Kirschner wire fixation of the distal interphalangeal joint in full extension.

Type 3 mallet fingers require soft-tissue coverage and pinning of the distal interphalangeal joint and possible primary arthrodesis. Pediatric mallet fingers or Seymour fractures should be treated with closed reduction and splinting of the distal interphalangeal joint in neutral or slight extension for 4 weeks. These fractures frequently are open fractures, as evidenced by fairly continuous bleeding around the nail base. The nail often is displaced out of the proximal eponychial fold and rests dorsally on the skin. After an adequate digital block (single injection at the palmar digital crease), the wound should be cleaned and irrigated by gently flexing the distal fragment. The nail is placed beneath the eponychial fold, and a splint and dressing are applied. Displaced Salter-Harris type III fractures are reduced closed with mild extension of the distal phalanx. Open reduction and Kirschner wire fixation

of the epiphyseal fragment are indicated if closed reduction cannot be obtained. Treatment of type 4B and type 4C mallet fingers is controversial. Operative treatment is associated with numerous complications, including infection, nail deformity, tender pulp scars, and loss of reduction and fixation. Nonoperative treatment by extension splinting is recommended by some for all mallet fractures, including the hyperextension type with subluxation of the distal phalanx. Joint congruity may not affect end results. For fractures involving more than one third of the articular surface and associated subluxation and dislocation, open reduction using a pull-out wire and transarticular Kirschner wire in extension is advised (Figs. 4.70 and 4.71). Painful chronic mallet fingers resulting from fracture-dislocation are probably better treated with distal interphalangeal joint arthrodesis.

OPEN REDUCTION AND FIXATION WITH A PULL-OUT WIRE AND TRANSARTICULAR KIRSCHNER WIRE

TECHNIQUE 4.25

(DOYLE)

- Expose the joint through a zigzag dorsal incision (Fig. 4.72A).
- Pass a 0.035-inch Kirschner wire longitudinally through the distal phalanx (Fig. 4.72B).
- Reduce the joint and manipulate the fracture fragment into place.
- Pass the Kirschner wire across the joint, holding it in full extension.
- Obtain radiographs in two planes to verify reduction.
- If the fracture fragment cannot be maintained in close apposition to the major fragment, use a pull-out suture to hold it in position (Fig. 4.72C).
- After closure, apply a splint to protect the transarticular Kirschner wire.

POSTOPERATIVE CARE The splint and Kirschner wire are removed at 6 weeks, and range-of-motion exercises are begun.

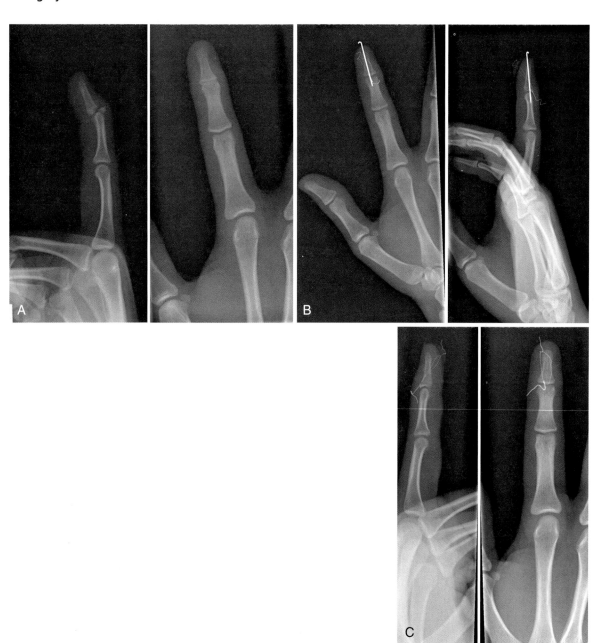

FIGURE 4.70   **A,** Type 4 mallet finger in high school basketball player. **B,** Results of pull-out wire and pin fixation of distal interphalangeal joint just before pin removal at 4 weeks. **C,** Pull-out wire left in until 6 weeks after surgery.

INTRAARTICULAR FRACTURES

Intraarticular fractures with a single fragment involving one third or more of the joint surface and that are accompanied by subluxation or dislocation require reduction and fixation with a suture or a Kirschner wire (see section on fracture-dislocation of the PIP joint). Closed reduction is sometimes accomplished by flexing the finger and apposing the larger fragment to the smaller; the joint is transfixed with a Kirschner wire. Another closed method is three-point skeletal traction using a vertical traction ring. Open reduction usually is preferred, however. A Kirschner wire is drilled into the smaller fragment, the fracture is reduced, and the wire is brought out through the larger fragment. The drill is attached to the opposite end of the wire and used to extract it until its

tip is just beneath the articular cartilage of the smaller fragment. Motion usually can be started at 2 weeks, and the wire can be removed at 4 weeks. As an alternative, a small AO screw (1.5 or 2 mm) can be used to fix an articular fragment, provided that the fragment's width is three times the diameter of the screw being used.

Impaction fractures with comminution may require supplemental bone grafting in addition to internal fixation after careful surgical elevation of the depressed articular fragments. Intraarticular fractures include avulsion fractures at the insertions of tendons and ligaments. The fragments usually are displaced widely by the pull of the tendon or ligament and should be reduced and fixed internally to restore tendon or ligament function and joint integrity (Fig. 4.73). When the

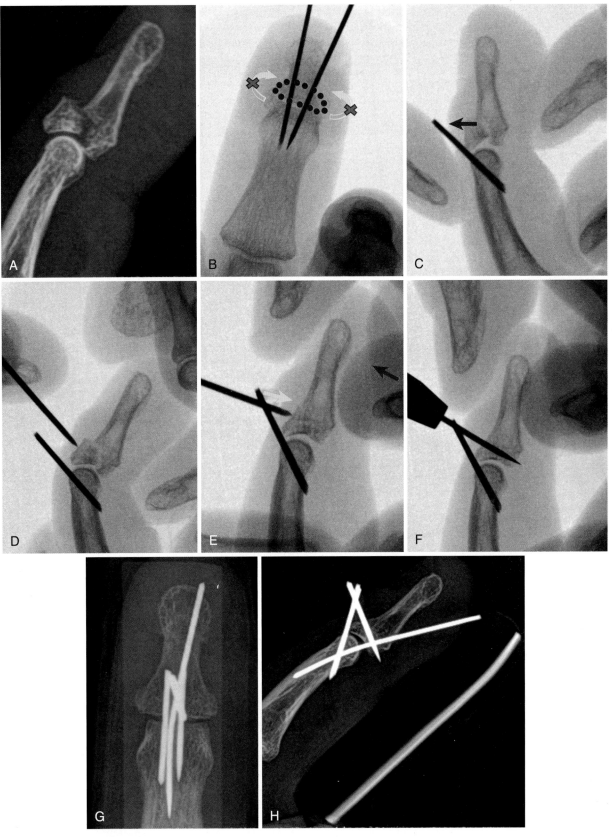

FIGURE 4.71 Mallet fracture of ring finger in 60-year-old man. (See complete legend on following page.)

FIGURE **4.71**   Mallet fracture of ring finger in 60-year-old man. **A,** Preoperative simple radiograph showing fracture fragment involving more than 50% of articular surface. **B,** Intraoperative anteroposterior C-arm image. Using modified two-extension block technique, two parallel block wires inserted 2 mm apart. Note two parallel block wires prevent rotation of dorsal fragment in axial plane *(yellow arrow)*. *Red circle,* fractured dorsal fragment. **C,** Intraoperative lateral C-arm image showing trial of closed reduction with traction and dorsal translation. *Red arrow* shows dorsal rotation of dorsal fragment in sagittal plane. **D,** Dorsal counterforce applied to dorsal fragment using 1.1-mm Kirschner wire. **E,** By applying dorsal counterforce to dorsal fragment, anatomic reduction with traction and dorsal translation of distal digit was achieved. *Red arrow* shows compressive force from volar side and yellow arrow shows dorsal counterforce by Kirschner wire. **F,** Due to large size of dorsal fragment, Kirschner wire used for dorsal counterforce was pushed into fragment for fixation. **G,** Postoperative anteroposterior radiograph. **H,** Postoperative lateral radiograph. Volar aluminum orthosis protects wire and limits excursion of extensors by blocking movement of distal interphalangeal joint. (From Lee SH, Lee JE, Lee KH, et al: Supplemental method for reduction of irreducible mallet finger fractures by the 2-extension block technique: the dorsal counterforce technique, *J Hand Surg Am* 2018 Nov. 5. Pii:S0363-5023(18)30406-4.)

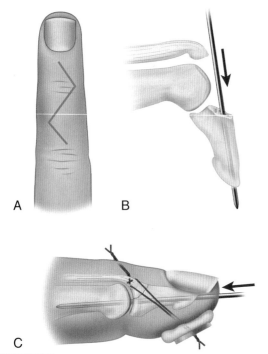

FIGURE **4.72**   Reduction and fixation for mallet fracture. **A,** Joint is exposed through dorsal zigzag incision. **B,** Kirschner wire is drilled longitudinally through distal phalanx. **C,** Joint is reduced, Kirschner wire is driven proximally across joint, and fracture fragment is reduced. If fracture fragment cannot be maintained in proper position, pull-out suture is passed through fragment and distal phalanx and tied over padded button. (From Green DP, editor: *Operative hand surgery*, ed 3, New York, 1993, Churchill Livingstone; redrawn after Elizabeth Roselius.) **SEE TECHNIQUE 4.25.**

fragment is small (less than one fourth of the joint surface), treatment is directed toward the soft-tissue avulsion and may consist of open reduction and splinting or splinting alone in the position of function.

Hemicondylar fractures produced by lateral stress (usually at the PIP joint) require internal fixation if displaced. Open reduction often is necessary, but closed reduction and percutaneous pinning (Fig. 4.74) can be attempted.

The outcome after intraarticular fractures of the interphalangeal joints of the hand depends on the patient's age, location of injury, degree of comminution, associated soft-tissue injuries, accuracy of reduction, and postoperative management. At long-term follow-up, pain usually diminishes and motion improves with time. According to O'Rourke, Gaur, and Barton, only 27% of their patients were pain free at early follow-up, but 66% reported no discomfort after 11 years. A gradual improvement in motion was observed, but only 60% regained a normal range of motion; 17% showed radiographic evidence of posttraumatic arthritis; however, radiographic findings did not correlate with pain.

COMPLICATIONS OF HAND FRACTURES

Complications of fractures include malunion, nonunion, adhesion of tendons to the fracture site, infection (see chapter 16), and limitation of joint motion. If multiple tissues must be reconstructed, the repair of bones and joints is third in the order of priority. If good skin coverage is absent, repair fails; if the hand is insensitive, repair is futile. Bone and joint reconstruction procedures are indicated only after good skin coverage can be obtained and when at least protective sensation is present or is forthcoming.

MALUNION

If fractures of one or more bones of the hand unite in poor position, the resulting disturbance of muscle balance causes weakness of grasp and pinch, especially if the metacarpals and proximal phalanges are involved. The kinesthetic sense also seems to be disturbed. Rotational malalignment and angulation can cause notable hand deformity, which usually is accentuated when a composite fist is made.

Not every malunited fracture requires intervention. The function of the fingers and the hand, not the radiographic appearance, determines whether treatment is necessary. Ill-advised treatment usually fails to improve function and sometimes makes it worse. Minor malunion deformities usually should be accepted when motion of the surrounding joints is satisfactory because treatment by osteotomy can lead not only to nonunion but also to difficulty in reestablishing satisfactory joint motion. This is especially true in patients beyond middle age.

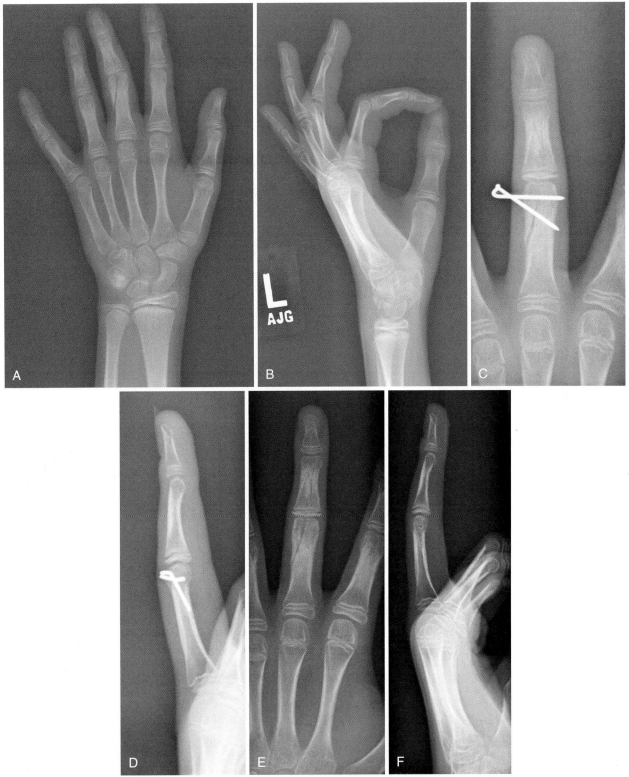

FIGURE 4.73 Closed reduction and pinning of displaced intraarticular fracture of proximal phalangeal head in 11-year-old girl. **A** and **B,** Anteroposterior and lateral images before reduction. **C** and **D,** Kirschner wire fixation. **E** and **F,** Final follow-up.

Most malunited fractures of the metacarpal neck should not be treated, particularly fractures of the neck of the fifth metacarpal. Flexion deformities of 40 degrees or more can easily be accepted with good function. When the fifth metacarpal head is displaced volarward, the carpometacarpal joint allows dorsal displacement of the distal end of the bone so that the palm can yield when a hard object is grasped; this also is true to less extent of the ring finger. For the second and third metacarpals, however, there is little or no motion in the carpometacarpal joints; and when the metacarpal head is displaced volarward, pain with firm grasp may occur. When a metacarpal head is markedly displaced, metacarpophalangeal joint hyperextension and secondary collateral ligament contracture often occur; a capsulotomy and an osteotomy may be necessary.

Certain malunions can be treated with corrective osteotomy (Fig. 4.75). When articular cartilage loss results in angular deformity, subluxation, dislocation, impending joint destruction, or pain, osteoarticular grafts may be useful (Fig. 4.76). Complex malunions can be approached by using CT images to generate patient-specific systems. The preliminary results reported by Hirsiger et al. for such a system indicate that a precise reduction for corrective osteotomies of metacarpal (six patients) and phalangeal (two patients) bones can be achieved by using three-dimensional (3D) planning and patient-specific guides.

CORRECTION OF METACARPAL NECK MALUNION

TECHNIQUE 4.26

- Make a longitudinal dorsal incision just proximal and lateral to the metacarpal head; expose the extensor hood, and

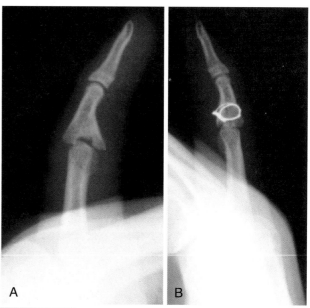

FIGURE 4.75   **A,** Malunited fracture of base of middle phalanx with splaying of volar and dorsal articular surfaces. **B,** After wedge resection of bone, volar and dorsal fragments were held securely with cerclage wire fixation.

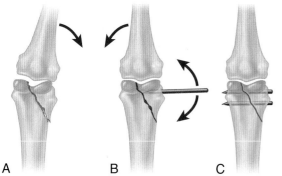

FIGURE 4.74   **A,** Displaced, unstable condylar fracture usually requires open reduction and fixation. **B,** Manipulation of fracture using intact collateral ligament may permit insertion of Kirschner wire to hold reduction. **C,** Two wires are necessary to avoid rotation and displacement of the reduced fragment.

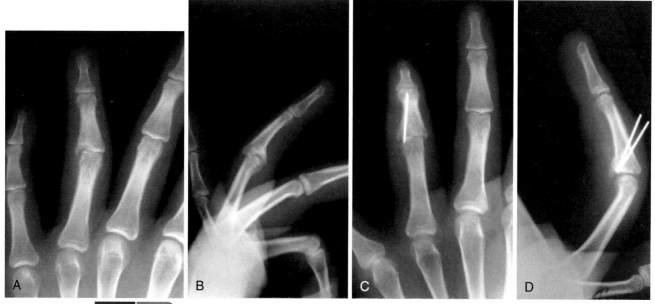

FIGURE 4.76   **A** and **B,** Destruction of middle phalanx ulnar base of golfer's ring finger resulted in ulnar deviation and pain. **C** and **D,** Osteoarticular graft fashioned from ipsilateral distal radius resulted in satisfactory correction of deformity.

free it on one side of the metacarpal neck with a sharp knife.

- Dissect the interosseous muscle from the lateral side of the neck and the extensor tendon and expansion from its dorsum as necessary for sufficient exposure.
- If the callus is hard, drill across the old fracture site transversely; otherwise, cut across it with an osteotome.
- Drill the medullary canal proximally and distally so that it accepts a medullary cortical bone peg a little larger than a matchstick. The peg can be obtained from the proximal ulna or proximal tibia.
- Insert it proximally into the medullary canal of the shaft and cap it with the metacarpal head.
- Carefully check rotational alignment, and impact the fragments.
- Pack cancellous bone chips around their juncture as needed. If the osteotomy is unstable despite the bone peg, insert a Kirschner wire across the osteotomy site (Fig. 4.77).
- Examine the metacarpophalangeal joint for passive flexion; when the collateral ligaments are contracted and allow little or no motion, capsulotomy may be indicated.
- Suture the lateral expansion of the extensor hood in place with fine suture.
- Hold the metacarpophalangeal joint in 60 to 70 degrees of flexion and apply a protective splint.

POSTOPERATIVE CARE A dorsal splint is worn for 2 weeks to maintain the metacarpophalangeal joints in 70 degrees of flexion, allowing some flexion of the interphalangeal joints. Sutures are removed at 2 weeks, and a lighter splint is applied that prevents extension of the metacarpophalangeal joint but allows flexion and extension of the interphalangeal joints. This splint is worn an additional 1 or 2 weeks.

Malunion of a metacarpal shaft or of a phalanx also can be treated with a medullary cortical bone peg; the peg must be shaped carefully to fit snugly (Fig. 4.78). Figure 4.79 illustrates malunited phalangeal fractures treated by osteotomy and fixation with Kirschner wires.

Malrotation of a proximal phalanx at any level should be treated by osteotomy at the base of the phalanx when possible. The base of the phalanx heals well and is cut with less difficulty than the hard cortical bone in the middle third. It is important to make an orientation mark on each side of the proposed osteotomy line so that these reference points can be used to determine the amount of change during the procedure.

NONUNION

Nonunion in the phalanges is caused most often by distraction of the fragments by traction; other causes are infection, lack of fixation resulting in motion, and gaps between bone ends from bone loss. If the nonunion is associated with nerve and tendon injuries that severely impair function, amputation must be considered; this is true especially if only one finger is involved. Nonunions of comminuted fractures of the distal phalangeal tuft usually require no treatment; the fragments commonly unite or finally are absorbed.

Nonunions of transverse distal phalangeal fractures may require surgical treatment to obtain union when they are painful. The differentiation between pain from the nonunion and pain from scar tissue around nerve endings is important because the nail plate usually provides sufficient protection. Lateral bending stress on the nonunion site should cause pain from a symptomatic nonunion. Simple tapping of the finger tuft when the nerve endings are tightly bound with dense scar tissue should cause pain similar to that of a neuroma.

Metacarpal nonunion is produced most often by bone loss. For a nonunion in which no bone substance is lost, the technique of repair is the same as that just described for

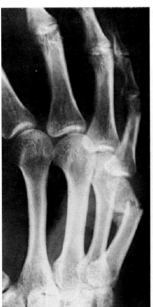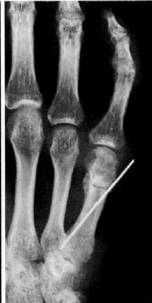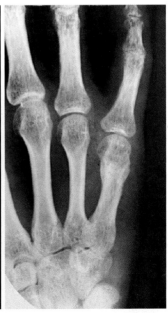

FIGURE 4.77   Malunited fracture of fifth metacarpal neck treated by open reduction and fixation with one Kirschner wire inserted obliquely. This rarely is necessary because normal motion of fifth carpometacarpal joint permits tolerance of 40 degrees or more of angulation at fracture site. **SEE TECHNIQUE 4.26.**

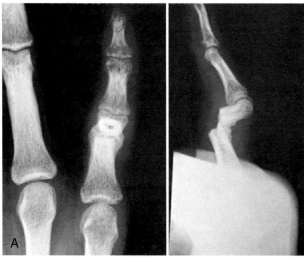

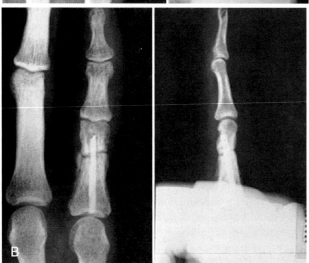

FIGURE 4.78 **A,** Malunited phalangeal fracture. **B,** Result is satisfactory after treatment by osteotomy and intramedullary fixation.

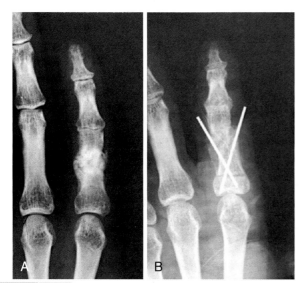

FIGURE 4.79 **A,** Malunited phalangeal diaphyseal fracture with rotational deformity. **B,** After treatment by proximal metaphyseal osteotomy with two Kirschner wires the healing was rapid.

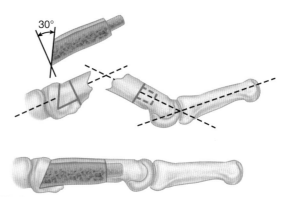

FIGURE 4.80 Littler technique for grafting metacarpal nonunion in which bone substance has been lost. **SEE TECHNIQUE 4.27.**

malunion. For a nonunion in which bone substance is lost, an interpositional corticocancellous bone graft, allograft, or synthetic bone graft substitute combined with plating usually is recommended. As an alternative, Littler's method can be used, provided that bony stability is achieved with the corticocancellous graft alone (Fig. 4.80).

CORRECTION OF NONUNION OF THE METACARPALS

The success of bone grafting metacarpal defects depends on soft-tissue and bony factors. First, the dorsum of the hand must be well covered by skin and subcutaneous tissue, even if local or remote flaps, such as an abdominal pedicle flap, are required (see chapter 2). Second, the fine details of what Bunnell called "bone carpentry" must be exact.

TECHNIQUE 4.27

(LITTLER)

- Expose the defective metacarpal with a longitudinal or curved dorsal incision, depending on the location of existing scars.
- Dissect all scar tissue from the extensor tendons, but preserve the paratenon intact.
- Dissect the fibrous tissue en bloc from between the fragments so that traction can restore normal finger length.
- Usually the proximal fragment must be sacrificed as far as its base; resect it with an osteotome at an angle of 30 degrees (Fig. 4.81), making a recess in the bone.
- Cut the end of the distal fragment transversely with a saw or rongeur and open the medullary canal to receive the doweled end of the graft.
- With traction on the finger, measure the defect between the fragments and take from the tibia (or other suitable site) a graft at least 1.3 cm longer than the defect.
- Fashion a dowel at one end of the graft and cut the other end obliquely at 30 degrees. Insert the doweled end into the medullary canal of the distal fragment, and press the proximal end into the prepared metacarpal or carpal

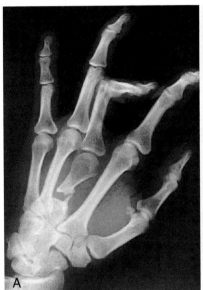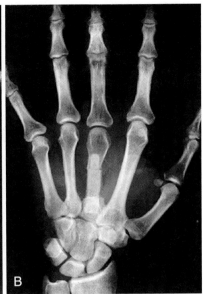

FIGURE 4.81 **A,** Metacarpal nonunion in which bone substance has been lost. **B,** After grafting by Littler technique.

recess. Compression of the graft between the two fragments holds it in place.

- If necessary, stabilize the graft by passing one or more Kirschner wires through it and into adjacent, uninvolved metacarpals.
- Close the periosteal sheath, if present, and the soft tissues over the graft with fine sutures.

POSTOPERATIVE CARE With the hand in the position of function, a plaster cast or splint is applied that extends to the PIP joints. This cast is immediately split to allow for postoperative swelling. On about the 12th day, a new cast is applied that immobilizes only the grafted metacarpal and the proximal phalanx; it is left in place for 2 months.

Administration of prophylactic antibiotics just before or during surgery should be considered. An antibiotic should be given for several days after surgery because the injury producing the bone defect is frequently open. The region is potentially infected even though the original wound has healed.

CONTRACTURE

If joint motion is limited because of secondary collateral ligament contracture, capsulotomy may be indicated.

METACARPOPHALANGEAL JOINT CAPSULOTOMY

When metacarpophalangeal joint motion is 60 degrees, capsulotomy is contraindicated because only 60 to 70 degrees of motion usually can be expected after surgery even if the soft tissues around the joint are normal.

TECHNIQUE 4.28

- Make a longitudinal incision 2.5 cm long over the affected joint. If a single joint is affected, make an incision over the joint.
- If two adjacent joints are affected, make either two incisions or one incision between the metacarpophalangeal joints. If multiple metacarpophalangeal joint contractures exist, longitudinal incisions between the metacarpophalangeal joints provide access to adjacent joints. Second and fourth web space dorsal longitudinal incisions can be used to release all four metacarpophalangeal joints if necessary.
- At a point 0.5 cm from the extensor tendon, incise the extensor hood on the dorsolateral and dorsomedial aspects of the joint. Alternately, if the common extensor tendon is well centered over the metacarpophalangeal joint, a longitudinal incision through the center of the tendon will allow closure of better tissue and maintain the integrity of the less substantive sagittal band tissue. The index and small finger exposures may be either through the common or proper extensor tendons, whichever appears to have more robust tendon structure.
- Retract the extensor hood and intrinsic tendons palmarward and expose the underlying dorsal capsule and collateral ligaments.
- Enter the joint by making a longitudinal incision centered over and through the joint capsule to expose the metacarpal head and proximal phalangeal base articular surfaces. Transect and remove the dorsal joint capsule and excise portions of the collateral ligaments from each side of the joint to gain passive flexion.
- Note that the collateral ligaments are merely specialized portions of joint capsule and often are not clearly distinguishable from the joint capsule, especially when the joint has been previously traumatized. Sequentially excise portions of these ligaments to gain passive flexion, taking

special care not to destabilize the joint. Moreover, passive metacarpophalangeal joint flexion can be achieved only if there is no extrinsic extensor tightness or proximal tendon adhesions. Evaluation and management of the extensor tendon tightness are prerequisites for satisfactory joint release.

- Flex the joint passively.
- Keep the joint surfaces in full contact and check that the proximal phalanx base remains seated on the metacarpal head during flexion and glides smoothly. Sometimes the volar pouch is scarred, and during attempted passive flexion the posterior joint opens from volar proximal phalanx lip impingement.
- If the volar plate is adherent, strip it from the anterior part of the metacarpal head with a probe or elevator. Release additional capsule and collateral ligament attachments to gain full passive flexion. Do not destabilize the joint, especially the radial side of the index finger.
- When satisfactory passive metacarpophalangeal joint motion is achieved, approximate the extensor tendon and close the skin edges. Do not close the dorsal capsule; often the dorsal capsule is thickened and contracted and its excision along with portions of the collateral ligaments has been done previously to achieve full passive flexion and maintain collateral ligament stability.
- Intraoperatively, inject a long-acting local anesthetic to help reduce postoperative pain.
- Apply a bandage incorporating a dorsal blocking splint, holding the wrist extended 15 to 20 degrees with the metacarpophalangeal joints in full flexion. Occasionally, it is necessary to pin the metacarpophalangeal joints in the achieved degree of passive flexion for several days to a week.

POSTOPERATIVE CARE Active flexion exercises of the metacarpophalangeal and interphalangeal joints are started immediately. If pins have been used, they are removed in 3 to 7 days, and daily supervised therapy is initiated. Continuous passive motion devices may be beneficial. Dynamic "knuckle-bender" splinting is used later to help mobilize the joint. These joint releases we prefer to do early in the week because supervised daily physical therapy is beneficial early in the postoperative recovery process.

PROXIMAL INTERPHALANGEAL JOINT CAPSULOTOMY

PIP joint capsulotomy is indicated only when the surrounding tissues are yielding, the joint surface integrity has been maintained, and extensor tendon adhesions, dorsal capsular tightness, and collateral ligaments are considered responsible for motion limitation. The following is a list of causes of limited motion in this joint, as outlined by Curtis.

Flexion may be limited by the following conditions:
- Contracture of skin on the dorsum of the finger.
- Contracture of long extensor muscle or adherence of tendon.
- Contracture of interosseous muscle or adherence of tendon.

- Contracture of capsular ligaments, especially the collateral ligaments.
- Bony block or exostosis.

Extension may be blocked by the following conditions:
- Scarring of skin on the volar surface of the digit.
- Contracture of the superficial fascia in the digit.
- Contracture of the flexor tendon sheath within the digit.
- Contracture of flexor muscle or tendon adherence.
- Contracture of the volar plate.
- Adherence of the collateral ligament with the finger in the flexed position.
- Bony block or exostosis.

These causes all must be considered and, except for those involving the collateral ligaments, carefully eliminated before capsulotomy. Ideally, capsulotomy is performed with the patient awake so that he or she can move the fingers and the surgeon can observe any improvement in motion during surgery. In this instance, proper sedation and a regional block at the wrist or a more distal level are used. Moreover, when a PIP joint is stiff and volar structures are concomitantly suspected of limiting motion either actively (such as flexor tendon adhesions or otherwise) or passively, the surgery should be staged such that the passive flexion is achieved first before proceeding to the second-stage flexor surface procedure(s).

TECHNIQUE 4.29

(CURTIS)
- Approach the interphalangeal joint through a midlateral or a curved dorsal incision. On one side, deepen the incision through the subcutaneous tissue to expose the transverse retinacular ligament (Fig. 4.82A and B).
- Expose the collateral ligament by approaching the joint from the base of the middle phalanx and elevating the transverse retinacular ligament; preserve this ligament for repair after capsulotomy.
- Starting at its distal attachment, excise en bloc as much of the collateral ligament as necessary to achieve the desired motion (Fig. 4.82C). Repeat the procedure on the opposite side of the joint.
- When the contracture is of long duration, the volar synovial pouch may have been obliterated; if so, restore it with a small curved elevator or by forcing the phalangeal base into flexion.
- When the interosseous muscle is contracted, lengthen its tendon by tenotomy and suture (Fig. 4.82D and E). If necessary, free the extensor tendon over the dorsum of the finger through the same approach.
- Satisfactory passive motion must be exhibited during surgery because no further active flexion motion can be anticipated after surgery. It also is important that the flexor tendons not be adherent in the palm. This can be shown by having the patient actively attempt to flex the finger. Flexor tendon adhesion at the forearm, wrist, palm, or finger can compromise active motion. When a flexor tenolysis in the finger is necessary to regain active flexion, it should be staged 10 to 12 weeks later, provided that adequate passive motion has been maintained.
- Close the wound. Apply a dressing and palmar and dorsal splints to keep the wrist extended, the metacarpophalangeal joints flexed, and the interphalangeal joints extended.

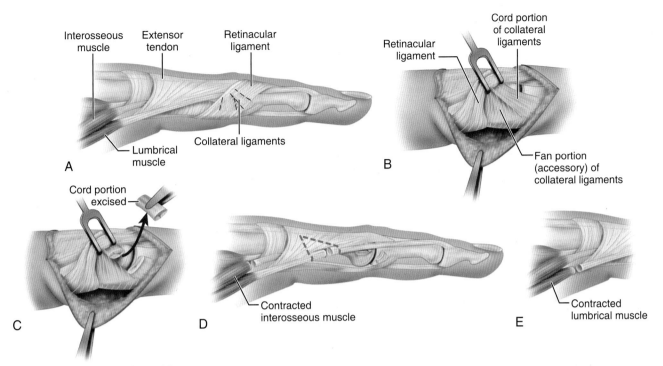

FIGURE 4.82 **A to E,** Curtis technique for capsulotomy of proximal interphalangeal joint. (Redrawn from Curtis RM: Management of the stiff hand. In: *The practice of hand surgery*, Oxford, Blackwell, 1981.) **SEE TECHNIQUE 4.29.**

POSTOPERATIVE CARE Motion is begun immediately under supervision. The joint is splinted alternately in flexion and extension. Splinting is continued until the range of motion obtained at surgery is possible. Splinting may be necessary at least part of the time for 3 or 4 months.

Sometimes, the capsulectomy recommended by Curtis is insufficient to allow full extension of the joint. Watson, Light, and Johnson emphasized the importance of the "check" ligaments in maintaining persistent flexion deformities of the PIP joint. These are normal structures consisting of fibers from the dorsal portion of the flexor sheath and reflections of the accessory ligament inserting in the lateral margins of the volar plate. These ligaments, designated "checkreins" by Watson et al., extend from thick attachments along the proximal edge of the volar plate and then diverge to insert separately along the volar-lateral periosteum of the proximal phalanx. These ligamentous structures may be significant in restricting PIP joint extension, and some authors have recommended that their resection should be part of all middle joint releases.

PROXIMAL INTERPHALANGEAL JOINT CAPSULOTOMY

TECHNIQUE 4.30

(WATSON ET AL.)
- With the patient under suitable anesthesia and with the pneumatic tourniquet inflated, approach the volar aspect of the PIP joint through a midlateral or volar incision. If the flexion deformity is severe and long standing, a longitudinal incision converted to a Z-plasty may be helpful. If a midlateral incision is selected, a second incision on the opposite side of the joint frequently is required.
- Dissect the subcutaneous tissue, preserving the cutaneous sensory nerves. Isolate the flexor sheath and tendon and resect portions of the flexor sheath that contribute to the flexion contracture. If possible, avoid injury to the annular portions of the flexor sheath.
- Using magnification, identify the vessels to the flexor tendons, and retract them to avoid injury.
- Identify the proximal edge of the volar plate and bluntly dissect the checkrein extensions proximally (Fig. 4.83A).
- Sharply excise the checkrein ligaments on both sides, avoiding injury to the volar plate (Fig. 4.83B and C).
- Extend the joint fully with a moderate amount of pressure to disrupt intraarticular adhesions to achieve full passive extension.
- If the deformity tends to recur in a "springy" fashion, fix the joint in extension with a transarticular Kirschner wire.
- Obtain satisfactory hemostasis, and close the wound in a routine manner.
- Apply a bulky dressing and splints to maintain the wrist in extension, the metacarpophalangeal joints in flexion, and the interphalangeal joints in full extension.

POSTOPERATIVE CARE The hand is immobilized in the bulky dressing and splint for 3 to 7 days. A light dressing is then applied, and active joint movement is begun. Subsequently, dynamic splints are used for at least 1 hour of maximal tension while the patient is awake, with less

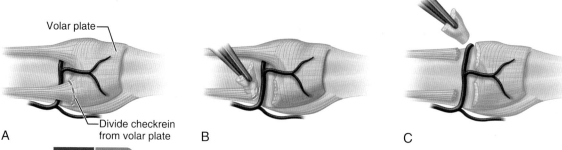

FIGURE 4.83   **A** to **C,** Technique of Watson et al. for capsulotomy of proximal interphalangeal joint. (Redrawn from Watson JK, Light TR, Johnson TR: Checkrein resection for flexion contracture of the middle joint, *J Hand Surg* 4A:67-71, 1979.) **SEE TECHNIQUE 4.30.**

tension throughout the night if tolerated. At times, palmar and dorsal plaster splints may be necessary for 2 to 3 days at a time to keep the joint in full extension. The sutures are removed at 12 to 14 days, and splinting is begun. Watson et al. recommended a screw-tension three-point splint with tension increased every 3 to 5 minutes for 1 hour before the patient retires for the night and then it is left in place overnight. Care should be taken when using such a splint because pressure necrosis of the dorsal skin may occur. Night splinting is continued until full extension is obtained. Dynamic splinting may be required for 4 months.

REFERENCES

GENERAL

Bernstein DT, McCulloch PC, Winston LA, Liberman SR: Early return to play with thumb spica gauntlet casting for ulnar collateral ligament injuries complicated by adjacent joint dislocations in collegiate, *Hand (N Y),* 2018. [Epub ahead of print].

Cheah AE, Yao J: Hand fractures: indications, the tried and true and new innovations, *J Hand Surg Am* 41(6):712, 2016.

Gajendran VK, Gajendran VK, Malone KJ: Management of complications with hand fractures, *Hand Clin* 31:165, 2015.

Giesen T, Neukom L, Fakin R, et al.: Modified Suzuki frame for the treatment of difficult Rolando fractures, hand Surg Rehabil, 35(5):335, 2016. Erratum in: *Hand Surg Rehabil* 36(3):230, 2017.

Goldfarb A, Puri SK, Carlson MG: Diagnosis, treatment, and return to play for four common sports injuries of the hand and wrist, *J Am Acad Orthop Surg* 24(12):853, 2016.

Halim A, Weiss AP: Return to play after hand and wrist fractures, *Clin Sports Med* 35(4):597, 2016.

Hammert WC: Treatment of non-union and malunion following hand fractures, *Clin Plast Surg* 38:683, 2011.

Hyatt BT, Rhee PC: Wide-awake surgical management of hand fractures: technical pearls and advanced rehabilitation, *Plast Reconstr Surg* 143(3):800, 2019.

Jameel SS, Thomas R: An extensile approach to the radial aspect of the carpus: "the link incision", *Tech Hand Up Extrem Surg* 2019. [Epub ahead of print].

Jupiter JB, Hastings 2nd H, Capo JT: The treatment of complex fractures and fracture-dislocations of the hand, *Instr Course Lect* 59:333, 2010.

Pulos N, Kakar S: Hand and wrist injuries: common problems and solutions, *Clin Sports Med* 37(2):217, 2018.

Rosenbaum YA, Awan HM: Acute hand injuries in athletes, *Phys Sportsmed* 45(2):151, 2017.

Rozmaryn LM: The collateral ligament of the digits of the hand: anatomy, physiology, biomechanics, injury, and treatment, *J Hand Surg Am* 42(11):904, 2017.

Tang JB, Blazar PE, Giddins G, et al.: Overview of indications, preferred methods and technical tips for hand fractures from around the work, *J Hand Surg Eur* 40:88, 2015.

Tulipan JE, Ilyas AM: Open fractures of the hand: review of pathogenesis and introduction of a new classification system, *Orthop Clin North Am* 47:245, 2016.

Warrender WJ, Lucasti CJ, Chapman TR, Ilyas AM: Antibiotic management and operative debridement in open fractures of the hand and upper extremity: a systematic review, *Hand Clin* 34(1):9, 2018.

Woo SH, Lee YK, Kim JM, et al.: Hand and wrist injuries in golfers and their treatment, *Hand Clin* 33(1):81, 2017.

THUMB

Alexander C, Abzug JM, Johnson AJ, et al.: Motorcyclist's thumb: carpometacarpal injuries of the thumb sustained in motorcycle crashes, *J Hand Surg Eur* 41(7):707, 2016.

Annappa R, Kotian P, Ja P, Mudiganty S: Ligamentous reconstruction of traumatic dislocation of thumb carpometacarpal joint: case report and review of the literature, *J Orthop Case Rep* 5(4):79, 2015.

Başar H, Başar B, Kaplan T, et al.: Comparison of results after surgical repair of acute and chronic ulnar collateral ligament injury of the thumb, *Chir Main* 33(6):384, 2014.

Carlson MG, Warner KK, Meyers KN, et al.: Anatomy of the thumb metacarpophalangeal ulnar and radial collateral ligaments, *J Hand Surg Am* 37A:2021, 2012.

Carlson MG, Warner KK, Meyers KN, et al.: Mechanics of an anatomical reconstruction for the thumb metacarpophalangeal collateral ligaments, *J Hand Surg Am* 38A:117, 2013.

Christensen T, Sarfani S, Shin AY, Kakar S: Long-term outcomes of primary repair of chronic thumb ulnar collateral ligament injuries, *Hand (N Y)* 11(3):3203, 2016.

Duan W, Zhang X, Yu Y, et al.: Treatment of comminuted fractures of the base of the thumb metacarpal using a cemented bone-K-wire frame, *Hand Surg Rehabil* 38(1):44, 2019.

El Shafie S, Menorca RMG, Elfar JC: Management of neglected Bennett fracture in manual laborers by tension fixation, *J Hand Surg Am* 39:1728, 2014.

Grawe KR, Griesser M, Cook PA: Palmar fracture-dislocation of the metacarpophalangeal joint of the thumb, *J Hand Surg Eur* 36:79, 2011.

Houshian S, Jing SS: Treatment of Rolando fracture by capsuloligamentotaxis using mini external fixator: a report of 16 cases, *Hand Surg* 18:73, 2013.

Huang JI, Fernandez DL: Fractures of the base of the thumb metacarpal, *Instr Course Lect* 59:343, 2010.

Iba K, Wada T, Hiraiwa T, et al.: Reconstruction of chronic thumb metacarpophalangeal joint radial collateral injuries with a half-slip of the abductor pollicis brevis tendon, *J Hand Surg Am* 38A:1945, 2013.

Kang JR, Behn AW, Messana J, Ladd AL: Bennett fractures: a biomechanical model and relevant ligamentous anatomy, *J Hand Surg Am* 44(2):154, 2019.

Kim DH, Kang HJ, Choi JW: The "fish-hook" technique for bony mallet finger, *Orthopedics* 39(5):295, 2016.

Lark ME, Maroukis BL, Chung KC: The Stener lesion: historical perspective and evolution of diagnostic criteria, *Hand (N Y)* 12(3):283, 2017.

Le M, Lourie GM, Gaston G: Relationship of surgically repaired ulnar collateral ligament injury of the thumb to the morphology of the metacarpophalangeal joint of the thumb, *J Hand Surg Eur* 43(2):214, 2018.

Leclère FM, Jenzer A, Hüsler R, et al.: 7-year follow-up after open reduction and internal screw fixation in Bennett fractures, *Arch Orthop Trauma Surg* 132(7):1045, 2012.

Mahmoud M, Middleton SD, McNiven N, et al.: Long-term patient-reported outcomes following Bennett's fractures, *Bone Joint J* 97B:1004, 2015.

Middleton SD, McNiven N, Griffin EJ, et al.: Long-term patient-reported outcomes following Bennett's fractures, *Bone Joint J* 97-B:1004, 2015.

Milner CS, Manon-Matos Y, Thirkannad SM: Gamekeeper's thumb—a treatment-oriented magnetic resonance imaging classification, *J Hand Surg Am* 40(1):90, 2015.

Mumtaz MU, Ahmad F, Kawoosa AA, et al.: Treatment of Rolando fractures by open reduction and internal fixation using mini T-plate and screws, *J Hand Microsurg* 8(2):80, 2016.

Owings FP, Calandruccio H, Mauck BM: Thumb ligament injuries in the athlete, *Orthop Clin North Am* 47(4):799, 2016.

Pulos N, Shin AY: Treatment of ulnar collateral ligament injuries of the thumb: a critical analysis review, *JBJS Rev* 5920:pii:01874474-201702000-0005, 2017.

Rhee PC, Kakar S: Chronic thumb metacarpophalangeal joint ulnar collateral ligament insufficiency, *J Hand Surg Am* 37A:346, 2012.

Schroeder NS, Goldfarb CA: Thumb ulnar collateral and radial collateral ligament injuries, *Clin Sports Med* 34(1):117, 2015.

Sochacki KR, Jack 2nd RA, Nauert R, et al.: Performance and return to sport after thumb ulnar collateral ligament surgery in National Football League players, *Hand (N Y)* 2018. [Epub ahead of print].

Tabrizi A, Afshar A: Hook plate fixation for the thumb ulnar collateral ligament fracture-avulsion, *J hand Microsurg* 9(2):95, 2017.

Tang P: Collateral ligament injuries of the thumb metacarpophalangeal joint, *J Am Acad Orthop Surg* 19:287, 2011.

Werner BC, Belkin NS, Kennelly S, et al.: Injuries to the collateral ligaments of the metacarpophalangeal joint of the thumb, including simultaneous combined thumb ulnar and radial collateral ligament injuries, in National Football League athletes, *Am J Sports Med* 45(1):195, 2017.

Zhang X, Shao X, Nhuang W, et al.: An alternative technqiue for stabilisation of the carpometacarpal joint of the thumb after dislocation or subluxation, *Bone Joint J* 97-B(11):1533, 2015.

METACARPALS AND PHALANGES (EXCLUDING THUMB)

Afifi A, Medoro A, Salas C, et al.: A cadaver model that investigates irreducible metacarpophalangeal joint dislocation, *Hand Surg* 34A:1506, 2009.

Balaram AK, Bednar MS: Complications after the fractures of metacarpal and phalanges, *Hand Clin* 26:169, 2010.

Barksfield RC, Bowden B, Chojnowski AJ: Hemi-hamate arthroplasty versus transarticular Kirschner wire fixation for unstable fracture-dislocation of the proximal interphalangeal joint in the hand, *Hand Surg* 20:115, 2015.

Barr C, Behn AW, Yao J: Plating of metacarpal fractures with locked or non-locked screws, a biomechanical study: how many cortices are really necessary? *Hand* 8:454, 2013.

Bear DM, Weichbrodt MT, Huang C, et al.: Unstable dorsal proximal interphalangeal joint fracture-dislocations treated with extension-block pinning, *Am J Orthop (Belle Mead NJ)* 44:122, 2015.

Cheah AEJ, Tan DMK, Chong AKS, Chew WYC: Volar plating for unstable proximal interphalangeal joint dorsal fracture-dislocations, *J Hand Surg Am* 37A:28, 2012.

del Piñal F, Moraleda E, Rúas JS, et al.: Minimally invasive fixation of fractures of the phalanges and metacarpals with intramedullary cannulated headless compression screws, *J Hand Surg Am* 40(4):692, 2015.

Dreyfuss D, Allon R, Izacson N, Hutt D: A comparison of locking plates and intramedullary pinning for fixation of metacarpal shaft fractures, *Hand (N Y)* 14(1):27, 2019.

Dukas AG, Wold JM: Management of complications of periarticular fractures of the distal interphalangeal, proximal interphalangeal, metacarpophalangeal, and carpometacarpal joints, *Hand Clin* 31:179, 2015.

El-saeed M, Sallam A, Radwan M, Metwally A: Kirschner wires versus titanium plates and screws in management of unstable phalangeal fractures: a randomized, controlled clinical trial, *J Hand Surg Am* e1, 2019.

Etier BE, Scillia A, Tessier DD, et al.: Return to play following metacarpal fractures in football players, *Hand (N Y)* 10(4):762, 2015.

Friedrich JB, Vedder NB: An evidence-based approach to metacarpal fractures, *Plast Reconstr Surg* 126:2205, 2010.

Gaheer RS, Ferdinand RD: Fracture dislocation of carpometacarpal joints: a missed injury, *Orthopedics* 34:399, 2011.

Galal S, Safwat W: Transverse pinning versus intramedullary pinning in fifth metacarpal's neck fractures: a randomized controlled study with patient-reported outcome, *J Clin Orthop Trauma* 8(4):339, 2017.

Giesen T, Gazzola R, Poggetti A, et al.: Intramedullary headless screw fixation for fractures of the proximal and middle phalanges in the digits of the hand: a review of 31 consecutive fractures, *J Hand Surg Eur* 41(7):688, 2016.

Greeven AP, Alta TD, Scholtens RE, et al.: Closed reduction intermetacarpal Kirschner wire fixation in the treatment of unstable fractures of the base of the first metacarpal, *Injury* 43:246, 2012.

Hiatt SV, Gegonia MT, Thiagarajan G, Hutchison RL: Biomechanical comparison of 2 methods of intramedullary K-wire fixation of transverse metacarpal shaft fractures, *J Hand Surg Am* 40(8):1586, 2015.

Hirsiger S, Schweizer A, Miyake J, et al.: Corrective ostetotomies of phalangeal and metacarpal malunions using patient-specific guides: CT-based evaluation of the reduction accuracy, *Hand (N Y)* 13(6):627, 2018.

Kappos EA, Esenwein P, Meoli M, et al.: Implantation of a denatured cellulose adhesion barrier after plate osteosynthesis of finger proximal phalangeal fractures: results of a randomized controlled trial, *J Hand Surg Eur* 41(4):413, 2016.

Kapur B, Paniker J, Casaletto J: An alternative technique for external fixation of traumatic intra-articular fractures of the proximal and middle phalanx, *Techn Hand Up Extrem Surg* 19(4):163, 2015.

Kim JK, Kim DJ: Antegrade intramedullary pinning versus retrograde intramedullary pinning for displaced fifth metacarpal neck fractures, *Clin Orthop Relat Res* 473:1747, 2015.

Kodama A, Sunagawa T, Nakashima Y, et al.: Joint distraction and early mobilization using a new dynamic external finger fixator for the treatment of fracture-dislocations of the proximal interphalangeal joint, *J Orthop Sci* 23(6):959, 2018.

Kostoris F, Addevico F, Murena L, et al.: Proposal of a new dynamic distraction device to treat complex periarticular fractures of the metacarpophalangeal joint of long finger, *Hand (N Y)* 2018, 1558944718787859.

Kralj R, Barcot Z, Vlahovic T, et al.: The patterns of phalangeal fractures in children and adolescents: review of 512 cases, *Handchir Mickrochir Plast Chir* 51(1):49, 2019.

Kural C, Başaran SH, Ercin E, et al.: Fourth and fifth carpometacarpal fracture dislocations, *Acta Orthop Traumatol Turc* 48(6):655, 2014.

Lee SH, Lee JE, Lee KH, et al.: Supplemental method for reduction of irreducible mallet finger fractures by the 2- extension block technique: the dorsal counterforce technique, *J Hand Surg Am* 2018. [Epub ahead of print].

Lin JS, Samora JB: Surgical and nonsurgical management of mallet finger: a systematic review, *J Hand Surg Am* 43(2):146, 2018.

Maalla R, Youssef M, Ben Jdidia GB, et al.: Extension-block pinning for fracture-dislocation of the proximal interphalangeal joint, *Orthop Traumatol Surg Res* 98:559, 2012.

Marsland D, Sanghrajka AP, Goldie B: Static monolateral external fixation for the Rolando fracture: a simple solution for a complex fracture, *Ann R Coll Surg Engl* 94:112, 2012.

Melamed E, Joo L, Lin E, et al.: Plate fixation versus percutaneous pinning for unstable metacarpal fractures: a meta-analysis, *J Hand Surg Asian Pac* 22(1):29, 2017.

Minhas SV, Catalano LW: Comparison of open and closed hand fractures and the effect of urgent operative intervention, *J Hand Surg Am* 44(10):65.e1, 2019.

Nikkhah D, Ruston J, Toft N: Refinements in dynamic external fixation for optimal fracture distraction in pilon-type fractures of the proximal interphalangeal joint, *J Plast Reconstr Aesthet Surg* 69(8):1153, 2016.

Pellatt R, Fomin I, Pienaar C, et al.: Is buddy taping as effective as plaster immobilization for adults with uncomplicated fifth metacarpal fracture? A randomized controlled trial, *Ann Emerg Med* 2019, pii: S0196-0644919)30059-9.

Potenza V, Caterini R, De Maio F, et al.: Fractures of the neck of the fifth metacarpal bone: medium-term results in 28 cases treated by percutaneous transverse pinning, *Injury* 43:242, 2012.

Rhee SH, Lee SK, Lee SL, et al.: Prospective multicenter trial of modified retrograde percutaneous intramedullary Kirschner wire fixation for displaced metacarpal neck and shaft fractures, *Plast Reconstr Surg* 129:694, 2012.

Soong M, Got C, Katarincic J: Ring and little finger metacarpal fractures: mechanisms, locations, and radiographic parameters, *J Hand Surg Am* 35A:1256, 2010.

Sraj S: A simple phalangeal external fixator using Kirschner wires and locking balls: no need for cement or rubber bands, *J Hand Surg Am* 41(7):e217, 2016.

Tajima K, Sato K, Sasaki T, Peimer CA: Vertical locking of the metacarpophalangeal joint in young adults, *J Hand Surg Am* 36A:1482, 2011.

Vitale MA, White NJ, Strauch RJ: Percutaneous technique to treat unstable dorsal fracture-dislocations of the proximal interphalangeal joint, *J Hand Surg Am* 36A:1453, 2011.

Zelken JA, Hayes AG, Parks BG, et al.: Two versus 3 lag screws for fixation of long oblique proximal phalanx fractures of the fingers: a cadaver study, *J Hand Surg Am* 40:1124, 2015.

Waris E, Mattila S, Sillat T, Karjalainen T: Extension block pinning for unstable proximal interphalangeal joint dorsal fracture dislocations, *J Hand Surg Am* 41(2):196, 2016.

Wollstein R, Trouw A, Carlson L, et al.: The effect of age on fracture healing time in metacarpal fractures, *Hand (N Y)* 2018, 1558944718813730. [Epub ahead of print].

Zelken JA, Hayes AG, Parks BG, et al.: Two versus three lag screws for fixation of long oblique proximal phalanx fractures of the fingers: a cadaver study, *J Hand Surg Am* 40(6):1124, 2015.

Zhang B, Hu P, Yu KL, et al.: Comparison of AO titanium locking plate and screw fixation versus anterograde intramedullary fixation for isolated unstable metacarpal and phalangeal fractures, *Orthop Surg* 8(3):316, 2016.

Zhang C, Whang H, Liang C, et al.: The effect of timing on the treatment and outcome of combined fourth and fifth carpometacarpal fracture dislocations, *J Hand Surg Am* 40:2169, 2015.

MALLET FINGER

Alla SR, Deal ND, Dempsey IJ: Current concepts: mallet finger, *Hand (N Y)* 9:138, 2014.

Georgescu AV, Capota IM, Matei IR: A new surgical treatment for mallet finger deformity: deepithelialised pedicled skin flap technique, *Injury* 44:351, 2013.

Imoto FS, Leão TA, Imoto RS, et al.: Osteosynthesis of mallet finger using plate and screws: evaluation of 25 patients, *Rev Bras Orthop* 5193:268, 2016.

Kanaya K, Wada T, Yamashita T: The Thompson procedure for chronic mallet finger deformity, *J Hand Surg Am* 38:1295, 2013.

Kim JY, Lee SH: Factors related to distal interphalangeal joint extension loss after extension block pinning of mallet finger fractures, *J Hand Surg Am* 41:414, 2016.

Lee SK, Kim KJ, et al.: Modified extension-block K-wire fixation technique for the treatment of bony mallet finger, *Orthopedics* 33:728, 2010.

Lee SH, Lee JE, Lee KH, et al.: Supplemental method for reduction of irreducible mallet finger fractures by the 2-extension block technique: the dorsal counterforce technique, *J Hand Surg Am* 2018. [Epub ahead of print].

Lin JS, Samora JB: Surgical nonsurgical management of mallet finger: a systematic review, *J Hand Surg Am* 43(2):146, 2018.

Lucchina S, Badia A, Mistor A, Fusetti C: Surgical treatment options for unstable mallet fractures, *Plast Reconstr Surg* 128:599, 2011.

Makhlouf VM, Deek NA: Surgical treatment of chronic mallet finger, *Ann Plast Surg* 66:670, 2011.

Pike J, Mulpuri K, Metzger M, et al.: Blinded, prospective, randomized clinical trial comparing volar, dorsal, and custom thermoplastic splinting in treatment of acute mallet finger, *J Hand Surg Am* 35A:580, 2010.

Shimura H, Wakabayashi Y, Nimura A: A novel closed reduction with extension block and flexion block using Kirschner wires and microscrew fixation for mallet fractures, *J Orthop Sci* 19:308, 2014.

Shin SH, Lee YS, Kang JWE, et al.: Tips under the skin: a simple modification of extension block pinning for mallet fractures, *Orthopedics* 41(2):e299, 2018.

Smit JM, Beets MR, Zeebregts CJ, et al.: Treatment options for mallet finger: a review, *Plast Reconstr Surg* 126:1624, 2010.

Toker S, Türkmen F, Pekince O, et al.: Extension block pinning versus hook plate fixation for treatment of mallet fractures, *J Hand Surg Am* 40(8):1591, 2015.

Usami S, Kawahara S, Kuno H, et al.: A retrospective study of closed extension block pinning for mallet fractures: analysis of predictors of postoperative range of motion, *J Plast Reconstr Aesthet Surg* 71(6):876, 2018.

Valdes K, Naughton N, Algar L: Conservative treatment of mallet finger: a systematic review, *J Hand Ther* 28:237, 2015.

Zhang X, Meng H, Shao X, et al.: Pull-out wire fixation for acute mallet finger fractures with k-wire stabilization of the distal interphalangeal joint, *J Hand Surg Am* 35A:1864, 2010.

The complete list of references is available online at Expert Consult com.

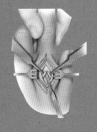

CHAPTER 5

NERVE INJURIES AT THE LEVEL OF THE HAND AND WRIST

Mark T. Jobe, William J. Weller

This chapter includes the essentials of treatment of nerve injuries in the digits, palm, and wrist. Although many of the principles discussed here can be applied to injuries in the forearm and arm, more detailed discussions of more proximal nerve injuries can be found in *Trauma and Amputations Volume* on peripheral nerve injuries. Nerve entrapments and compression neuropathies also are discussed in detail in *Trauma and Amputations Volume*. Reconstructive procedures including tendon transfers are discussed in *Pediatric Orthopaedics Volume*, and an expansion of the discussion of microsurgical technique can be found in *Arthroscopy and Microsurger Volume*.

EVALUATION
PREOPERATIVE ASSESSMENT

At times, it is difficult to evaluate the extent of nerve injury in the hand. Factors that interfere with the examination of the nerves in the hand include other injuries that may be life threatening or limb threatening, patient intoxication, anxiety or lack of cooperation of the patient, and injury in a child. These factors and others, including an extensive injury to the hand, may cause nerve injuries to be overlooked during the initial or preliminary examination. If the conditions are not satisfactory for a thorough examination during the initial evaluation, the hand should be reexamined within a reasonable period to determine the extent of nerve and other injuries sustained. An injury to the digital nerves frequently is overlooked; however, if a flexor tendon function deficit is present after a finger laceration, at least one digital nerve probably has been injured as well. A high index of suspicion is necessary in the evaluation of patients with hand injuries. At least four areas of consideration are important when evaluating a patient with an injury to a nerve in the hand: (1) type of injury, (2) sensibility evaluation, (3) motor function, and (4) sudomotor function (sweating).

■ TYPE OF INJURY

Nerve injuries seen in a civilian practice commonly are caused by one of several mechanisms, including direct trauma (blow to the limb, fracture, missile wound), laceration, traction or stretching, and entrapment or compression. To determine the type of treatment and to arrive at tentative prognostic projections, it is helpful to recall the classification of nerve injuries according to Seddon and Sunderland (Table 5.1). Common injuries such as bumping the "funny bone" (ulnar nerve at the elbow) fall easily into the category of neurapraxia (type I injuries), and lacerations are classified as neurotmesis (type V injuries); however, closed injuries with partial nerve deficits are not as easily classified, and the prognosis may not be as well defined. The extent to which the nature of the injuring agent determines primary and secondary repair is discussed in this chapter under their respective headings. Additional discussion of extent of injury may be found in *Trauma and Amputations Volume*.

■ SENSIBILITY EVALUATION

When evaluating the injured hand for sensibility, in addition to an awareness of the classic sensory distribution of the median, radial, and ulnar nerves, it is helpful to recall the autonomous sensory distributions of the median, radial, and ulnar nerves in the volar pulp of the index finger, the volar pulp of the little finger, and the thumb-index web space. If the injury is a laceration, and the nerve has been transected, the examination usually is more definitive than in closed injuries or in lacerations in which the depth may not be fully known. Even if a wound is to be explored to determine the extent of the nerve injury, it is helpful to document the clinical deficit before surgical exploration. Careful evaluation, especially in the presence of a closed injury, defines the initial deficit, allowing for assessment of progress if observation of the injury is elected rather than exploration of the nerve. Closed partial rupture of a

	TABLE 5.1	
Classification of Nerve Injury		
SEDDON	**SUNDERLAND (DEGREES)**	
Neurapraxia	I	
Axonotmesis	II	
	III	VI (combination of any of Sunderland I–V)
	IV	
Neurotmesis	V	

From MacKinnon SF, Dellon AL: *Surgery of the peripheral nerve*, New York, 1988, Thieme.

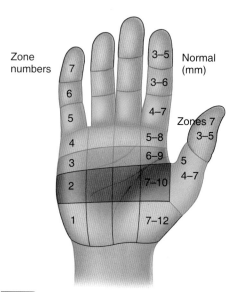

FIGURE 5.1 Two-point discrimination of hand sensibility, palmar surface. Dorsal surface averages 7 mm distally to 12 mm proximally.

common digital nerve in the palm requiring MRI and surgical exploration for diagnosis has been described. Additionally, magnetic resonance neurography (MRA) and ultrasound have been used in these scenarios. The MRA, although still in the development phase, is reported to be able to provide details regarding nerve anatomic relationships, fascicular pattern, intraneural swelling, and evaluation of downstream muscle injury. Although compelling, the authors of this chapter do not have any experience with this diagnostic modality.

The customary methods used to evaluate damaged sensory nerves include the use of a sharp pin to assess pain, a cotton-tipped applicator or a finger eraser to assess light touch, and the tips of a paper clip or commercially prepared tool to assess two-point discrimination. Normal two-point discrimination usually is 6 mm or less. If the nerve is transected, a patient would not feel light touch, would not appreciate the pin as a sharp stimulus, and would be unable to discriminate between one and two points. Patients with closed injuries or partial injuries to nerves may show spotty appreciation of light touch and pain and have markedly widened two-point discrimination (Fig. 5.1).

◼ MOTOR FUNCTION

Although the function in the hand served by the underlying median nerve includes the proximally innervated pronator teres, flexor carpi radialis, palmaris longus, flexor digitorum sublimis, index and middle flexor digitorum profundus, flexor pollicis longus, and pronator quadratus, the usual median-innervated muscles of concern in the hand include the lumbricals to the index and long fingers, the opponens pollicis, the abductor pollicis brevis, and the superficial portion of the flexor pollicis brevis. The single median nerve–mediated motor function that usually is checked is apposition of the tip of the thumb to the pulp of the ring or little finger with palpation of active contraction of the abductor pollicis brevis muscle belly to supplement the visual inspection. Anatomic variations that cause cross-innervation of the muscles usually innervated by the median nerve should be kept in mind.

The muscles proximally innervated by the ulnar nerve include the flexor carpi ulnaris and flexor digitorum profundus tendons to the ring and little fingers. In the hand, the ulnar-innervated muscles of interest include the flexor pollicis brevis, adductor pollicis, abductor digiti minimi, flexor digiti minimi, opponens digiti minimi, and all the interosseous muscles. When testing for motor function of the ulnar nerve in the hand, the

usual motions mediated by the ulnar intrinsic muscles include active abduction of the middle finger from the ulnar to the radial side with the palm resting on a flat surface. This motion should be observed carefully to exclude the functions of the long flexor tendons, which tend to converge the digits and confuse accurate interpretation of the function of the volar interosseous muscles, and the long extensor tendons, which tend to diverge the fingers and confuse accurate interpretation of the dorsal interosseous muscles. Additionally, thumb adduction usually is tested by having the patient maintain a piece of paper tightly in the thumb-index web, squeezing the paper between the thumb interphalangeal joint and the base of the index finger proximal phalanx. If the adductor is weak or paralyzed, the patient is unable to hold the piece of paper against resistance. The function of the abductor digiti minimi also may be tested by having the patient abduct the little finger against resistance and by palpating the muscle belly of the abductor digiti minimi (Fig. 5.2). Although clawing of the little and ring fingers may not be seen at the time of an acute injury, it is present sometimes, and careful observation of the hand should reveal this finding. The first dorsal interosseous muscle may receive an anomalous innervation from the median nerve in about 10% of hands. The posterior interosseous or superficial branches of the radial nerve also may supply the first dorsal and the second and third dorsal interosseous muscles in some hands.

Proximal muscles innervated by the radial nerve include the triceps, brachioradialis, supinator, and anconeus. The radially innervated muscles having influence on the hand include the extensor carpi radialis longus and brevis, the extensor carpi ulnaris, the extensor digitorum communis, the extensor indicis proprius, the extensor digiti minimi, the abductor pollicis longus, the extensor pollicis longus, and the extensor pollicis brevis. The motions that can be examined and that are mediated by the radial nerve in the hand and wrist include wrist dorsiflexion and radial and ulnar deviation and thumb abduction and extension. Metacarpophalangeal extension, mediated by the radial nerve, should be evaluated carefully so

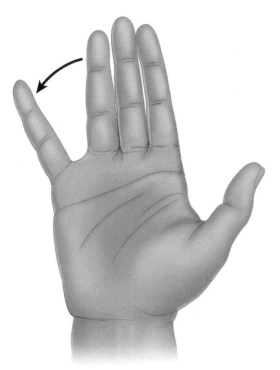

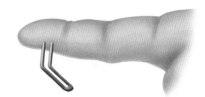

FIGURE 5.3   Two-point discrimination testing. **SEE TECHNIQUE 5.1.**

- Apply a blunt, two-pointed caliper or paper clip distally over the distal pulp in the longitudinal axis on the radial or ulnar side (Fig. 5.3). The pressure applied should be just slightly less than blanching pressure. Test each area three times. Start at a width of 10 mm and gradually decrease the distance.
- Perform the moving two-point discrimination test in a similar fashion. Apply the caliper in an axial direction and move it from proximal to distal along the digital pad. Two of three correct answers are considered proof of perception with either test.

FIGURE 5.2   Testing of function of abductor digiti minimi. Patient abducts little finger against resistance while muscle belly is palpated.

that the examiner is not confused by extension of the proximal and distal interphalangeal joints of the fingers, controlled by the intrinsic muscles.

■ SUDOMOTOR FUNCTION

Usually a denervated area shows no sweating within about 30 minutes after a nerve injury. It is helpful to compare the normal and suspected injured areas by palpation with a dry fingertip.

POSTOPERATIVE ASSESSMENT

In evaluating the progress of peripheral nerve injury and repair sensibility testing, motor testing, subjective evaluation, and sudomotor function are important.

■ SENSIBILITY EVALUATION

The basic minimum tests recommended for sensibility evaluation are stationary two-point discrimination and moving two-point discrimination.

TWO-POINT AND MOVING TWO-POINT DISCRIMINATION TESTING

TECHNIQUE 5.1

- The hand should be warm, and the instrument should be at room temperature.
- Rest the hand on a flat surface, palm up.

■ MOTOR FUNCTION

Three basic tests are recommended for motor function: grip strength, key pinch, and tip pinch strength. The squeeze grip dynamometer should be used, and the results should be recorded at all five positions with three successive determinations. This reflects the overall integrated function of the hand, in addition to areas of extrinsic and intrinsic muscle deficits.

Pinch strength is measured using a pinch dynamometer. Applying the thumb tip to the radial aspect of the middle phalanx of the index finger measures key pinch. Three successive determinations should be made, and the opposite hand should be measured as well. Pinching with the index tip to the ulnar side of the tip of the thumb allows measurement of tip pinch values. Three measurements should be made.

■ SUBJECTIVE EVALUATION

Subjective evaluation refers to the patient's evaluation of current status and includes symptoms such as the presence of pain, cold intolerance, dysesthesias, and functional disabilities.

■ SUDOMOTOR FUNCTION

The loss of sweating is an indicator of nerve disruption and loss of sympathetic function. Sweating may return without a return of two-point discrimination; however, usually it returns with the return of two-point discrimination. A statement relative to sweating should be included in the evaluation.

NERVE REGENERATION

After a nerve injury, the response in the proximal elements of the peripheral nerve includes an increased rate of metabolic activity and proliferation from the nerve cell bodies distally, resulting in the sprouting of axonal processes at the injury site within the first 1 to 3 weeks. The response distally consists of the elements of wallerian degeneration, including disruption of the myelin sheath and phagocytosis, and preparation of the distal segment to receive the regenerating elements of the proximal axons. A more detailed discussion of this response is presented in *Trauma and Amputations Volume.*

Usually, after repair of a sensory nerve (digital, pure sensory, mixed motor, and sensory), the area of anesthesia decreases in size as regeneration progresses and the quality of sensation changes. In 2 to 3 months, the entire area supplied by the nerve may become paresthetic. It then becomes hyperesthetic to light touch or cold. Firm pressure usually is less painful. With time and the use of various physical and occupational therapy techniques, the hyperesthesia resolves. Patients usually have less objectionable sensation after the period of hyperesthesia.

With progression of regeneration, the quality of sensation improves significantly within the first 1.5 to 2 years with additional gradual improvement thereafter. Fully normal sensation with appreciation of functional two-point discrimination rarely is expected in adults. Although the functional result after digital nerve regeneration usually is better than that seen for injuries to nerves more proximally and to mixed motor and sensory nerves (e.g., the ulnar nerve), age seems to have an influence on the final functional result after peripheral nerve repair. A fully functional hand with minimal loss of power can be expected in children after epineurial repair. Studies suggest that patients younger than age 20 can be expected to have a better prognosis for return of functional two-point discrimination than can older patients. Patients younger than age 40 have been shown to have better sensibility recovery than patients older than age 40. Although exceptions may be encountered, it is rare for patients older than age 50 to regain more than protective sensation.

In considering the repair of multiple digital nerves in an injured hand, the location of the injured nerves should be considered. Although it is general practice to repair all digital nerves, the most important areas of sensory innervation of the digits include the ulnar side of the thumb, the radial side of the index and middle fingers, and the ulnar side of the little finger. These areas are important for pinch and for ulnar border contact of the hand. These nerves should be given priority if there are limiting factors, such as prolonged operative time in a patient with multiple injuries, multiple soft-tissue problems on the various fingers, or segmental nerve loss.

PRIMARY AND DELAYED PRIMARY NERVE REPAIR
TIMING OF REPAIR

The controversy regarding the timing of nerve repairs in general is unresolved. The terms applied to the timing of the nerve repair include *primary repair* (immediately after injury, or within 6 to 12 hours), *delayed primary repair* (usually within the first 2 to 2.5 weeks), and *secondary repair* (after 2.5 to 3 weeks). Advocates of primary repair are supported by experimental work, which suggests that the results may be better after primary repair. Authors

advocating a delay in repair are supported by the clinical observations after nerve injuries that occurred during wars. Generally, however, the longer the delay in repair, the poorer the return of motor function that can be expected. The reinnervation of denervated muscle may occur 12 months later; however, after that period, irreversible changes occur in the muscle cells and there is little hope of recovery of motor function after reinnervation. The return of sensation has been observed when nerve repair has been performed 2 years after injury. Satisfactory return of function can occur after nerve repair performed within 3 months of injury. Delay in nerve repair assumes the following: (1) muscle atrophy occurs, (2) contraction in the endoneural tubules of the distal segment progresses, (3) retraction of the nerve ends may occur, (4) joint contractures may develop, (5) a second operation is involved, and (6) intraneural alignment of fascicles may be more difficult. Additional factors to consider in the timing of peripheral nerve repairs include the condition of the patient and the state of preparedness of the surgeon and the institution, including the availability of instruments and personnel to allow a satisfactory primary repair.

Regardless of the timing of repair, tension should be avoided at the site of nerve repair. Nerve grafts accomplished without tension heal and function better than nerve repairs performed with tension, despite the need for regeneration to occur across two suture lines with a nerve graft.

INDICATIONS

In general, a nerve repair can be done immediately after injury or within the first 2 to 2.5 weeks in the presence of a clean, sharp injury. A delay of 2 to 2.5 weeks can be caused by a variety of factors, including the condition of the patient and the availability of appropriate personnel, including a surgeon to treat the wound. We repair injured nerves, if the wound is clean and sharp, either on the day of injury or in the first 5 to 7 days.

SECONDARY NERVE REPAIR
INDICATIONS

Several conditions should influence the surgeon to delay the repair of injured peripheral nerves, including (1) the existence of extensive soft-tissue injury and loss with extensive trauma to the nerve, (2) the presence of extensive wound contamination, (3) the presence of multiple limb injuries requiring aggressive and expeditious management in preference to the nerve injury, (4) the existence of extensive crush injury, (5) the presence of an extensive traction injury, and (6) a nerve injury that has been treated by another surgeon, in which the extent and nature of the nerve repair are unknown to the second treating surgeon.

If multiple tissue injuries have occurred, especially in the presence of soft-tissue loss, the nerve repair is secondary and is indicated only after good skin coverage has been obtained. After satisfactory and complete healing of all wounds and the establishment of satisfactory nutrition to the skin and other tissues of the hand, common and proper digital nerves usually can be sutured as a secondary procedure 3 weeks or more after injury. Although most reports suggest that the results after secondary repair are similar to, if not better than, the results after primary repair, the best results seem to occur if repairs are done within the first 3 months of injury. The reports of patients treated after World War II suggest that useful sensation can occur after repairs 2 years after injury. This is not the normal expectation, however. Return of motor function after excessive delay is even more unpredictable.

With a severe soft-tissue injury, skin coverage is a priority. The extent of intraneural injury is unknown. It is best to wait 3 to 6 weeks to allow clear demarcation of intraneural scar to have a better chance at more precise nerve apposition at the time of repair.

An extensively contaminated wound may require a delay in nerve repair because infection may supervene and delay not only definitive treatment of the nerve but also wound closure itself. Although initial debridement may remove significant wound contamination and allow delayed primary repair, if wound contamination and necrotic material persist, additional debridements of necessity interpose a delay until definitive nerve repair later.

Multiple limb injuries may create priorities of wound cleansing, bone stabilization, vascular repair, and soft-tissue coverage. Segmental injury to nerves also might dictate secondary repair. Crush and traction injuries cause intraneural damage that cannot be assessed accurately at the time of primary wound evaluation. When the nerve has sustained extensive intraneural or extensive segmental intraneural injury or loss because of crush or traction, it is best to wait 3 to 6 weeks to allow clear demarcation between scar and normal nerve to become established. If the extent of intraneural injury is unclear, or if extensive segmental loss of nerve requires grafting, primary repair should not be done and secondary repair or nerve reconstruction by graft should be considered.

A special situation occurs when the patient's initial and primary care have been accomplished by another surgeon. Frequently, one does not know the extent of the initial injury and has no awareness of the nature of the repair. At times, it may be necessary to consider exploration of the nerve, possibly considering secondary repair. Exploration of the nerve may reveal that secondary repair is unnecessary. The exploration of a nerve injury in such a situation may help ensure that a skillful nerve repair has been done, which is one important determinant of outcome.

SUTURING OF NERVES

For additional discussion of surgical techniques, see other Volumes on peripheral nerve injuries and on microsurgery. Generally, the principles that apply to the suture of other peripheral nerves also apply to suturing of the peripheral nerves of the hand. Important considerations include (1) mixed versus pure motor or sensory nerves, (2) internal arrangement of the nerves, (3) incisions to be used, (4) amount of mobilization and limb positioning required for tension-free apposition, (5) suture materials to be used, (6) nature of the suture arrangement, (7) magnification, and (8) postoperative management.

Careful technique is crucial to provide the best restoration and repair of the anatomy. The internal arrangement of the nerve in the palm and digits usually is oligofascicular as described by Millesi (Fig. 5.4). In the median and ulnar

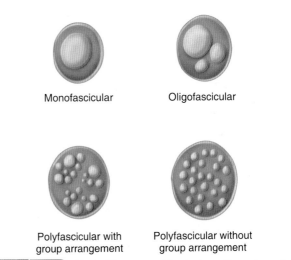

Monofascicular Oligofascicular

Polyfascicular with group arrangement Polyfascicular without group arrangement

FIGURE 5.4 Typical intraneural fascicular patterns in peripheral nerves.

nerves at the wrist, an intraneural polyfascicular or group arrangement is found. The outlook is better after repair of common digital and proper digital nerves because of their internal arrangement, their pure sensory function, and the short distance from the injury to the end organ.

Incisions to expose the nerve and mobilize it proximally and distally should be made in accordance with proven principles of skin incisions in the palm. They should not cross flexion creases at right angles, skin flaps should not be devascularized, and additional neurovascular injury should not be created in extending the skin incisions. The exact extent to which a nerve can be mobilized without creating ischemia is unknown. Generally, within the digits, palm, and wrist, extensive mobilization of the nerve from its surrounding tissues is insufficient to cause harm. Magnification is extremely helpful to permit the most precise and accurate restoration of the anatomy. In the palm and fingers, the magnification achieved by 2.5× to 4.5× magnifying loupes usually is sufficient to allow accurate repair. More proximally, magnification achieved with an operating microscope is more helpful in allowing satisfactory anatomic repair. The operating microscope also may be extremely helpful in repair of the terminal branches of the proper digital nerves distal to the distal flexion crease of the finger. Suture materials reflect the amount of tension to be applied to the nerve repair. Generally, in the forearm, wrist, and hand, 8-0 and 9-0 monofilament nylon sutures are used. Nylon suture of 9-0 caliber has been found to have more predictable failure via *breakage* with a failure threshold of 5% to 8% strain as compared to 8-0 nylon, which failed more often at higher strain and with suture pullout from the epineurium in a cadaveric median nerve model. Thus, this finding suggests that 9-0 nylon is most optimal for setting tension in nerve repairs at the wrist and hand level. In the past a perineurial neurorrhaphy (fascicular) (Fig. 5.5) or a combination epiperineurial-perineurial neurorrhaphy (Fig. 5.6) has been utilized. The literature, however, has not shown perineurial repair to be superior to a simpler epineural repair and thus at our institution an epineural repair is pursued in order to limit the trauma from suture bulk.

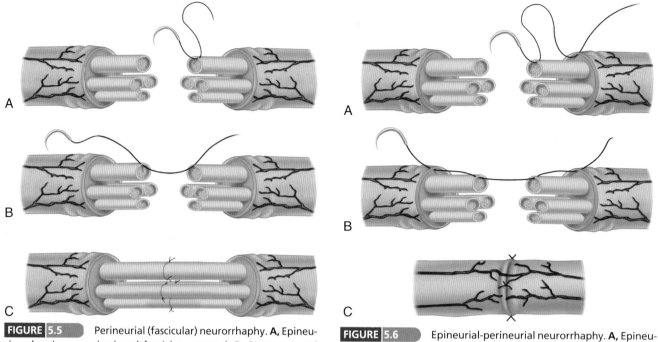

FIGURE 5.5 Perineurial (fascicular) neurorrhaphy. **A,** Epineurium has been excised and fascicles exposed. **B,** Suture passed through corresponding fascicles on either side of cut surface of nerve. **C,** Neurorrhaphy completed, usually with two 10-0 nylon sutures in each fascicle.

FIGURE 5.6 Epineurial-perineurial neurorrhaphy. **A,** Epineurium has been excised and retracted. Suture has been placed through epineurium, near large fascicle at periphery of nerve, and then through perineurium of fascicle. **B,** Suture passed through epineurium of matching fascicle on opposite side of cut surface of nerve, and then out through epineurium. **C,** Repair completed, after suturing other suitably matched fascicles.

NERVE GRAFTS
INDICATIONS

At times, as a result of extensive destruction, a segmental nerve defect is created that cannot be overcome through nerve mobilization, joint flexing, or rerouting of a nerve. A principal indication for nerve grafting in the hand is the bridging of defects after segmental nerve injury if a tension-free neurorrhaphy cannot be accomplished. Less commonly seen indications include nerve grafts to innervate free vascularized muscle grafts and to innervate free neurovascular island flaps.

Before performing a nerve graft, other techniques for closing the small gaps between nerve endings should be considered because they frequently solve the problem of closing small gaps in nerves. These techniques include mobilization of the nerve ends over a distance of a few centimeters proximally and distally, positioning of the joints near the nerve injury in less-than-awkward positions, and transposing or changing the course of nerve endings.

SOURCES OF NERVE GRAFTS

Donor nerves for nerve grafts in the upper extremities include the sural nerve; lateral antebrachial cutaneous and medial antebrachial cutaneous nerves; anterior and posterior interosseous nerves; digital nerves from an amputated finger; and a segment of a severed nerve from the opposite, but less critical, side of a single digit to repair the digital nerve on the opposite side. (For example, for lacerations of both nerves of the long finger requiring grafting, the ulnar digital nerve can be used to graft the radial digital nerve gap.) An anatomic study determined that the sural nerve best matches the common digital nerve. The lateral antebrachial cutaneous nerve best matches the digital nerve proximal to the level of the distal trifurcation. The posterior interosseous nerve, the anterior interosseous nerve, and the medial antebrachial cutaneous nerve best match the digital nerve distal to the trifurcation.

ALTERNATIVE NERVE GRAFT MATERIAL

Alternatives to autogenous nerve graft are available, and their use avoids sacrificing donor site sensation and saves surgical time. Options include silicone tubes or conduits made of polyglycolic acid, bovine collagen, processed porcine submucosa, or polycaprolactone. Historically conduits have been indicated for nerve gaps less than 3 cm. In addition to conduits, decellularized or processed nerve allograft (PNA) has seen increased utilization in recent years.

Processed nerve allografts are available in lengths up to 7 cm and are useful in restoring sensation in the hand. Although clear evidence-based guidelines are not yet in place, due to the lack of rigorous prospective randomized studies, the use of nerve allograft and conduits is probably best indicated in the pure sensory nerves of the common and proper digital nerves. Several studies have suggested that with modest nerve gaps of less than 10 mm in digital nerve injuries acceptable recovery of static two-point discrimination (S3+) is possible with nerve conduits. PNA may be better indicated for digital nerve gaps greater than 10 mm, although the maximal nerve gap at which no meaningful recovery can be attained has yet to be fully elucidated by the current body of literature. The Comparative Study of Hollow Nerve Conduit and Avance Nerve Graft Evaluation Recovery Outcomes of the Nerve Repair in the Hand (*CHANGE*) pilot study first attempted to answer this question. This AxoGen Incorporated sponsored study was one of the first to publish results of a double-blind, prospective, multicenter, randomized study comparing PNA to bovine type I collagen-based hollow nerve conduits. The average gap length before repair was 12 mm ± 4 mm (5 to 20 mm range). Their results were promising, with the PNA having a significantly better static 2-point discrimination (S2PD) of 5 mm ± 1 mm compared to 8 mm ± 5 mm for nerve conduit at 12 months post-operative. Although the patient numbers were low (PNA n = 6, conduit n = 9) because of attrition, for patients who reached 12-month follow-up the final results showed 100% of PNA recovered at least S3+ Medical Research Council Classification (MRCC) of sensory function compared to 75% of the conduits attaining S3+ function. Additionally, return to S4 level for patients reaching 12-month follow-up was 80% in the PNA group compared to 50% in the conduit cohort; however, this did not reach statistical significance. Further smaller case series have added support of PNA in digital nerve gaps >10 mm. A case series of eight digital nerves with PNA reconstruction of mean nerve gaps of 21 mm (range 5 to 30 mm) reported return of S2PD to S4 function in all. Another small case series of five digital nerve defects of 23 mm (range 18 to 28 mm) reconstructed with PNA reported that 4 patients recovered S2PD of S4 function with the lone outlier having S2PD of 7 mm. Taras et al. published a larger prospective PNA study of 18 digital nerve injuries with an average gap length of 11 mm (range 5 to 30 mm). The authors developed their own classification system for outcomes, which makes it difficult to compare outcomes to other published metrics. However, by extrapolating their S2PD results to MRCC classification for the sake of comparison, this study found that 12 of the 18 patients recovered S3+ function and an additional six patients recovered S4 function.

The AxoGen Incorporated sponsored Retrospective Study of Avance Nerve Graft Utilization, Evaluations and Outcomes in Peripheral Nerve Injury Repair (RANGER) database has subsequently been developed to try to answer the question of the upper limit nerve gap length of the processed nerve allograft. The first *RANGER* database study was published in 2012 by Cho et al. This multicenter retrospective study looked at 71 nerve PNA reconstructions for mixed, motor, and sensory nerves, 35 of which were digital nerve reconstructions. The mean digital nerve gap length was 19 mm (range 5 to 50 mm), and 31 patients (89%) with digital nerve PNA reconstructions achieved S3 or S4 sensory function, or what they defined as "meaningful recovery on the MRCC scale." The subsequent *RANGER* database study published in 2016 comprised 50 digital nerve injuries with an average gap length of 35 mm (range 27 to 50). To evaluate the outcomes of PNA at larger gap lengths, the authors queried the database for gaps of more than 25 mm. They reported that 43 (86%) reconstructions achieved S3 function or greater, with 32 (64%) reconstructions achieving S3+ or S4 levels of recovery. These values were found to be consistent independent of the gap range up to 50 mm. They reported no adverse events and found the outcomes to be comparable to historical studies for autografting.

Autogenous veins with or without intraluminal muscle also have been used to repair or reconstruct nerves. In a randomized prospective study, Rinker and Liau compared autogenous vein graft and woven polyglycolic acid conduits in 76 acute digital nerve repairs. They found mean static two-point discrimination was 7.5 mm for both test groups at 12 months follow-up with an average nerve gap

length of 10 mm reconstructed. There were comparable costs between the autogenous vein graft versus the polyglycolic acid conduits, however, the vein graft had less complications.

In summary, the literature is only beginning to elucidate the best indications for processed nerve allograft compared to nerve conduits in digital nerve injuries. Based on the current available data, the use of nerve conduits or autogenous vein grafts for digital nerve gaps of less than 10 mm can provide meaningful sensory recovery. The use of processed nerve allograft for providing meaningful sensory recovery is supported by the current body of literature for digital nerve gaps of 10 mm or more. The maximal digital nerve gap at which no meaningful recovery can be attained has yet to be determined; however, with further studies this question may be answered.

CONDUIT-ASSISTED DIGITAL NERVE REPAIR

TECHNIQUE 5.2

(WEBER ET AL.)

- Before nerve repair, trim the ends back to the level at which there was no intraneural hemorrhage for the primary cases and no interfascicular scarring for the secondary cases.
- Measure the distance or gap length between the two nerve ends at rest.
- Intussuscept the nerve end into the conduit
- Pull the proximal end of the nerve into the conduit with an 8-0 nylon suture, such that 5 mm of the nerve lies within the tube (Fig. 5.7).
- Because blood clots are an impediment to axonal regeneration, fill the tube with a solution containing 1000 U of heparin per 100 mL of normal saline.
- Insert the distal end of the nerve into the conduit using the same technique.
- Leave a minimum space of 5 mm between nerve ends even in cases in which there is only a 0- to 10-mm nerve tissue deficit.
- Inject additional heparinized saline into the tube to fill any remaining space.
- Repair any concomitant injuries to bone or tendon and reconstruct any vascular interruptions.
- Close the soft tissue using whatever tissue is necessary and splint the hand and finger as appropriate for the overall hand surgery.

POSTOPERATIVE CARE Sensory reeducation should be started 6 weeks after surgery. Exercises that focus on localization and pressure versus movement are done 5-10 minutes twice a day until sensation to the fingertip is recovered. Thereafter, late-phase sensory reeducation is begun, which consists of tactile discrimination between grades of sandpaper, textured cloth, and small objects.

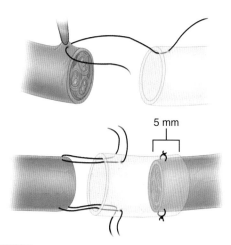

(MILLESI, MODIFIED)

- In the digits, hand, and distal forearm, use a pneumatic tourniquet to allow dissection of the injured nerve in a bloodless field.
- Make appropriate extensile skin incisions to locate and expose the distal glioma and the proximal neuroma on the injured nerve.
- Open the epineurium proximal to the neuroma in near-normal tissue on the proximal stump, and in the distal segment dissect proximally toward the scarred distal stump.
- At the wrist and in the distal forearm, identify the major fascicle groups within the nerve and, using sharp dissection with microscissors or a diamond knife for thicker scar, transect the fascicle groups so that a step-cut results (Fig. 5.8A and B). Such fascicular dissection is unnecessary in the common and proper digital nerves because of their pure sensory and oligofascicular nature. In a polyfascicular nerve, such as the median and ulnar nerves at the wrist, individual fascicle groups of different lengths protrude from the nerve stump after completion of the interfascicular dissection.
- Carry out similar dissection on the proximal and distal stumps. In a polyfascicular nerve, it is helpful to sketch the ends of the two nerve stumps with their fascicular patterns to allow matching of the respective fascicles, depending on the size, number of fascicles, and their arrangement within the proximal and distal stumps of the nerve (Fig. 5.8C). This clinical estimation is easier over short distances and more difficult over longer defects.
- Select a donor site that is appropriate for the size of the nerve and the gap to be filled. Generally, for common and proper digital nerves, the antebrachial cutaneous nerves are satisfactory. If a great deal of nerve tissue is required, the sural nerve is best in our experience.
- After the nerve graft has been harvested, place it between the proximal and distal nerve stumps.
- In the polyfascicular nerves, such as the median and ulnar nerves at the wrist, attempt to use the sketch of the fascicle groups to allow appropriate placement of the graft.
- When coaptation of the graft has been achieved, suture the graft with 10-0 monofilament nylon through the epineurium of the graft and the perineurium of one of the fascicles in the group or in the interfascicular connective tissue. Multiple sutures may not be required with satisfactory coaptation of the graft to the nerve stump ends.
- Insert Silastic drains as needed. Avoid the use of suction drainage.
- Close the skin so that the graft is not displaced during wound closure by shearing forces.
- Immobilize the extremity in a padded dorsal splint in as near an anatomic position as possible.

POSTOPERATIVE CARE   The part is immobilized for about 10 days, the splint is removed, and free movement of the joints is allowed. Hematomas that develop early in the postoperative period are removed, unsatisfactory or necrotic skin is debrided, and local flaps or skin grafts are used to cover a nerve graft that may have become exposed as a result of wound necrosis. At about 2 weeks, physical therapy is begun with supervised active and active-assisted range-of-motion exercises. The progress of regeneration is followed

FIGURE 5.7   Weber et al. conduit repair technique. Minimal distance between nerve stumps is 5 mm, even in instances in which ends can be coapted without tension. (Redrawn from Weber RA, Breidenach WC, Brown RE, et al: A randomized prospective study of polyglycolic acid conduits for digital nerve reconstruction in humans, *Plast Reconstr Surg* 106:1036, 2000.) **SEE TECHNIQUE 5.2.**

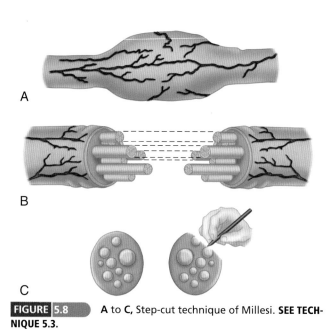

FIGURE 5.8   **A** to **C,** Step-cut technique of Millesi. **SEE TECHNIQUE 5.3.**

TENSION-FREE NERVE GRAFT

The experimental and clinical observations in reports of Millesi and of Millesi and Meissl suggest that a nerve repaired with a tension-free nerve graft has a better prognosis than end-to-end nerve repair done under excessive tension. In general, we have had satisfactory results with nerve grafts, particularly regarding sensory return, using the technique of Millesi. It is a technique that requires microsurgical experience. Nerve gaps of greater than 20 cm have been bridged using this technique.

using the Tinel sign. If the Tinel sign stops with no further progression for 3 to 4 months at the distal end of the graft, the nerve graft should be explored with resection of the distal suture line and another end-to-end repair.

MANAGEMENT OF SPECIFIC NERVE INJURIES
DIGITAL NERVES

Distal to the wrist, the digital nerves are the most frequently severed. It is important to repair the digital nerves, particularly the thumb ulnar digital nerve; the radial digital nerve to the index, long, ring, and little fingers; and the ulnar digital nerve to the little finger. Knowledge of the anatomy of the cutaneous sensory branches of the nerves on the dorsum of the hand allows repair of these nerves as well.

Digital nerves can be repaired distal to the distal volar flexion crease of the fingers in the region of the terminal branches of the nerves. If digital nerves are repaired secondarily, the suture line should lie in a well-vascularized bed free of scar. Before secondary repair, the proximal end of the nerve often can be located by passing a firm object, such as a paper clip, gently distally along the course of the nerve. On reaching the terminal neuroma, the patient indicates exquisite tenderness.

SUTURE OF DIGITAL NERVES
TECHNIQUE 5.4

- The digital nerves lie to the radial and ulnar sides of the volar aspect of the finger and can be exposed through the same midradial or midulnar incision when necessary.
- Begin proximally and dissect a normal segment of the nerve from its investing fascia (part of the Cleland ligament) (Fig. 5.9); proceed distally to the scar at the site of injury.
- Begin distal to the site of injury and dissect proximally to the scar.
- With scissors or a diamond knife, remove the neuroma from the proximal end of the nerve and the glioma from the distal end. Use loupe magnification for dissection and repair.
- Always suture divided tendons before suturing any nerve to avoid disrupting the delicate repair.
- Approximate the nerve ends without tension; flex the finger joints minimally if necessary. If a large gap requires extreme flexion, consider a nerve graft.
- Use an 8-0 or 9-0 monofilament nylon suture on an atraumatic curved needle (Fig. 5.10).
- Use 10-0 or 11-0 nylon to repair the terminal branches distal to the distal interphalangeal joint. If necessary, the nerve ends can be held in place temporarily by passing the smallest straight Bunnell needle transversely through

them into the adjoining soft tissue to avoid tension while the sutures are placed and tied.
- Pass a suture through the epineurium of the nerve about 1 mm from its edge and again in a similar manner through the epineurium of the other end of the nerve; tie the knot with at least five loops to prevent its slipping or untying.
- Place a second suture on the exact opposite side of the nerve. Leave these first two sutures long so that they can be used as traction sutures to rotate the nerve 180 degrees, making accessible all of its surfaces.
- Place a total of four sutures.
- After the repair, slowly extend the joints and observe the suture line for tension; note the optimal position of the joints for this purpose and maintain it by splinting after closure.

POSTOPERATIVE CARE After 3 weeks, the finger joints are allowed gradual active extension beyond the optimal position noted at surgery. If the defect in the nerve is large, active extension cannot be permitted before 4 weeks and a proximal interphalangeal (PIP) joint flexion contracture is likely to result. In this circumstance, it is best to perform a nerve graft and allow early digital motion. Immediate flexion exercises can be allowed within an extension block splint that prevents tension on the repair site. Although the suture line must be protected, active finger motion must be started as soon as possible to avoid stiffness and neural adhesions. The difference in sensibility recovery between patients who had immobilization and those who were allowed early protected motion has not been found to be significant. Likewise, no difference in clinical outcomes after digital nerve repair has been found between those who were and those who were not splinted postoperatively.

While major nerves are regenerating after repair, the hand may assume an unnatural posture because of changes in muscle balance. Even when the nerve lesion is proximal to the wrist, the hand suffers most and may incur fixed contractures before nerve function returns. Proper splinting (see chapter 1) is necessary to prevent contractures during this period. The patient should be warned that until sensation returns, the anesthetic skin can become infected after even minor trauma or can be burned, frostbitten, cut, or blistered by friction unless properly protected. The patient should be instructed to inspect the insensitive areas routinely and to avoid friction and extremes of heat and cold.

◼ NERVE TRANSFERS TO RESTORE DIGITAL SENSATION

Nerve transfers can be used to restore critical and noncritical sensation in the hand. Its role at our facility is limited to high nerve lesions when significant recovery is unlikely. Nerve defects in the hand are routinely repaired with grafting to avoid sacrifice of intact sensibility. The common digital nerve to the fourth web space arising from the ulnar nerve can be transferred end-to-end into the common digital nerve to the first web space for an irreparable median nerve injury. The superficial radial and dorsal cutaneous branch of the ulnar nerve can be transferred to common or proper digital nerves. Digital nerve defects located between

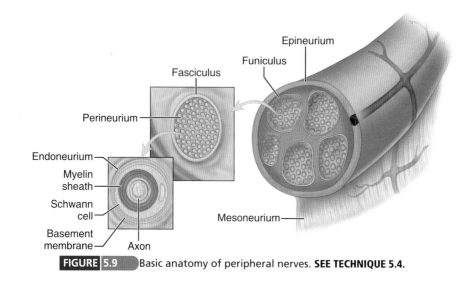

FIGURE 5.9 Basic anatomy of peripheral nerves. **SEE TECHNIQUE 5.4.**

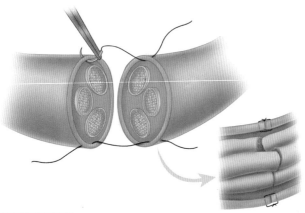

FIGURE 5.10 Basic suture technique for laceration of peripheral nerves should result in no tension at suture line, and each small fascicle should be aligned to match opposing, mirror image. **SEE TECHNIQUE 5.4.**

the PIP flexion crease and its takeoff from the common digital nerve can be reconstructed using a dorsal digital branch transfer from the involved or adjacent digit (Fig. 5.11). Chen et al. reported their experience with this technique in 17 patients and found it to be useful and superior to sural nerve grafting.

TRANSFER OF THE PROPER DIGITAL NERVE DORSAL BRANCH

TECHNIQUE 5.5

(CHEN ET AL.)

- With the use of an axillary block, tourniquet control, and operating microscope, determine the site and size of the proper digital nerve defect.

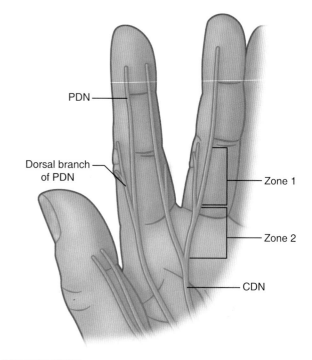

FIGURE 5.11 Anatomic zone system of the proper digital nerve (PDN) defects. Zone 1, the origin of the dorsal branch of the PDN to the proximal interphalangeal joint; zone 2, the origin of the dorsal branch to the common digital nerve (CDN) bifurcation. (Redrawn from Chen C, Tang P, Zhang X: Finger sensory reconstruction with transfer of the proper digital nerve dorsal branch, *J Hand Surg Am* 38:82, 2013.)

- For nerve gaps in zone 1, use the uninjured dorsal branch of the other proper digital nerve of the same digit as a donor nerve (Fig. 5.12A).
- Dissect the donor nerve and isolate it to its full extent as it courses to the PIP joint line.
- Isolate the distal end of the proper digital nerve in preparation for neurorrhaphy.

- Transect the dorsal branch, allowing enough length to reach the distal nerve end. To obtain maximal length of the donor nerve, the dorsal branch can be transected as far distally as the PIP joint.
- For nerve gaps in zone 2, use the dorsal branch of the proper digital nerve of an adjacent digit as the donor nerve.
- In zone 2, the distal nerve stump includes the proper digital nerve and the dorsal sensory branch. To obtain a better size match, separate the dorsal branch by splitting the nerve distally from the fascicles (Fig. 5.12B). Retain the remaining distal nerve stump that innervates the pulp and retain the volar aspect of the digit and suture it with the donor nerve.
- Perform neurorrhaphy with 10-0 nylon in an end-to-end fashion with the aid of the operating microscope.
- Cover the remaining proximal nerve stump of the proper digital nerve with normal soft tissue or bury it into the interosseous muscle to prevent neuroma irritation.

POSTOPERATIVE CARE The injured finger is kept in an extension block splint with the interphalangeal joints in full extension and the metacarpophalangeal joint in 70 degrees of flexion for 3 weeks.

ULNAR NERVE AT THE WRIST

If the ulnar artery and the tendon of the flexor carpi ulnaris are severed at the wrist, the ulnar nerve usually is severed, too. At this level, it is motor and sensory, and proper rotational alignment of the ends is important at the time of suture.

REPAIR OF THE ULNAR NERVE

TECHNIQUE 5.6

- With a pneumatic tourniquet inflated, make proximal and distal extensile skin incisions. Expose the proximal and distal segments of the nerve, but do not yet remove them from their normal beds.
- With a suture through the epineurium, mark exactly the most anterior aspect of each segment some distance from the scarred area.
- Free each segment from the surrounding soft tissues. Use loupe magnification for dissection and the operating microscope for repair.
- With microscissors or a diamond knife, make clean transverse cuts and excise the neuroma from the proximal segment and the glioma from the distal segment.
- Inspect each cut end for a pattern of large and small bundles. By matching these patterns and using the two epineurial sutures just described, proper rotational alignment should be possible.
- When further length is needed for suture without tension, dissect and mobilize the nerve more proximally or, if

necessary, transplant it anteriorly from behind the medial epicondyle of the humerus.
- Extensive freeing of a nerve may damage its blood supply. When advancing the nerve distally, do not divide its branches to the muscles in the proximal forearm.
- Careful intraneural dissection of the branches may allow mobilization of the nerve. Flex the elbow as necessary to avoid tension, but avoid excessive flexion of the elbow.
- Use the operating microscope to help align major groups of fascicles. Although four-quadrant traction sutures may be sufficient, it is sometimes easier to start with the deep surface and close the cut surface like a book, using a combination of 8-0 or 9-0 nylon epiperineurial and 10-0 perineurial (fascicular) sutures to complete the repair.
- When the ulnar nerve is severed near but just distal to its division into its volar (palmar) superficial sensory branch and its deep motor branch, identify the two small proximal segments and dissect them apart in a proximal direction for ease of mobilization; suture each branch separately.

DEEP BRANCH OF THE ULNAR NERVE

Boyes noted the feasibility of repairing the important deep branch of the ulnar nerve, which supplies the intrinsic muscles of the hand not supplied by the median nerve: the medial two lumbricals, all interossei, the hypothenar muscles, and the adductor pollicis. These are among the muscles most responsible for the quick and skillful movements of the fingers. Many tendon transfers have been devised to restore motor function lost by interruption of the ulnar nerve, but, if possible, direct repair of the nerve is desirable.

REPAIR OF THE DEEP BRANCH OF THE ULNAR NERVE

TECHNIQUE 5.7

(BOYES, MODIFIED)
- Use loupe magnification for dissection and the operating microscope for repair.
- Expose the nerve from its origin as a branch of the main trunk at the wrist to its midpalmar part through a curved incision distal and parallel to the thenar crease; extend it over the hook of the hamate to the flexion crease of the wrist; proceed proximally and medially, crossing the crease obliquely; and proceed to the ulnar aspect of the distal forearm.
- Reflect the skin, divide the palmaris brevis muscle at its insertion, and reflect it ulnarward so as not to disturb its nerve supply.
- Retract the ulnar vessels toward the thumb and divide the origins of the abductor digiti quinti, flexor digiti quinti, and opponens digiti quinti muscles. Retract the tendons of the flexor digitorum.

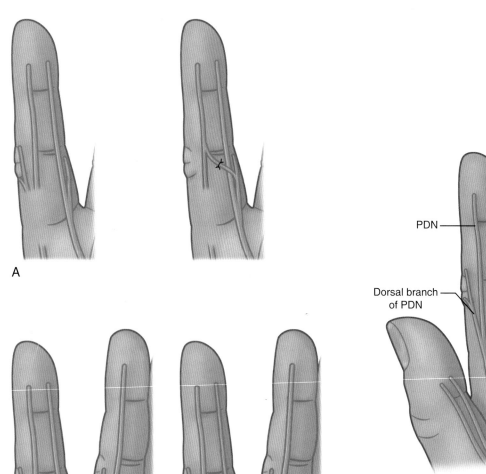

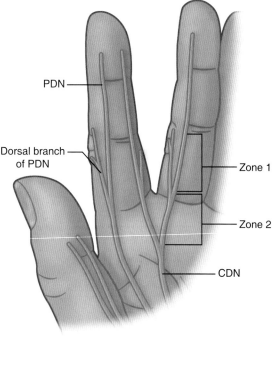

A

B

FIGURE 5.12   **A,** Proper digital nerve defect involving zone 2. **B,** Donor nerve is harvested from dorsal branch of the proper digital nerve of adjacent digit. To achieve a good size match of donor nerve, the dorsal branch *(arrowhead)* is separated from stump of distal nerve and remaining nerve stump is sutured with donor nerve.   (Redrawn from Chen C, Tang P, Zhang X: Finger sensory reconstruction with transfer of the proper digital nerve dorsal branch, *J Hand Surg Am* 38:82, 2013.) **SEE TECHNIQUE 5.5.**

- The course of the nerve is now exposed from the pisiform to the midpalm (Fig. 5.13A). If necessary, the nerve can be exposed farther distally by extending the incision to the index metacarpal and by retracting the flexor tendons with the lumbrical muscles. If these are displaced ulnarward, the nerve can be identified and followed where it passes through the transverse fibers of the adductor pollicis.
- When the nerve has been divided by a sharp instrument, gently free it proximally and distally to the point of damage. This usually allows enough length for suture without tension.

- If a gap exists as a result of gunshot wounds or other severe injuries in which nerve substance has been lost, consider a nerve graft or reroute the nerve (Fig. 5.13C and D).
- Dissect its motor component from the trunk well into the distal forearm. Divide the volar carpal ligament and free from the ulnar side of the carpus the ulnar bursa that lines the carpal tunnel; displace the proximal end of the nerve into the tunnel.
- Bring the proximal end to the midpalm by flexing the wrist. In some instances, when branches to the hypothenar muscles are still intact, gentle dissection and mobilization of

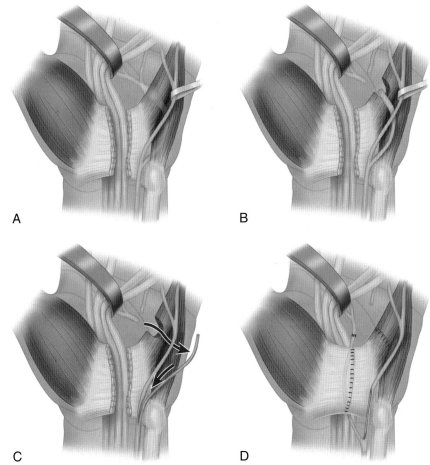

FIGURE 5.13 Boyes technique of repairing deep branch of ulnar nerve. **A,** Main trunk and deep branch of ulnar nerve have been exposed, and volar carpal ligament has been divided. **B,** Ends of deep branch have been freshened. **C,** Deep branch has been split intraneurally into distal forearm. **D,** Deep branch has been rerouted through carpal tunnel, and its ends have been sutured. **SEE TECHNIQUE 5.7.**

the bundles allow branches to be saved and yet permit the nerve to be rerouted.

- Use microscissors or a diamond knife to freshen the ends of the nerve (Fig. 5.13B).
- Repair the nerve using an epiperineurial or combination of epiperineurial and perineurial repairs with 8-0 or 9-0 nylon externally and 10-0 nylon within the nerves as needed.
- Suture the volar carpal ligament, replace the insertion of the palmaris brevis, and close the wound.
- According to Boyes, the results are proportional to the accuracy of the approximation and inversely proportional to the scarring and fibrosis. Regeneration occurs in an orderly way; the recovery of nerve function can be tested by noting voluntary activity of the first dorsal interosseous muscle (Fig. 5.14).

DORSAL BRANCH OF THE ULNAR NERVE

The dorsal branch of the ulnar nerve is large enough at the wrist and just distal to it to be repaired similar to a digital nerve. It crosses the ulnar styloid superficially, although it

may have branched from the trunk 5 cm or more proximal to the wrist. If extra length is needed to oppose the ends, it may be made to branch from the main trunk more proximally by intraneural dissection and is then routed more directly to the dorsum of the hand. The wrist should be held in extension for 3 to 4 weeks after surgery, following which gradual protected motion is begun, and a progressive exercise program is followed.

MEDIAN NERVE AT THE WRIST

Division of the median nerve at the wrist is not unusual, and the vital sensory function of the hand depends on its successful repair. It is important to emphasize the following: (1) the neuroma must be carefully excised from the proximal end, and the glioma must be excised from the distal end; (2) surrounding scar must be excised to provide a vascular bed; (3) the repair must be accurate, with the ends in proper rotation, for the nerve contains motor and sensory fibers; and (4) tension on the repair must be avoided.

The following points are helpful. A vessel usually lies on the anterior surface of the median nerve parallel with its long axis; this vessel may be helpful in securing proper rotational alignment, or it may be obliterated by scar when the repair is

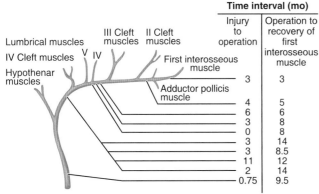

			Time interval (mo)	
			Injury to operation	Operation to recovery of first interosseous muscle
			3	3
			4	5
			6	6
			3	8
			0	8
			3	14
			3	8.5
			11	12
			2	14
			0.75	9.5

FIGURE 5.14 Rate of recovery of voluntary function of first dorsal interosseous muscle after repair of deep branch of ulnar nerve in 10 patients. (Modified from Boyd JH: Repair of the motor branch of the ulnar nerve in the palm, *J Bone Joint Surg* 37A:920, 1955.) **SEE TECHNIQUE 5.7.**

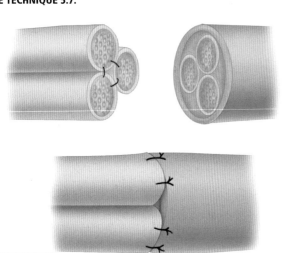

FIGURE 5.15 Bundle suture for segmental gap (see text).

late. An epineurial suture in each segment as described for the ulnar nerve at the wrist (see Technique 5.5) may aid in obtaining proper rotation. Tension can be reduced by dissecting and mobilizing the nerve proximally in the forearm and by flexing the wrist and elbow.

REPAIR OF THE MEDIAN NERVE

TECHNIQUE 5.8

- Expose the median nerve at the wrist using a palmar incision parallel to the thenar crease, extending proximally and crossing the wrist flexion crease obliquely and medially. Extend the incision proximal to the nerve transection in the volar midline of the forearm.
- Use magnifying loupes and the operating microscope as needed for dissection and repair.
- Use 8-0, 9-0, and 10-0 nylon on an atraumatic curved needle to place epiperineurial and perineurial (fascicular) sutures as needed to complete the repair.

- When a flexor tendon and the median nerve are sutured secondarily, release of the transverse carpal ligament may be needed to help prevent scar adhesions.

MEDIAN NERVE IN THE PALM

If the median nerve is divided where it branches in the palm, it occasionally can be repaired with a bundle suture (Fig. 5.15). This suture gathers the several branches of the nerve into a single trunk so that it can be sutured to the proximal segment of the nerve.

Every effort should be made to repair the recurrent branch of the median nerve. It may be difficult to find because of surrounding fascia and scar tissue, but when it is seen it can be identified readily by its yellow fibers running transversely toward the base of the thumb. This branch usually projects from the main trunk radially and superficially, passing just over the distal margin of the transverse carpal ligament. It courses slightly posteriorly and laterally to innervate the thenar muscles. Several important anatomic variations exist, so this recurrent branch may be represented by two branches instead of one; it may come off the ulnar side of the trunk, and it may perforate the distal portion of the transverse carpal ligament. It is repaired with the technique described for digital nerves (see Technique 5.4); the prognosis is good if careful attention is given to anatomic detail. If the median nerve cannot be repaired, a neurovascular island free graft may be indicated.

SUPERFICIAL RADIAL NERVE

Disability after interruption of the superficial radial nerve at the wrist is less than that after interruption of sensory nerves on the volar surface of the hand; there is anesthesia over a variable area on the dorsum of the thumb and index finger. Sometimes the ulnar side of the area of pinch of the thumb receives its major innervation from this nerve. Neuromas caught in dorsal scars are particularly painful because they are stimulated not only by direct touch but also by stretching of the surrounding skin, nerve, and scar when the wrist and fingers are flexed.

Unless there is some unusual reason for repairing the nerve or one of its branches, it should be resected proximal to its site of severance to permit it to lie in an area of minimal scar. It is so common to have a painful and, at times, disabling neuroma after repair that the small area of lost sensibility is a small disability in comparison.

REPAIR OF THE SUPERFICIAL RADIAL NERVE

TECHNIQUE 5.9

- The suture technique is as described for digital nerves. Locate the nerve proximally and dissect it distally to the scar; a consistent anatomic landmark proximally is the exit of the nerve from beneath the tendon of the brachioradialis muscle, usually about 5 cm proximal to its insertion into the radial styloid.

- Locate the nerve distally and dissect it proximally toward the scar. At the base of the thumb, the nerve usually already has divided into two major branches; each is larger than a digital nerve and when severed can be repaired (for the technique of suture, see Technique 5.4).
- If the wrist must be extended to appose the nerve ends, it should be maintained in this position for 4 or 5 weeks to prevent tension on the repair.
- If the distal branch or branches cannot be found, release the nerve proximally from the scar to relieve pain; resect some of it if necessary.

TRAUMATIC NEUROMAS

The treatment of traumatic neuromas is discussed in chapter 15.

NEUROVASCULAR ISLAND GRAFTS

Any digit deprived of sensibility is selectively and unconsciously avoided during use of the hand. Restoration of sensibility to a selected area of a given digit by transfer of a neurovascular island graft is useful at times. In permanent nerve damage, sensibility can be restored to critical areas, especially on the thumb or index finger. Transfer of a neurovascular island graft is essential to innervate an osteoplastic reconstruction of the thumb. Sensibility in the graft is never normal after transfer, however. In grafts critically examined at some time after surgery, sensibility usually is abnormal in all. More than half of patients have persistently hyperesthetic skin. All patients lack precise sensory reorientation. Although it need not be normal for a good functional result, reorientation seems to improve with time and with use of the part.

Transfer of a neurovascular island graft may be indicated to treat permanent sensory deficits on the radial side of an otherwise normal index finger or on the area of pinch on the distal ulnar aspect of the thumb. Before the decision for surgery is made, the following factors must be considered: (1) the dominance of the involved hand, (2) the presence of any scarring in the palm through which an incision must be made for channeling of the neurovascular bundle, (3) the status of the ipsilateral ulnar nerve, (4) the condition of the opposite hand, (5) the age of the patient, and (6) the experience of the surgeon.

Early descriptions of the operation suggested transfer of skin from just the ulnar side of the distal phalanx of the ring finger. Experience has shown, however, that most of the skin from an entire side of the donor finger should be included in the transfer. This larger transfer increases the area of sensitive skin on the recipient digit and causes no wider sensory loss on the donor digit; usually the larger free graft required to cover the donor area is of little consequence.

In the usual case, death of the transferred neurovascular island pedicle graft is unlikely, but even temporary impairment of the circulation can cause permanent sensory deficit in the graft and a partial failure of the operation. In handling the neurovascular bundle, several points in technique must be emphasized: (1) the bundle, including all veins, should be dissected from proximally to distally so that any anomalies of the vessels can be treated properly; (2) the bundle should not be completely freed from the surrounding fatty tissue, especially at the base of the finger, but should be transferred along with some attached tissue; and (3) the bundle should be channeled through an incision large enough to show the entire bundle to prevent kinking, twisting, or stretching of the nerve or vessels.

This procedure can be altered as necessary to meet other given requirements. In complete median nerve paralysis, if sensibility on the ulnar edge of the thumb pulp is reasonably good as a result of overlap of innervation from the radial nerve, transfer of the island graft to the radial side of the proximal and middle phalanges of the index finger may be desirable. This area of the finger is used especially in strong pinch.

NEUROVASCULAR ISLAND GRAFT TRANSFER

TECHNIQUE 5.10

- Using a skin pencil, accurately outline the area of sensory deficit on the thumb and prepare to remove skin from a similar area on the ulnar side of the ring finger. Alternative donor sites include the radial side of the little finger or, in the absence of median nerve damage, the ulnar side of the middle finger.
- If the entire palmar surface of the thumb is insensitive, outline on the ring finger the maximal donor area for transfer. Shape the donor area to include most of the ulnar side of the finger, with darts to near the midline on the palmar and dorsal surfaces between the finger joints. The area outlined includes skin supplied by the dorsal branch of the proper digital nerve and is shaped to prevent tension on the resulting scars during finger movements.
- Exsanguinate the limb by wrapping or elevation and inflate a pneumatic tourniquet on the arm.
- Beginning proximally near the base of the palm, make a zigzag incision distally to the fourth web (Fig. 5.16).
- Identify and dissect free, along with some surrounding tissue, the common volar digital artery and nerve to the ring and little fingers and the proper digital artery and nerve to the ulnar side of the ring finger. Loupe magnification is helpful in this dissection.
- Ligate and divide the proper digital artery to the radial side of the little finger.
- Carefully dissect and split proximally from the common volar digital nerve the proper digital nerve to the ulnar side of the ring finger.
- Continue the dissection distally and excise, with this attached neurovascular bundle, the previously outlined area of skin from the ulnar side of the ring finger; do not damage the artery, and preserve as many veins as possible.

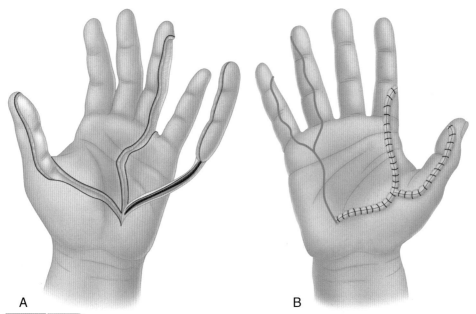

A   B

FIGURE 5.16 Technique of transferring neurovascular island graft. **A,** Palmar incision has been made, neurovascular island graft has been excised from ulnar surface of ring finger and its bundle has been freed proximally, and insensitive skin has been excised from palmar surface of thumb (see text). **B,** Alternative technique in which neurovascular island graft includes adjacent surfaces of ring and little fingers, and area covered by it is larger as shown. **SEE TECHNIQUE 5.10.**

- Use bipolar cautery to divide any small branches of the artery as necessary.
- Free the composite graft and carry the island graft across the palm to the recipient area on the thumb; ensure that the neurovascular bundle is long enough to permit the transfer without causing tension on the bundle. The island graft should cover most of the pulp area on the palmar aspect of the thumb and should extend to the ulnar aspect of the digit, but not to the distal edge of the nail.
- Beginning at the proximal end of the original incision and proceeding to the thumb, make a second zigzag incision across the palm conforming to the skin creases.
- Excise from the thumb the previously outlined area of skin, and if large enough, save it to be used later as a free skin graft on the donor finger.
- Suture the island graft in place on the thumb.
- Carefully check the entire neurovascular bundle for stretching, kinking, or twisting, and close the palmar incisions.
- Cover the donor area of the finger with a full-thickness graft from the recipient thumb, free of fat, or with a thick split graft obtained elsewhere; cover this graft with a stent dressing.
- Release the tourniquet and hold the wrist in slight flexion and the thumb in the best position to eliminate tension on the transferred bundle. Carefully observe the island graft for evidence of return of circulation. Vascular spasm can cause ischemia of the graft for a few minutes. The graft eventually should become pink; if it does not, check the positions of the wrist and thumb again and, if necessary, reopen part of the palmar incision and explore the transferred neurovascular bundle for kinking.

POSTOPERATIVE CARE A bulky dressing and a dorsal plaster splint are applied, holding the wrist, thumb, and fingers in flexion. The hand is elevated constantly for 4 or 5 days after surgery. After suture removal at 10 to 14 days, gentle, protected motion exercises are begun. Use of the splint can be discontinued at 3 to 4 weeks, depending on the needs of the thumb and donor finger.

REFERENCES

DIAGNOSTIC AIDS, MANAGEMENT PLAN, AND RESULTS
Cunningham ME, Potter HG, Weiland AJ: Closed partial rupture of a common digital nerve in the palm: a case report, *J Hand Surg* 30A:100, 2005.

TECHNIQUES OF REPAIR
Boyd KU, Nimigan AS, Mackinnon SE: Nerve reconstruction in the hand and upper extremity, *Clin Plast Surg* 38:643, 2011.

Isaacs J: Treatment of acute peripheral nerve injuries: current concepts, *J Hand Surg* 35A:491, 2010.

Vipond N, Taylor W, Rider M: Postoperative splinting for isolated digital nerve injuries in the hand, *J Hand Ther* 20:222, 2007.

Yu RS, Catalano LW, Barron A, et al.: Limited, protected postsurgical motion does not affect the results of digital nerve repair, *J Hand Surg* 29A:302, 2004.

NERVE GRAFTS
Bertleff MJ, Meek MF, Nicolai JPA: A prospective clinical evaluation of biodegradable Neurolac nerve guides for sensory nerve repair in the hand, *J Hand Surg* 30A:513, 2005.

Bushnell BD, McWilliams AD, Whitener GM, Messer TM: Early clinical experience with collagen nerve tubes in digital nerve repair, *J Hand Surg* 33A:1081, 2008.

Chen C, Tang P, Zhang X: Finger sensory reconstruction with transfer of the proper digital nerve dorsal branch, *J Hand Surg Am* 38:82, 2013.

Cho MS, Rinker BD, Weber RV, et al.: Functional outcome following nerve repair in the upper extremity using processed nerve allograft, *J Hand Surg Am* 37:2340, 2012.

Higgins JP, Fisher S, Serlett JM, et al.: Assessment of nerve graft donor sites used for reconstruction of traumatic digital nerve defects, *J Hand Surg* 27A:286, 2002.

Karabekmez FE, Duymaz A, Moran SL: Early clinical outcomes with the use of decellularized nerve allograft for repair of sensory defects within the hand, *Hand* 4:245, 2009.

Lee YH, Shieh SJ: Secondary nerve reconstruction using vein conduit grafts for neglected digital nerve injuries, *Microsurgery* 28:436, 2008.

Marcoccio I, Vigasio A: Muscle-in-vein nerve guide for secondary reconstruction in digital nerve lesions, *J Hand Surg* 35A:1418, 2010.

Meek MF, Coert JH: Clinical use of nerve conduits in peripheral-nerve repair: review of the literature, *J Reconstr Microsurg* 18:97, 2002.

Rinker B, Liau JY: A prospective randomized study comparing woven polyglycolic acid and autogenous vein conduits for reconstruction of digital nerve gaps, *J Hand Surg* 36A:775, 2011.

Rivlin M, Sheikh E, Isaac R, Beredjiklian PK: The role of nerve allografts and conduits for nerve injuries, *Hand Clin* 26:435, 2010.

Taras JS, Jacoby SM, Lincoski CJ: Reconstruction of digital nerves with collagen conduits, *J Hand Surg* 36A:1441, 2011.

Weber RA, Breidenach WC, Brown RE, et al.: A randomized prospective study of polyglycolic acid conduits for digital nerve reconstruction in humans, *Plast Reconstr Surg* 106:1036, 2000.

NEUROLYSIS, NEUROMAS, AND PAIN CONTROL

Atherton DD, Leong JC, Anand P, Elliot D: Relocation of painful end neuromas and scared nerves from the zone II territory of the hand, *J Hand Surg Eur* 32:38, 2007.

Thomsen L, Bellemere P, Loubersac T, et al.: Treatment by collagen conduit of painful post-traumatic neuromas of the sensitive digital nerve: a retrospective study of 10 cases, *Chir Main* 29:255, 2010.

The complete list of references is available online at Expert Consult.com.

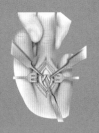

CHAPTER **6**

WRIST DISORDERS

William J. Weller

This chapter includes a discussion of anatomic, biomechanical, and kinematic aspects of wrist function and diagnostic methods, treatment options, and procedures for various wrist conditions. A considerable body of information on the wrist has developed in recent years. No attempt is made to resolve all controversies or to define narrowly the place of new procedures or technologies.

ANATOMY

The wrist is the anatomic region between the forearm and the hand. For the purposes of this discussion, the wrist includes the distal radioulnar, radiocarpal, and ulnocarpal joints and the eight carpal bones and their proximal and distal articulations and attached ligaments.

The eight carpal bones include the scaphoid, lunate, triquetrum, and pisiform in the proximal row and the trapezium, trapezoid, capitate, and hamate in the distal row (Fig. 6.1). They vary in size from the smallest, the pisiform and trapezoid, to the largest, the capitate, and in the amount of articular cartilage allowing for articulation, with one bone by the pisiform (the triquetrum) to seven bones by the capitate.

Viegas emphasized the considerable variation found in the fourth carpometacarpal articulation and in the scaphotrapeziotrapezoid, capitolunate, and hamatolunate articulations. Awareness of these variations may lead to better understanding of the normal kinematics of the wrist and the various injury patterns that are encountered.

The radiocarpal joints are formed by the articulation of the distal radius with the scaphoid and lunate through their respective concave facets on the distal radius and the triquetrum on the triangular fibrocartilage. The distal concave articular surfaces of the proximal carpal row form the midcarpal articulations with the distal row. The distal row articulates with the metacarpals, allowing mobility in the thumb, stability in the index and long finger metacarpals, and increased mobility in the ring and little finger metacarpals.

The distal ulnar convexity articulates at the lesser sigmoid notch of the distal radius. The sigmoid notch articular surface accommodates the ulnar head through two thirds of its arc. There is about a 20-degree inclination of the distal ulna at its articulation with the radius. The ulnar styloid lies dorsal to the ulnar head and extends distally. The triangular fibrocartilage attaches to the base of the ulnar styloid and

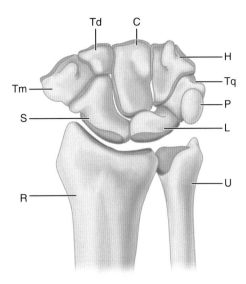

FIGURE 6.1 Radiocarpal joint. *C*, Capitate; *H*, hamate; *L*, lunate; *P*, pisiform; *R*, radius; *S*, scaphoid; *Td*, trapezoid; *Tm*, trapezium; *Tq*, triquetrum; *U*, ulna.

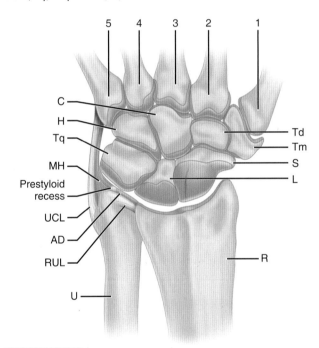

FIGURE 6.2 Components of triangular fibrocartilage complex. *AD*, Articular disc; *MH*, meniscus homologue; *RUL*, dorsal and volar radioulnar ligaments; *UCL*, ulnar collateral ligament. Other structures shown are metacarpal bones (*1*, *2*, *3*, *4*, and *5*), carpal bones (*C*, capitate; *H*, hamate; *L*, lunate; *S*, scaphoid; *Td*, trapezoid; *Tm*, trapezium; *Tq*, triquetrum), radius *(R)*, and ulna *(U)*.

separates the hyaline cartilage–covered ulnar head from the styloid (Fig. 6.2).

The chondroligamentous supports attaching the distal radius and ulnar side of the carpus to the distal ulna are designated as the *triangular fibrocartilage complex* (TFCC). Attaching to the ulnar margin of the lunate fossa of the radius, these supports include the ulnar collateral ligament, the dorsal and volar radioulnar ligaments, the articular disc, the meniscal homologue, the extensor carpi ulnaris sheath, and the ulnolunate and ulnotriquetral ligament. Additional

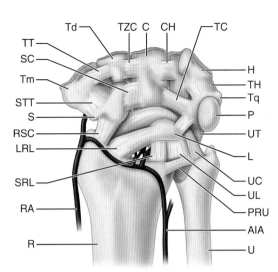

FIGURE 6.3 Wrist from palmar perspective. Bones: *C*, capitate; *H*, hamate; *L*, lunate; *P*, pisiform; *R*, radius; *S*, scaphoid; *Td*, trapezoid; *Tm*, trapezium; *Tq*, triquetrum; *U*, ulna. Arteries: *AIA*, anterior interosseous artery; *RA*, radial artery. Ligaments: *CH*, capitohamate; *LRL*, long radiolunate; *PRU*, palmar radioulnar ligament; *RSC*, radioscaphocapitate; *SC*, scaphocapitate; *SRL*, short radiolunate; *STT*, scaphotrapeziotrapezoid; *TZC*, trapezocapitate; *TC*, triquetrocapitate; *TH*, triquetrohamate; *TT*, trapeziotrapezoid; *UC*, ulnocapitate; *UL*, ulnolunate; *UT*, ulnotriquetral.

ligaments are found in two locations: (1) between the carpal bones (interosseous intrinsic ligaments) connecting the carpal bones in the proximal and distal carpal rows and (2) extending from the radius and ulna distally across the carpal rows (extrinsic ligaments). The interosseous ligaments include the scapholunate and lunotriquetral interosseous ligaments connecting the proximal carpal row and the ligaments connecting the trapezium to the trapezoid, the trapezoid to the capitate, and the capitate to the hamate in the distal carpal row. The extrinsic or crossing ligaments include the radial collateral ligament from the radial styloid to the scaphoid waist, the ulnar collateral ligament from the base of the ulnar styloid attaching to the pisiform, and the transverse carpal ligament. The volar extrinsic or crossing ligaments also include the radioscaphocapitate ligament, the radiolunotriquetral ligament, and the radioscapholunate ligament on the radial side and the ulnolunate and ulnotriquetral components of the TFCC on the ulnar side. On the palmar side of the carpus, between the radiolunotriquetral ligament and the radioscaphocapitate ligament, is a relatively thin area, the space of Poirier, overlying the palmar surface of the lunate (Fig. 6.3).

Dorsally, the identifiable extrinsic ligaments include the dorsal radiocarpal and the dorsal intercarpal ligaments. The trapezoidal dorsal radiocarpal ligament attaches along the dorsal radial articular margin of the lunate fossa, from the Lister tubercle to the lesser sigmoid notch. It spans the lunotriquetral joint and inserts on the dorsal surface of the triquetrum. There are four types of dorsal radiocarpal ligaments (Fig. 6.4). The dorsal intercarpal ligament, which is attached to the distal, dorsal surface of the triquetrum, passes across the midcarpal joint to attach to the dorsal surfaces of the scaphoid waist and the trapezoid. The dorsal intercarpal ligaments have variations in thickness and

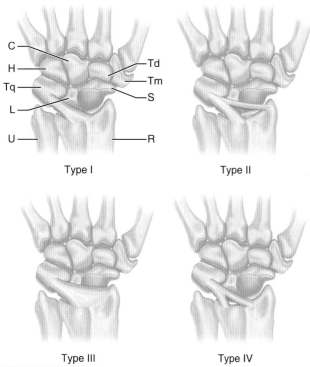

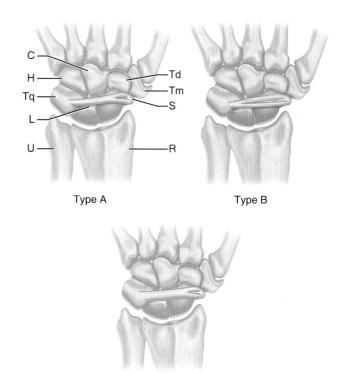

FIGURE 6.4 Four types of dorsal radiocarpal ligaments. *C,* Capitate; *H,* hamate; *L,* lunate; *R,* radius; *S,* scaphoid; *Td,* trapezoid; *Tm,* trapezium; *Tq,* triquetrum; *U,* ulna.

FIGURE 6.5 Three types of dorsal intercarpal ligament. *C,* Capitate; *H,* hamate; *L,* lunate; *R,* radius; *S,* scaphoid; *Td,* trapezoid; *Tm,* trapezium; *Tq,* triquetrum; *U,* ulna.

attachments (Fig. 6.5). The laminated structure of the dorsal intercarpal ligament allows for changing shape with wrist movement (Fig. 6.6).

CIRCULATION

The terminal branches of the radial, ulnar, and anterior interosseous arteries provide extraosseous blood supply to the carpus through three dorsal and three palmar transverse arterial arches with longitudinal connections (Fig. 6.7). The dorsal arches are (1) the dorsal radiocarpal at the radiocarpal joint, supplying the lunate and triquetrum; (2) the dorsal intercarpal (the largest) between the proximal and distal carpal rows, supplying the distal carpal row and, through anastomoses with the radiocarpal arch, the lunate and triquetrum; and (3) the basal metacarpal arch at the base of the metacarpals (the most variable) to supply the distal carpal row. The palmar arches are (1) the palmar radiocarpal at the level of the radiocarpal joint to the palmar surfaces of the lunate and triquetrum, (2) the intercarpal arch between the proximal and distal carpal rows, which is the most variable and does not contribute to nutrient vessels in the carpus, and (3) the deep palmar arch at the level of the metacarpal bases, which is consistent and communicates with the dorsal basal metacarpal arch and the palmar metacarpal arteries. Additional descriptions of the intraosseous circulation of certain carpal bones (especially the scaphoid, lunate, and capitate) are found with the discussions of afflictions of those bones and in the references listed at the end of the chapter.

BIOMECHANICS AND KINEMATICS

The stability of the wrist during motion and interrelated motions depends on capsuloligamentous integrity and contact

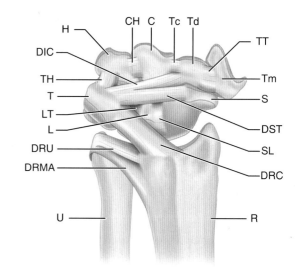

FIGURE 6.6 Wrist from dorsal perspective. Bones: *C,* capitate; *H,* hamate; *L,* lunate; *R,* radius; *S,* scaphoid; *T,* triquetrum; *Td,* trapezoid; *Tm,* trapezium; *U,* ulna. Ligaments: *CH,* capitohamate; *DIC,* dorsal intercarpal; *DRC,* dorsal radiocarpal; *DRMA,* dorsal radial metaphyseal; *DRU,* dorsal radioulnar; *LT,* lunotriquetral; *SL,* scapholunate; *Tc,* trapezocapitate; *TH,* triquetrohamate; *TT,* trapeziotrapezoid.

surface contours of the carpal bones. The center of rotation for most wrist motions generally is considered to be located in the proximal capitate. During flexion and extension, most motion occurs at the radiocarpal joint, with some occurring through the midcarpal area. Using ultrafast CT in vivo kinematic studies, the radiocarpal and midcarpal joints were

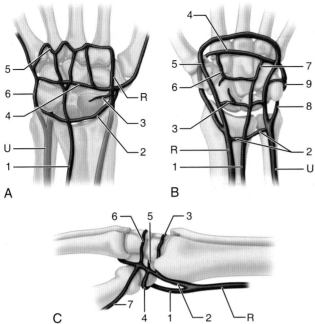

FIGURE 6.7 **A,** Arterial supply of dorsum of wrist. *1,* Dorsal branch of anterior interosseous artery; *2,* dorsal radiocarpal arch; *3,* branch to dorsal ridge of scaphoid; *4,* dorsal intercarpal arch; *5,* basal metacarpal arch; *6,* medial branch of ulnar artery; *R,* radial artery; *U,* ulnar artery. **B,** Arterial supply of palmar aspect of wrist. *1,* Palmar branch of anterior interosseous artery; *2,* palmar radiocarpal arch; *3,* palmar intercarpal arch; *4,* deep palmar arch; *5,* superficial palmar arch; *6,* radial recurrent artery; *7,* ulnar recurrent artery; *8,* medial branch, ulnar artery; *9,* branch off ulnar artery contributing to dorsal intercarpal arch; *R,* radial artery; *U,* ulnar artery. **C,** Arterial supply of lateral aspect of wrist. *1,* Superficial palmar artery; *2,* palmar radiocarpal arch; *3,* dorsal radiocarpal arch; *4,* branch to scaphoid tubercle and trapezium; *5,* artery to dorsal ridge of scaphoid; *6,* dorsal intercarpal arch; *7,* branch to lateral trapezium and thumb metacarpal; *R,* radial artery.

found to contribute equally to wrist flexion and the midcarpal joint contributed more to extension. During radial-to-ulnar deviation, the proximal carpal row rotates dorsally and the proximal row translocates or shifts radially at the midcarpal and radiocarpal joints, with motion occurring at the radiocarpal and intercarpal joints. During ulnar-to-radial deviation, the proximal carpal row tends toward palmar rotation, with most of the motion occurring in the intercarpal joints. The proximal carpal row is considered to be an intercalated segment in the forearm-to-hand connection, with the scaphoid functioning to stabilize the wrist.

For purposes of understanding the ways in which forces are transmitted and motions and positions of the carpal bones are controlled by ligaments and contact surface contours, the concept of a wrist consisting of three columns was popularized by Novarro: the central (force-bearing) column, the radial column, and the ulnar (control) column. The central column includes the distal articular surface of the radius, the lunate, and the capitate, and some would add the proximal two thirds of the scaphoid, the trapezoid, and the articulations with the second and third metacarpal bases. The radial column includes the radius, the scaphoid, the trapezium, the trapezoid, and the thumb carpometacarpal joint. The ulnar column includes the triangular fibrocartilage (articular disc), the hamate, the triquetrum, and the articulations of the carpometacarpal joints of the ring and little fingers. Taleisnik proposed that the central column includes the entire distal row and the lunate. According to his concept, the scaphoid is included as the lateral column and the triquetrum as a rotary medial column (Fig. 6.8A). Lichtman proposed a ring concept of wrist kinematics (Fig. 6.8B). According to this concept, the interosseous ligaments stabilize the semirigid proximal and distal carpal rows. Limited mobility occurs between the scaphotrapezial joints and the triquetrohamate joints. Bone or ligament disruption of the ring creates instability deformities, with the lunate tilting either dorsally (dorsal intercalated

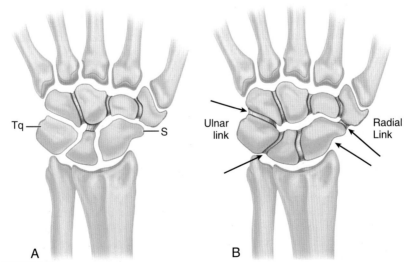

FIGURE 6.8 **A,** Taleisnik's concept of central (flexion-extension) column involves entire distal row and lunate: scaphoid *(S)* is lateral (mobile) column, and triquetrum *(Tq)* is rotary medial column. **B,** Lichtman's ring concept of carpal kinematics: proximal and distal rows are semirigid posts stabilized by interosseous ligaments; normal controlled mobility occurs at scaphotrapezial and triquetrohamate joints. Any break in ring, either bony or ligamentous *(arrows),* can produce dorsal intercalated segmental instability or volar intercalated segmental instability deformity.

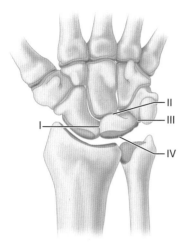

FIGURE 6.9   Stages of perilunar instability.

segmental instability) or toward the volar aspect (volar intercalated segmental instability).

Studies of transmission of forces suggest that the distal carpal row may bear more than 10 times the force applied to the fingertips. About 55% to 60% of the load on the distal row is transmitted through the capitate, scaphoid, and lunate. At the radiocarpal level, the load on the radioscaphoid joint varies from 50% to 56%; on the radiolunate joint, 29% to 30%; and on the ulnolunate joint, 10% to 21%.

DIAGNOSIS OF WRIST CONDITIONS

HISTORY

The usual historical information is documented, including age, hand dominance, occupation, hobbies, date of injury or onset of symptoms, correlation of symptoms with activities and modifying factors (e.g., medications, cold, heat), and previous injury or surgery. Current work status and the existence of various legal concerns (e.g., lawsuits, workers' compensation, or disability claims) are helpful in assessing the overall situation.

When obtaining the history of traumatic conditions, the mechanism of injury frequently is unknown. The various carpal injuries represent a spectrum of injury. The extent of injury depends on (1) loading in three dimensions, (2) duration and amount of forces, (3) hand position at impact, and (4) mechanical properties of the ligaments and bones. A pattern can be seen in which carpal dislocations result from ulnar deviation and intercarpal supination, and scaphoid fractures result from wrist extension with the dorsal articular margin of the radius serving as a fulcrum (Fig. 6.9). Flexion and pronation injuries, conversely, may contribute more to ligament injuries on the ulnar side of the wrist, especially the lunotriquetral ligament. It is important to be able to document swelling, bruising, local areas of pain, point tenderness, and sensations of grating, popping, and crunching.

For long-standing problems, it is important to correlate the problem with the factors that cause worsening or improvement. The relationship to work and recreational activities; the presence and location of swelling and aching with mechanical symptoms, such as clicking, popping, snapping, and grating; and the response to treatment are important. Other joint involvement and the possible presence of various arthritides in the patient or family members also should be considered.

PHYSICAL EXAMINATION

A careful, detailed examination is conducted with the forearm and hand supported whether the examination is done immediately after injury or for chronic problems. In addition to the usual assessment of motor, sensory, and circulatory integrity, it is important to try to correlate the patient's complaints with the underlying muscles, tendons, tendon sheaths, bones, joints, ligaments, and capsules. Scars, bruises, and other skin findings and the ranges of active and passive motion should be documented and compared with the uninjured side.

The underlying anatomy can be correlated with easily identified and palpable bony structures, including the radial styloid, Lister tubercle, ulnar styloid, pisiform, and scaphoid tuberosity. Overlying superficial tenosynovitis, such as that seen in the first dorsal compartment (de Quervain), must be differentiated from conditions related to deeper structures or problems related to ligamentous and bony structures (e.g., thumb carpometacarpal arthritis; tenosynovitis in the extensor compartments, the flexor carpi radialis tunnel, and the carpal tunnel; masses such as ganglions; and underlying compression neuropathies of the radial, median, and ulnar nerves in their respective areas of compression).

RADIOGRAPHIC TECHNIQUES

After the history and physical examination, radiographic evaluation is helpful in determining the diagnosis, prognosis, and management of wrist problems. Gilula et al. proposed a useful algorithm detailing one approach to the radiographic assessment of a painful wrist (Fig. 6.10). MRI should be added for evaluation of the triangular fibrocartilage; the distal radioulnar joint (DRUJ); and vascularity of the various carpal bones, extrinsic ligaments, joint surfaces, and surrounding soft tissues to confirm clinical suspicion and correlate with physical examination findings. A high rate of false-positive findings on MR images of normal subjects has been reported. A dedicated wrist coil provides enhanced resolution of wrist structures.

Various radiographic techniques useful in evaluating a painful wrist include the following:
1. Routine radiographic series consisting of four views
   - Posteroanterior
   - Lateral
   - Oblique
   - Ulnar-deviated posteroanterior scaphoid view
2. Spot views of the carpal bones for detail (carpal tunnel view) (Fig. 6.11)
3. Fluoroscopic spot views of the wrist (Fig. 6.12)
4. Series of views for instability
   - Anteroposterior clenched fist
   - Posteroanterior in neutral, radial, and ulnar deviation
   - Lateral in neutral and full flexion and extension
   - Semipronated oblique 30 degrees from the postero-anterior
   - Semisupinated oblique 30 degrees from the lateral

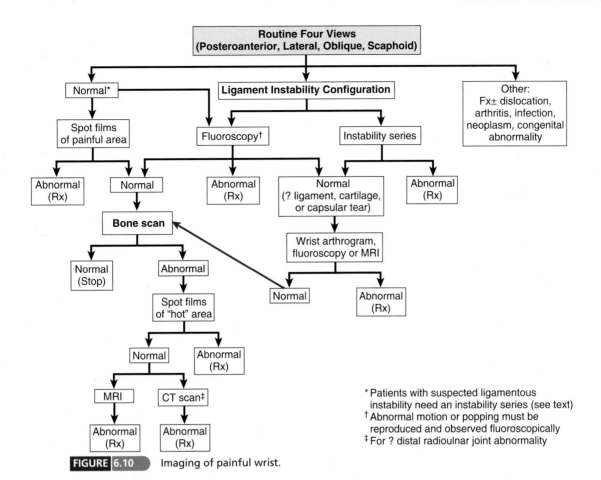

FIGURE 6.10 Imaging of painful wrist.

Chart text:

Routine Four Views
(Posteroanterior, Lateral, Oblique, Scaphoid)

Normal*

Ligament Instability Configuration

Other:
Fx± dislocation, arthritis, infection, neoplasm, congenital abnormality

Spot films of painful area

Fluoroscopy†

Instability series

Abnormal (Rx)

Normal

Abnormal (Rx)

Normal (? ligament, cartilage, or capsular tear)

Abnormal (Rx)

Bone scan

Normal (Stop)

Abnormal

Wrist arthrogram, fluoroscopy or MRI

Spot films of "hot" area

Normal

Abnormal (Rx)

Normal

Abnormal (Rx)

MRI

CT scan‡

Abnormal (Rx)

Abnormal (Rx)

* Patients with suspected ligamentous instability need an instability series (see text)
† Abnormal motion or popping must be reproduced and observed fluoroscopically
‡ For ? distal radioulnar joint abnormality

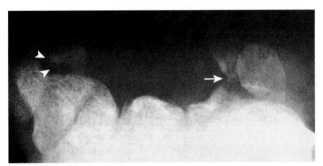

FIGURE 6.11 Carpal tunnel view shows avulsion fracture of hamate hook *(arrow)* and trapezium *(arrowheads).*

5. Diagnostic ultrasound
6. Cine or video fluoroscopy
7. Bone scanning
8. Arthrography of the wrist (triple injection when indicated) (Fig. 6.13)
9. CT
10. MRI

Other radiographic techniques relevant to specific problems are discussed later.

OTHER DIAGNOSTIC TECHNIQUES

Other clinical methods for determining the specific anatomic location of a problem include (1) differential local anesthetic injection, (2) wrist arthroscopy, and (3) various other operative procedures. If the specific structure causing the pain cannot be precisely identified (e.g., extensor carpi ulnaris versus underlying ulnocarpal joint), it is sometimes useful to inject a small amount (<3 mL) of local anesthetic into the most likely site. This helps in the localization of the pain. Sterile technique is used, and the patient is always advised of the benefits and risks.

ARTHROSCOPY OF THE WRIST

From a mostly diagnostic tool, wrist arthroscopy has developed into an effective therapeutic tool, useful for the treatment of a variety of wrist disorders from arthritis to acute fractures. It has produced new arthroscopic classifications of disorders such as Kienböck disease, TFCC injuries, and interosseous ligament tears that can help guide treatment. Arthroscopic assessment of intercarpal ligament injuries and instability is considered by many the "gold standard" for evaluation of these conditions, as well as for examination of patients who have wrist pain of unknown origin.

INDICATIONS

Indications for wrist arthroscopy include the evaluation of ligamentous injuries, examination of joint articular surfaces, removal of loose bodies, biopsy of synovium, irrigation and debridement of joints, and confirmation and supplementation of wrist arthrography. Arthroscopy has been found to be more accurate than arthrography in identifying the location and size of triangular fibrocartilage and interosseous ligament injuries and more accurate than triple-injection cinearthrography in detecting tears of the

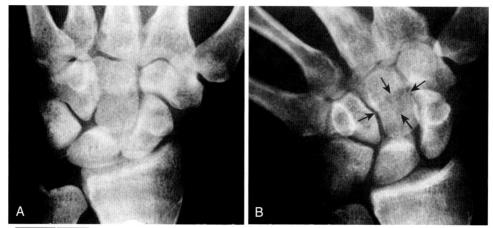

FIGURE 6.12 **A,** Posteroanterior view of capitate shows no definite abnormality. **B,** On angled view, cystic defect with fracture is seen in capitate waist *(arrows).*

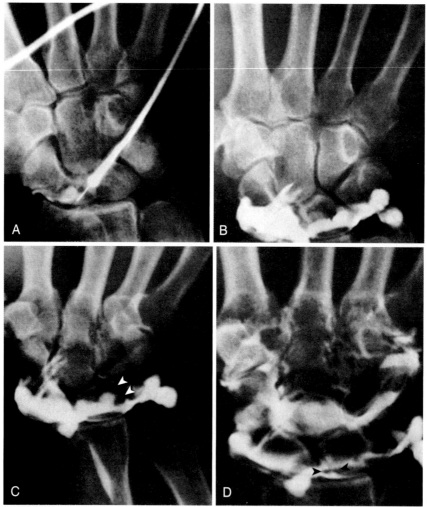

FIGURE 6.13 Fluoroscopic spots during arthrogram. **A,** Needle in place, start of contrast injection. **B,** End of contrast injection, at point of slight patient discomfort; contrast material is confined to radiocarpal joint. **C,** With ulnar deviation, contrast material passes into midcarpal joint between lunate and triquetrum *(arrowheads),* indicating lunotriquetral ligament tear. **D,** On follow-up overhead view, contrast material fills midcarpal joints, including scapholunate joint from its distal aspect, making it difficult to see whether scapholunate or lunotriquetral ligament is torn. Small defect *(arrowheads)* between contrast material in scapholunate space and radiocarpal space indicates intact scapholunate ligament.

Arthroscopic Procedures of the Wrist

Triangular Fibrocartilage Complex
Repair
Debridement

Carpal Instability
Debridement of scapholunate interosseous ligament/lunotri-
    quetral interosseous ligament
Scapholunate/lunotriquetral percutaneous pinning

Wrist Fractures
Distal radial fractures
Scaphoid fractures

Chondral Lesions
Dorsal ganglion excision

Bone Excision Procedures
Radial styloidectomy
Excision of distal ulna
Partial resection (wafer procedure)
Proximal row carpectomy
Excision of proximal pole of scaphoid
Lunate excision for Kienböck disease
Loose body removal

Miscellaneous
Synovectomy
Intraarticular adhesion release
Lavage of septic wrist

From Gupta R, Bozentka DJ, Osterman AL: Wrist arthroscopy: principles and clinical applications, *J Am Acad Orthop Surg* 9:200, 2001.

scapholunate and lunotriquetral ligaments and the triangular fibrocartilage.

Wrist arthroscopy has been found to be useful in diagnosing and treating wrist cartilage lesions, synovitis, TFCC disorders, and scapholunate and lunotriquetral ligament injuries. Debridement of osteochondritic lesions; reduction and fixation of carpal fractures, distal radial intraarticular fractures, and perilunate injuries; distal ulnar resection; and dorsal ganglion excision can be added to the growing list of indications for wrist arthroscopy (Box 6.1).

COMPLICATIONS

Complication rates for wrist arthroscopy vary from 1.2% to 5.2%. A systematic analysis of the literature identified a 4.7% complication rate in 895 procedures reported in 11 studies. Complications of wrist arthroscopy can be divided into four categories:

1. Complications related to traction and arm position—skin injury, joint stiffness, and peripheral nerve injury
2. Portal and instrument insertion complications—injury to cutaneous nerves, vascular structures, flexor and extensor tendons, ligaments, and articular cartilage
3. Procedure-related complications—forearm compartment syndrome caused by fluid extravasation during fracture treatment, injury of the

dorsal sensory branch of the ulnar nerve during arthroscopic repair of the triangular fibrocartilage, and injury to sensory nerves during insertion of Kirschner wires
4. General arthroscopic complications (equipment failure and infection)

A knowledge of wrist anatomy, the use of correct technique, and an understanding of the equipment and its use may help to avoid significant complications. This section covers the basics of diagnostic wrist arthroscopy. The use of arthroscopy in the treatment of various wrist conditions is included in the discussions of specific conditions.

EQUIPMENT

Equipment for wrist arthroscopy includes the following:
Arthroscope
    Diameter: 2.5 to 3 mm best for routine use; 1.7 to 4 mm
        optional
    Length: 50 to 60 mm
    Lens-offset angle: 30 to 70 degrees
Effective light source
High-definition (HD) video camera system/imaging console
Liquid crystal display (LCD) or light-emitting diode (LED)
    video monitor
Image capture system/digital video recorder
Irrigation system: gravity feed usually satisfactory; pumps
    (mechanical and manual) allow better irrigation and use
    of suction and cutting tools
    18-gauge needles
    Sterile tubing
    Limb-positioning attachments
    Ceiling hook or overhead pole and pulley
    Robotic devices, convenient and easily adjustable (trac-
        tion "tower")
    Fingertraps
    Forearm and wrist stabilizers
    Traction weights: 4 to 7 lb
    Scalpel blades
    Arthroscopy instruments
    Radiofrequency probes
    Basket forceps: 2 to 3 mm in diameter, 40 to 60 mm long
    Cutting tools
    Four-jaw, shallow probe: 40 mm long, 1.5 to 2.0 mm in
        diameter
    Grasping forceps with thin jaws: straight and curved
    Resector: full radius and 2 to 3 mm in diameter usually
        best
Power source

POSITIONING AND PREPARATION OF THE PATIENT

Wrist arthroscopy can be done with the patient under regional block anesthesia or general anesthesia. If multiple procedures are to be done, or if the patient is uncomfortable, a general anesthetic usually is best. The use of a pneumatic arm tourniquet is optional but may be helpful when treating an intraarticular fracture. With the patient supine and the shoulder abducted on a hand table, arthroscopy can be done with the elbow flexed and the hand pointing toward the ceiling. Extension of the elbow (horizontal position) to allow pronation of the forearm may facilitate the treatment of intraarticular fractures.

PATIENT POSITIONING FOR WRIST ARTHROSCOPY

TECHNIQUE 6.1

- With the patient under a suitable anesthetic, suspend the hand from the traction beam with sterile fingertraps and rope through an overhead pulley to use traction to move weight out and away from the operative field (Fig. 6.14). An arthroscopy tower can be used in the place of overhead traction. Include the thumb, index, and long fingers in the fingertraps.
- Maintain the elbow in 80 to 90 degrees of flexion. Flex the wrist about 20 degrees.
- If a tourniquet is to be used, exsanguinate the limb and inflate the tourniquet.
- Stabilize the forearm by securing it to a mechanical well-padded forearm clamp.
- Apply 4 to 10 lb of traction weight through the fingertraps for distraction of the wrist.

GENERAL PRINCIPLES

The usual arthroscopic portals are located between the extensor compartments of the wrist (Fig. 6.15). The portals are numbered according to the compartments on either side of the portal (Fig. 6.16). There are 11 dorsal portals, 9 for radiocarpal and intercarpal access and 2 for the DRUJ. An additional volar portal can be made lateral to the flexor carpi radialis tendon at the proximal wrist flexion crease. Slutsky described success using a volar ulnar approach between the flexor tendons and the ulnar neurovascular bundle and flexor carpi ulnaris. Portals most often used for evaluation of the radiocarpal and ulnocarpal joints are portal 3-4 (between the third and fourth extensor dorsal compartments) and portal 4-5 (between the fourth and fifth compartments). The midcarpal joint radial portal lies to the radial side of the third metacarpal axis proximal to the capitate in a soft depression between the capitate and scaphoid. It is in line with Lister tubercle (Fig. 6.17) at the scaphocapitate and scapholunate joint. The midcarpal ulnar portal is about 1 cm distal to the 4-5 portal, aligned with the fourth metacarpal, at the lunotriquetral-capitate-hamate joint. A portal between the fifth and sixth compartments, the 6R portal, is located on the dorsoradial aspect of the extensor carpi ulnaris tendon. The 6U portal is located to the ulnar side of the extensor carpi ulnaris tendon. The triangular fibrocartilage and the ulnolunate, ulnotriquetral, and lunotriquetral ligaments can be seen from the 6R portal. The scapholunate interosseous ligament, a potential origin for a dorsal ganglion, also can be seen from this portal.

In addition to the frequently used 3-4 and 6 portals, other portals allow inspection of other parts of the wrist. Portal 4-5 permits better inspection of the TFCC and the ulnocarpal ligament on the palmar side. Portal 2-3 allows inspection of the radial palmar ligaments. A probe placed through portal 1 can help to evaluate the articular surface

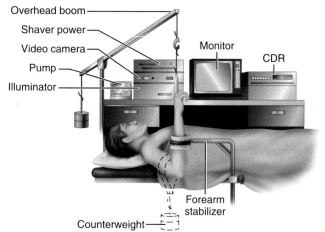

FIGURE 6.14 Positioning of patient and equipment for wrist arthroscopy. *CDR*, Compact disc recorder. **SEE TECHNIQUE 6.1.**

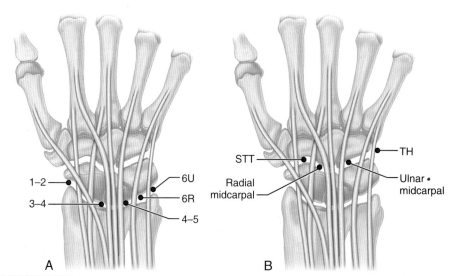

FIGURE 6.15 **A,** Standard radiocarpal portals. **B,** Standard midcarpal portals. *STT*, Scaphotrapeziotrapezoid; *TH*, triquetrohamate. (From Gupta R, Bozentka DJ, Osterman AL: Wrist arthroscopy: principles and clinical applications, *J Am Acad Orthop Surg* 9:200, 2001.)

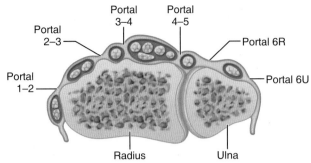

FIGURE 6.16 Cross section of wrist at level of distal radius showing compartments and portals used for examination of radiocarpal and ulnocarpal joints.

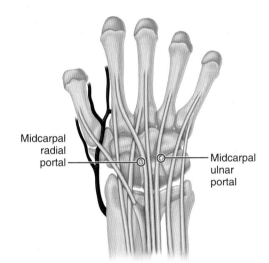

FIGURE 6.17 Midcarpal radial and ulnar arthroscopic portals on radial side (proximal to capitate "soft spot") and ulnar side (1 cm distal to 4-5 portal) of the third metacarpal.

of the distal radius. Use of needles, such as 20-gauge and 22-gauge hypodermic needles, in the various portals before placement of the probe or other instruments helps determine which portal would work best. Portals for the DRUJ are located just proximal and distal to the ulnar head. The posterior interosseous nerve is at risk when the proximal portal is used, whereas the triangular fibrocartilage may be injured by instruments entering the distal portal. The use of a blunt trocar helps avoid injury to the joint surface when inserting the arthroscope sheath.

Although larger arthroscopes provide better fields of vision, they usually are too large and difficult to manipulate. If continuous inflow irrigation is used, an efficient drainage system also must be used to avoid fluid extravasation and complications in the forearm. Pumps with automatic monitoring of pressure and flow also help to avoid such complications. Continuous fluid infusion and positioning the arthroscope with the camera end toward the ceiling helps avoid air bubble accumulation. Dry wrist arthroscopy also is feasible and helps avoid some of the complications associated with fluid extravasation. The use of a probe for triangulation is helpful in examining the ligaments and cartilage surfaces. To see in the joint satisfactorily, joint distraction should be maintained with weight to allow distention with saline and frequent irrigation.

RADIOCARPAL EXAMINATION

TECHNIQUE 6.2

- Identify and mark the skin at the sites of the arthroscopic portals to be used. Mark the distal radial joint margin and the location of Lister tubercle (Fig. 6.18A).
- Distend the radiocarpal joint by locating the portal between the third and fourth extensor compartments just distal to the extensor pollicis longus and Lister tubercle. Insert an 18-gauge needle into this portal, inclining the needle from dorsal-distal to palmar-proximal 12 to 15 degrees to follow the normal distal radial joint palmar tilt (Fig. 6.18B). Distend the joint with 5 to 10 mL of normal saline.
- Remove the needle, incise the skin over the portal, use a small hemostat to dissect gently down to and through the capsule, insert a cannula and blunt obturator, and establish inflow irrigation through the arthroscope.
- As an alternative, a continuous inflow system can be established through the ulnocarpal joint through portal 6 to the ulnar side of the extensor carpi ulnaris. Avoid the dorsal sensory branch of the ulnar nerve.
- Outflow can occur through the arthroscope or with gravity drainage through a tube. An irrigation pump that maintains constant pressure and flow may be helpful. Avoid extravasation.
- Introduce the arthroscope into the radiocarpal joint at portal 3 through a small skin incision.
- Use a small hemostat to dissect bluntly and spread the subcutaneous soft tissues to retract the extensor pollicis longus tendon to the radial side.
- Use the hemostat or a no. 11 blade to open the dorsal capsule. Avoid tendon injury.
- Insert the arthroscope with a proximal palmar inclination to accommodate the palmar tilt of the distal radius.
- Incline the arthroscope so that the proximal end is toward the ceiling to help remove air bubbles.
- At this point, identify the palmar capsule of the wrist and the distal radial articular concavity.
- Insert a probe through portal 4-5 through a skin incision or between the extensor digiti quinti and the extensor carpi ulnaris (6R portal). This portal can be used as an inflow or outflow portal during radiocarpal examination or as a portal for the arthroscope during ulnocarpal examination.
- Follow an organized pattern of identifying structures within the wrist. Direct the arthroscope toward the distal end of the radius, follow it along the scaphoid and lunate fossae, and examine them. Move the arthroscope in the radial direction to identify the distal radius and the proximal margin of the scaphoid. Note the scapholunate articulation, which is a small crease between the scaphoid and lunate with intimate blending of the ligament with the articular cartilage.
- Extend the wrist to expose the dorsal surfaces of the scaphoid and lunate and flex the wrist to examine the palmar surfaces of these bones. Identify the palmar carpal ligaments (Fig. 6.19).

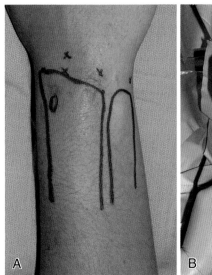
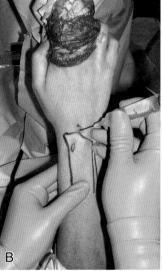
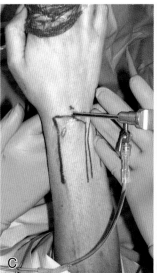
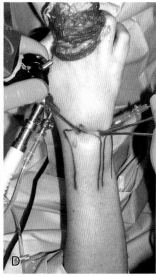

FIGURE 6.18   **A,** Radial and ulnar styloid are marked, and distal radius and ulna are outlined. **B,** Twenty-gauge needle with bevel parallel to extensor tendons is inserted through 3-4 portal. **C,** Blunt trocar is removed and arthroscope inserted. **D,** 6U portal is established slightly ulnar to extensor carpi ulnaris tendon. **SEE TECHNIQUE 6.2.**

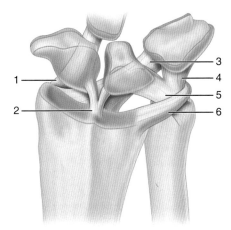

FIGURE 6.19   Ligaments of radiocarpal joint: *1,* radioscapho-capitate; *2,* radioscapholunate; *3,* radiolunotriquetral; *4,* ulnotriquetral; *5,* ulnolunate; *6,* triangular fibrocartilage. **SEE TECHNIQUE 6.2.**

- The radioscapholunate and radiotriquetral ligaments can be identified, as can the radiocapitate ligament (Fig. 6.20). Use a probe to stress the ligaments and evaluate their integrity.
- Move the arthroscope to the 4-5 or 6R portal and exchange the inflow or outflow cannula to the 3-4 portal for examination of the ulnar aspect of the joint and the TFCC.
- With a probe, palpate the TFCC to determine its integrity, especially its attachment to the ulnar margin of the radius.
- Moving toward the ulnar side of the wrist, identify the ulnocarpal ligaments and the proximal articular surface of the triquetrum.
- Insert a probe in portal 4 or 5 to evaluate the palmar carpal ligaments and the scapholunate and lunotriquetral interosseous ligaments. It may be necessary to move the probe into a more radial portal to examine the TFCC.

MIDCARPAL EXAMINATION

TECHNIQUE 6.3

- The portal for entry into the radial side of the midcarpal joint is located about 1 cm distal to the 3-4 portal for radiocarpal examination. It is located to the radial side of the third metacarpal and proximal to the soft area between the scaphoid and capitate.
- Insert an 18-gauge needle into this portal and distend the joint with 5 to 7 mL of saline, incise the skin over this area, dissect bluntly to the capsule, and insert a cannula and obturator, permitting inflow through the arthroscope.
- The ulnar midcarpal portal is located in the center of the axis of the fourth metacarpal and proximal to the capitohamate joint. Enter this joint with an 18-gauge needle, distend the joint, and verify the position of the needle by direct vision of the needle with the arthroscope remaining in the radial midcarpal portal to the radial side of the extensor tendons.
- The scaphocapitate and capitohamate joints can be examined through these portals. The scaphotrapezial-trapezoid joint also can be examined through the midcarpal radial portal.
- Place the arthroscope through a skin incision into this portal to view the capitate distally and the scaphoid proximally.
- Moving the arthroscope toward the radial side along the scaphocapitate joint, examine the scaphotrapezial-trapezoid joint.
- Moving in an ulnar direction along the scaphocapitate joint, examine the scapholunate, lunotriquetral, and capitohamate joints. Traction and manipulation of the wrist allow better inspection of these joints.

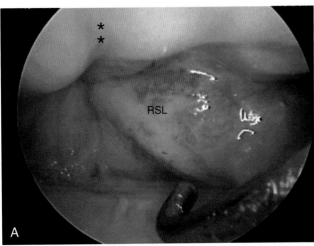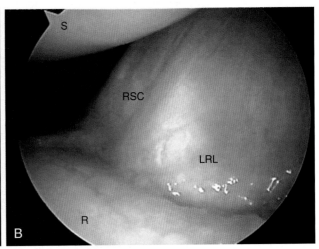

FIGURE 6.20 **A,** Normal arthroscopic appearance of radioscapholunate (*RSL*) and scapholunate interosseous *(asterisks)* ligament. **B,** Normal appearance of radioscaphocapitate (*RSC*) and long radiolunate (*LRL*) ligaments. *R,* Radius; *S,* scaphoid. (From Slutsky D: Wrist arthroscopy. In Wolfe SW, editor: *Green's operative hand surgery,* 6th ed, Philadelphia, Elsevier, 2011.) **SEE TECHNIQUE 6.2.**

- After the examination and operative procedures have been completed, determine that no loose objects are left within the joint and remove the arthroscope, instruments, and drainage tubing.
- Remove the tourniquet, obtain hemostasis, and close the portal incisions with staples or skin sutures. Infiltration of the joint with a local anesthetic agent helps minimize postoperative pain. Apply a bulky hand dressing with a splint.

DISTAL RADIOULNAR EXAMINATION

TECHNIQUE 6.4

- Distend the DRUJ by inserting an 18- or 20-gauge needle into the joint just lateral and dorsal to the ulnar head and inject a small amount of normal saline. The joint is best located by palpation of the distal radioulnar area with the forearm supinated.
- Proximal and distal radioulnar portals have been described by Whipple. The proximal portal is safer because it presents less risk to the articular cartilage of the ulnar head and to the triangular fibrocartilage.
- To establish the proximal portal, incise the dorsal skin just proximal to the dorsal prominence of the ulnar head, centered between the distal ulna and the medial (ulnar) side of the radius.
- Bluntly dissect with a hemostat to avoid injury to the extensor carpi ulnaris tendon and the dorsal sensory branch of the ulnar nerve.
- Enter the joint with the hemostat.
- Pass the arthroscopic cannula with a blunt obturator from proximal to distal.
- Remove the obturator and insert the arthroscope to determine entry into the joint.

- Establish a working portal 5 to 10 mm distal to the proximal radioulnar portal by making a small skin incision and bluntly dissecting to pass an 18-gauge needle. Use the arthroscope to ensure that the needle is in the joint. This portal can be used as needed for the insertion of instruments such as forceps and shavers.
- To establish the DRUJ portal, make an incision over the fifth and sixth extensor compartments, dissecting to enter the joint just proximal to the triangular fibrocartilage, between the fibrocartilage and the ulnar head. As noted previously, the proximal portal allows safer inspection of the lesser sigmoid notch, the ulnar head, and the proximal surface of the triangular fibrocartilage.
- After thorough arthroscopic examination, remove the arthroscope, instruments, and cannulas.
- Suture the wounds and apply a compressing bandage and supporting splint.

POSTOPERATIVE CARE Depending on the nature of the procedure, the splint is removed and mobilization is begun in the first 7 to 10 days after arthroscopy. After fracture reduction and ligament repairs, immobilization and rehabilitation may be prolonged.

Arthroscopic procedures for specific conditions are described in the sections discussing those conditions.

FRACTURES AND DISLOCATIONS OF THE CARPAL BONES, INCLUDING KIENBÖCK DISEASE

The diagnosis of fractures and dislocations of the carpal bones can be difficult for several reasons. The outlines of the eight bones are superimposed in most radiographic views. Even in the anteroposterior view, at least one bone overlies another. All views must be interpreted with an understanding of the normal bone contours, the relationships between the

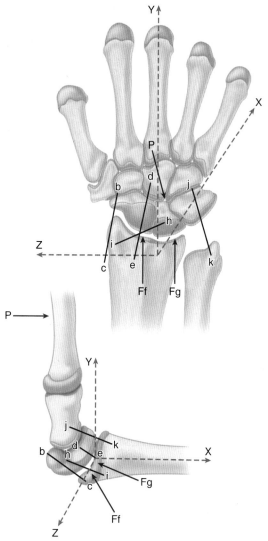

Representation of potential load-carrying structures involved in proximal carpal articulation as described by Weber and Chao. Four ligamentous components (*cb, ed, ih, kj*) potentially transmit tensile loads when wrist is in strong dorsiflexion. Dorsal ligamentous structures eliminated from analysis because in dorsiflexion structures would be lax. Articular surface between radius and scaphoid and between radius and lunate potentially transmit compressive forces *Ff* and *Fg*. These forces are related to fixed coordinate system (*XYZ*) and to vector representation of applied load (*P*). *cb*, Radiocollateral ligament complex; *ed*, radiocapite ligament; *Ff*, radioscaphoid contact force; *Fg*, radiolunate contact force; *ih*, radiolunate ligament; *kj*, ulnar capsular ligament; *XYZ*, cartesian coordinate system.

bones, and the changing relationships during the various arcs of wrist motion.

Because of the difficulty in recognizing fractures in acute injuries, fractures in this region may not be seen at initial examination. Articular damage and ligament injuries are even more difficult to evaluate. The latter may permit abnormal rotations and subluxations of the various bones. Special radiographic techniques are helpful. Scaphoid fracture displacement may be more readily detected and distinct with three-dimensional CT than with plain CT. Even though special techniques are used, establishing a precise diagnosis can

be difficult. Often prognosis is uncertain because of the peculiarities of the blood supply of these bones, especially of the scaphoid and lunate. Compared with plain radiographs, CT scans, and the surgeon's operative impression in the assessment of scaphoid nonunions, MRI was more accurate than the other techniques in predicting the vascularity of scaphoid nonunions.

FRACTURES OF THE SCAPHOID

Fracture of the carpal scaphoid bone is the most common fracture of the carpus, and frequently diagnosis is delayed. A delay in diagnosis and treatment of this fracture may alter the prognosis for union. A wrist sprain that is sufficiently severe to require radiographic examination initially should be treated as a possible fracture of the scaphoid, and radiographs should be repeated in 2 weeks even though initial radiographs may be negative.

■ ETIOLOGY

This fracture has been reported in individuals ranging from 10 to 70 years old, although it is most common in young men. It is caused by a fall on the outstretched palm, resulting in severe hyperextension and slight radial deviation of the wrist. The scaphoid usually fractures in tension with the wrist extended, concentrating the load on the radial-palmar side. The proximal pole locks in the scaphoid fossa of the radius, and the distal pole moves excessively dorsal (Fig. 6.21). Of scaphoid fractures, 60% to 80% occur at the scaphoid waist or midportion. Seventeen percent of patients have other fractures of the carpus and forearm, including transscaphoid perilunar dislocations, fractures of the trapezium, Bennett fractures, fractures of the radial head, dislocations of the lunate, and fractures at the distal end of the radius. When other injuries of carpal bones require open reduction, the fractured scaphoid also should be reduced accurately.

■ ANATOMY AND BLOOD SUPPLY OF THE SCAPHOID BONE

The unique anatomy of the scaphoid predisposes fracture of this carpal bone to delayed union or nonunion and to disability of the wrist. Because it articulates with the distal radius and with four of the remaining seven carpal bones, the scaphoid moves with nearly all carpal motions, especially volar flexion. Any alteration of its articular surface through fracture, dislocation, or subluxation or any alteration of its stability by ligamentous rupture can cause severe secondary changes throughout the entire carpus.

The blood supply of the scaphoid is precarious. Only 67% of scaphoid bones have arterial foramina throughout their length, including the distal, middle, and proximal thirds. Of the remaining bones, 13% have blood supply predominantly in the distal third and 20% have most of the arterial foramina in the waist area of the bone with no more than a single foramen near the proximal third. One third of scaphoid fractures occurring in the proximal third may be without adequate blood supply. This seems to be borne out clinically; the prevalence of osteonecrosis can be 35% in fractures at this level. Fractures in the proximal pole can be expected to take longer to heal and usually have higher rates of nonunion.

Vessels enter the scaphoid from the radial artery laterovolarly, dorsally, and distally. The laterovolar and dorsal systems share in the blood supply to the proximal two thirds of the scaphoid. Vascularity of the proximal pole and 70% to 80% of the interosseous circulation are provided through branches of the radial artery, entering through the dorsal ridge. In the distal tuberosity region, 20% to 30% of the bone receives its blood supply from volar branches of the radial artery.

◼ DIAGNOSIS AND TREATMENT

Treatment of scaphoid fractures is determined by displacement and stability of the fracture. Scaphoid fractures are generally classified as either undisplaced and stable or displaced and unstable (Fig. 6.22). Although this classification remains useful, fractures of the tuberosity, the distal articular surface, and the proximal pole may require special management decisions. For nondisplaced fractures, radiographic diagnosis can be difficult initially. A posteroanterior plain radiograph with the wrist slightly

Scaphoid nonunion associated with the location of fracture and amount of displacement		
Location	**Number of fractures**	**Percentage of union**
Distal third	2	100
Middle third	56	80
Proximal third	32	64
Displacement	**Number of fractures**	**Percentage of union**
Stable	48	85
Unstable	42	65

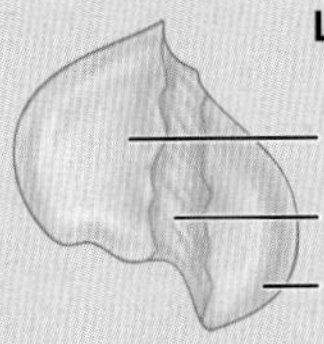

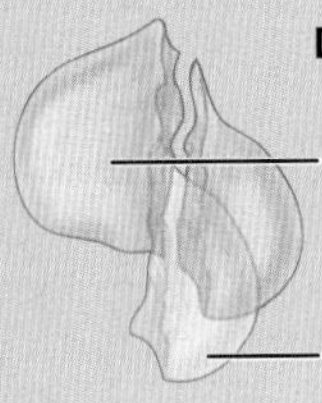

FIGURE 6.22 Union of scaphoid after bone grafting is influenced significantly by location of fracture and amount of displacement.

extended in ulnar deviation is helpful. Although repeating radiographs after 2 weeks of immobilization in a cast is a time-honored method for evaluation of a suspected nondisplaced scaphoid fracture, technetium bone scan, MRI, and CT (in the longitudinal axis of the scaphoid with 1 mm cuts as described by Sanders) provide diagnostic information sooner. Although bone scan has been considered the most sensitive study, Gaebler et al. reported 100% sensitivity and specificity using MRI to diagnose "occult" scaphoid fractures at an average of 2.8 days after injury (Fig. 6.23A). MRI, especially with gadolinium enhancement, also is useful in assessing the vascularity of a fractured scaphoid (Fig. 6.23B). Some reports have suggested that an MRI or CT scan should be obtained early so that patient downtime is decreased and productivity is increased.

▌NONDISPLACED, STABLE SCAPHOID FRACTURES

Nonoperative treatment usually is successful for acute nondisplaced, stable fractures through the scaphoid waist and in the distal pole without other bony or ligamentous injury and for scaphoid fractures in children. The prognosis is better if the fracture is diagnosed early. Controversies continue regarding the position of the wrist, the proximal and distal length of the cast, and elbow and thumb immobilization. There are clinical and experimental data to support most aspects of the controversies. Although some studies have found the incidence of nonunion to be no greater in patients treated by a removable short arm thumb spica cast than in patients treated by a long arm thumb spica cast, others have found that the time to union was earlier in patients treated initially for 6 weeks in a long arm thumb spica cast. A meta-analysis of randomized controlled trials of nonoperative treatment that involved below-elbow and above-elbow casting, casting with or without the thumb included, and casting with the wrist in 20 degrees of flexion to 20 degrees of extension found no significant differences in union rate, pain, grip strength, time to union, or osteonecrosis for the various nonoperative treatment methods. In an experimental scaphoid fracture model, displacement of more than 3 mm occurred between fracture fragments during pronation and supination with the forearm in a short arm thumb spica cast.

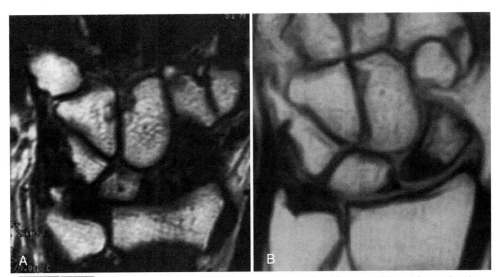

FIGURE 6.23 MRI is useful for diagnosis of "occult" scaphoid fractures **(A)** and for evaluation of vascularity of fractured scaphoid **(B)**. (From Segalman KA, Graham TJ: Scaphoid proximal pole fractures and nonunions, *J Am Soc Surg Hand* 4:233, 2004.)

We use a forearm cast from just below the elbow proximally to the base of the thumbnail and the proximal palmar crease distally (thumb spica) with the wrist in slight radial deviation and in neutral flexion. The thumb is maintained in a functional position, and the fingers are free to move from the metacarpophalangeal joints distally. Using nonoperative casting techniques, the expected rate of union is 90% to 95% within 10 to 12 weeks. During this time, the fracture is observed radiographically for healing. If collapse or angulation of the fractured fragments occurs, surgical treatment usually is required.

Fractures at and distal to the scaphoid waist are expected to heal sooner than fractures in the proximal pole. If the diagnosis is delayed, or the fracture is in the proximal third, the prognosis is less favorable, and an initial long arm thumb spica cast for 6 weeks may be justified. If the diagnosis of a nondisplaced fracture of the scaphoid has been delayed for several weeks, treatment usually begins with cast immobilization. Mack et al., reviewing scaphoid fractures diagnosed 1 to 6 months after injury, found that stable middle-third scaphoid fractures healed with cast immobilization but required an average of 19 weeks to heal, compared with a similar group of acute fractures that healed in an average of 10 weeks. As is reflected in the subsequent discussion of surgical treatment, there is a well-established trend toward earlier operative fixation of nondisplaced fractures. Surgery may be considered if new healing activity is not evident and if union is not apparent after a trial of cast immobilization for about 20 weeks.

Because of the potential for joint stiffness, muscle atrophy, or the inability to use the hand during and after prolonged immobilization, special nonoperative or operative treatment may be considered in certain patients (e.g., young laborers or athletes). Operative techniques, including percutaneous fixation with cannulated screws, are used with increasing frequency. Prospective, randomized studies comparing percutaneous screw fixation with cast immobilization showed that patients in the screw fixation groups were able to regain movement and return to most activities earlier than patients in the casted groups. No harmful effects on fracture healing were seen. In a prospective randomized study of nondisplaced scaphoid waist fractures, there were no nonunions in the 44 patients treated with Herbert screw fixation without postoperative immobilization, but 10 nonunions were present at 12 weeks in the 44 treated with cast immobilization. Several studies have reported healing of all fractures treated with "limited access," percutaneous, and arthroscopic percutaneous fixation. Advantages of this technique, according to its proponents, include less risk to neurovascular structures and intercarpal ligaments, earlier bone healing, and earlier return to activities. Patients considering such treatment should understand that acute, nondisplaced scaphoid fractures have a high probability of healing with cast treatment and that complex and demanding surgical procedures may have complications.

For some athletes, the use of padded casts during competition may be considered. The advantages and disadvantages of various treatment modifications should be considered in each patient.

DISPLACED, UNSTABLE SCAPHOID FRACTURES

A different course of treatment is required for a displaced, unstable fracture in which the fragments are offset more than 1 mm in the anteroposterior or oblique view, or lunocapitate angulation is greater than 15 degrees, or the scapholunate angulation is greater than 45 degrees in the lateral view (range 30 to 60 degrees). Other criteria for evaluating displacement include a lateral intrascaphoid angle greater than 45 degrees, an anteroposterior intrascaphoid angle less than 35 degrees (Amadio et al.), and a height-to-length ratio of 0.65 or greater (Bain et al.). Because the range of lunocapitate and scapholunate angulation can vary, comparison views of the opposite wrist can be helpful. Reduction can be attempted initially by longitudinal traction and percutaneous joystick Kirschner wires. If the reduction attempt is successful, percutaneous fixation with a cannulated screw or pins and application of a thumb spica cast may suffice. Otherwise, open reduction and internal fixation may be required.

For a displaced or unstable recent fracture of the scaphoid, the best method of fixation depends on the surgeon's experience and the equipment available. In some fractures, adequate internal fixation can be obtained with Kirschner wires. The AO cannulated screw, the Herbert differential pitch bone screw, and other more recently designed headless screws have been used to advantage in displaced and unstable scaphoid fractures. According to a cadaver comparison study, the AO screw, the Acutrak screw, and the Herbert-Whipple screw showed better resistance to cyclical bending load than the noncannulated Herbert screw. In a comparison study of patients with scaphoid fractures, one treated with AO cannulated screws and the other with Herbert-Whipple cannulated screws, the union rate was 100% in both groups. Cannulated bone screws are useful because the screw can be placed accurately over a guide pin with video fluoroscopic control. Cited advantages of screw fixation are that it (1) reduces the time of external immobilization, (2) provides relatively strong internal fixation, and (3) produces compression at the fracture site. In addition, because the headless screw remains below the bone surface, removal is usually unnecessary. These screws can be used with a bone graft to correct scaphoid angulation.

Regardless of the fixation device used, preoperative review and practice of the details of the procedure for the planned fixation are necessary. Careful intraoperative attention to the details of the procedure, the achievement of as near an anatomic reduction as possible, and precise placement of the fixation device are of utmost importance.

OPEN REDUCTION AND INTERNAL FIXATION OF ACUTE DISPLACED FRACTURES OF THE SCAPHOID— VOLAR APPROACH WITH ILIAC CREST BONE GRAFTING

TECHNIQUE 6.5

- With the patient supine and under preferably regional anesthesia, prepare the hand and wrist and inflate a pneumatic tourniquet.

- The volar approach usually gives the best exposure for scaphoid fractures at and distal to the waist. Make a longitudinal skin incision over the palmar surface of the wrist, beginning 3 to 4 cm proximal to the wrist flexion crease over the flexor carpi radialis.
- Extend the incision distally to the wrist flexion crease and angle it radially toward the scaphotrapezial and trapeziometacarpal joints in a hockey-stick configuration.
- Protect terminal branches of the palmar cutaneous branch of the median nerve and the superficial radial nerves.
- Reflect skin flaps at the level of the forearm fascia.
- Open the sheath of the flexor carpi radialis, retract the tendon ulnarly, and open the deep surface of its sheath.
- Expose the palmar capsule of the joint over the radioscaphoid joint.
- Extend the wrist in ulnar deviation and open the capsule in the longitudinal axis of the scaphoid bone, obliquely extending the incision toward the scaphotrapezial joint.
- With sharp dissection, expose the fracture, incise the long radiolunate and radioscaphocapitate ligaments, preserving each leaf of these capsuloligamentous structures for later repair. Inspect the fracture to determine the need for bone grafting.
- If comminution is absent or minimal, reduction and fixation suffice. If comminution is extensive, especially on the palmar surface, with a tendency to flexion of the scaphoid at the fracture, obtain an iliac crest bone graft. (See Techniques 6.14 through 6.17 and Fig. 6.40.)
- Kirschner wires placed in the distal and proximal poles as toggle levers ("joysticks") help to manipulate the fragments.
- Reduce the fracture and fix it with Kirschner wires or a screw technique (e.g., cannulated screws), avoiding rotation or angulation. If a cannulated device is used, ensure that the guidewire is centered in the proximal and distal poles. Image intensification with C-arm fluoroscopy is helpful for this step.
- For fractures through the waist and in the distal pole, insert the fixation device through a distal entry point. Create the distal entry point by opening the scaphotrapezial joint with a longitudinal capsular incision.
- Remove a portion of the trapezium with a rongeur to allow placement of the guidewire from distal to proximal to better place the wire in a more center-center position.
- Insert the screw until the trailing end (head) is flush with subchondral bone, countersunk beneath the articular cartilage.
- Placement of Kirschner wires down the long axis of the scaphoid is made easier by gentle radial deviation of the wrist, aligning the scaphoid vertically and placing a towel bump at the dorsal wrist flexion crease. Fingertrap traction on the thumb and index finger also can be helpful. With the wrist in this position, direct the wires almost dorsally into the scaphoid.
- After stable reduction and fixation are obtained, check the position and alignment of the reduction and the placement of the internal fixation with image intensification or radiographs.
- Deflate the tourniquet and obtain hemostasis.
- Close the wrist capsule with nonabsorbable sutures or long-lasting absorbable sutures.
- Close the skin and apply a dressing that includes either a thumb spica splint or thumb spica cast.

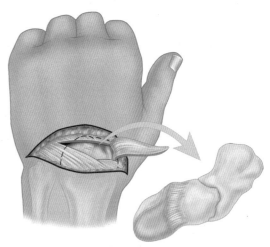

FIGURE 6.24   Dorsal approach to wrist. Transverse incision of skin. Radial-based capsular flap between dorsal radiotriquetral and dorsal intercarpal ligaments (enlargement shows proximal one third fracture of scaphoid). **SEE TECHNIQUE 6.6.**

OPEN REDUCTION AND INTERNAL FIXATION OF ACUTE DISPLACED FRACTURES OF THE SCAPHOID—DORSAL APPROACH

TECHNIQUE 6.6

- For noncomminuted fractures in the proximal pole of the scaphoid, exposure of the fracture site and placement of internal fixation can be done through a dorsal approach.
- Make a dorsal transverse incision 5 to 10 mm distal to the radiocarpal joint; localization with an image intensifier often is useful (Fig. 6.24). Protect the sensory branches of the radial and ulnar nerves. Preserve, cauterize, or ligate and divide dorsal veins.
- Extend the skin incision from the radial styloid to the ulnar styloid.
- Make parallel incisions in the extensor retinaculum on each side of the extensor digitorum communis tendons. Protect the extensor tendons, especially the extensor pollicis longus tendon as it exits the third dorsal retinacula compartment. Connect the parallel incisions proximally to create a flap to allow access to the dorsal wrist capsule.
- Pass a loop of Penrose drain around the extensor tendons, and retract them ulnarly.
- Open the dorsal capsule by creating a radially based flap, incising along the dorsal intercarpal ligament and the dorsal radiotriquetral ligament.
- Retract the capsular flap radially and expose the fracture.
- Insert a Kirschner wire into the proximal fragment parallel to the central axis of the scaphoid. Use this wire as a toggle lever ("joystick") to manipulate the proximal fragment into a reduced position.
- When the fracture is reduced, pass the first wire across the fracture for temporary interfragmentary fixation. Insert an additional Kirschner wire, or screw fixation, as the fracture configuration permits.

- If a cannulated screw is used, center the guidewire in the proximal and distal poles, monitoring this placement with C-arm fluoroscopy.
- Determine the appropriate length of the screw to be used. Drill and tap the bone, according to the device being used, and insert the screw of appropriate length (often subtracting 4 mm from the initial length measured). Ensure that the guidewire or screw fixation is placed in the center of the long axis of the proximal and distal poles of the scaphoid, using C-arm fluoroscopy. Either leave the initial Kirschner wire as supplemental fixation, or remove it if screw fixation has been selected.
- Close the capsular flap and repair the retinacula flap.
- Close the skin and apply a thumb spica cast or splint. See also Video 6.1.

POSTOPERATIVE CARE The sutures are removed, and the splint or cast is changed at 2 weeks. Some authors advocate transitioning directly to a removable splint once sutures are removed, whereas others recommend an additional 2 to 4 weeks of short arm thumb spica cast immobilization. As healing progresses as shown by radiographic examination, a short arm thumb spica brace is worn until bone healing is ensured. If healing cannot be determined with certainty, CT oriented in the longitudinal axis of the scaphoid with 1-mm cuts can be helpful to evaluate for bridging trabeculae. Finger, thumb, and shoulder motion is encouraged throughout convalescence, and, after cast removal, wrist motion and elbow motion are increased gradually, followed by strengthening exercises.

OPEN REDUCTION AND INTERNAL FIXATION OF ACUTE DISPLACED FRACTURES OF THE SCAPHOID— VOLAR APPROACH WITH DISTAL RADIAL AUTOGRAFT

TECHNIQUE 6.7

- Make a straight incision in the distal forearm between the distal portion of the flexor carpi radialis and the radial artery. Carry the incision across the distal wrist crease using a hockey-stick incision that angles toward the base of the thumb (Fig. 6.25A).
- Open the flexor carpi radialis tendon sheath and subsheath and retract it ulnarly, developing the interval between the flexor carpi radialis ulnarly and the radial artery radially.
- Enter the wrist capsule through a longitudinal incision from the volar lip of the radius to the proximal tubercle of the trapezium (Fig. 6.25B). Carefully divide the capsule and intracapsular ligament and reflect them sharply off the scaphoid with a scalpel. Take care to preserve the

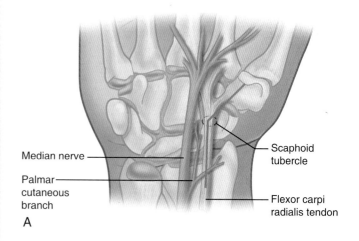

A

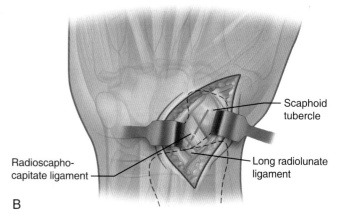

B

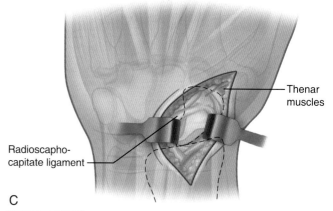

C

FIGURE 6.25 **A,** "Hockey-stick" incision for volar approach for open reduction and internal fixation of acute displaced scaphoid fractures. **B,** Longitudinal capsular incision. **C,** Approach to scapho-trapezial joint for placement of guidewire. **SEE TECHNIQUE 6.7**

capsule because it contains the radioscaphoid capitate ligament and will be repaired at the end of the procedure.
- Expose the entire volar scaphoid. Reduce the fracture with manipulation or joysticks and insert Kirschner wires for provisional fixation.
- If bone grafting is required for volar comminution or a subacute fracture, harvest grafts from the volar radius beneath the pronator quadratus by extending the incision

an additional 2 to 3 cm proximally or make a separate incision dorsally and just proximal to Lister's tubercle where cancellous autograft can be obtained through a cortical window.

- Open the scaphotrapezial joint and place a central guidewire in preparation for final fixation (Fig. 6.25C). If necessary, excise a small amount of the proximal trapezium with a rongeur to clear an unobstructed path for the implant.
- Obtain rigid internal fixation with the implant of choice (see Technique 6.6).

POSTOPERATIVE CARE Postoperative care is as described for Technique 6.6.

PERCUTANEOUS FIXATION OF SCAPHOID FRACTURES

TECHNIQUE 6.8

(SLADE ET AL.)
- Slade et al. recommended the following equipment for this technique: (1) headless cannulated compression screw (standard Acutrak screw), (2) minifluoroscopy unit, (3) Kirschner wires, and (4) equipment for small joint arthroscopy.
- If arthroscopy is to be used to check the fracture reduction and to place internal fixation, have the operating room prepared for wrist arthroscopy.
- Position the patient supine, with the upper extremity extended.
- After the induction of appropriate anesthesia and sterile preparation and draping procedures, flex the elbow 90 degrees.
- Use a C-arm fluoroscopic unit or mini C-arm fluoroscope to evaluate the fracture position and alignment and to determine if there are other bone or ligament injuries.
- Use a skin marking pen to indicate the best surface location for a dorsal skin incision and entry of the guidewire, drills, and screw.
- "Target" the scaphoid by locating the central axis of the scaphoid on the posteroanterior view of the reduced scaphoid (Fig. 6.26A).
- Gently pronate and flex the wrist until the proximal and distal poles of the scaphoid are aligned and confirmed with fluoroscopy. When the poles are aligned, the scaphoid has a "ring" appearance on the fluoroscopic monitor (Fig. 6.26B and C). The center of the "ring" circle is the central axis of the scaphoid, the best location for screw placement (Fig. 6.27).
- For ease of insertion, make a skin incision at the previously marked location to allow blunt dissection to the capsule of the wrist joint.
- With a double-point 0.045-inch (1.14-mm) Kirschner wire in a powered wire driver, insert the wire starting in the proximal pole of the scaphoid under fluoroscopic control.
- If there is uncertainty about wire placement, make the previously mentioned incision distal and medial (ulnar)

to the Lister tubercle, opening the dorsal wrist capsule lateral (radial) to the scapholunate interval, exposing the proximal pole of the scaphoid.
- Pass the guidewire from dorsally down the central axis of the scaphoid and out through the trapezium (Fig. 6.28A,B). Use a 12-gauge angiocatheter to assist with positioning of the guidewire. Keep the wrist flexed to avoid bending the guidewire.
- Advance the wire through the distal pole out the palmar surface. Check the position of the wire with the fluoroscope.
- Reverse the wire driver to pull the wire far enough distally to allow the dorsal, trailing end of the wire to clear the radiocarpal joint dorsally and to allow full wrist extension.
- With C-arm fluoroscopy, confirm scaphoid fracture alignment and correct positioning of the guidewire (Fig. 6.28C).
- If a correct path cannot be created with the 0.045-inch wire, use a 0.062-inch (1.57-mm) wire to create the correct path. Exchange the larger wire for the 0.045-inch wire before drilling the scaphoid.
- Check for wire position and fracture alignment with the fluoroscope. If the fracture reduction is unsatisfactory, and for displaced fractures, place a 0.062-inch Kirschner wire into each fracture fragment, perpendicular to the axis of the scaphoid, as toggle levers ("joysticks") to manipulate the fracture fragments (Fig. 6.29). If needed, place the proximal lever wire in the lunate.
- With the wire driver on the distal end of the guidewire, withdraw the wire distally across the fracture site, leaving the wire in the central axis of the distal fragment.
- Align the fracture fragments with the "joysticks."
- Pass the guidewire from distal to proximal across the fracture site to hold the reduction.
- If needed for stability and rotational control, insert another 0.045-inch wire, entering the proximal pole of the scaphoid, from dorsal to palmar, parallel to the first guidewire to control rotation. Leave the wire levers and the antirotational wire in place during screw insertion.
- Confirm the reduction and wire placement with fluoroscopy.
- If the fracture is difficult to reduce, percutaneously insert a small curved hemostat to assist with the reduction.
- If the fracture cannot be reduced, or if the guidewire cannot be properly placed, abandon the percutaneous technique and open the fracture, using either the volar or the dorsal approach (see Techniques 6.5 and 6.6).
- Determine the scaphoid length using two wires. To determine the scaphoid length, adjust the guidewire position so that the distal end is against the distal cortex of the scaphoid. Place a second wire of the same length as the guidewire parallel to the guidewire so the tip of the second wire is against the cortex of the proximal scaphoid pole. The difference in length is the length of the scaphoid (Fig. 6.30).
- To allow for countersinking the screw fully within the scaphoid, select a screw length that is 4 mm shorter than the scaphoid length.
- Determine dorsal or palmar insertion of the screw depending on the fracture location. For fractures of the proximal pole, insert the screw dorsally. For fractures of the waist, insert the screw from either the dorsal or the volar side. For fractures of the distal pole, insert the screw from the volar side.

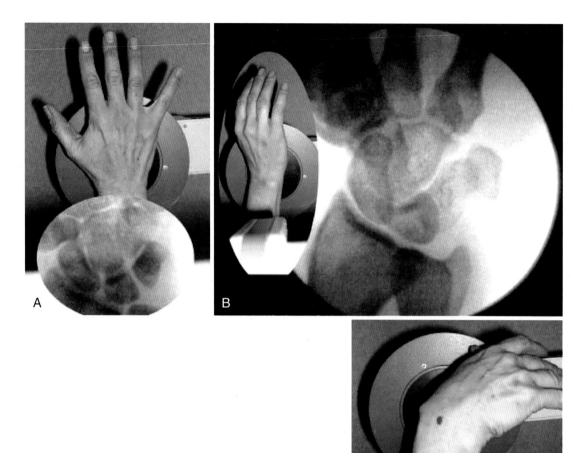

FIGURE 6.26 Percutaneous fixation of scaphoid fracture. **A,** Central axis of scaphoid is located on posteroanterior view. **B,** Wrist is pronated until scaphoid poles are aligned. **C,** Wrist is flexed until scaphoid has "ring" appearance on fluoroscopy. (From Slade JF III, Gutow AP, Geissler WB: Percutaneous internal fixation of scaphoid fractures via an arthroscopically assisted dorsal approach, *J Bone Joint Surg* 84A[Suppl 2]:21, 2002.) **SEE TECHNIQUE 6.8.**

- Drill the screw channel 2 mm short of the opposite scaphoid cortex, using a cannulated hand drill, always avoiding contact with the opposite cortex (Fig. 6.31).
- Check the position and depth of the drill with fluoroscopy.
- Use a standard Acutrak screw, 4 mm shorter than the scaphoid length. Advance the screw, monitoring with fluoroscopy, until the screw is within 1 to 2 mm of the opposite cortex (Fig. 6.32A).
- Verify fracture reduction and screw placement with final fluoroscopic images (Fig. 6.32B and C).
- If ligament injury or other carpal injuries are suspected, add arthroscopic examination to the fracture management.
- Apply longitudinal traction through the fingers.
- Locate the midcarpal and radiocarpal portals with fluoroscopy.
- Insert the arthroscope into the radial midcarpal portal to inspect the fracture reduction.
- Remove clot and synovium with the full radius shaver.
- Examine the scapholunate and lunotriquetral ligaments.

- Inspect the proximal pole through the 3-4 portal to confirm countersinking of the screw into the proximal pole.
- If ligament tears are encountered, treat them with debridement, intercarpal pinning, or open dorsal ligament repair.

POSTOPERATIVE CARE (MODIFIED) Apply a postoperative splint, depending on the extent of soft-tissue injury. If no ligament injury is present, apply a thumb spica splint. If there is ligament injury, apply a sugar-tong thumb spica splint of the Munster type, extending above the elbow. For fracture management, remove skin sutures at about 2 weeks and change the splint to a short arm thumb spica cast. Remove any remaining pins at 6 to 8 weeks. Continue with casting or removable thumb spica splinting until radiographic healing has occurred, changing the cast monthly. CT can help in determining if bridging trabeculae are present. After healing has occurred, begin a therapist-supervised rehabilitation program.

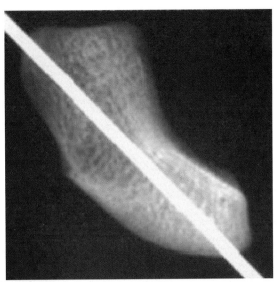

FIGURE 6.27 Percutaneous fixation of scaphoid fracture. Guidewire in central axis of scaphoid for placement of screw. (From Slade JF III, Gutow AP, Geissler WB: Percutaneous internal fixation of scaphoid fractures via an arthroscopically assisted dorsal approach, *J Bone Joint Surg* 84A[Suppl 2]:21, 2002.) **SEE TECHNIQUE 6.8.**

NONUNION OF SCAPHOID FRACTURES

Nonunion of scaphoid fractures is influenced by delayed diagnosis, gross displacement, associated injuries of the carpus, and impaired blood supply. Of these fractures, an estimated 40% are undiagnosed at the time of the original injury. Displaced scaphoid fractures have been suggested to have a nonunion rate of 92%. The incidence of osteonecrosis is approximately 30% to 40%, occurring most frequently in fractures of the proximal third.

Cystic changes in the scaphoid and the adjoining bones followed by osteonecrosis can occur after untreated fractures, but this is not an absolute indication for surgery. Nonunion is expected more often if the scaphoid fracture is untreated for 4 or more weeks. Delayed treatment can result in a nonunion rate of 88%.

Treatment options for nonunions of proximal pole fractures depend on the blood supply to the proximal pole and the size of the fragments. Nonunions involving the proximal third or more can be treated with nonvascularized bone grafts if circulation is satisfactory as determined by preoperative gadolinium-enhanced MRI and by intraoperative assessment of bone bleeding. Vascularized bone grafts are indicated when circulation to the proximal pole is poor. For very small, avascular, ununited fragments, the proximal pole can be excised if the scapholunate ligament integrity is still intact.

Electrical and ultrasound stimulation methods have been found to be of variable effectiveness for the treatment of scaphoid nonunions. Reports suggest that bone grafting should be considered a better option than pulsed electromagnetic field treatment of scaphoid nonunions. There is no conclusive information at this time to recommend the use of low-intensity ultrasound for scaphoid nonunions. More information is needed to define further the place of these technologies in the treatment of nonunions and acute fractures.

Many nonunions of the scaphoid have minimal symptoms and can be tolerated well by patients with sedentary occupations. Patients should be informed that some degenerative arthritis of the wrist probably is inevitable, but this can take years to develop, depending on the amount of chronic stress applied and the activity of the wrist. Radiographic findings of arthritis usually seen with scaphoid nonunion include radioscaphoid narrowing, capitolunate narrowing, cyst formation, and pronounced dorsal intercalated segment instability. This is the so-called scaphoid nonunion advanced collapse pattern (Fig. 6.33). The radiolunate joint usually is spared in early stages but may show degenerative changes as the arthritis becomes more diffuse. Jupiter et al. observed that ununited fractures of the scaphoid fall into three groups, depending on the extent of arthrosis: established nonunions without arthrosis, nonunions with radiocarpal arthrosis, and nonunions with advanced radiocarpal and intercarpal arthrosis. Although bone healing is needed for nonunions without arthrosis, additional procedures, including salvage operations, may be required for patients with more extensive arthrosis. Some nondisplaced scaphoid nonunions may heal after rigid internal fixation without bone grafting. Knoll and Trumble proposed a protocol for scaphoid nonunion treatment, including the consideration of osteonecrosis (Fig. 6.34). In old fractures with arthritis, symptoms can be decreased by excision of the radial styloid just proximal to the fracture in middle-third fractures; however, other reconstructive surgery, especially for severe arthritic degeneration, may be indicated, and proximal row carpectomy or arthrodesis of the wrist joint may prove to be more dependable. The following operations can be useful for nonunions of the scaphoid: (1) traditional bone grafting, (2) vascularized bone grafting, (3) excision of the proximal fragment, the distal fragment, and, occasionally, the entire scaphoid, (4) radial styloidectomy, (5) proximal row carpectomy, and (6) partial or total arthrodesis of the wrist.

Preiser disease (osteonecrosis of the scaphoid) usually manifests as wrist pain. Plain radiographs, MRI, and CT may help in assessing the circulation to the scaphoid and the extent of fragmentation. If symptoms and disability are not relieved with nonoperative methods, revascularization techniques similar to those used for Kienböck disease may preserve the scaphoid architecture. If there is significant scaphoid collapse or radioscaphoid arthrosis, scaphoid excision combined with capitate-lunate-triquetrum-hamate fusion or with proximal row carpectomy may be required.

STYLOIDECTOMY

Styloidectomy alone probably is of little value in treating nonunions of the scaphoid. If arthritic changes involve only the scaphoid fossa of the radiocarpal joint, however, styloidectomy is indicated in conjunction with any grafting of the scaphoid or excision of its ulnar fragment.

In older patients in whom radioscaphoid arthritis predominates, and the proximal fragment is not loose, styloidectomy alone can provide pain relief. A study of the amount of styloid to be resected found that ulnar and palmar displacement of the carpus increased significantly with resections of more than 4 mm of the radial styloid. Current recommendations are to resect no more than 4 mm of the styloid to preserve the radioscaphocapitate ligament integrity.

EXCISION OF THE PROXIMAL FRAGMENT

Excising both fragments of the scaphoid as the only procedure is unwise; although the immediate result may be satisfactory,

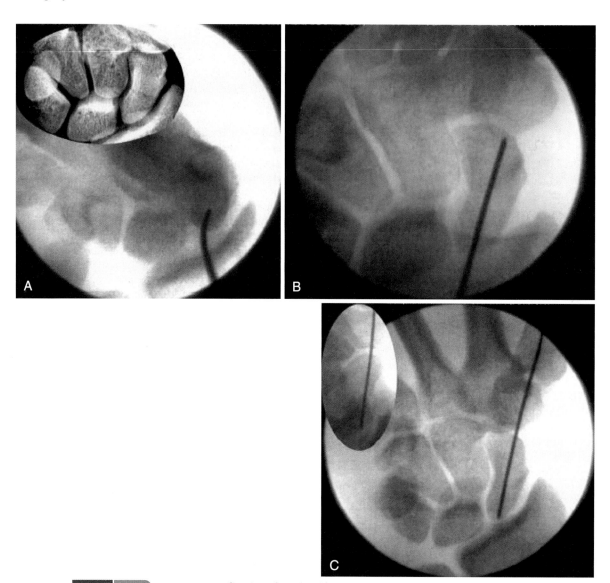

FIGURE 6.28   Percutaneous fixation of scaphoid fracture. **A** and **B,** Guidewire is placed at base of proximal pole of scaphoid **(A)** and driven along central axis **(B)**. **C,** Wrist is extended, and fracture alignment and guidewire position are confirmed with fluoroscopy. (From Slade JF III, Gutow AP, Geissler WB: Percutaneous internal fixation of scaphoid fractures via an arthroscopically assisted dorsal approach, *J Bone Joint Surg* 84A[Suppl 2]:21, 2002.) **SEE TECHNIQUE 6.8.**

eventual derangement of the wrist is likely. Soto-Hall and Haldeman reported gradual migration of the capitate into the space previously occupied by the scaphoid, although disability was not apparent for 5 to 7 years. If excision of both fragments is considered, it is preferable to add some other procedure to stabilize the capitolunate joint (e.g., capitolunate or capital-lunate-triquetral-hamate fusions).

When indicated, excising the proximal scaphoid fragment usually is satisfactory; the loss of one fourth or less of the scaphoid usually causes minimal impairment of wrist motion. Because postoperative immobilization is brief, function usually returns rapidly. Strength in the wrist usually is decreased to some extent. The following are indications for excising the proximal fragment of a scaphoid nonunion:

1.   The fragment is one fourth or less of the scaphoid. Regardless of its viability, grafting of such a small fragment frequently fails.

2.   The fragment is one fourth or less of the scaphoid and is sclerotic, comminuted, or severely displaced. The comminuted fragments usually should be excised early to prevent arthritic changes; a severely displaced fragment also should be excised early if it cannot be accurately replaced by manipulation. In the past, Silastic implants have been used to act as "space fillers." Because of the possibility of silicone synovitis, we prefer to leave the space empty or we use a folded or rolled tendon graft to fill the defect.

3.   The fragment is one fourth or less of the scaphoid, and grafting has failed. If a nonviable proximal fragment consists of more than one fourth of the scaphoid, some other treatment is preferable to excision alone.

4.   Arthritic changes are present in the region of the radial styloid. Styloidectomy is indicated in conjunction with excision of the proximal fragment.

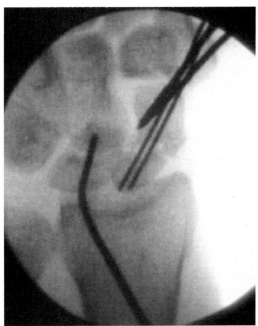

FIGURE 6.29 Percutaneous fixation of scaphoid fracture. Fracture reduction with two 0.062-inch Kirschner wires used as "joysticks" to manipulate fracture fragments. (From Slade JF III, Gutow AP, Geissler WB: Percutaneous internal fixation of scaphoid fractures via an arthroscopically assisted dorsal approach, *J Bone Joint Surg* 84A[Suppl 2]:21, 2002.) **SEE TECHNIQUE 6.8.**

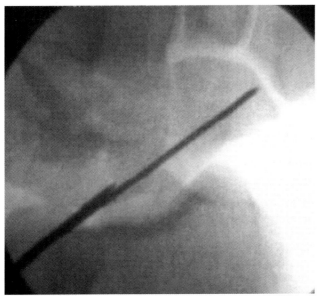

FIGURE 6.30 Percutaneous fixation of scaphoid fracture. Scaphoid length is determined. (From Slade JF III, Gutow AP, Geissler WB: Percutaneous internal fixation of scaphoid fractures via an arthroscopically assisted dorsal approach, *J Bone Joint Surg* 84A[Suppl 2]:21, 2002.) **SEE TECHNIQUE 6.8.**

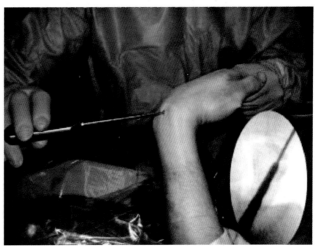

FIGURE 6.31 Percutaneous fixation of scaphoid fracture. Screw channel is created with cannulated hand drill and confirmed with fluoroscopy. (From Slade JF III, Gutow AP, Geissler WB: Percutaneous internal fixation of scaphoid fractures via an arthroscopically assisted dorsal approach, *J Bone Joint Surg* 84A[Suppl 2]:21, 2002.) **SEE TECHNIQUE 6.8.**

EXCISION OF THE PROXIMAL FRAGMENT

TECHNIQUE 6.9

- At the level of the styloid process of the radius, make a transverse skin incision 5 cm long on the dorsoradial aspect of the wrist, centered over the scaphoid.
- Protect the superficial radial nerve and its terminal branches.
- Release the radial side of the extensor retinaculum with a longitudinal incision along the radial border of the first dorsal compartment.
- Reflect the flap medially toward the second and third compartments.
- Protect and retract the tendons of the thumb abductors in a palmar direction and the tendon of the extensor pollicis longus in a dorsal and ulnar direction.
- Create a radially based triangular flap of dorsal capsule, incising along the distal border of the dorsal radiotriquetral and dorsal intercarpal ligaments to expose the scaphoid.
- To avoid excising a normal carpal bone, place a Kirschner wire in the proximal fragment of the scaphoid and identify the fragment in an anteroposterior radiograph.
- Grasp the fragment to be excised with a towel clip, apply traction, and remove the fragment by dividing its soft-tissue attachments.
- As an alternative, remove the proximal pole with a rongeur.
- If it seems that there is sufficient laxity in the wrist to allow the capitate to migrate into the defect left by proximal pole excision, proceed to a scaphocapitate fusion (see Technique 6.50).

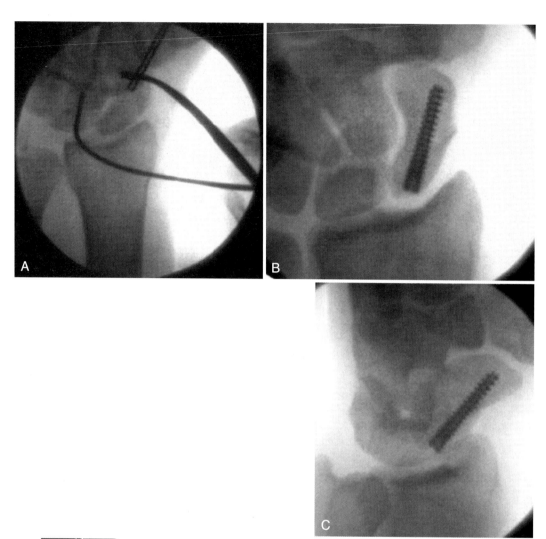

FIGURE 6.32 Percutaneous fixation of scaphoid fracture. **A,** Joysticks and antiglide wires are maintained during drilling and dorsal implantation of screw. **B** and **C,** Fluoroscopy confirms placement of headless compression screw. (From Slade JF III, Gutow AP, Geissler WB: Percutaneous internal fixation of scaphoid fractures via an arthroscopically assisted dorsal approach, *J Bone Joint Surg* 84A[Suppl 2]:21, 2002.) **SEE TECHNIQUE 6.8.**

- Close the capsular flap and repair the retinaculum with absorbable sutures.
- Close the skin and apply an anterior splint, extending from the palm to the elbow.

POSTOPERATIVE CARE The wrist is immobilized in the postoperative splint for 2 weeks. Sutures are removed at 10 to 14 days. A removable splint is used while the patient transitions to a program of active exercises, which is continued until satisfactory function is restored. If a limited intercarpal arthrodesis has been done, the postoperative care is the same as that described after Technique 6.51.

EXCISION OF THE DISTAL SCAPHOID

Satisfactory results have been reported with distal scaphoid resection for the treatment of scaphoid nonunions with radioscaphoid arthritis treated with distal scaphoid resection.

If capitolunate arthritis is present, an additional procedure (e.g., limited intercarpal arthrodesis) should be added to distal scaphoid excision. The technique and the postoperative care are similar to those described earlier for proximal pole excision.

PROXIMAL ROW CARPECTOMY

Proximal row carpectomy is used as a reconstructive procedure for posttraumatic degenerative conditions in the wrist, especially conditions involving the scaphoid and lunate. Reports support its use as an alternative to arthrodesis. Reports comparing proximal row carpectomy with limited intercarpal fusion confirmed that satisfactory relief of pain and preservation of motion and strength can be achieved. It is considered to be a satisfactory procedure in patients who have limited requirements, desire some wrist mobility, and accept the possibility of minimal persistent pain (Fig. 6.35). If a proximal row carpectomy fails to meet the patient's needs, arthrodesis remains an option. Manual laborers usually are better candidates for a wrist arthrodesis. Chen et al. also found that posterior and anterior interosseous neurectomy reduced the risk for reoperation and lessened the rate of conversion to wrist fusion after proximal row carpectomy.

When proximal row carpectomy is done for degenerative changes, healthy articular surfaces should be present in the lunate fossa of the radius and the proximal articular surface of the capitate to allow for satisfactory articulation between these surfaces. Arthrosis at the capitolunate joint does not *absolutely* contraindicate proximal row carpectomy because the proximal pole of the capitate can be excised and covered with a dorsal capsular flap with satisfactory function. If significant degenerative changes on these articular surfaces can be seen radiographically or by direct vision at the time of procedure, consideration should be given to an alternative procedure, such as arthrodesis. Primary proximal row carpectomy can be useful in treating severe open carpal fracture-dislocations characterized by significant disruption of

the bony architecture, comminuted fractures of the scaphoid and lunate, and disruption of the blood supply to the lunate and scaphoid.

Excision of the triquetrum, lunate, and entire scaphoid usually is recommended. The distal pole of the scaphoid at its articulation with the trapezium can be left, however, to provide a more stable base for the thumb. If the distal scaphoid pole is left, radial styloidectomy should be done to avoid impingement of the distal scaphoid pole and trapezium on the radial styloid. When a radial styloidectomy is done during proximal row carpectomy, care should be taken to avoid injury to the volar radioscaphocapitate ligament. Excision of the pisiform is unnecessary because of its location in the flexor carpi ulnaris tendon as a sesamoid. The bones usually are removed piecemeal; threaded Kirschner wires or screws used as "joysticks" or handles are helpful to lever the bone out at the wrist.

Proximal row carpectomy traditionally is reserved for patients over 35 to 40 years of age, and four-corner fusion is indicated for younger patients and those involved in heavy labor. Wagner et al., however, compared proximal row carpectomy and four-corner fusions in patients under the age of 45 with satisfactory results with both procedures at a mean follow-up of 11 years. They found no differences in patient-rated wrist evaluation scores (27 for proximal row carpectomy compared to 28 for four-corner fusion). Those with proximal row carpectomy had more range of motion and fewer complications, while those with four-corner fusion had better grip strength (65%) and DASH scores (19 for four-corner fusion compared to 32 for proximal row carpectomy) compared to proximal row carpectomy (54%).

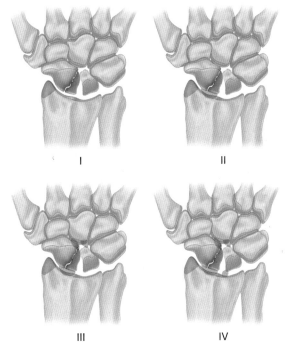

FIGURE 6.33 Stages of scaphoid nonunion advanced collapse. Stage I, arthritis at radial styloid. Stage II, scaphoid fossa arthritis. Stage III, capitolunate arthritis. Stage IV, diffuse arthritis of carpus.

PROXIMAL ROW CARPECTOMY

TECHNIQUE 6.10

- Make a longitudinal incision on the dorsum of the wrist in line with the third metacarpal. Longitudinal incisions are preferred because of the potential for future wrist fusion procedures.
- Deepen the incision to the extensor retinaculum, preserving the sensory branches of the radial and ulnar nerves.

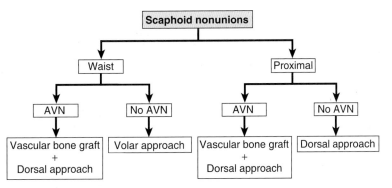

FIGURE 6.34 Algorithm for treatment of scaphoid nonunion developed by Knoll and Trumble. *AVN*, Avascular necrosis (osteonecrosis).

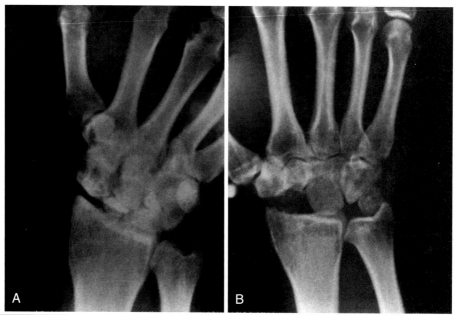

FIGURE 6.35   **A,** Long-standing scaphoid nonunion with arthritis, osteonecrosis, collapse of proximal pole, and settling of capitate into proximal row. **B,** After proximal row carpectomy with radial styloidectomy.

- Ligate and divide the superficial veins.
- Open the extensor retinaculum in a Z-shaped fashion to help facilitate closure; consider transposing the extensor pollicis longus tendon radially.
- Expose the dorsum of the proximal row of carpal bones through two longitudinal incisions in the capsule, one in the interval between the extensor digitorum communis tendons and the extensor carpi ulnaris and one between the extensor carpi radialis brevis tendon and the extensor digitorum communis.
- If the capitate articular surface shows erosion, fashion a capsular flap, based distally, by connecting the parallel capsular incisions with a transverse incision, proximally, near the dorsum of the distal radial articular surface.
- Expose the lunate by elevating the capsule of the wrist beneath the extensor digitorum communis tendons; insert a threaded pin into the lunate, apply traction to the bone through the pin, and excise the bone by dividing its capsular attachments with a scalpel. A small, angled cleft palate blade also is helpful.
- Insert the pin into the triquetrum and excise it in a similar manner (Fig. 6.36B). (The lunate and triquetrum are excised first to provide more space for the more difficult excision of the scaphoid.)
- Carefully fragment the scaphoid with a small bone cutter, osteotome, or saw to facilitate removal (Fig. 6.36A). A burr also can be helpful in removing the distal pole of the scaphoid.
- Align the capitate with the lunate fossa. Use a Steinmann pin to stabilize the capitate if needed. If the palmar radiocapitate ligament is preserved, this may be unnecessary.
- If the capitate head shows significant signs of degenerative changes, consider interposing the capsular flap between the capitate head and lunate fossa. Secure the proximal aspect of the flap to the volar lip of the distal ra-

dius with small bone anchors. Additionally, the technique of using a dermal allograft anchored to the degenerative capitate head or lunate fossa has been described.
- Obtain hemostasis or drain the wound as needed and close the wound in layers.
- Apply a sugar-tong splint with the hand and wrist in a functional position.

POSTOPERATIVE CARE   The wrist is immobilized in slight extension and with the hand in the functional position in a plaster short arm splint for 2 weeks. If a Steinmann pin has been used, it is removed at about 4 weeks. Active motion of the digits is encouraged soon after surgery and is continued throughout the convalescence. When the soft tissues have healed, active motion of the wrist is increased gradually, usually after 6 weeks of immobilization. Active exercises to strengthen grip are instituted 3 months postoperatively.

ARTHROSCOPIC PROXIMAL ROW CARPECTOMY

TECHNIQUE 6.11

(WEISS ET AL.)
- Carry out routine radiocarpal and midcarpal arthroscopic examinations (see Techniques 6.2 and 6.3), using the 3-4, 4-5, 6R, 6U, midcarpal radial, and midcarpal ulnar portals as needed.

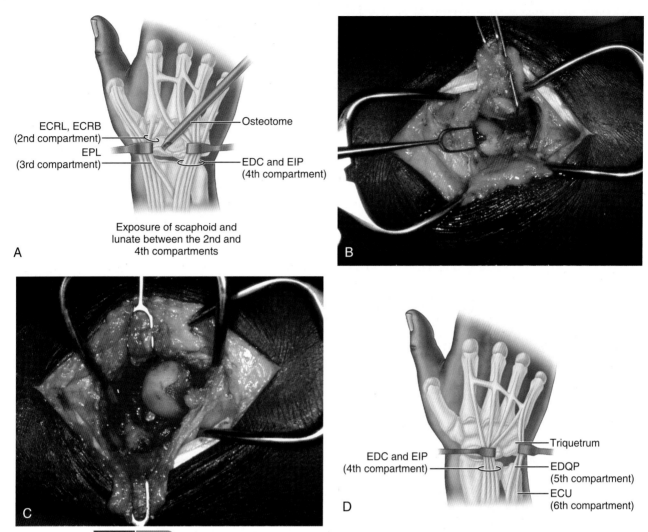

A

ECRL, ECRB (2nd compartment)
EPL (3rd compartment)
Osteotome
EDC and EIP (4th compartment)

Exposure of scaphoid and lunate between the 2nd and 4th compartments

B

C

D

EDC and EIP (4th compartment)
Triquetrum
EDQP (5th compartment)
ECU (6th compartment)

FIGURE 6.36 Proximal row carpectomy through dorsal approach. **A** and **B,** Exposure and morcellation of scaphoid and lunate between second and fourth dorsal compartments. **C** and **D,** Exposure of triquetrum between fourth and fifth extensor compartments for triquetrum excision. *ECRB,* Extensor carpi radialis brevis; *ECRL,* extensor carpi radialis longus; *ECU,* extensor carpi ulnaris; *EDC,* extensor digitorum communis; *EPL,* extensor pollicis longus; *EDQP,* extensor digiti quinti proprius; *EIP,* extensor indicis proprius. (From Calandruccio JH: Proximal row carpectomy, *J Am Soc Surg Hand* 1:112, 2001.) **SEE TECHNIQUE 6.10.**

- Introduce a small joint arthroscopic burr or shaver into the midcarpal joint through the midcarpal radial portal, with the scope in the midcarpal ulnar portal for viewing.
- Use the burr or shaver to decorticate the medial corner of the scaphoid at the midcarpal scapholunate joint. Take care not to injure the articular cartilage of the head of the capitate.
- Once an adequate portion of the corner of the scaphoid is removed, slightly enlarge the midcarpal radial portal with careful dissection, and introduce a 4.0-mm hooded burr into the midcarpal joint. Again, take care not to injure the articular cartilage of the head of the capitate.
- Remove the scaphoid from ulnar to radial and distal to proximal (Fig. 6.37A) through the scaphotrapezial trapezoid (STT) portal while viewing through the midcarpal radial portal.

- After scaphoid excision, place the arthroscope in the STT or midcarpal radial portal and a burr in an enlarged midcarpal radial or midcarpal ulnar portal and sequentially remove the lunate (distal to proximal) and triquetrum (distal to proximal) (Fig. 6.37B).
- Under arthroscopic vision, use a fine synovial rongeur to remove tiny fragments of bone or cartilage that remain adherent to the capsule.
- Confirm complete proximal row carpectomy with fluoroscopy.
- Release traction and use arthroscopy and fluoroscopy to confirm seating of the head of the capitate in the lunate fossa (Fig. 6.37C).
- If sufficient radiocarpal impaction is observed with radial deviation of the wrist, perform arthroscopic radial styloidectomy with the burr in the 1-2 portal and the arthroscope in the 3-4 portal.

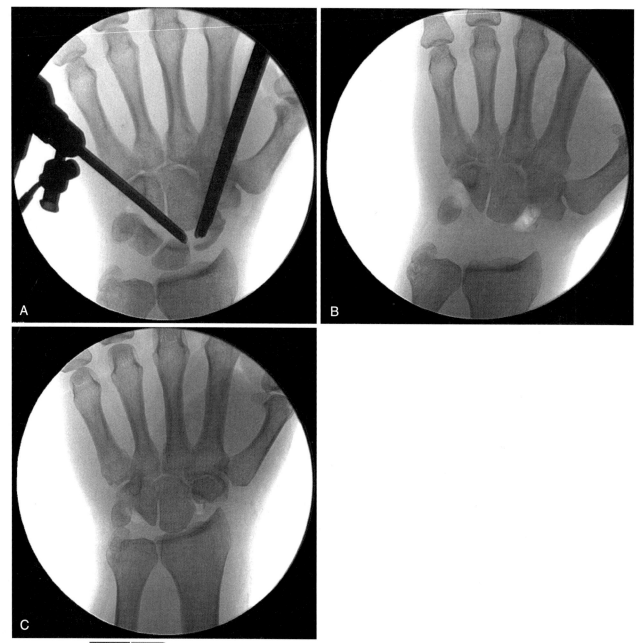

FIGURE 6.37 Arthroscopic proximal row carpectomy (see text). **A,** Initial removal of distal ulnar pole of scaphoid. **B,** Entire proximal row has been excised. **C,** After release of traction. (From Weiss ND, Molina RA, Gwin S: Arthroscopic proximal row carpectomy, *J Hand Surg* 36A:577, 2011.) **SEE TECHNIQUE 6.11.**

POSTOPERATIVE CARE A bulky dressing and volar splint are applied, and immediate finger range of motion is allowed. Two days after surgery, the bandage is removed and a removable volar splint is applied for comfort. Early active and passive range of motion of the wrist and fingers is encouraged, and return to activity is allowed within the limits of comfort. Formal physical therapy is prescribed on an individual basis as needed.

GRAFTING OPERATIONS

Cancellous bone grafting for scaphoid nonunion, as first described by Matti and modified by Russe, has proved to

be a reliable procedure, producing bony union in 80% to 97% of patients. Cohen et al. reported success with this technique even for scaphoid nonunions with "humpback deformity."

TECHNIQUE 6.12

(MATTI-RUSSE)

- With the patient supine and under general anesthesia, prepare the injured limb and prepare one iliac crest for possible bone graft harvest.
- Under pneumatic tourniquet control, make a longitudinal incision 3 to 4 cm long on the volar aspect of the wrist slightly to the radial side of the flexor carpi radialis tendon.

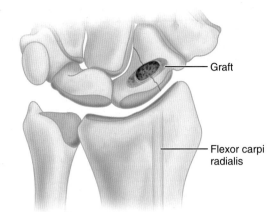

Graft

Flexor carpi radialis

FIGURE 6.38 Matti-Russe technique of bone grafting for nonunion of carpal scaphoid. **SEE TECHNIQUE 6.12.**

- Protect the palmar cutaneous branch of the median nerve and the terminal branches of the superficial radial nerve.
- Retract the flexor carpi radialis tendon ulnarward. Incise the wrist capsule, reflecting the radiocarpal ligaments as medial and lateral flaps to be repaired.
- Identify the scaphoid bone and expose the nonunion. It can be seen more clearly with dorsiflexion and ulnar deviation of the wrist.
- Freshen the sclerotic bone ends with a small gouge and form a cavity that extends well into each adjacent fragment. The cavity can be formed with a high-speed burr; however, thermal bone injury can occur. As an alternative, outline a rectangular trough with drill holes and connect the holes with a thin osteotome or a powered thin saw blade (Linscheid and Weber).
- From the iliac crest, obtain a piece of cancellous bone and shape it into a large lozenge-shaped peg to fit into the preformed cavity and stabilize the two fragments (Fig. 6.38). If a rectangular trough has been formed, shape the bone graft to fit the cancellous portion into the trough.
- Place multiple small bone chips around the peg. Use intraoperative C-arm fluoroscopy to verify filling of the cavity.
- Although the fragments can be stabilized by the corticocancellous bone graft, stability can be improved with a Kirschner wire inserted from distal to proximal across the fracture. Leave the wire either just beneath the skin or protruding from the palmar skin.
- After removing the tourniquet, suture the capsule and close the skin.
- Apply a sugar-tong splint with a thumb spica extension, from above the elbow to the palm with the wrist in neutral position.

POSTOPERATIVE CARE The sutures are removed at 10-14 days, and a new cast is applied. If a Kirschner wire is used, it is removed at 4 to 6 weeks. Casting is continued until radiographic healing, around the tenth to twelfth postoperative week.

MALPOSITIONED NONUNION OF SCAPHOID FRACTURES ("HUMPBACK" DEFORMITY)

Established nonunions of scaphoid fractures can be seen in preoperative radiographs to have resorption or comminution, with resulting shortening and angulation, with its convexity dorsal and radial ("humpback" deformity). Preoperative CT in the sagittal and coronal planes shows this deformity best when oriented in the longitudinal axis of the scaphoid. Correct orientation of the CT scan can be confirmed by viewing the orientation of the wrist on the scout images. The forearm is angled roughly 45 degrees relative to the frame of the image and scout cuts appear to traverse directly through the long axis of the scaphoid (Fig. 6.39). The deformity includes extension of the proximal pole of the scaphoid, resulting extension of the lunate, and a form of dorsal intercalated instability pattern seen on lateral plain radiographs. Fisk emphasized that interposition bone grafting allows restoration of length and correction of malalignment. Amadio et al. and Cooney et al. proposed anterior wedge grafting for angulation resulting in a scapholunate angle of more than 60 degrees or an intrascaphoid angle of more than 45 degrees. Modifications proposed by Fernandez emphasized careful preoperative planning, comparison radiographs of the uninjured side, the use of a bone graft fitted to the defect, and Kirschner wire fixation. Tomaino et al. treated persistent lunate extension after interposition grafting of the scaphoid by radiolunate pinning to stabilize the lunate in a neutral position before correcting the scaphoid "humpback" deformity. The cannulated Herbert-Whipple screw was found to be effective fixation. According to Manske, McCarthy, and Strecker, the double-threaded Herbert screw was most effective in nonunions with evidence of osteonecrosis, nonunions involving the proximal third, or nonunions having had previous failed bone grafts. Stark et al. recommended Kirschner wire fixation with an iliac bone graft for all nonunions because judging stability with bone grafting alone was difficult, and because the technique was technically easy and added little to the operating time. They achieved union in 97% of 151 old ununited fractures of the scaphoid. More recently, the use of two headless microscrews combined with bone grafting was reported to obtain a 100% union rate in 19 patients with scaphoid nonunions. Combining volar wedge grafting with Herbert screw fixation in 26 scaphoid nonunions, Daly et al. reported a union rate of 95%. Of the five methods he had used, Barton reported a 74% union rate, his best results, using the "wedge" graft and the Herbert screw. The meta-analysis of 1121 articles reported by Merrell, Wolfe, and Slade included 36 eligible reports indicating that grafting with screw fixation produced better healing rates (94% union) than Kirschner wires and wedge grafting (74%). Vascularized grafts provided a better union rate (88%) than wedge grafting and screw fixation (47%) in cases with osteonecrosis of the proximal pole.

GRAFTING OPERATIONS

TECHNIQUE 6.13

(FERNANDEZ)
- Preoperatively, calculate the amount of resection, size of graft, and angular deformity on tracing paper by using the radiographic findings of the uninjured wrist as a guide (Fig. 6.40).

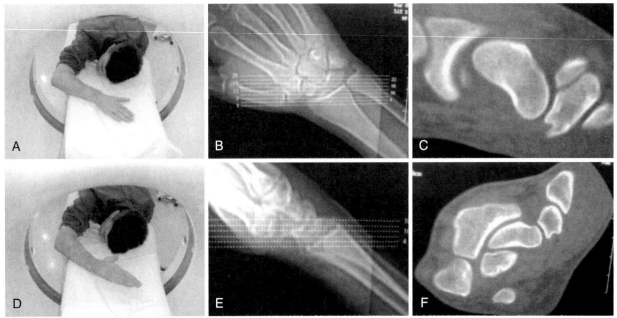

FIGURE 6.39   **A,** For sagittal plane images, forearm is held pronated and hand lies flat on table. Forearm crosses gantry at angle of approximately 45 degrees (roughly in line with abducted thumb metacarpal). **B,** Scout images are obtained to confirm appropriate orientation and to ensure that entire scaphoid is imaged. Sections are obtained at 1-mm intervals. **C,** Images obtained in sagittal plane are best for measuring intrascaphoid angle. **D,** For coronal plane images, forearm is in neutral rotation. **E,** Scout images show alignment of wrist through gantry of scanner. **F,** Interpretation of images obtained in coronal plane is straightforward. (Copyright 1999 by Jesse B. Jupiter, MD.)

- Approach the scaphoid between the flexor carpi radialis and the radial artery according to the classic Russe procedure.
- Incise the palmar capsule of the wrist longitudinally in line with the skin incision and extend it to the scaphoid tubercle for exposure of the nonunion, the proximal and distal fragments, and the scapholunate junction.
- Using an oscillating saw, carry out resection according to the preoperative plan.
- If signs of osteonecrosis of the proximal fragment are apparent, place multiple 1-mm drill holes within the sclerotic cancellous bone.
- Correct the flexion deformity and shortening by distracting the osteotomy site on the palmar-radial aspect with two small bone hooks or a spreader clamp. As this is done, have an assistant simultaneously correct the dorsal rotation of the lunate by pushing the palmar pole toward the radius with a fine bone spike.
- Shape the corticocancellous graft from the iliac crest to fit the defect with a saw, rongeur, or bone cutter. If considerable lengthening is necessary, the graft would need to be trapezoidal to bridge the defect that appears on the dorsal aspect of the navicular (see Fig. 6.40). Orient the graft so that its cortical part is palmar.
- After insertion of the graft, shape the protruding edges flush with the proximal and distal fragments.
- Use image intensification to control correction of lunate rotation.
- Fix the scaphoid with two or three 0.05-in (1.2-mm) Kirschner wires, which are power driven percutaneously into the palmar aspect of the distal fragment across the graft into the dorsal aspect of the proximal fragment (see Fig. 6.37). Use

image intensification to ensure correct placement of the internal fixation material.
- Carefully close the palmar capsule and cut the Kirschner wires short, 3 mm below the palmar skin of the thenar area.

POSTOPERATIVE CARE A palmar plaster splint that includes the thumb is applied for 2 weeks, at which time the sutures are removed. The wrist and thumb are immobilized in a short navicular cast for 6 weeks. Immobilization is discontinued after 8 weeks, and a palmar thermoplastic removable splint is applied with which the patient can perform active exercises of the wrist three times a day for 15 minutes. CT scans of the navicular are obtained at 12 weeks, and if bony union is confirmed, the internal fixation material is removed through a small incision under local anesthesia.

Defining union on CT scan is controversial. It has been defined as 50% to 75% bridging trabeculae. Sommerkamp et al. described a "cross-section trabeculation score" in scaphoid nonunions. This is calculated by estimating the percentage of cross-sectional trabecular bridging at the fracture site on a series of longitudinally oriented 1-mm CT scans along the scaphoid axis. This is done for both the coronal and sagittal planes, and the two percentages are averaged to provide an overall percentage or cross-section trabeculation score. The value of 50% scaphoid healing as being adequate is supported by a biomechanical model that showed the native failure strength of the scaphoid with cantilever bending applied was 610 N and the failure strength of the scaphoid with a compression screw and half of the scaphoid waist excised was 666 N.

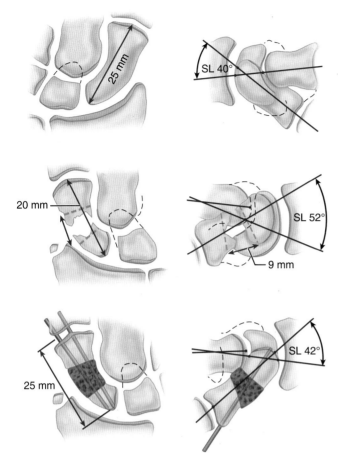

FIGURE 6.40 Preoperative planning. *Top,* Tracing of uninjured wrist and measurement of scaphoid length and scapholunate (SL) angle. *Middle,* Calculation of size of resection area and form of graft. *Bottom,* Definitive diagram of operation. **SEE TECHNIQUE 6.13.**

GRAFTING OPERATIONS

TECHNIQUE 6.14

(TOMAINO ET AL.)
- With the patient supine and under appropriate anesthesia, and after preparation of the skin and one iliac crest, exsanguinate the limb with an elastic wrap and inflate the pneumatic tourniquet.
- Make a palmar skin incision between the flexor carpi radialis and the radial artery, extending from about 2 cm proximal to the radial styloid to about 1 cm distal to the scaphoid tuberosity.
- Incise the palmar capsule and radioscaphocapitate ligament longitudinally in line with the skin incision. Extend the incision distally, exposing the proximal trapezium and the scaphotrapezial joint.
- Correct lunate extension by maximally flexing the wrist joint to derotate the extended lunate (Fig. 6.41A).
- Fix the lunate in the flexed position by percutaneously passing a 0.045-in (1.1-mm) Kirschner wire through the radius from its lateral surface into the lunate fossa

of the articular surface of the radius (Figs. 6.41A and 6.42A,B).
- Protect the superficial radial nerve during the wire passage.
- Use the C-arm fluoroscope to obtain a lateral image to ensure neutral alignment of the lunate (Fig. 6.42C).
- Supinate the forearm and maximally extend the wrist to open up the scaphoid nonunion site (Fig. 6.41B).
- Using a microsagittal saw or rongeur, resect the nonunion to viable bleeding bone proximally and distally.
- Measure the gap in the scaphoid (length, width, and depth) to determine the dimensions of the wedge graft.
- Distally, notch the trapezium with a rongeur to allow for placement of a cannulated screw (Herbert-Whipple).
- Obtain a tricortical corticocancellous graft from the iliac crest using a microsagittal saw, irrigating with saline to avoid thermal bone injury (Fig. 6.41C).
- Sculpt the graft to fit the defect.
- Gently impact the graft into place with the inner (cancellous) surface facing the capitate (Fig. 6.41D). Avoid prominence of the graft on the dorsal and ulnar surfaces.
- Pass a single 0.045-in (1.1-mm) Kirschner wire eccentrically down the long scaphoid axis to hold the scaphoid and graft in place.
- Remove the radiolunate wire to allow movement of the wrist to obtain satisfactory images of guidewire placement.
- Using C-arm fluoroscopic images, place the guidewire for the Herbert-Whipple screw. Ascertain with the fluoroscopic images that the guidewire is centrally placed.
- Insert a screw of appropriate length. Anticipate that it might be necessary to reduce the screw length 4 to 6 mm from the length obtained from the guidewire.
- Using the fluoroscope, ascertain central placement of the guidewire and screw.
- Use a small burr to remove prominent graft on the radial and volar surfaces.
- Assess wrist flexion and extension and radial and ulnar deviation to ensure that the graft is not impinging on the distal radius. If there is impingement, perform a limited radial styloidectomy.
- Repair the palmar capsule, the radioscaphocapitate ligament, and the sheath of the flexor carpi radialis.
- Deflate the pneumatic tourniquet, obtain hemostasis, and close the skin.
- Apply a short arm thumb spica splint.

POSTOPERATIVE CARE The splint and sutures are removed at 2 weeks. A removable short arm thumb spica splint is provided. Activities are limited and casting is continued until bone union has occurred, usually at 10 to 12 weeks.

GRAFTING OPERATIONS

TECHNIQUE 6.15

(STARK ET AL.)
- Expose the scaphoid through a straight or zigzag volar incision.

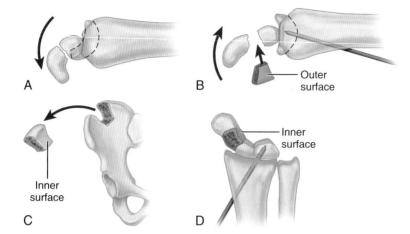

FIGURE 6.41 **A,** Lunate extension (dorsal intercalated segment instability deformity) accompanies scaphoid nonunion with humpback deformity because of carpal collapse. **B,** With wrist extension, radiolunate joint is pinned and scaphoid opens at nonunion site. Microsagittal saw is used to smooth ends of bone at nonunion. **C,** Tricortical iliac crest graft is harvested. **D,** Graft is pinned in place before insertion of Herbert-Whipple screw. Lunate transfixion pin is removed before screw placement to facilitate accurate imaging of scaphoid and guidewire. (Redrawn from Tomaino MM, King J, Pizillo M: Correction of lunate malalignment when bone grafting scaphoid nonunion with humpback deformity: rationale and results of a technique revisited, *J Hand Surg* 25A:322, 2000.) **SEE TECHNIQUE 6.14.**

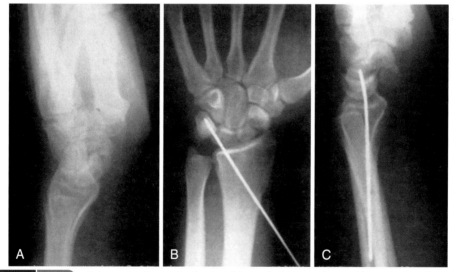

FIGURE 6.42 **A,** Lateral radiograph of wrist with scaphoid nonunion and humpback deformity shows lunate extension because of collapse. **B,** Posteroanterior radiograph shows Kirschner wire that has been placed percutaneously through radial side of radius into lunate after correcting lunate extension. **C,** Normal radiolunate angle has been restored. (From Tomaino MM, King J, Pizillo M: Correction of lunate malalignment when bone grafting scaphoid nonunion with humpback deformity: rationale and results of a technique revisited, *J Hand Surg* 25A:322, 2000.) **SEE TECHNIQUE 6.14.**

- After the wrist capsule is incised longitudinally and the wrist is dorsiflexed, both parts of the scaphoid and the articular surface of the radius can be seen readily.
- Remove a small, rectangular window of bone from the volar aspect of the distal fragment immediately adjacent to the fracture. Through this opening, clear fragments of fibrous tissue and dead bone using a low-speed power burr or curet.

- Fashion a large cavity in the proximal and distal parts of the scaphoid.
- Use a Chandler retractor to protect the articular cartilage of the radioscaphoid joint (Fig. 6.43A). It also helps to correct angulation, malrotation, and displacement of the fragments.
- The volar part of the cortex of the scaphoid often is deficient, and this deficiency permits an exaggerated volar

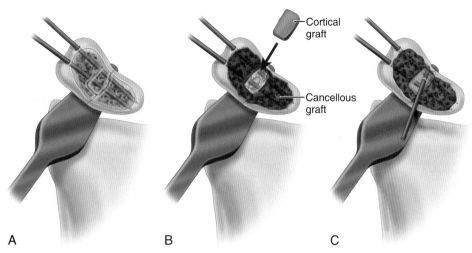

FIGURE 6.43   Technique for scaphoid nonunion (Stark et al.). **A,** Excavation of scaphoid and placement of Kirschner wires; Chandler retractor is used to protect articular cartilage of radioscaphoid joint. **B,** Cortical graft is inserted into cavity. **C,** Kirschner wire is inserted to stabilize bone graft. **SEE TECHNIQUE 6.15.**

tilt of the distal fragment, creating the "humpback" deformity of the scaphoid.

- Realignment and reduction of the fracture and restoration of the bone to the proper length are difficult parts of the procedure. Intraoperative radiographs usually are necessary.
- Transfix the scaphoid with two 0.035-inch (0.9-mm) Kirschner wires by inserting them through the distal fragment into the proximal one; protect the articular cartilages of the scaphoid and radius with the retractor. Observe correct placement of the wires through the volar window.
- Pack cancellous bone from the ilium into the cavity (Fig. 6.43B).
- The wires can be inserted after packing the cavity with bone, but it is easier to verify their location before inserting the graft.
- Often a cortical bone graft can be fashioned to fit snugly into the volar window; stabilize it with one additional 0.028-inch (0.7-mm) Kirschner wire (Fig. 6.43C).
- Cut the wires off beneath the skin.
- Approximate the capsule with absorbable sutures, close the skin, and immobilize the extremity in a long arm thumb spica splint with the forearm in supination, the wrist in neutral, and the thumb in abduction.

POSTOPERATIVE CARE The sutures are removed at 2 weeks, and a long arm thumb spica cast is applied and is worn for 6 additional weeks. The Kirschner wires are removed after the fracture has united. When immobilization is discontinued, patients are permitted to use the wrist and hand for light activities, but strenuous and forceful activity is discouraged for an additional 2 months.

VASCULARIZED BONE GRAFTS

The use of vascularized bone grafts has proved to be an effective method for treating scaphoid nonunions, especially nonunions with an avascular proximal pole and those that have failed to heal after previous procedures. Since Braun's 1983 report of success with a pronator quadratus pedicle graft from the distal radius, other sources of pedicle flaps from the distal radius and ulna and the metacarpals have been described, including an iliac crest free flap with microvascular techniques, a vascularized bone graft from the distal dorsolateral radius, and pedicle bone grafts based on the 1,2 intercompartmental supraretinacular artery. Although vascularized pedicle grafts are useful for promoting healing, the presence of established radiocarpal arthrosis may compromise the functional outcome. Additional studies have also shown success with the medial femoral condyle osteochondral free flap in scaphoid nonunions, with reported union rates of 89% at 16 weeks.

PRONATOR-BASED GRAFT

TECHNIQUE 6.16

(KAWAI AND YAMAMOTO)
- Make a volar zigzag incision over the scaphoid tuberosity and the distal radius to expose the site of nonunion.
- Divide the radioscaphocapitate ligament complex but retain it for later repair to the muscle pedicle.
- Excise the sclerotic bone ends and freshen them with a power burr to form an oval cavity 10 to 20 mm long and parallel to the axis of the scaphoid.
- Identify the pronator quadratus and outline a block of bone graft 15 to 20 mm long at its distal insertion on the distal radius close to the abductor pollicis longus tendon (Fig. 6.44). Outline the margin of the graft with Kirschner wire holes to facilitate separation with a fine osteotome.
- Ensure that the pronator quadratus is not detached from the harvested bone graft; dissect the muscle toward the ulna to secure a pedicle 20 mm thick. The anterior interosseous vessels need not be identified.

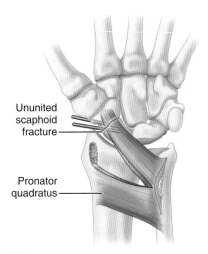

FIGURE 6.44 Pronator quadratus pedicle bone graft for scaphoid nonunion. Graft fills excavated site of nonunion and is fixed with Kirschner wires. **SEE TECHNIQUE 6.16.**

- If the muscle is too tight to allow easy transfer of the pedicled bone, dissect the ulnar origin of the pronator quadratus subperiosteally from the ulna through an additional incision over the distal ulna.
- Align the proximal and distal scaphoid segments carefully as a traction force is applied to the thumb. This maneuver corrects any intercalated segment instability and allows the grafted bone to be inserted snugly into the cavity in the scaphoid.
- Fix the proximal and distal scaphoid segments and the graft with two 0.045-inch (1.16-mm) Kirschner wires introduced at the scaphoid tuberosity. Do not cross the radiocarpal joint with a Kirschner wire.
- Close the skin and apply a long arm thumb spica cast.

POSTOPERATIVE CARE The arm is immobilized in a short arm cast until healing has occurred, usually at 10 to 12 weeks. When stable bony union is certain, the Kirschner wires are removed, usually about 3 to 4 months after surgery.

VASCULARIZED BONE GRAFTS— 1,2 INTERCOMPARTMENTAL SUPRARE- TINACULAR ARTERY GRAFT (1,2 ICSRA)

TECHNIQUE 6.17

(ZAIDEMBERG ET AL.)
- Place the patient supine on the operating table with the hand pronated on the hand table. Prepare the arm to use the pneumatic tourniquet.
- After skin preparation, draping, limb exsanguination, and tourniquet inflation, with the forearm pronated, make an oblique skin incision on the dorsoradial side of the wrist, centered on the radiocarpal joint. Avoid injury to the branches of the superficial radial nerve.
- Incise the extensor retinaculum of the first dorsal extensor compartment.

- Retract the extensor pollicis brevis and the abductor pollicis longus in a palmar direction.
- Retract the wrist and finger extensors toward the ulna.
- On the distal radial periosteum, identify the longitudinal course of the ascending irrigating branch of the radial artery (Fig. 6.45A). Design a bone graft with the longitudinal vessel as its center.
- Identify and protect the branches of the superficial branch of the radial nerve (Fig. 6.45B).
- Expose the scaphoid nonunion and freshen the sclerotic bone ends with curets or a power burr.
- Reduce the fracture. A Kirschner wire used as a "joystick" can be helpful.
- If the fracture cannot be reduced, approach the scaphoid through a second, palmar incision over the distal flexor carpi radialis, retracting its tendon and entering the wrist through the volar capsule.
- Make a 15- to 20-mm long trough in the scaphoid parallel to its long axis.
- Use narrow osteotomes or a small gouge to harvest a bone graft from the distal radius, beneath the periosteal vessel (Fig. 6.45C). Avoid comminution of the cortex and injury to the vessel. Make the bone graft about the size of the defect in the scaphoid and transpose it to the defect in the scaphoid (Fig. 6.45D).
- Stabilize the bone graft with Kirschner wires.
- Obtain additional cancellous bone from the same radial donor site, if needed.
- Deflate the tourniquet, ensure hemostasis, and close the capsule; avoid strangulating the vessel.
- Close the skin and apply a bulky bandage supported by a long arm thumb spica cast.

POSTOPERATIVE CARE The sutures are removed at 2 weeks, and the short arm thumb spica cast is worn until radiographic healing. Wrist motion and forearm rehabilitation are begun when union is established.

VASCULARIZED BONE GRAFTS— PROXIMAL RADIOCARPAL ARTERY GRAFT (PRCA GRAFT)

TECHNIQUE 6.18

(SOMMERKAMP ET AL.)
- Approach the wrist volarly through the flexor carpi radialis approach, as previously described (Technique 6.17), but extend it more proximally to complete a roughly 8-cm incision.
- Take care not to extend the dissection in a radial direction when proximal or at the distal radial rim to preserve the proximal radiocarpal artery pedicle. Carefully dissect to expose the volar rim of the distal radius and the distal half of the pronator quadratus.
- Debride the scaphoid nonunion site and assess the proximal pole bleeding with the tourniquet down for avascularity.
- Use 0.0625 (1.5 mm) Kirschner wires as joysticks to correct the humpback deformity; measure the defect needed

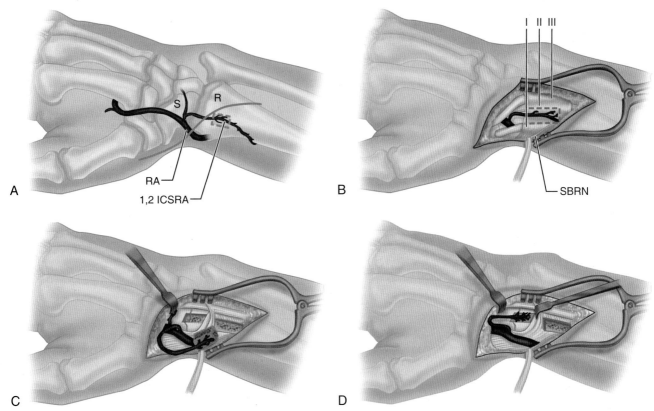

FIGURE 6.45 Pedicled vascularized bone graft for scaphoid nonunion. **A,** Incision *(solid green line)* exposes scaphoid and bone graft donor site. Subcutaneous tissues are raised from extensor retinaculum, and *1,2* intercompartmental supraretinacular artery (*ICSRA*) is identified. R, radius; RA, radial artery; S, scaphoid. **B,** Branches (I, II, III) of superficial branch of the radial nerve (SBRN) are identified and protected. *Dashed lines* indicate incisions of first and second extensor compartments. **C,** With graft levered out, tourniquet is deflated, and vascularity of graft is checked. **D,** Graft is gently press-fit into scaphoid nonunion site. Supplemental fixation with Kirschner wires or placement of scaphoid screws can be done at this time. (Redrawn from Shin AY, Bishop AT: Pedicled vascularized bone grafts for disorders of the carpus: nonunion and Kienböck's disease, *J Am Acad Orthop Surg* 10:210, 2002. Adapted with permission from the Mayo Foundation, Rochester, MN.) **SEE TECHNIQUE 6.17.**

for the vascularized graft (maximum size obtainable: 12 mm long, 10 mm wide, 13 mm deep).

- For harvest of the graft, carry out the dissection ulnar to the flexor carpi radialis. Retract the median nerve and flexor tendons ulnarly with a wide Penrose drain and slightly flex the wrist to relax the tendons and widen the view. The Penrose drain can be used to retract the carpal tunnel contents radial or ulnar, whichever provides better exposure of the donor site or pedicle.
- The proximal radiocarpal artery (PRCA) pedicle can now be seen at the distal edge of the pronator quadratus, often surrounded by fat.
- Identify the lunate fossa and place Kirschner wires to match the volar tilt of the articular surface to prevent penetration into the joint when harvesting.
- Gently dissect the pronator from the PRCA pedicle along the ulnar side of the radius. Carefully avoid skeletonizing the pedicle in the mid to radial part of the distal radius.
- Mark the desired graft size on the volar ulnar aspect of the exposed distal radius with the pedicle centered in the

graft templating. Ligate the ulnar continuation of the PRCA pedicle as it crosses the distal radioulnar joint.

- Complete distal, ulnar, and proximal cuts along the markings of the donor graft site with a 7-mm oscillating saw under continuous irrigation, avoiding penetration into the lunate fossa or distal radioulnar joint.
- Complete the graft harvest with a radial osteotomy using 2-mm osteotomes on either side of the pedicle. Lift the graft out of the donor site with a Freer elevator.
- Mobilize the PRCA radially by keeping a wide cuff of tissue and dissecting in a subperiosteal manner.
- Rotate the pedicle 30 to 40 degrees to inset into the scaphoid nonunion defect. The proximodistal and radioulnar parts of the graft correspond identically to the scaphoid recipient site.
- Complete fixation with either Kirschner wires or a cannulated compression screw in a retrograde manner, according to surgeon preference.
- Take care when performing the radioscaphocapitate ligament repair to not compress the pedicle.

POSTOPERATIVE CARE The sutures are removed at 2 weeks, and the short arm thumb spica cast is worn until radiographic healing, often confirmed on CT scanning at 3 months postoperatively. Wrist motion and forearm rehabilitation are begun when union is established.

▌ARTHRODESIS OF THE WRIST

Arthrodesis should be considered a salvage procedure for old ununited or malunited fractures of the scaphoid with associated radiocarpal traumatic arthritis. Wrist arthrodesis is discussed later in this chapter.

WRIST DENERVATION

Wrist denervation has been described for the treatment of chronic wrist pain with a variety of etiologies. Good results have been reported in 12% to 95% of patients after total wrist denervation. To avoid multiple incisions and extensive dissection, partial neurectomies have been used, but their results have been inconsistent. Berger described denervation of the anterior and posterior interosseous nerve through a single dorsal incision, and Weinstein and Berger reported improvement in 76% of patients with chronic wrist pain after this procedure.

TECHNIQUE 6.19

- Make a longitudinal 3- to 4-cm dorsal incision centered between the radius and ulna, just proximal to the proximal edge of the distal radioulnar joint (Fig. 6.46A).
- Expose the floor of the fourth compartment and the posterior interosseous nerve; remove a 1-cm portion of the posterior interosseous nerve (Fig. 6.46B).
- Incise the interosseous membrane, identify the distal sensory portion of the anterior interosseous nerve, and remove a 1-cm section (Fig. 6.46C).
- Close the skin and apply a bulky hand dressing with a volar plaster splint.

POSTOPERATIVE CARE A short arm splint is worn for 2 weeks, and sutures are removed between 10 and 14 days. At the end of 2 weeks of immobilization, a range-of-motion and strengthening protocol is initiated.

NAVICULOCAPITATE FRACTURE SYNDROME AND CAPITATE FRACTURES

Although naviculocapitate fracture syndrome is rare, it should be considered among the associated injuries that can occur with a fracture of the scaphoid. Axial compression of a dorsiflexed wrist forces further dorsiflexion, and after the scaphoid fractures, the dorsal lip of the radius forcefully impacts the head of the capitate, causing it to fracture. As the wrist continues into further dorsiflexion, after the scaphoid and the capitate are fractured, the

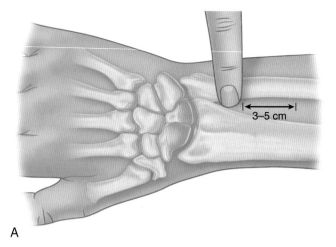

A

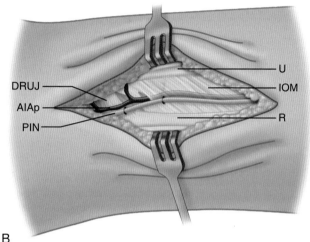

B

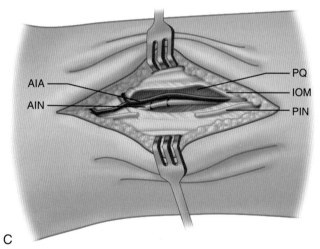

C

FIGURE 6.46   Wrist denervation. **A,** Incision. **B,** Removal of 1-cm section of posterior interosseous nerve. **C,** Removal of 1-cm section of anterior interosseous nerve. *AIA,* anterior interosseous artery; *AIAp,* posterior division of the anterior interosseous artery; *AIN,* anterior interosseous nerve; *DRUJ,* distal radioulnar joint; *IOM,* interosseous membrane; *PIN,* posterior interosseous nerve, *PQ,* pronator quadratus. (Redrawn from Hofmeister EP, Moran SL, Shin AY: Anterior and posterior interosseous neurectomy for the treatment of chronic dynamic instability of the wrist, *Hand* 1:63, 2006.) **SEE TECHNIQUE 6.19.**

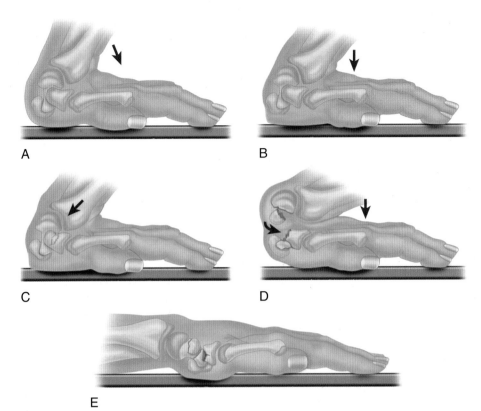

FIGURE 6.47 Mechanism of carpal fractures from falls on outstretched hand with wrist going into marked dorsiflexion. **A,** Wrist in marked dorsiflexion. Capitate is at 90-degree angle to radius. **B,** Scaphoid fractures as result of increased dorsiflexion at midcarpal joint. **C,** Dorsal lip of radius strikes capitate, causing it to fracture. **D,** Proximal fragment of capitate is rotated 90 degrees. **E,** Return of wrist to neutral position. Proximal fragment of capitate is now rotated 180 degrees.

capitate head rotates 90 degrees. The hand, when returned to neutral position, brings the proximal fragment of the capitate into 180 degrees of rotation (Fig. 6.47). This injury can be associated with dorsal perilunate dislocation (see Fig. 6.88B) or fractures of the distal end of the radius. Open reduction is necessary to derotate the capitate fragment. Some surgeons have excised this fragment, but others have replaced it, reduced the scaphoid and capitate fractures, and maintained them with internal fixation or cast immobilization. Osteonecrosis of the capitate may follow such injuries. If sufficiently symptomatic, osteonecrosis of the capitate can be treated with excisional-interposition arthroplasty or midcarpal or capitate-hamate arthrodesis. Isolated fractures of the capitate are unusual. Nondisplaced fractures of the body of the capitate are treated nonoperatively. Displaced fractures, especially fractures involving the joint, usually require open reduction and internal fixation with Kirschner wires or screws.

FRACTURES OF OTHER CARPAL BONES

Putman and Meyer tabulated the types of fractures of carpal bones other than the scaphoid, the most common treatment methods, associated injuries, and treatment tips (Table 6.1).

FRACTURE OF THE HAMATE

Fractures of the hamate can involve the hamulus or hook, the body, and various articular surfaces. Fractures of the hook can be treated with casting, open reduction, or excision of the hook. Fractures of the body usually are treated with casting unless displacement is significant. Articular fractures require open reduction and internal fixation if displacement of the articular surface is 1 mm or more.

A fracture of the hook of the hamate is sometimes difficult to show. Pain is elicited at the heel of the hand with firm grasp and with pressure against the bony prominence just lateral and slightly distal to the pisiform. A carpal tunnel view (Fig. 6.48A) or salute view (90-degree orthogonal from carpal tunnel view) may show the fracture, but some are better shown by CT (Fig. 6.48B). When using the latter technique, placing the patient's hands together in the praying position makes the diagnosis easier because the view of both wrists rules out congenital variation of the hamate, which usually is bilateral. Occasionally, the body of the hamate is fractured, but this rarely requires surgery.

A stress fracture may develop in the hook of the hamate with some repetitive activities, such as golf. Initial diagnosis can be difficult. Transient ulnar nerve motor palsy can be caused by an undiagnosed stress fracture of the hook of the hamate. In most instances, unless the diagnosis is delayed, union is likely after immobilization, but excision of the fragment may be necessary for nonunion, persistent pain, or ulnar nerve palsy.

TABLE 6.1

Patterns of Carpal Fractures

BONE (NORMAL RIGHT POSTEROANTERIOR AND LATERAL)	FRACTURE TYPES	MOST COMMON TREATMENT	COMMON ASSOCIATED INJURIES	TREATMENT PEARLS
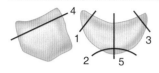	Palmar pole Osteochondral (chip) Dorsal pole	Closed treatment and casting for 4-6 weeks if minimally displaced or small fragments ORIF for intraarticular incongruity or associated instability	Lunotriquetral or radiolunate ligament tears Kienböck disease	Beware Kienböck disease if fracture presents independent of significant trauma. Consider MRI for evaluation of vascularity. Injury may suggest carpal instability pattern.
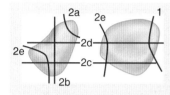	Dorsal rim chip fractures Body fractures: Medial tuberosity Sagittal Transverse proximal pole Transverse body Palmar radial Comminuted	Closed treatment with casting for 4-6 weeks of small chip (type 1) or minimally displaced If large type 1 or significantly displaced body type, may require ORIF	Dorsal avulsion may represent avulsion from DRC and DIC ligament. Triquetrum and lunate may secondarily flex if DRC ligament torn. Ulnar impaction/TFCC injury may accompany body fracture.	Stabilization of DRC and DIC ligament may be required if large dorsal avulsion. Arthroscopy may be necessary to evaluate ulnar/TFCC injury after healing of body fracture.
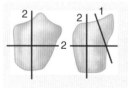	Vertical transarticular Horizontal Dorsoradial tuberosity Anteromedial ridge Comminuted	Thumb spica casting 4-6 weeks for minimally displaced fractures Spanning external fixation if comminuted ORIF vs. Kirschner wires for displaced intraarticular fractures Ridge excision for symptomatic type 4 Trapezium excision or carpometacarpal fusion for late arthrosis	First metacarpophalangeal fractures are common. Ridge fractures may secondarily cause carpal tunnel syndrome. Late first carpometacarpal arthritis may develop after intraarticular injury. FCR/FPL rupture is possible if medial irregularity.	Anatomic reduction for intraarticular fractures. May consider primary fusion for combined trapezium and proximal first metacarpophalangeal intraarticular fractures.
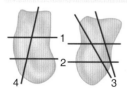	Dorsal rim Body	Cast immobilization for 4-6 weeks for minimally displaced fractures May require closed reduction of fracture or second metacarpophalangeal pinning for stabilization ORIF rarely necessary	Unusual as an isolated injury Usually associated with second metacarpophalangeal dorsal dislocation	Often requires CT or MRI to diagnose Recurrence of posterior subluxation of second metacarpophalangeal joint must be carefully followed. Fusion of trapezoid-second metacarpophalangeal may be necessary for late arthrosis and pain.
	Transverse (axial) body Transverse proximal pole Coronal oblique	Cast immobilization for 4-6 weeks for minimally displaced fractures Closed reduction and Kirschner wires for extraarticular reducible fractures ORIF for irreducible displaced, intraarticular, or proximal pole fractures	"Scaphocapitate syndrome"—including scaphoid fracture and lunotriquetral ligament injury Osteonecrosis (late) of proximal capitates	Proximal capitate is mostly intraarticular—leading to poor vascular supply. Urgent ORIF of displaced or rotated proximal pole fractures Beware associated (but not apparent) scaphoid fracture, lunotriquetral ligament injury, or other perilunate injury.

Continued

TABLE 6.1

Patterns of Carpal Fractures—cont'd

BONE (NORMAL RIGHT POSTEROANTERIOR AND LATERAL)	FRACTURE TYPES	MOST COMMON TREATMENT	COMMON ASSOCIATED INJURIES	TREATMENT PEARLS
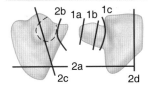	Hook Avulsion (tip) Waist Base Body Proximal pole Medial tuberosity Sagittal oblique Dorsal coronal	Cast immobilization for 4-6 weeks for minimally displaced fractures Hamate hook excision if continued pain after period of immobilization Rest, equipment adaptation, and immobilization for stress or repetitive injury fracture ORIF of displaced body or intraarticular fractures	Irritation and eventual rupture of ulnar finger flexors may occur with displaced hook fracture May be associated with fourth or fifth metacarpophalangeal dislocation May occur with avulsion of FCU	Cast immobilization in slight radial deviation minimizes deforming force of ulnar finger flexors. Hamate hook provides mechanical advantage of ulnar finger flexors. Hook has watershed blood supply at waist with feeding vessels through tip and base. Consider hamate hook lateral or carpal tunnel view radiograph for visualization.
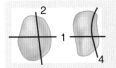	Transverse (common) Parasagittal	Immobilization for 2-4 weeks for minimally displaced or comminuted fractures Consider ORIF or excision and tendon reconstruction if FCU disrupted Excision and tendon reconstruction for arthrosis related to healed (or unhealed) fracture	FCU disruption (partial or complete)	Best visualized on lateral radiograph

CT, Computed tomography; DIC, dorsal intercarpal; DRC, dorsal radiocarpal; FCR, flexor carpi radialis; FCU, flexor carpi ulnaris; FPL, flexor pollicis longus; MRI, magnetic resonance imaging; ORIF, open reduction and internal fixation; TFCC, triangular fibrocartilage complex.

From Putnam MD, Meyer NJ: Carpal fractures excluding the scaphoid. In Trumble TE, editor: *Hand surgery update 3*, American Society for Surgery of the Hand, 2003.

EXCISION OR REDUCTION AND FIXATION OF THE HOOK OF THE HAMATE

TECHNIQUE 6.20

- With the patient supine and under appropriate anesthesia, prepare the skin and exsanguinate the limb with a pneumatic tourniquet.
- Make an incision parallel to the thenar crease, extending distally into the palm and proximally, obliquely, and medially across the wrist flexion crease to expose the hook of the hamate at the medial distal margin of the carpal tunnel. Incise the palmar fascia longitudinally, exposing the underlying transverse carpal ligament over the carpal tunnel. For excision of the hook, it is not necessary to open the carpal tunnel.
- Palpate the hook of the hamate with the tip of an instrument.

- Incise the ligament and periosteal cover over the tip of the hook.
- Expose the hook subperiosteally, "shucking" the soft-tissue covering of the hook until the fracture line can be seen.
- Grasp the tip of the hook with a Kocher clamp and mobilize the fracture site. Fibrosis at the base of an ununited hamate hook may make it difficult to move. Incise the fibrous attachments at the nonunion at the base of the hook.
- Avoid injury to the ulnar nerve as it passes from medial to distal and laterally around the hook.
- Remove the hook and smooth any rough surfaces at the base with a rongeur.
- If possible, cover the exposed fracture site with ligament and periosteal flaps.
- After release of the tourniquet, ensure hemostasis is obtained and close the skin with fine nonabsorbable sutures.
- If open reduction and internal fixation is selected, approach the hook of the hamate as described for excision. In this case, release of the transverse carpal ligament can make the fracture site easier to see.

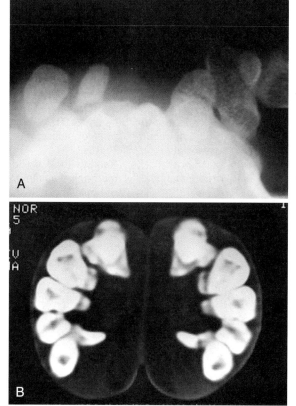

FIGURE **6.48** Carpal tunnel view **(A)** and CT scan **(B)** of patient with fracture of hook of hamate. Patient injured his left hand on full-swing foul ball. (From Egawa M, Asai T: Fracture of the hook of the hamate: report of six cases and the suitability of computerized tomography, *J Hand Surg* 8A:393, 1983.)

TRAPEZIUM AND TRAPEZOID FRACTURES

Fractures of the trapezium and trapezoid are rare and may be comminuted when seen in conjunction with radial fracture-dislocations and other carpal bone fractures. These fractures usually can be seen radiographically on the carpal tunnel view of the wrist and with CT. Fractures typically occur through the body or the trapezial ridge. Fractures through the body may be seen with fracture-dislocation of the trapeziometacarpal joint. Palmer classified trapezial ridge fractures into two types: type I is a fracture of the base of the ridge, and it may heal when treated by immobilization in plaster (Figs. 6.49 and 6.50); type II is an avulsion at the tip of the ridge, and it usually fails to heal when immobilized.

Displaced trapezial fractures require open reduction. Fractures of the body can be exposed through a J-shaped incision along the dorsum of the thumb metacarpal, curving medially at the wrist flexion crease. Ununited fragments of the trapezial ridge can be excised using the proximal limb of the J-shaped incision or through a longitudinal incision in the thenar crease, as when approaching the carpal tunnel. Care should be taken to avoid injury to the palmar cutaneous branch of the median nerve.

The trapezoid is fractured least often of the carpal bones and usually is injured at the time of other carpometacarpal injuries, especially injuries to the index metacarpal. Displaced fractures usually require reduction and fixation.

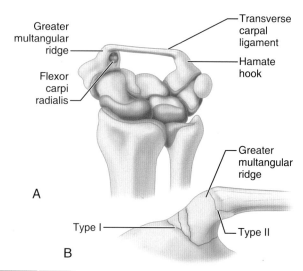

FIGURE **6.49** **A,** Carpal tunnel view showing flexor carpi radialis cradled by palmar ridge of trapezium. **B,** Type I fracture at base of volar ridge of trapezium (direct loading) and type II fracture at tip (avulsion).

FRACTURES OF THE LUNATE AND KIENBÖCK DISEASE

Fractures of the lunate can be difficult to detect on plain radiography. CT or MRI may be required to see the fracture (Fig. 6.51). Fractures of the lunate may be nondisplaced; displaced with large fragments; avulsed, especially the dorsal pole; or comminuted. Nondisplaced and nondisplaced comminuted fractures can be treated with cast immobilization. Fractures with more than 1 mm offset and avulsion fractures usually require open reduction. Internal fixation techniques vary depending on the requirements of the individual situation and may include Kirschner wires, small cannulated screws, and suture anchors. Trauma to the lunate may be sufficient to damage the circulation, leading to osteonecrosis of the lunate. Gelberman et al. described three patterns of vessels entering the lunate (Fig. 6.52). The lunates believed to be most at risk for osteonecrosis are those with a single vessel or one surface exposed to the blood supply, representing about 20% of lunates.

Kienböck disease is a painful disorder of the wrist of unknown cause in which radiographs eventually show osteonecrosis of the carpal lunate. It occurs more frequently between the ages of 15 and 40 years and in the dominant wrist of men engaged in manual labor. Armistead et al., using CT, showed occult fractures of the lunate in some patients (Fig. 6.53A). If untreated, the disease usually results in fragmentation of the lunate, collapse with shortening of the carpus (Fig. 6.53B), and secondary arthritic changes throughout the proximal carpal area. Symptoms can develop 18 months before radiographs show evidence of the disease. MRI can be helpful in the diagnosis of early avascular changes in the lunate. Correlation of the patient's clinical and plain radiographic findings with MRI helps to differentiate Kienböck disease from ulnar impaction (see later section "Ulnar Impaction-Abutment and Distal Radioulnar Joint Arthritis").

The staging classification of Kienböck disease proposed by Lichtman et al., based on radiographs and MRI, has been useful when planning treatment (Fig. 6.54 and Table 6.2). More recently, Bain and Beggs classified Kienböck disease

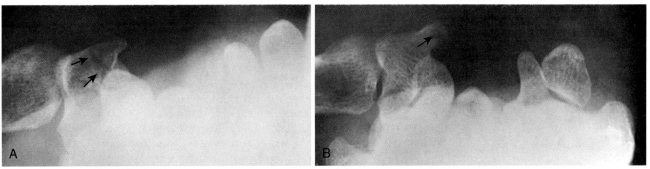

FIGURE 6.50 **A,** Carpal tunnel view shows fracture of base of palmar ridge of trapezium *(arrows).* This is designated as type I greater multiangular ridge fracture. **B,** Type II fracture of tip of palmar ridge of trapezium *(arrow)* caused by fall on dorsiflexed wrist. (From Palmer AK: Trapezial ridge fractures, *J Hand Surg* 6A:561, 1981.)

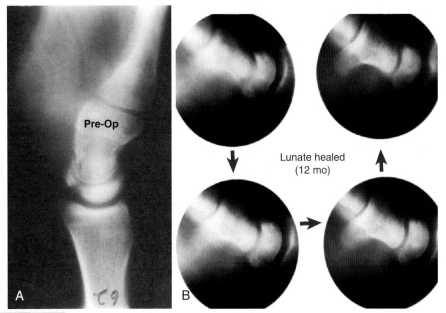

FIGURE 6.51 **A,** Lateral tomogram of wrist, showing typical anterior pole fracture. **B,** Lunate shows no further collapse 12 months after ulnar lengthening, and early healing is suggested. (From Armistead RB, Linscheid RL, Dobyns JH, et al: Ulnar lengthening in the treatment of Kienböck's disease, *J Bone Joint Surg* 64A:170, 1982. By permission of Mayo Foundation.)

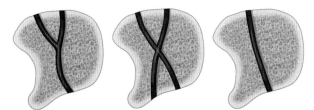

FIGURE 6.52 Three patterns of vessels entering lunate. Patterns with single vessel or one surface exposed to blood supply (approximately 20%) are believed to be most at risk for osteonecrosis.

based on arthroscopic determination of the functional status of the involved articular surfaces (Table 6.3 and Fig. 6.55).

Because the natural course of Kienböck disease is unpredictable, the treatment of established Kienböck disease cannot be rigidly prescribed. Immobilization in a cast has been recommended if the disease is considered to be quite early

(stage I or II, before sclerosis, fragmentation, or collapse occurs). Such management includes casting of the wrist for several weeks, if warranted, followed by repeated radiographs in search of occult fracture or avascular changes of the lunate or other disorders that become apparent later, including previously undiagnosed fractures of the carpal scaphoid. This treatment generally may be difficult for patients to accept because it requires 4 months or more of immobilization with an uncertain outcome. Reports regarding nonoperative treatment are difficult to evaluate because staging at the time of diagnosis often is unspecified.

Hultén described a condition known as the *ulna-minus variant.* He found in 78% of patients with Kienböck disease that the ulna was shorter than the radius at their distal articulation (Persson). This was true in only 23% of normal wrists. In no patient with Kienböck disease was the ulna longer than the radius at the distal articulation, but 16% of the control group had a so-called ulna-plus variant. Contrary to this, a more recent study by Ring et al. compared 166 wrists with

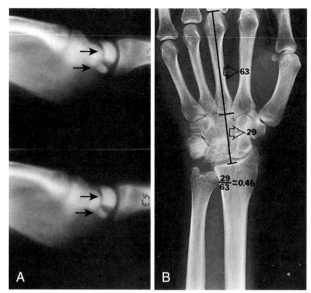

Kienböck disease to a similar number of control wrists without the disease. Measurement of ulnar variance determined that the prevalence of ulna minus variance was high in both the Kienböck and control groups. The authors concluded that the precise role of the ulna minus variance in Kienböck disease is unknown because those with the disease can be ulnar positive or negative. Additionally, there is a high number of ulna minus variance in the normal population, yet Kienböck disease is rare in the general population.

Numerous surgical procedures have been described for Kienböck disease. Joint "leveling" procedures include ulnar lengthening and radial shortening and usually are indicated for Lichtman stage I through IIIA Kienböck disease, with an ulnar-minus variation and without degenerative changes in the radiolunate or capitolunate joints. Wedge osteotomies have been used to decrease the load on the lunate by decreasing the radioulnar inclination of the distal radius. Capitate shortening, with and without capitate-hamate fusion, has also been used to decrease the load on the lunate in those with ulnar neutral variance. In a retrospective review of case series, Mansour et al. found that distal capitate shortening with arthrodesis of the third metacarpal base improved visual analog scores, functional outcomes, and grip strength in patients with stage II disease. They also found that identical treatment for stage IIIA disease did not prevent carpal collapse and did not improve pain scores, grip, or functional outcomes significantly. They recommended against capitate shortening

in stage IIIA disease. Lunate revascularization using a variety of pedicled bone grafts has been effective in preserving the lunate architecture. These revascularization procedures usually require protection of the lunate with pinning of the scaphocapitate or scaphotrapeziotrapezoid joint or with an external fixator. Excision of the lunate can give short-term relief. Prosthetic lunate replacement also may provide relief. Limited intercarpal fusions can prevent proximal carpal migration after lunate excision and can help decrease pressure on lunate prostheses. When secondary arthritic changes have developed throughout the wrist (stage IV), treatment usually is proximal carpal row resection or wrist arthrodesis.

JOINT LEVELING PROCEDURES

Persson, in 1945, reported a series of patients in whom he lengthened the ulna for Kienböck disease. Axelsson and Moberg observed these patients for several years. They found 16 patients who had been operated on some 20 years previously, and all but one had been able to continue with manual labor after the operation. Even in one who had pain, the disease process seemed to have been halted. Subsequently, Armistead et al. performed the ulnar lengthening operation for Kienböck disease, reporting 20 cases in 1982. Three non-unions required a second plating and bone grafting; 18 of the 20 patients had pain relief.

To minimize the chance of ulnar nonunion and the need for an iliac crest bone graft and implant removal, radial shortening osteotomy is the preferred joint leveling procedure for many surgeons. Shortening of the radius consists of making a transverse osteotomy about 3 inches (7.6 cm) proximal to the distal articular surface, shortening the radius by 2 mm, and fixing the bone with a compression plate.

CAPITATE SHORTENING

Capitate shortening was first described by Almquist, who reported an 83% lunate revascularization rate. This technique, combined with capitate-hamate fusion and carpometacarpal fusion of the distal capsule, has been used to unload the lunate in ulnar neutral wrists. Afshar described partial revascularization of the lunate at an average of approximately 5 months in 9 patients; he considered this the beginning of the revascularization process. Hegazy et al. found that capitate shortening worked best in patients with stage II disease, with improved visual analog scores, range of motion, and grip strength; however, the stage IIIA group did not show significant improvements and carpal collapse was not prevented.

CAPITATE SHORTENING WITH CAPITATE-HAMATE FUSION

TECHNIQUE 6.21

- Make a dorsal incision from the base of the third metacarpal to the Lister tubercle.
- Release the fifth dorsal compartment and retract the extensor digiti quinti tendon.
- Retract the fourth dorsal compartment radially and open the dorsal capsule. Take care not to elevate the fourth compartment and disrupt vascular supply.

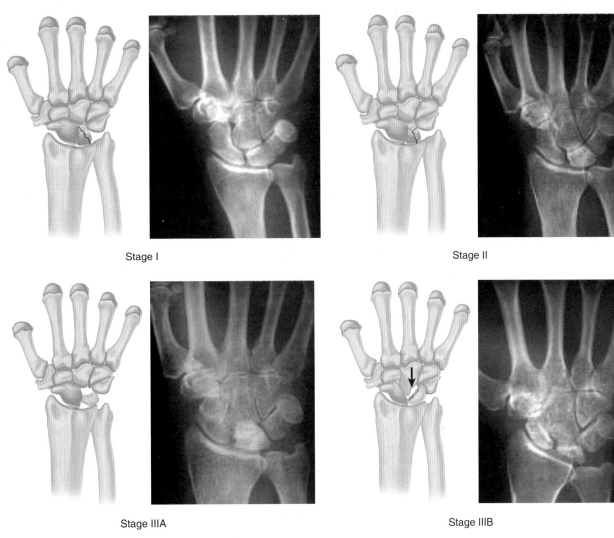

Stage I

Stage II

Stage IIIA

Stage IIIB

Stage IV

FIGURE 6.54 Staging of Kienböck disease according to Lichtman classification system (see Table 6.2). (From Allan CH, Joshi A, Lichtman DM: Kienböck's disease: diagnosis and treatment, *J Am Acad Orthop Surg* 9:128, 2001.)

- Incise the capitate-hamate joint from proximal to distal and identify the waist of the capitate; this level should correspond to the distal pole of the scaphoid.
- Use a sharp, thin osteotome to make the osteotomy to avoid disruption of the volar capsule blood supply.

- Carefully insert a small, curved elevator into the capitolunate joint, avoiding injury to the articular surface. Use the elevator to compress the capitate head against the distal segment and use two crossed 0.062-inch (1.6 mm) Kirschner wires to stabilize the osteotomy.

TABLE 6.2

Lichtman Classification and Treatment Recommendations

STAGE	DESCRIPTION	TREATMENT
I	No visible changes on radiograph; changes seen on MRI	Immobilization and NSAIDs. If no improvement, treat as stage II.
II	Sclerosis of lunate	Joint leveling procedure: radial shortening or ulnar lengthening in patients who are ulnar negative
IIIA	Fragmentation of lunate	Radial wedge osteotomy or STT fusion in patients who are ulnar neutral Distal radial core decompression to create local vascular healing response Revascularization procedures promising but long-term results not available
IIIB	Fixed rotation of scaphoid	Proximal row carpectomy or STT fusion; must treat internal collapse pattern
IV	Degeneration of adjacent intercarpal joints	Wrist fusion, proximal row carpectomy, or limited intercarpal fusion; must remove arthritic part of joint

MRI, Magnetic resonance imaging; *NSAID*, nonsteroidal antiinflammatory drug; *STT*, scaphoid, trapezoid, trapezium.

TABLE 6.3

Bain and Begg Classification of Kienböck Disease

GRADE	DESCRIPTION	RECOMMENDED TREATMENT
0	All articular surfaces are functional.	Extra articular procedure; radial shortening osteotomy for negative ulnar variance; capitate shortening procedure for neutral or positive ulnar variance; revascularization procedure
1	One non functional articular surface, typically the proximal articular surface of the lunate.	Proximal row carpectomy or radioscapholunate fusion
2	Two non functional articular surfaces. Grade 2A: proximal lunate and lunate facet of the radius. Grade 2B: proximal articular surface of the lunate, distal articular surface of the lunate.	2A: Radioscapholunate fusion 2B: Proximal row carpectomy
3	Three non functional articular surfaces: lunate facet of the radius, proximal and distal articular surfaces of the lunate; capitate is preserved.	Hemiarthroplasty, total wrist fusion or arthroplasty
4	All four articular surfaces are non functional.	Total wrist fusion or arthroplasty

Modified from Bain GI, Begg M: Arthroscopic assessment and classification of Kienbock's disease, *Tech Hand Up Extrem Surg* 10:8, 2006.

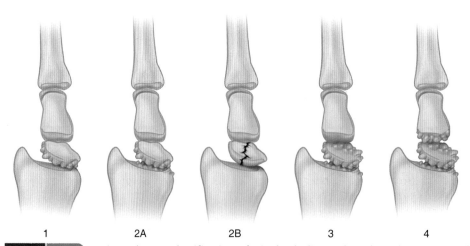

| 1 | 2A | 2B | 3 | 4 |

FIGURE 6.55 Bain and Begg classification of Kienböck disease based on the number of nonfunctional articular surfaces (see also Table 6.3). (Redrawn from Bain GI, Begg M: Arthroscopic assessment and classification of Kienbock's disease, *Tech Hand Up Extrem Surg* 10:8, 2006.)

- If capitate-hamate fusion is to be performed, remove all subchondral bone at the capitate-hamate interface. Harvest bone from the osteotomy or from a separate distal radial graft site and pack it into the space.
- Place Kirschner wires or headless cannulated screws percutaneously from the hamate into each of the capitate fragments.
- If the tip of the hamate becomes prominent proximally, preventing the unloading effect of the capitate-shortening osteotomy, remove the tip of the hamate to correct this problem.
- Alternatively, perform the osteotomy across both the capitate and the hamate, reduce it, and secure it with Kirschner wires or buried headless screws inserted from proximal to distal.

POSTOPERATIVE CARE Cast immobilization is continued for 6 weeks, followed by splinting. Range-of-motion and strengthening exercises are begun when fusion is seen on radiographs.

■ OSTEOTOMIES OF THE DISTAL RADIUS

For patients with stage II or III Kienböck disease and ulnar-neutral wrists, a radial closing wedge osteotomy has been proposed to shift pressure from the lunate by decreasing the radioulnar inclination. Reports verify that this technique can be effective in relieving symptoms. Closing wedge osteotomy has been reported to be useful in patients with stage IIIB and IV changes, but there is not universal agreement regarding the effects of such osteotomies. A biomechanical analysis of radial closing wedge osteotomies showed that force on the lunocapitate joint was decreased (23%), as were the forces on the radiolunate (10%) and ulnolunate (36%) joints, whereas another biomechanical evaluation showed that *lateral opening* or *medial closing* radial wedge osteotomies unloaded the radial lunate fossa. Similarly, another biomechanical analysis showed a decrease in lunate cortical strain with the radial opening wedge osteotomy and an increase with the radial closing wedge osteotomy.

■ CORE DECOMPRESSION

In 2001, Illarramendi et al. introduced the concept of metaphyseal core decompression of the radius and ulna as a less invasive treatment option for Kienböck disease. Decompression involved curettage of the distal radius and ulna through a small cortical window. The authors developed the procedure after noting spontaneous resolution of Kienböck disease after a nondisplaced distal radial fracture and credited the healing response after decompression to the response of the local vascular environment after trauma. A biomechanical study by Sherman et al. found that core decompression of the radius did not alter the load on the radiolunate fossa and postulated that the observed clinical effect of the procedure may be more a result of increased vascularity into the region of the lunate than a result of biomechanical unloading as obtained by joint-leveling procedures. Cited advantages of metaphyseal core decompression include simplicity of the procedure, no invasion of the wrist joint, and no need for any form of internal fixation. In a later report, Illarramendi et al. indicated that decompression of the radius alone did not affect

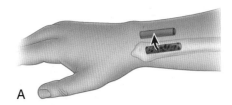

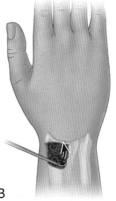

FIGURE 6.56 Core decompression for treatment of Kienböck disease. **A,** Cortical window. **B,** Cancellous bone impaction into metaphysis. (Redrawn from Illarramendi AA, De Carli P: Radius decompression for treatment of Kienböck disease, *Tech Hand Up Extrem Surg* 7:110, 2003.) **SEE TECHNIQUE 6.22.**

outcomes. They reported satisfactory results in 43 (90%) of 48 patients and no complications. A more recent study by De Carli et al. analyzed outcomes an average of 13 years after core decompression for stage IIIA lunates and found that only two of 15 patients had radiographic progression. Believing that it could decrease the intraosseous pressure in the lunate as occurs with decompression for femoral head osteonecrosis, Mehrpour et al. performed lunate core decompression in 20 patients, 18 of whom had good results. Bain et al. described an arthroscopic-assisted technique of lunate core decompression in two patients.

RADIAL DECOMPRESSION FOR TREATMENT OF KIENBÖCK DISEASE

TECHNIQUE 6.22

(ILLARRAMENDI AND DE CARLI)
- With the patient supine and the hand and arm resting on a hand table, apply and inflate a pneumatic tourniquet.
- Approach the radius through a 3- to 4-cm longitudinal incision along the radial border of the distal metaphysis, beginning 1 cm proximal to the radial styloid.
- Identify and protect the radial nerve branches.
- Separate the extensors with blunt dissection.
- Incise the periosteum and elevate it widely to expose the bone and to simulate a reactive healing response.
- With osteotomes or a small bone saw, make a window approximately 2.0 × 0.5 cm beginning 2.0 cm proximal to the radial styloid (Fig. 6.56A).

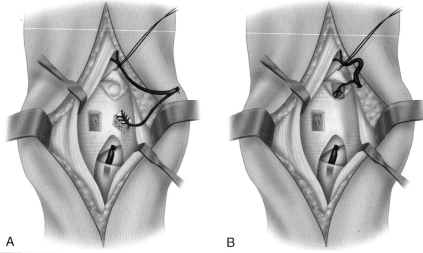

A   B

FIGURE 6.57   Pedicled vascularized bone graft of Kienböck disease. **A,** Anterior interosseous artery is ligated proximal to fourth and fifth extensor compartment arteries, and graft is elevated. After verifying blood flow, graft is shaped to fit dorsal opening to lunate. **B,** Cancellous bone is packed into lunate. Bone graft is inserted with pedicle placed vertically and cortical surface oriented proximal-distal. (From Shin AY, Bishop AT: Pedicled vascularized bone grafts for disorders of the carpus: nonunion and Kienböck's disease, *J Am Acad Orthop Surg* 10:210, 2002.)

- Through this window, curet and impact the cancellous bone of the distal metaphysis without removing bone. Impacting of the cancellous bone should take place only in the metaphysis, without compromising the cortex of the opposite side of the radius.
- Either break the removed bone cortex into 5-mm² fragments or maintain it as a single piece and leave it impacted in the metaphysis (Fig. 6.56B).
- Leave the periosteum open and close the skin in routine fashion.

POSTOPERATIVE CARE The arm is immobilized in a below-elbow cast for 2 weeks, with free active range of motion encouraged. Strenuous activities are avoided for 3 months.

▣ LUNATE REVASCULARIZATION PROCEDURES

Transplantation of an arteriovenous pedicle into normal and avascular bone has been shown to result in the formation of new bone. Other sources of vascularized grafts include the distal radius based on the pronator quadratus, the pisiform as a pedicle graft, and various other grafts from the distal radius, second metacarpal, and pisiform. A fourth and fifth extensor compartment artery graft from the distal radius also has been used for revascularizing the lunate (Fig. 6.57). Restoration of the lunate architecture and revascularization are reported to occur in 60% to 95% of lunates treated with revascularization techniques. These procedures also are effective in relieving pain and improving function in approximately 90% of patients. Most reports reflect that the promising early radiographic changes may not persist over time, and in many patients there is further deterioration in radiographic and clinical results.

▣ PROSTHETIC LUNATE REPLACEMENT

Replacement of the lunate with a hand-carved silicone rubber spacer has been recommended if there is no significant alteration in the shape of the bone (Fig. 6.58), and a previously molded, lunate-shaped silicone block has been used, followed by careful repair of the capsule to avoid dislocation of the block. This ligamentous and capsular reconstruction is crucial and has been emphasized by many authors.

Troublesome complications of the silicone lunate prosthesis, including silicone synovitis and foreign body cysts, are more likely to occur if the implant is oversized or malpositioned, if carpal instability is present, or if motion or occupational stress of the wrist is excessive. Because of this possibility, some surgeons have abandoned or limited this technique and have suggested intercarpal fusion (scaphoid-capitate, capitate-hamate, or hamate-triquetrum). These procedures are described later in this chapter.

Simple excision of the lunate, although controversial, has been shown to produce satisfactory results with continued pain relief at an average follow-up of 12 years. In 18 patients, the carpus rearranged itself with proximal migration of the capitate, triquetrum, and palmar-flexed scaphoid, but a good range of motion was preserved, and degenerative changes were less than anticipated. The procedure is not recommended for individuals who do heavy work.

The most recent addition to procedures for Kienböck disease is the medial femoral condyle osteochondral free flap. Pet et al. described using this in wrists with stage IIIA and IIIB involvement; at short-term follow-up (less than 2 years) the procedure appeared to halt further carpal collapse.

RADIAL SHORTENING

TECHNIQUE 6.23

- With the patient supine and under satisfactory anesthesia and after limb exsanguination and tourniquet inflation, make an incision on the palmar aspect of the distal forearm extending distally to the wrist flexion crease.

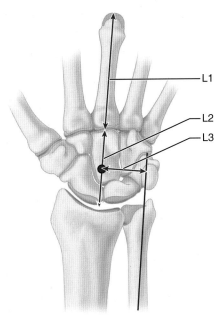

FIGURE 6.58 Three kinematic indices: center of rotation, carpal height *(L2)*, and carpal-ulnar distance *(L3)*. *L1*, length of third metacarpal. Carpal height ratio is L2/L1, and carpal-to-ulnar distance ratio is L3/L1.

- To protect the radial artery, incise the superficial surface of the sheath of the flexor carpi radialis. Retract the flexor carpi radialis radiolaterally and incise the dorsal surface of the sheath of the flexor carpi radialis. Carefully retract the radial artery laterally and identify the radial insertion of the pronator quadratus.
- Dissect proximally and identify the flexor pollicis longus.
- Elevate the pronator quadratus and flexor pollicis longus subperiosteally proximally so that the distal diaphysis and metaphyseal-diaphyseal junction of the radius can be easily identified.
- Based on preoperative radiographs and the amount of ulnar-minus variation, make an osteotomy in the metaphyseal-diaphyseal junction of the radius. A diaphyseal osteotomy, as recommended by Almquist and Burns, usually is required to allow enough length on the distal segment to place two or three screws. Placement of a plate in the metaphyseal-diaphyseal junction might be more difficult because of the palmar flare of the radial metaphysis, even though healing might be more predictable.
- Make the osteotomy proximal enough to allow placement of three screws in the distal fragment.
- Measure preoperative radiographs for the amount of shortening required.
- Fix the distal two screws to the distal radial fragment before osteotomy.
- Remove the plate and screws, perform the osteotomy with a thin-bladed oscillating saw, and shorten the radius by the appropriate amount, usually 2 to 3 mm.
- Reattach the plate to the distal fragment with screws.
- Before placing the proximal screws, compress the osteotomy and hold it with reduction forceps.
- Obtain C-arm fluoroscopic images to check radioulnar length.

- Fix the radius with a compression plate technique, deflate the tourniquet, obtain satisfactory hemostasis, and drain the wound if needed.
- Replace the pronator quadratus over the plate and close the subcutaneous tissues and skin, leaving the forearm fascia open to minimize the chances of compartment syndrome.
- Immobilize the forearm in a sugar-tong splint.

POSTOPERATIVE CARE The drain is removed after 1 or 2 days. Finger motion and wrist motion are encouraged. The sugar-tong splint is removed after approximately 10 days to allow inspection of the wound, and the sutures are removed at 10 to 14 days. A solid forearm cast is worn for another 4 weeks. After 8 to 10 weeks, additional casting depends on the radiographic appearance of the osteotomy. Exercise and light use of the hand are encouraged throughout convalescence.

DISTAL RADIOULNAR AND ULNOCARPAL JOINT INJURIES
ANATOMY

The structures causing pain on the ulnar side of the wrist include the DRUJ and the distal ulnocarpal joint and the ligamentous and cartilaginous structures attaching the distal ulna to the distal radius and ulnar side of the carpus, known as the triangular fibrocartilage complex or TFCC of Werner and Palmer. The TFCC includes the dorsal and volar radioulnar ligaments, ulnar collateral ligament, meniscal homologue, articular disc, ulnolunate ligaments, ulnotriquetral ligaments, and extensor carpi ulnaris sheath. The deep and superficial fibers of the TFCC begin on the ulnar side of the lunate fossa of the radius. The deep fibers of the TFCC then attach ulnarly at the head of the ulna called the "fovea," and the superficial fibers of the TFCC attach to the ulnar styloid tip where it joins with the ulnar collateral ligaments. Articular surface contact in the shallow sigmoid notch accounts for about 20% of DRUJ stability and allows dorsopalmar translation of about 1 cm with the forearm in neutral position. During forearm rotation, the ulnar head at its articulation with the sigmoid notch appears to move from dorsal and distal in full pronation to proximal and palmar in full supination. Additional DRUJ stability is provided through the dorsal and palmar margins and their attachments to the radioulnar ligaments. The extensor carpi ulnaris sheath and part of the distal radioulnar ligaments attach to the ulnar styloid, which extends 2 to 6 mm distal to the ulnar head. Most of the distal radioulnar ligaments and the ulnocapitate ligament attach to the fovea at the base of the ulnar styloid. The articular disc has attachments to the distal radioulnar ligaments and passes from the distal margin of the sigmoid notch to the fovea at the base of the ulnar styloid. The thickness of the articular disc has an inverse relationship to the amount of ulnar variance. Palmer et al. cited cadaver studies showing that loads applied to the distal radiocarpal and ulnocarpal joints are distributed about 80% to the distal radius and 20% to the ulna.

DIAGNOSIS AND TREATMENT

When evaluating patients with painful wrists, it is important to try to localize the anatomic source of pain. History, physical examination, radiography, arthrography, and, in the case of the DRUJ, CT are especially helpful. To assess radioulnar variance, a "neutral position" plain posteroanterior view is obtained with the shoulder abducted 90 degrees, the elbow flexed 90 degrees, the wrist in neutral flexion-extension and radioulnar deviation, and the forearm and hand flat on the cassette. A satisfactory lateral projection is obtained with the arm by the side, the elbow flexed 90 degrees, and the wrist in a neutral position. Arthrographic findings of TFCC perforation do not correlate with clinical findings. Patients with normal wrist radiographs, normal arthrogram, and inconclusive physical findings tend to do well without further invasive treatment. CT may clarify fractures of the sigmoid notch and is helpful in assessing DRUJ instability. Bone scanning provides minimal information about the DRUJ. Improvements in imaging techniques have increased the usefulness of MRI in the evaluation of the DRUJ, especially tears of the TFCC. Arthroscopy allows accurate diagnosis of readily seen lesions such as lesions in the central portion of the fibrocartilaginous disc and carpal bone osteocartilaginous lesions. Some peripheral ligament and cartilage damage may be more difficult to show. In some patients, although pain complaints may persist, conservative management usually is best until a clear indication for invasive treatment is established.

DRUJ conditions have been categorized as acute and chronic problems. Acute conditions include fractures of the ulnar head, styloid, radius, and carpal bones and dislocations or subluxations involving the DRUJ, carpal bones, and the TFCC and extensor carpi ulnaris subluxation. Chronic conditions include bony nonunions and malunions and incongruities of the wrist joint, including subluxation and dislocation of the DRUJ, the ulnocarpal region, the various carpal bones, and the TFCC, and localized arthritis of the pisotriquetral, lunotriquetral, and radioulnar joints and extensor carpi ulnaris subluxation related to arthritis. Procedures helpful in managing these problems include arthroscopic debridement and repair, limited ulnar head excision, ulnar shortening, and ulnar pseudarthrosis with distal radioulnar arthrodesis and distal ulnar excision (Darrach).

■ LESIONS OF THE TRIANGULAR FIBROCARTILAGE COMPLEX, INCLUDING TRAUMATIC DISTAL RADIOULNAR JOINT INSTABILITY
▌PHYSICAL EXAMINATION

Patients with a TFCC injury usually report a fall or some other trauma to the wrist that resulted in ulnar-sided wrist pain and mechanical symptoms (e.g., clicking) that improve with rest and worsen with activity, as well as weakness of grasp. High-demand athletes, such as tennis players or gymnasts, also are at risk of TFCC injuries. Physical examination may find painful grinding or clicking of the wrist with a range of motion. Ulnar deviation of the wrist with the forearm in neutral produces ulnar wrist pain and occasional clicking. A painful click may be elicited by having the patient clench and ulnarly deviate the wrist and then repeatedly pronate and supinate the wrist. In contrast, patients with scapholunate instability usually have pain and clicking when the clenched fist is moved from ulnar to radial deviation. The ulnar impaction test—wrist hyperextension and ulnar deviation with axial compression—also will elicit pain. The "press test" is another useful provocative test: the seated patient is asked to push the body weight up off a chair using the affected wrist, creating an axial ulnar load. If this reproduces the patient's pain, the test is considered positive; however, this is not highly specific and may indicate DRUJ instability or ulnar impaction. With the wrist in pronation, an unstable distal ulna may translate dorsally and can be manually reduced with dorsal thumb pressure ("piano key test"). Tenderness and pain identified when external pressure is applied to the area of the fovea (fovea sign) is indicative of an ulnocarpal ligament lesion. TFCC instability also is suggested by excessive motion with the "shuck test"—with the radial aspect of the wrist stabilized, anteroposterior stress is applied to the ulnar side of the wrist.

▌RADIOGRAPHIC EVALUATION

Anteroposterior and lateral views of the wrist and a pronated grip view should be obtained to determine ulnar variance. Whereas MRI has a sensitivity and specificity for TFCC tears approaching 100%, many asymptomatic wrists have positive MRI findings. CT arthrography is highly sensitive for detecting central TFCC tears but is not accurate for detecting peripheral tears. Some recommend proceeding directly to wrist arthroscopy for evaluation of the TFCC if the clinical examination and plain radiographs are suggestive of a TFCC lesion.

▌ARTHROSCOPIC EVALUATION

Arthroscopic examination of the DRUJ and the radiocarpal joint allows evaluation of the proximal and distal components of the TFCC, respectively. With the arthroscope in the standard 3-4 portal (see Fig. 6.15), a probe inserted through the 6R (or 4-5) portal is used to test the resilience of the TFCC by applying a compressive load (trampoline test) (Fig. 6.59A). A lack of normal resilience indicates a tear of the TFCC, although interobserver and intraobserver reliability of this test are only around 67%. The hook test is performed with a probe inserted through the 6R portal into the prestyloid recess and used to attempt to pull the TFCC in multiple directions (Fig. 6.59B). The hook test has roughly 90% agreement among observers. The TFCC can be displaced toward the center of the radiocarpal joint only when the proximal component is torn or avulsed from the fovea. According to Atzei and Luchetti, with an isolated distal TFCC tear, the trampoline test is positive and the hook test is negative. With proximal tears or complete tears, both tests are positive.

▌CLASSIFICATION

Palmer divided TFCC lesions into traumatic (class 1) and degenerative (class 2) groups, further subdividing the groups according to the location and severity of the changes encountered (Box 6.2). Lesions in class 1 may be caused by injuries to the DRUJ secondary to forced pronation or supination. Class 1 lesions also are likely to occur with distal radial fractures, especially if there is significant shortening of the radius. In most injuries, other structures supporting the DRUJ (lunotriquetral and ulnar lunotriquetral ligaments, extensor carpi ulnaris subsheath, and interosseous membrane) remain intact. Disruption of these structures is more likely with more severe injuries. Persistent instability is unusual if the fracture is reduced and heals satisfactorily. Younger patients with

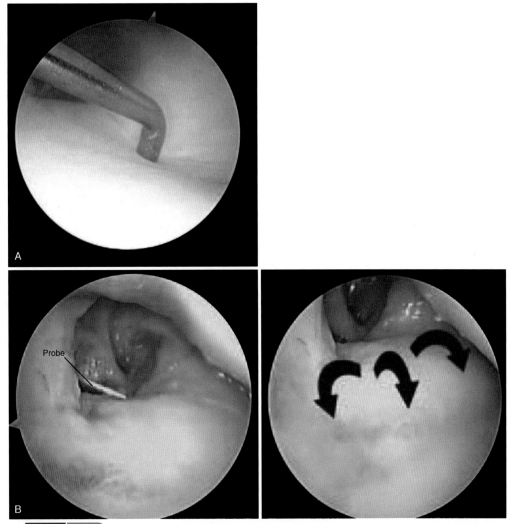

FIGURE 6.59 Resilience of triangular fibrocartilage complex (TFCC) is tested by applying compressive load (trampoline test) **(A)** and by attempting to pull TFCC in multiple directions (hook test) **(B)**. (**A** from Carlsen BT, Rizzo M, Moran SL: Soft-tissue injuries associated with distal radius fractures, *Oper Tech Orthop* 19:107, 2009; **B** from Atzei A: New trends in arthroscopic management of type 1-B TFCC injuries with DRUJ instability, *J Hand Surg Eur* 34:582, 2009.) **SEE TECHNIQUE 6.25.**

distal radial fractures and TFCC tears may be more likely to have significant late DRUJ instability. Other associated injuries that may contribute to DRUJ instability include displaced ulnar styloid fractures, fractures of the sigmoid notch, ulnar head fractures, and Galeazzi fracture-dislocations of the distal radius. Closed, nonoperative treatment, when possible, usually results in a stable DRUJ. If significant instability is present, early treatment may include pinning of the DRUJ combined with the appropriate management of the associated fractures. DRUJ instability associated with a comminuted fracture-dislocation of the radial head (Essex-Lopresti) may be extremely difficult to manage. If DRUJ instability persists, the procedures described may be appropriate. If chronic instability develops, DRUJ ligament reconstruction may be necessary.

Currently, management of class 1A TFCC (central perforation) lesions includes nonoperative measures initially. If significant symptoms persist, arthroscopic debridement may provide relief. For class 1B lesions (avulsion from the ulna, with or without ulnar styloid fracture), immobilization for 6

weeks followed by rehabilitation may be sufficient. There is a tendency for more severe peripheral tears to be associated with late instability in a younger population. If symptoms persist, and if there is DRUJ instability, arthroscopic repair using either an inside-out or an outside-in technique may produce satisfactory relief of pain and improvement of grip strength and wrist motion. For class 1C lesions (distal avulsion of ulnocarpal ligaments), which result in a volar ulnar "sag" of the carpus, late open or arthroscopic repair may relieve symptoms of pain and instability. Class 1D lesions (avulsions of the TFCC from the radius, with or without sigmoid notch fracture) may occur with fractures of the distal radius and ulna. If the ligament injury is unstable after reduction of the associated fracture, or if the notch fracture requires further treatment, detachment of the ligament from the radius can be repaired with open or arthroscopic techniques.

Class 2 degenerative lesions may be asymptomatic. In a cadaver study of wrist interosseous ligament and triangular fibrocartilage articular disc disruptions in specimens averaging 75 years of age, 60% had triangular fibrocartilage

Abnormalities of the Triangular Fibrocartilage Complex

Class 1: Traumatic
A. Central perforation
B. Ulnar avulsion
   With distal ulnar fracture
   Without distal ulnar fracture
C. Distal avulsion
D. Radial avulsion
   With sigmoid notch fracture
   Without sigmoid notch fracture

Class 2: Degenerative (Ulnocarpal Abutment Syndrome)
A. TFCC wear
B. TFCC wear
   + Lunate and/or ulnar chondromalacia
C. TFCC perforation
   + Lunate and/or ulnar chondromalacia
D. TFCC perforation
   + Lunate and/or ulnar chondromalacia
   + Lunotriquetral ligament perforation
E. TFCC perforation
   + Lunate and/or ulnar chondromalacia
   + Lunotriquetral ligament perforation
   + Ulnocarpal arthritis

TFCC, Triangular fibrocartilage complex.
From Palmer AK, Werner FW: Triangular fibrocartilage of the wrist: anatomy and function, *J Hand Surg* 6A:153, 1981.

articular disc disruptions. The most common lesions were linear defects at the radial attachment of the disc and central oval defects. Sixty-four percent of specimens with triangular fibrocartilage lesions had no arthrosis.

Palmer classified degenerative changes in the triangular fibrocartilage, lunate, triquetrum, lunotriquetral ligament, and ulnocarpal joints according to extent and severity (class 2A-E). These lesions usually are included in the "ulnar impaction syndrome" or "ulnar abutment syndrome." Triangular fibrocartilage perforation related to ulnar impaction may occur in 73% of ulnar-positive and ulnar-neutral wrists; it is unusual in ulnar-negative wrists (17%) according to cadaver studies by Palmer and Werner. The thinner articular disc in the ulnar-positive wrist may make it more susceptible to wear changes. Injuries to the distal radial physis, radial shortening after fracture of the distal radius, and shortening after radial head and elbow injuries (Essex-Lopresti) are acquired causes of ulnar-positive changes that may contribute to ulnar impaction symptoms. Symptoms of ulnar impaction include ulnar-sided wrist pain that is worsened by ulnar deviation with pronation and supination. Swelling and restriction of motion may be present. Physical findings also include pain on passive ulnar deviation and passive depression of the ulnar head with the wrist stabilized. Infiltration of a local anesthetic may help locate the source of the pain. Radiographic techniques mentioned previously assist in showing ulnar-positive relationships and ulnolunate changes. Surgical treatment may be considered when splinting, medications, and injections have failed. Unloading of the ulnocarpal joint may be

accomplished with open or arthroscopic intraarticular procedures and extraarticular procedures such as ulnar shortening.

TREATMENT OF TRAUMATIC LESIONS OF THE TRIANGULAR FIBROCARTILAGE COMPLEX (PALMER CLASS 1)

Class 1A lesions are traumatic central tears of the TFCC with no instability. Initial treatment is nonoperative for about 4 weeks. Persistent pain may be relieved by arthroscopic debridement of the flap portion of the tear. No more than two thirds of the central disc should be excised, and 2 mm of the TFCC peripheral rim should be preserved to avoid instability of the DRUJ. Preoperative evaluation should indicate the presence of an ulnar-positive variation. With an ulnar-positive wrist, the possible presence of degenerative changes in the ulnocarpal joint should be considered; these can be treated with arthroscopic "wafer" resection of the ulnar head (see Technique 6.3) or ulnar shortening osteotomy (see Technique 6.32).

ARTHROSCOPIC DEBRIDEMENT OF TRIANGULAR FIBROCARTILAGE TEARS

TECHNIQUE 6.24

- Follow the procedures for patient preparation; anesthetic management; and radiocarpal, ulnocarpal, and midcarpal examination outlined in Techniques 6.1 through 6.4.
- Inflate a pneumatic tourniquet as needed, especially when shaving or burring bone or soft tissue.
- Repeat the clinical examination for crepitus, "clicks," extensor carpi ulnaris tendon abnormalities, and DRUJ instability.
- Through the 3-4 portal, examine the radiocarpal and ulnocarpal joints.
- Use the 6R and 6U portals for further ulnocarpal examination.
- Examine the midcarpal joints.
- After the midcarpal examination, insert an 18-gauge needle to find the best working portals.
- Use the 6R portal for insertion of a full-radius suction shaver (2 to 3 mm). Debride synovium as needed to allow inspection of the joint.
- Use a probe to assess the central portion of the TFCC and the surrounding structures. Inspect and probe the ulnar lunotriquetral and the dorsal and palmar radioulnar ligaments.
- Use the full-radius shaver, suction punches, or small blades to excise only the flap portion of the tear. Trim the margin of the tear carefully, leaving the peripheral 2 mm of the rim of the TFCC.
- Close the portal sites with 4-0 or 5-0 nylon suture.
- Apply a volar, short arm splint.

POSTOPERATIVE CARE Sutures are removed at 10 to 14 days, and protected range-of-motion exercises are begun. Splint wear is continued for 4 weeks, depending on symptoms. Strenuous pronation-supination and grasping activities should be avoided during the first 4 weeks. Therapist-supervised rehabilitation is added as needed.

Class 1B lesions are traumatic detachments of the TFCC from the ulna, with or without ulnar styloid fracture. The deeper fibers of the radioulnar ligaments attach to the fovea at the base of the ulnar styloid. Fractures through the base may indicate more significant detachment of the TFCC than fractures at the tip of the styloid. If the ulnar styloid is fractured, open reduction and internal fixation of the fracture or excision of a small fragment is the usual treatment. Open repair of the TFCC injury is done at the time of ulnar styloid fixation. Significant injury to the extensor carpi ulnaris sheath also may occur with traumatic TFCC injuries. Extensor carpi ulnaris tendon subluxation may be a preoperative indicator of such an additional injury. If such a combination is encountered, arthroscopic repair of the triangular fibrocartilage and open extensor carpi ulnaris sheath reconstruction may be necessary.

ARTHROSCOPIC REPAIR OF CLASS 1B TRIANGULAR FIBROCARTILAGE COMPLEX TEARS FROM THE ULNA

TECHNIQUE 6.25

- Follow the procedures for patient preparation; anesthetic management; and radiocarpal, ulnocarpal, and midcarpal examination outlined in Techniques 6.1 through 6.4.
- Inflate a pneumatic tourniquet as needed, especially when shaving or burring bone or soft tissue.
- After the usual examination of the wrist joints, evaluate the TFCC from the 3-4 portal. Establish 4-5 and 6R portals. Remove any synovium that obstructs the view. Examine the dorsal and palmar radioulnar ligaments; the ulnar lunotriquetral ligaments; the lunate, triquetral, and, if visible, ulnar articular surfaces; and the ulnar foveal attachment of the triangular fibrocartilage.
- Place a probe through the 6R portal to assess the tautness of the triangular fibrocartilage (see Fig. 6.59A). The normal triangular fibrocartilage has a tension resembling a trampoline. Loss of the normal tension indicates an ulnar-side foveal tear.
- Make a counter incision directly ulnar to the distal ulna down to bone. Under fluoroscopic guidance, use an anterior cruciate ligament–type drill guide through the 6R portal or a free-hand technique to drill two bone tunnels parallel and obliquely at a 45-degree angle toward the fovea. Use a 0.0787-in (2-mm) Kirschner wire or drill for drilling.
- Load a 2-0 polyethylene braided suture into the Arthrex Micro SutureLasso; remove the nitinol to load the suture.
- Under arthroscopic view, pass a 2-0 polyethylene braided suture through one of the bone tunnels and pierce the TFCC. Viewing from the 3-4 portal and instrumenting through the 6R portal, grasp the suture and pull it out of the 6R portal.
- Load the nitinol loop back into the Micro SutureLasso and pass this through the opposite bone tunnel. Pierce the TFCC adjacent to the previously placed suture, keeping a good bridge of the TFCC between the two sutures to fix the TFCC well.

- Viewing from the 3-4 portal, pull the nitinol lasso out of the 6R portal; outside the joint, loop the polyethylene braided suture through the nitinol lasso and then pull the nitinol lasso out of the bone tunnel, bringing the suture with it. This should create a horizontal mattress-type repair of the TFCC.
- Tie the two polyethylene braided suture tails together over the bone bridge. Inspect the repair, pin the DRUJ in supination with 0.0625-in Kirschner wires, and leave in place for 4 weeks if there is concern about the strength of repair or patient compliance. Otherwise, splint in supination for 4 to 6 weeks.

POSTOPERATIVE CARE Sutures are removed at 10 to 14 days, and the cast is changed. The pins are removed at 4 weeks, and the cast is changed again at 4 weeks after surgery. The cast is removed after a total of 4-6 weeks. A therapist-supervised rehabilitation program is begun at 6 weeks. Forceful pronation-supination and grasping should be avoided for 10 to 12 weeks.

Nakamura et al. described an arthroscopic technique for repair of foveal detachment of the TFCC using transosseous sutures similar to that described above. They recommended this technique for complete or partial ulnar disruption of the TFCC at the fovea in wrists with an ulnar neutral or minus variance; in wrists with a positive ulnar variance, shear stress between the ulnar head and the suture site of the TFCC may rupture the sutures. The concept of this repair is based on the anatomic characteristics of the TFCC. A line drawn between a point on the ulnar cortex of the ulnar shaft 15 mm proximal to the tip of the ulnar styloid and the ulnar half of the triangular fibrocartilage passes through the foveal insertion. Sutures placed into this area can attach the TFCC to the fovea with an outside-in pull-out technique.

OPEN REPAIR OF CLASS 1B INJURY

TECHNIQUE 6.26

- After induction of an appropriate anesthetic, with the patient supine and the extremity on a hand table, exsanguinate the limb with an elastic wrap, and inflate a well-padded pneumatic tourniquet.
- Make a hockey-stick skin incision between the extensor digiti quinti (fifth extensor compartment) and the extensor carpi ulnaris (sixth extensor compartment). Center the incision on the ulnar head and extend the incision for 5 to 6 cm; angle the incision distal to the pole of the ulna in a radial direction to avoid injuring the dorsal sensory branch of the ulnar nerve.
- Open the fifth extensor compartment and retract the extensor digiti quinti tendon radially.
- Through the floor of the fifth compartment and protecting the radial border of the extensor carpi ulnaris, open the DRUJ with a transverse capsular incision beginning proximal to the TFCC fibers and just distal to the ulnar head articular surface. Preserve the radial attachment of the TFCC on the dorsal ulnar corner of the distal radius.

- Just distal to the transverse incision make an inverted T incision; this will gain visualization of the triquetrum and articular disc TFCC surface. The TFCC can now be seen between the two transverse incisions.
- Pass a Freer elevator from the distal ulna articular surface in an ulnar direction. If the Freer is able to be passed without impediment (or very little impediment) from the articular surface up and onto the ulnar styloid, then the TFCC deep foveal attachment has been disrupted. Roughen the bone at the fovea with a curet to produce a bleeding bone surface.
- Remove remnants of an ununited ulnar styloid, if present.
- Place a bone anchor or suture anchor into the fovea; a G2 Mitek/Dupuy anchor is often used. Alternatively, bone tunnels can be used similar to that described in the arthroscopic technique above; this way knots are kept out of the joint.
- Take the needles from the anchor and pass them from proximal to distal through the TFCC separately. Position the forearm in neutral and tie this down snugly.
- Close the longitudinal portion of the joint capsule, repair the extensor retinaculum. The extensor digiti quinti is often left transposed.
- To support the repair, especially in a patient of uncertain compliance, pin the ulna to the radius proximal to the sigmoid notch with two divergent 0.0625-in (1.6 mm) Kirschner wires in supination.
- Close the skin.
- Apply a sugar-tong splint.

POSTOPERATIVE CARE Sutures are removed at 2 weeks, and the splint is changed. The radioulnar pins are removed at 4 weeks. Splinting is discontinued at 6 weeks after the operation. A therapist-supervised rehabilitation program is begun after removal of the short arm cast. Forceful rotational and grasping activities should be avoided until comfortable, satisfactory motion and strength have been achieved.

OPEN REPAIR OF CLASS 1C INJURY

Class 1C lesions represent disruptions of the ulnocarpal ligaments in the substance of the ligaments or from the distal lunate and triquetral insertions. Associated injuries include lunotriquetral and class 1B tears. Class 1C injuries can be difficult to diagnose, may heal satisfactorily, and usually are treated without surgery unless significant instability develops. Carpal supination with a "sagging" of the ulnar side of the carpus is a helpful sign of instability.

TECHNIQUE 6.27

(CULP, OSTERMAN, AND KAUFMANN, MODIFIED)
- Follow the procedures for patient preparation; anesthetic management; and radiocarpal, ulnocarpal, and midcarpal examination outlined in Techniques 6.1 through 6.4.
- Use a pneumatic tourniquet as needed, especially when shaving or burring bone or soft tissue.

- If arthroscopic examination reveals clear exposure of the pisotriquetral joint, significant disruption of the ulnocarpal ligaments is likely. If the ligaments appear reparable, make a 1-cm or larger incision, distal to the ulnar head and volar to the extensor carpi ulnaris tendon. Avoid injury to the dorsal sensory branch of the ulnar nerve and the ulnar nerve and artery.
- Pass two needles through the volar capsule and, under arthroscopic control, through the ulnocarpal ligaments.
- Pass a 2-0 or 3-0 absorbable polydioxanone suture through one needle into the joint.
- Pass a nylon or wire suture loop through the second needle.
- Position the first needle so that the suture can be captured by the loop in the second needle.
- Remove the needles, retrieve the suture ends, and tie the ends over the capsule, creating a horizontal mattress suture through the ligament and out through the capsule.
- If a class 1B lesion is present, or if there is dorsoulnar laxity, secure the triangular fibrocartilage to the fovea as described for class 1B injuries.
- For large defects, use an open technique; consider approaching the ulnocarpal joint from the volar side, imbricate the ulnocarpal ligaments, and augment with a distally based strip of flexor carpi ulnaris secured to the dorsum of the ulnocarpal capsule.
- Close the wound and apply an above-elbow cast.

POSTOPERATIVE CARE The sutures are removed, and the cast is changed at 10 to 14 days. An above-elbow cast is worn for 4 weeks and is then changed to a short arm cast for another 3 to 4 weeks, followed by a removable splint for 2 to 4 weeks. A therapist-supervised rehabilitation program is begun at 6 to 8 weeks.

ARTHROSCOPIC REPAIR OF CLASS 1D INJURY

Class 1D injuries are tears of the triangular fibrocartilage from the radius at the distal end of the sigmoid notch. The tear usually is oriented in the anteroposterior direction, may involve dorsal and palmar radioulnar ligaments, and frequently is associated with distal radial fractures with extension into the sigmoid notch. Satisfactory reduction of the radial fracture may result in healing with a stable DRUJ. Open or arthroscopic repair may be required if there is instability after fracture reduction. Displaced fragments of the sigmoid notch may contribute to instability and require open repair. Ulnar shortening or recession at the time of triangular fibrocartilage repair improves results in patients with an ulna-positive variation and in patients with a chronic, retracted triangular fibrocartilage. Arthroscopic repair of the triangular fibrocartilage in patients with ulna-plus variation should be used with caution because the triangular fibrocartilage may be too thin to repair. If the triangular fibrocartilage is retracted more than 5 mm, open reconstruction of the triangular fibrocartilage, using a flap of the extensor retinaculum placed between the ulna and triquetrum and sutured to the radius and palmar and dorsal wrist capsule, may be more appropriate.

TECHNIQUE 6.28

(SAGERMAN AND SHORT; TRUMBLE ET AL.; JANTEA ET AL., MODIFIED)

- Follow the procedures for patient preparation; anesthetic management; and radiocarpal, ulnocarpal, and midcarpal examination outlined in Techniques 6.1 through 6.4.
- Inflate a tourniquet as needed, especially when shaving or burring to bleeding bone or soft tissue.
- Place the arthroscope in the 3-4 portal and a probe in the 6R portal to inspect and clarify the tear of the triangular fibrocartilage from the margin of the sigmoid notch of the radius.
- Through the 6R portal, remove synovium with the full-radius shaver as needed.
- Insert a motorized burr or the shaver through the 6R portal and debride the distal rim of the sigmoid notch down to bleeding bone (Fig. 6.60A).
- If they are intact, avoid injury to the dorsal and palmar radioulnar ligaments.
- Determine the best location for the insertion of sutures using a 20-gauge hypodermic needle placed through the ulnar side of the wrist proximal to the triquetrum. Through the arthroscope, probe the triangular fibrocartilage to estimate the best location for drilling for placement of the sutures.
- Make a small skin incision between the extensor carpi ulnaris and flexor carpi radialis tendon sheaths to avoid injury to the dorsal cutaneous branch of the ulnar nerve and the ulnar nerve and artery.
- Using the power drill and entering the 6R or 6U portal, use a 0.045-inch (1.2-mm) Kirschner wire to make two parallel channels in the distal radius, beginning side-by-side at the distal margin of the sigmoid notch and passing from the ulnar to radial direction (Fig. 6.60B). This allows the use of one suture. If two sutures are planned, three channels are required.
- After passing one wire, leave it in place and pass the second wire. Aim the wires to exit the radius in the distal metaphysis, between the first and second extensor compartments.
- Make a 1- to 2-cm skin incision at the exit point of the wires and with blunt dissection expose the exit sites of the wires. Protect the superficial radial nerve and the tendons of the first and second extensor compartments.
- Remove the wires one at a time.
- Pass the sutures in one of the following ways.
- After drilling the channels, use long meniscal repair needles, passed through an arthroscopic cannula from the ulnar side, through the triangular fibrocartilage, and then through the radius, from ulnar to radial, and out the lateral (radial) side of the radius, tying the knots on the radius, after arthroscopic evaluation of satisfactory tension on the repair (Fig. 6.60C,D).
- Pass an 18-gauge spinal needle through the first channel from radial (lateral) to ulnar (medial). Leave the obturator

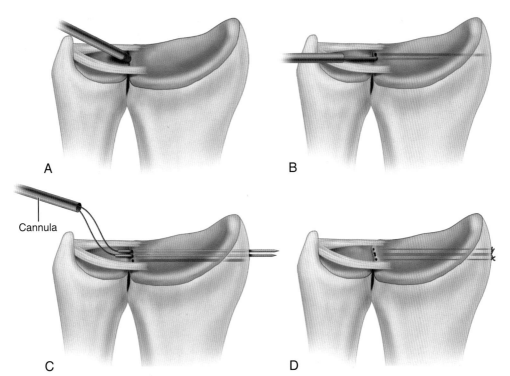

A

B

Cannula

C

D

FIGURE 6.60   Arthroscopic repair of class 1D injury of triangular fibrocartilage complex. **A,** Edge of sigmoid notch is abraded with motorized burr. **B,** Holes are drilled through radius with Kirschner wire. **C,** Sutures are placed into triangular fibrocartilage complex through drill holes with long meniscal repair needles. **D,** Sutures are tied on surface of radius. (Redrawn from Sagerman SD, Short W: Arthroscopic repair of radial-sided triangular fibrocartilage complex tears, *Arthroscopy* 12:339, 1996.) **SEE TECHNIQUE 6.28.**

(trocar) in the needle. Remove the obturator after needle passage. After the needle has been passed through the radius and the proximal undersurface of the free margin of the triangular fibrocartilage, insert a 2-0 or 0 polydioxanone suture into the needle and pass the suture through the free margin of the triangular fibrocartilage under arthroscopic control. Leave the first needle in place. Pass another 18-gauge spinal needle through the second channel and through the proximal undersurface of the free margin of the triangular fibrocartilage, adjacent to the suture. Remove the obturator from the needle. Pass a wire loop through the second needle to retrieve the end of the suture from the first needle. Withdraw the suture from the second needle. Apply tension to the suture ends and determine the tension of the triangular fibrocartilage against the distal radius. If the tension is satisfactory, tie the suture knot on the radial (lateral) surface of the radius. If the tension and apposition are unsatisfactory, another set of sutures might be needed, requiring another drilled channel. If possible, it is helpful to determine the need for the second suture before suture passage.

- Trumble et al. described the following suture passage technique.
- Insert a straight 12-French suction cannula through the 6R or 6U portal.
- Pass 2-0 Maxon (Davis and Geck) meniscal repair sutures through the cannula and through the triangular fibrocartilage, drilling the suture needles through the radius at the distal margin of the sigmoid notch, from the ulnar to the radial direction (Fig. 6.61). If the radius is predrilled, the needle passage is facilitated and drilling the needles might not be required.
- Tie the sutures over the radius.
- Jantea et al. described another option for suture passage. A combination drill guide-tissue protector jig is used for pin placement and more precise location of the channels drilled for suture passage (Fig. 6.62).
- Insert the first 0.045-in (2-mm) Kirschner wire from the ulnar side of the wrist, entering between the extensor carpi ulnaris and the flexor carpi ulnaris.
- Through the arthroscope, verify that this wire marks the insertion of the triangular fibrocartilage at the distal end of the sigmoid notch.
- Slide one barrel of the guide over the first wire and place the guide over the dorsum of the wrist so that the second barrel is against the distal radial metaphysis between the first and second extensor compartments.
- Make a small skin incision over this area, to dissect bluntly down to the radial cortex between the first and second extensor compartments.
- Protect the superficial radial nerve, radial artery, and abductor pollicis longus, extensor pollicis longus, and extensor pollicis brevis tendons.
- Insert the second 1.2-mm Kirschner wire into the barrel of the guide and drill this second wire across the radius. This wire should be seen through the arthroscope to penetrate the ulnar side of the radius at the distal end of the sigmoid notch, at the end of the first pin.
- Withdraw the first pin in the drill guide barrel sufficiently to move it to an adjacent site on the triangular fibrocartilage for drilling of another channel for another wire.

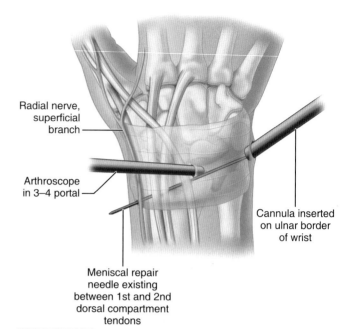

FIGURE 6.61 Passage of sutures through cannula in ulnar aspect of wrist between flexor carpi ulnaris and extensor carpi ulnaris just proximal to triquetrum. (Redrawn from Division of Hand and Microvascular Surgery, University of Washington, School of Medicine, Seattle, WA.) **SEE TECHNIQUE 6.28.**

Labels: Radial nerve, superficial branch; Arthroscope in 3–4 portal; Meniscal repair needle existing between 1st and 2nd dorsal compartment tendons; Cannula inserted on ulnar border of wrist

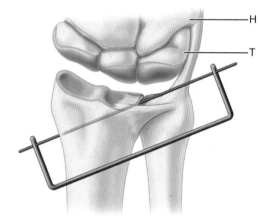

FIGURE 6.62 Use of combination drill guide-tissue protector jig for pin placement and precise location of channels for suture passage. *H*, Hamate; *T*, triquetrum. (From Jantea CL, Baltzer A, Rüther W: Arthroscopic repair of radial-sided lesions of the fibrocartilage complex, *Hand Clin* 11:31, 1995.) **SEE TECHNIQUE 6.28.**

- Pass another wire into the drill guide barrel and drill the wire from the radial side of the radius, across the radius, to exit at the distal margin of the sigmoid notch adjacent to the exit site of the previous channel.
- Remove the Kirschner wires and the drill guide.
- After predrilling, keep the obturator (trocar) in an 18-gauge spinal needle and insert the 18-gauge spinal needle through the first channel in the radius from the radial side toward the ulna, exiting at the triangular fibrocartilage insertion and passing through the proximal undersurface of the triangular fibrocartilage.

- Pass another 18-gauge spinal needle through the adjacent, parallel channel in the radius.
- Exit through the second opening at the distal end of the sigmoid notch.
- Pass this needle through the proximal undersurface of the triangular fibrocartilage.
- Remove the obturators (trocars) of the spinal needles.
- Ensure that the needles remain protruding through the triangular fibrocartilage.
- Pass a 2-0 or 0 polydioxanone suture through one needle and out through the triangular fibrocartilage.
- Pass a wire loop through the second spinal needle and through the triangular fibrocartilage.
- Position the end of the first needle and the suture end to facilitate passing the suture end through the loop.
- Carefully remove the spinal needles.
- Retrieve the suture ends and tie them over the radius between the first and second extensor compartments.
- Verify that there is satisfactory tension on the triangular fibrocartilage against the distal end of the sigmoid notch.
- Use a 0.062-inch (2-mm) Kirschner wire to pin the ulna to the radius from ulnar (medial) to radial (lateral) in midposition.
- Close the arthroscopic portals and incisions as needed.
- Apply a long arm cast.

POSTOPERATIVE CARE The sutures are removed at 10 to 14 days, and the cast is changed. The radioulnar pin is removed at 6 to 8 weeks. The forearm and wrist are supported with a removable splint for another month. Active motion and a therapist-supervised rehabilitation program are begun. Strenuous, forceful grasping and rotational activities should be avoided until motion and strength have returned.

OPEN REPAIR OF CLASS 1D INJURIES

TECHNIQUE 6.29

(COONEY ET AL.)
- With the patient supine and under an appropriate anesthetic, apply a well-padded pneumatic tourniquet to the upper arm. Extend the extremity on the hand table. After sterile skin preparation and draping, exsanguinate the limb and inflate the pneumatic tourniquet.
- Make a straight, dorsoulnar skin incision between the fourth and fifth extensor compartments. Make the incision long enough to gain access to the DRUJ and the ulnocarpal joint, usually 8 to 10 cm.
- Open the extensor retinaculum in a Z-shaped configuration to allow use of the flaps for retinacula repair or triangular fibrocartilage reconstruction.
- Retract the extensor carpi ulnaris tendon laterally (radially).
- Incise the radioulnar joint capsule longitudinally, beginning proximal to the DRUJ, extending to the dorsal radioulnar ligament, and then turn the incision medially (ulnarward) along the proximal edge of the dorsal radioulnar ligament to make an L-shaped capsular flap.

- Beginning just distal to the dorsal radioulnar ligament, extend the capsular incision transversely to expose the ulnocarpal joint, the lunate fossa, the lunate, the triquetrum, the ulnar lunotriquetral ligament complex, and the triangular fibrocartilage.
- Use small periosteal elevators and probes to determine the extent of triangular fibrocartilage damage.
- Detach the dorsal radioulnar ligament from the dorsal surface of the distal radius.
- Reflect the periosteum from the distal radius just proximal to the lunate fossa to expose the dorsoulnar cortex of the distal radius (Fig. 6.63A).
- Inspect the triangular fibrocartilage and radiocarpal joint for other injuries.
- Use a 0.045-in (1.2-mm) Kirschner wire or drill point of similar size to drill a line of four holes, side-by-side, from the dorsal surface of the distal radius from dorsoradial to palmar-ulnar, with the wire or drill point exiting at the distal margin of the sigmoid notch, at the ulnar (medial) border of the lunate fossa.

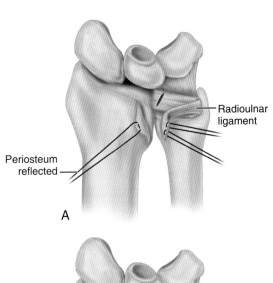

A

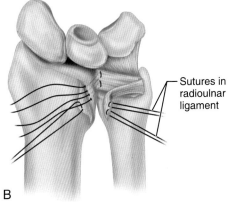

B

FIGURE 6.63 Open repair of class 1D injuries of triangular fibrocartilage complex (TFCC). **A,** Approach to TFCC, reflection of dorsal radioulnar ligament and periosteum over lunate fossa. **B,** Suture placement into TFCC through holes drilled in dorsoulnar aspect of distal radius; sutures are directed in palmar and ulnar direction to exit at edge of lunate fossa and sigmoid notch. Horizontal mattress sutures are placed in TFCC. (Redrawn from Cooney WP, Linscheid RL, Dobyns JH: Triangular fibrocartilage tears, *J Hand Surg* 19A:143, 1994. Copyright of the Mayo Clinic.) **SEE TECHNIQUE 6.29.**

- Debride the distal margin of the sigmoid notch and the torn margin with a rongeur or powered burr to bleeding bone.
- Insert a small lamina spreader to improve exposure. If satisfactory exposure of the triangular fibrocartilage cannot be achieved, especially with an ulnar-positive variation, osteotomy of the ulna, with recession and plate fixation, is recommended by Cooney et al.
- Use 2-0 or 3-0 polyglactin 910 (Vicryl) suture or a polydioxanone suture on a small, round needle to place horizontal mattress sutures in the triangular fibrocartilage, passing the suture from the proximal undersurface to the distal surface of the triangular fibrocartilage (Fig. 6.63B).
- Remove the small needles. Pass a straight needle, without suture, reversed into the drill holes to retrieve the ends of the pairs of suture. Other satisfactory methods of suture retrieval include the use of a wire loop or a suture passer.
- Flex the elbow and maintain the forearm in neutral to slight supination to reduce the DRUJ.
- Stabilize the DRUJ by placing a 0.045-inch, 0.062-inch, or 2-mm Kirschner wire from the ulna into the radius, proximal to the sigmoid notch.
- Tighten the repair sutures and tie the knots on the dorsal surface of the distal radius, just proximal to the lunate fossa.
- Reattach the dorsal edge of the triangular fibrocartilage (dorsal radioulnar ligament) to the dorsoulnar distal radius, suturing it to the reflected flap of periosteum with 3-0 or larger absorbable suture.
- If the dorsal radioulnar ligament is attenuated, reinforce it with a flap of the extensor retinaculum, based at the dorsoradial margin of the extensor carpi ulnaris sheath.
- Close the ulnocarpal joint capsule, extensor retinaculum, and skin in layers.
- Apply a long arm cast.

POSTOPERATIVE CARE The cast is changed and skin sutures and pin sites are checked at about 2 weeks. The radioulnar pins are removed between 4 and 6 weeks. The long arm cast is worn 8 weeks from the time of repair. At 8 weeks, a long arm thermoplastic splint is applied and a therapist-supervised rehabilitation program is begun, starting with gentle, active forearm pronation-supination exercises. The long arm splint is worn for an additional 6 weeks. A strengthening program is begun as motion improves, usually about 10 weeks from the time of repair. Return to work and sports is delayed until grip strength is about 80% of the uninjured extremity.

■ CHRONIC INSTABILITY OF THE DISTAL RADIOULNAR JOINT

Symptomatic chronic instability of the DRUJ may occur after isolated trauma to the DRUJ, after fractures of the distal radius and ulna, after unsuccessful attempts to repair the TFCC, and in inflammatory arthritis. Cadaver studies have shown that angulation of radial fractures with volar convexity of more than 20 or 30 degrees contributes to DRUJ incongruity. Radial shortening disturbs radioulnar kinematics, and more than 5 mm of radial shortening implies significant damage to the TFCC. A clinical study of 166 distal radial fractures by May et al. suggested that displaced fractures through the base of the ulnar styloid may contribute to DRUJ instability. Most acute injuries, with appropriate treatment, result in a stable DRUJ. Patients with symptomatic DRUJ instability usually have symptoms related to dorsal displacement of the distal ulna.

PROCEDURES TO STABILIZE THE DISTAL RADIOULNAR JOINT

DRUJ instability related to malunited distal radial fractures can be treated with distal radial osteotomy and bone grafting to correct shortening and angulation. Ununited, displaced ulnar styloid fractures can be treated with open reduction and internal fixation.

Many soft-tissue techniques have been proposed to stabilize the DRUJ and the unstable distal ulna. Bowers emphasized the importance of repairing or reconstructing the TFCC. Late repair of the TFCC may be possible. If the TFCC cannot be repaired, but the articular surfaces are in good condition, and the sigmoid notch is competent, reconstruction of the ligaments around the DRUJ may stabilize the joint satisfactorily. Adams identified three categories of soft-tissue reconstruction for chronic DRUJ instability: (1) distal ulnar tenodesis, with the extensor carpi ulnaris or flexor carpi ulnaris tendon, (2) ulnocarpal tether, and (3) radioulnar tether. Although the ulnocarpal techniques described by Hui and Linscheid and by Boyes and Bunnell may be effective, a cadaver study by Gupta et al. suggested that the ulnocarpal ligaments may not require reconstruction in all patients with DRUJ instability. The difficulty of restoring the smooth carpal articulation, a flexible rotational radioulnar tether, an ulnocarpal suspension from the radius, an ulnocarpal cushion, and an ulnar shaft to the ulnar carpal connection is recognized. Many complex radioulnar tethering procedures proximal to the radioulnar joint have been described. Hermansdorfer and Kleinman found reattachment of the TFCC effective for minimal subluxation. The reports of Bach et al. and of Scheker et al. suggested that tenodesis augmentation of TFCC repair with extensor carpi ulnaris (Bach) or tendon graft reconstruction through radioulnar drill holes (Scheker) helped to stabilize the DRUJ. Adams emphasized the importance of reconstruction of the distal radioulnar ligaments to restore DRUJ stability and to preserve DRUJ motion. In a retrospective study of 95 Adams-Berger reconstructions, 90% of patients had a stable DRUJ with a mean follow-up of 65 months. Grip strength increased while pronosupination decreased. Pain was either zero or mild in 76%. The procedure was deemed "successful" in 86% of the cohort. Although this is a complex procedure, it provides an answer to a very difficult problem. Additional studies in cadaver models have found the distal oblique bundle reconstruction of the interosseous membrane to have stability similar to the Adams-Berger procedure. The authors suggest that there is less morbidity with the distal oblique bundle reconstruction.

ANATOMIC RECONSTRUCTION OF THE DISTAL RADIOULNAR LIGAMENTS

TECHNIQUE 6.30

(ADAMS AND BERGER)

- Before induction of the anesthetic, determine if a palmaris longus tendon is present on either upper extremity. Prepare the extremities accordingly. If a palmaris longus is unavailable, consider harvesting a tendon graft from another location or using an allograft tendon.
- With the patient supine and under the appropriate anesthetic, apply a well-padded tourniquet to the upper arm, prepare the skin, and apply drapes with the arm positioned on the hand table.
- Make a longitudinal 4-cm incision between the fifth and sixth extensor compartments. Begin the incision at the level of the ulnar styloid and extend it proximally.
- Open the fifth compartment except for the distal retinaculum over the ulnocarpal joint.
- Retract the extensor digiti quinti tendon laterally (radially).
- Open the DRUJ capsule with an L-shaped incision. Make the capsular incision extending longitudinally along the dorsal rim of the sigmoid notch, then transversely, proximal and parallel to the normal location of the dorsal radioulnar ligament.
- Retract the capsular flap proximally and medially (ulnarward) to expose the articular surface of the DRUJ and the proximal surface of the TFCC remnant (Fig. 6.64A).
- Determine whether the TFCC can be repaired. If the TFCC cannot be repaired or used to stabilize the DRUJ, proceed with reconstruction of the radioulnar ligaments.
- Debride granulation tissue from the fovea of the ulnar head. Leave any functioning remnants of the TFCC, including the palmar radioulnar and ulnocarpal ligaments, if they are intact.
- Debride a central tear in the triangular fibrocartilage disc to make the edges smooth.
- Leave the extensor carpi ulnaris sheath intact during the procedure. Do not open the extensor carpi ulnaris sheath or dissect the sheath from the ulnar groove during this procedure.
- If an ulnar styloid nonunion is encountered, remove the styloid fragment with sharp, subperiosteal dissection.
- Harvest a palmaris longus tendon graft from the same side, if present. Use a 1- to 2-cm transverse incision at the wrist flexion crease to identify the palmaris longus tendon and mobilize it with blunt dissection. Protect the median nerve. Leave the palmaris attached distally.
- In the mid-to-proximal forearm, make another 1- to 2-cm longitudinal incision over the palmaris longus musculotendinous junction and transect the tendon in the proximal incision. Avoid injury to the median nerve.
- Deliver the tendon in the distal incision, transect the tendon distally, and place the graft in a safe location. Close the donor incisions.
- Prepare the site for the tunnel in the radius by elevating the periosteum from the dorsal radius at the margin of the sigmoid notch.

- Using C-arm fluoroscopy, drive a guidewire for a 2- to 4-mm cannulated drill through the radius from dorsal to palmar, beginning far enough proximal to the lunate fossa and lateral (radial) to the articular surface of the sigmoid notch that a tunnel about 5 mm in diameter can be created without fracturing into the lunate fossa or the sigmoid notch.
- Use posteroanterior and lateral fluoroscopy to confirm that the guidewire is safely and accurately placed without passing completely through the palmar cortex (Fig. 6.64B).
- Use a cannulated 2- or 3-mm drill to create a pilot tunnel. Progressively enlarge the radial tunnel with noncannulated drill bits sufficiently to allow passage of the tendon graft (Fig. 6.64C).
- If radial osteotomy is planned to correct a malunion at the time of radioulnar ligament reconstruction, make the radial tunnel before doing the osteotomy to facilitate the drilling of the tunnel. If a radial malunion is present, avoid penetration of the lunate fossa by making the tunnel so that it is parallel to the malaligned lunate fossa as determined on fluoroscopy.
- Make an obliquely directed tunnel in the distal ulna from the fovea to the ulnar neck. Use the same guidewire, cannulated drill, and noncannulated drill sequence as that used in making the tunnel in the radius.
- Expose the fovea at the base of the ulnar styloid by flexing the wrist and retracting the TFCC remnants distally.
- Insert the guidewire through the fovea and direct it to exit the ulnar neck medially and just palmar to the extensor carpi ulnaris (Fig. 6.64D). To avoid fracture of the ulnar neck and injury to the carpus, place the 2- or 3-mm cannulated drill over the guidewire from the medial ulnar neck cortex so that reaming is done from the superficial ulnar neck in a retrograde direction toward the fovea.
- Carefully enlarge the tunnel in the ulna with noncannulated drill bits, to make an opening large enough for passage of both limbs of the graft (Fig. 6.64C,E).
- Make a 3-cm longitudinal incision on the volar side of the wrist, between the ulnar neurovascular bundle and the flexor tendons to the fingers. Begin the incision at the proximal wrist flexion crease.
- Retract the ulnar neurovascular bundle medially (ulnar) and the finger flexors laterally (radial) to expose the area of the palmar opening of the tunnel.
- Pass a suture retriever through the tunnel from dorsal to palmar. Pull one end of the tendon graft from the palmar side to the dorsum with the suture retriever.
- Pass a straight hemostat from dorsal to palmar over the ulnar head and proximal to any TFCC remnant. Push the straight hemostat through the palmar DRUJ capsule. Grasp the palmar end of the graft and pull it into the ulnocarpal joint, proximal to the TFCC remnant. Avoid catching tendons and the neurovascular bundle as the palmar end of the graft is delivered from palmar to dorsal and out the dorsal incision.
- Use the suture retriever to pull both limbs of the graft proximally through the tunnel in the distal ulna, passing the grafts from the fovea distally to the cortex of the ulnar neck proximally.

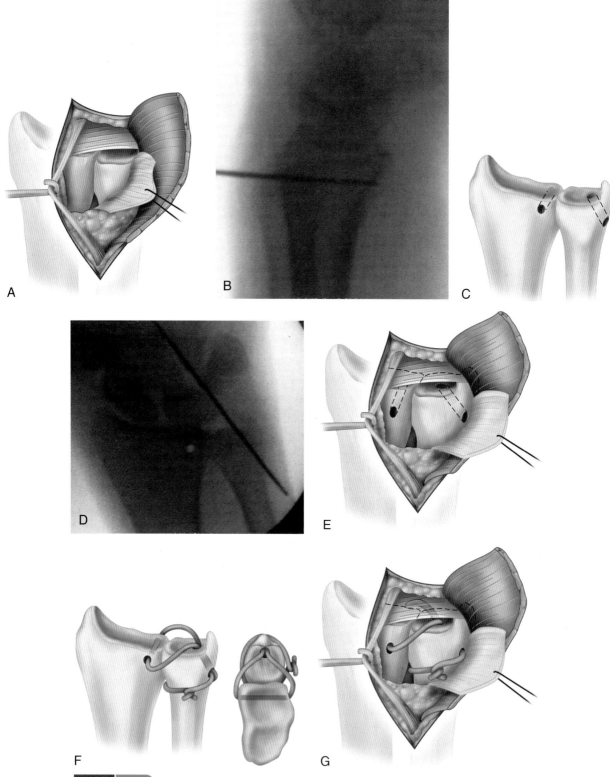

FIGURE 6.64   Anatomic reconstruction of distal radioulnar ligaments. **A,** Retraction of capsular flap to expose articular surface of distal radioulnar joint and proximal surface of triangular fibrocartilage complex. **B,** Position of guidewire for creating radial tunnel. **C,** Location of radial and ulnar tunnels. **D,** Position of guidewire for creating tunnel through ulnar head and neck (radial tunnel also can be seen). **E,** Deep exposure and location of bone tunnels for tendon graft. **F,** Tendon graft passed through bone tunnels and volar capsule of distal radioulnar joint. **G,** Completed passage of tendon graft. (**A, C, E-G,** redrawn from and **B** and **D** from Adams BD, Berger RA: An anatomic reconstruction of the distal radioulnar ligaments for posttraumatic distal radioulnar joint instability, *J Hand Surg* 27A:243, 2002.) **SEE TECHNIQUE 6.30.**

- At the ulnar neck, pass a hemostat from the interosseous space, radial to ulnar under the extensor carpi ulnaris sheath, dorsal to the ulna. Grasp one limb of the graft with this hemostat and deliver it dorsal to the ulna, beneath the extensor carpi ulnaris sheath, into the dorsal incision.
- Pass a medium-sized right-angle clamp (Kantrowicz) from the dorsal incision, between the radius and ulna, around the neck of the ulna, deep to the flexor carpi ulnaris, to the palmar medial (ulnar) side of the neck of the ulna to retrieve the other limb of the tendon graft. Pass this limb of the tendon graft around the ulnar neck from palmar to dorsal, avoiding the ulnar neurovascular bundle and flexor tendons.
- Deliver this limb of the tendon graft into the dorsal incision. Both limbs of the tendon graft are now in the dorsal incision and should lie at the ulnar neck.
- Place the forearm in neutral rotation.
- Pull both limbs of the tendon graft taut and manually compress the DRUJ. Place a "half-hitch" in the two limbs of the graft at the ulnar neck. Maintain maximal tension on the graft and suture the limbs of the graft together at the half-hitch with 3-0 nonabsorbable sutures (Fig. 6.64F,G).
- Close the dorsal DRUJ capsule and extensor retinaculum in layers with 3-0 sutures. Leave the extensor digiti quinti in the subcutaneous tissue over the DRUJ. Close the palmar skin in layers.
- If there is concern about the durability of the repair or patient compliance, pin the ulna to the radius with a pin of sufficient size to stabilize the DRUJ and to minimize the chance of pin breakage. To avoid fracture through the ulnar tunnel, place the pin at least 2 cm proximal to the ulnar tunnel. In anticipation of possible pin breakage, advance the pin through the lateral radial cortex and through the skin on the lateral (radial) side, and cut the point of the pin off beneath the skin. Cut the trailing shaft of the pin beneath the skin on the medial (ulnar) side of the forearm.
- Apply a long arm cast with the forearm in neutral rotation to control rotation sufficiently and protect the repair.

POSTOPERATIVE CARE If nonabsorbable skin closure is used, the sutures or staples are removed and the cast is changed at 10 to 14 days. If the pin causes irritation of the superficial radial nerve, it can be backed out enough to relieve the irritation. The long arm cast is worn for 6 weeks. The pin is removed at 6 weeks. A well-molded, ulnar-gutter wrist splint is applied to prevent extreme forearm rotation and wrist deviation; this splint is worn for another 4 weeks. During the 4 weeks of removable splinting, active wrist motion, gentle hand strengthening, and active forearm rotation are begun but passive motion exercises are avoided. Supination and pronation may be regained gradually over 4 to 6 months. If grip strength and wrist motion have recovered, most activities are permitted after 4 months, but heavy lifting and impact loading should be avoided for 6 months.

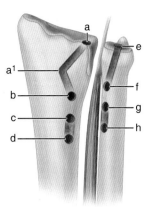

FIGURE 6.65 Scheker technique. Two tunnels each are made in radius and ulna. See text for description. (From the Christine M. Kleinert Institute for Hand and Microsurgery, Inc.) **SEE TECHNIQUE 6.31.**

RECONSTRUCTION OF THE DORSAL LIGAMENT OF THE TRIANGULAR FIBROCARTILAGE COMPLEX

TECHNIQUE 6.31

(SCHEKER ET AL.)
- With a proximal tourniquet inflated and the forearm in pronation, make an angled incision in the skin overlying the junction between the fourth and fifth extensor compartments.
- Open the deep fascia between the extensor digitorum and extensor carpi radialis brevis tendons proximal to the extensor retinaculum.
- Retract the musculotendinous units, exposing the dorsoulnar aspect of the distal radius, just distal to the extensor pollicis brevis.
- Perform a small capsulotomy between the fourth and fifth compartments, exposing the dorsal corner of the sigmoid notch (Fig. 6.65).
- Use a heavy Kirschner wire to drill a tunnel in the distal radius, starting from the dorsal lip of the sigmoid notch and proceeding in a proximal, radial, and palmar direction into the medullary cavity (Fig. 6.65, a-a^1).
- Make a second tunnel in the metaphysis of the radius, starting about 3 cm proximal and radial to the lip of the sigmoid notch and proceeding in a distal radial and palmar direction to meet the previous tunnel in the medullary cavity (Fig. 6.65, b-a^1). This creates an angulated tunnel in the distal radius, which is enlarged with a hand drill using a 3-mm drill bit (Fig. 6.65, a-a^1-b).
- Make two more unicortical holes, measuring 3.0 to 3.5 mm in diameter in the radial metaphysis at 1-cm intervals each (Fig. 6.65, c and d). Connect these two holes within the medulla with a large tendon hook and smooth the tunnel to facilitate passage of the tendon graft.
- Approach the radial aspect of the distal ulna between the fifth and sixth compartment muscles and retract the soft tissues.

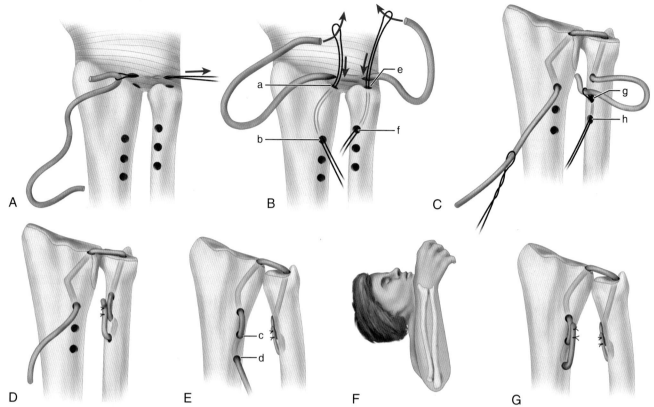

FIGURE 6.66   Scheker technique. **A,** Tendon graft is drawn through capsulotomies. **B,** Ends of tendon graft inserted into loops of wire emerging from tunnels in ulnar fovea and dorsal lip of sigmoid notch of radius. **C,** Tendon graft is drawn through two distal tunnels. **D,** Ulnar end of tendon graft is threaded through second tunnel and sutured to itself. **E,** Tendon graft is pulled between middle and distal hole in metaphysis of radius to ensure that full tension has been applied between fovea and sigmoid notch. **F,** With tension applied to radial end of tendon graft while forearm is supinated, joint stability is tested through full range of motion. **G,** On radial side, graft is sutured to itself with forearm in supination, completing reconstruction of dorsal ligament. (From the Christine M. Kleinert Institute for Hand and Microsurgery, Inc.) **SEE TECHNIQUE 6.31.**

- Open the capsule at the level of the ulnar styloid just radial to the tendon of the extensor carpi ulnaris.
- Use a heavy Kirschner wire to make a tunnel from the fovea within the medulla to the dorsoradial side of the ulnar cortex (Fig. 6.65, e and f). Enlarge this tunnel with a 3-mm drill.
- Make two more drill holes 1 cm apart along the distal ulna and connect to form a tunnel within the medullary canal (Fig. 6.65, g and h).
- Use small angulated mosquito forceps to pass a loop of "O" wire into the radial capsulotomy, through the DRUJ, and out of the ulnar capsulotomy. Draw a palmaris longus tendon graft through using the wire loop (Fig. 6.66A).
- Using the wire loop technique, pull the radial end of the tendon graft into hole *a* and out of hole *b*. Pull the ulnar end of the tendon graft into hole *e* and out of hole *f* (Fig. 6.66B). Route this tendon end into the medulla of the ulna through hole *g* and out through hole *h* (Fig. 6.66C).
- Suture the ulnar end of the tendon to itself with 3-0 braided Ticron suture (Fig. 6.66D). Attach the ulnar side first because when the hand is supinated the ulnar tunnel rotates toward the volar aspect and disappears from

view. Using a similar technique, pull the radial end of the tendon graft into hole *c* and out of hole *d* (Fig. 6.66E).
- Place the forearm in full supination (Fig. 6.66F). Apply tension to the radial end of the tendon graft and assess the stability of the DRUJ in pronation and supination. Tighten the radial end of the tendon in supination and suture to itself (Fig. 6.66G). During wound closure, maintain the forearm in supination.

POSTOPERATIVE CARE   The forearm is immobilized in neutral rotation in a long arm cast for 3 weeks. At that time, the sutures are removed and a new cast is applied with the forearm in 20 to 30 degrees of pronation for an additional 3 weeks. Active range-of-motion exercises begin at 6 weeks, followed by passive motion at 10 weeks.

■ ULNAR IMPACTION-ABUTMENT AND DISTAL RADIOULNAR JOINT ARTHRITIS

Symptoms of ulnar wrist pain aggravated by ulnar deviation with forearm rotation may be caused by ulnocarpal impaction. Ulnocarpal loads may be increased by 42% for a positive ulnar variation of 2.5 mm and 65% with a 45-degree dorsal tilt of the distal radius. Patients with acquired or developmental ulnar-positive variation may develop degenerative changes in the triangular fibrocartilage, ulnar head, articular surfaces of the lunate and triquetrum, and lunotriquetral interosseous ligament.

Ulnocarpal abutment/impaction should be differentiated from ulnostyloid abutment/impaction. Patients with ulnostyloid abutment experience pain with ulnar deviation and forearm supination, whereas those with ulnocarpal abutment experience pain with ulnar deviation and forearm pronation or with the forearm in a neutral position. An old styloid nonunion is a frequent cause. Operative management of ulnostyloid impaction is styloidectomy, and for ulnocarpal impaction, arthroscopic TFCC debridement and ulnar wafer resection are indicated.

Positive ulnar variation may be a normal finding or may be part of a developmental abnormality such as Madelung deformity (see chapter 17). Shortening of the radius after fracture, radial head fracture-dislocation with interosseous membrane injury (Essex-Lopresti), and traumatic growth arrest of the distal radius are causes of acquired ulnar-positive variation. Physical findings may include ulnocarpal pain aggravated by passive ulnar deviation. Passive dorsal translation of the ulnar side of the carpus by pushing dorsally against the palmar surface of the pisiform while stabilizing the distal ulna also may produce pain. Arthritis in the DRUJ and pisotriquetral joints may coexist and produce similar symptoms and findings.

Routine, neutral rotation radiographs may show ulnar-positive variation without stress. Tomaino reported that the pronated grip view showed an average increased ulnar-positive variation of 2.5 mm, suggesting that dynamic changes may contribute to symptoms in a patient with indefinite static radiographs. Radiographic findings, in addition to an ulnar-positive variation, include cystic changes in the lunate and ulnar head. DRUJ arthritis also may be shown by DRUJ narrowing and osteophyte formation.

Operative treatment may be needed if there is no improvement in symptoms with activity modification, splinting, oral medications, and injections of corticosteroids. Arthroscopic joint debridement, open or arthroscopic distal ulnar resection, and ulnar shortening osteotomy may be effective in reducing symptoms of ulnocarpal impaction-abutment, especially if there is no DRUJ arthritis. For an ulnar-neutral to slightly positive wrist, arthroscopic joint debridement may suffice. Pain may persist if there is significant ulnar-positive change. For ulnar-positive variation caused by radial shortening after fracture, open or arthroscopic distal ulnar resection provides satisfactory results without risks of nonunion and implant complications. Ulnar shortening osteotomy also restores joint congruity, and a high rate of bone healing is expected with current fixation techniques.

Arthritic changes in the DRUJ may be attributed to osteoarthritis, posttraumatic changes secondary to fractures or instability, and rheumatoid arthritis. Operative treatment options for arthritis of the DRUJ include excisional or implant arthroplasty and modified arthrodesis. No single procedure is always successful. Salvage procedures for a painful distal ulnar stump after resection include tethering procedures, excision of much of the ulna, and radioulnar fusion to create a "one-bone" forearm.

ULNAR SHORTENING OSTEOTOMY

TECHNIQUE 6.32

(CHUN AND PALMER)

- Preoperative planning includes estimation of ulnar-positive variation radiographically. Plan to achieve a final ulnar variation of 0 or −1 mm.
- After the induction of satisfactory anesthesia, with the patient supine and the extremity on a hand table, apply a well-padded tourniquet to the upper arm, prepare the skin, and arrange the drapes. Exsanguinate the limb and inflate the tourniquet as needed. Use intraoperative C-arm fluoroscopy to verify satisfactory shortening of the ulna and placement of plate and screws.
- Beginning at the ulnar neck, make a longitudinal incision on the ulnar (medial) side of the distal forearm, over the subcutaneous surface of the ulna, long enough to allow for completion of the osteotomy, manipulation of the fragments, and placement of a six-hole plate. Protect the dorsal sensory branch of the ulnar nerve.
- Open the fascia between the flexor carpi ulnaris and the extensor carpi ulnaris.
- Expose the dorsum of the ulna subperiosteally. Avoid wide stripping of the periosteum distally.
- Align a six-hole, 3.5-mm dynamic compression plate on the dorsum of the distal ulna so that the distal end is at about the ulnar neck, just proximal to the sigmoid notch. Contour the plate to fit the ulna and secure it to the dorsum of the ulna with a plate clamp.
- Insert the two distal screws in the plate.
- Locate an osteotomy site at the middle of the plate. At the osteotomy site, use an electric cautery to make a longitudinal mark on the ulna for rotational orientation. Loosen the distal screw and remove the second screw. Hinging on the distal screw, swing the plate out of the way (Fig. 6.67A).
- Use the oscillating saw to make an oblique osteotomy through 70% of the ulna (Fig. 6.67B). Osteotomize the ulna from the medial (ulnar) side from proximal-medial, to distal-lateral. Make the osteotomy sufficiently oblique that a screw would fit across the osteotomy. Measure the thickness of the bone to be removed.
- Place a free saw blade in the first cut. Make a second cut parallel to the first cut (Fig. 6.67B).
- Remove the resected bone and reduce the ulnar osteotomy.
- Rotate the plate into position over the ulna, tighten the first screw, and replace and tighten the second screw. Secure the plate to the proximal fragment with a bone clamp. Use fluoroscopy to assess the ulnar length. Secure the plate to the ulna by inserting the remaining screws, using a dynamic compression technique.
- Place a separate, independent, interfragmentary screw at 90 degrees to the plate (Fig. 6.67C).
- Apply a short arm cast.

POSTOPERATIVE CARE The cast is changed and sutures are removed at about 2 weeks. The cast is worn for at least 4 weeks. Range-of-motion exercises are begun at 4 weeks. The limb is maintained in a removable splint, and strenuous activities are limited until bone healing has been achieved (Fig. 6.68).

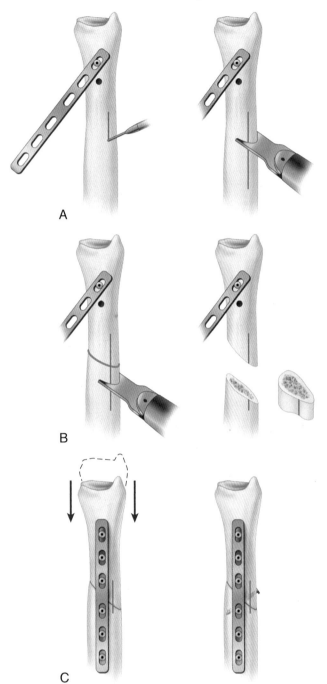

A

B

C

FIGURE 6.67 Ulnar shortening osteotomy. **A,** Six-hole 3.5-mm AO plate is placed on dorsal surface of ulna, and two most distal screws are inserted. Longitudinal mark is made with electrocautery for rotational orientation. **B,** Oscillating saw is used to make oblique osteotomy through 70% of ulna. **C,** Plate is secured to ulna with dynamic compression technique. **SEE TECHNIQUE 6.32.**

LIMITED ULNAR HEAD EXCISION: HEMIRESECTION INTERPOSITION ARTHROPLASTY

The TFCC provides (1) a stable radioulnar connection, (2) a stable ulnocarpal connection, (3) a mechanism for transmitting forces from the hand, (4) a suspensory ligament function for the ulnar side of the carpus from the radius, and (5) an extended dividing surface for the proximal row across the distal end of the forearm bones. A DRUJ arthroplasty involving partial ulnar head resection was developed by Bowers to maintain the triangular fibrocartilage function. This technique is indicated for (1) unreconstructable fractures of the ulnar head, (2) ulnocarpal impingement syndrome with incongruity of the DRUJ, (3) rheumatoid arthritis involving the DRUJ, (4) posttraumatic arthritis and osteoarthritis of the DRUJ, and (5) chronic painful triangular fibrocartilage tear. The procedure is contraindicated if there is no reconstructable TFCC. Without the TFCC, the hemiresection interposition technique is not believed to have a significant advantage over ulnar shortening techniques.

TECHNIQUE 6.33

(BOWERS)

- Begin the incision 5 to 7 cm proximal to the ulnocarpal joint on the dorsal aspect of the distal ulna. Extend the incision distally and at the level of the ulnocarpal joint curve or angle palmarward for 1 to 2 cm.
- Carefully protect the cutaneous nerves to the skin in the area and expose the extensor retinaculum and the distal ulnocarpal area to the fascia.
- Elevate retinacular flaps, raising a proximal flap based laterally and a distal flap based medially. Develop these flaps for exposure and for tissue for extensor carpi ulnaris stabilization or triangular fibrocartilage augmentation. Otherwise, reattach the flaps, use them for coverage of the arthroplasty, or excise them.
- If the extensor carpi ulnaris is stable, reflect it laterally with subperiosteal dissection to expose the distal ulna.
- If the extensor carpi ulnaris is unstable, mobilize it distally to its insertion on the fifth metacarpal. Use the proximal flap to fashion a sling, pass it around the extensor carpi ulnaris, and suture it to the fourth extensor compartment (Fig. 6.69).
- After the retinacular flaps have been elevated, detach the radioulnar joint capsule distally, laterally (radially), and proximally and reflect it medially (ulnarward) to expose the articular surface.
- Remove the synovium, ulnar head articular surface, and subchondral bone with osteotomes and rongeurs.
- Remove osteophytes around the sigmoid notch and remove all subchondral bone of the ulnar head. Leave the styloid axis and ulnar shaft resembling a tapering, 1-cm dowel (Fig. 6.70).
- Inspect the triangular fibrocartilage carefully. Central perforation repairs are unnecessary.
- With the wrist in ulnar deviation, compress and rotate the radial and ulnar shafts. If there is ulnocarpal abutment or impingement, consider ulnar shortening. If it cannot be determined preoperatively or during surgery, fill the radioulnar space with a ball of tendon or muscle and stabilize the tendon to dorsal and volar capsules with sutures. Use tendon from the palmaris longus, extensor carpi ulnaris, or flexor carpi ulnaris. This interposition helps prevent radioulnar shaft approximation and stylocarpal impingement.

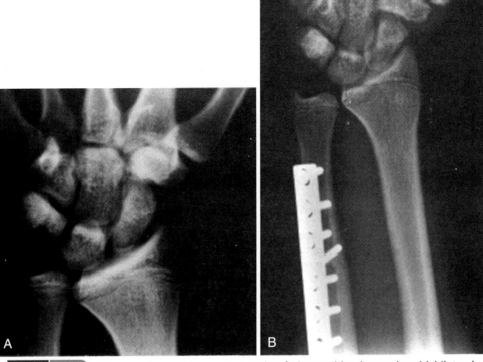

FIGURE 6.68 Ulnar shortening osteotomy. **A,** Wrist of 16-year-old male wrestler with bilateral ulnar wrist pain and positive ulnar variance of 2 mm. **B,** Four weeks after surgery, wrist is in ulnar neutral variance and osteotomy is healed. (From Chun S, Palmer AK: The ulnar impaction syndrome: follow-up of ulnar shortening osteotomy, *J Hand Surg* 18A:46, 1993.) **SEE TECHNIQUE 6.32.**

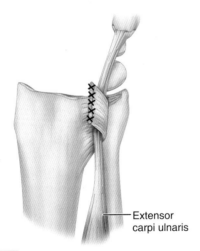

Extensor carpi ulnaris

FIGURE 6.69 Stabilization of extensor carpi ulnaris with retinacular sling. Flap is based on fibrous wall between compartments four and five. **SEE TECHNIQUE 6.33.**

- Close the wound by first replacing the extensor carpi ulnaris compartment, or use a retinacular flap. If shortening is not required, close the wound and apply a short arm bulky dressing with dorsal and palmar splints. If ulnar shortening has been done, use a sugar-tong splint to control rotation.

POSTOPERATIVE CARE The splint and sutures are removed at 2 weeks. A wrist splint is worn for an additional 2 weeks, and finger motion is encouraged. If ulnar shortening was done, a short arm cast is worn for another

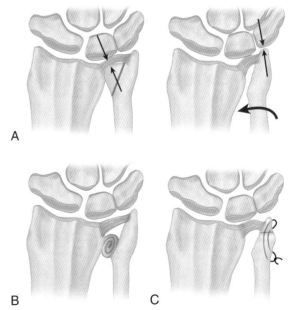

FIGURE 6.70 Bowers technique of hemiresection arthroplasty. **A,** Because ulna is too long, it impinges on stylocarpal ligament. **B** and **C,** This problem can be corrected by interposition **(B)** or shortening **(C)**. **SEE TECHNIQUE 6.33.**

2 weeks and then a short arm wrist splint is worn until healing is complete. If shortening was done in the ulnar shaft, a splint or cast is worn for 8 to 12 weeks.

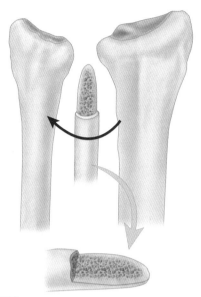

FIGURE 6.71   Matched distal ulnar resection. Ulna is resected 5 to 6 cm and shaped to match contour of radius through full supination and pronation. Distal resected ulna should be at level of radial articular surface. Large cancellous surface adheres to ulnar sling mechanism. **SEE TECHNIQUE 6.35.**

ULNAR SHORTENING PROCEDURES

Numerous ulnar shortening procedures have been described, including the Darrach resection of the distal ulna, the "matched resection" (Watson et al.), the "wafer resection" (Feldon et al.), and a combined distal radioulnar ankylosis (Baldwin) with formation of a pseudarthrosis of the distal ulna (Sauvé-Kapandji and Lauenstein).

"MATCHED" DISTAL ULNAR RESECTION

Watson et al. described matched ulnar arthroplasty for treating patients with distal radioulnar problems caused by rheumatoid arthritis and trauma. Resection of the distal ulna matches the distal radius, and according to the description allows full supination and pronation without impingement, and permits the distal ulna to adhere to the ulnar "sling" mechanism.

TECHNIQUE 6.34

(WATSON ET AL.)
- Place the patient supine on the operating table. After limb exsanguination and tourniquet application, prepare and drape the hand and forearm. Fully pronate the forearm on the hand table.
- Incise the skin dorsally in a transverse straight line or in a zigzag about 2.5 cm proximal to the distal end of the ulna.
- Open the proximal edge of the extensor retinaculum.
- Use rongeurs to resect the distal ulna in a long, sloping shape over 5 to 6 cm so that the distal ulna resembles an eccentrically sharpened pencil (Fig. 6.71).

- Supinate the forearm and palpate between the radius and ulna to ensure parallel matching surfaces.
- Usually, resect the ulnar styloid, leaving the distal ulnar tip at or just proximal to the articular surface of the radius.
- Leave the deep fascia of the extensor carpi ulnaris sheath attached to the periosteum of the ulna because this helps stabilize the ulna during healing. Do not interpose soft tissues because the distal ulna would adhere to the ulnar sling mechanism.
- If the ulna abuts against the articular sulcus in the distal radius, remove a sufficient amount of this part of the radius to allow free movement.
- Confirm free forearm rotation.
- Deflate the tourniquet, obtain adequate hemostasis, and close the skin.
- Apply a bulky hand dressing, supported with a splint.

POSTOPERATIVE CARE   After about 7 days, the splint is removed and a course of rehabilitation directed at achieving full mobilization is begun. Sutures are removed at 10 to 14 days. Most activities can be resumed in 4 to 6 weeks, although it may take longer to return to activities requiring heavy labor and some activities may be permanently restricted.

"WAFER" DISTAL ULNAR RESECTION

Partial ("wafer") excision of the distal ulna has been described for patients with symptomatic tears of the TFCC or ulnar impaction syndrome or both and has been found to provide pain relief and restoration of function equal or superior to those obtained with ulnar shortening osteotomy. Enough of the ulna can be removed arthroscopically to unload the ulnocarpal joint, and combined arthroscopic TFCC debridement and wafer resection of the distal ulna provides pain relief in patients who had TFCC tears and ulnar-positive variation. The procedure preserves the ulnar styloid process and attached ligaments. It is not indicated for distal radioulnar instability, distal radioulnar degenerative arthritis, or carpal instability.

TECHNIQUE 6.35

(FELDON, TERRONO, AND BELSKY)
- Place the patient supine on the operating table. Apply a pneumatic tourniquet and prepare and drape the forearm and hand. Pronate the forearm on the hand table and approach the DRUJ as described for the Bowers procedure (see Technique 6.33).
- Make a dorsal skin incision extending 5 to 7 cm proximal to the distal ulnocarpal joint. Protect the dorsal sensory branch of the ulnar nerve. Leave the extensor carpi ulnaris sheath intact.
- Make a U-shaped incision in the DRUJ capsule, leaving the capsule attached to the radius.
- Expose the DRUJ, the TFCC, and the proximal articular surfaces of the lunate and triquetrum. Inspect the exposed structures to determine the extent of damage.

- Using a narrow osteotome or a small rongeur, remove the distal 2 to 4 mm of the ulnar head, including articular cartilage and subchondral bone (Fig. 6.72).
- Preserve the ulnar styloid and triangular fibrocartilage attachments and the articular cartilage of the ulna at its articulation with the sigmoid notch of the radius.
- Debride flap tears and abrasions of the proximal surface of the triangular fibrocartilage.
- Deflate the tourniquet and ensure hemostasis.
- Close the capsule carefully, suspending the dorsal edge of the TFCC with a row of interrupted sutures. Tightly close the capsule of the DRUJ.
- Close the extensor retinaculum and the skin.
- Apply a bulky compression dressing, supported by a sugar-tong splint, extending above the elbow and holding the forearm in midsupination to relax the capsule.

POSTOPERATIVE CARE The skin sutures are removed at 10 to 14 days; the supination splint is worn for 3 weeks. Gentle motion exercises are begun after 3 weeks, and progression to normal use and activities is encouraged after 6 weeks. Maximal recovery should not be expected for 3 to 6 months.

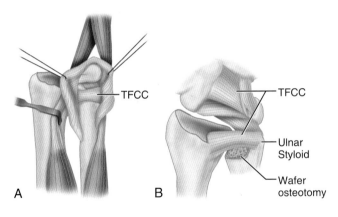

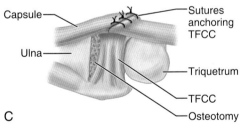

FIGURE 6.72 Wafer distal ulnar resection. **A,** Distally, 2 to 4 mm of ulna is resected to decompress triangular fibrocartilage complex (TFCC), lunate, and triquetrum; styloid process and ligament insertions are preserved. **B,** In left wrist, probe passes through TFCC tear, which can be seen easily after wafer resection. **C,** Sagittal view of ulnocarpal junction, showing triquetrum on right and distal ulna on left. Triangular fibrocartilage, which appears as vertical structure between these two bones, is sutured to dorsal capsule with row of sutures to suspend TFCC under normal tension. **SEE TECHNIQUE 6.35.**

COMBINED ARTHROSCOPIC "WAFER" DISTAL ULNAR RESECTION AND TRIANGULAR FIBROCARTILAGE COMPLEX DEBRIDEMENT

TECHNIQUE 6.36

(TOMAINO AND WEISER)
- After patient preparation and arthroscopic examination as outlined in Techniques 6.1 through 6.3, maintain traction of 4.5 to 5.5 kg (10 to 12 lb) through fingertraps on the index and middle fingers.
- Distend the wrist with 5 to 10 mL of sterile saline solution.
- Insert a 2.7-mm arthroscope through the 3-4 portal. Obtain outflow through an 18-gauge needle in the radiostyloid-scaphoid joint.
- Use the 6R and the 4-5 portals for instrumentation.
- Excise enough of the triangular fibrocartilage central disc to expose the ulnar head. Avoid injury to the dorsal and volar radioulnar ligaments and their attachment to the base of the ulnar styloid (Fig. 6.73A,B).
- Through the 6R portal, insert a 2-mm burr to remove the cartilage of the ulnar head and subchondral bone. Begin on the radial side of the ulnar head and remove the radial portion of the ulnar head the width of the 2-mm burr beneath the margin of the sigmoid notch at the medial (ulnar) edge of the lunate fossa of the radius.
- Move the burr more medially, toward the base of the ulnar styloid, carefully removing the ulnar head.
- Place the burr beneath the triangular fibrocartilage to allow removal of the ulnar head proximal to (beneath) the triangular fibrocartilage to the fovea at the base of the ulnar styloid but do not debride the fovea.
- Passively pronate the forearm to expose the portion of the ulnar head that is most prominent in pronation. Monitor the position of instruments and the location of the bone removal with C-arm fluoroscopy.
- Move the arthroscope to the 6R portal to ensure that the ulnar recession is done to a level about 2 mm proximal to the margin of the lunate fossa of the radius, from dorsal to palmar with the wrist in neutral rotation (Fig. 6.73C).
- Use the tip of a 2-mm arthroscopic probe to evaluate the extent of bone removal. Usually, remove no more than 4 mm of bone. Check the amount of bone removal with C-arm fluoroscopy.
- Close the skin with 5-0 nonabsorbable suture.
- Apply a compressive dressing and short arm wrist splint.

POSTOPERATIVE CARE The sutures and wrist splint are removed at about 2 weeks. A removable wrist splint is applied, and motion exercises and a therapist-supervised program of rehabilitation are begun.

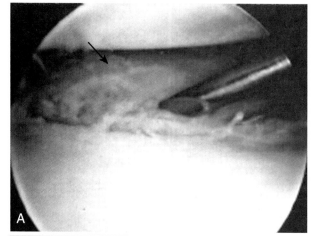

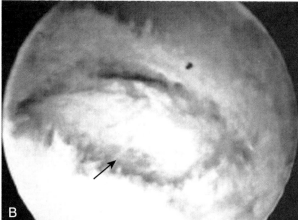

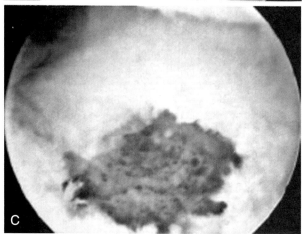

FIGURE 6.73 Combined arthroscopic "wafer" distal ulnar resection and triangular fibrocartilage complex (TFCC) debridement. **A,** Central perforation of TFCC *(arrow).* **B,** After excision of central disc, wafer resection of 2 mm of ulnar head is done *(arrow).* **C,** After completion of TFCC debridement and wafer resection. (From Tomaino MM, Weiser RW: Combined arthroscopic debridement and wafer resection of the distal ulna with triangular fibrocartilage complex tears and positive variance, *J Hand Surg* 26A:1047, 2001.) **SEE TECHNIQUE 6.36.**

DISTAL RADIOULNAR ARTHRODESIS WITH DISTAL ULNAR PSEUDARTHROSIS (BALDWIN; SAUVÉ-KAPANDJI; LAUENSTEIN)

Sauvé and Kapandji and Goncalves found that fusion of the DRUJ combined with the intentional formation of a distal ulnar pseudarthrosis was effective in resolving a variety of problems at the DRUJ. This technique has been used successfully to salvage painful wrists caused by previous surgery, traumatic arthritis, and rheumatoid arthritis. It is effective in providing ulnar-side support to the wrist with extensive distal radioulnar destruction from rheumatoid arthritis. Although a stable DRUJ with ulnocarpal support is achieved, the potential for an unstable proximal ulna remains, leaving few satisfactory solutions for a symptomatic unstable proximal ulnar stump. To reduce the potential for painful instability of the proximal ulnar stump, Lamey and Fernandez modified the technique. They used a distally based slip of flexor carpi ulnaris as a tenodesis through drill holes in the distal end of the proximal ulnar segment, placing the pronator quadratus in the osteotomy ("nonunion") site and suturing it to the sheath of the extensor carpi ulnaris (Fig. 6.74). Johnson and Ruby et al. reported that attaching the ulnar portion of the pronator quadratus through a drill hole in the proximal ulna was effective. In addition to the development of a painful pseudarthrosis, ankylosis or healing of the pseudarthrosis can occur, defeating the purpose of the procedure.

TECHNIQUE 6.37

(SANDERS ET AL.; VINCENT ET AL.; LAMEY AND FERNANDEZ)

- Position the patient supine on the operating table; apply a well-padded tourniquet; extend the arm on the hand table; prepare the skin; and apply drapes to expose the elbow, forearm, and hand. Exsanguinate the limb with an elastic wrap and inflate a pneumatic tourniquet.
- The location of the incision may vary slightly if the patient has rheumatoid arthritis with extensor tenosynovitis. For rheumatoid patients, make a dorsal longitudinal incision to allow extensor tenosynovectomy and repair, grafting, or tendon transfers for ruptured tendons.
- For nonrheumatoid patients, make a dorsoulnar incision centered over the ulnar head. Avoid injury to the dorsal sensory branch of the ulnar nerve.
- Identify the interval between the extensor carpi ulnaris and the extensor digiti minimi.
- Open the extensor retinaculum, forming a proximal flap based laterally (radially) and a distal flap based medially (ulnarward). Use these flaps later to reinforce the extensor retinaculum and the capsule, or they can be discarded.
- Decorticate the radial and ulnar articular surfaces of the DRUJ with narrow osteotomes and a narrow rongeur.
- Temporarily stabilize the DRUJ with a 0.045-inch Kirschner wire.

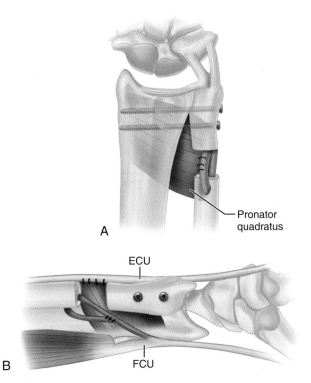

A

ECU

B   FCU

Pronator
quadratus

FIGURE 6.74 Distal radioulnar arthrodesis with distal ulnar pseudarthrosis (modified Sauvé-Kapandji procedure). **A,** Posterior view of wrist with two screws fixing ulnar head to sigmoid notch; after resection, gap, which measures 10 mm, is filled with pronator quadratus. **B,** Lateral view of wrist showing stabilization of proximal ulnar segment with distally based slip of flexor carpi ulnaris tendon (*FCU*). Nonunion gap is filled with pronator quadratus, which is sutured to tendon sheath of extensor carpi ulnaris muscle (*ECU*). (From Lamey DM, Fernandez DL: Results of the modified Sauvé-Kapandji procedure in the treatment of chronic posttraumatic derangement of the distal radioulnar joint, *J Bone Joint Surg* 80A:1758, 1998.)

- Just proximal to the ulnar neck and proximal to the DRUJ, make an ulnar osteotomy with an oscillating saw.
- For patients with neutral or negative ulnar variance, remove a 15-mm segment of ulna with its surrounding periosteum. For patients with positive ulnar variance, remove a larger segment of ulna to allow radioulnar arthrodesis at neutral variance and to allow removal of sufficient bone to allow pain-free rotation, a 15-mm gap, and stabilization by the pronator quadratus.
- Remove the temporary fixation from the DRUJ, and obtain permanent fixation with a 3.5-mm bone screw, using a "lag" technique (Fig. 6.75). Use a washer if needed in poor-quality bone, or use Kirschner wires for permanent fixation.
- Use bone from the excised segment of ulna to graft the arthrodesis.
- Drill holes in the proximal ulnar stump to secure the pronator quadratus from the excised ulnar segment to the proximal segment for stabilization.
- To include the modifications of Lamey and Fernandez, perform the following:

- Remove a 10-mm segment of the distal ulna or sufficient ulna to create a neutral ulnar variance, with a sufficient gap in the bone to create a nonunion.
- Remove all bone debris.
- To be able to resect the bone more distally, leaving a smaller head-neck segment, use a 3.5-mm cortical screw as the lag screw through the ulnar head into the sigmoid notch and a 2.7-mm cortical screw for the more proximal screw.
- Create a slip of the flexor carpi ulnaris, leaving it attached distally to the pisiform. Make the slip about one half the width of the tendon and 8 to 10 cm long.
- Drill a 4.0- to 4.5-mm hole in the volar cortex of the proximal segment of the ulna, about 1 cm proximal to the osteotomy site. Drill the hole obliquely from distal to proximal, through the medullary canal from dorsal to volar.
- Pass the flexor carpi ulnaris tendon slip through the drill hole in the distal end of the proximal ulnar segment from outside the bone, into the bone, and out the distal end of the osteotomy site.
- With the forearm in neutral rotation and the wrist in neutral flexion-extension, suture the tendon loop to itself with nonabsorbable suture (Fig. 6.74B).
- Mobilize the pronator quadratus muscle from the distal segment of the ulna, pull it into the gap between the ulnar segments, and suture it to the volar aspect of the sheath of the extensor carpi ulnaris.
- Use the retinacula flaps to stabilize the extensor carpi ulnaris, especially in patients with rheumatoid arthritis, and to reinforce the capsule.
- Deflate the pneumatic tourniquet, ensure hemostasis, and close the skin.
- Apply a bulky compression dressing, supported by an above-elbow or below-elbow splint or cast. If a patient with rheumatoid arthritis has had other procedures, such as a tendon transfer, more immobilization may be required.

POSTOPERATIVE CARE The skin sutures are removed at 10 to 14 days, and the splint or cast immobilization is continued for about 4 weeks. The wrist is protected with a removable splint for comfort for another 3 to 4 weeks or until healing of the arthrodesis has stabilized. The hand and forearm are gradually rehabilitated with motion and strengthening exercises.

■ PROCEDURES TO STABILIZE THE UNSTABLE PROXIMAL ULNAR SEGMENT AFTER DISTAL ULNAR EXCISION

Instability of the proximal ulna after distal ulnar excision can cause discomfort and a feeling of weakness with grasp and forearm rotation. Various structures, in various combinations, have been used to stabilize the distal end of the proximal ulnar segment, including a volar, distally based capsular flap attached to the ulna proximally; alignment of the extensor carpi ulnaris dorsally beneath a retinacular flap; a slip of the extensor carpi ulnaris tendon, based proximally or distally, passed through drill holes in the ulna or wrapped around the ulna; the pronator quadratus as a combination interposition-stabilizer; a slip

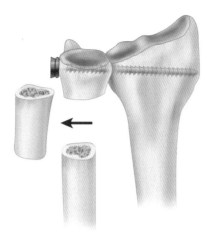

FIGURE 6.75 Sauvé-Kapandji procedure. Distal radioulnar arthrodesis and creation of pseudarthrosis in distal ulna. **SEE TECHNIQUE 6.37.**

of flexor carpi ulnaris tendon, usually distally based and passed through drill holes in the ulna, and a combination of extensor carpi ulnaris tenodesis and dorsal transfer of the pronator quadratus (Fig. 6.76). Breen and Jupiter described a technique that incorporated three components of previously described procedures. They included a distally based slip of the flexor carpi ulnaris tendon, a proximally based slip of the extensor carpi ulnaris tendon, and dorsal stabilization of the extensor carpi ulnaris with a retinacular flap.

Sotereanos et al. have described success with interposition of an Achilles allograft between the distal ulna stump and medial aspect of the radius after failed Darrach resection. The allograft is secured between the two bones with suture anchors (Technique 6.5). A retrospective study of this technique by Sotereanos et al. showed improvement in grip strength of 72%, increased pronation and supination, improvement in pain scores, and no complications with average follow up of 79 months.

Laboratory analysis of two ulnar head prosthetic designs by Masaoka et al. suggested that a satisfactory prosthesis maintains "near-normal" DRUJ mechanics compared with distal ulnar excision. Reports suggest that distal ulnar implant arthroplasty may be an effective solution to failed distal ulnar excision (Darrach). The experiences of more patients with long-term outcome studies will help clarify the proper use of the evolving technology of distal ulnar prosthetic implants. Silicone ulnar head implants have not been found to be durable enough for use in active patients applying significant forces to the ulnocarpal and radioulnar joints.

TENODESIS OF THE EXTENSOR CARPI ULNARIS AND TRANSFER OF THE PRONATOR QUADRATUS

TECHNIQU5E 6.38

(KLEINMAN AND GREENBERG)
- With the patient supine, apply a well-padded tourniquet, prepare the skin, and apply drapes to the hand and arm on the hand table. Sit on the cephalad side of the hand table and pronate the patient's forearm for ease of access to the ulnar side of the forearm and wrist. Exsanguinate the extremity, and inflate the tourniquet.
- Make a curvilinear dorsoulnar skin incision at the wrist level. Extend the incision proximally along the distal ulnar shaft; avoid injury to the dorsal sensory branches of the ulnar nerve. Approach the ulna between the extensor carpi ulnaris and the flexor carpi ulnaris.
- Identify and expose the distal end of the previous Darrach resection of the distal ulna.
- Contour the distal end of the ulna with a burr or rongeur as needed.
- Dissect the pronator quadratus free from its palmar-medial attachment to the ulna (Fig. 6.76A). Mobilize the pronator quadratus radially with its ulnar border tendon to allow its passage from palmar to dorsal through the interosseous space to the dorsomedial aspect of the ulna (Fig. 6.76B).
- Use a side-cutting power burr to ream the ulnar medullary canal for later intramedullary passage of the extensor carpi ulnaris tendon.
- Make an exit hole for the tendon 1.5 cm proximal to the end of the ulna.
- Dissect the extensor carpi ulnaris tendon from the musculotendinous junction distally to, but not into, the sixth dorsal compartment. Split the tendon longitudinally, detaching half from the muscle and leaving the fifth metacarpal attachment and the sixth dorsal compartment intact (Fig. 6.76C).
- Pass the distally based half of the extensor carpi ulnaris tendon through the cortical drill hole in the ulna.
- Use a lamina spreader to maintain the interosseous space between the radius and the ulna.
- Flex the elbow to 90 degrees with the forearm in neutral rotation and the fingers pointing toward the ceiling.
- Pass two divergent 0.062-inch Kirschner wires percutaneously through the medial border of the ulna into the radius. Place the wires in divergent directions to prevent postoperative migration of the radius and ulna; place them proximal to the proximal margin of the pronator quadratus to allow pronator quadratus transfer.
- Pass the pronator quadratus dorsally between the forearm bones and anchor it to the medial periosteum of the ulna.
- Position the hand and forearm in 10 degrees of ulnar deviation and tighten the extensor carpi ulnaris tendon to support the radioulnar interosseous space.
- Deflate the tourniquet, ensure hemostasis, and close the skin.
- Apply a bulky dressing, supported by a long arm splint.

POSTOPERATIVE CARE The postoperative dressing and skin sutures are removed at 2 weeks. A long arm cast is applied and is worn for 4 weeks. The Kirschner wires are removed at 6 weeks, and rehabilitation exercises are begun with active, active-assisted, and passive wrist and elbow range of motion. Splinting is continued as needed for comfort until satisfactory motion and strength have been regained.

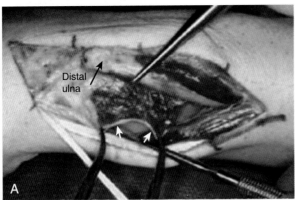
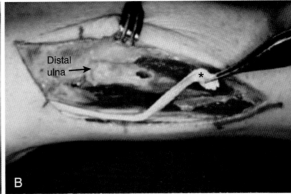
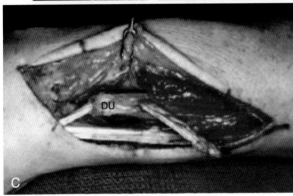
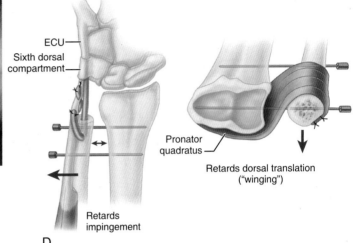

FIGURE 6.76 Reconstructive salvage technique after failed Darrach procedure. **A,** Pronator quadratus *(white arrows),* held by hemostats, is mobilized free from its palmar-medial insertion on ulna in preparation for interosseous transfer to dorsomedial aspect of ulna. **B,** Hole is drilled approximately 1.5 cm proximal to distal end of ulna, through which harvested half of extensor carpi ulnaris (ECU) *(asterisk)* is passed in preparation for longitudinal tenodesis. **C,** Half of ECU prepared for longitudinal tenodesis of distal ulna *(DU);* free end is reflected distally and anchored to itself under appropriate tension before pronator quadratus transposition. **D,** Diagrammatic representation of components of salvage reconstruction. ECU longitudinal tenodesis retards radioulnar impingement, and pronator quadratus transfer retards dorsal translation. Temporary percutaneous pinning of distal radioulnar joint allows complete soft-tissue healing; by 6 weeks, stability can be maintained independently of hardware. **(A-C,** From Kleinman WB: Salvage procedures for the distal end of the ulna: there is no magic, *Am J Orthop* 38:172, 2009. **D,** Redrawn from Kleinman WB, Greenberg JA: Salvage of the failed Darrach procedure, *J Hand Surg* 20A:951, 1995.) **SEE TECHNIQUE 6.38.**

COMBINATION TENODESIS OF THE FLEXOR CARPI ULNARIS AND THE EXTENSOR CARPI ULNARIS

TECHNIQUE 6.39

(JUPITER AND BREEN, MODIFIED)
- With the patient supine, after anesthetic induction, with the upper extremity on a hand table, apply a well-padded tourniquet, prepare the skin, and arrange drapes to expose the limb distal to the tourniquet. Exsanguinate the limb and inflate the tourniquet.

- Use two incisions, one dorsal and the other palmar (Fig. 6.77A,B). Make a 10-cm, dorsal, S-shaped incision, beginning over the carpus, distal to the wrist extension crease, and extending proximally over the ulna. Carefully avoid the dorsal sensory branches of the ulnar nerve.
- Expose the extensor retinaculum and make a Z-shaped incision in the retinaculum, preserving a retinacula flap to create a stabilizing sling for the extensor carpi ulnaris tendon (Fig. 6.77C).
- If the ulnar head is present and a distal ulnar excision is planned, expose the distal ulna subperiosteally or extraperiosteally.
- Protect the flexor carpi ulnaris and the extensor carpi ulnaris with retractors.

- Perform a transverse osteotomy of the ulna at the neck or just proximal to the level of the sigmoid notch. Depending on the size of the patient, the length of the ulna to be excised is 1.5 to 2.0 cm.
- Mark the ulna with an osteotome and proceed with the osteotomy in either of two ways. In the first, use an oscillating saw with a small blade to cut the ulna at about the neck. In the second, drill a transverse line of holes through the ulnar neck and complete the osteotomy with a bone-cutting forceps.
- Expose the extensor carpi ulnaris and create a proximally based slip of the tendon 9 to 10 cm long (Fig. 6.78).
- Supinate the hand, and, beginning at the pisiform, make a 10-cm curved incision, extending proximally along the palmar and ulnar side of the forearm (see Fig. 6.77B).
- Protect the ulnar neurovascular bundle and expose the flexor carpi ulnaris. Leaving it distally based and attached

to the pisiform, create a tendon slip of the flexor carpi ulnaris 8 to 10 cm long.
- Starting 1.5 to 2.0 cm proximal to the cut end of the ulna, use a ¼-inch (6- to 7-mm) drill point to make a transverse tunnel from the dorsal cortex of the ulna, passing through the medullary canal and out the volar cortex, slanting slightly from proximal-dorsal to distal-palmar.
- Starting at the distal, cut end of the ulna, make another tunnel, drilling proximally, up the medullary canal of the ulna to connect with the first, transverse tunnel (Fig. 6.78).
- Use a suture passer or 20-gauge wire loop to pass the flexor carpi ulnaris slip into the medullary canal tunnel, from the distal, cut end of the ulna and out through the dorsal tunnel.
- In a similar way, pass the extensor carpi ulnaris slip through the dorsopalmar tunnel, entering dorsally and passing the slip out the palmar side of the ulna (Fig. 6.79A,B).
- Supinate the forearm. Pull both of the tendon slips taught and suture them to each other with nonabsorbable suture (Fig. 6.80).
- Stabilize the extensor carpi ulnaris dorsally with the loop of extensor retinaculum (see Fig. 6.77C).
- Close the incisions and apply a long arm cast or splint with the elbow flexed to 90 degrees and the forearm supinated.

POSTOPERATIVE CARE If removable sutures or staples have been used, they are removed at 10 to 14 days and the long arm cast or splint is changed. Immobilization is continued for 6 weeks after the operation. A program of therapist-supervised rehabilitation is begun, advancing through a program of range-of-motion and strengthening exercises to unrestricted activity.

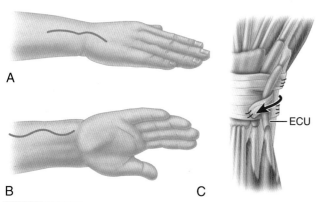

FIGURE 6.77 **A,** Dorsal skin incision. **B,** Palmar skin incision. **C,** Extensor carpi ulnaris *(ECU)* stabilized by sling created from retinaculum. **SEE TECHNIQUE 6.39.**

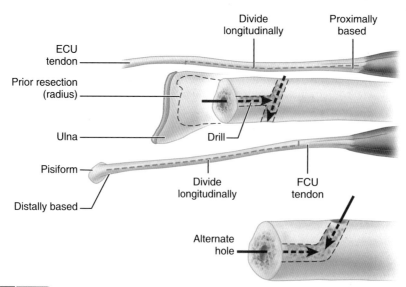

FIGURE 6.78 Combination tenodesis of flexor carpi ulnaris *(FCU)* and extensor carpi ulnaris *(ECU)*. Passage of ECU through holes drilled in medullary canal of ulna. (Redrawn from Breen TF, Jupiter JB: Extensor carpi ulnaris and flexor carpi ulnaris tenodesis of the unstable distal ulna, *J Hand Surg* 14A:612, 1989.) **SEE TECHNIQUE 6.39.**

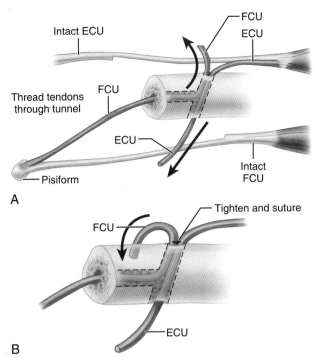

FIGURE 6.79 Combination tenodesis of flexor carpi ulnaris (*FCU*) and extensor carpi ulnaris (*ECU*). **A** and **B,** Tendons threaded through tunnel for start of tenodesis weave. (Redrawn from Breen TF, Jupiter JB: Extensor carpi ulnaris and flexor carpi ulnaris tenodesis of the unstable distal ulna, *J Hand Surg* 14A:612, 1989.) **SEE TECHNIQUE 6.39.**

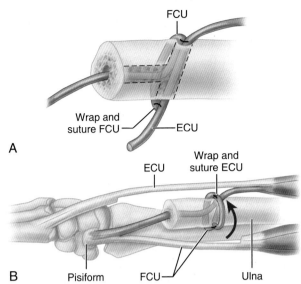

FIGURE 6.80 Combination tenodesis of flexor carpi ulnaris (*FCU*) and extensor carpi ulnaris (*ECU*). **A** and **B,** Completion of weave and suturing of ECU and FCU tendons. **SEE TECHNIQUE 6.39.**

INTERPOSITION FOR FAILED ULNA RESECTION

TECHNIQUE 6.40

(SOTEREANOS ET AL.)

- With the patient supine, after anesthetic induction and with the upper extremity on a hand table, apply a well-padded tourniquet, prepare the skin, and arrange drapes to expose the limb distal to the tourniquet. Exsanguinate the limb and inflate the tourniquet.
- Incorporate previous incisions or incise via the fifth compartment to provide exposure of both the distal ulna and radius.
- Expose the distal stump of the ulna and the ulnar border of the radius; try to preserve distal ulna stump length as much as possible.
- Place three or four suture anchors into the medial border of the radius spaced out by 1 cm each starting just proximal to the sigmoid notch.
- Drill a corresponding number of holes across from these anchors in the ulna.
- Obtain an Achilles allograft, fold it into a rectangle 5 cm × 3 cm and suture it into this configuration.
- Place the allograft between the radius and ulna bones, pass the sutures from the anchors through the graft and then through the holes previously drilled into the ulna. The allograft should be interposed between the two

bones acting as a bumper or cushion. The sutures are then tied over the ulna to stabilize the reconstruction.
- Close capsule if possible; perform standard skin closure.
- Place in a long arm splint in neutral forearm rotation.

POSTOPERATIVE CARE Sutures are removed at 10 to 14 days. A long arm cast is worn until 6 weeks postoperatively and is followed by interval splinting and motion exercises, which are continued for 6 more weeks.

ARTHRODESIS OF THE WRIST

Fusion of the wrist is done most often for ununited or malunited fractures of the carpal scaphoid with associated radiocarpal traumatic arthritis and for severely comminuted fractures of the distal end of the radius. It also is useful for rheumatoid arthritis, for positioning the wrist after Volkmann ischemic paralysis, for stabilization of the wrist in poliomyelitis and cerebral palsy of the spastic type, and for tuberculosis. The wrist should be fused in a position that would not be fatiguing and that would allow maximal grasping strength in the hand. This usually is 10 to 20 degrees of extension, with the long axis of the third metacarpal shaft aligned with the long axis of the radial shaft. Clinically, it is determined by the position that the wrist normally assumes with the fist strongly clenched.

In patients with arthritis limited to the radiocarpal joint, without midcarpal involvement, proximal row fusion (radioscapholunate) was successful in relieving pain in 29 of 31 patients reported by Bach et al. For patients with ulnar translation of the carpus resulting from rheumatoid arthritis, radiolunate fusion has been found to be an effective method to prevent further translation.

Of the many techniques that have been described, most include the use of a bone graft. In some, the graft bridges from the radius to the proximal carpal bones, but in others it extends distally to the base of the third metacarpal. The carpometacarpal joints may be preserved, retaining a small amount of "wrist" motion. Haddad and Riordan recommended, however, that the second and third carpometacarpal joints always be included in the fusion to prevent development of painful motion in them. The disease of the wrist frequently extends into these joints, making a complete fusion necessary.

Because the distal radial physis does not close until approximately 17 years of age, care should be taken not to damage it in patients younger than 17. After partial destruction of the physis by disease or trauma, however, the remaining part can be excised to prevent unequal growth. Fusion of the wrist in children is difficult to secure because of the amount of cartilage in the joint. If possible, operation should be postponed until the patient is 10 to 12 years old.

In addition to many other useful procedures for rheumatoid arthritis of the upper extremity, Smith-Petersen reported a method of fusing the wrist suggested by the exposure of the wrist after resection of the distal end of the ulna. This technique should not be used unless there is disease or derangement of the DRUJ because the procedure uses the distal ulna as a bone graft inserted between the radius and the carpus. It has the disadvantage of allowing limited access to the radiocarpal joint.

Although pseudarthrosis rates for wrist fusions generally range from 8% to 29%, the addition of a plate and screws, as in the AO/ASIF technique (Heim and Pfeiffer), yields fusion rates from 93% to 100%. Modification of the plate (Weiss and Hastings) minimizes the need for plate removal.

Haddad and Riordan described a technique of arthrodesis of the wrist through a radial or lateral approach. It has the following advantages: the DRUJ is not entered, the extensor tendons to the digits are not disturbed, and, because dorsal thickening is avoided, the appearance of the wrist is not altered. These authors reported only one failure in 24 wrists using this technique.

ARTHRODESIS OF THE WRIST

TECHNIQUE 6.41

(HADDAD AND RIORDAN)
- Begin a J-shaped skin incision 2.5 to 3.8 cm proximal to the radial styloid on the midlateral aspect of the forearm, extend it distally across the styloid, and curve it dorsally to end at the base of the second metacarpal.
- Mobilize and retract the superficial branch of the radial nerve. Identify the interval between the first and second dorsal compartments and incise the dorsal carpal ligament in this interval, leaving it attached to the volar aspect of the radius.
- Mobilize subperiosteally and retract the abductor pollicis longus, extensor pollicis brevis, and wrist and finger extensors.
- Divide the extensor carpi radialis longus tendon just proximal to its insertion on the base of the second metacarpal, leaving a stump distally so that it can be sutured later.
- Remove the capsule from the radiocarpal, the intercarpal, and the second carpometacarpal joints.
- Locate the dorsal branch of the radial artery and ligate and divide its dorsal branch to the dorsal carpal arch.

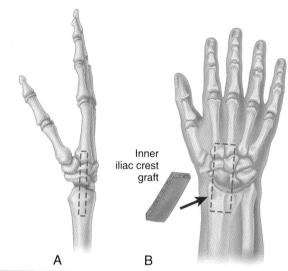

Inner iliac crest graft

FIGURE 6.81   Haddad and Riordan arthrodesis of wrist. **A,** Radial view showing slot cut in distal radius, carpal bones, and bases of second and third metacarpals. **B,** Dorsal view showing shape of graft and its final position *(broken line)* in slot. **SEE TECHNIQUE 6.41.**

- Denude the radiocarpal joint of articular cartilage and subchondral bone.
- Using an oscillating saw and osteotomes, obtain from the inner table of the iliac crest a graft about 3.8 cm long × 2.5 cm wide.
- With the wrist in 15 degrees of dorsiflexion, cut a slot, using an oscillating saw, in the distal end of the radius, the carpal bones, and the bases of the second and third metacarpals. Do not cut through the medial cortex of the radius and enter the DRUJ. Place the graft in the prepared bed (Fig. 6.81).
- If the wrist is unstable, insert a smooth Kirschner wire obliquely or longitudinally to engage the base of the second metacarpal and the distal radius; cut off the wire under the skin at the palm (remove it 6 to 8 weeks later).
- Close the dorsal carpal ligament deep to the abductor pollicis longus and extensor pollicis brevis.
- Suture the extensor carpi radialis longus tendon and close the wound.
- Apply a sugar-tong splint.

POSTOPERATIVE CARE The bandage is changed and the sutures are removed at 10 to 14 days. A solid sugar-tong cast is applied and is worn for another 4 weeks; a short arm cast is worn until healing is evident clinically and radiographically. Exercises are encouraged throughout the healing phase.

The compression plate technique has proved beneficial in providing excellent internal fixation and eliminating the need for prolonged immobilization. In their review of complications after AO/ASIF wrist arthrodesis, Zachary and Stern stressed the importance of preoperative clinical and radiographic evaluation of the DRUJ to minimize postoperative radioulnar and ulnocarpal complications. The fusion techniques with a standard plate and with a specially contoured wrist fusion plate are described.

COMPRESSION PLATE TECHNIQUE

TECHNIQUE 6.42

- Between the third and fourth compartments, make a 10- to 15-cm longitudinal dorsal incision centered over the radiocarpal joint.
- Expose the extensor tendons with their retinaculum, retracting the finger extensors medially.
- Open the wrist capsule with an H-shaped incision to expose the radiocarpal and intercarpal joints.
- Denude the radiocarpal and intercarpal joint surfaces of cartilage and subchondral bone and fill the gaps with cancellous iliac bone.
- Place a 3.5-mm cortex lag screw through the radial styloid into the capitate to pull the carpus against the radial styloid to avoid impingement of the DRUJ.
- Inlay a flat rectangular corticocancellous graft from the ilium into a prepared bed between the metacarpal bases and the distal radius.
- Place a seven-hole or eight-hole, 3.5-mm dynamic compression plate over the graft.
- Compress the radiocarpal joint with one screw in the capitate and one screw proximal to the bone graft in the radius.
- Attach the plate to the third metacarpal (or occasionally the second metacarpal) with two or three screws and to the radius with three or four screws (Fig. 6.82).
- Close the wound over drains as needed and apply a compression dressing, supported by a sugar-tong splint.

POSTOPERATIVE CARE The hand is kept elevated, and finger motion is encouraged from the first postoperative day. The bandage is changed, and the splint and sutures are removed at 10 to 14 days. Above-elbow immobilization is continued for 4 to 6 weeks; a short arm cast is applied and is worn until healing is evident clinically and radiographically. Plate removal is optional, depending on the patient.

ARTHRODESIS OF THE WRIST

TECHNIQUE 6.43

(WEISS AND HASTINGS)
- Make a 10- to 15-cm dorsal longitudinal incision centered over the radiocarpal joint. Incise the subcutaneous tissues sharply, protecting sensory nerves. Incise the extensor retinaculum between the third and fourth extensor compartments. Expose the distal radius and the dorsum of the carpus and long finger metacarpal subperiosteally.
- Use an osteotome to remove Lister tubercle from the distal radius and to decorticate the dorsal fourth of the scaphoid, lunate, capitate, and long finger carpometacarpal joint (Fig. 6.83). Do not include the ulnar midcarpal joints and the second (index) carpometacarpal joints unless they have arthritic changes.

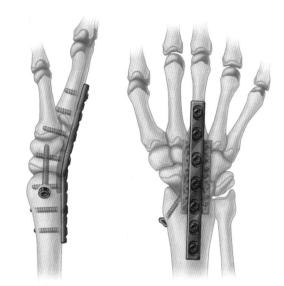

FIGURE 6.82 Arthrodesis of wrist with lag screw and dynamic compression plate fixation. **SEE TECHNIQUE 6.42.**

- Use a large (6-mm cup) curet to obtain bone from the distal radius slightly to the lateral (radial) side of Lister tubercle.
- Use a contoured dynamic compression plate to stabilize the long finger metacarpal-carpal-radius together. Select a plate of sufficient length so that six bone cortices are included in the distal metacarpal, six bone cortices are included in the distal radius, and one or two cancellous lag screws in the midportion fit into selected carpal bones, such as the capitate.
- After placement of the plate, secure the distal screws to the metacarpal first.
- Pack the cancellous bone graft from the distal radius into the denuded bone surfaces.
- Fix the plate to the distal radius, and use a cancellous screw to fix the plate to the capitate. Unless the DRUJ is symptomatic, do not include it in the procedure.
- Use intraoperative radiographs to ensure that the plate holds the wrist in 10 to 15 degrees of extension.
- Deflate the tourniquet, ensure hemostasis, and place drains as needed.
- Close the capsule over the plate with interrupted sutures, close the extensor retinaculum, and close the skin.
- Apply a bulky compressive dressing, supported by a short arm splint.

POSTOPERATIVE CARE With the hand elevated, finger, elbow, and shoulder motion is begun immediately. The splint and skin sutures are removed at 2 weeks, and a molded plastic splint is applied to be worn at all times except during bathing and exercising. In a noncompliant patient, a short arm cast is more reliable immobilization for another month. Hand therapy is begun at 2 weeks. Protective immobilization is discontinued when bone union is shown radiographically, usually at 6 to 8 weeks.

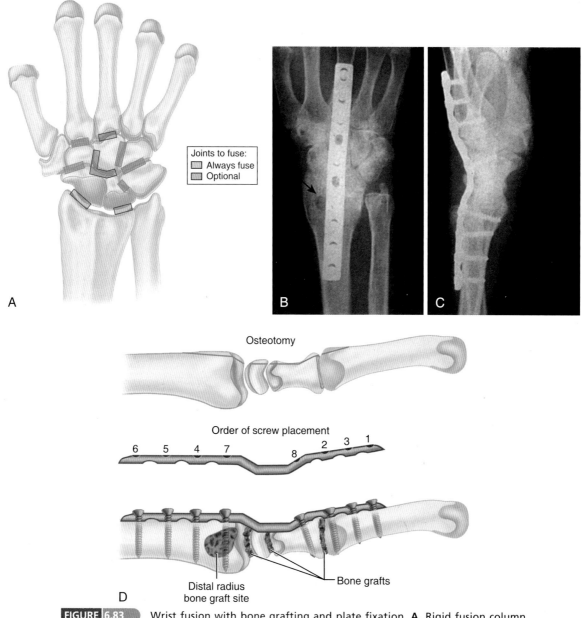

A

B

C

Osteotomy

Order of screw placement

6   5   4   7   8   2   3   1

Distal radius
bone graft site

Bone grafts

D

FIGURE 6.83 Wrist fusion with bone grafting and plate fixation. **A,** Rigid fusion column through carpus to metacarpal must coincide with plate placement. All joints spanned directly by plate should be fused; adjacent joints can be fused if desired. **B** and **C,** Placement of 3.5-mm dynamic compression plate; note local distal radial bone graft portal *(arrow)* and thickness of plate distally. **D,** Dorsal cartilage is denuded, and plate is applied from distal to proximal, spanning local radial bone graft augmentation. (From Weiss APC, Hastings H II: Wrist arthrodesis for traumatic conditions: a study of plate and local bone graft application, *J Hand Surg* 20A:50, 1995.) **SEE TECHNIQUE 6.43.**

Joints to fuse:
☐ Always fuse
☐ Optional

CARPAL LIGAMENT INJURIES AND INSTABILITY PATTERNS

Describing posttraumatic loss of alignment of the carpal bones, Linscheid et al. grouped carpal instabilities into four types: (1) dorsiflexion instability, (2) palmar-flexion instability, (3) ulnar translocation, and (4) dorsal subluxation. Instability in the carpus is considered static if the radiographic intercarpal relationships do not change with motion and dynamic if the intercarpal relationships change with manipulation and motion. Linscheid et al. stressed radiographic evaluation of the proximal carpal row in the lateral projection in which the radius, lunate, capitate, and third metacarpal should have collinear axes within an approximately 15-degree tolerance. On this projection, the wrist-collapse patterns include (1) patterns in which the distal articular surface of the lunate is tilted to face dorsally, known as dorsal intercalated segment instability; and (2) patterns in which the distal articular surface of the lunate faces toward the palm, known as volar intercalated segment instability. In addition, Linscheid et al. advocated

TABLE 6.4

Classification of Carpal Instability

TYPE, SITE, NAME	RADIOGRAPHIC PATTERN
I. CID (CARPAL INSTABILITY—DISSOCIATIVE)	
1.1 Proximal carpal row CID	
a. Unstable scaphoid fracture	DISI
b. Scapholunate dissociation	DISI
c. Lunotriquetral dissociation	VISI
1.2 Distal carpal row CID	
a. Axial radial disruption	RT or PT
b. Axial ulnar disruption	UT or PT
c. Combined axial radial and axial ulnar disruption	
1.3 Combined proximal and distal CID	
II. CIND (CARPAL INSTABILITY—NONDISSOCIATIVE)	
2.1 Radiocarpal CIND	
a. Palmar ligament rupture	DISI, UT of entire proximal carpal row UT with increased scapholunate space PT (actually is a combined carpal instability)
b. Dorsal ligament rupture	VISI, DT
c. After "radial malunion," Madelung deformity, scaphoid malunion, lunate malunion (see "Adaptive carpus")	
2.2 Midcarpal CIND	
a. Ulnar midcarpal instability from palmar ligament damage	VISI
b. Radial midcarpal instability from palmar ligament damage	VISI
c. Combined ulnar and radial midcarpal instability, palmar ligament	VISI
d. Midcarpal instability from dorsal ligament damage	DISI
2.3 Combined radiocarpal-midcarpal CIND	
a. Capitolunate instability pattern	VISI, DISI, alternating
b. Disruption of radial and central ligaments	UT with or without VISI or DISI
III. CIC (CARPAL INSTABILITY COMBINED OR COMPLEX—DISSOCIATIVE AND NONDISSOCIATIVE)	
a. Perilunate with radiocarpal instability	DISI and UT
b. Perilunate with axial instability	AxUI and UT
c. Radiocarpal with axial instability	AxRI and UT
d. Scapholunate dissociation with ulnar translation	DISI and UT
IV. "ADAPTIVE CARPUS"	
a. Malposition of carpus with distal radial malunion	DISI or DT
b. Malposition of carpus with scaphoid nonunion	DISI
c. Malposition of carpus with lunate malunion	DISI or VISI
d. Malposition of carpus with Madelung deformity	UT, DISI, PT

From Dobyns JH, Cooney JP: Classification of carpal instability. In Cooney WP, Linscheid RL, Dobyns JH, editors: *The wrist*, St. Louis, 1998, Mosby.

AxRI, Axial radial instability; *AxUI*, axial ulnar instability; *DISI*, dorsal intercalated segment instability; *DT*, dorsal translation; *PT*, proximal translation; *RT*, radial translation; *UT*, ulnar translation; *VISI*, volar intercalated segment instability.

the concept of dissociative and nondissociative instabilities in the wrist. Dissociative carpal instabilities are those in which there is disruption of the intrinsic interosseous ligaments between the bones of the proximal carpal row. Nondissociative instabilities are those in which the extrinsic radiocarpal ligaments may be disrupted, with intact intrinsic ligaments between the carpal bones.

INSTABILITY CLASSIFICATION

A number of classifications of carpal instability have been suggested, based on anatomic, mechanical, and kinematic

aspects of carpal instability. The classification system developed by Dobyns and Cooney is shown in Table 6.4.

PROGRESSIVE PERILUNAR INSTABILITY

Mayfield, Johnson, and Kilcoyne described four stages of progressive disruption of ligament attachments and anatomic relationships to the lunate resulting from forced wrist hyperextension (Fig. 6.9). Stage I represents scapholunate injury; stage II, capitolunate failure; stage III, lunotriquetral ligament failure; and stage IV, dorsal radiocarpal ligament failure, allowing lunate dislocation from the lunate fossa.

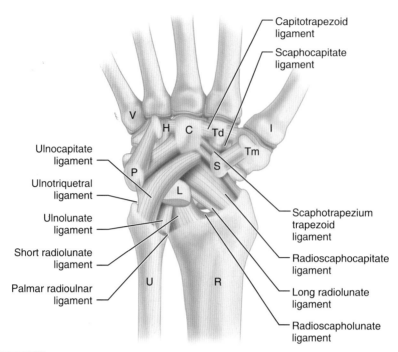

FIGURE 6.84 Interosseous wrist ligaments and palmar radiocarpal ligaments. Key ligaments are radioscaphocapitate, long and short radiolunate, and ulnar carpal ligaments (ulnolunate, ulnotriquetral, and ulnocapitate ligaments). *C*, Capitate; *H*, hamate; *I*, first metacarpal, *L*, lunate; *P*, pisiform; *R*, radius; *S*, scaphoid; *Td*, trapezoid; *Tm*, trapezium; *U*, ulna; *V*, fifth metacarpal. (From Mayo Foundation.)

ROTARY SUBLUXATION OF THE SCAPHOID

Injuries to the dorsal and volar portions of the scapholunate interosseous ligament (Fig. 6.84), the long radiolunate ligament, and the radioscaphocapitate ligament (Fig. 6.3) allow the proximal pole of the scaphoid to rotate dorsally. The scaphoid assumes a more vertical orientation, and eventually the scaphoid separates from the lunate (scapholunate dissociation). Watson and Black observed that rotary subluxation of the scaphoid may manifest in four types: (1) dynamic, (2) static, (3) with degenerative arthritis, and (4) secondary to a condition such as Kienböck osteochondrosis. Although a patient may not recall the specific injury, a fall on the extended wrist is the usual cause. The severity of the initial injury may not be appreciated, leading to the mistaken diagnosis of an uncomplicated wrist sprain. Other causes include fracture-dislocations of the wrist, rheumatoid arthritis, and degenerative changes in the ligaments. Typically, patients report pain with activity followed by aching. On examination, pain and tenderness are present along the dorsal radiocarpal articulation at the scapholunate area. Edema may be present with limitation of motion, particularly in flexion. The following maneuvers are considered to be helpful in evaluating rotary instability of the scaphoid. Watson and Black described a "scaphoid test," in which the examiner places four fingers on the dorsum of the radius with the thumb on the scaphoid tuberosity, using the right hand for the right wrist and the left hand for the left wrist. Ulnar deviation of the wrist aligns the scaphoid with the long axis of the forearm. Applying thumb pressure to the scaphoid tuberosity, the wrist is returned to radial deviation, maintaining the thumb pressure on the scaphoid tuberosity. If the scaphoid is sufficiently unstable, the proximal pole is driven dorsally, and pain results.

Watson also found the "catch-up clunk" to be helpful in evaluating rotary instability of the scaphoid. As the wrist under load progresses from radial deviation to ulnar deviation, the scaphoid normally moves smoothly into extension, aligning with the forearm axis. If scaphoid rotary subluxation is present, the lunate remains in a volar-flexed and dorsal position until sufficient pressure is applied, so that it suddenly shifts from the volar-flexed position and "catches up" with the scaphoid with a "clunking" sensation. Although dynamic rotary subluxation of the scaphoid usually cannot be shown radiographically, the diagnosis of static rotary subluxation of the scaphoid can be made on an anteroposterior radiographic view when a gap of more than 2 mm is noted between the scaphoid and the lunate bones. This gap is seen to increase with an anteroposterior view taken with the fist clenched. Other findings on the anteroposterior view include apparent shortening of the scaphoid and the so-called cortical ring appearance of the axial projection of the scaphoid.

A separation of 2 mm at the scapholunate articulation is not always symptomatic. The affected wrist should be compared with the opposite normal wrist. The lateral view of the wrist shows the more vertical orientation of the rotated scaphoid. The normal scapholunate angle is 30 to 80 degrees (mean 47 degrees), and the normal capitolunate angle is less than 20 degrees (Fig. 6.85A). The scaphoid rotation leads to the development of dorsal intercalated segment instability, in which the scapholunate angle is more than 60 degrees and the capitolunate angle is more than 20 degrees (Fig. 6.85B). Occasionally, the capitate migrates proximally into the gap created by the separation of the scaphoid and lunate, especially when an axial force is exerted on the capitate, as when making a fist. Degenerative arthritic changes may eventually

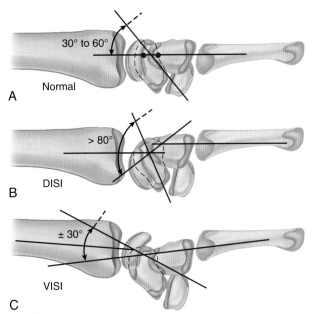

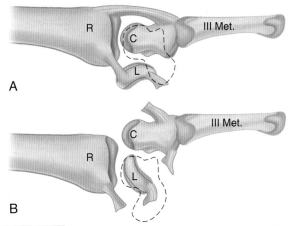

FIGURE 6.86 Anterior dislocation of lunate and perilunar dislocation of carpus. **A,** Anterior dislocation of lunate (*L*). **B,** Dorsal perilunar dislocation of carpus (*C*). *III Met,* Third metacarpal; *R,* radius.

FIGURE 6.85 **A,** Normal scapholunate and capitolunate angles. **B,** Dorsal intercalated segmental instability (DISI) deformity of wrist. Concave surface of lunate points dorsally, scapholunate angle is greater than 80 degrees, and capitolunate angle is greater than 20 degrees. **C,** Volar intercalated segmental instability (VISI) deformity of wrist. Concave surface of lunate points palmarly, and scapholunate angle is less than 30 degrees.

develop. Closed treatment of acute rotary subluxation of the scaphoid consists of attempting reduction by placing the wrist in neutral flexion and a few degrees of ulnar deviation. Percutaneous pinning can be done with one 0.045-inch (1.16-mm) Kirschner wire placed through the scaphoid into the capitate and a second placed through the scaphoid into the lunate. If closed reduction is unsuccessful, arthroscopic reduction and percutaneous pin fixation can be attempted; however, open reduction through a dorsal approach with closure of the scapholunate gap, Kirschner wire internal fixation of the lunate to the scaphoid, and ligament repair usually are indicated. Management of an old rotary subluxation of the scaphoid may require reconstruction of the scapholunate interosseous ligament with a segment of the extensor carpi radialis brevis tendon plus Kirschner wire fixation after the graft has been passed through the scaphoid into the adjoining lunate. Insufficient experience with this procedure has been reported in the literature to provide data for comparing results with nontreatment.

ANTERIOR DISLOCATION OF THE LUNATE

The most common carpal dislocation is anterior dislocation of the lunate. On a lateral radiographic view of the normal wrist, the half-moon–shaped profile of the lunate articulates with the cup of the distal radius proximally and with the rounded proximal capitate distally. On an anteroposterior view, the normal rectangular profile of the lunate when dislocated becomes triangular because of its tilt. An anteriorly dislocated lunate can cause acute compression of the median nerve (Fig. 6.86A), which if prolonged can result in a permanent palsy. If a patient's condition permits, and if swelling is not excessive, the lunate bone should be reduced promptly. Because an open release of the transverse carpal ligament

may be required, every effort should be made to reduce and control the swelling to permit wound closure. When the injury is treated early, manipulative reduction usually is possible. This is followed by open repair of the scapholunate and lunotriquetral ligaments via a dorsal approach. Supplemental pinning of the scaphocapitate, scapholunate, lunotriquetral, and hamocapitate articulations is done as well in a diamond configuration to stabilize the repair. When treated after 3 weeks, the injury can be difficult to reduce by manipulation, and open reduction may be necessary. A dorsal approach has been recommended to clean out the space to receive the lunate, whereas a palmar approach has been recommended to decompress the median nerve as the lunate is reduced. At times, a combined dorsal and palmar approach may be required. When the lunate cannot be reduced by open reduction, a reconstructive procedure, such as proximal row carpectomy or arthrodesis, may be necessary.

PALMAR TRANSSCAPHOID PERILUNAR DISLOCATIONS

Palmar transscaphoid perilunar fracture dislocations are extremely rare and usually result from a fall on the dorsum of the flexed wrist. This is directly opposite to the mechanism that produces a dorsal perilunar dislocation (Fig. 6.86B).

DORSAL TRANSSCAPHOID PERILUNAR DISLOCATIONS

Similar to the isolated scaphoid fracture, diagnosis of this injury may be overlooked and delayed. It can be associated with other injuries of the upper extremity. Early reduction by closed manipulation is best. When accurate reduction of the scaphoid fracture is not obtained, open reduction, internal fixation, and, when indicated, bone grafting may be necessary.

Closed reduction may be possible up to 3 weeks after injury. Most of these injuries later require open reduction and internal fixation with Kirschner wires for stability unless the patient is not a surgical candidate. Although Boyes reported successful open reduction 6 weeks after injury, after 2 months, open reduction may not be possible. Proximal row carpectomy or arthrodesis of the wrist may be indicated.

TRIQUETROLUNATE AND MIDCARPAL INSTABILITIES

Axial loading of a hyperextended pronated wrist contributes to injury of the ligamentous supports of the triquetrolunate and midcarpal joints. Disruption of the triquetrolunate, dorsal intercarpal, and radiotriquetral ligaments leads to laxity on the ulnar side of the wrist. Patients with triquetrolunate instability usually report pain on the ulnar aspect of the wrist, with or without an associated wrist click in radial and ulnar deviation. Usually a traumatic event can be described. The physical examination usually reveals tenderness over the ulnar aspect of the wrist in the region of the triquetrolunate joint, and a click usually can be reproduced in radial and ulnar deviation. Ballottement of the lunotriquetral joint can help in diagnosing this instability. The lunate is stabilized with the thumb and index finger of one hand, and an attempt is made to displace the triquetrum and pisiform dorsally and palmarward with the opposite hand. Usually, excessive laxity, pain, and crepitance constitute a positive test. If the triquetrolunate injury is a tear or sprain, the usual static radiographs are normal. If there is triquetrolunate dissociation, the triquetrum may be displaced proximally on the anteroposterior view. This displacement may be exaggerated with ulnar deviation, creating overlapping of the lunate and triquetrum. Although arthrography can be helpful in evaluating triquetrolunate ligament injuries, arthroscopic examination usually is diagnostic.

Lichtman et al. believed palmar instability in the midcarpal region (capitolunate) to be a manifestation of laxity of the ulnar arm of the arcuate ligament. This laxity allows the proximal carpal row to develop a palmar-flexed position (volar intercalated segment instability). Defects in the dorsal intercarpal and radiotriquetral ligaments may contribute to static malpositioning. Most patients have the sensation of a painful "clunk" with ulnar deviation and pronation of the wrist. A palmar sag can be identified at the level of the midcarpal joint on physical examination. The clunk can be reproduced by passively moving the hand from the relaxed neutral position into ulnar deviation. As the wrist reaches its extreme of ulnar deviation, a palpable sensation, or a "clunk," is noted. At this time, the volar sag is corrected. The radiographic examination usually reveals volar intercalated segmental instability. With the wrist in neutral position and unsupported, the scapholunate angle decreases to less than 30 degrees in the lateral projection (Fig. 6.85C). Video fluoroscopy or cineradiography can be helpful in assessing wrist instability.

OTHER INSTABILITY PATTERNS

Other instability patterns have been described and may require treatment, including dorsal instability patterns related to malunited fractures of the distal radius or lax ligaments (nondissociative), capitolunate instability patterns ("CLIP" wrist), volar instability related to laxity in the triquetrohamate ligament, ulnar translocation of the carpus resulting from severe traumatic or inflammatory (rheumatoid) disruption of the dorsal and volar radiocarpal ligaments, scapholunate advanced collapse (SLAC), and scaphoid nonunion advanced collapse. Triquetrohamate instability usually is associated with other significant ligament injuries in the wrist. Ulnar translocation of the carpus, usually seen in patients with rheumatoid arthritis, also may be present after major ligament disruptions in the wrist. The SLAC pattern usually is seen after conditions that lead to rotary subluxation of the scaphoid, resulting in loss of cartilage and degenerative changes in the radioscaphoid and capitolunate joints with sparing of the radiolunate joint.

TREATMENT OPTIONS FOR WRIST LIGAMENT INJURIES AND INSTABILITY

For acute wrist ligament injuries, options include closed or arthroscopically controlled manipulation and percutaneous pinning. If closed methods are unsuccessful, open repair or reconstruction of ligaments may be required. For instability problems that are seen later and have no significant arthrosis, ligament reconstruction, capsular imbrication, and limited intercarpal arthrodesis are considered. Dorsal capsulodesis can be added to limit scaphoid flexion. If there is fixed deformity, arthrosis, pain, or interference with function, excisional arthroplasty (e.g., proximal row carpectomy), limited intercarpal arthrodesis, and wrist fusion can preserve function and relieve pain. Geissler et al. proposed a classification of carpal instabilities and treatment options, based on arthroscopic findings (Table 6.5).

LIGAMENT REPAIR

Ligament repairs can be made if closed reduction of rotary subluxation of the scaphoid and other carpal instability patterns cannot be accomplished satisfactorily. For primary rotary subluxation of the scaphoid and other carpal instabilities seen acutely, closed manipulation and arthroscopic pinning may be successful as noted in Table 6.5. For rotary subluxation of the scaphoid, Taleisnik suggested that the scaphoid be reduced with the wrist in dorsiflexion and that the scaphoid be pinned to the capitate and lunate with three 0.045-inch (1.16-mm) Kirschner wires. After the scaphoid has been stabilized, the wrist is flexed, allowing approximation of the volar wrist ligaments. Yao also described a case series of 9 patients with Geissler stage I, II, and III addressed with arthroscopic thermal treatment and found good outcomes in regard to grip strength, range of motion, VAS scores, and quick DASH out to 5 years.

TECHNIQUE 6.44

- If open reduction is required, make a longitudinal incision dorsally, to the medial (ulnar) side of Lister tubercle. On the palmar aspect, make the incision parallel to the thenar crease and extend it proximally to cross the volar wrist crease obliquely medially.
- Expose the radiovolar aspect of the wrist by retracting the digital flexor tendons to see the volar wrist capsule.
- Carefully incise the volar radioscaphocapitate and radiolunate ligaments to allow repair at the time of closure.
- Expose the dorsum of the wrist through a longitudinal skin incision centered over the finger extensors. Avoid injury to branches of the superficial radial nerve, and the median nerve and flexor tendons through the palmar approach.
- Open the distal half of the extensor retinaculum, raising a retinacular flap based on the ulnar or the radial side of the fourth extensor compartment.

TABLE 6.5

Classification of Carpal Instability

GRADE	DESCRIPTION	TREATMENT
I	Attenuation or hemorrhage of interosseous ligament as seen from radiocarpal space. No incongruency of carpal alignment in midcarpal space.	Immobilization in cast
II	Attenuation or hemorrhage of interosseous ligament as seen from radiocarpal space. Incongruency or step-off seen in midcarpal space. Slight gap (less than width of probe) may be present between carpal bones.	Arthroscopic pinning
III	Incongruency or step-off of carpal alignment as seen from radiocarpal and midcarpal space. Probe may be passed through gap between carpal bones.	Arthroscopic pinning or open repair
IV	Incongruency or step-off of carpal alignment as seen from radiocarpal and midcarpal space. Gross instability with manipulation. A 2.7-mm arthroscope may be passed through gap between carpal bones.	Open repair

From Geissler WB, Freeland AE, Weiss A-P, et al: Techniques of wrist arthroscopy, *Instr Course Lect* 49:225, 2000.

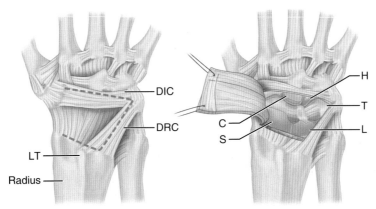

FIGURE 6.87 Alternative capsular incision, radially based between dorsal intercarpal ligament and dorsal radiotriquetral ligament. *C*, Capitate; *DIC*, dorsal intercarpal ligament; *DRC*, dorsal radiocarpal ligament; *H*, hamate; *L*, lunate; *LT*, Lister tubercle; *S*, scaphoid; *T*, triquetrum. **SEE TECHNIQUE 6.44.**

- Retract the finger extensors ulnarward and the extensor pollicis longus radially. Wide exposure of the dorsum of the carpal bones can be attained by raising a radially based capsular flap, using an incision that follows the dorsal radial articular margin proximally, the dorsal radiocarpal ligament medially, and the dorsal intercarpal ligament distally (Fig. 6.87).
- Reduce the scapholunate disruption and fix it with three 0.045-inch (1.16-mm) Kirschner wires directed from the scaphoid into the lunate and capitate.
- Although frequently difficult, attempt to repair the dorsal scapholunate interosseous ligament. This is easier if a small osteochondral fragment of bone has been avulsed. At times, such a fragment can be stabilized with small Kirschner wires, very small suture anchors, or sutures placed through holes drilled in the scaphoid.
- Close the wound and immobilize the limb with a thumb spica splint.

POSTOPERATIVE CARE Remove the sutures in 10 to 14 days, and change the cast. At the end of 8 to 10 weeks, remove all Kirschner wires and begin range-of-motion exercises followed by progressive strengthening exercises.

LIGAMENT RECONSTRUCTION

Ligament reconstruction can be accomplished with free tendon grafts or tenodesis using prolonged slips of wrist flexors and extensors. Complications make ligament reconstruction satisfactory for some patients but unpredictable for others. Tendons, used as substitute ligaments, may stretch and become lax. Bone tunnels for passage of tendon slips may lead to fracture and possibly avascular changes. Taleisnik pointed out that satisfactory results have been achieved; however, the procedures are technically demanding, patient satisfaction is unpredictable, and the tightness required to maintain apposition of the bones limits eventual wrist motion. Palmer, Dobyns, and Linscheid reported satisfactory results using a distally attached slip of the flexor carpi radialis tendon (Fig. 6.88). They recommended that ligament reconstruction be reserved for patients whose ligament ruptures cannot be maintained with closed reduction or patients who have their diagnosis made after about 1 month. Ligament reconstruction is not indicated in patients with associated degenerative joint disease for whom other procedures, such as radial styloidectomy, wrist arthrodesis, or wrist arthroplasty, should be

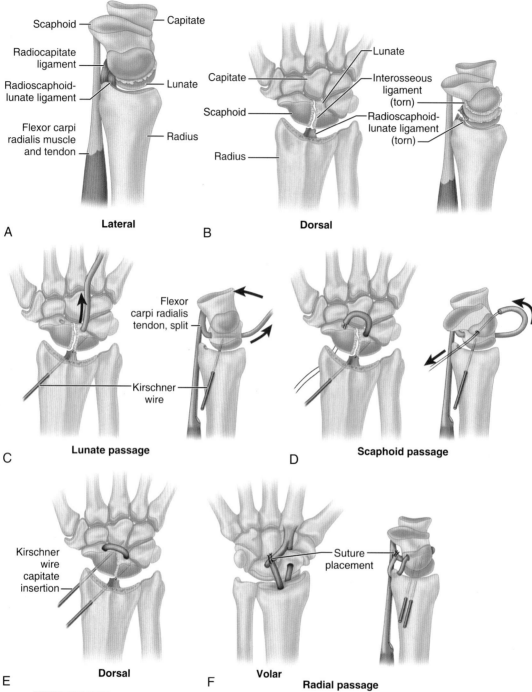

FIGURE 6.88   Repair of scapholunate dissociation as described by Palmer, Dobyns, and Linscheid. **A,** Radial view of wrist showing position of flexor carpi radialis muscle-tendon unit. **B,** Dorsal view of wrist with overhang of radius cut away shows tear of radioscapholunate ligament and separation of scaphoid and lunate. **C,** Both views show tunnels in scaphoid and lunate for tendon passage; first, or lunate, passage (volar to dorsal) of flexor carpi radialis tendon graft slip, and first Kirschner wire stabilization of lunate to radius, done after tendon graft is passed. **D,** Second, or scaphoid, passage (dorsal to volar) of flexor carpi radialis tendon graft. **E,** Carpals aligned in slightly overreduced position with each other and with radius. Position of scaphoid had been stabilized by Kirschner wire through radius into scaphoid and capitate. **F,** Volar and lateral views of wrist showing third, or radial, passage (volar and intraarticular to volar and extraarticular) of tendon graft, which is sutured to itself. **SEE TECHNIQUE 6.45.**

considered. All patients can expect to have a loss of wrist motion after most of the procedures described and advocated for these problems. Almquist et al. achieved success in 36 patients with chronic scapholunate separation, using a four-bone ligament weave reconstruction incorporating the extensor carpi radialis brevis tendon (Fig. 6.89). With an average follow-up of 4.8 years, 86 patients returned to preinjury activities. Criteria for this procedure include complete scapholunate separation (no intact ligaments, widely separated, freely movable scapholunate joint) and no sign of arthrosis. Brunelli and Brunelli stabilized rotary subluxation of the scaphoid with a distally based slip of the flexor carpi radialis, achieving satisfactory results in 13 patients (Figs. 6.90 and 6.91). Kakar et al. described a 360-degree tenodesis for reconstructing the scapholunate interval in patients who have a reducible deformity. A harvested palmaris longus is used to reconstruct both the dorsal and volar scapholunate ligaments through bone tunnels and dual volar/dorsal approaches. Additionally, a suture tape is used to brace the construct internally. The authors of the study suggest that this obviates the need for Kirschner wires, thus allowing earlier rehabilitation.

TECHNIQUE 6.45

(PALMER, DOBYNS, AND LINSCHEID)

- After induction of anesthesia, application of the tourniquet, and preparation and draping of the arm with the patient supine, approach the wrist through dorsal and palmar incisions, allowing sufficient exposure to identify the scapholunate articulations on the palmar and dorsal surfaces (Fig. 6.88A,B).
- Dorsally, the interval between the wrist extensors and the finger extensors usually is satisfactory, although tendons might require retraction radially or ulnarward for exposure. On the palmar surface, approaching the radiovolar wrist capsule through the flexor carpi radialis sheath or to the ulnar side of the flexor carpi radialis, retract the flexor carpi radialis radially and enter the capsule at the scapholunate interval.

- Carefully incise the volar radioscaphocapitate and radiolunate ligaments to allow repair with capsular closure.
- Holding the scapholunate interval reduced with Kirschner wires as toggle levers, carefully drill holes in the scaphoid and lunate for tendon passage; avoid fracturing through the cortical surfaces between the scaphoid and lunate (Fig. 6.88B,C). Start with small drill points and enlarge the holes gradually with larger drill points and curets.
- Longitudinally incise the flexor carpi radialis and split a tendon slip 2 to 4 mm wide from the musculotendinous junction proximally to distally, leaving the distal insertion.
- Pass the flexor carpi radialis tendon slip first through the lunate from palmar to dorsal (Fig. 6.88C).
- With the wrist reduced, stabilize the lunate with a 0.062-inch (1.59-mm) Kirschner wire drilled from proximally through the radial metaphysis into the lunate through the distal radial articular surface (Fig. 6.88C). Secure the Kirschner wire stabilization after the tendon graft has been passed.
- Using wire loops and sutures, pass the tendon slip from dorsal to palmar through the scaphoid drill hole (Fig. 6.88D). Try to overreduce the carpal bones in their alignment with each other and with the radius.
- Stabilize the scaphoid with a 0.062-inch Kirschner wire through the radial metaphysis into the scaphoid (Fig. 6.88E).
- Drill a hole in the distal radius at the level of the radioscapholunate ligament and pass the tendon from palmar to dorsal from within the joint on the palmar surface to extraarticular on the dorsal surface (Fig. 6.88F). Suture the flexor carpi radialis back to itself dorsally.
- An alternative technique described by Palmer, Dobyns, and Linscheid involves passing the flexor carpi radialis tendon slip dorsally through the scaphoid initially, then palmarward through the lunate from dorsal to palmar, and then through a drill hole in the distal radius, and suturing the flexor carpi radialis slip to itself near its insertion.
- Apply a long arm thumb spica cast.

POSTOPERATIVE CARE The sutures are removed at 10 days to 2 weeks. The cast is changed and left in place

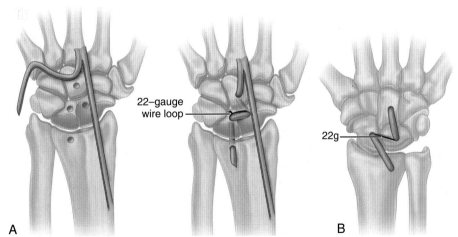

FIGURE 6.89 **A,** Four-bone ligamentous repair. Half of extensor carpi radialis brevis is used for new ligament. Holes are drilled from dorsal to palmar on nonarticular surfaces of capitate, lunate, scaphoid, and radius. **B,** Scapholunate dissociation reduced by 22-gauge wire loop, which is sole internal fixation. **SEE TECHNIQUE 6.46.**

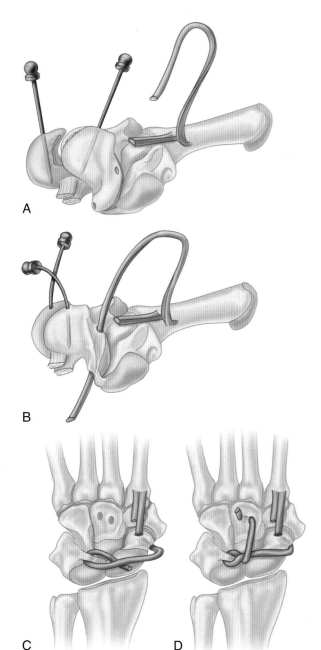

FIGURE 6.90 **A,** Ligamentous augmentation. Some laxity of scaphotrapezial joint is apparent. Strip of extensor carpi radialis longus can be passed through drill hole that is directed through tuberosity. **B,** Tendon is pulled through hole and passed into joint capsule over scaphoid waist. **C,** Tendon is passed through dorsal aspect of lunotriquetral ligament after producing hole with tendon passer. **D,** This is looped under itself and passed distally into hole in capitate. Scaphoid and lunate are reduced and fixed. Tendon can be pulled taut and sutured to itself. Line of pull tends to depress proximal pole of scaphoid, elevate distal pole correcting rotatory subluxation, and rotate lunotriquetral joint into flexion. If ligamentous repair between scaphoid and lunate is not possible, drill hole can be made directly through scaphoid and lunate in oblique directions so that hole perforates midportion of their contiguous articular surfaces. Wire loop using 20-gauge wire passed through parallel dorsal palmar holes in scaphoid and lunate provides internal suture that gives measure of security for repairs of this type.

for 6 weeks, and then the cast is changed to a short arm cast, which is worn for an additional 4 weeks. The pins are removed at 8 to 10 weeks, and range-of-motion and strengthening exercises are begun.

LIGAMENT RECONSTRUCTION

TECHNIQUE 6.46

(ALMQUIST ET AL.)

- With the patient supine on the operating table, the forearm resting on the hand table, and a tourniquet in place, make a straight dorsal longitudinal incision over the fourth dorsal compartment.
- Reflect the extensor retinaculum radially from the fifth dorsal compartment to the third dorsal compartment. Leave the retinaculum attached radially.
- Divide the end of the posterior interosseous nerve proximal to the wrist joint.
- Open the wrist capsule longitudinally, exposing the scaphoid, lunate, and capitate.
- Make a palmar incision parallel to the thenar crease, extending proximally in a zigzag several centimeters proximal to the wrist flexion crease.
- Drill small holes from dorsal to palmar in the proximal neck of the capitate, the nonarticular surface of the lunate, and the nonarticular proximal pole of the scaphoid, 5 to 7 mm from the proximal articular surface.
- Penetrate the palmar capsule without stripping it. Reduce the rotary subluxation of the scaphoid before passing the drill through the palmar capsule.
- To avoid uncertainty in placing the drill hole, use a Kirschner wire as a guide. Enlarge the small drill holes to about 3.5 mm with a larger drill, burr, or curet. Make the holes large enough to accommodate the tendon without stripping or shredding.
- Extend the dorsal incision proximally along the course of the radial wrist extensor tendons.
- Split the extensor carpi radialis brevis tendon in half by cutting into the musculotendinous junction and stripping it distally to its insertion (Fig. 6.89A). If the musculotendinous junction is too far distal, use the extensor carpi radialis longus tendon.
- Pass a locking zigzag suture in the distal end of the tendon, leaving suture ends freely extending from the tendon end.
- Pass a 22-gauge stainless steel wire through the holes in the scaphoid and lunate. Use a wire tightener to tighten the wire loop dorsally, reducing the scaphoid rotation, and securing the scaphoid and lunate firmly together.
- Use another loop of 22-gauge wire as a tendon passer, first passing the loop from palmar to dorsal through the hole in the capitate to retrieve the suture in the extensor carpi radialis brevis tendon.

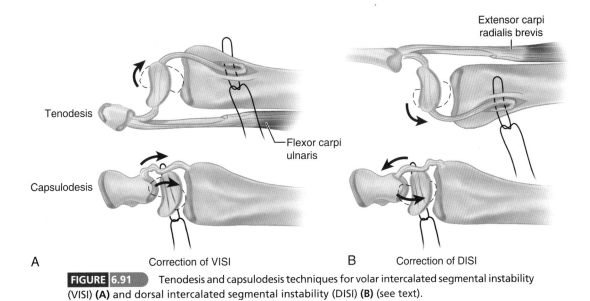

Tenodesis

Capsulodesis

Flexor carpi
ulnaris

Extensor carpi
radialis brevis

A   Correction of VISI   B   Correction of DISI

FIGURE 6.91 Tenodesis and capsulodesis techniques for volar intercalated segmental instability (VISI) **(A)** and dorsal intercalated segmental instability (DISI) **(B)** (see text).

- Using the wire loop, pass the tendon from dorsal to palmar, through the capitate and out through the palmar capsule in the carpal canal.
- Thread the tendon through the palmar surface of the lunate, out dorsally, and over to the scaphoid, passing dorsally through the scaphoid and exiting the palmar surface of the scaphoid, outside the capsule without stripping the capsule.
- Expose the palmar surface of the radius to the ulnar side of the exit hole of the scaphoid to tether the proximal pole of the scaphoid in the ulnar direction.
- Drill a hole in the radius from the palmar surface, exiting in the fourth dorsal compartment. Enlarge the hole sufficiently to allow free passage of the tendon.
- Pass the tendon from palmar to dorsal and pull the tendon as taut as possible through the radial hole. Suture the tendon dorsally to the periosteum, the capsule, or both and to the palmar capsule with nonabsorbable sutures (Fig. 6.89B).
- Close the dorsal capsule and retinaculum and then the skin.
- Apply a nonadherent dressing and a long arm splint.

POSTOPERATIVE CARE The long arm splint and sutures are removed after 7 to 10 days. A long arm cast is applied and worn for an additional 7 weeks. At about 8 weeks, the cast is removed and a removable long arm plaster splint is applied and is worn at all times except while exercising. Range-of-motion exercises are begun after cast removal. At 12 weeks, a short arm splint is applied. Resistive exercises are begun at 16 weeks and are progressed to strengthening exercises.

Taleisnik and Linscheid described another simplified palmar repair technique, using the flexor carpi radialis. This procedure requires dorsal and palmar incisions; tunnels made in the scaphoid, lunate, and distal radius; and the passage of a distally based, longitudinally split slip of the flexor carpi radialis (Fig. 6.90).

LIGAMENT RECONSTRUCTION

TECHNIQUE 6.47

(BRUNELLI AND BRUNELLI)

- With the patient supine, the arm on a hand table, and the tourniquet appropriately padded, placed, and inflated, make a straight longitudinal, 4-cm dorsal incision. Section and reflect the extensor retinaculum.
- Enter the wrist joint through a longitudinal capsular incision between the extensor carpi radialis brevis and the extensor pollicis longus tendons.
- Incise the capsuloligamentous structures between the scaphoid and lunate. Remove scar between the scaphoid and lunate, sparing the articular cartilage.
- Identify the scaphotrapeziotrapezoid joint distal to the scaphoid. Excise capsular scar or thickening in this area to allow reduction of the scaphoid.
- Make a palmar skin incision over the flexor carpi radialis tendon. Avoid injury to the radial artery, median nerve, and palmar cutaneous branch of the median nerve by entering the wrist through the flexor carpi radialis sheath. Remove scar between the scaphoid and lunate so that the interval between the bones can be seen clearly from dorsal to palmar.
- Incise the flexor carpi radialis sheath to the trapezium and trapezoid, preserving its deep insertion. Prepare the flexor carpi radialis tendon by splitting it longitudinally, leaving a 7-cm tendon slip attached to the palmar base of the second metacarpal.
- Drill a small hole in the distal pole of the scaphoid parallel to its distal articular surface. Enlarge the hole to about 2.5 mm in diameter.
- Pass the flexor carpi radialis tendon slip from palmar to dorsal through the prepared tunnel. Pull the tendon slip dorsally, reducing the scaphoid and correcting the proximal pole subluxation and the scapholunate dissociation.

- Temporarily fix the scaphoid, using a Kirschner wire through the distal scaphoid into the capitate.
- Suture the tendon slip to the fibrous remnant of the lunate ligament and to the fibrous tissue at the dorsoulnar margin of the radius.
- Close the capsular incision and the skin.
- Apply a nonadherent dressing and a sugar-tong splint.

POSTOPERATIVE CARE The splint is removed in 7 to 10 days for wound inspection and suture removal. A solid sugar-tong cast is applied and is worn for 4 weeks. At 4 weeks, the cast and Kirschner wire are removed. Active mobilization of the wrist is begun, using a short arm plastic splint. Resistive exercises are begun at 8 or 9 weeks and are progressed with strengthening at 10 to 12 weeks.

For lunate stabilization in patients with triquetrolunate instability (static volar intercalated segmental instability collapse patterns and dynamic dorsal intercalated segmental instability collapse patterns), in whom the instability of the lunate contributes to medial carpal instability, Taleisnik recommended use of the lateral half of the flexor carpi ulnaris in a strip left attached distally and threaded from the palm through to the dorsal aspect of the lunate and secured to the dorsal surface of the distal radius (Fig. 6.91A). For dynamic dorsal intercalated segmental instability deformities, the medial half of the extensor carpi radialis brevis is left attached distally, threaded through the lunate from dorsal to palmar, and anchored under the pronator quadratus on the anterior surface of the distal radius (Fig. 6.91B).

■ CAPSULODESIS

Blatt found capsulodesis useful for two conditions causing impairment of wrist function: scapholunate dissociation and the caput ulnae syndrome caused by DRUJ incongruity. Blatt found it particularly useful in patients with symptomatic dynamic instability and a static deformity and applied it to all patients with reducible scapholunate dissociations.

DORSAL CAPSULODESIS

TECHNIQUE 6.48

(BLATT WITH BERGER MODIFICATION)
- Before the operative procedure, thoroughly evaluate the radiographs to determine the nature and extent of the scapholunate dissociation and rotary subluxation of the scaphoid. Blatt stated, "a single criterion for this procedure is the ability to anatomically reduce the scaphoid at the time of surgery."
- After achieving satisfactory anesthesia and appropriate skin preparation and draping of the extremity and with the well-padded tourniquet inflated, make a longitudinal dorsoradial incision.
- Retract the wrist and finger extensors laterally (wrist) and medially (finger).
- Make a longitudinal incision through the capsule near the axis of the scaphoid. Expose the full length of the scaphoid.

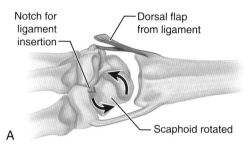

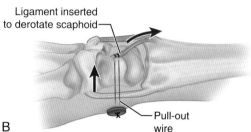

FIGURE 6.92 Dorsal capsulodesis (Blatt). **A,** Proximal-based ligamentous flap is developed from dorsal wrist capsule. Notch for ligament insertion is created in dorsal cortex of distal scaphoid pole. **B,** Scaphoid has been derotated, and ligament has been inserted with pull-out wire suture. **SEE TECHNIQUE 6.48.**

- Preserve a 1-cm–wide flap of dorsal wrist capsule and develop it from the ulnar side of the capsular incision (Fig. 6.92A). This flap is released distally, and the proximal origin on the dorsum of the distal radius is left attached.
- Inspect the interosseous and dorsal scapholunate ligaments to ascertain their rupture and irreparability.
- Reduce the scaphoid with thumb pressure on the scaphoid tubercle on the palm side, bring the wrist into slight ulnar deviation, and transfix the scaphoid with 0.045-inch (1.16-mm) Kirschner wires placed from the distal pole of the scaphoid into the capitate and base of the third metacarpal.
- Make a notch in the dorsum of the distal pole of the scaphoid proximal to the distal articular surface and distal to the midaxis of rotation of the scaphoid with a narrow osteotome or small rongeur.
- Trim the dorsal capsuloligamentous flap to attach into the distal pole of the scaphoid with a 4-0 stainless steel pull-out wire suture. Pass this wire suture through fine drill holes to the volar tubercle of the scaphoid and tie it at the level of the skin over felt and a button (Fig. 6.92B).
- Deflate the tourniquet, obtain hemostasis, and close the skin.
- A variation in technique described by Berger can be used instead of that just described. Detach the proximal half of the dorsal intercarpal ligament, incising down the length of the ligament. Leave the lateral (scaphoid) insertion attached, and detach the medial (triquetral) end of the ligament. Reduce the scaphoid into an extended position and suture the free, triquetral end of the ligament to the dorsal rim of the distal radius. Make this attachment to bone or to the dorsal radiocarpal ligament (Fig. 6.93). Apply a thumb spica cast.

POSTOPERATIVE CARE The cast is changed at 10 to 14 days. Sutures are removed, and another cast is applied and is left in place for an additional 6 weeks. After 2 months,

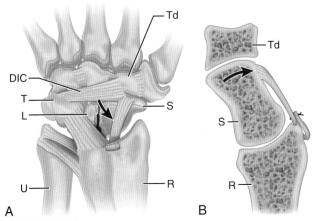

FIGURE 6.93 **A,** Dorsal capsulodesis in which dorsal intercarpal ligament *(DIC)* is detached (50%) from dorsal aspect of triquetrum *(T)* and dissected radially to distal scaphoid *(S)*, where it is firmly attached; then with scaphoid extended to neutral position, DIC is sutured to dorsal rim of distal radius *(R)*, either through bone or to origin of dorsal radiocarpal ligament. *L,* Lunate; *Td,* trapezoid; *U,* ulna. **B,** Lateral view shows scaphoid extension position achieved with dorsal capsulodesis using DIC. **SEE TECHNIQUE 6.48.**

> the cast is removed, as is the pull-out wire. Kirschner wires are left in place. A removable splint is provided, and progressive range-of-motion exercises are started. The Kirschner wires are removed 3 months postoperatively, and range of motion progresses with no forceful stress activities permitted for about 4 months.

LIMITED WRIST ARTHRODESIS

Limited wrist arthrodesis has been used in various forms for rotary subluxation of the scaphoid since the 1950s. In 1967, Peterson and Lipscomb described successful fusion of the scaphoid, trapezium, and trapezoid. Subsequently, Watson and Hempton found the triscaphe arthrodesis to be an effective procedure to resist the forces of movement, tending to keep the scaphoid in a perpendicular position relative to the forearm. Kleinman carefully reviewed the results of scaphotrapezial-trapezoid fusion for rotary subluxation of the scaphoid and found the carpal mechanics to be disturbed by loss of the carpal shift relationship of the scaphoid and lunate. Between 70% and 75% of the dorsiflexion-palmar flexion motion was preserved. In 41 cases reviewed, 11 patients had major surgical complications. The development of postoperative arthrosis, on retrospective review, seemed to be related to imperfect reduction of the scaphoid. This procedure achieved pain relief and preserved a functional arc of motion. Other limited wrist arthrodeses have been reported on an anecdotal basis and include fusions of the capitate and lunate; scaphoid, lunate, and capitate; capitate, hamate, lunate, and triquetrum; and radioscaphoid and radiolunate arthrodeses.

INDICATIONS FOR TRISCAPHE ARTHRODESIS

Watson initially considered three indications for triscaphe arthrodesis: (1) degenerative arthritis of the scaphotrapezial-trapezoid joint with normal thumb carpometacarpal joint, (2) radial hand dislocations, and (3) rotary subluxation of the scaphoid. Subsequently, he added the existence of the dorsal intercalated segmental instability pattern with disruption of the volar ligaments tethering the lunate, allowing the scaphoid to assume a static rotary instability. He also advocated this arthrodesis for resistant scaphoid nonunions, combining the triscaphe arthrodesis with bone grafts. Kleinman considered the clinical indications to be pain at the end arcs of motion, especially in radial deviation; weakness caused by instability of the proximal carpal row at the scapholunate joint; and loss of motion secondary to pain. Radiographic criteria included a scapholunate diastasis more than 2 mm; scaphoid angle of greater than 60 degrees on the true lateral view of the wrist; and foreshortening of the scaphoid seen on the anteroposterior view, in which the inferior margin of the distal scaphoid pole to the proximal pole at the radioscaphoid joint is shortened to less than 7 mm.

CONTRAINDICATIONS FOR TRISCAPHE ARTHRODESIS

Scaphotrapezial-trapezoid arthrodesis is contraindicated in patients with radioscaphoid arthritis or early phases of degenerative changes in the wrist progressing to SLAC.

SCAPHOTRAPEZIAL-TRAPEZOID FUSION

TECHNIQUE 6.49

(WATSON)

- After satisfactory induction of anesthesia, prepare the hand, wrist, and forearm and apply drapes in the routine manner.
- Make a transverse incision in the skin on the dorsum of the wrist over the area of fusion.
- Retract the branches of the superficial radial nerve and the veins.
- Open the extensor retinaculum along the tendon of the extensor pollicis longus.
- Approach the wrist between the tendons of the extensor carpi radialis longus and the extensor carpi radialis brevis, or, as recommended by Kleinman, expose the wrist capsule between the first and second dorsal tendon compartments, exposing the adjacent surfaces of the scaphotrapezial-trapezoid joint and retracting the radial artery.
- Open the scaphotrapezial-trapezoid joint and open the capsule of the wrist to expose the proximal articular surface of the scaphoid. Triscaphe arthrodesis is contraindicated in the presence of significant radioscaphoid arthritis. If this is found, SLAC wrist reconstruction should be done. Observe the following principles as recommended by Watson: (1) careful planning is essential; (2) the minimum necessary joints should be fused; (3) packed, cancellous bone graft arthrodesis with sufficient graft should be used; (4) the external dimensions of the fused unit must equal the external dimensions of the same bones in their normal state; and (5) only the joints to be fused should be pinned.
- Careful attention to the reduction of the scaphoid is required to avoid fixing the scaphoid in an excessively longitudinal or dorsiflexed position. Kleinman recommended

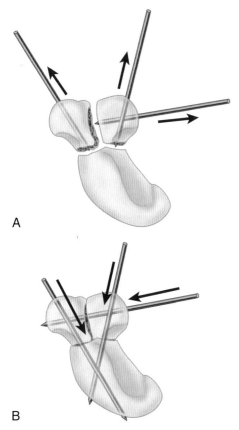

A

B

FIGURE 6.94 Limited wrist (triscaphe) arthrodesis. **A,** Articular surfaces have been removed, and three pins have been "preset" in retrograde fashion. **B,** Cancellous bone grafts have been packed between bones, external shape of triscaphoid unit is maintained, and pins are driven across arthrodesis sites. **SEE TECHNIQUE 6.49.**

introducing a curved instrument palmar to the distal neck of the rotated scaphoid and dorsiflexing the distal pole with it. This allows reduction of the scaphoid to its anatomic position with the proximal pole secured in the scaphoid fossa of the radius.
- Insert 0.045-in (1.1-mm) Kirschner wires through the scaphoid into the carpus to maintain this reduction and correlate the reduction by inspecting the reduced dorsal surface of the proximal pole of the scaphoid and the dorsal aspect of the lunate. The longitudinal axis attitude of the scaphoid should be 30 degrees or more to avoid excessive longitudinal orientation of the scaphoid and subsequent radioscaphoid impingement.
- Remove the articular surfaces of the trapezium, trapezoid, and scaphoid to cancellous bone. Kleinman's modification of removing only the dorsal two thirds of the articular surfaces allows preservation of the carpal height, maintaining the contact surfaces of the palmar one third.
- Obtain anteroposterior and lateral radiographs to confirm acceptable reduction of the scaphoid and closure of the preoperative scapholunate diastasis.
- Usually three 0.045-in (1.1-mm) Kirschner wires are used to secure the scaphoid, trapezium, and trapezoid (Fig. 6.94A). Two pins pass from the trapezoid toward the scaphoid, and one pin passes across the trapezium-trapezoid joint. Remove all hyaline cartilage and subchondral bone.

- Bone graft can be obtained from the distal radius or from the iliac crest. If the distal radius is selected, retract the skin proximally, or use a second proximal transverse incision over the distal radial metaphysis, exposing the radius between the extensor carpi radialis longus and the extensor pollicis brevis. Incise the periosteum, and elevate it between these compartments, exposing the flat area of cortical bone in the distal dorsoradial metaphysis. The use of small gouges allows the removal of corticocancellous bone, and the remaining cancellous bone can be harvested with curets. Control bleeding, close the donor site wound, and pack the cancellous bone into the defect left in the scaphotrapezial-trapezoid joint (Fig. 6.94B).
- Watson recommended placing pins by passing 0.045-inch Kirschner wires retrograde out through the raw bony surfaces. After the scaphoid, trapezium, and trapezoid are positioned for fusion, the pins are drilled across the fusion site in an antegrade direction. To maintain the proper position of the scaphoid with the proximal pole depressed into the radial articular surface, the distal pole is elevated, as noted previously, and two pins can be used to secure the scaphoid to the capitate for temporary maintenance of reduction. Avoid passing the pins from the intercarpal arthrodesis into the radius or ulna. Ascertain that the spaces between the bones have been thoroughly packed with bone graft and that the external dimensions of the fusion unit are the same as the external dimensions of bones in the normal wrist.
- As an addition to the technique, a cortical bone graft can be used to bridge the fusion site on the dorsal surface; this requires mortise fitting or notching into position. Pins are driven across the surfaces previously prepared. Check wrist motion to ensure that no pins obstruct radiocarpal motion, and cut the pins off just beneath the skin.
- Deflate the tourniquet, obtain hemostasis, insert drains as needed, and close the wound.
- Apply a bulky compression dressing with a long arm plaster splint.

POSTOPERATIVE CARE The compression dressing is left in place for 7 to 10 days. After this time, the bandage is changed, the sutures are removed, and a long arm cast is applied. Watson recommended volar extension of the cast to support the index and long fingers in the intrinsic-plus position; however, Kleinman did not find this to be necessary, substituting a thumb spica cast at the time of suture removal. The second cast is left in place for another 4 to 6 weeks. Kirschner wires are removed at 6 to 8 weeks, using radiographs to determine healing. After about 8 weeks, either a short arm cast or a short arm splint can be applied for 1 or 2 more weeks, depending on the radiographs and the patient's compliance. When satisfactory healing has occurred, the hand and wrist are fully mobilized with gradual progression. Although motion usually is limited initially, it should increase within the first year after surgery. The patient is observed closely to avoid stiffness or dystrophic complications, and intervention with physical therapy is instituted immediately if problems such as complex regional pain syndrome develop.

■ OTHER LIMITED WRIST ARTHRODESES

Arthrodesis of the scaphoid, capitate, and lunate; capitate, hamate, lunate, and triquetrum; hamate and triquetrum; radius to lunate; and radius to scaphoid can be done in a manner similar to that described previously. McAuliffe et al. found complications in 36 of 50 patients treated with a variety of limited intercarpal fusions. Nonunion was the most frequent problem. Fortin and Louis reported complications in 11 of 14 patients after scaphoid-trapezium-trapezoid arthrodesis. Among the significant problems were radiocarpal arthrosis, trapeziometacarpal arthrosis, and nonunion. Included here are techniques for scaphocapitate arthrodesis (Sennwald and Ufenast), scaphocapitolunate arthrodesis (Rotman et al.), and lunotriquetral arthrodesis (Kirschenbaum et al., Nelson et al.).

SCAPHOCAPITATE ARTHRODESIS

TECHNIQUE 6.50

(SENNWALD AND UFENAST)
- With the patient supine, the hand on the hand table, and the tourniquet inflated, make a straight dorsal longitudinal incision over the wrist. Incise and reflect the extensor retinaculum. Retract the fourth compartment extensor tendons.
- Make a longitudinal incision in the dorsal wrist capsule, dissecting distally and radially to identify the scaphocapitate joint.
- Remove the articular cartilage between the scaphoid and capitate with a burr.
- Remove a corticocancellous bone graft from the distal dorsoradial metaphysis. Mobilize the skin to allow exposure of the dorsoradial aspect of the radius to harvest the bone graft from the radius between the first and second extensor compartments.
- Place the bone graft in the space between the scaphoid and the capitate.
- Use two lag screws to secure the scaphocapitate arthrodesis with the radioscaphoid angle at about 50 degrees. Obtain radiographs to ascertain satisfactory bone and screw position.
- Close the dorsal capsule and the extensor retinaculum and the skin.
- Apply a nonadherent dressing and a short arm cast.

POSTOPERATIVE CARE The cast and sutures are removed at 2 weeks. A new short arm cast is applied and is worn for 8 weeks. After cast removal, a removable protective splint is worn for another 2 weeks. A graduated exercise program is begun.

SCAPHOCAPITOLUNATE ARTHRODESIS

TECHNIQUE 6.51

(ROTMAN ET AL.)
- With the patient supine and the hand on the hand table, inflate the tourniquet after elastic wrap limb exsanguination.

- Make an oblique dorsal wrist incision, extending from the ulnar aspect of the distal radius to the distal pole of the scaphoid (Fig. 6.95A).
- Expose the wrist capsule in the interval between the third and fourth extensor compartments. Open the wrist capsule with an inverted-T–shaped incision.
- Expose the adjoining articular surfaces of the scaphoid, capitate, and lunate (Fig. 6.95B). Remove the articular cartilage and subchondral bone from the adjoining articular surfaces with rongeurs and curets. Preserve the architecture of the articular spaces and fill them with cancellous bone graft taken from the distal radius or the iliac crest (Fig. 6.95C).
- Reduce any instability pattern that may be present.
- Place four or five intercarpal Kirschner wires in a triangular configuration to fix the arthrodesis (Fig. 6.95D). Place no wires across the radiocarpal joint. Cut off all wires beneath the skin.
- Obtain radiographs to ascertain satisfactory position of the bones and the internal fixation.
- Close the wrist capsule and the skin and apply a nonadherent dressing and a long arm thumb spica cast.

POSTOPERATIVE CARE The cast and skin sutures are removed in 2 weeks. A new long arm thumb spica cast is applied and is worn for 4 weeks. At 4 weeks, a short arm thumb spica cast is applied and worn until there is radiographic evidence of bone union (4 to 6 weeks). A removable molded plastic thumb spica splint is applied, and gentle motion exercises are begun, followed by strengthening exercises. The Kirschner wires are removed at about 3 months.

LUNOTRIQUETRAL ARTHRODESIS

TECHNIQUE 6.52

(KIRSCHENBAUM ET AL.; NELSON ET AL.)
- With the patient supine and the hand on the hand table, after elastic wrap exsanguination of the limb, inflate the pneumatic tourniquet.
- Make a dorsal transverse or a curved longitudinal incision in the region of the lunotriquetral joint.
- Incise and reflect the extensor retinaculum between the fourth and fifth extensor compartments.
- Enter the wrist capsule through a longitudinal incision and identify the lunotriquetral joint.
- Use a rongeur and curets to remove the articular cartilage and subchondral bone down to cancellous bone on each side of the joint. Leave the most palmar portion of the joint intact to maintain joint alignment and to hold the graft in place (Fig. 6.96A).
- Obtain cancellous bone graft from the distal radius or the iliac crest if the distal radius has been used as a bone graft donor previously.
- Use multiple Kirschner wires for lunotriquetral fixation (Fig. 6.96B). Tightly pack the cancellous bone graft into

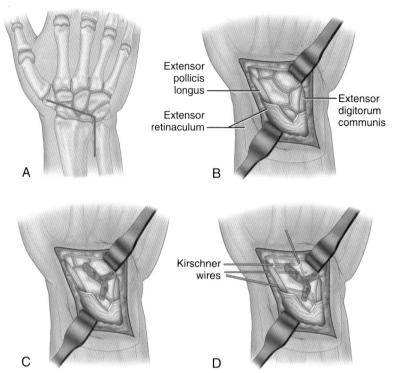

FIGURE 6.95 Scaphocapitolunate arthrodesis. **A,** Skin incision *(line)* extending from ulnar aspect of distal radius to distal pole of scaphoid. **B,** Scaphocapitolunate articulation exposed between third and fourth dorsal compartments. Retractors on capsule opened in inverted-T fashion. **C,** Scaphocapitolunate articulation filled with cancellous bone graft after decortication to cancellous bone. **D,** Fixation with Kirschner wires; note triangular configuration. **SEE TECHNIQUE 6.51.**

the lunotriquetral space (Fig. 6.96C). A Herbert screw or other lag screw can be used for fixation. If a screw is to be used, make another incision over the ulnar margin of the triquetrum to allow placement of the screw.

- After fixation and packing of the bone graft, obtain radiographs to ascertain satisfactory position of the bone and fixation.
- Close the capsule, retinaculum, and skin.
- Apply a nonadherent dressing and a short arm volar splint.

POSTOPERATIVE CARE The skin sutures are removed about 2 weeks after surgery. Protective splinting is continued for about 12 weeks. Protected motion exercises are allowed at about 8 weeks. The Kirschner wires are removed after union is shown radiographically, usually at 8 to 12 weeks. Strengthening exercises are begun at about 3 months after operation. Sports and heavy lifting should be avoided for at least 4 months.

TRIQUETROHAMATE ARTHRODESIS

Arthrodesis of the triquetrohamate joint can be accomplished through the same incision used for the lunotriquetral

arthrodesis described earlier. Decortication of the articular surfaces, bone grafting and Kirschner wire fixation techniques, and postoperative care are similar to those used for other intercarpal arthrodeses.

OSTEOARTHRITIS OF THE WRIST

Degenerative arthritis developing in the wrist (SLAC wrist) frequently seems to be related to instability around the scaphoid. The instability usually is a posttraumatic change, although primary degenerative changes are seen. The end result is a wrist with narrowing of the radioscaphoid joint, widening of the scapholunate gap, narrowing of the capitolunate joint, and remarkable preservation of the radiolunate joint (Fig. 6.97). The surgical treatment of this problem involves limited intercarpal arthrodesis of the capitohamate and triquetrolunate joints or wrist arthrodesis. Reports suggest that motion-preserving procedures, such as wrist neurectomy, proximal row carpectomy, or capitate-hamate-triquetrum-lunate (four corner) fusion with scaphoid excision, are satisfactory methods for dealing with this troublesome problem.

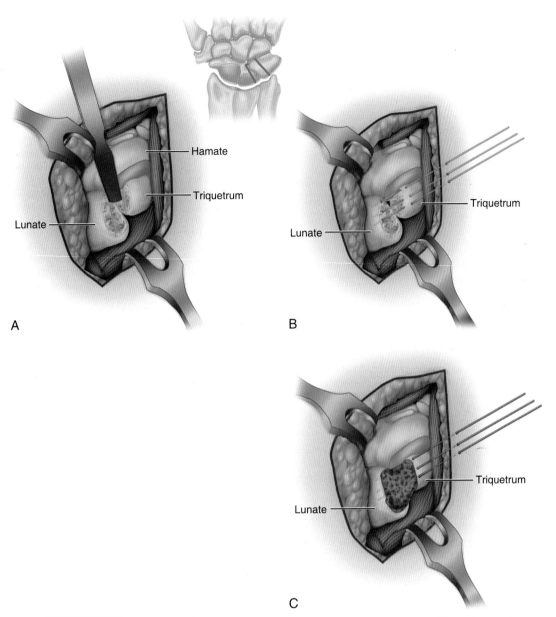

FIGURE 6.96 Lunotriquetral arthrodesis. **A,** Decortication of both surfaces of lunotriquetral joint. **B,** Kirschner wire fixation of lunotriquetral joint. **C,** Bone graft packed into lunotriquetral space. **SEE TECHNIQUE 6.52.**

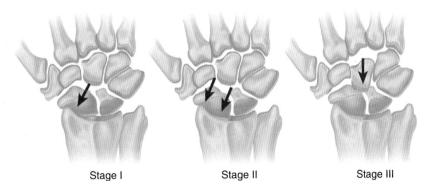

Stage I   Stage II   Stage III

FIGURE 6.97 Scapholunate advanced collapse wrist stages I, II, and III. In stage I, changes are limited to radial styloid. In stage II, scaphoid fossa is involved. In stage III, capitolunate joint is additionally narrowed and sclerotic.

REFERENCES

ANATOMY AND BIOMECHANICS

Brody MJ, Merrell GA: The effect of progressive extensor retinaculum excision on wrist biomechanics and bowstringing, *J Hand Surg Am* 40:2388, 2015.

Buijze GA, Dvinskikh NA, Strackee SD, et al.: Osseous and ligamentous scaphoid anatomy, part II: evaluation of ligament morphology using three-dimensional anatomical imaging, *J Hand Surg Am* 36A:1936, 2011.

Buijze GA, Iørgsholm P, Thomsen NO, et al.: Diagnostic performance of radiographs and computed tomography for displacement and instability of acute scaphoid waist fractures, *J Bone Joint Surg* 94A:1967, 2012.

Buijze GA, Lozano-Calderon SA, Strackee SD, et al.: Osseous and ligamentous scaphoid anatomy, part I: a systematic literature review highlighting controversies, *J Hand Surg Am* 36A:1926, 2011.

Cardoso R, Szabo RM: Wrist anatomy and surgical approaches, *Hand Clin* 26:1, 2010.

Catalano LW, Zlotolow DA, Purcelli Lafter M, et al.: Surgical exposures of the wrist and hand, *J Am Acad Orthop Surg* 20:48, 2012.

Ek ET, Suh N, Carlson MG: Vascular anomalies of the hand and wrist, *J Am Acad Orthop Surg* 22:352, 2014.

Garcia-Elias M, Hagert E: Surgical approaches to the distal radioulnar joint, *Hand Clin* 26:477, 2010.

Gurses IA, Coskun O, Gayretli O, et al.: The anatomy of the fibrous and osseous components of the first extensor compartment of the wrist: a cadaveric study, *Surg Radiol Anat* 37:773, 2015.

Hagert E, Hagert CG: Understanding stability of the distal radioulnar joint through an understanding of its anatomy, *Hand Clin* 26:459, 2010.

Huang JI, Hanel DP: Anatomy and biomechanics of the distal radioulnar joint, *Hand Clin* 28:157, 2012.

Kijima Y, Viegas SF: Wrist anatomy and biomechanics, *J Hand Surg Am* 34A:1555, 2009.

Ombaba J, Kuo M, Rayan G: Anatomy of the ulnar tunnel and the influence of wrist motion on its morphology, *J Hand Surg Am* 35A:760, 2010.

Pulos N, Bozentka DJ: Carpal ligament anatomy and biomechanics, *Hand Clin* 31:381, 2015.

Rainbow MJ, Kamal RN, Leventhal E, et al.: In vivo kinematics of the scaphoid, lunate, capitate, and third metacarpal in extreme wrist flexion and extension, *J Hand Surg Am* 38:278, 2013.

Rajan PV, Day CS: Scapholunate interosseous ligament anatomy and biomechanics, *J Hand Surg Am* 40:1692, 2015.

Stromps JP, Eschweiler J, Knobe M, et al.: Impact of scapholunate dissociation on human wrist kinematics, *J Hand Surg Eur* 43:179, 2018.

DIAGNOSIS AND EVALUATION

Andersson JK, Andernord D, Karlsson J, Fridén J: Efficacy of magnetic resonance imaging and clinical tests in diagnostics of wrist ligament injuries: a systematic review, *Arthroscopy* 31:2014, 2015.

Dornberger JE, Rademacher G, Mutze S, et al.: Accuracy of simple plain radiographic signs and measures to diagnose acute scapholunate ligament injuries of the wrist, *Eur Radiol* 25:3488, 2015.

Kleinan WB: Physical examination of the wrist: useful provocative maneuvers, *J Hand Surg Am* 40:1486, 2015.

Lee Master D, Yao J: The wrist insufflation test: a confirmatory test for detecting intercarpal ligament and triangular fibrocartilage complex tears, *Arthroscopy* 30:451, 2014.

Moritomo H: Radiographic clues for determining carpal instability and treatment protocol for scaphoid fractures, *J Orthop Sci* 19:379, 2014.

Murthy NS: The role of magnetic resonance imaging in scaphoid fractures, *J Hand Surg Am* 38:2047, 2013.

Rhee PC, Sauvé PS, Lindau T, Shin AY: Examination of the wrist: ulnar-sided pain due to ligamentous injury, *J Hand Surg Am* 39:1859, 2014.

Squires JH, England E, Mehta K, Wissman RD: The role of imaging in diagnosing diseases of the distal radioulnar joint, triangular fibrocartilage complex, and distal ulna, *AJR Am J Roentgenol* 203:146, 2014.

Vezeridis PS, Yoshioka H, Han R, Blazar P: Ulnar-sided wrist pain, part I: anatomy and physical examination, *Skeletal Radiol* 39:733, 2010.

Young D, Papp S, Giachino A: Physical examination of the wrist, *Hand Clin* 26:21, 2010.

RADIOGRAPHIC TECHNIQUES

Allainmat L, Aubault M, Noël V, et al.: Use of hybrid SPECT/CT for diagnosis of radiographic occult fractures of the wrist, *Clin Nucl Med* 38:e246, 2013.

Cerezal L, de Dios Berná-Mestre J, Canga A, et al.: MR and CT arthrography of the wrist, *Semin Musculoskelet Radiol* 16:27, 2012.

Coggins CA: Imaging of ulnar-sided wrist pain, *Clin Sports Med* 25:505, 2006.

Dewan AK, Chhabra AB, Khanna AJ, et al.: Magnetic resonance imaging of the hand and wrist: techniques and spectrum of disease: AAOS exhibit selection, *J Bone Joint Surg* 95A:e68, 2013.

Edlund R, Skorpil M, Lapidus G, Bäcklund J: Cone-beam CT in diagnosis of scaphoid fractures, *Skeletal Radiol* 45:197, 2016.

Fotiadou A, Patel A, Morgan T, Karantanas AH: Wrist injuries in young adults: the diagnostic impact of CT and MRI, *Eur J Radiol* 77:235, 2011.

Haugstvedt JR, Langer MF, Berger RA: Distal radioulnar joint: functional anatomy, including pathomechanics, *J Hand Surg Eur* Vol 42:338, 2017.

Iida A, Omokawa S, Akahane M, et al.: Distal radioulnar joint stress radiography for detecting radioulnar ligament injury, *J Hand Surg Am* 37A:968, 2012.

Langner I, Fischer S, Eisenschenk A, Langner S: Cine MRI: a new approach to the diagnosis of scapholunate dissociation, *Skeletal Radiol* 44:1103, 2015.

Lee SK, Desai H, Silver B, et al.: Comparison of radiographic stress views for scapholunate dynamic instability in a cadaver model, *J Hand Surg Am* 36A:1149, 2011.

Lee RK, Griffith JF, Ng AW, Wong CW: Imaging of radial wrist pain. I. Imaging modalities and anatomy, *Skeletal Radiol* 43:713, 2014.

Lee RK, Ng AW, Tong CS, et al.: Intrinsic ligament and triangular fibrocartilage complex tears of the wrist: comparison of MDCT arthrography, conventional 3-T MRI, and MR arthrograpy, *Skeletal Radiol* 42:1277, 2013.

Ramdhian-Wihlm R, Le Minor JM, Schmittbuhl M, et al.: Cone-beam computed tomography arthrography: an innovative modality for the evaluation of wrist ligament and cartilage injuries, *Skeletal Radiol* 41:963, 2012.

Ringler MD: MRI of wrist ligaments, *J Hand Surg Am* 38:2034, 2013.

Sandow MJ: 3D analysis of the wrist, *Hand Surg* 20:366, 2015.

Stein JM, Cook TS, Simonson S, Kim W: Normal and variant anatomy of the wrist and hand on MR imaging, *Magn Reson Imaging Clin N Am* 19:595, 2011.

ARTHROSCOPY OF THE WRIST

Adolfsson L: Arthroscopic synovectomy of the wrist, *Hand Clin* 27:395, 2011.

Ahsan BS, Yao J: Complications of wrist arthroscopy, *Arthroscopy* 28:855, 2012.

Aslani H, Najafi A, Zaaferani Z: Prospective outcomes of arthroscopic treatment of dorsal wrist ganglia, *Orthopedics* 35:e365, 2012.

Atzei A, Luchetti R: Foveal TFCC tear classification and treatment, *Hand Clin* 27:263, 2011.

Azbug JM, Osterman AL: Arthroscopic hemiresection for stage II-III trapeziometacarpal osteoarthritis, *Hand Clin* 27:347, 2011.

Bain GI, Durrant AW: Arthroscopic assessment of avascular necrosis, *Hand Clin* 27:323, 2011.

Bain GI, Smith ML, Watts AC: Arthroscopic core decompression of the lunate in early stage Kienböck disease of the lunate, *Tech Hand Up Extrem Surg* 15:66, 2011.

Bednar JM: Acute scapholunate ligament injuries: arthroscopic treatment, *Hand Clin* 31:417, 2015.

Burn MB, Sarkissian EJ, Yao J: Long-term outcomes for arthroscopic thermal treatment for scapholunate ligament injuries, *J Wrist Surg* 8:403, 2019.

Colantoni J, Chadderdon C, Gaston RG: Arthroscopic wafer procedure for ulnar impaction syndrome, *Arthrosc Tech* 3:e123, 2014.

El-Gazzar Y, Baker 3rd CL, Baker Jr CL: Complications of elbow and wrist arthroscopy, *Sports Med Arthrosc* 21:80, 2013.

Gallego S, Mathoulin C: Arthroscopic resection of dorsal wrist ganglia: 114 cases with minimum follow-up of 2 years, *Arthroscopy* 26:1675, 2010.

Geissler WB: Arthroscopic knotless peripheral ulnar-sided TFCC repair, *Hand Clin* 27:273, 2011.

Geissler WB: Arthroscopic management of scapholunate instability, *J Wrist Surg* 2:129, 2013.

Herzberg G, Burnier M, Marc A, et al.: The role of arthroscopy for treatment of perilunate injuries, *J Wrist Surg* 4:101, 2015.

Iwasaki N, Nishida K, Motomiya M, et al.: Arthroscopic-assisted repair of avulsed triangular fibrocartilage complex to the fovea of the ulnar head: a 2- to 4-year follow-up study, *Arthroscopy* 27:1371, 2011.

Kakar S, Burnier M, Atzei A, et al.: Dry wrist arthroscopy for radial-sided wrist disorders, *J Hand Surg Am* 45:341, 2020.

Kim JP, Lee JS, Park MJ: Arthroscopic reduction and percutaneous fixation of perilunate dislocations and fracture-dislocations, *Arthroscopy* 28:196, 2012.

Kim JP, Seo JB, Yoo JY, Lee JY: Arthroscopic management of chronic unstable scaphoid nonunions: effects on restoration of carpal alignment and recovery of wrist function, *Arthroscopy* 31:460, 2015.

Kovachevich R, Elhassan BT: Arthroscopic and open repair of the TFCC, *Hand Clin* 26:485, 2010.

Mathoulin C, Darin F: Arthroscopic treatment of scaphotrapeziotrapezoid osteoarthritis, *Hand Clin* 27:319, 2011.

Meftah M, Keefer EP, Panagopoulos G, Yang SS: Arthroscopic wafer resection for ulnar impaction syndrome: prediction of outcomes, *Hand Surg* 15:89, 2010.

Nakamura T, Sato K, Okazaki M, et al.: Repair of foveal detachment of the triangular fibrocartilage complex: open and arthroscopic transosseous techniques, *Hand Clin* 27:281, 2011.

Papapetropoulos PA, Wartinbee DA, Richard MJ, et al.: Management of peripheral triangular fibrocartilage complex tears in the ulnar positive patient: arthroscopic repair versus ulnar shortening osteotomy, *J Hand Surg Am* 35A:1607, 2010.

Park A, Lutsky K, Matzon J, et al.: An evaluation of the reliability of wrist arthroscopy in the assessment of tears of the triangular fibrocartilage complex, *J Hand Surg Am* 43:545, 2018.

Sammer DM, Shin AY: Comparison of arthroscopic and open treatment of septic arthritis of the wrist: surgical technique, *J Bone Joint Surg* 92A(Suppl 1 Pt 1):107, 2010.

Shimizu T, Omokawa S, del Pinal F, et al.: Arthroscopic partial capitate resection for type Ia avascular necrosis: a short-term outcome analysis, *J Hand Surg Am* 40:2393, 2015.

Shyamalan G, Jordan RW, Kimani PK, et al.: Assessment of the structures at risk during wrist arthroscopy: a cadaveric study and systematic review, *J Hand Surg Eur* Vol 41:852, 2016.

Slutsky DJ: Arthroscopic evaluation of the foveal attachment of the triangular fibrocartilage, *Hand Clin* 27:255, 2011.

Slutsky DJ: Current innovations in wrist arthroscopy, *J Hand Surg Am* 37:1932, 2012.

Slutsky DJ, Trevare J: Use of arthroscopy for the treatment of scaphoid fractures, *Hand Clin* 30:91, 2014.

Stuffmann ES, McAdams TR, Shah RP, Yao J: Arthroscopic repair of the scapholunate interosseous ligament, *Tech Hand Up Extrem Surg* 14:204, 2010.

Trehan SK, Wall LB, Calfee RP, et al.: Arthroscopic diagnosis of the triangular fibrocartilage complex foveal tear: a cadaver assessment, *J Hand Surg Am* 43:680–e1, 2018.

Van Meir N, Degreef I, De Smet L: The volar portal in wrist arthroscopy, *Acta Orthop Belg* 77:290, 2011.

Wagner J, Ipaktchi K, Livermore M, Banegas R: Current indications for and the technique of wrist arthroscopy, *Orthopedics* 37:251, 2014.

Waterman SM, Slade D, Masini BD, Owens BD: Safety analysis of all-inside arthroscopic repair of peripheral triangular fibrocartilage complex, *Arthroscopy* 26:1474, 2010.

Weiss ND, Molina RA, Gwin S: Arthroscopic proximal row carpectomy, *J Hand Surg Am* 36:577, 2011.

Yamamoto M, Koh S, Tatebe M, et al.: Importance of distal radioulnar joint arthroscopy for evaluating the triangular fibrocartilage complex, *J Orthop Sci* 15:210, 2010.

Yao J: All-arthroscopic repair of peripheral triangular fibrocartilage complex tears using Fas T-Fix, *Hand Clin* 27:237, 2011.

TRAUMA (FRACTURES AND DISLOCATIONS)

Adams JE, Steinmann SP: Acute scaphoid fractures, *Hand Clin* 26:97, 2010.

Bain GI, Turow A, Phadnis J: Dorsal plating of unstable scaphoid fractures and nonunions, *Tech Hand Up Extrem Surg* 19:95, 2015.

Brogan DM, Moran SL, Shin AY: Outcomes of open reduction and internal fixation of acute proximal pole scaphoid fractures, *Hand (N Y)* 10:227, 2015.

Buijze GA, Doornberg JN, Ham JS, et al.: Surgical compared with conservative treatment for acute nondisplaced or minimally displaced scaphoid fractures: a systematic review and meta-analysis of randomized controlled trials, *J Bone Joint Surg* 92A:1534, 2010.

Chen AC, Lee MS, Ueng SW, Chen WJ: Management of late-diagnosed scaphoid fractures, *Injury* 41:e10, 2010.

Clementson M, Jørgsholm P, Besjakov J, et al.: Conservative treatment versus arthroscopic-assisted screw fixation of scaphoid waist fractures—a randomized trial with minimum 4-year follow-up, *J Hand Surg Am* 40:1341, 2015.

Cohen MS, Jupiter JB, Fallahi K, et al.: Scaphoid waist nonunion with humpback deformity treated without structural bone graft, *J Hand Surg Am* 38:701, 2013.

Devers BN, Douglas KC, Naik RD, et al.: Outcomes of hook of hamate fracture excision in high-level amateur athletes, *J Hand Surg Am* 38:72, 2013.

Doornberg JN, Buijze GA, Ham SJ, et al.: Nonoperative treatment for acute scaphoid fractures: a systematic review and meta-analysis of randomized controlled trials, *J Trauma* 71:1073, 2011.

Duckworth AD, Ring D, McQueen MM: Assessment of the suspected fracture of the scaphoid, *J Bone Joint Surg* 93:713, 2011.

Eastley N, Singh H, Dias JJ, Taub N: Union rates after proximal scaphoid fractures: meta-analyses and review of available evidence, *J Hand Surg Eur* 38:888, 2013.

Ferguson DO, Shanbhag V, Hedley H, et al.: Scaphoid fracture non-union: a systematic review of surgical treatment using bone graft, *J Hand Surg Eur* 41:492, 2016.

Garcia RM, Leversedge F, Aldridge JM, et al.: Scaphoid nonunions treated with 2 headless compression screws and bone grafting, *J Hand Surg Am* 39:1301, 2014.

Garcia RM, Ruch DS: Management of scaphoid fractures in the athlete: open and percutaneous fixation, *Sports Med Arthrosc* 22:22, 2014.

Gaston RG, Chadderdon RC: Management of complications of wrist fractures, *Hand Clin* 31:193, 2015.

Geissler WB, Adams JE, Bindra RR, et al.: Scaphoid fractures: what's hot, what's not, *Instr Course Lect* 61:71, 2012.

Guss MS, Mitgang JT, Sapienza A: Scaphoid healing required for unrestricted activity: a biomechanical cadaver model, *J Hand Surg Am* 43:134, 2018.

Hovius SE, de Jong T: Bone grafts for scaphoid nonunions: an overview, *Hand Surg* 20:222, 2015.

Kang HJ, Chun YM, Koh IH, et al.: Is arthroscopic bone graft and fixation for scaphoid nonunions effective? *Clin Orthop Relat Res* 474:204, 2016.

Kang L: Operative treatment of acute scaphoid fractures, *Hand Surg* 20:210, 2015.

Kakar S, Greene RM: Scapholunate ligament internal brace 360-degree tenodesis (SLITT) procedure, *J Wrist Surg* 7:336, 2018.

Krief E, Appy-Fedida B, Rotari V, et al.: Results of perilunate dislocations and perilunate fracture dislocations with a minimum 15-year follow-up, *J Hand Surg Am* 40:2191, 2015.

Mallee W, Doornberg JN, Ring D, et al.: Comparison of CT and MRI for diagnosis of suspected scaphoid fractures, *J Bone Joint Surg* 93A:20, 2011.

Meyer C, Chang J, Stern PJ, et al.: Complications of distal radial and scaphoid fracture treatment, *Instr Course Lect* 63:113, 2014.

Moon ES, Dy CJ, Derman P, et al.: Management of nonunion following surgical management of scaphoid fractures: current concepts, *J Am Acad Orthop Surg* 21:548, 2013.

Muppavarapu RC, Capo JT: Perilunate dislocations and fracture dislocations, *Hand Clin* 31:399, 2015.

Obert L, Loisel F, Jardin E, et al.: High-energy injuries of the wrist, *Orthop Traumatol Surg Res* 102(Suppl 1):S81, 2016.

Papp S: Carpal bone fractures, *Hand Clin* 26:119, 2010.

Pinder RM, Brkljac M, Rix L, et al.: Treatment of scaphoid nonunion: a systematic review of the existing evidence, *J Hand Surg Am* 40:1797, 2015.

Ruch DS, Papadonikolakis A: Resection of the scaphoid distal pole for symptomatic scaphoid nonunion after failed previous surgical treatment, *J Hand Surg Am* 31A:588, 2006.

Ruch DS, Wray 3rd WH, Papadonikolakis A, et al.: Corrective osteotomy for isolated malunion of the palmar lunate facet in distal radius fractures, *J Hand Surg Am* 35A:1779, 2010.

Slutsky DJ, Trevare J: Scapholunate and lunotriquetral injuries: arthroscopic and open management, *Sports Med Arthrosc* 22:12, 2014.

Sommerkamp TG, Hastings 2nd H, Greenberg JA: Palmar radiocarpal artery vascularized bone graft for the unstable humpbacked scaphoid nonunion with an avascular proximal pole, *J Hand Surg Am* 45:298, 2020.

Suh N, Benson EC, Faber KJ, et al.: Treatment of acute scaphoid fractures: a systematic review and meta-analysis, *Hand (N Y)* 5:345, 2010.

Suh N, Ek ET, Wolfe SW: Carpal fractures, *J Hand Surg Am* 39:785, 2014.

Tang P, Fischer CR: A new volar vascularization technique using the superficial palmar branch of the radial artery for the collapsed scaphoid nonunion, *Tech Hand Up Extrem Surg* 14:160, 2010.

Verstreken F, Meermans G: Transtrapezial approach for fixation of acute scaphoid fractures: rationale, surgical techniques, and results: AAOS exhibit selection, *J Bone Joint Surg* 97A:850, 2015.

Walenkamp MM, Aydin S, Mulders MA, et al.: Predictors of unstable distal radius fractures: a systematic review and meta-analysis, *J Hand Surg Eur* 41:501, 2016.

Wijffels MM, Keizer J, Buijze GA, et al.: Ulnar styloid process nonunion and outcome in patients with a distal radius fracture: a meta-analysis of comparative clinical trials, *Injury* 45:1889, 2014.

Williksen JH, Frihagen F, Hellund JC, et al.: Volar locking plates versus external fixation and adjuvant pin fixation in unstable distal radius fractures: a randomized, controlled study, *J Hand Surg Am* 38:1469, 2013.

Wong WYC, Ho PC: Minimal invasive management of scaphoid fractures: from fresh to non-union, *Hand Clin* 27:291, 2011.

PROXIMAL ROW CARPECTOMY

De Carli P, Zaidenberg EE, Alfie V, et al.: Radius core decompression for Kienböck disease stage IIIA: outcomes at 13 years follow-up, *J Hand Surg Am* 42:752.e1, 2017.

DiDonna ML, Kiefhaber TR, Stern PJ: Proximal row carpectomy: study with a minimum of 10 years of follow-up, *J Bone Joint Surg Am* 86:2359, 2004.

Elfar JC, Stern PJ: Proximal row carpectomy for scapholunate dissociation, *J Hand Surg Eur* vol 36:111, 2011.

Gaspar MP, Pham PP, Pankiw CD, et al.: Mid-term outcomes of routine proximal row carpectomy compared with proximal row carpectomy with dorsal capsular interposition arthroplasty for the treatment of late-stage arthropathy of the wrist, *Bone Joint J* 100-B:197, 2018.

Green DP, Perreira AC, Longhofer LK: Proximal row carpectomy, *J Hand Surg Am* 40:1672, 2015.

Russchen M, Kachooei AR, Teunis T, Ring D: Acute proximal row carpectomy after complex carpal fracture dislocation, *J Hand Microsurg* 7:212, 2015.

van Hernen JJ, Lans J, Garg R, et al.: Factors associated with reoperation and conversion to wrist fusion after proximal row carpectomy or 4-corner arthrodesis, *J Hand Surg Am* 45:85, 2020.

Wagner ER, Bravo D, Elhassan B, Moran SL: Factors associated with improved outcomes following proximal row carpectomy: a long-term outcome study of 144 patients, *J Hand Surg Eur* 41:484, 2016.

Wagner ER, Werthel JD, Elhassan BT, et al.: Proximal row carpectomy and 4-corner arthrodesis in patients younger than age 45 years, *J Hand Surg Am* 42:428, 2017.

Wall LB, Stern PJ: Proximal row carpectomy, *Hand Clin* 29:69, 2013.

Weiss ND, Molina RA, Gwin S: Arthroscopic proximal row carpectomy, *J Hand Surg Am* 36:577, 2011.

KIENBÖCK DISEASE

Arnaiz J, Peidra T, Cerezal L, et al.: Imaging of Kienböck disease, *AJR Am J Roentgenol* 203:131, 2014.

Bain GI, Durrant A: An articular-based approach to Kienböck avascular necrosis of the lunate, *Tech Hand Up Extrem Surg* 15:41, 2011.

Bain GI, Smith ML, Watts AC: Arthroscopic core decompression of the lunate in early stage Kienböck disease of the lunate, *Tech Hand Up Extrem Surg* 15:66, 2011.

Bain GI, Yeo CJ, Morse LP: Kienböck disease: recent advances in the basic science, assessment and treatment, *Hand Surg* 20:352, 2015.

Buijze GA, Goslings JC, Rhemrey SJ, et al.: Cast immobilization with and without immobilization of the thumb for nondisplaced and minimally displaced scaphoid waist fractures: a multicenter, randomized, controlled trial, *J Hand Surg Am* 39:621, 2014.

Calfee RP, Van Steyn MO, Gyuricza C, et al.: Joint leveling for advanced Kienböck's disease, *J Hand Surg Am* 35A:2010, 1947.

Citlak A, Akgun U, Bulut T, et al.: Partial capitate shortening for Kienböck's disease, *J Hand Surg Eur* 40:957, 2015.

De Carli P, Zaidenberg EE, Alfie V, et al.: Radius core decompression for Kienböck disease stage IIIA: outcomes at 13 years follow-up, *J Hand Surg Am* 42:752–e1, 2017.

Fujiwara H, Oda R, Morisaki S, et al.: Long-term results of vascularized bone graft for stage III Kienböck disease, *J Hand Surg Am* 38:904, 2013.

Hegazy G, Akar A, Abd-Elghany T, et al.: Treatment of Kienböck's disease with neutral ulnar variance by distal capitate shortening and arthrodesis to the base of the third metacarpal bone, *J Hand Surg Am* 44:518–e1, 2019.

Innes L, Strauch RJ: Systematic review of the treatment of Kienböck's disease in its early and late stages, *J Hand Surg Am* 35A:713, 2010.

Kakar S, Giuffre JL, Shin AY: Revascularization procedures for Kienböck disease, *Tech Hand Up Extrem Surg* 15:55, 2011.

Lichtman DM, Lesley NE, Simmons SP: The classification and treatment of Kienböck's disease: the state of the art and a look at the future, *J Hand Surg Eur* 35:549, 2010.

Lluch A, Garcia-Elias M: Etiology of Kienböck disease, *Tech Hand Up Extrem Surg* 15:33, 2011.

Matsuhashi T, Iwasaki N, Kato H, et al.: Clinical outcomes of excision arthroplasty for Kienböck's disease, *Hand Surg* 16:277, 2011.

Matsui Y, Funakoshi T, Motomiya M, et al.: Radial shortening osteotomy for Kienböck disease: minimum 10-year follow-up, *J Hand Surg Am* 39:679, 2014.

Mehrpour SR, Kamrani RS, Aghamirsalim MR, et al.: Treatment of Kienböck disease by lunate core decompression, *J Hand Surg Am* 36A:1675, 2011.

Mozaffarian K, Namzi H, Namdari A: Radial shortening osteotomy in advanced stages of Kienbock disease, *Tech Hand Up Extrem Surg* 16:242, 2012.

Nakagawa M, Omokawa S, Kira T, et al.: Vascularized bone grafts from the dorsal wrist for the treatment of Kienböck disease, *J Wrist Surg* 5:98, 2016.

Nakamura R, Nakao E, Nishizuka T, et al.: Radial osteotomy for Kienböck disease, *Tech Hand Up Extrem Surg* 15:48, 2011.

Pegoli L, Ghezzi A, Cavalli E, et al.: Arthroscopic assisted bone grafting for early stages of Kienböck's disease, *Hand Surg* 16:172, 2011.

Pet MA, Assi PE, Giladi AM, et al.: Preliminary clinical, radiographic, and patient-reported outcomes of the medial femoral trochlea osteochondral free flap for lunate reconstruction in advanced Kienböck disease, *J Hand Surg Am*, 2020, Mar 5. [Epub ahead of print].

Rodrigues-Pinto R, Freitas D, Costa LD, et al.: Clinical and radiological results following radial osteotomy in patients with Kienböck's disease: four- to 18-year follow-up, *J Bone Joint Surg* 94B:222, 2012.

Saunders BM, Lichtman D: A classification-based treatment algorithm for Kienböck disease: current and future considerations, *Tech Hand Up Extrem Surg* 15:38, 2011.

Shin M, Tatebe M, Hirata H, et al.: Reliability of Lichtman's classification for Kienböck's disease in 99 subjects, *Hand Surg* 16:15, 2011.

Tatebe M, Hirata H, Shinohara T, et al.: Arthroscopic findings of Kienböck's disease, *J Orthop Sci* 16:745, 2011.

Tatebe M, Koh S, Hirata H: Long-term outcomes of radial osteotomy for the treatment of Kienböck's disease, *J Wrist Surg* 5:92, 2016.

van Leeuwen WF, Janssen SJ: Ring D: Radiographic progression of Kienböck disease: radial shortening versus no surgery, *J Hand Surg Am* 41:681, 2016.

van Leeuwen WF, Janssen SJ, Ter Meulen DP, Ring D: What is the radiographic prevalence of incidental Kienböck disease? *Clin Orthop Relat Res* 474:808, 2016.

van Leeuwen WF, Oflazoglu K, Menendez ME, et al.: Negative ulnar variance and Kienböck disease, 41:214, 2016.

Viljakka T, Tallroth K, Vastamäki M: Long-term outcome (20 to 33 years) of radial shortening osteotomy for Kienböck's lunatomalacia, *J Hand Surg Eur* vol 39:761, 2014.

RADIOULNAR JOINT

Ahmed SK, Cheung JP, Fung BK, Ip WY: Long term results of matched hemiresection interposition arthroplasty for DRUJ arthritis in rheumatoid patients, *Hand Surg* 16:119, 2011.

Ahsan ZS, Song Y, Yao J: Outcomes of ulnar shortening osteotomy fixed with a dynamic compression system, *J Hand Surg Am* 38:1520, 2013.

Atzei A, Luchetti R: Foveal TFCC tear classification and treatment, *Hand Clin* 27:263, 2011.

Boardman MJ, Imbriglia JE: Surgical management of ulnocarpal impaction syndrome, *J Hand Surg Am* 35A:649, 2010.

Ehman EC, Hayes ML, Berger RA, et al.: Subluxation of the distal radioulnar joint as a predictor of foveal triangular fibrocartilage complex tears, *J Hand Surg Am* 36A:1780, 2011.

Fujitani R, Omokawa S, Akahane M, et al.: Predictors of distal radioulnar joint instability in distal radius fractures, *J Hand Surg Am* 36A:2011, 1919.

Gillis JA, Soreide E, Khouri JS, et al.: Outcomes of the Adams–Berger ligament reconstruction for the distal radioulnar joint instability in 95 consecutive cases, *J Wrist Surg* 8:268, 2019.

Grawe B, Heincelman C, Stern P: Functional results of the Darrach procedure: a long-term outcome study, *J Hand Surg Am* 37:2475, 2012.

Griska A, Feldon P: Wafer resection of the distal ulna, *J Hand Surg Am* 40:2283, 2015.

Hammert WC, Williams RB, Greenberg JA: Distal metaphyseal ulnar-shortening osteotomy: surgical technique, *J Hand Surg Am* 37:1071, 2012.

Iordache SD, Rowan R, Garvin GJ, et al.: Prevalence of triangular fibrocartilage abnormalities on MRI scans of asymptomatic wrists, *J Hand Surg Am* 37A:98, 2012.

Kakar S, Carlsen BT, Morgan SL, Berger RA: The management of chronic distal radioulnar instability, *Hand Clin* 26:517, 2010.

Katz JI, Seiler 3rd JG, Bond TC: The treatment of ulnar impaction syndrome: a systematic review of the literature, *J Surg Orthop Adv* 19:218, 2010.

Khouri JS, Hammert WC: Distal metaphyseal ulnar shortening osteotomy: technique, pearls, and outcomes, *J Wrist Surg* 3:175, 2014.

Koh KH, Lee HL, Chang YS, Park MJ: Arthroscopy during ulnar shortening for idiopathic ulnar impaction syndrome, *Orthopedics* 36:e1495, 2013.

Lluch A: The Sauvé-Kapandji procedure: indications and tips for surgical success, *Hand Clin* 26:559, 2010.

Low SL, Clippinger BB, Landfair GL, et al.: A biomechanical evaluation of the DRUJ after distal oblique bundle reconstruction, *J Hand Surg Am*, Dec 20 2019, [Epub ahead of print].

Manz S, Wolf SB, Leclere FM, et al.: Capsular imbrication for posttraumatic instability of the distal radioulnar joint, *J Hand Surg Am* 36A:1170, 2011.

McBeath R, Katlik LI, Shin EK: Ulnar shortening osteotomy for ulnar impaction syndrome, *J Hand Surg Am* 38:379, 2013.

Meftah M, Keefer EP, Panagopoulos G, Yang SS: Arthroscopic wafer resection for ulnar impaction syndrome: prediction of outcomes, *Hand Surg* 15:89, 2010.

Moritomo H, Masatomi T, Murase T, et al.: Open repair of foveal avulsion of the triangular fibrocartilage complex and comparison by types of injury mechanism, *J Hand Surg Am* 35A:2010, 1955.

Murray D, Javed S, Hayton M: Mini dorsal incision to the triangular fibrocartilage complex: a new surgical approach, *Hand (N Y)* 10:717, 2015.

Murray PM, Adams JE, Lam J, et al.: Disorders of the distal radioulnar joint, *Instr Course Lect* 59:295, 2010.

Nakamura T, Cooney 3rd WP, Lui WH, et al.: Radial styloidectomy: a biomechanical study on stability of the wrist joint, *J Hand Surg Am* 26:85, 2001.

Nikkhah D, Rodrigues J, Dejager L: Do patients really do better after the Sauvé-Kapandji procedure when compared to the Darrach procedure? A systematic review, *J Hand Surg Eur* 36:615, 2011.

Papapetropoulos PA, Wartinbee DA, Richard MJ, et al.: Management of peripheral triangular fibrocartilage complex tears in the ulnar positive patient: arthroscopic repair versus ulnar shortening osteotomy, *J Hand Surg Am* 35A:1607, 2010.

Park MJ, Jagadish A, Yao J: The rate of triangular fibrocartilage injuries requiring surgical intervention, *Orthopedics* 33:806, 2010.

Protopsaltis TS, Ruch DS: Triangular fibrocartilage complex tears associated with symptomatic ulnar styloid nonunions, *J Hand Surg Am* 35A:1251, 2010.

Rajgopal R, Roth J, King G, et al.: Outcomes and complications of ulnar shortening osteotomy: an institutional review, *Hand (N Y)* 10:535, 2015.

Roenbeck K, Imbriglia JE: Peripheral triangular fibrocartilage complex tears, *J Hand Surg Am* 36A:1687, 2011.

Sachar K: Ulnar-sided wrist pain: evaluation and treatment of triangular fibrocartilage complex tears, ulnocarpal impaction syndrome, and lunotriquetral ligament tears, *J Hand Surg Am* 37:1489, 2012.

Sotereanos DG, Papatheodorou LK, Williams BG: Tendon allograft interposition for failed distal ulnar resection: 2- to 14-year follow-up, *J Hand Surg Am* 39:443, 2014.

Stockton DJ, Pelletier ME, Pike JM: Operative treatment of ulnar impaction syndrome: a systematic review, *J Hand Surg Eur* 40:470, 2015.

Strauss ML, Goldfarb CA: Arthrosopic management of traumatic peripheral triangular fibrocartilage complex tears, *J Hand Surg Am* 36A:136, 2011.

Tatebe M, Nishizuka T, Hirata H, Nakamura R: Ulnar shortening osteotomy for ulnar-sided wrist pain, *J Wrist Surg* 3:77, 2014.

Vandenberghe L, Degreef I, Didden K, et al.: Ulnar shortening or arthroscopic wafer resection for ulnar impaction syndrome, *Acta Orthop Belg* 78:323, 2012.

Waterman SM, Slade D, Masini BD, Owens BD: Safety analysis of all-inside arthrosocopic repair of peripheral triangular fibrocartilage complex, *Arthroscopy* 26:1474, 2010.

Watts AC, Hayton MJ, Stanely JK: Salvage of failed distal radioulnar joint reconstruction, *Hand Clin* 26:529, 2010.

Wolff AL, Garg R, Kraszewski AP, et al.: Surgical treatments for scapholunate advanced collapse wrist: kinematics and functional performance, *J Hand Surg Am* 40:1547, 2015.

Zahiri H, Zahiri CA, Ravari FK: Ulnar styloid impingement syndrome, *Int Orthop* 34:1233, 2010.

ARTHRODESIS

Allison DM: A new plate for partial wrist fusioins: results in midcarpal arthrodesis, *J Hand Surg Eur* 36:315, 2011.

Bedford B, Yang SS: High fusion rates with circular plate fixation for four-corner arthrodesis of the wrist, *Clin Orthop Relat Res* 468:163, 2010.

Berkhout MJ, Bachour Y, Zheng KH, et al.: Four-corner arthrodesis versus proximal row carpectomy: a retrospective study with a mean follow-up of 17 years, *J Hand Surg Am* 40:1349, 2015.

Debottis DP, Werner FW, Sutton LG, Harley BJ: 4-corner arthrodesis and proximal row carpectomy: a biomechanical comparison of wrist motion and tendon forces, *J Hand Surg Am* 38:893, 2013.

Delattre O, Goulon G, Vogels J, et al.: Three-corner arthrodesis with scaphoid and triquetrum excision for wrist arthritis, *J Hand Surg Am* 40:2176, 2015.

Green DP, Henderson CJ: Modified AO arthrodesis of the wrist (with proximal row carpectomy), *J Hand Surg Am* 38:388, 2013.

Iorio ML, Kennedy CD, Hunag JI: Limited intercarpal fusion as a salvage procedure for advanced Kienbock disease, *Hand (N Y)* 10:472, 2015.

Kitzinger HB, Karle B, Prommersberger KJ, et al.: Four-corner arthrodesis—does the source of graft affect bony union rate? Iliac crest versus distal radius bone graft, *J Plast Reconstr Aesthet Surg* 65:379, 2012.

Kraisarin J, Dennison DG, Berglund LJ, et al.: Biomechanical comparison of three fixation techniques used for four-corner arthrodesis, *J Hand Surg Eur* 36:560, 2011.

Lamas Gomez C, Proubasta Renart I, Llusa Perez M: Relationship between wrist motion and capitolunate reduction in four-corner arthrodesis, *Orthopedics* 38:e1040, 2015.

Lautenbach M, Millrose M, Langner I, Eisenschenk A: Results of Mannerfelt wrist arthrodesis for rheumatoid arthritis in relation to the position of the fused wrist, *Int Orthop* 37:2409, 2013.

Luegmair M, Saffar P: Scaphocapitate arthrodesis for treatment of scapholunate instability in manual workers, *J Hand Surg Am* 38:878, 2013.

Luegmair M, Saffar P: Scaphocapitate arthrodesis for treatment of late stage Kienbock disease, *J Hand Surg Eur* 39:416, 2014.

Neubrech F, Mühldorfer-Fodor M, Pillukat T, et al.: Long-term results after midcarpal arthrodesis, *J Wrist Surg* 1:123, 2012.

Raven EE, Ottink KD, Doets KC: Radiolunate and radioscapholunate arthrodeses as treatments for rheumatoid and psoriatic arthritis: long-term follow-up, *J Hand Surg Am* 37A:55, 2012.

Rhee PC, Linn IC, Moran Sl, et al.: Scaphocapitate arthrodesis for Kienböck disease, *J Hand Surg Am* 40:745, 2015.

Rizzo M, Ackerman DB, Rodrigues RL, Beckenbaugh RD: Wrist arthrodesis as a salvage procedure for failed implant arthroplasty, *J Hand Surg Eur* 36:29, 2011.

Singh HP, Dias JJ, Phadnis J, Bain G: Comparison of the clinical and functional outcomes following 3- and 4-corner fusions, *J Hand Surg Am* 40:1117, 2015.

Trail JA, Murali R, Stanley JK, et al.: The long-term outcome of four-corner fusion, *J Wrist Surg* 4:128, 2015.

Wysocki RW, Cohen MS: Complications of limited and total wrist arthrodesis, *Hand Clin* 26:221, 2010.

INSTABILITY

Cizmar I, Ira D, Bisna P, Pilny J: Early results of reconstruction of the dorsal scapholunate ligament, *J Plast Surg Hand Surg* 44:245, 2010.

De Carli P, Donndorff AG, Gallucci GL, et al.: Chronic scapholunate dissociation: ligament reconstruction combining a new extensor carpi radialis longus tenodesis and a dorsal intercarpal ligament capsulodesis, *Tech Hand Up Extrem Surg* 15:6, 2011.

Ellanti P, Sisodia G, Al-Ajami A, et al.: The modified Brunelli procedure for scapholunate instability: a single centre study, *Hand Surg* 19:39, 2014.

Gray A, Cuénod P, Papaloïzos MY: Midterm outcome of bone-ligament-bone graft and dorsal capsulodesis for chronic scapholunate instability, *J Hand Surg Am* 40:1540, 2014.

Harwood C, Turner L: Conservative management of midcarpal instability, *J Hand Surg Eur* 41:102, 2016.

Ho PC, Wong CW, Tse WL: Arthroscopic-assisted combined dorsal and volar scapholunate ligament reconstruction with tendon graft for chronic SL instability, *J Wrist Surg* 4:252, 2015.

Kitay A, Wolfe SW: Scapholunate instability: current concepts in diagnosis and management, *J Hand Surg Am* 37:2175, 2012.

Luchetti R, Zorli IP, Atzei A, Fairplay T: Dorsal intercarpal ligament capsulodesis for predynamic and dynamic scapholunate instability, *J Hand Surg Eur* 35:32, 2010.

Nicaris T, Ming BW, Lichtman DM: Midcarpal instability: a comprehensive review and update, *Hand Clin* 31:487, 2015.

Pollock PJ, Seig RN, Baechler MF, et al.: Radiographic evaluation of the modified Brunelli technique versus the Blatt capsulodesis for scapholunate dissociation in a cadaver model, *J Hand Surg Am* 35A:1589, 2010.

Rohman EM, Agel J, Putnam MD, Adams JE: Scapholunate interosseous ligament injuries: a retrospective review of treatment and outcomes in 82 wrists, *J Hand Surg Am* 39:2020, 2014.

Toms AP, Chojnowski A, Cahir JG: Midcarpal instability: a radiological perspective, *Skeletal Radiol* 40:533, 2011.

van de Grift TC, Ritt MJ: Management of lunotriquetral instability: a review of the literature, *J Hand Surg Eur* 41:72, 2016.

Ward PJ, Fowler JR: Scapholunate ligament tears: acute reconstructive options, *Orthop Clin North Am* 46:551, 2015.

White NJ, Rollick NC: Injuries of the scapholunate interosseous ligament: an update, *J Am Acad Orthop Surg* 23:691, 2015.

Wolfe SW, Garcia-Elias M, Kitay A: Carpal instability nondissociative, *J Am Acad Orthop Surg* 20:575, 2012.

WRIST ARTHRITIS

Braga-Silva J, Román JA, Padoin AV: Wrist denervation for painful conditions of the wrist, *J Hand Surg Am* 36A:961, 2011.

Katayama T, Ono H, Suzuki D, et al.: Distribution of primary osteoarthritis in the ulnar aspect of the wrist and the factors that are correlated with ulnar wrist osteoarthritis: a cross-sectional study, *Skeletal Radiol* 42:1253, 2013.

Kluge S, Schindele S, Henkel T, Herren D: The modified Clayton-Mannerfelt arthrodesis of the wrist in rheumatoid arthritis: operative technique and report on 93 cases, *J Hand Surg Am* 38:999, 2013.

Lane LB, Daher RJ, Leo AJ: Scapholunate dissociation with radiolunate arthritis without radioscaphoid arthritis, *J Hand Surg Am* 35A:1075, 2010.

Lee HJ, Lee KH, Koh KH, Park MJ: Long-term results of arthroscopic wrist synovectomy in rheumatoid arthritis, *J Hand Surg Am* 39:1295, 2014.

Nacke E, Paksima N: The evaluation and treatment of the arthritic distal radioulnar joint, *Bull Hosp Jt Dis* 73:141, 2015.

Vermeulen GM, Brink SM, Slijper H, et al.: Trapeziometacarpal arthrodesis or trapeziectomy with ligament reconstruction in primary trapeziometacarpal osteoarthritis: a randomized controlled trial, *J Bone Joint Surg* 96A:726, 2014.

Wang ML, Bednar JM: Lunatocapitate and triquetrohamate arthrodeses for degenerative arthritis of the wrist, *J Hand Surg Am* 37:1136, 2012.

Zimmerman RM, Kim JM, Jupiter JB: Arthritis of the distal radioulnar joint: from Darrach to total joint arthroplasty, *J Am Acad Orthop Surg* 20:623, 2012.

The complete list of references is available online at expertconsult.inkling.com.

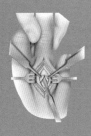

CHAPTER 7

SPECIAL HAND DISORDERS

Mark T. Jobe

ANEURYSM, THROMBOSIS, AND EMBOLISM IN RADIAL, ULNAR, AND DIGITAL ARTERIES

Through the continuation of the radial artery into the hand as the deep palmar arch and the ulnar artery as the superficial palmar arch, circulation to the hand is usually sufficient to allow the digits to remain viable despite most disease and injury. The superficial arch is complete in almost 80% of hands and incomplete in about 20%. The deep arch is complete in about 98% of hands. The radial artery usually provides most of the flow to three or more digits in 57% of hands, whereas the ulnar artery provides flow to three or more digits in almost 22%. Flow provided from both arteries equally is provided in almost 22%.

Ischemic problems in the hand can result from an aneurysm, thrombosis, or embolism in the radial, ulnar, or digital arteries. Arterial occlusive ischemia is associated with trauma from direct blows, instrumentation of the vascular tree for angiography, vascular access procedures, and systemic illnesses, such as atherosclerosis and various collagen vascular diseases.

Symptoms of ischemia, pain, sensory changes, skin discoloration, ulceration, and necrosis can be aggravated by smoking, activity, and exposure to cold. Physical findings include hand or digital pallor or cyanosis, skin ulceration, necrosis distal to areas of occlusion, sensory and possibly motor changes of affected nerves, coolness to palpation, tenderness over an aneurysmal or thrombotic mass, a palpable thrill through an aneurysm, and lack of flow through the affected artery, which is shown by the Allen test (Figs. 7.1 and 7.2). Because of spasms in the distal vessels, this condition can be confused with other conditions, such as Raynaud disease. Plain radiographs, Doppler flow assessment, ultrasonography, pulse volume recordings, segmental arterial measurement, skin temperature measurement, radionuclide scanning, magnetic resonance angiography, and contrast angiography are helpful diagnostic measures. Angiography provides definitive information about the location and extent of the principal lesion and the presence of other circulatory problems in the upper extremity and in the face of ischemia should be the first choice of imaging technique. If no ischemia exists then Doppler ultrasound, CT angiography, and MR angiography are useful.

Although aneurysms may have atherosclerotic, mycotic, metabolic, and congenital origins, aneurysms seen in the hand and wrist usually are the result of trauma. Blunt trauma can cause true and false aneurysms (see Fig. 13.12), whereas penetrating trauma usually causes false aneurysms to form. The patient will present with a pulsatile and painful mass as well as possible cold intolerance.

Preoperative and intraoperative evaluations of the anatomy of the palmar vascular arch and of the quality of distal circulation are important when deciding between aneurysm excision alone and aneurysm excision with end-to-end repair and reversed vein graft arterial reconstruction. If the palmar arterial arch is complete, and distal circulation is adequate, as determined by pink distal skin color after release of the tourniquet or by pulse volume recordings showing a digital-brachial index of more than 0.7, repair or reconstruction usually is unnecessary. Conversely, if the palmar arterial arch is incomplete, or if the distal circulation is inadequate, the artery should be repaired or reconstructed with a reversed segmental vein graft (Fig. 7.3).

Although usually related to occupational or recreational trauma, arterial thrombosis in the wrist, palm, and fingers also can result from arterial cannulation in the forearm. The ulnar artery is the vessel most commonly affected by trauma-related thrombosis, probably because of a relative lack of protection at the wrist and its exposure to repeated forceful impacts, such as when the ulnar side of the wrist is used as a hammer. Occupations in which this may be seen include auto mechanics, machinists, miners, butchers, and even firearm use in police officers. Sometimes the pain is severe, and sensibility is lost over the distribution of the ulnar nerve in the hand. Tenderness is present over the artery, and occasionally a feeling of fullness is described in the wrist and hand. Although possible, it rarely causes digital ischemia. The Allen test (see Figs. 7.1 and 7.2) is helpful in diagnosing thrombosis, but arteriography is diagnostic.

Treatment options include exploration of the artery and resection of the entire thrombotic mass, arterial reconstruction with artery or vein grafts, local and regional sympathectomy, and palliation with medical and psychological

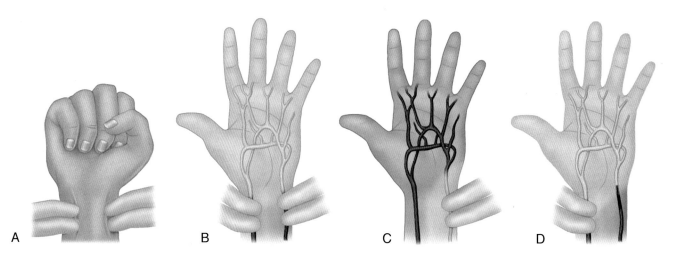

A   B   C   D

FIGURE 7.1 Allen test for patency of radial and ulnar arteries. **A,** Patient elevates hand and makes fist while examiner occludes radial and ulnar arteries. **B,** Patient extends fingers, and blanching of hand is seen. **C,** Radial artery alone is released, and color of hand returns to normal. **D,** In thrombosis of ulnar artery, test is positive (hand remains blanched) when this artery alone is released.

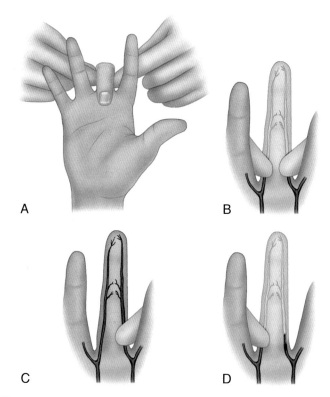

A   B

C   D

FIGURE 7.2 Allen test applied to digital arteries. **A,** Examiner occludes both digital arteries, and patient flexes finger. **B,** Patient extends finger, and blanching of finger is seen. **C,** When either artery is patent and it alone is released, color of finger returns to normal. **D,** When either artery is thrombosed and it alone is released, finger remains blanched. (From Ashbell TS, Kutz JE, Kleinert HE: The digital Allen test, *Plast Reconstr Surg* 39:311, 1967.)

methods. The history, physical examination, and Allen test determine the initial diagnosis. If the Allen test is positive, thermography, temperature probes, Doppler studies, and pulse volume recordings are used to confirm the diagnosis. If a stellate ganglion or brachial block relieves symptoms, treatment is observation. A stellate or brachial block may relieve vasospasm in acute thrombosis threatening digital survival. If symptoms are not relieved, arteriography is done, and, at the same time, intraarterial medications (reserpine or tolazoline) usually are given. Arteriography establishes the

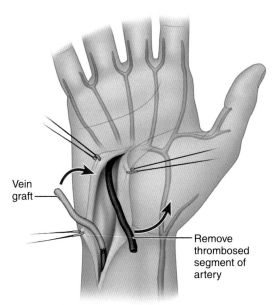

FIGURE 7.3 Resection of thrombosed segment and replacement with reversed vein graft. (Redrawn from Koman LA, Urbaniak JR: Thrombosis of ulnar artery at the wrist. In *American Academy of Orthopaedic Surgeons: Symposium on microsurgery: practical use in orthopaedics*, St. Louis, 1979, Mosby.)

diagnosis, identifies the extent of the thrombosis and vascular disease, and determines the probable success of surgery. Symptomatic treatment is indicated if vascular disease is generalized. If symptoms diminish after arteriography, the patient can be observed. Surgery is indicated if symptoms persist and if digital survival is in question. After the thrombosed segment has been resected, the proximal end is clamped and the tourniquet is released. If backflow is good and pulse volume recordings of the ulnar digits are normal, the vessel is ligated, and the wound is closed. If backflow is poor, with no pulsatile flow on digital plethysmography, vein grafting should be considered. Contraindications to vein grafting include erythrocytosis, patient refusal to modify the environment, and patient refusal to discontinue smoking. If vein grafting is indicated, the entire thrombosed segment should be resected until normal intima is seen with the operating microscope. A reversed vein graft harvested from the forearm is inserted (see Fig. 7.3). Vein grafting is contraindicated if there is inadequate peripheral "runoff" on the arteriogram. Persistent symptoms after surgery can be controlled conservatively by cessation of smoking, biofeedback techniques, and intermittent administration of intraarterial medications; sympathectomy can be used as a last resort.

The thrombosed mass may extend proximally in the forearm but rarely distally across the palmar arch to involve the more distal vessels; in the latter instance, complete resection may be impossible. Adequate resection relieves the spasm of the distal vessels, and symptoms usually improve; the circulation in the hand depends entirely on the radial artery, which usually is sufficient.

Radial artery thrombosis after cannulation has an incidence of about 10% to 18% after removal of the cannula; however, it is only symptomatic in about 5%. Spontaneous recanalization has been reported to occur in 35% of patients.

If significant ischemia is present surgical thrombectomy and repair with a vein patch or graft is performed.

In rare cases, thrombosis of a patent median artery may cause pain of median nerve compression within the carpal tunnel. It should be considered in the diagnosis when acute pain in the hand is limited to the distribution of the median nerve.

Arterial lacerations in the wrist and hand are discussed in chapter 2. Arterial emboli in the upper extremity account for 15% to 20% of all emboli. About 70% of emboli in the upper extremity are believed to be of cardiac origin (e.g., through atrial fibrillation or as postmyocardial infarction mural thrombi); the remainder are related to the subclavian artery. Usually, acute arterial embolism is signaled by pallor, cold sensation, ischemic pain, paresthesia, occasional paralysis, and loss of palpable or Doppler-sensed pulses. Treatment includes intravenous administration of heparin, Fogarty catheter embolectomy, and warfarin (Coumadin) therapy. If the embolus significantly obstructs flow and cannot be removed, intraarterial administration of streptokinase has been effective if given within 36 hours of thrombosis and if not contraindicated. Newer thrombolytic agents, such as reteplase and TPA, are also effective in the management of this problem.

THERMAL BURNS

Hands are involved in 80% of severe burns; however, life-threatening injuries and extensive body burns take precedence over hand burns. Assessment for inhalation injury is essential because mortality from burns with associated inhalation injury approaches 35%, whereas mortality from burns without inhalation injury is only approximately 4%. Burns are best managed in a specialized burn center and specific indications for transfer to a burn center are burns involving greater than 20% of total body surface area, inhalation injury, involvement of face, hands, feet, perineum, genitalia, and major joints. The rule of nines is used in estimation of burn size, with the surface area of the palm and fingers being 1% of the total body surface area. Other measures essential to early management include taking appropriate radiographs, establishing intravenous lines, administering tetanus prophylaxis and antibiotics, preparing for blood transfusion, and conducting a careful physical examination. Preserving viable tissue, preventing infection, controlling fibrosis, and avoiding deforming contractures also take high priority in the management of a burn injury in the hand.

Although the initial examination may be difficult because of pain and other injuries, an estimation of burn depth is necessary. Wilhelm Fabry in 1607 classified burns into first degree involving epidermis only, second degree involving the dermis, and third degree involving full-thickness skin. Tissue depth classification divided second degree burns into superficial second degree involving the papillary layer and deep involving the reticular layer. Fourth degree burns involve muscle, tendon, and/or bone (Fig. 7.4). The judgment of the treating surgeon usually determines the estimation of burn depth. Superficial burns (first degree) produce no blisters; although they are erythematous, capillary refill is good, sensation is intact, and the dermis is unharmed. Treatment is symptomatic with soothing lotions and the burns usually heal spontaneously in 2 to 3 days without scarring. In superficial

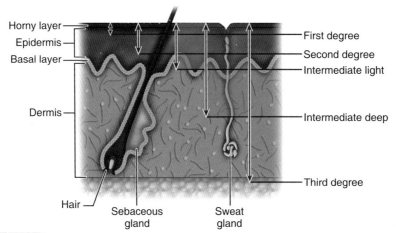

Horny layer
Epidermis
Basal layer

Dermis

Hair
Sebaceous gland
Sweat gland

First degree
Second degree
Intermediate light

Intermediate deep

Third degree

FIGURE 7.4 **Classification of burns by anatomic depth.** (From Baux S: Thermal and chemical burns. In Tubiana R, editor: *The hand*, vol 3, Philadelphia, 1988, Saunders.)

partial-thickness burns, some of the dermis is left intact, blisters may form, and capillary refill and sensation usually are present. They are quite painful since they involve nerve endings in the dermis; however, the blisters that are formed heal spontaneously in 10 to 14 days via re-epithelialization. Deep partial-thickness burns usually involve the entire dermis with minimal epithelial elements preserved. Capillary refill may or may not be present, but there should be some bleeding with pinprick; sensation usually is not intact; and thrombosed veins may be seen. These burns may heal spontaneously but very slowly and with considerable scarring. In deep burns (third and fourth degree) with dermal and subcutaneous necrosis, the skin appears leathery, brown to black, and no circulation or sensation to the skin is present. These cannot heal spontaneously.

The most important determination for limb survival is the adequacy of distal circulation, especially if the burn has a circumferential component. Interdisciplinary involvement is necessary and may include a burn team, pediatric surgeon, plastic surgeon, and hand therapist. Circulation of the upper extremity is considered adequate if the hand and fingers have rapid capillary refill and are pink, warm, and soft, and if pulsatile flow can be shown in the palmar and digital vessels with a Doppler probe. If the burn has a circumferential component with decreased distal perfusion (pale hand and fingers; decreased capillary refill; firm, cool hand and fingers; diminished flow shown by Doppler probe), immediate escharotomy should be considered. Intracompartmental pressures also should be measured, and if these are elevated, fasciotomies may be required. While perfusion is being assessed, the patient should receive adequate hydration with appropriate intravenous fluid replacement and monitoring of urinary output.

The depth of the burn, infection, and early management are major determinants of the functional and cosmetic outcome of hand burns. Other important factors are the location of the burn, the patient's age, and the patient's compliance with a rehabilitation program. There is agreement regarding the management of superficial hand burns and full-thickness and deeper burns. Superficial second-degree burns, if protected from additional injury and infection, should heal within 10 to 14 days with no significant impairment of hand function or cosmesis. Outpatient treatment usually is appropriate for

these injuries. For partial-thickness burns (deep dermal, superficial full thickness), two approaches are advocated: (1) a "wait-and-see" method, with conservative treatment consisting of hydrotherapy, topical chemotherapy, and physiotherapy, and (2) an "operative" approach (in the first 3 to 5 days, as soon as practical), with tangential or full-thickness burn excision and early skin grafting (Fig. 7.5). Advocates of conservative treatment believe that with close follow-up and good patient cooperation patients who are treated with topical antimicrobials (silver nitrate, silver sulfadiazine, mafenide acetate, povidone-iodine), hydrotherapy, and an organized rehabilitation program may achieve long-term functional and cosmetic results similar to patients who undergo early surgical treatment. The risks and discomfort of the surgical route are avoided. Falcone and Edstrom proposed an algorithm for management of hand burns that allows flexibility for appropriate, timely treatment, depending on burn depth and apparent wound healing (Fig. 7.6).

Proponents of surgical treatment of partial-thickness hand burns cite as advantages (1) accurate determination of burn depth early in treatment, (2) earlier physiologic healing achieved by definitive debridement, closure, and skin grafting, (3) early and quicker rehabilitation, and (4) avoidance of excessive scarring and contractures associated with the "failed" conservative method. Tangential excision with skin grafting and full-thickness excision with skin grafting are two techniques used for treatment of partial-thickness hand burns. The advent of vacuum-assisted closure (VAC), with and without the use of skin substitutes, has made early surgical intervention a better choice.

The special characteristics of the soft tissues in the hand allow for what might be considered a combined approach to partial-thickness burns of the hand. Dorsal burns may benefit from early excision (within 14 days) allowing for protective coverage and early mobilization of the superficial extensor tendon mechanism and interphalangeal joints where extension contractures can be devastating to hand function. On the flexor surface, the flexor mechanism and joints are deeper and relatively better protected and may tolerate a delay of 3 weeks better than the dorsal structures.

For deep full-thickness burns (third and fourth degree), primary full-thickness excision of the burn wound with skin grafting is the appropriate treatment (Fig. 7.7). For palmar

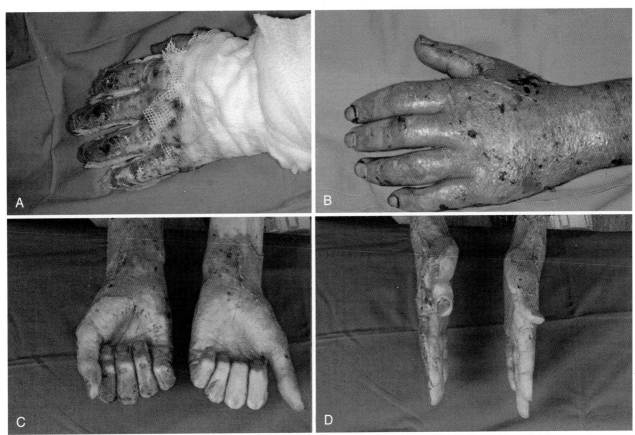

FIGURE 7.5   **A,** Biobrane glove (Smith and Nephew, New Zealand) fitted to superficially burned hand. **B-D,** Excellent cosmetic and functional result after spontaneous healing. (From Germann G, Weigel G: The burned hand. In Wolfe SW, editor: *Green's operative hand surgery*, ed 6, Philadelphia, 2011, Elsevier.)

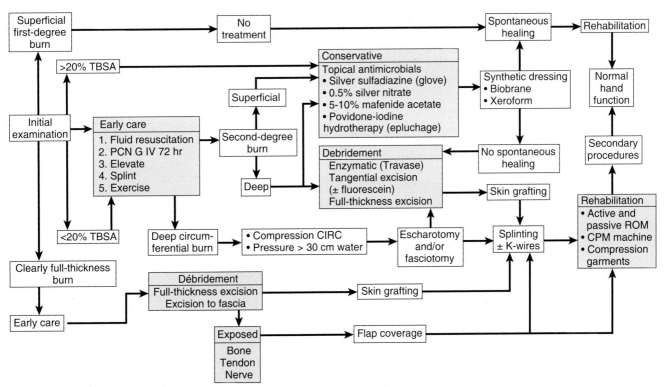

FIGURE 7.6   Algorithm for treatment of burned hand. *CIRC,* Circulation; *CPM,* continuous passive motion; *PCN,* penicillin; *ROM,* range of motion; *TBSA,* total body surface area. (From Falcone PA, Edstrom LE: Decision making in the acute thermal hand burn: an algorithm for treatment, *Hand Clin* 6:233, 1990.)

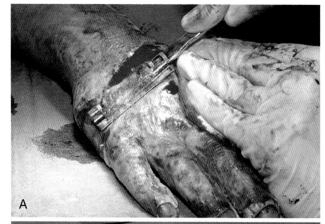

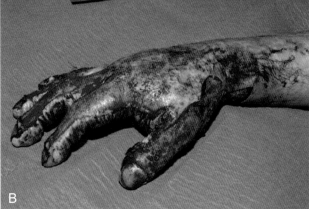

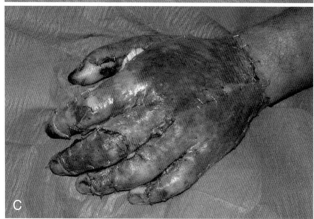

FIGURE 7.7 **A,** Tangential excision of deep partial-thickness burn on dorsum of hand. **B,** Sheet graft transplantation to excised areas. **C,** Short-term postoperative result. (From Germann G, Weigel G: The burned hand. In Wolfe SW, editor: *Green's operative hand surgery*, ed 6, Philadelphia, 2011, Elsevier.)

hand burns, full-thickness skin grafts offer improved durability and elasticity with less scar contracture than split-thickness skin grafts. Plantar glabrous skin grafts have been shown to offer reliable coverage in pediatric patients. Split-thickness skin grafting meshed 1 to 1 is preferred for dorsal coverage. When tendons, nerves, vessels, ligaments, bones, and joints are damaged by thermal injury, measures in addition to burn wound excision and split skin grafting may be required. Dermal substitutes such as Integra followed by skin grafting at 2 to 4 weeks has proved useful. Stabilization of bones and

joints with Kirschner wires, arthrodesis of destroyed joints, local and remote pedicled skin flaps, and free tissue transfers may be needed to preserve a viable, functioning hand. (For additional information, see chapter 4 for fractures, Chapter 10 for arthrodesis, Chapter 2 for flaps, and *Arthroscopy and Microsurgery Volume* for microvascular flaps.)

An organized plan of rehabilitation is important to the success of the treatment of the burned hand. The focus of rehabilitation in the early acute stage is wound care, edema control, and preservation of motion. After closure of the burn wound, a program including static and dynamic splinting, active and passive range-of-motion exercises, and control of scar and edema is pursued. Scar contractures may severely limit hand function, so rehabilitation should be aimed at prevention. Puri et al. recommended the preoperative use of splints in certain patients with thermal burn contractures. The rehabilitation plan depends on the needs of the individual patient and requires the participation of hand therapists, occupational and physical therapists, and physical medicine consultants. Many patients with severe and disfiguring burns require the emotional support of psychiatric and psychologic consultants.

ESCHAROTOMY

TECHNIQUE 7.1

(SHERIDAN ET AL.)

- Prepare the patient preoperatively for blood transfusion.
- With the patient supine, usually under general anesthesia and with the upper extremity extended on the hand table, thoroughly clean the extremity with an antiseptic and drape it.
- Make medial and lateral midaxial longitudinal incisions through the eschar using an electrocautery cutting current. At the elbow, make the medial incision anterior to the medial epicondyle to avoid the ulnar nerve. Stop the incisions at the metacarpophalangeal joints.
- If muscle compartments are tense, or if intracompartmental pressures are elevated, perform fasciotomies on the forearm and hand compartments (see chapters 11 and 12).
- Evaluate the adequacy of distal perfusion (skin color, warmth, and pulsatile flow in the hand and digits with the Doppler probe). If finger perfusion is unsatisfactory, perform digital escharotomies on the involved fingers, using pinpoint electrocautery along only the ulnar sides of the digits from the distal phalanges to the finger web spaces.
- Make a longitudinal incision between the digital neurovascular bundles and the extensor tendons.
- Make the incision for thumb escharotomy along the radial side of the thumb from the distal phalanx to the base of the thumb, avoiding the digital neurovascular bundle.
- Additional dorsal longitudinal intermetacarpal incisions between the index-middle and the ring-little metacarpals allow access for release of the interosseous fascia, if needed.
- Obtain meticulous hemostasis with electrocautery.
- Use a Doppler probe to assess distal flow.

- Apply a nonadhering, medicated gauze and a bulky, non-constricting dressing.

POSTOPERATIVE CARE The limb is elevated, and circulation is monitored. Finger movement is encouraged. Treatment after escharotomy depends on the extent and depth of the burn. If the burn is extensive and deep enough to require escharotomy, additional debridement and skin graft coverage may be required.

TANGENTIAL EXCISION

Tangential excision allows removal of dead tissue, while preserving viable deep dermis and superficial subcutaneous tissue. Tangential excision and grafting usually are done in the first 3 to 5 days after the burn injury occurs.

TECHNIQUE 7.2

(RUOSSO AND WEXLER MODIFIED)

- After inducing general anesthesia, place the patient supine and support the upper limb on the hand table. Apply a well-padded pneumatic tourniquet. Thoroughly clean the limb with antiseptic soap solution, with attention to the nails and removal of blebs and loose surface debris. The tourniquet can be used intermittently to control bleeding and to allow inspection for bleeding during the excision.
- Suspend the hand to an overhead pulley if needed for excision of the forearm and arm wounds. Usually this is unnecessary for hand excision.
- Exsanguinate the limb and inflate the tourniquet.
- Using a guarded knife or a dermatome, shave the burned areas tangentially in layers about 0.010-inch thick until punctate bleeding is encountered when the tourniquet is deflated. Shave the dermal and subcutaneous tissues containing venous thrombosis until healthy, bleeding tissue is encountered.
- Deflate the tourniquet and obtain hemostasis by electrocautery.
- Apply topical thrombin and cover the hand with warm, saline-soaked sponges.
- If satisfactory hemostasis has been achieved and if there are no areas of questionable viability, apply a split-thickness skin graft as a sheet or meshed and unopened.
- Place darts in skin folds at the interdigital webs and in the thumb-index web.
- Suture or staple the graft in place.
- Apply a dressing of nonadherent gauze covered with a synthetic compress (Acrilan) soaked in saline or glycerin.
- Support the hand in a fiberglass or plaster splint with the wrist extended, the metacarpophalangeal joints flexed, the interphalangeal joints slightly flexed, and the thumb in palmar abduction.
- If excessive bloody oozing occurs, or if tissue viability is uncertain, apply a saline-moistened dressing or a biologic dressing (Biobrane, heterograft, allograft), and support the hand with a splint. Repeat the process in 24 to 48 hours.

POSTOPERATIVE CARE The hand is elevated, and the patient is encouraged to begin active isometric exercises the first postoperative day. The wound is inspected at 3 to 4 days and at 7 to 10 days. If the graft is healthy in 7 to 10 days, hand therapy is begun, including gentle bathing of the hand, elastic compression, static and dynamic splinting, and active and assisted exercises. Sutures are removed in 10 to 14 days. Large areas of graft necrosis may require regrafting. Small areas may be left and treated with topical antimicrobials (silver sulfadiazine, mafenide acetate) until covered with epithelium. Splinting and therapy may require many months to reach a satisfactory functional end point.

FULL-THICKNESS EXCISION

Full-thickness excision involves excision of the entire layer of necrotic tissue superficial to the dorsal veins and extensor tenosynovium dorsally and superficial to the flexor tenosynovium and digital neurovascular bundles on the palmar surface.

TECHNIQUE 7.3

- Position and prepare the patient as for tangential excision. Inflate the pneumatic tourniquet just before excision, and deflate it when the excision is completed. Cleanse the limb, including the nails, with antiseptic soap.
- With the limb supported on a hand table, identify the boundaries of the burn wound to be excised. Mark the boundaries of burn excision with a skin pencil, making a pattern that conforms to the skin creases, avoiding tension lines at the skin-graft and graft-graft junctures. Extend the excision pattern into the finger and thumb-index webs to prevent finger scar syndactyly and thumb-index web contracture.
- Exsanguinate the limb with an elastic wrap and inflate the pneumatic tourniquet.
- Incise through the marked borders of the burn wound into the subcutaneous tissues. Identify and dissect in an edematous plane superficial to the dorsal veins and extensor tenosynovium dorsally and superficial to the flexor tenosynovium and digital neurovascular bundles on the palmar surface.
- After all necrotic skin has been removed, apply topical thrombin to the wound and wrap the hand in warm, saline-moistened gauze sponges.
- Deflate the tourniquet and remove it from the arm to prevent a venous tourniquet effect.
- Maintain the hand under compression and elevation for a sufficient time to achieve hemostasis or to minimize significant bleeding—usually 10 to 15 minutes or longer.
- Remove the wrap and obtain hemostasis with electrocautery.
- If satisfactory hemostasis can be achieved, position the metacarpophalangeal joints in flexion with transarticular Kirschner wires, if necessary, for dorsal burns and apply a sheet of split-thickness skin graft or mesh the graft (1:1 or 1:1.5) and apply it unopened to the dorsum of the hand. Suture the graft with interrupted 5-0 chromic gut suture or with small skin staples.

- If the burn is on the palmar surface, the metacarpophalangeal joints can be splinted in extension to avoid flexion contractures.
- Apply a nonadhering gauze pad covered with a soft compression bandage of synthetic material (Acrilan).
- Support the hand with a plaster or fiberglass splint or, if conditions permit, a previously fabricated thermoplastic splint with the wrist extended, the metacarpophalangeal joints flexed (dorsal burn), the interphalangeal joints slightly flexed, and the thumb in palmar abduction.
- If the bleeding cannot be satisfactorily controlled, wrap the wound with a saline-moistened dressing or biologic dressing (Biobrane, heterograft, allograft) and return in 24 to 48 hours to apply a graft.

POSTOPERATIVE CARE The extremity is elevated for the first 3 to 5 days. In 2 to 3 days, if necessary, the outer bandage is removed in the operating room to inspect the graft and remove any fluid collections. For small areas on the hand, the dressing can be changed in the patient's room. For large areas on the hand and forearm, sedation or an anesthetic frequently is required. Although the graft can be left open and exposed, it frequently is helpful to apply a light bandage of nonadhering gauze covered with gauze wrap to protect the graft from bumping and abrasion. Staples or Kirschner wires are removed in 10 to 14 days. After 7 days, or when the graft seems to be satisfactory, a hand therapy program is begun that includes gentle washing of the hand, dynamic and static splinting, elastic compression, and active and active-assisted exercises. Large areas of graft necrosis may require regrafting. Small areas can be treated with topical antimicrobials (silver sulfadiazine, mafenide acetate) until covered with epithelium. Splinting and therapy require many months to reach a satisfactory functional end point.

ELECTRICAL BURNS

Electrical burns frequently involve the upper extremity and involve working age males 95% of the time. The dominant hand frequently is injured, and 50% of these injuries result in amputation. Tissue damage can result from a combination of thermal, electrical, and metabolic cellular factors. The extent of injury is determined by the characteristics of the injuring current, including the voltage, amperage, and resistance of the tissues; the duration of contact with the current; and the patient's susceptibility to it (Fig. 7.8). Exposure to 1 to 2 mA causes a tingling sensation, 8 to 12 mA causes muscle contraction, and greater than 20 mA causes tetanic contractions exceeding the let-go threshold, causing prolonged exposure with dislocations and fractures. Although the skin damage caused by electrical injury may be the most impressive presenting finding, significant deep injury may be present as determined by the route the electrical current takes through the body. Maximal damage occurs in narrow anatomic zones such as the elbow, wrist, and fingers, which are called choke points. Electrical injuries may involve the central and peripheral nervous systems, the cardiopulmonary and peripheral vasculature, the musculoskeletal system, the kidneys, and the skin. Initial management is directed at resuscitation. Appropriate diagnostic measures

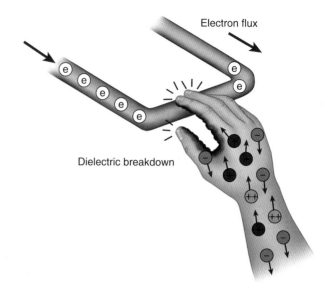

FIGURE 7.8 Electrical contact. Various damaging forces involved in high-energy electrical shock. With voltages greater than 1000 volts, electrical contact (arc mediated) precedes mechanical contact. High surface temperatures at contact points produce deep burns. Current passage through extremity leads to electrical breakdown of muscle and nerve membranes. Prolonged contacts of several seconds result in substantial deep tissue burning. High-energy arcs produce shock waves that can cause blunt trauma. (From Danielson JR, Capelli-Schellpfeffer M, Lee RC: Upper extremity electrical injury, *Hand Clin* 16:225, 2000.)

include radiographs of potential fractures and dislocations; electrocardiogram; and serum chemistries to assess electrolytes and liver, renal, cardiac, and skeletal muscle injury. Urine myoglobin levels and arterial blood gases are measured as well. The extent of injury to all systems should be evaluated, ensuring satisfactory hydration and urinary output, because patients with electrical burns may require more fluid resuscitation than might be calculated based on the injury to the total body surface area. Urinary output of 50 to 100 mL/hr is preferable. Recognizing, stabilizing, and reversing the effects of cardiac injury and the nephrotoxic effects of myoglobinuria and hemoglobinuria also are important. Because of the potential for hemorrhage from damaged vessels, a tourniquet should be kept near the patient's bedside.

In electrical burns of the hand and upper extremity, the initial evaluation should include a thorough examination of the entire body for skin and neuromuscular injury. Evaluation of circulation includes examination of skin color and warmth, palpation of peripheral pulses, and flow assessment with a Doppler probe. Skin burns may be the result of contact, flame, flash, or electrical arcing, or all of these may be factors. Contact burns have a central charred area surrounded by erythema. Flash and flame burns are thermal injuries, having the appearance of other thermal burns. Arcing burns usually are seen in the axilla, the antecubital fossa, and the distal forearm. There is no correlation between the size of the skin injury and the actual extent of injury.

Muscle injury is assessed clinically using the usual methods of palpation and evaluation of active motion and measurement of tissue compartment pressures. Extensive muscle damage may be undetectable in a clinical examination, and myoglobinuria may be a clue as to the extent of muscle injury.

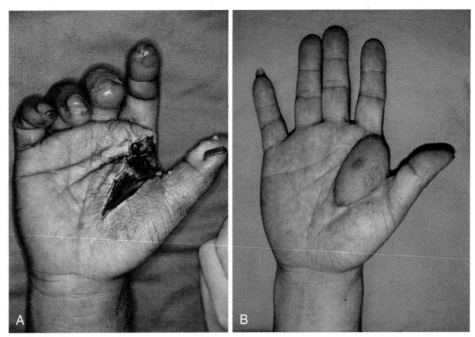

FIGURE 7.9 **A,** Electrical burn contracture of first webspace. **B,** After release and resurfacing with free lateral arm flap. (From Fufa DT, Chuang SS, Yang JY: Postburn contractures of the hand, *J Hand Surg Am* 39:1869, 2014.)

Other techniques that have been studied include technetium-99m pyrophosphate scanning, arteriography, and a xenon-133 washout technique. Deep injury also may be shown with gadolinium-enhanced MRI.

Patients with relatively minor electrical injuries may not require surgical treatment. For the management of more severe electrical injuries of the upper extremity, two methods are advocated. One method is immediate escharotomy, fasciotomy, and debridement of necrotic tissue, followed by repeat debridement until the wound is suitable for closure with skin grafts, remote flaps, or free tissue transfer. Decompression of peripheral nerves, including the median nerve at the carpal tunnel, is included in this initial procedure. Because tissue necrosis may not be clearly detectable for 24 to 48 hours after injury, some prefer a second approach in which decompression procedures are delayed unless decreased perfusion or increasing compartment pressures are clearly evident. The extent and severity of the injury may make amputation inevitable. Mann et al. reported an amputation rate of 45% in patients who had decompression within 24 hours and a rate of 10% in patients undergoing delayed decompression and debridement. Management of severe injuries should proceed in a progressive manner. Decompression by escharotomy and fasciotomy, when indicated, should be performed, followed by thorough debridement of necrotic tissue, usually in a serial fashion, and coverage by means of skin grafting, a remote flap technique, or free tissue transfer. After a course of healing and rehabilitation, patients with electrical burns may require additional reconstructive procedures (Fig. 7.9).

RADIATION BURNS

In radiation burns or dermatitis caused by overexposure to roentgen rays, the skin becomes pale, dry, atrophic, and wrinkled, and scattered keratoses develop; the fingernails split longitudinally. Within weeks of exposure, itching, erythema, and blistering may be seen; later, painful ulcers may develop. The skin can become increasingly painful, and eventually narcotics may be indicated. Multiple squamous cell carcinomas may develop and cause ulceration. Such burns have caused physicians and other medical professionals to lose digits. These burns, typically on the dorsum of the fingers of the left hand, presumably are caused in the medical profession by holding roentgen cassettes or using the fluoroscope without protection. When breakdown of tissue, pain, or malignant change makes resurfacing of the hand necessary, the damaged skin is excised and split-thickness grafts are applied simultaneously. The area of excision should be generous, including even questionably involved skin; usually all dorsal skin from the wrist distally should be replaced. Malignant changes in the hand may require amputation.

CHEMICAL BURNS

Chemical burns to the hand usually result from spills, splashing, or immersion. Most chemical burns to the hand are superficial, requiring only first aid management, and the prognosis is good. It is important to remember, however, that certain chemicals carry a risk of systemic toxicity and even death. Circumferential burns of the hand are unusual. Sulfuric acid and alkali account for most chemical injuries. Acid burns usually progress until damaged tissue neutralizes the acid or the acid is neutralized by lavage or a neutralization treatment. Injury caused by alkaline substances may progress for long periods, resulting in extensive and deep liquefaction necrosis. Jelenko and Reilly and Garner reviewed the chemicals that burn and their recommended emergency treatment (Fig. 7.10). Prolonged water lavage is best for most chemical burns, avoiding attempts to neutralize with either alkaline or acidic solutions. It should be started at the scene of

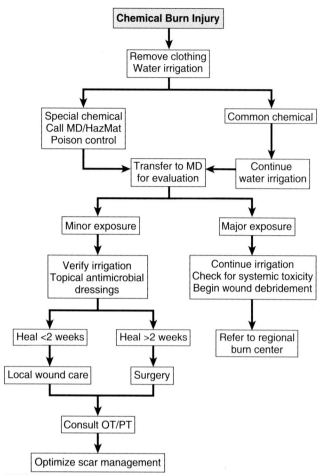

Chemical Burn Injury

Remove clothing
Water irrigation

Special chemical
Call MD/HazMat
Poison control

Common chemical

Transfer to MD
for evaluation

Continue
water irrigation

Minor exposure

Major exposure

Verify irrigation
Topical antimicrobial
dressings

Continue irrigation
Check for systemic toxicity
Begin wound debridement

Heal <2 weeks

Heal >2 weeks

Refer to regional
burn center

Local wound care

Surgery

Consult OT/PT

Optimize scar management

FIGURE 7.10 Critical pathway for treatment of chemical burn injury. (From Reilly DA, Garner WL: Management of chemical injuries to the upper extremity, *Hand Clin* 16:215, 2000.)

TABLE 7.1

Common Chemicals

COMMERCIAL TYPES	CHEMICAL COMPOUND	TREATMENT
Batteries	Sulfuric acid, Li^{2+}	Water irrigation
Toilet bowl cleaners	HSO_4 HCl (muriatic acid)	Water irrigation
Pool cleaners	HCl	Magnesium oxide, soaps
Rust removers	HFl (H^+/F1), chromic acid	Water irrigation, calcium/magnesium ($Ca^{2+}Mg^{2+}$) slurry
Petroleum solvents	Organics	Dilute soaps, water irrigation
Bleach	Sodium hypochlorite	Water irrigation
Drain unclog-gers, oven cleaners	Lye (sodium hypo-chlorite), NaOH	Water irrigation
Tile cleaners*	Ammonium chloride (alkali)	Water irrigation
Cement	Lye	Water irrigation

*Brand-name companies make multiple products—some acid, some alkali. It is not enough to have patients tell you what brand-name chemical they came into contact with; the exact product name must be known to treat an injury adequately.
From Reilly DA, Garner WL: Management of chemical injuries to the upper extremity, *Hand Clin* 16:215, 2000.

injury and should last 20 to 30 minutes to bring the skin pH to near neutral. Lavage for longer periods of time may be necessary for severe acid burns and for alkali burns. Chemical injury from some agents requires specific management (Table 7.1). Exposure of elemental lithium, potassium, and sodium to water causes ignition. Initial management includes mineral oil application, followed by water irrigation of particles remaining in the skin. Hydrofluoric acid, which is used in glass etching and petrochemical refining, results in continuing tissue damage because of the fluoride ion, which combines with calcium and magnesium in the tissues. Hypocalcemia may result if it involves more than 2.5% total body surface area. After initial water irrigation, application of a 2.5% calcium gluconate gel may be sufficient. If pain is not relieved promptly, injection of 10% calcium gluconate or magnesium sulfate deep to the lesions may be beneficial. For persistent pain, 10 cc of 10% calcium gluconate in 40 cc saline can be delivered as Bier block or intraarterially over 4 hours or until the pain is eliminated. Because phenol is not water soluble, removal with glycerol or polyethylene glycol has been recommended. White phosphorus particles may continue to smoke as long as they are exposed to air. Initial irrigation with a solution of 1% to 3% copper sulfate blackens the phosphorus particles so that they can be removed under water in a water bath. If the phosphorus is not irrigated first with copper sulfate, it may ignite on contact with water. Tar burns are best treated with an emulsifying agent such as Neosporin cream. Significant chemical burns seen late may require hospitalization and monitoring of the hand and digital circulation with Doppler probes and digital oximetry. If circulatory compromise results from a circumferential burn, decompression is indicated. Deeper chemical burns may require debridement and closure with skin grafts, pedicle flaps, or free tissue transfer. Recovery usually is prompt if surgical treatment is combined with a hand therapy rehabilitation program.

FROSTBITE

Frostbite injuries to the hands and feet account for about 90% of frostbite cases. Frostbite tissue damage seems to arise from direct cell death owing to freezing and anoxia caused early by vascular constriction and later by vascular thrombosis. Research by Heggers et al. found elevation of thromboxane and prostaglandin metabolites in frostbite blister fluid. In order of increasing degrees of damage, the following conditions develop: erythema, edema, vesiculation, necrosis of the skin, necrosis of deeper soft tissue, and necrosis of bone (Fig. 7.11). Superficial frostbite results in relatively clear blisters, and deeper injuries may be anesthetic after thawing and form hemorrhagic blisters. The traditional categorization of frostbite into four degrees has not been as useful in determining results of treatment as has the designation of the injuries as *superficial* and *deep* (Box 7.1).

Regardless of the depth of injury, the initial treatment of frostbite is the same. In the field, there should be no attempt at rewarming because of the risk of refreezing and consequently

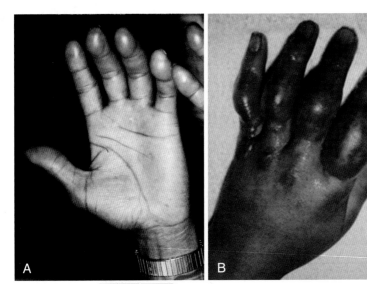
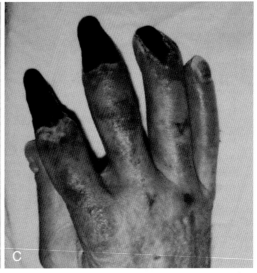

FIGURE 7.11 Frostbite injuries. **A** and **B**, Superficial (first and second degree frostbite). **C**, Deep frostbite 3 weeks after injury. (From Hutchison RL: Frostbite of the hand, *J Hand Surg Am* 39:1863, 2014.)

more injury. Splinting the part and support of the patient with prompt transfer to a hospital is recommended. The immediate basic care of frostbite, whether the tissue is blistered or discolored, is warming in a water bath and cleaning, followed by minimal debridement and watchful waiting for necrosis. A widely accepted treatment protocol has been developed to include later management (Fig. 7.12). Rewarming is done gradually. The patient is placed in a tub or whirlpool bath with the temperature at about 38°C. The bath temperature is slowly increased to about 40°C. The goal is to bring the skin temperature to normal in 15 to 20 minutes. Care is taken to support the circulation with intravenous infusions and to minimize systemic acidosis, which may occur. Sodium bicarbonate should be given as needed. After warming, the hand should be washed daily. A Hubbard tank usually is satisfactory for washing. Blisters are debrided if they rupture spontaneously, become too tight and uncomfortable, or become infected; otherwise, they should not be disturbed. Active motion should be encouraged, and frequent washings should be continued. Amputation should be delayed until there is definite demarcation; this may require several weeks or a few months. Radiographic techniques, including technetium-99m–labeled methylene diphosphonate bone scanning, MRI, and magnetic resonance angiography, can be helpful in identifying demarcation of tissue necrosis. Splinting and an organized program of hand therapy may be needed to assist in fully rehabilitating the patient. In contrast to thermal burns, there is no place for early excision and grafting in the treatment of frostbite. If there is extensive tissue loss, coverage may require skin grafts, pedicle skin flaps, and free tissue transfer.

Physeal arrest has been described in several children with severe frostbite (Fig. 7.13); the index and little fingers were involved more frequently than the middle and ring fingers, and the thumb was involved least of all. Disturbance in growth develops gradually. Later in life, procedures may be needed to correct angular deformities; these should be delayed as long as possible to obtain maximal growth.

BOX 7.1

Classification of Cold Injury According to Severity

Superficial

First Degree
Partial skin freezing
Erythema, edema, and hyperemia
No blisters or necrosis
Occasional skin desquamation (5-10 days later)

Second Degree
Full-thickness skin freezing
Erythema and substantial edema
Vesicles with clear fluid
Blisters that desquamate and form blackened eschar

Deep

Third Degree
Full-thickness skin and subcutaneous tissue freezing
Violaceous/hemorrhagic blisters
Skin necrosis
Blue-gray discoloration

Fourth Degree
Full-thickness skin, subcutaneous tissue, muscle, tendon, and bone
Freezing
Little edema
Initially mottled, deep red or cyanotic
Eventually dry, black, and mummified

From McAdams TR, Swenson DR, Miler RA: Frostbite: an orthopedic perspective, *Am J Orthop* 28:23, 1999.

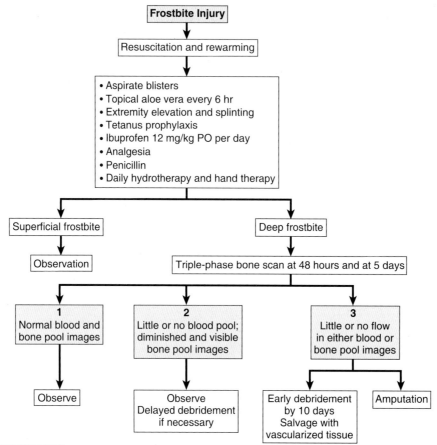

FIGURE 7.12   Treating frostbite injuries of upper extremity. After initial resuscitation and rewarming, clinical assessment of injury severity is made. Triple-phase bone scan is performed in deep injuries at 48 hours and repeated 72 hours later if no flow is seen in delayed images. Vascularized tissue transfer is performed if patient is candidate for salvage. (From Su CW, Lohman R, Gottlieb LJ: Frostbite of the upper extremity, *Hand Clin* 16:235, 2000.)

INJECTION INJURIES

High-pressure injection injuries can be devastating, frequently resulting in functional loss or amputation. Nozzle pressure as low as 100 psi can penetrate the skin, and some materials are sprayed at a pressure as high as 10,000 psi. The main determinants of outcome are location of the injection, pressure of injection, the material injected, and the time to surgical debridement. Fluids that have been accidentally injected into the hand through high-pressure guns include water, lubricating grease, diesel fuel, brake fluid, dry cleaning solvents, insecticides, paint, turpentine, cement, molten metal, and plastics. Oil-based substances are particularly hazardous. Paints have been found to be more toxic than grease, and oil-based paints are more damaging than latex paints. Dry cleaning solvents (hydrocarbons, methoxypropanol, and dichlorofluoroethane) may cause tissue necrosis owing to local toxicity, at times resulting in amputation of the digit.

The nozzle pressure in paint guns may reach 5000 psi. Paint gun injuries usually are caused by wiping the jet opening of a high-pressure gun with the index fingertip. The stream of paint strikes the part with such pressure that it penetrates the skin and spreads widely throughout the underlying fascial planes and tendon sheaths. The resulting distention of tissues and the inflammatory reaction cause marked ischemia of tissue; tissue necrosis, fever, and leukocytosis follow. Immediate incision and drainage of the injured part, with the patient under general anesthesia, are recommended to relieve pressure and to remove as much of the foreign material as possible; delay in such treatment can result in loss of the part. Amputation rates reported for injection injuries range from 16% to 49%. Higher amputation rates have been associated with organic and caustic materials.

Grease gun injuries (Fig. 7.14), similar to paint gun injuries, are caused by penetration of the tissues by grease or diesel fuel under high pressure. The grease or fuel balloons the soft tissues and follows the planes of least resistance; it causes ischemia and chemical irritation, but the inflammation is not as severe as that caused by paint. Treatment consists of relieving ischemia by decompression and, if possible, preventing infection; the distended tissues are opened immediately through bold incisions that follow the principles given for placing hand incisions (see chapter 1), and the foreign material is evacuated. The incisions are closed loosely, if at all; antibiotics are administered, and the hand is immobilized and elevated.

SHOTGUN INJURIES

Shotgun injuries are low-velocity missile wounds, are multiple, and often are contaminated by such foreign material as clothing and wadding from the shotgun shell. The wadding

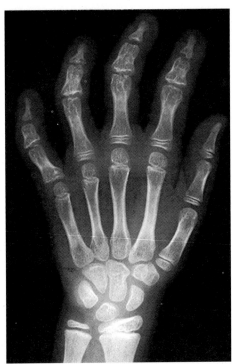

FIGURE 7.13 Deformities of fingers in 12-year-old girl caused by frostbite incurred at age 2 years. Note destruction of epiphyses of middle and distal phalanges of all fingers and deformity of epiphysis of proximal phalanx of little finger. Osseous changes in right hand were similar. (From Bigelow DR, Ritchie GW: The effects of frostbite in childhood, *J Bone Joint Surg* 45B:122, 1963.)

usually is made of paper or plastic and represents a dangerous foreign body contaminating the wound. In the upper extremity, such injuries usually occur at close range and the clustered shots cause destruction of multiple tissues; often the skin surrounding the wound is burned by powder (Fig. 7.15).

The wound should be thoroughly debrided of foreign material, devitalized muscle, fat, and skin. Nerves, although damaged, should not be excised. Removing every piece of shot is unnecessary, but attempts should be made to remove any that are lodged within joints. Pellets lying just beneath the skin often erode it, are painful, and require removal later. All free osseous fragments should be removed, and any segmental defects in bones should be bridged by Kirschner wires to prevent collapse of the bony architecture. External fixation may be required to maintain skeletal alignment if there are large bone defects. When the patient's condition permits and when joints, nerves, and tendons are exposed, the wound can be closed primarily or with skin grafts. A remote pedicle flap or free tissue transfer may be necessary. A filleted finger is useful. The wound can be left open for a few days but should not be allowed to fill in slowly by granulation tissue and heal spontaneously. A healed, stable wound is necessary before any reconstructive surgery is possible.

WRINGER INJURIES

The term *wringer injury* was first used by MacCollum in 1938 to designate a crushing injury of the upper extremity caused by its passage between the rollers of the wringer on an electric washing machine. Similar injuries continue to occur in industrial workers. Early examination may reveal only abrasions or tears of the skin or occasionally a fracture. This first examination often is misleading, however, because severe swelling caused by hemorrhage and edema may occur hours later. If the injury is severe, the skin and deep tissues are burned by the rollers, often at one level where the extremity is blocked from entering farther between the rollers, usually at the base of the thumb, the antecubital fossa, or the axilla. Some of the skin avulsion may be caused by the patient's vigorous attempts to free the limb while the rollers are still in motion. These injuries typically include bursting of the skin at the thumb web, with the thenar muscles protruding through the opening. Hospitalization usually is required. The limb is cleaned with soap and water, and any open wounds are debrided and closed loosely or left open for delayed closure or skin grafting. A pressure dressing that includes the entire hand is applied immediately, with care taken to distribute the pressure evenly. First, the area is covered by finely woven, nonadherent gauze, and flat gauze pads are applied; next, large masses of cotton and an elastic bandage are rolled on evenly. The extremity is elevated and is kept so throughout treatment. At 24 hours, the dressing is removed; the wound then is inspected for blisters, hematomas, and necrosis and the dressing is reapplied. This is repeated every 24 hours until the injury becomes stabilized. If necessary, any devitalized tissue is excised, and the wound is closed appropriately.

EXTRAVASATION INJURIES

Extravasation of numerous intravenously administered medications can cause deep necrosis and morbidity. Problems related to the extravasation of chemotherapeutic agents and radiographic contrast materials have been reported frequently in recent years. Effects of some extravasated substances may be minimal, whereas others may cause extensive tissue necrosis. These substances may be grouped into vesicants and irritants. Vesicants may cause full-thickness tissue death, pain, and redness. Irritants cause pain without an inflammatory component.

With an incidence of 0.5% to 6% or more, extravasation of chemotherapeutic agents is a leading cause of tissue injury. Causative agents include doxorubicin, bleomycin, nitrogen mustards, bacille Calmette-Guérin, and 5-fluorouracil. Lesions caused by their extravasation range from deep tissue necrosis to perivenous hyperpigmentation. Postextravasation necrosis is determined by several factors, including the agent extravasated, the extravasation site, the host response, the delay in recognition and treatment, and the type of treatment administered. Box 7.2 lists risk factors involved in extravasation injuries. Pathophysiologic mechanisms of injury secondary to extravasation include ischemic necrosis, cell toxicity, mechanical compression, osmotic damage, and bacterial proliferation beneath an eschar. In a report of doxorubicin extravasation injuries, Linder et al. found that factors causing extravasation included infusion under pressure, failure to release a proximal tourniquet, use of inadequate veins, thrombosis of proximal veins, spasm at previous venipuncture sites, active thrombophlebitis, and veins with multiple holes near the infusion site.

Most authors recommend immediate treatment. There is no universal agreement on pharmacologic treatment. Reported antidotes include hydrocortisone, hyaluronidase,

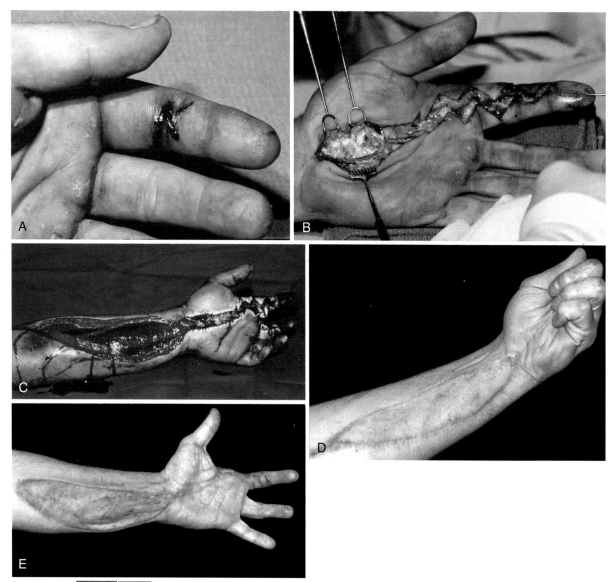

FIGURE 7.14 **A,** Site of high-pressure injection of unknown substance. Patient complained of pain and numbness of digit and palm. **B,** Extensive debridement was done through modified Brunner incision. **C,** Two days after surgery, compartment syndrome necessitated fasciotomies. Repeated debridements of devitalized tissue were required, including amputation of left index finger. **D** and **E,** Hand function at 7 months after injury.

propranolol, sodium bicarbonate, isoproterenol, topical dimethyl sulfoxide, vitamin E, and heat packs. Clinical studies support early debridement, drainage, irrigation, repeat debridement, and delayed closure as methods that consistently yield the best results. Ultraviolet light has been found to be useful in locating and removing fluorescent doxorubicin-containing tissue. After removing the extravasated fluid, intravenous fluorescein can be injected to determine the demarcation between viable and nonviable tissue for debridement. A comparison of various antidotes with early surgical treatment in rats found early surgical debridement most effective in decreasing the size of vesicant ulcers and speeding the healing of ulcers. In treating phenytoin extravasation in the hand, elevation and splinting with a compression dressing were effective in the absence of cellulitis, abscess, skin loss, or compartment pressure elevation. For treatment of upper extremity injuries from medications, the best results have

been obtained with immediate discontinuation of the intravenous line, elevation of the part, avoidance of antidotes, late debridement and coverage, and incorporation of a rehabilitation program early in the recovery. Healing without soft-tissue injury has been reported in 86% to 96% of patients with the use of liposuction and saline flush to remove extravasated material, preserving the overlying skin.

Although extravasation of radiographic contrast materials probably occurs more often than literature reports suggest, skin necrosis as a complication has been reported in 0.5% of radiographic contrast studies. The incidence increased with the introduction of automatic power injectors that allowed for less radiation exposure to the technician. Tissue response varies depending on whether iodinated high osmolar contrast is used versus noniodinated low osmolar contrast. The noniodinated contrast is more commonly used and causes much less tissue damage if extravasated. Local inflammation may be

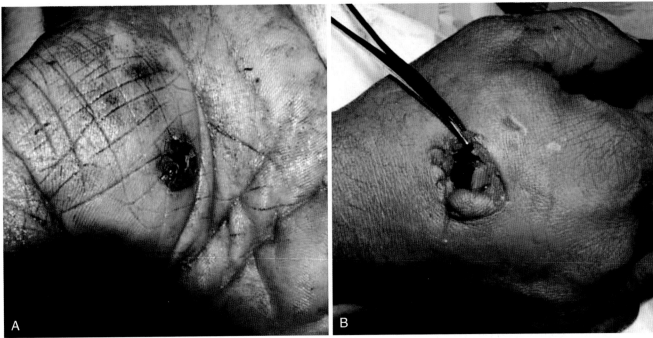

FIGURE 7.15 Close range gunshot injury shows tattooing from gunpowder **(A)** and exit wound **(B)**. (From Eardley WGP, Stewart MPM: Early management of ballistic hand trauma, *J Am Acad Orthop Surg* 18:118, 2010.)

the only response to extravasation of small amounts of contrast solutions. Large extravasations can result in skin necrosis, producing painful ulcers that are slow to heal. Historically, Loth and Jones reported that early surgical debridement, wound lavage, and delayed closure produced "excellent" functional and cosmetic results. Their management of patients with these injuries was determined by the amount of solution extravasated. Radiographs were used to estimate the volume and extent of extravasation. Insignificant extravasations (<5 mL) were treated with elevation in warm compressive dressings. Significant extravasations (>20 mL) were treated with emergency surgical drainage and wound lavage, preferably within 6 hours of extravasation. Intraoperative radiographs were used to ensure complete removal of contrast solution. When tissue necrosis was found, closure was delayed 3 to 5 days. Treatment of extravasation of 5 to 20 mL was based on the clinical presentation; severe soft-tissue reaction, swelling, and pain were indications for surgery. Less invasive surgical techniques are currently used for large (>50 mL) extravasations. Tsai et al. in 2007 described the manual squeeze technique in which multiple punctures or stab incisions are created and the contrast is expressed with squeezing or milking. Kim et al. in 2017 reported 23 patients in whom large volume extravasations were successfully treated with this squeezing technique.

FOCAL DYSTONIA OF THE HAND

Idiopathic focal hand dystonia is characterized by muscle cramps that accompany execution of specific tasks. These task-specific dystonias involving the hand are referred to as writer's cramp, keyboarder's cramp, occupational hand cramp, musician's cramp, or golfer's "yip." Unfortunately 1% to 2% of professional musicians are affected and may be forced to alter their career. Although there are cases reported

after musculoskeletal injury or paravertebral or central nerve injury, most are believed to involve dysfunction in integration or circuitry of the basal ganglia, sensory thalamus, and the somatosensory and sensorimotor cortices. A thorough history and physical examination will help differentiate focal dystonia from other diagnoses such as peripheral neuropathy, radiculopathy, plexopathy, thoracic outlet syndrome, repetitive overuse injury, focal seizures, medication effects, and psychogenic movement disorders. This condition often is treated with injection of botulinum toxin, but this is not a cure and merely targets the symptoms. Because this is a neurologic problem, sensorimotor retraining and proprioceptive activities generally are recommended.

PSYCHOFLEXED AND PSYCHOEXTENDED HANDS (DYSFUNCTIONAL POSTURES)

At least two typical postures of the hand are associated with psychiatric disorders. One is the psychoflexed hand or clenched fist syndrome (Figs. 7.16 and 7.17), in which either all or only the ulnar three digits are severely flexed and contracted. The clenched fist syndrome was first described by Simmons and Vasile in 1980 and the psychoflexed hand by Frykman et al. in 1983. These were thought to be different manifestations of the same disorder. It is generally considered a conversion disorder in which it is unconsciously motivated and unconsciously produced. Often this disorder is associated with depression, schizophrenia, or obsessive-compulsive disorders. It interferes with hygiene of the hand and may cause an offensive odor and palmar skin maceration. In addition, secondary infection can occur from pressure of the fingernails in the palm. There is no predilection for the minor or dominant hand. The psychoflexed hand should

Risk Factors in Extravasation Injuries

Patient Factors

- Increased age associated with greater likelihood of sustaining injury because of:
  Fragile skin and vessels
  Low muscle to subcutaneous tissue mass ratio
  Inability to report pain at infusion site
- Vascular compromise associated with reduced tolerance to injury
- Peripheral neuropathy associated with inability to detect pain upon extravasation

Mechanism of Injection and Infusion Site

- Use of power injectors instead of plastic cannulae
- Periarticular infusion sites more prone to injury because of movement
- Cannulae placed near tendons or nerves increases risk for severe complications
- Multiple previous venous punctures along a vein compromise venous wall

Type of Injected Drug

- Volume and concentration of drug injected
- Cytotoxicity
  Vesicant (DNA binding and non-DNA binding)
  Exfoliant
  Irritant
  Inflammatory
  Neutral
- Extremes of pH (agents with pH values over 5.5-8.5 are particularly harmful)
- Osmolality (hypertonic solutions cause tissue damage by cell implosion; hypotonic solutions cause tissue damage by cell explosion)
  Glucose (>10%)
  Sodium bicarbonate (>1.8%)
  Potassium/sodium chloride, calcium gluconate, magnesium sulfate
  Mannitol infusions
  Parenteral nutrition preparations (650 mOsm/L)
  Ionic, high osmolarity radiologic contrast media
- Vasoconstrictor agents
  Adrenaline
  Noradrenaline

Data from Goutos I, Cogswell LK, Giele H: Extravasation injuries: a review, *J Hand Surg Eur Vol* 39E:808, 2014.

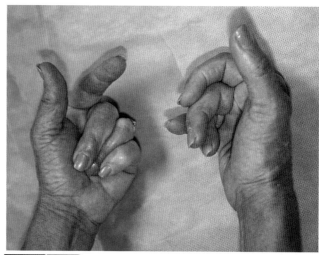

FIGURE 7.16 Psychoflexed hands. Patient had flexion contractures of ulnar three fingers of both hands with palmar maceration.

of a pinch mechanism preserved between the thumb and index finger. The index finger metacarpophalangeal joint is held in flexion, but active flexion and extension are preserved at the proximal interphalangeal joint, permitting opposition to the thumb pulp. Sometimes these patients permit passive extension at the metacarpophalangeal joint and passive flexion at the proximal interphalangeal joint, but after release the posture quickly recurs. Increased hyperextension is eventually possible at the proximal interphalangeal joints by persistent stretching. These patients rarely are distressed by their problems and rarely demand treatment to correct the posture. They may permit surgery to be performed, but it should be avoided. The treatment should involve physical therapy and psychotherapy, although these may be unsuccessful.

FACTITIOUS HAND SYNDROMES

Factitious lymphedema, Secretan syndrome, factitious ulcerations, subcutaneous emphysema, wound manipulation, pachydermodactyly, self-mutilation, and self-induced nail dystrophies may be encountered by physicians in all fields and occasionally are referred to an orthopaedic specialist. It is important to recognize the warning signs that the patient may be causing the presenting illness through a careful history and physical examination. Unlike the clenched fist syndrome, which is unconsciously motivated and produced, fictitious hand syndrome is unconsciously motivated but consciously produced. Also, in comparison malingering is consciously motivated and produced.

Grunert et al. identified three types of factitious hand syndromes, depending on the physical presentation: (1) self-mutilation and wound mutilation, (2) edema, and (3) finger and hand deformities. These patients had two distinct psychologic diagnoses: factitious disorder with physical symptoms and conversion disorder. Of two personality profiles identified with the Minnesota Multiphasic Personality Inventory, the emotionally dependent group responded to behavioral treatment, whereas the angry, hostile, and self-mutilating patients had the poorest response to treatment.

Self-induced injury should be suspected when there is a history of prolonged edema, lack of wound healing, or a deformity without a plausible explanation. Further suspicion

be differentiated carefully from such disorders as Dupuytren contracture, arthrogryposis multiplex congenita, and certain spastic hand deformities that occur secondary to stroke or cerebral palsy. Extensive workup may be necessary including electromyography and MRI to rule out other disorders. An experienced surgeon usually can distinguish these conditions easily.

The second posture is the psychoextended hand. It is similar to the psychoflexed hand except that the ulnar three digits are held in rigid hyperextension at the proximal interphalangeal joints and in flexion at the metacarpophalangeal joints. This seems to permit a partially functioning hand consisting

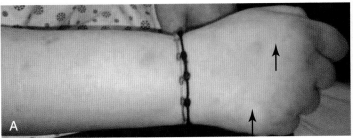
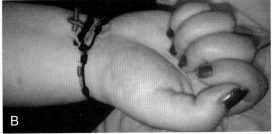

FIGURE 7.17 Clenched fist syndrome. Dorsal **(A)** and volar **(B)** aspects of hand with clenched fist syndrome in 28-year-old woman with history of multiple hospital admissions for headaches and arm pain. (From Birman MV, Lee DH: Factitious disorders of the upper extremity, *J Am Acad Orthop Surg* 20:78, 2012.)

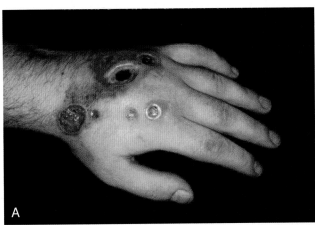
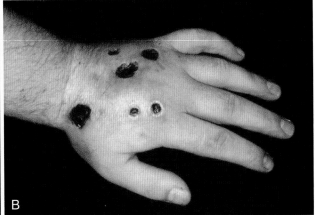

FIGURE 7.18 **A,** A 22-year-old man developed lesions that would not heal after trivial trauma at work. They regressed under cast immobilization **(B)** but reappeared after cast removal. They were presumed to be cigarette burns. (From Louis DS, Kasdan ML: Factitious disorders. In Wolfe SW, editor: *Green's operative hand surgery*, ed 6, Philadelphia, 2011, Elsevier.)

should be aroused when the patient gives a history of having seen several competent physicians who were unable to establish an organic diagnosis after multiple diagnostic procedures. Casting the edematous part or wound may be of diagnostic value if the cast is worn long enough for a wound to heal or for edema to resolve. Reappearance of the wound or edema after the cast has been removed helps to establish the diagnosis. Most of these patients do not wear the cast long enough to make a difference (Fig. 7.18).

Secretan disease was described in 1901 as an edematous process over the dorsal metacarpal area. It also has been called peritendinous fibrosis and factitious lymphedema. Although the cause is controversial, it has been considered to be a result of self-inflicted injury for the purpose of secondary gain or as a conversion reaction. Conservative, nonoperative care and psychiatric counseling generally are the best treatments for these patients.

The entire extremity should be inspected for evidence of some type of constricting band proximally. The edema varies in severity depending on the length of time and the frequency with which and how recently the limb has been constricted. The constriction usually is applied when the individual is alone. As with any patient, it is important to rule out an organic, anatomic basis for the complaint; however, surgery is rarely beneficial in these patients. Psychologic assistance should be obtained early in the course of evaluation and management.

REFERENCES

ANEURYSM, THROMBOSIS, AND EMBOLISM

Bouvet C, Bouddabous S, Beaulieu J-Y: Aneurysms of the hand: imaging and surgical technique, *Hand Surg Rehabil* 37:186, 2018.

Finke-Fyffe S, Regan J, Golan J, et al.: Hypothenar hammer syndrome: an uncommon cause of secondary syndrome and digital ischemia, *JAAPA* 32(9):33, 2019.

Fung A, Culig J, Taylor DC: Firearm-related hypothenar hammer syndrome in a police officer, *J Vasc Surg Cases Innov Tech* 4(3):223, 2018.

Kanei Y, Kwan T, Nakra NC, et al.: Transradial cardiac catheterization: a review of access site complications, *Catheter Cardiovasc Interv* 78(6):840, 2011.

Kim D, Arbra CA, Ivey S, et al.: Iatrogenic radial artery injuries: variable injury patterns, treatment times, and outcomes, *Hand (N Y)* May 1, 2019, 1558944719844348.

Kumar S, Jitendra M, Mishra V, et al.: Radial arter occlusion – incidence, predictors, and long-term outcome after transradial catheterization: clinic-Doppler ultrasound-based study (RAIL-TRAC study), *Acta Cardiol* 72(3):318, 2017.

Larsen BT, Edwards WD, Jensen MH, et al.: Surgical pathology of hypothenar hammer syndrome with new pathogenetic insights: a 25-year institutional experience with clinical and pathologic review of 67 cases, *Am J Surg Pathol* 37:1700, 2013.

Pasha AK, Elder MD, Malik UE, et al.: Symptomatic radial artery thrombosis successfully treated with endovascular approach via femoral access route, *Cardiovasc Revasc Med* 15:357, 2014.

Sheikh Z, Selvakumar, Goon P: True aneurysm of the digital artery: a case report and systematic review of the literature, *J Surg Case Rep* 2(1), 2020.

THERMAL BURNS

Askari M, Cohen MJ, Grossman PH, Kulber DA: The use of acellular dermal matrix in release of burn contracture in the hand, *Plast Reconstr Surg* 127:1593, 2011.

Cowan AC, Stegink-Jansen CW: Rehabilitation of hand burn injuries: current updates, *Injury* 44:391, 2013.

Davami B, Pourkhameneh G: Correction of severe postburn claw hand, *Tech Hand Up Extrem Surg* 15:260, 2011.

Friel MT, Duquette SP, Ranganath B, et al.: The use of glabrous skin grafts in the treatment of pediatric palmar hand burns, *Ann Plast Surg* 75:153, 2015.

Fufa DT, Chuang SS, Yang JY: Postburn contractures of the hand, *J Hand Surg Am* 39:1869, 2014.

Fufa DT, Chuang SS, Yang JY: Prevention and surgical management of postburn contractures of the hand, *Curr Rev Musculoskelet Med* 7(53), 2014.

Hundeshagen G, Warsawski J, Tapking C, et al.: Concepts in early reconstruction of the burned hand, *Ann Plast Surg* 84(3):276, 2020.

Kreymerman PA, Andres LA, Lucas HD, et al.: Reconstruction of the burned hand, *Plast Reconstr Surg* 127:752, 2011.

Liodaki E, Kisch T, Mauss KL, et al.: Management of pediatric hand burns, *Pediatr Surg Int* 31:397, 2015.

McKee DM: Acute management of burn injuries to the hand and upper extremity, *J Hand Surg Am* 35:1542, 2010.

McKee DM: Reconstructive options of burn injuries to the hand and upper extremity, *J Hand Surg Am* 36:922, 2011.

Pan BS, Vu AT, Yakuboff KP: Management of the acutely burned hand, *J Hand Surg Am* 40:1477, 2015.

Parcells AL, Karcich J, Granick MS, Marano MA: The use of fetal bovine dermal scaffold (primatrix) in the management of full-thickness hand burns, *Eplasty* 14:336, 2014.

Park YS, Lee JW, Huh GY, et al.: Algorithm for primary full-thickness skin grafting in pediatric hand burns, *Arch Plast Surg* 39:483, 2012.

Puri V, Khare N, Venkateshwaran N, et al.: Serial splintage: preoperative treatment of upper limb contracture, *Burns* 39(6):1096, 2013.

Richards WT, Vergara E, Dealaly DG, et al.: Acute surgical management of hand burns, *J Hand Surg Am* 39:2075, 2014.

Williams N, Stiller K, Greenwood J, et al.: Physical and quality of life outcomes of patients with isolated hand burns—a prospective audit, *J Burn Care Res* 33:188, 2012.

ELECTRICAL BURNS

Jeevaratnam JA, Nikkhah D, Nugent NF, Blackburn AV: The medial sural artery perforator flap and its application in electrical injury to the hand, *J Plast Reconstr Aesthet Surg* 67:1591, 2014.

Karunadasa KP, Beneragama TS, Dissanayake DA, Perera D: Dorsal metacarpal artery flap for resurfacing of fourth-degree electrical burns of fingers, *J Burn Care Res* 31:674, 2010.

Lee GK, Suh KJ, Kang IW, et al.: MR imaging findings of high-voltage electrical burns in the upper extremities: correlation with angiographic findings, *Acta Radiol* 52:198, 2011.

CHEMICAL BURNS

Robinson EP, Chhabra AB: Hand chemical burns, *J Hand Surg Am* 40:604, 2015.

FROSTBITE

Chandran GJ, Chung B, Lalonde J, Lalonde DH: The hypothermic effect of a distal volar forearm nerve block: a possible treatment of acute digital frostbite injuries? *Plast Reconstr Surg* 126:946, 2010.

Grasu BL, Jones CM, Murphy MS: Use of diagnostic modalities for assessing upper extremity vascular pathology, *Hand Clin* 31(1), 2015.

Hutchison RL: Frostbite of the hand, *J Hand Surg Am* 39:1863, 2014.

Kiss TL: Critical care for frostbite, *Crit Care Nurs Clin North Am* 24:581, 2012.

Kloeters O, Ryssel H, Suda AJ, Lehnhardt M: Severe frostbite injury in a 19-year-old patient requiring amputation of both distal forearms and lower legs due to delayed rescue: a need for advanced accident collision notification systems? *Arch Orthop Trauma Surg* 131:875, 2011.

Knobloch K, Ipaktchi R, Rennekampff HO, Vogt PM: Hand and facial burns related to liquefied petroleum gas (LPG) refuelling and cigarette smoking—an underestimated risk? *Burns* 36, 2010:e140.

Sever C, Kulachi Y, Acar A, Duman H: Frostbite injury of hand caused by liquid helium: a case report, *Eplasty* 10:e35, 2010.

Sever C, Kulachi Y, Acar A, Karabacak E: Unusual hand frostbite caused by refrigerant liquids and gases, *Ulus Travma Acil Cerrahi Derg* 16:433, 2010.

Wisler JW, Wisler JR, Coffey R, Miller SF: The diversity of wound presentation associated with Freon contact frostbite injury, *J Burn Care Res* 31:809, 2010.

INJECTION INJURIES

Amsdell SL, Hammert WC: High-pressure injection injuries in the hand: current treatment concepts, *Plast Reconstr Surg* 132:586e, 2013.

Rosenwasser MP, Wei DH: High-pressure injection injuries to the hand, *J Am Acad Orthop Surg* 22:38, 2014.

SHOTGUN INJURIES AND GUNSHOT

Al-Qattan MM: Air gun pellet injuries of the hand, *J Hand Surg Am* 31B:178, 2006.

Eardley WG, Stewart MP: Early management of ballistic hand trauma, *J Am Acad Orthop Surg* 18:118, 2010.

WRINGER INJURIES

Sever C, Külahci Y, Noyan N, Acar A: Thermal crush injury of the hand caused by roller type ironing press machine, *Acta Orthop Traumatol Turc* 44:496, 2010.

EXTRAVASATION INJURIES

Breguet R, Terraz S, Righini M, Didier D: Acute hand ischemia after unintentional intraarterial injection of drugs: is catheter-directed thrombolysis useful? *J Vasc Interv Radiol* 25:963, 2014.

Di Costanzo G, Loquercio G, Marcacci G, et al.: Use of allogeneic platelet gel in the management of chemotherapy extravasation injuries: a case report, *OncoTargets Ther* 8:401, 2015.

Goutos I, Cogswell LK, Giele H: Extravasation injuries: a review, *J Hand Surg Eur* 39:808, 2014.

Hahn JC, Safritz ZB: Chemotherapy extravasation injuries, *J Hand Surg Am* 37:360, 2012.

Hannon MG, Lee SK: Extravasation injuries, *J Hand Surg Am* 36A:2060, 2011.

Kim SM, Cook KH, Lee IJ, et al.: Computed tomography contrast media extravasation: treatment algorithm and immediate treatment by squeezing with multiple slit incisions, *Int Wound J* 14:430, 2017.

PSYCHOLOGICAL CONDITIONS

Birman MV, Lee DH: Factitious disorders of the upper extremity, *J Am Acad Orthop Surg* 20:78, 2012.

Byl NN: Diagnosis and management of focal hand dystonia in a rheumatology practice, *Curr Opin Rheumatol* 24:222, 2012.

Frykman GK, Wood VE, Miller EB: The psycho-flexed hand, *Clin Orthop Relat Res* 174:153, 1983.

Iroozabadi A, Seifsafari S, Mozafarian K, Bahredar MJ: Psychopathological hand disorders: a rare somatoform reaction to psychological conflicts, *Hand* 7(2):181, 2012.

Lungu C, Karp BI, Alter K, et al.: Long-term follow-up of botulinum toxin therapy for focal hand dystonia: outcome at 10 years or more, *Mov Disord* 26:750, 2011.

Opsteegh L, Reinders-Messelink HA, Groothoff JW, et al.: Symptoms of acute posttraumatic stress disorder in patients with acute hand injuries, *J Hand Surg Am* 35A:961, 2010.

Potter P: Task specific focal hand dystonia: understanding the enigma and current concepts, *Work* 41:61, 2012.

The complete list of references is available online at ExpertConsult.com.

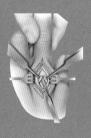

CHAPTER 8

PARALYTIC HAND

Norfleet Thompson

Sensation, mobility, and strength are required for the highly adaptive functions of pinch, grasp, and hook. Positional changes and delicate movements also are made possible by the many joints of the 29 hand, wrist, and forearm bones and by the 50 muscles that act as motors and stabilizers. To be purposeful, motion must be controlled, and joints crossed by moving tendons must be stabilized by balanced antagonistic muscles.

The normal upper extremity can rhythmically position the hand through varied concerted extrinsic and intrinsic phasic muscle activity. Muscle activities are controlled at the unconscious and conscious level and become patterned by repetition. Some patterns of muscle group movement act in such endless coordinated repetition that they are said to be synergistic or working together (Fig. 8.1). The wrist extensors, finger flexors, and digital adductors act together with ease and are synergistic; similarly, the wrist flexors, finger extensors, and digital abductors are synergistic. Beginning with the wrist flexed and the fingers extended and abducted, the wrist can be extended and the fingers can be flexed, and then the original position can be resumed with ease. With the wrist and fingers extended, however, flexing the wrist and fingers and then resuming the original position involves slower, more awkward movements that must be directed consciously.

When a major hand muscle is paralyzed, hand balance is disrupted. Unopposed antagonist muscle contraction often leads to fixed contractures. Although contractures may increase the stability of the hand, they usually increase its disability.

A common imbalance resulting in predictable contractures follows a low ulnar nerve paralysis leading to a clawhand deformity (Fig. 8.2). Paralysis of the intrinsic metacarpophalangeal joint flexors and intrinsic interphalangeal joint extensors (interossei and lumbricals) leads to characteristic deformities of the fingers, wrist, and thumb. In clawhand the extrinsic digital extensors and flexors are unopposed. The metacarpophalangeal joints extend and the interphalangeal joints flex at the fingers. The wrist is pulled into flexion by the strong finger flexors, which, by a tenodesis effect, worsens the metacarpophalangeal joint hyperextension. Even the thumb may assume a typical deformity.

The extensor pollicis longus adducts the thumb as it is unopposed by the intrinsic muscles of opposition and abduction. This adducted position is accompanied by extension of the carpometacarpal joint and flexion of the interphalangeal joint.

The hand position just described is known as the *intrinsic minus* or *clawhand deformity*. Whether the loss of intrinsic function is caused by disease or trauma, the results of dynamic muscle imbalance are the same. Sensation in clawhand varies according to the cause of imbalance. In poliomyelitis, sensation is normal; in peripheral nerve lesions, sensory deficits depend on the nerve lesion and level; in Hansen disease, sensation is absent, sometimes in a glovelike distribution; and in syringomyelia, sensation is partly absent.

Muscle spasticity also can disrupt hand balance, and muscle tension may not be controlled and balanced effectively by the opposing normal muscles. Such a situation is sometimes seen in cases of cerebral palsy, and it can cause overstretching of muscles and dislocation of joints.

PRINCIPLES OF TENDON TRANSFER

Tendon transfers are useful in restoring hand and upper extremity functions. Some basic principles must be followed if transfers are to be successful and if an increase in imbalance and deformity is to be avoided. After these principles are discussed, some specific tendon transfers are suggested for patterns of functional loss.

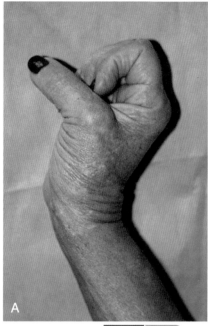
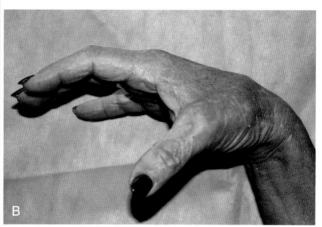

FIGURE 8.1   Synergistic muscle movement of hand (see text).

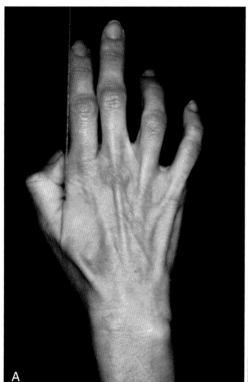
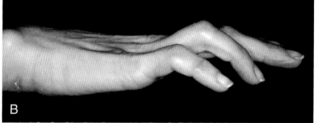

FIGURE 8.2   Clawing of hand caused by paralysis of intrinsic muscles. **A,** Long finger extensors cannot extend interphalangeal joints because metacarpophalangeal joints are hyperextended. **B,** Long finger extensors can extend interphalangeal joints because hyperextension of metacarpophalangeal joints has been prevented.

PLANNING TENDON TRANSFER

Regardless of the cause of the imbalance (traumatic, congenital, infectious, or vascular) the extremity must be evaluated in terms of function lost, function retained, and function possible through reconstruction. Muscles to be transferred must be expendable and have sufficient strength and appropriate amplitude of excursion. Moreover, the muscle should be synergistic, have appropriate alignment, and perform one function. Ideal timing of tendon transfers should consider the condition of the soft tissue and the mobility of adjacent joints. Transfers are best performed after reaching favorable soft-tissue conditions (not in the context of severe swelling or scarring) and after restoring passive motion of adjacent joints. Sometimes it is helpful to list in one column functions that are needed and in an opposite column the muscles available for transfer. Transfers can be planned with more ease and accuracy by matching these columns.

■ EVALUATING MUSCLES FOR TENDON TRANSFER

The two most important points in considering a muscle for transfer are its expendability and its strength. Restoring one major function, such as finger extension, is contraindicated if done at the expense of another major function, such as finger flexion. The strength of a muscle is graded from 0 to 5 as follows:

    0, zero—no contraction
    1, trace—palpable contraction only
    2, poor—moves joint but not against gravity
    3, fair—moves joint against gravity
    4, good—moves joint against gravity and resistance
    5, normal—normal strength

A muscle usually loses strength by one grade when transferred and should be good or normal if the transfer is to be satisfactory. In addition to expendability and strength, the synergy and the amplitude of excursion of its tendon should be considered. Rehabilitation of a muscle whose tendon has been transferred is less difficult when the transfer is synergistic (e.g., a wrist flexor transfer to restore finger extension). The amplitude of excursion of the tendon should be sufficient for satisfactory function, although it may not be as great as that of the tendon or tendons it is to replace. The brachioradialis, an expendable muscle for transfer, is capable of pulling its tendon through only a short excursion, but sometimes it can be useful, if not ideal, as a transfer to the long thumb flexor because even limited flexion of the interphalangeal joint of the thumb is useful.

The excursion of the brachioradialis can be increased by dissecting its tendon proximally and freeing all of its fascial attachments. The muscle is not useful as a transfer for finger flexion because its excursion cannot be increased enough.

■ TIMING OF TENDON TRANSFER

The transfer of tendons is the final step in rehabilitation of the hand. It should not be done until scar tissue has been satisfactorily replaced because transferred tendons must be surrounded by fat to prevent them from adhering to raw bone or subcutaneous scar; consequently, a flap or graft containing fat is necessary to replace scar. A satisfactory range of passive joint motion is also necessary before the transfer; proper splinting or ligamentous release is done as needed. Stiffness or contracture of joints cannot be corrected by tendon transfers alone; if left uncorrected, stiffness or contracture prevents a transferred tendon from moving at the proper time after surgery, so the tendon becomes permanently adherent to the surrounding tissues. Malalignment of bone must be corrected by osteotomy, and any necessary bone grafting must be accomplished before transfer. Necessary operations to restore any loss of sensibility should also precede tendon transfer.

In poliomyelitis, some recovery of muscle power can be expected until 18 months after the acute stage of the disease, and consequently this much time must pass before an accurate evaluation is possible; any further recovery cannot be expected to improve muscle strength more than one grade, if at all. During this waiting period, parts must be splinted properly to improve available muscle function and to prevent fixed deformity. In congenital anomalies, the relative muscle strength does not change. In syringomyelia, weakness may increase even after transfer. Peripheral nerve injuries must be considered individually; in division of the radial nerve at the midhumerus, transfers for finger and thumb extension and for thumb abduction should be delayed for 6 months or longer after neurorrhaphy. Certain nerve transfers also may be useful to restore function either alone or concomitantly with tendon transfers. Early transfer to restore wrist extension should be considered an internal splint for the wrist; this immediately improves the function of the hand. Transfer of the pronator teres to the extensor carpi radialis brevis is recommended. In high median nerve lesions, some function should return in the most proximal muscles in 4 months (3 months in low median nerve lesions); if it has not, the nerve should be explored, or tendon transfers should be considered.

TECHNICAL CONSIDERATIONS FOR TENDON TRANSFER

Although the strength of a muscle is evaluated clinically before surgery, its color at the time of tendon transfer provides a further check. A muscle suitable for transfer is dark pink or red, indicating satisfactory nutrition and the presence of normal muscle fibers. A weak or paralyzed muscle is pale pink and is smaller than normal, and its amplitude of excursion (Table 8.1) is less than normal when tested at surgery; such a muscle is unsuitable for transfer (Fig. 8.3). Muscles that do not contract with a stimulus (pinch or electrocautery) are probably nonfunctional and should not be chosen as active donor muscles.

A muscle that has been detached from its insertion some time before transfer will have developed a contracture, and consequently its tendon should be anchored under more tension than usual because it will stretch and regain some of its excursion. A muscle and its tendon should not make an acute angle between the origin of the muscle and the new attachment of the tendon—the straighter the muscle, the more efficient its action. If an acute angle is necessary, a pulley must be created, but efficiency of the muscle is diminished by friction at the pulley. In freeing a muscle for transfer, care must be taken to avoid stretching or otherwise damaging the neurovascular bundle, which usually enters the proximal third of the muscle belly. A transferred tendon cannot be expected to glide properly when it crosses raw bone, passes through fascia without a sufficient opening, or is buried within scarred

TABLE 8.1	
Amplitude of Excursion	
TENDONS	AMPLITUDE (MM)
Wrist tendons	33
Flexor profundus	70
Flexor sublimis	64
Extensor digitorum communis	50
Flexor pollicis longus	52
Extensor pollicis longus	58
Extensor pollicis brevis	28
Abductor pollicis longus	28

From Curtis RM: Fundamental principles of tendon transfer, *Orthop Clin North Am* 2:231, 1974.

tissue; with a few exceptions, transferred tendons should be passed subcutaneously. Should it be necessary to split a transferred tendon and anchor it to two or more separate points, the muscle acts primarily on the slip of tendon under greatest tension; great care must be taken to equalize tension on the slips at the time of attachment.

The more distal to a given joint a tendon is anchored, the more power the muscle can exert across the joint, but also the more excursion is required of the tendon to provide normal motion. The greater the angle of approach of a tendon to bone, the greater the force the muscle can exert on the bone and across the joint. Most muscles lie almost parallel to the bones whose joints they act on, and few approach a bone at close to a right angle; the pronator quadratus and the supinator are notable exceptions.

RESTORATION OF PINCH
RESTORATION OF THUMB OPPOSITION

Thumb opposition is necessary for pinch. Frequently, opposition is either partially or totally lost in poliomyelitis or median nerve palsy. Opposition depends primarily on function of the thumb intrinsic muscles, especially the abductor pollicis brevis. Extrinsic muscles also are necessary to stabilize dynamically the thumb metacarpophalangeal and interphalangeal joints, or these joints must be stabilized by arthrodesis or tenodesis. At the same time, the thumb carpometacarpal joint must be freely movable, unrestricted by contracture of the joint capsule or other structures of the thumb web.

Thumb opposition is a complex motion made by coordination of (1) abduction of the thumb from the palmar surface of the index finger, (2) flexion of the metacarpophalangeal joint, (3) internal rotation or pronation, (4) radial deviation of the proximal phalanx, and (5) thumb motion toward the fingers (see Fig. 8.13). Although opposition is the result of coordinated function of all of the long and short muscles that act on the thumb, the abductor pollicis brevis is the most important single muscle that participates in this complex movement; it rotates internally and abducts the thumb away from the index metacarpal, internally rotates and abducts the proximal phalanx of the thumb on its metacarpal, and assists the extensor pollicis longus in extending the interphalangeal

joint of the thumb. For these reasons, in restoring opposition by tendon transfer, the transferred tendon can be inserted into the tendon of the abductor pollicis brevis.

■ CORRECTION OF THUMB DEFORMITY

To restore thumb function properly, deformities or disabilities of the digit other than those corrected by the operation designed primarily to restore opposition frequently must be corrected either before or during such surgery. As a substitute for opposition, adduction of the thumb by the long thumb extensor may have become a habit; in these instances, adduction and extension of the thumb occur as a single function in which the flexed tip of the thumb is brought against the base of the proximal phalanx of the index finger by the pull of the long thumb extensor toward Lister's tubercle. Pinch occurs at the base of a finger instead of at its tip, and to pick up an object, the point of contact between the thumb and the finger must be rotated downward; this is accomplished by pronating the wrist, elevating the elbow, and abducting the shoulder. As the substitution patterns become more firmly established after paralysis of the intrinsic muscles of the thumb, the long thumb extensor tendon, acting as an adductor, gradually migrates into the web space between the thumb and index finger.

Any fixed adduction and external rotational deformity of the thumb must be corrected; this usually can be accomplished by dividing the fascia in the web space between the index and thumb metacarpals and by subperiosteal stripping of the ulnar side of the first metacarpal. If the deformity is severe, a Z-plasty of the web also may be required (see section on restoration of adduction of the thumb); if the deformity is so severe that it cannot be corrected by rotational osteotomy and release of the web space, arthrodesis of the first carpometacarpal joint may be indicated. A tendon transfer for opposition still may be useful after such an arthrodesis because the more proximal joints may allow some motion. If mobility is more desirable than stability, however, excising the trapezium may release the soft tissues enough to make arthrodesis unnecessary.

Tendon transfers to the long thumb flexor, long thumb extensor, or long thumb abductor may be necessary to stabilize the thumb dynamically if the transfer to restore opposition is to function satisfactorily. Arthrodesis of the metacarpophalangeal joint of the thumb may be necessary if available muscle power is insufficient to stabilize it dynamically, or if the joint is made unstable by relaxation of its ligaments or capsule. (Arthrodesis of this joint also may be indicated after tendon transfer to restore opposition when the tendon has been anchored in an incorrect location and hyperextends or hyperflexes the joint.) The joint is arthrodesed in 15 degrees of flexion and slight internal rotation to allow pinch between the thumb and index fingertip. Arthrodesis of the thumb interphalangeal joint is indicated occasionally for a fixed flexion contracture; it is arthrodesed in 20 degrees of flexion.

■ TENDON TRANSFERS TO RESTORE OPPOSITION

Multiple tendon transfer techniques to restore elongated pinch in paralytic hands have been devised. Common to all techniques is the selection of one extrinsic, expendable, healthy muscle-tendon unit motor and its transfer to a suitable point

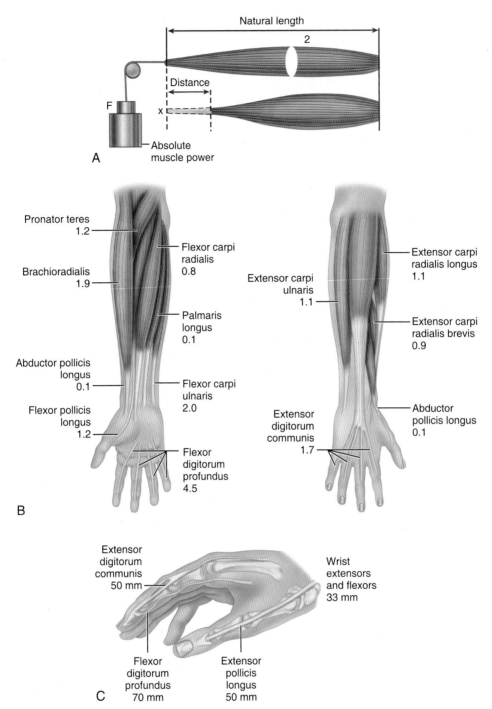

FIGURE 8.3 Power of muscle transfer. **A,** Working capacity of muscle. W = F × d, where F (force) = absolute muscle power, 3.65 × cm² of physiologic cross section, and d (distance) = amplitude or displacement. **B,** Working capacity of muscle in mkg (meter-kilograms). **C,** Muscle amplitude in millimeters. (Redrawn from Curtis RM: Fundamental principles of tendon transfer, *Orthop Clin North Am* 2:231, 1974.)

and angle to pull the thumb into opposition. The direction in which the transferred tendon approaches the thumb usually has been from the ulnar side of the wrist or palm; sometimes the tendon has been brought around a pulley to provide this direction. A pulley often is needed, and some authors prefer a static pulley created by making a loop at the distal end of the flexor carpi ulnaris tendon, whereas others prefer a dynamic pulley formed by looping the transfer around this tendon.

A proper muscle for a motor is selected after carefully evaluating the strength of available units. The ring finger flexor digitorum sublimis usually is the muscle of choice and often is used if it is strong enough to function as the transfer and if its associated flexor digitorum profundus is strong enough alone to flex the finger satisfactorily; the second choice is the sublimis to the middle finger. If the preferred flexor tendons of the digits are unsuitable for transfer, the extensor indicis proprius is an acceptable alternative. All other muscles require tendon grafting to reach the point of attachment on the thumb. The extensor carpi ulnaris is the next choice, followed by the palmaris longus or extensor carpi radialis longus. A wrist extensor should be transferred, however, only if the other wrist extensors are strong and have not been or will not be transferred elsewhere.

TRANSFER OF THE SUBLIMIS TENDON

TECHNIQUE 8.1

(RIORDAN)

- Expose the ring finger sublimis tendon through an ulnar midlateral incision over the proximal interphalangeal joint and divide the tendon at the level of the joint or just proximal to it.
- Divide the chiasm, separating the two slips of tendon at the level of the joint so that they pass around the profundus and can be withdrawn easily at the wrist.
- Expose the flexor carpi ulnaris tendon through an L-shaped incision that proximally extends along the flexor carpi ulnaris tendon and distally turns radialward parallel to the flexor creases of the wrist. To make a pulley, cut halfway through the flexor carpi ulnaris tendon at a point approximately 6.0 cm proximal to the pisiform (Fig. 8.4).
- Strip the radial half of the tendon distally almost to the pisiform and create a loop large enough for the sublimis tendon to pass through easily; carry the radial segment of the flexor carpi ulnaris through a split in the remaining half of the tendon, loop it back, and suture it to the remaining half.
- Make a wide C-shaped incision on the thumb as follows: Begin on the thumb dorsum just proximal to the interphalangeal joint and proceed proximally and volarward around to the radial aspect of the thumb. At a point just proximal to the metacarpophalangeal joint, curve the incision dorsalward in line with the major skin creases of the thenar eminence. On the dorsoradial aspect of the thumb, preserve the fine sensory nerve from the superficial branch of the radial nerve. Expose and define the extensor pollicis longus tendon over the proximal phalanx, the extensor aponeurosis over the metacarpophalangeal joint, and the abductor pollicis brevis tendon.
- At the wrist, identify the ring finger sublimis tendon and withdraw it into the forearm incision. Pass the tendon through the loop fashioned from the flexor carpi ulnaris.
- With a small hemostat or preferably a tendon carrier, pass the tendon subcutaneously across the thenar eminence in line with the fibers of the abductor pollicis brevis.
- Make a small tunnel for insertion of the transfer by burrowing between two small parallel incisions in the abductor pollicis brevis tendon.
- Split the end of the sublimis tendon for approximately 2.5 cm, or more if necessary, and pass one half of it through the tunnel.
- Separate the extensor aponeurosis from the thumb proximal phalanx periosteum, make a small incision in it 6 mm

distal to the first tunnel, and pass the same strip of sublimis through it. Bring the slip out from beneath the aponeurosis through a small longitudinal slit in the long extensor tendon about 3 mm proximal to the interphalangeal joint.
- Determine the proper tension for the transfer. Grasp the two slips of sublimis with small hemostats and cross them. With the thumb in full opposition and the wrist in a straight line, place the two overlapping slips of sublimis under some tension. Releasing the thumb and passively flexing the wrist should completely relax the transfer so that the thumb can be brought into full extension and abduction; extending the wrist 45 degrees should place enough tension on the transfer to bring the thumb into complete opposition and the tip of the thumb into complete extension.
- If the tension is insufficient, increase it and repeat the test.
- When the correct tension has been determined, suture the slips of sublimis together with the cut ends buried (Fig. 8.4).
- Anchor the transfer and the tendon of the abductor pollicis brevis to the joint capsule with a single nylon or wire suture so that the transfer passes over the middle of the metacarpal head; this prevents later displacement of the tendon toward the palmar aspect of the joint during opposition.
- Close the wound with nonabsorbable sutures and immobilize the hand in a pressure dressing and a dorsal plaster splint as follows: place the wrist in 30 degrees of flexion, the fingers in the functional position, and the thumb in full opposition with the distal phalanx extended; place a few layers of gauze between the individual fingers to prevent maceration of the skin.

POSTOPERATIVE CARE At 4 weeks, the dressing and splint are removed and active motion is begun, but the

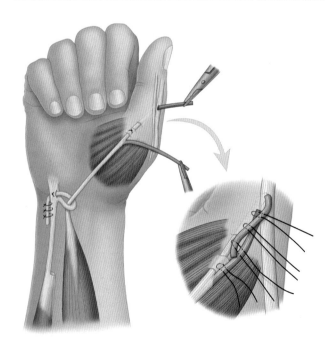

FIGURE 8.4   Riordan transfer to restore opposition (see text).
SEE TECHNIQUE 8.1.

thumb is supported with an opponens splint for an additional 6 weeks. Many patients can oppose the thumb as soon as the splint is removed. When the ring finger sublimis has been used for the transfer, as in the Riordan technique, training in its use can be facilitated by asking the patient to place the tip of the thumb against the ring finger; this maneuver produces flexion of the ring finger and an automatic attempt to oppose the thumb with the transferred sublimis. In patients with weak quadriceps muscles who habitually rise from a sitting position by pushing up with the flattened hands or in patients who use crutches, the transfer must be protected for 3 months or longer or it will be overstretched and cease to function.

TRANSFER OF THE SUBLIMIS TENDON

TECHNIQUE 8.2

(BRAND)
- Expose and divide the ring finger sublimis tendon and make the incision over the thumb as just described in the Riordan technique.
- Withdraw the sublimis tendon through a small transverse incision about 5 cm proximal to the flexor crease of the wrist.
- Make a small longitudinal incision just to the radial side of and about 6 mm distal to the pisiform. Deepen this incision until the quality of fat changes from the fibrous superficial type to a soft, loose, free type that bulges into the wound. This change in the fat marks the entry into a tunnel that runs proximally and contains a branch of the ulnar nerve.
- In this loose fat, make a tunnel in the proximal direction to the forearm incision, grasp the end of the sublimis tendon, and pull it through into the palmar incision. The tunnel is superficial to the hook of the hamate, and the fibrous septa in the fat compose the pulley.
- Pass the tendon to the thumb metacarpophalangeal joint and attach it proximal and distal to the joint after splitting its end; attach the proximal slip of the tendon to the ulnar side of the joint and the distal slip to the tendons of the abductor pollicis brevis and the extensor pollicis longus (Fig. 8.5). This dual insertion of the tendon may prevent the tendon from shifting in position as it crosses the metacarpophalangeal joint. (If an unsplit tendon shifts dorsally over the metacarpophalangeal joint, it is likely to hyperextend the joint; if it shifts anteriorly from the radial side of the joint, it is likely to flex the joint.)

POSTOPERATIVE CARE Postoperative care is similar to that described after the Riordan technique (see Technique 8.1).

If the ring or long finger sublimis is unsuitable for transfer, the extensor indicis proprius can be rerouted around the ulnar aspect of the wrist to provide opposition, as described by Burkhalter et al. (see Technique 8.3). For high median nerve

palsy or brachial plexus paralysis, a technique described by Groves and Goldner (see Technique 8.4) employing the flexor carpi ulnaris as a motor for a transferred sublimis tendon unit can be used.

TRANSFER OF THE EXTENSOR INDICIS PROPRIUS

TECHNIQUE 8.3

(BURKHALTER ET AL.)
- Through a short, curved incision on the radial side of the dorsum of the index metacarpophalangeal joint, identify the extensor indicis proprius tendon.
- Divide its insertion and a small portion of the extensor hood by sharp dissection and repair the hood with interrupted suture (Fig. 8.6A).
- If necessary, make a short incision over the midportion of the dorsum of the hand to withdraw the extensor tendon.
- Make a longitudinal incision about 2 cm long proximal to the wrist crease on the ulnar aspect of the forearm, and through it extract the tendon (Fig. 8.6B).
- Cut the fascia as necessary to reroute the muscle.
- Make another small incision in the area of the pisiform bone and pass through it the tendon unit, creating a gradual curve from the dorsum of the forearm to this

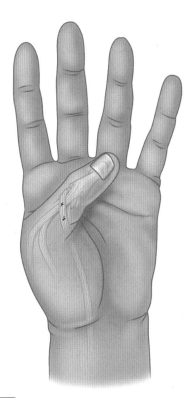

FIGURE 8.5 Brand transfer to restore opposition. (Redrawn from White WL: Restoration of function and balance of the wrist and hand by tendon transfers, *Surg Clin North Am* 40:427, 1960.) **SEE TECHNIQUE 8.2.**

point. From the pisiform area, pass the tendon unit subcutaneously to the tendinous portion of the abductor pollicis brevis just proximal to the metacarpophalangeal joint (Fig. 8.7A).

■ Make another incision over the palmar side of the radial aspect of the metacarpophalangeal joint to expose the site of attachment.
■ At this distal insertion, employ the technique of Riordan by splitting the tendon, or simply pass it into the tendinous portion of the abductor pollicis brevis and suture it with several interrupted sutures (Fig. 8.7B).
■ Suture the tendon under maximal tension with the thumb in full abduction but with the wrist in only slight volar flexion.

POSTOPERATIVE CARE Postoperative care consists of maintaining the wrist in flexion with a splint for a minimum of 4 weeks.

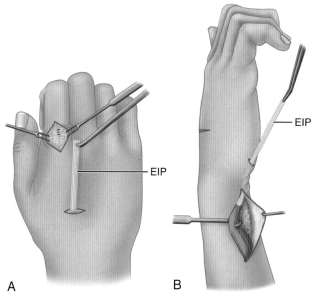

A   B

FIGURE 8.6 **A,** Tendon of the extensor indicis proprius (EIP) has been severed from extensor hood, and hood is carefully repaired. **B,** Through incision on ulnar aspect of forearm, wide fascial excision is carried out, and EIP muscle is transposed superficial to extensor carpi ulnaris through subcutaneous tissue. (Redrawn from Burkhalter WE, Christensen RJ, Brown P: Extensor indicis proprius opponensplasty, *J Bone Joint Surg* 55A:725, 1973.) **SEE TECHNIQUE 8.3.**

TRANSFER OF THE FLEXOR CARPI ULNARIS COMBINED WITH THE SUBLIMIS TENDON

TECHNIQUE 8.4

(GROVES AND GOLDNER)
■ Make volar and ulnar incisions at the wrist as shown in Figure 8.8A–C. The volar incision exposes the flexor sublimis tendon to the ring finger and the flexor carpi ulnaris, and the ulnar incision exposes the extensor carpi ulnaris.

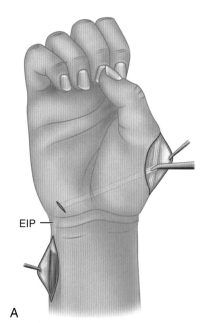

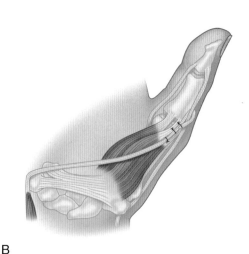

A   B

FIGURE 8.7 **A,** Tendon of extensor indicis proprius (EIP) is brought out in area of pisiform and passed again subcutaneously across palm to thumb. **B,** Method of attachment to thumb using abductor pollicis brevis tendon, metacarpophalangeal joint capsule, and extensor pollicis longus tendon over proximal phalanx. (Redrawn from Burkhalter WE, Christensen RJ, Brown P: Extensor indicis proprius opponensplasty, *J Bone Joint Surg* 55A:725, 1973.) **SEE TECHNIQUE 8.3.**

- Divide the ring finger sublimis tendon insertion from the middle phalanx and bring it out at the wrist.
- Sever the flexor carpi ulnaris tendon, leaving a distal segment of this tendon sufficiently long to bring around the extensor carpi ulnaris tendon to create a pulley.

- Pass the sublimis tendon through this pulley and continue it subcutaneously to the proximal end of the proximal phalanx of the thumb. Insert one split portion of this tendon into the bone with a pull-out wire and another into the bone by direct attachment (Fig. 8.8D).

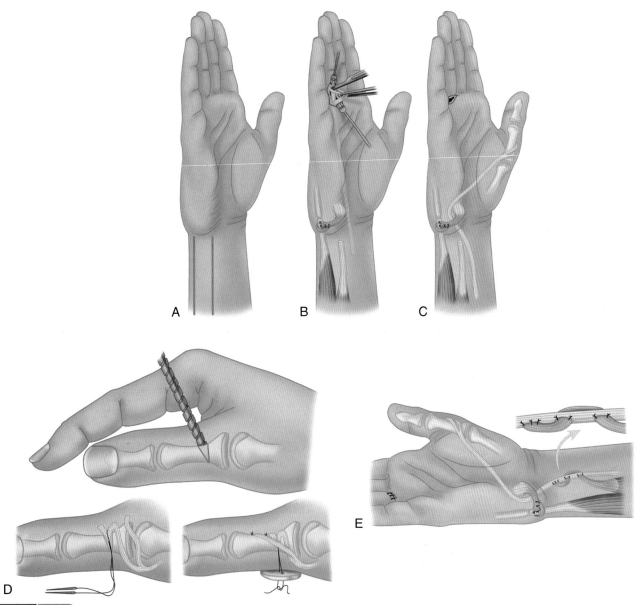

FIGURE 8.8   **A,** Two incisions made at wrist. **B,** Through volar incision, flexor sublimis tendon to ring finger and flexor carpi ulnaris tendon are exposed. Through ulnar incision, extensor carpi ulnaris is exposed. Flexor carpi ulnaris tendon is divided 4 cm from its insertion, and free end of distal segment is sutured to extensor carpi ulnaris. Flexor digitorum sublimis tendon to ring finger is exposed through transverse incision at proximal flexor crease of finger, and its two slips are divided. **C,** Tendon of flexor digitorum sublimis to ring finger is drawn proximally through volar incision at wrist, threaded through pulley, and passed through subcutaneous tissue to metacarpophalangeal joint of thumb. **D,** Two slips of transferred tendon are secured to base of proximal phalanx. Hole is made through proximal phalanx in ulnar-to-radial direction and is enlarged on ulnar side to accept loop of one tendon slip, which is secured with pull-out suture. **E,** After transfer has been secured to thumb phalanx, tension is adjusted (see text), and proximal segment of flexor carpi ulnaris tendon is sutured to transferred tendon. (Redrawn from Groves RJ, Goldner JL: Restoration of strong opposition after median-nerve or brachial plexus paralysis, *J Bone Joint Surg* 57A:112, 1975.) **SEE TECHNIQUE 8.4.**

- Suture the proximal functioning segment of the flexor carpi ulnaris and its tendon into the sublimis tendon unit under sufficient tension that dorsiflexion of the wrist provides full thumb opposition (Fig. 8.8E).

TRANSFER OF THE PALMARIS LONGUS TENDON TO ENHANCE OPPOSITION OF THE THUMB

Transfer of the palmaris longus tendon to enhance opposition of the thumb has been recommended if the abductor pollicis brevis has weakened and atrophied from a partial median nerve palsy, which may accompany severe carpal tunnel syndrome. An advantage of the operation is its close proximity to the median nerve, which may require repair or release that can be done at the same time without much additional surgery. It does not produce true opposition but rather elevates the thumb toward the flexed and abducted position. Presence of a palmaris longus must be confirmed before this procedure. This transfer is not a viable option for high median nerve palsies.

TECHNIQUE 8.5

(CAMITZ)
- Make a curved incision parallel to the base of the thenar crease and extend it proximally 4 cm up the forearm.
- Isolate the palmaris longus tendon in the distal forearm and preserve its insertion on the deep palmar fascia.
- Dissect the palmar fascia fibers in continuity with the palmaris longus tendon to obtain a strip of fascia long enough to reach the distal part of the abductor pollicis brevis tendon.
- Pass the lengthened tendon into a small skin incision made over the thumb metacarpal and suture it to the tendon of the abductor pollicis brevis under appropriate tension with the thumb in full opposition and the wrist in neutral position.

MUSCLE TRANSFER (ABDUCTOR DIGITI QUINTI) TO RESTORE OPPOSITION

If other motors are unavailable or must be transferred elsewhere, the abductor digiti quinti muscle can be utilized to restore opposition. Such transfer has been described by Huber and by Littler and Cooley as presented here. Because its mass and excursion are similar to those of the abductor pollicis brevis, this muscle is an excellent substitute for it. Cosmetically, the transfer is helpful because it fills the space left by the wasted thenar muscles. It does not require a pulley.

TECHNIQUE 8.6

(LITTLER AND COOLEY)
- Make a curved palmar incision along the radial border of the abductor digiti quinti muscle belly extending from the proximal side of the pisiform proximally to the ulnar border of the little finger distally (Fig. 8.9A).
- Free both tendinous insertions of the muscle, one from the extensor expansion and the other from the base of the proximal phalanx.
- Lift the muscle from its fascial compartment and carefully expose its neurovascular bundle. Isolate the bundle, taking care not to damage the veins.
- Free the origin of the muscle from the pisiform, but retain the origin on the flexor carpi ulnaris tendon; now the muscle can be mobilized enough for its insertion to reach the thumb (Fig. 8.9B).
- Make a curved incision on the radial border of the thenar eminence and create across the palm a subcutaneous pocket to receive the transfer.
- Fold the abductor digiti quinti muscle over about 170 degrees (like a page of a book) and pass it subcutaneously to the thumb (Fig. 8.9C).
- Suture its tendons of insertion to the abductor pollicis brevis insertion. Throughout the procedure, avoid compression of and undue tension on the muscle and its neurovascular pedicle.
- Apply a carefully formed light compression dressing and a volar plaster splint to hold the thumb in abduction and the wrist in slight flexion.

RESTORATION OF ADDUCTION OF THE THUMB

Strong pinch requires both thumb opposition and adduction. Opposition is the refined, unique movement that positions the thumb so that its tip can oppose the fingertips throughout their flexion arcs. Once the tips are opposed, especially that of the thumb and index finger, thumb adduction force is necessary for performing work activities. If the adductor pollicis is paralyzed, as in ulnar nerve palsy, firm index and middle finger pinch is impossible, and the thumb cannot be brought across the palm for pinch with the ring and little fingers. The flexor pollicis longus can provide some adduction power when the thumb is held in slight adduction so that the muscle flexes the digit through an arc parallel to the plane of the palm. Eventually, the interphalangeal joint of the thumb becomes hyperflexed as the flexor pollicis longus attempts to produce pulp pinch (Froment sign) and the metacarpophalangeal joint becomes hyperextended secondary to unbalanced extensor forces (Jeanne sign) (Fig. 8.10).

Several transfers have been devised to restore adduction. If adduction alone is absent, the brachioradialis or one of the radial wrist extensors can be lengthened by a graft, transferred palmarward through the third interosseous space, and carried across the palm to the tendon of the adductor pollicis. Such a transfer provides adduction only and this in the direction normally provided by the adductor pollicis. It is most often indicated in ulnar nerve palsy because in this instance restoring thumb abduction is unnecessary; however, it should be combined with some procedure to restore index finger abduction. If adduction and opposition of the thumb are absent, unless some other provision is made to restore adduction, a single tendon transfer to restore opposition should have its pulley located not near the pisiform, but more distally so that some adduction also is restored. One technique meeting this requirement is the Royle-Thompson transfer in which the ring finger flexor digitorum sublimis is carried across the palm and anchored to the adductor pollicis tendon and the transverse carpal ligament serves as a pulley. To restore abduction of the index finger and adduction of the thumb, the sublimis tendon can be split and one slip anchored to the tendon of the adductor pollicis and the other to the insertion of the first dorsal interosseous.

Opposition is only partially restored by Royle-Thompson transfer, and thumb metacarpophalangeal abduction and pronation remain limited. An alternative adductorplasty to correct these deficiencies was described by Brand in which the ring finger sublimis is used as a motor (Fig. 8.11). It traverses the palm superficially and is inserted on the radial aspect of the thumb. The sublimis is sectioned at the proximal phalanx through a short incision and is brought out at the midpalm just ulnar to the thenar crease. This tendon is passed through the natural openings of the fascia between the ring and long fingers at the distal third of the palm. It is passed subcutaneously to be inserted radial and distal to the metacarpophalangeal joint, which pronates the thumb and restores adduction power.

TRANSFER OF THE BRACHIORADIALIS OR RADIAL WRIST EXTENSOR TO RESTORE THUMB ADDUCTION

TECHNIQUE 8.7

(BOYES)

- Detach the brachioradialis tendon at its radial styloid insertion and carefully free the tendon proximally of all fascial attachments to increase its excursion.
- Anchor a tendon graft (plantaris or palmaris longus) to the adductor tubercle of the thumb by a pull-out wire, or suture the graft to the tendon of insertion of the adductor pollicis.
- Pass the graft along the adductor muscle belly and through the third interosseous space to the dorsum of the hand (Fig. 8.12).
- Pass it subcutaneously in a proximal and radial direction and suture it to the end of the brachioradialis tendon. If a radial wrist extensor is used, pass the tendon graft deep to the extensor digitorum communis tendons and attach it to the wrist extensor. The tension should be set maximally with the thumb in radial and palmar abduction and the wrist in neutral position.
- Apply a plaster splint while holding the thumb in adduction and the wrist in extension.

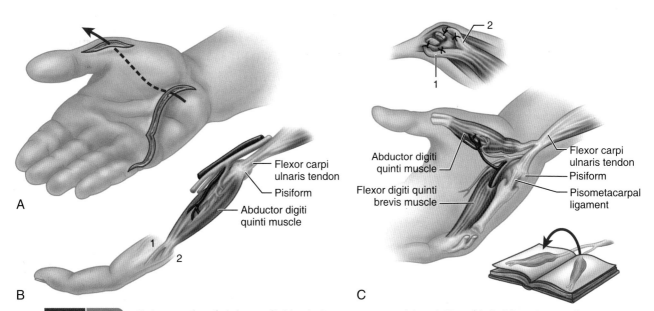

FIGURE 8.9 Littler transfer of abductor digiti quinti to restore opposition. **A,** Two skin incisions. Intervening skin *(shaded area)* is undermined, creating pocket to receive transfer. **B,** Anatomy of abductor digiti quinti. Neurovascular bundle is located proximally on deep surface of muscle. Muscle inserts on proximal phalanx *(1)* and extensor tendon *(2)* of little finger. **C,** Origin of muscle is freed from pisiform but not from flexor carpi ulnaris tendon. Muscle is folded over about 170 degrees and is passed subcutaneously to thenar area, and its two tendons of insertion (1 and 2) are sutured to abductor pollicis brevis tendon. (Modified from Littler JW, Cooley SGE: Opposition of the thumb and its restoration by abductor digiti quinti transfer, *J Bone Joint Surg* 45A:1389, 1963.) **SEE TECHNIQUE 8.6.**

Labels in figure:
- Flexor carpi ulnaris tendon
- Pisiform
- Abductor digiti quinti muscle
- Abductor digiti quinti muscle
- Flexor digiti quinti brevis muscle
- Flexor carpi ulnaris tendon
- Pisiform
- Pisometacarpal ligament

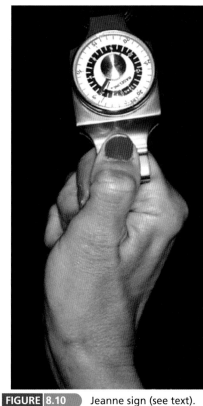

FIGURE 8.10   Jeanne sign (see text).

- Make a third incision between the second and third meta-carpals and remove a window of tissue from the paralyzed interosseous muscles.
- Make a longitudinal incision on the ulnar side of the metacarpophalangeal joint of the thumb.
- With a curved hemostat, tunnel deep to the adductor pollicis muscle and through the window in the second interosseous space. Secure an appropriate tendon graft (usually the palmaris longus tendon).
- Draw the graft through the tunnel from the thumb to the dorsum of the hand (Fig. 8.14C) and suture it to the tendon of the adductor pollicis (Fig. 8.14D).
- Pass the proximal end of the graft subcutaneously to the most proximal incision (Fig. 8.14E) and suture it to the extensor carpi radialis brevis tendon, taking up all slack but with no tension so that the thumb lies just palmar to the index finger with the wrist in neutral position (Fig. 8.14F).
- Dorsiflex the wrist and note that the thumb is pulled into adduction. Flex the wrist and note that the thumb lies firmly against the palm.

POSTOPERATIVE CARE The hand is immobilized in a cast with the thumb in neutral position and the wrist in 40 degrees of dorsiflexion. The cast is removed in 4 weeks, and active motion is encouraged.

POSTOPERATIVE CARE At 4 weeks, the splint is removed and active exercises are begun with a removable protective forearm-based thumb spica preventing thumb hyperextension for the next 2 weeks.

TRANSFER OF THE EXTENSOR CARPI RADIALIS BREVIS TENDON TO RESTORE THUMB ADDUCTION

Smith described transfer of the extensor carpi radialis brevis tendon to provide strong thumb adduction. To extend the tendon, he used a tendon graft and passed it through the second interosseous space. On average, pinch was reported to have doubled in strength after the transfer (Figs. 8.13 and 8.14).

TECHNIQUE 8.8

(SMITH)
- Make two dorsal transverse incisions over the extensor carpi radialis brevis tendon proximal to its insertion (Fig. 8.14A).
- Divide the tendon near its insertion on the third metacarpal base and withdraw it through the incision proximal to the dorsal retinaculum (Fig. 8.14B).

ROYLE-THOMPSON TRANSFER (MODIFIED)

TECHNIQUE 8.9

- Make a midlateral incision over the ulnar aspect of the ring finger and free the insertion of the flexor digitorum sublimis tendon (Fig. 8.15).
- Bring the tendon out of the palm through a short transverse incision and split it into two slips.
- Make a curved incision on the dorsoradial aspect of the thumb as described earlier for the Riordan transfer (see Technique 8.1). Tunnel the slips of the sublimis tendon radially into this incision.
- Suture one slip to the extensor pollicis longus tendon distal to the metacarpophalangeal joint; tunnel the other slip dorsally over the metacarpal, and suture it on the ulnar side of the thumb to the tendon of insertion of the adductor pollicis.
- Close the wounds and apply a forearm-based thumb splint holding the thumb in adduction and the wrist in moderate flexion.

POSTOPERATIVE CARE At 4 weeks, the splint is removed and active exercises are begun with a removable protective forearm-based thumb spica preventing thumb hyperextension for the next 2 weeks.

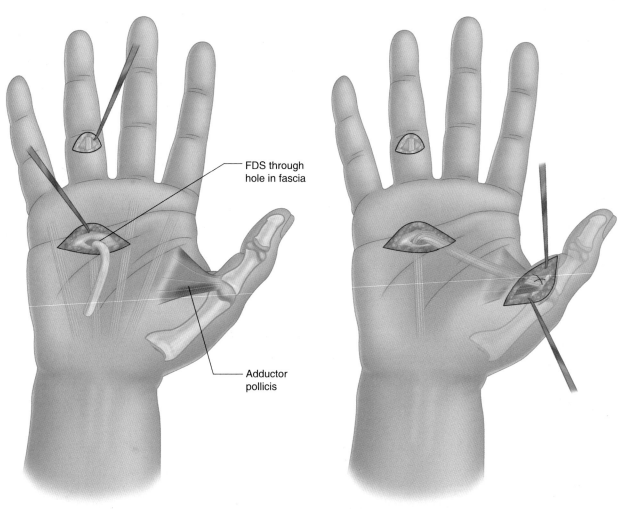

FDS through
hole in fascia

Adductor
pollicis

FIGURE 8.11   Brand transfer (see text).

■ RESTORATION OF ABDUCTION OF THE INDEX FINGER

The index finger is against which the thumb is brought most frequently in pinch. Strong index finger-thumb pinch relies on stability of the index finger metacarpophalangeal joint. Abduction of the index finger also is especially useful in such activities as playing a piano or using a typewriter or keyboard. In poliomyelitis, abduction of the index finger is lost so frequently that its restoration is considered here separately from that of the intrinsic functions of the other fingers.

A transfer to restore index finger abduction is a substitute chiefly for the first dorsal interosseous muscle and, therefore, the transferred tendon is attached to the first dorsal interosseous tendon insertion, which is primarily on the radial base of the index proximal phalanx. The tendons most frequently transferred are those of the extensor indicis proprius, extensor pollicis brevis, and palmaris longus; any of these when transferred abducts the index finger but does not stabilize it for strong pinch. A sublimis tendon also has been used, but this generally is contraindicated unless the hand is otherwise strong. If thumb opposition also must be restored, the sublimis to the ring finger often is used for this transfer (see Techniques 8.1 and 8.2).

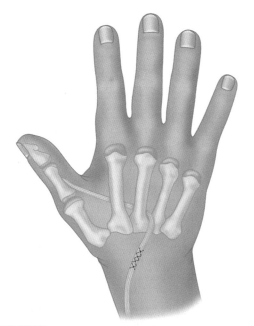

FIGURE 8.12   Boyes transfer of brachioradialis or radial wrist extensor to restore thumb adduction (see text). **SEE TECHNIQUE 8.7.**

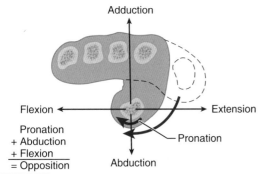

FIGURE 8.13 Adduction and abduction of thumb are in plane perpendicular to palm. Flexion and extension of thumb are in palmar plane. Pronation and supination are rotation of thumb around its longitudinal axis. Opposition is complex of abduction, flexion, and pronation of first metacarpal (and flexion and abduction of proximal phalanx and extension of distal phalanx). (Redrawn from Smith RJ: Extensor carpi radialis brevis tendon transfer for thumb abduction: a study of power pinch, *J Hand Surg* 8A:4, 1983.)

TRANSFER OF THE EXTENSOR INDICIS PROPRIUS TENDON

TECHNIQUE 8.10

- Begin a curved incision at the midlateral point on the radial side of the index finger proximal phalanx; carry it proximally over the radial aspect of the metacarpophalangeal joint, and curve it dorsally to end at the middle of the index metacarpal.
- To add length to the extensor indicis proprius tendon, elevate a small flap of the dorsal expansion over the metacarpophalangeal joint where it is attached to the insertion of the tendon.
- Withdraw the tendon proximally, free it throughout the wound, and close the defect in the expansion.
- Pass the tendon radially in a gentle curve, roughen the tendon of the first dorsal interosseous muscle, and securely suture the transferred tendon.
- If fusion of the thumb metacarpophalangeal joint is necessary (global thumb metacarpophalangeal instability or degenerative disease), the extensor pollicis brevis tendon can be transferred to the first dorsal interosseous.

TRANSFER OF A SLIP OF THE ABDUCTOR POLLICIS LONGUS TENDON

Neviaser, Wilson, and Gardner suggested transfer of a slip of the abductor pollicis longus tendon to replace the first dorsal interosseous muscle. In most patients, the abductor

pollicis longus tendon consists of two or more slips; only 20% or fewer have a single tendon. The normal insertions are the thumb metacarpal base, trapezium, and abductor pollicis brevis thenar fascia. One of these extra slips is used in this transfer.

TECHNIQUE 8.11

(NEVIASER, WILSON, AND GARDNER)

- Make a transverse incision near the insertion of the abductor pollicis longus.
- Identify the slips of the abductor tendon at the level of the radial styloid and note their insertions. Avoid the branches of the superficial radial nerve. Apply traction to each of the slips to determine which insert on the metacarpal and which insert elsewhere. Select a slip that does not insert on the metacarpal and divide it at its insertion (Fig. 8.16A).
- Make a second incision over the radial side of the metacarpophalangeal joint of the index finger and identify the tendon of the first dorsal interosseous muscle (Fig. 8.16B).
- Make a subcutaneous tunnel from the radial styloid to the base of the index finger.
- Obtain a tendon graft from the palmaris longus or elsewhere and weave it into the first dorsal interosseous tendon distal to the metacarpophalangeal joint (Fig. 8.16C and D).
- Pass the graft subcutaneously into the area of the radial styloid without disturbing the first dorsal compartment.
- At the level of the radial styloid, with the index finger and the wrist in neutral position, suture the graft to the selected slip of the abductor pollicis longus. The tension should not be so tight as to overabduct the resting index finger posture.

POSTOPERATIVE CARE The wrist is immobilized for 3 to 4 weeks, and then active exercise is begun.

RESTORATION OF INTRINSIC FUNCTION OF THE FINGERS

Loss of intrinsic muscle function of the fingers may result from paralytic disease or low median and ulnar nerve lesions; low lesions of these nerves cause selective paralysis of the intrinsic muscles but spare the long extrinsics to act unopposed and produce a clawhand. The mechanics of development of this deformity are discussed at the beginning of this chapter.

Loss of intrinsic muscle power may cause hyperextension of the metacarpophalangeal joints in a mobile hand; however, this deformity usually is not the primary or most disabling aspect of this paralysis. It has been shown that with intrinsic paralysis, grasp is diminished 50% or more because of the lack of power of flexion at the metacarpophalangeal joints. In addition, there is asynchronous movement in flexion of the fingers themselves. The roll-up maneuver of the fingers in the intrinsically paralyzed hand shows this characteristic. The interphalangeal joints must flex first, followed next by

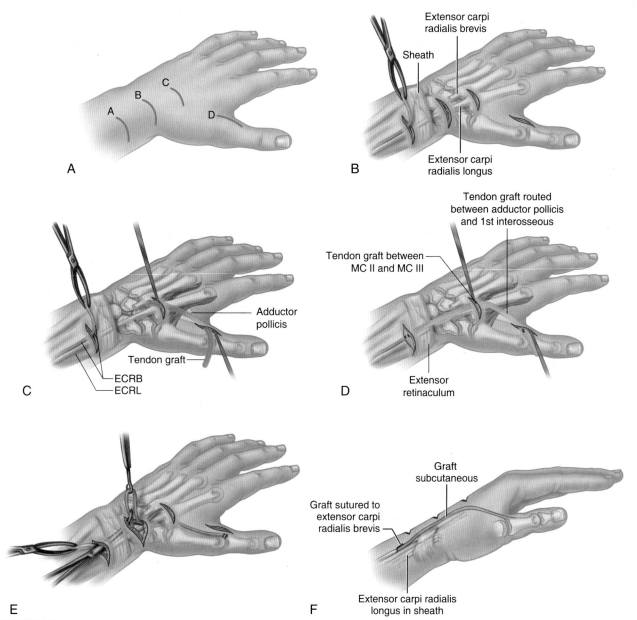

A

B

Extensor carpi
radialis brevis

Sheath

Extensor carpi
radialis longus

C

Adductor
pollicis

Tendon graft

ECRB
ECRL

D

Tendon graft routed
between adductor pollicis
and 1st interosseous

Tendon graft between
MC II and MC III

Extensor
retinaculum

E

F

Graft
subcutaneous

Graft sutured to
extensor carpi
radialis brevis

Extensor carpi radialis
longus in sheath

FIGURE 8.14   Smith transfer of extensor carpi radialis brevis tendon. **A,** Usual incisions (*A* and *B*) for detaching and withdrawing extensor carpi radialis brevis, channeling tendon graft through second interspace (*C*), and attaching graft to tendon of adductor pollicis (*D*). **B,** Extensor carpi radialis brevis is transected distally and withdrawn proximal to dorsal retinacular ligament ("sheath"). **C,** Tendon graft (palmaris longus or plantaris) is passed deep to adductor pollicis and between second and third metacarpals. **D,** Tendon graft is sutured to adductor tendon. **E,** Proximal end of tendon graft is passed subcutaneously to proximal incision. **F,** Tendon graft sutured proximally to extensor carpi radialis brevis with thumb adducted and wrist at 0 degrees of extension. Extensor carpi radialis brevis is at resting length. Graft is made slightly longer if thenars are paralyzed.(Redrawn from Smith RJ: Extensor carpi radialis brevis tendon transfer for thumb abduction: a study of power pinch, *J Hand Surg* 8A:4, 1983.) **SEE TECHNIQUE 8.8.**

the metacarpophalangeal joints and ultimately by full flexion of the fingers. In-phase flexion of the metacarpophalangeal joints is lost with the loss of intrinsic muscle power; the hand is unable to grasp a large object, which is pushed out of the palm by the asynchronous motion (Fig. 8.17). As previously mentioned, it also lacks power of grasp because metacarpophalangeal flexion depends entirely on the long flexors in the absence of intrinsics. Power of pinch also is diminished

in addition to the effects of paralysis of the thenar muscles because the collateral ligaments of the metacarpophalangeal joints of the fingers are lax in extension and the stabilizing intrinsic musculature that would ordinarily give lateral stability is paralyzed. Divergence of the fingers is automatic with extension produced by the long extensor tendons, and as a result of the alignment of the finger flexors, convergence of the tips on grasping is automatic. To stabilize the fingers in

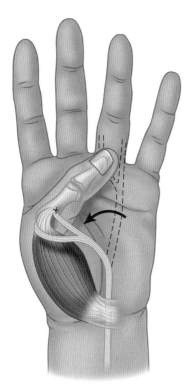

FIGURE 8.15 Modified Royle-Thompson transfer to restore thumb adduction (see text). **SEE TECHNIQUE 8.9.**

extension at the metacarpophalangeal joint, especially for the resistance of the index finger to the pinch pressure of the thumb, the intrinsics are essential.

Many procedures have been devised to block hyperextension of the metacarpophalangeal joints, but stabilizing these joints at a selected position and permitting controlled deviation from side to side requires functioning intrinsic muscles. The restoration of grasping power should be sought if suitable muscles are available for the reconstruction, but this depends on individual circumstances.

In this section, detailed knowledge of the anatomy and function of the intrinsic muscles is assumed and is not reviewed. The interosseous and lumbrical muscles flex the metacarpophalangeal joints and extend the interphalangeal joints of the fingers, but the long finger extensors are capable of extending the interphalangeal joints if the metacarpophalangeal joints are stabilized and cannot hyperextend (see Fig. 8.2). This principle (that the long finger extensors can extend interphalangeal joints, provided that hyperextension of the metacarpophalangeal joints is prevented) is the basis for many of the operations for intrinsic paralysis. The metacarpophalangeal joints can be stabilized by capsuloplasty (Zancolli), tenodesis (Riordan), bone block (Mikhail), arthrodesis, or tendon transfers that actively extend the interphalangeal joints and flex the metacarpophalangeal joints. The proper operation for a given hand depends on the muscles available for transfer, the amount of passive motion present in the finger and wrist joints, and the opinion and experience of the surgeon. Transfers to replace intrinsic function of the fingers are the most variable, complicated, and surgically difficult procedures. Several different transfers have been devised, but no one procedure predictably compensates for the deformities that follow intrinsic paralysis. The Bouvier maneuver is

an examination technique used to assess the competency of the extensor apparatus. If active extension of the interphalangeal joints is present with mechanical block to metacarpophalangeal hyperextension, the Bouvier test is positive and the extensor mechanism is competent. Static procedures to block metacarpophalangeal hyperextension may be sufficient. If active extension of the interphalangeal joints is lacking with mechanical block to metacarpophalangeal hyperextension, the Bouvier test is negative and the extensor mechanism is incompetent. Dynamic procedures to restore interphalangeal extension will be needed in addition to correction of metacarpophalangeal hyperextension.

Bunnell, in a modification of an earlier technique, detached the sublimis tendon from each finger, split it, and passed one slip to each side of the extensor aponeurosis of each finger by way of the lumbrical canals, removing the powerful flexor of the proximal interphalangeal joints and converting it into an extensor of the same joints. However, this transfer often is too strong and pulls the proximal interphalangeal joints into extension, producing an intrinsic-plus deformity that appears several months to many years after the transfer. A modification of this procedure in which only one sublimis is transferred to all fingers may be useful; however, setting and maintaining proper tension in this method are difficult (Fig. 8.18).

Flexing the wrist in an attempt to extend the interphalangeal joints often becomes a necessary habit after intrinsic paralysis. Its objective is to create a tenodesing effect on the long extensor tendons. If this flexion is too marked, the Bunnell transfer is rendered ineffective, but if the intrinsics are weak but not paralyzed, the transfer may be useful if the wrist extensors are strong enough to prevent flexion of the wrist. When flexing the wrist is a chronic habit and a wrist flexor can be spared, Riordan transferred the flexor carpi radialis (see Fig. 8.25).

Fowler split the extensor proprius tendons of the index and little fingers to form four slips and attached one each to the extensor aponeuroses on the radial side of the index and middle fingers and on the ulnar side of the ring and little fingers. In a later modification, the tendons are split as described but the slips are passed to the volar side of the deep transverse metacarpal ligament and are attached to the radial side of the extensor aponeurosis of each finger (Figs. 8.19 and 8.20). This is a more efficient transfer and has the advantage of a tenodesing effect when the wrist is flexed. The ends of the tendon slips must be advanced about 2.5 cm to reach their destinations on the extensor aponeuroses, however, and are under considerable tension; sometimes an intrinsic overpull or intrinsic-plus deformity develops. This excessive tension may be avoided as follows. The detached end of the extensor indicis proprius tendon is split into two slips, passed volar to the deep transverse metacarpal ligament, and attached to the radial side of the ring and little fingers. One end of a free tendon graft is attached to the musculotendinous junction of the extensor indicis proprius, and the other end is split into two slips that are passed distally in a similar manner and attached to the radial side of the middle and index fingers. Riordan further modified this procedure by attaching the tendon graft to the freed insertion of the palmaris longus tendon instead of to the musculotendinous junction of the extensor indicis proprius (Fig. 8.21).

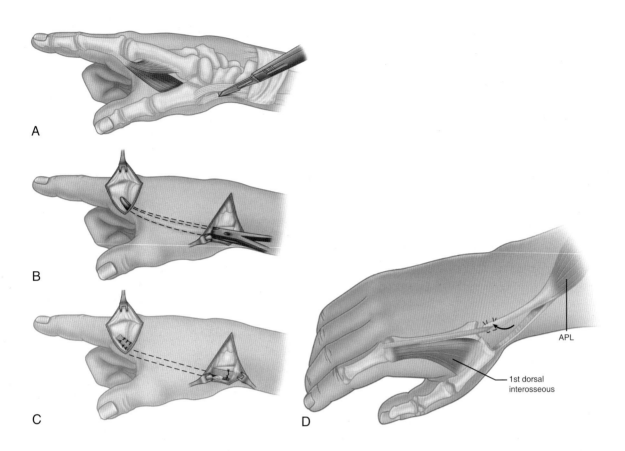

FIGURE 8.16   **A,** Accessory slip inserting into trapezium is detached distal to retinaculum. Functional slip, inserting into metacarpal, is preserved. **B,** Subcutaneous tunnel is created from radial styloid to insertion of first dorsal interosseous. **C and D,** Tendon graft is woven into tendon of first dorsal interosseous and sutured to accessory slip. (Redrawn from Neviaser RJ, Wilson JN, Gardner MM: Abductor pollicis longus transfer for replacement of first dorsal interosseus, *J Hand Surg* 5A:53, 1980.) **SEE TECHNIQUE 8.11.**

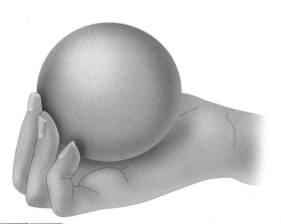

FIGURE 8.17   Intrinsic paralysis results in failure to grasp large objects.

Brand devised a technique using the extensor carpi radialis brevis tendon lengthened by a free graft from the plantaris tendon (Fig. 8.22); the distal end of the graft is split into four slips, or tails, and each tail is passed to the volar side of the deep transverse metacarpal ligament and is attached on the radial side of each proximal phalanx to the extensor aponeurosis, except in the index finger, where it is attached on the ulnar side. In his opinion, index finger pinch can be secured more firmly when the finger is in adduction rather than in abduction (Fig. 8.23). Brand advised transferring the extensor carpi radialis longus or brevis to the volar side of the forearm and extending it by a four-tailed graft through the carpal tunnel and the lumbrical canals and finally to the extensor aponeuroses as before (Fig. 8.24). This transfer crowds the carpal tunnel and may cause symptoms of median nerve compression should the nerve be functioning. For severe clawing of the hand with wrist flexion, Riordan advised freeing the insertion of the flexor carpi radialis and transferring it to the dorsum of the wrist; here it is prolonged with a four-tailed graft, each tail of which is passed volar to the deep transverse metacarpal ligament and is attached to the radial sides of the extensor aponeuroses (Fig. 8.25).

The procedures just described require that muscles strong enough for transfer be available. If they are not, a Zancolli capsuloplasty or a tenodesing procedure to stabilize the metacarpophalangeal joints may be indicated (Fig. 8.26). Riordan devised a tenodesing procedure in which the extensor carpi radialis brevis and extensor carpi ulnaris tendons are each cut halfway through at about the level of the junction of the middle and distal thirds of the forearm; one half of each tendon is

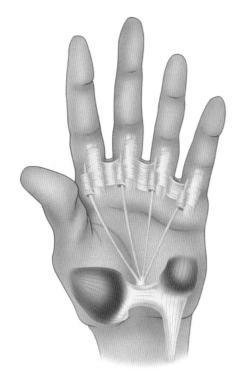

FIGURE 8.18 Modification of Bunnell transfer to restore intrinsic function of fingers (see text). **SEE TECHNIQUE 8.12.**

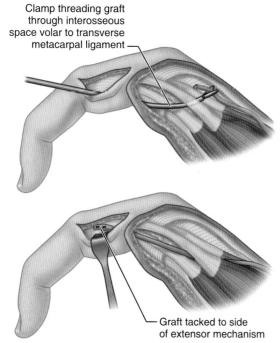

Clamp threading graft
through interosseous
space volar to transverse
metacarpal ligament

Graft tacked to side
of extensor mechanism

FIGURE 8.19 Any tendons transferred from dorsum of hand to restore intrinsic function of fingers must pass to volar side of deep transverse metacarpal ligament.

stripped distally and is left attached at its insertion on a metacarpal base. Each strand of tendon is split into two strips, forming four slips; each slip is passed through an interosseous space and along the volar side of the deep transverse metacarpal ligament to a finger and is attached to the radial side of its extensor

aponeurosis. The disadvantage of this tenodesis is that it cannot be activated by wrist motion, as can the Fowler tenodesis. Fowler used a free tendon graft attached to the fingers as in the Riordan technique but anchored proximally in the area of the dorsal carpal ligament proximal to the wrist. When the wrist is flexed, the tenodesis is activated (Fig. 8.27).

If the finger flexors and the wrist flexors and extensors are strong, and if there is no habitual wrist flexion, the operation of choice to restore finger intrinsic function is the modified Bunnell procedure, in which the flexor digitorum sublimis of the ring finger is transferred (see Fig. 8.18). If flexing the wrist is habitual, or there is a flexion contracture of the joint and if a wrist flexor can be spared, Riordan recommended transfer of the flexor carpi radialis to the dorsum of the wrist prolonged by tendon grafts (see Fig. 8.25); however, at least one strong wrist flexor should remain after the transfer. If the wrist extensors are strong, and the flexors are weak, the Brand transfer of the extensor carpi radialis longus volarward and prolonged by a free graft through the carpal tunnel (see Fig. 8.24) may be indicated. The Brand transfer of the extensor carpi radialis brevis prolonged by a free graft carried between the metacarpals and attached to the extensor aponeuroses (see Fig. 8.22) may be complicated by difficulty in reeducation. If a flexor digitorum sublimis or a wrist flexor or extensor is unavailable for transfer or cannot be spared, the extensor proprius tendons of the index and little fingers can be transferred by the Fowler technique (see Figs. 8.19 and 8.20), or the Riordan modification of the Fowler technique in which the palmaris longus tendon is one of the transfers (see Fig. 8.21) can be used. If no muscle is available for transfer, and if the joints are supple, the Zancolli capsulodesis of the metacarpophalangeal joints (see Fig. 8.26), a Fowler tenodesis (see Fig. 8.27), or a Riordan tenodesis may be indicated.

The tendency to overload the extensor mechanism by routine attachment of transferred tendons to the lateral bands has been noted; this means that the desirable flexor power to the metacarpophalangeal joints is not obtained; Brooks and Jones suggested attaching the transfers to the flexor tendon sheath (Fig. 8.28) and, depending on the intact extensor power, extending the proximal interphalangeal joints with the metacarpophalangeal joints stabilized. Likewise, Burkhalter and others suggested a bony attachment of the transferred tendon to the midportion of the proximal phalanx to provide leverage for flexion at the metacarpophalangeal joint and a better restoration of grip (see Fig. 8.33). We have found, however, the Zancolli tendon insertion into the flexor sheath to be much less time-consuming than insertion into bone. It also eliminates the tendency for hyperextension of the proximal interphalangeal joint, as occurs sometimes when the tendon is inserted into the extensor mechanism.

TRANSFER OF THE FLEXOR DIGITORUM SUBLIMIS OF THE RING FINGER

TECHNIQUE 8.12

(BUNNELL, MODIFIED)

- Transfer either the ring or the long finger sublimis tendon. Make a midlateral incision about 4.0 cm long on the radial

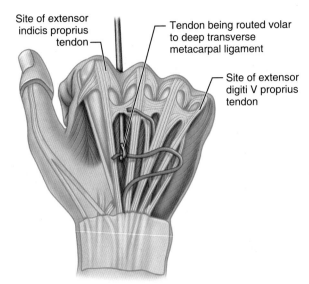

FIGURE 8.20 Fowler transfer to restore intrinsic function of fingers (see text). **SEE TECHNIQUE 8.14.**

Site of extensor indicis proprius tendon

Tendon being routed volar to deep transverse metacarpal ligament

Site of extensor digiti V proprius tendon

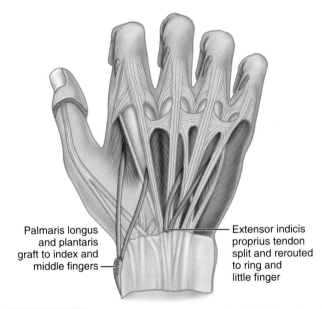

FIGURE 8.21 Riordan transfer to restore intrinsic function of fingers (see text). **SEE TECHNIQUE 8.14.**

Palmaris longus and plantaris graft to index and middle fingers

Extensor indicis proprius tendon split and rerouted to ring and little finger

side of the selected finger, beginning at the midshaft of the proximal phalanx and extending distally to beyond the proximal interphalangeal joint.

- Deepen the incision to the flexor tendon sheath, open the sheath laterally, and identify and divide the sublimis tendon at the level of the proximal interphalangeal joint.
- Separate the two slips of the tendon so that the tendon can be withdrawn into the palm.
- Make a transverse incision about 4.0 cm long at the level of the proximal palmar crease. Identify the sublimis tendon, withdraw it through the palmar incision, and split it into four equal tails.
- Make a longitudinal incision about 2.5 cm long on the radial side (and slightly dorsal) of the proximal phalanx of each finger except the donor finger and identify the extensor aponeuroses.
- With a narrow instrument, a wire loop, or a tendon carrier, pass each tail of tendon through the lumbrical canal of a finger and over the oblique fibers of the extensor aponeurosis to its dorsum (see Fig. 8.18). Passage through the lumbrical canals should be easy; if any obstruction is met, redirect the instrument.
- With the metacarpophalangeal joint at 80 or 90 degrees of flexion, the interphalangeal joints at neutral, and the wrist at 30 degrees of flexion, suture each tail to the aponeurosis under some tension with interrupted sutures and bury its end. Usually 2.5 cm or more of redundant tendon must be excised.
- Close the incisions and immobilize the hand with the wrist in neutral position, the metacarpophalangeal joints in flexion, and the interphalangeal joints in extension.
- Brooks recommended attaching each transfer to the flexor pulley at the level of the proximal phalanx, preventing the development of hyperextension deformities of the proximal interphalangeal joints.

POSTOPERATIVE CARE At 3 weeks, the cast is removed and each finger is splinted with a plaster or plastic gutter splint in a neutral position. Movement of the metacarpophalangeal joints and resisted active extension of the wrist are encouraged. The finger splints are removed and are reapplied daily until reeducation is complete.

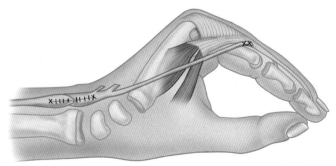

FIGURE 8.22 Brand transfer of extensor carpi radialis brevis tendon prolonged with free graft to restore intrinsic function of fingers (see text).

TRANSFER OF THE EXTENSOR CARPI RADIALIS LONGUS OR BREVIS TENDON

TECHNIQUE 8.13

(BRAND)

- Divide the distal end of the extensor carpi radialis brevis tendon of the radius through a short dorsal transverse incision.
- Make a second incision 9.0 cm proximal to the first, withdraw the tendon through it, and place the tendon on a wet towel. Remove a plantaris tendon for a graft, and divide it in half or double it on itself to make two grafts. Split open the end of the motor tendon along the natural plane of cleavage, spread it out, and suture the graft to it.
- Introduce a tendon-tunneling forceps at the first incision, pass it subcutaneously to the second, grasp the ends of the tendon grafts, and pull them under intact skin.
- Split the end of each graft into two parts to form a total of four slips or tails.
- Make a longitudinal dorsoulnar incision over the proximal phalanx of the index finger and dorsoradial incisions over the proximal phalanx of the long, ring, and little fingers.
- Identify the lumbrical tendon and lateral band of the extensor aponeurosis in each finger, tunnel from this point on each finger through the palm and appropriate interosseous space, grasp a strand of tendon graft, and withdraw it into the finger. Tunnel to the volar side of the deep transverse metacarpal ligament and then between the appropriate metacarpal shafts.
- When all tendon grafts are in position, suture them one by one under equal tension to the dorsal expansion lateral band of each finger—first the index, then the little, and finally the intermediate ones (Fig. 8.29). The transfers should be relaxed completely when the wrist is extended 45 degrees, the metacarpophalangeal joints are flexed 70 degrees, and the interphalangeal joints are in neutral. Close the wounds and apply a light plaster cast.
- As an alternative method, use the extensor carpi radialis longus tendon. Through a dorsal transverse incision,

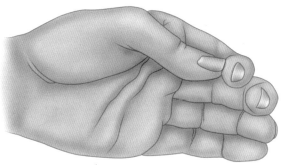

FIGURE 8.23 When firm pinch would be more useful than abduction of index finger, transferred tendon is attached to ulnar lateral band of extensor hood rather than to insertion of first dorsal interosseous muscle. During pinch, index finger is in adduction, rather than in abduction. (Redrawn from White WL: Restoration of function and balance of the wrist and hand by tendon transfers, *Surg Clin North Am* 40:427, 1960.)

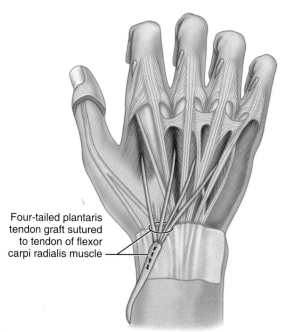

Four-tailed plantaris tendon graft sutured to tendon of flexor carpi radialis muscle

FIGURE 8.25 Riordan transfer to restore intrinsic function of fingers (see text).

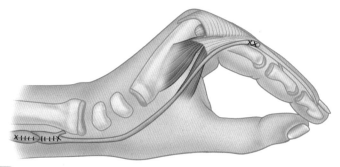

FIGURE 8.24 Brand transfer of extensor carpi radialis longus or brevis, first to volar side of forearm and then, after prolongation with free graft, to extensor aponeuroses to restore intrinsic function of fingers (see text).

free its insertion and withdraw it through a second incision at the middle of the forearm. Make an incision on the anterior aspect of the forearm 7.5 cm proximal to the wrist, tunnel from the anterior incision deep to the brachioradialis to the proximal incision, and draw the tendon into the anterior incision. Suture the grafts to the motor tendon as described previously. Through a midpalmar incision, pass it through the carpal tunnel into the forearm and draw the grafts into the palm, leaving the tendon junctions proximal to the carpal tunnel. Pass each strand of the graft separately to its finger destination.

POSTOPERATIVE CARE Postoperative care is as described for the modified Bunnell technique (see Technique 8.12).

TRANSFER OF THE EXTENSOR INDICIS PROPRIUS AND EXTENSOR DIGITI QUINTI PROPRIUS

TECHNIQUE 8.14

(FOWLER)
- In this transfer, the extensor indicis proprius and the extensor digiti quinti proprius are used as motors (see Fig. 8.20).
- Make a dorsal incision over the radial aspect of the index finger metacarpophalangeal joint and identify the exten-

sor indicis proprius tendon, which should be deep and ulnar to the common extensor tendon.
- Dissect the tendon from the extensor aponeurosis, obtaining as much length as possible by excising a part of the aponeurosis with it; otherwise, the tendon could be too tight after transfer.
- Suture the residual defect in the aponeurosis.
- Split the extensor indicis proprius into two equal parts, pass each volar to the deep transverse metacarpal ligament, and attach one each to the extensor aponeurosis

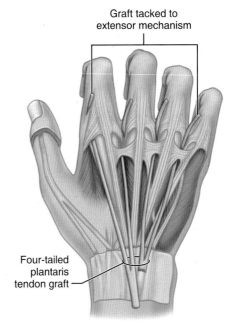

FIGURE 8.27 Fowler tenodesis for intrinsic paralysis (see text). **SEE TECHNIQUE 8.16.**

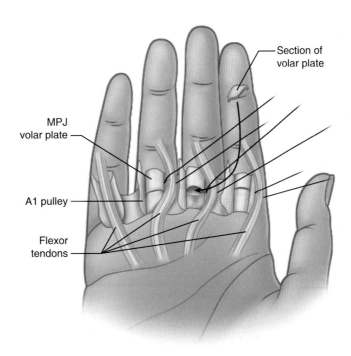

FIGURE 8.26 Zancolli capsulodesis for intrinsic paralysis (see text). **SEE TECHNIQUE 8.15.**

on the radial side of the index and middle fingers, as in the Bunnell technique.

- Make a dorsal incision over the little finger, identify the extensor digiti quinti proprius tendon, and free its insertion; split this tendon also into two equal parts, pass each volar to the deep transverse metacarpal ligament, and attach one each to the radial side of the ring and little fingers. Ensure that this tendon is not too tight.

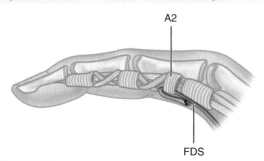

FIGURE 8.28 Flexor digitorum sublimis (FDS) inserted into strip of annular ligament (A2) at middle of proximal phalanx. (Redrawn from slide supplied by Brooks. *In* Riordan DC: Tendon transfers in hand surgery, *J Hand Surg* 8:748, 1983.)

- The Riordan modification of this operation (see Fig. 8.21) does not use the extensor digiti quinti proprius.

POSTOPERATIVE CARE Postoperative care is as described for after the modified Bunnell technique.

CAPSULODESIS

TECHNIQUE 8.15

(ZANCOLLI)
- Make a transverse incision in the palm at the level of the distal crease. Undermine widely the skin and fat and expose the flexor tendon sheaths, taking care to protect the neurovascular bundles.
- Over each metacarpophalangeal joint, make a longitudinal incision in the paratendinous fascia and tendon sheath and expose the flexor tendons.

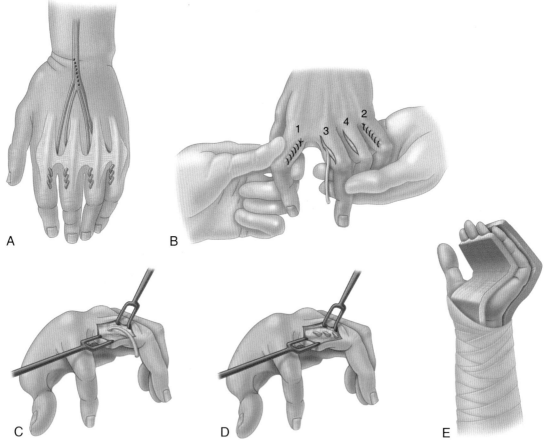

FIGURE 8.29 **A,** One slip of tendon graft is sutured to appropriate lateral band of each finger. **B,** First, one slip of graft is sutured to ulnar lateral band of index finger (1), and then one each to radial lateral band of little (2), long (3), and ring (4) fingers in that order. **C** and **D,** Method of weaving slip of graft into lateral band. **E,** Wrist is immobilized in 45 degrees of dorsiflexion, and metacarpophalangeal joints are immobilized in 70 degrees of flexion. (Redrawn from White WL: Restoration of function and balance of the wrist and hand by tendon transfers, *Surg Clin North Am* 40:427, 1960.) **SEE TECHNIQUE 8.13.**

- Carefully retract the tendons and expose the underlying metacarpophalangeal joint (Fig. 8.26).
- Resect an elliptical segment of the volar fibrocartilaginous plate, including the vertical septum and its deep origin. Resect enough tissue to produce a 10- to 30-degree flexion contracture when the plate is closed. Alternatively, the volar plate can be imbricated or its proximal attachment advanced proximally and secured with a bone anchor.
- Close the volar plates with nonabsorbable sutures placed laterally in its thickest part, this being at the insertion of the accessory collateral ligaments. If desired, insert transarticular Kirschner wires to maintain the metacarpophalangeal joint positions.
- Close the wound and apply a dorsal plaster splint, holding the metacarpophalangeal joints in flexion and the wrist in extension.

POSTOPERATIVE CARE Movements of the interphalangeal joints are continued after surgery. At 3 weeks, the cast and any Kirschner wires are removed and metacarpophalangeal joint exercises are begun.

TENODESIS

TECHNIQUE 8.16

(FOWLER)

- In this operation, a tendon graft is substituted for the finger intrinsics; the graft is activated by wrist flexion (see Fig. 8.27).
- Obtain a tendon graft twice as long as the distance from the dorsum of the wrist to the proximal interphalangeal joints.
- Make a transverse incision on the dorsum of the wrist and expose the wrist extensor retinaculum.
- Pass the graft through the retinaculum just distal to its proximal edge.
- Split each end of the graft into two equal slips and transfer each slip to a finger, as in the Fowler transfer previously described.
- Suture the graft under proper tension so that when the wrist is flexed, force is exerted on the extensor mechanism to extend the interphalangeal joints without hyperflexing the metacarpophalangeal joints.

PERIPHERAL NERVE PALSIES
RADIAL NERVE PALSY

Radial nerve injuries rarely occur at sites other than the humeral shaft or the proximal third of the dorsoradial forearm. Injuries to the radial nerve at this high level typically do not affect triceps function, and elbow extension is preserved; however, in high radial nerve palsy, the pattern of motor paralysis includes loss of wrist extension, thumb extension and abduction, and finger metacarpophalangeal joint extension. Wrist extension is necessary for proper flexor tendon tensioning, and grasp is profoundly reduced and represents a significant functional deficit after high radial nerve paralysis. More distal nerve injuries affect the posterior interosseous nerve and result in a low radial nerve palsy. Wrist extension is preserved with a tendency toward radial deviation secondary to preserved extensor carpi radialis longus function. However, loss of thumb extension and abduction and finger metacarpophalangeal joint extension prevents appropriate grasp posture, and awkwardness and clumsiness of the hand is striking.

Observation is indicated in most nerve palsies associated with closed humeral fractures because return of normal function can be anticipated at 3 to 6 months after fracture. Early surgical exploration for the Holstein-Lewis fracture pattern (spiral fracture of the middle-distal third junction) may not be indicated. A series of patients with this pattern were noted to have full recovery regardless of surgical intervention. Indications for open reduction and fixation of acute closed humeral fractures should rely more on factors other than the status of the radial nerve. The timing for nerve exploration in closed injuries varies. Surgical exploration in the absence of nerve recovery or advancing Tinel sign may be indicated at 3 months after injury. The results of nerve repair seem to be better when done before rather than after 6 months. Nerve exploration should accompany management of open humeral fractures and lacerations associated with nerve deficit. Radial nerve neurorrhaphy should be performed when possible; outcomes theoretically are favorable because the nerve is largely motor and the distances between the sites of injury and reinnervation are short. When a nerve repair is performed, and suitable recovery is anticipated, tendon transfers generally should be delayed for 6 months. Burkhalter outlined three indications, however, for early tendon transfer: (1) to act as a substitute during regrowth of the nerve, avoiding use of external splints, (2) to act as a helper as reinnervation proceeds, and (3) to intervene when the results of the nerve repair are considered poor or the nerve is irreparable. Burkhalter contended that transfer of the pronator teres to establish wrist extension early creates no disability and that the transferred unit still functions as a forearm pronator. Radial nerve injuries in the proximal third of the forearm result in low radial nerve palsy in which finger metacarpophalangeal joint extension and thumb extension and radial abduction are lost. Procedures for low radial nerve palsy are derived from the more common procedures used for high radial nerve palsy. The synergistic wrist flexors, long finger flexors, palmaris longus, and pronator teres commonly are used for transfer, and numerous combinations of these transfers have been described.

Despite numerous tendon transfer variations for radial nerve paralysis, several tendon transfer combinations are commonly used. One strong wrist flexor should be retained to prevent wrist hyperextension. Scuderi modified Starr's transfer of the palmaris longus to the extensor pollicis longus to provide thumb extension and abduction. Most surgeons prefer the flexor carpi radialis over the flexor carpi ulnaris to establish metacarpophalangeal joint extension. The flexor carpi ulnaris is the major wrist flexor and the only remaining ulnar deviator of the wrist because the extensor carpi ulnaris is lost in

TABLE 8.2

Tendon Transfers for Radial Nerve Palsy

TENDON TRANSFER	RESTORATION OF WRIST EXTENSION	RESTORATION OF THUMB EXTENSION	RESTORATION OF FINGER EXTENSION
Brand	PT to ECRB	PL to EPL	FCR to EDC
Jones	PT to ECRB	PL to EPL	FCR to EDC
Boyes superficialis	PT to ECRB	FDS of ring finger to EPL	FDS of long finger to EDC

ECRB, Extensor carpi radialis brevis; EDC, extensor digitorum communis; EPL, extensor pollicis longus; FCR, flexor carpi radialis; FDS, flexor digitorum superficialis; PL, palmaris longus; PT, pronator teres.
From Seiler JG, Desai MJ, Payne SH: Tendon transfers for radial, median, and ulnar nerve palsy, J Am Acad Orthop Surg 21:675, 2013.

high and low radial nerve paralyses. In addition, the normal wrist motion is from dorsoradial extension to volar-ulnar flexion as in a dart-throwing motion. Elimination of this balancing force may accentuate hand radial deviation and disturb the more normal wrist flexion-extension arc. The wrist position for power grip also is one of ulnar deviation, and sacrificing the flexor carpi ulnaris may compromise grip strength. In patients in whom significant wrist radial deviation exists before tendon transfer, use of the flexor carpi ulnaris is contraindicated. Moreover, the flexor carpi ulnaris has muscular attachments all along the ulnar shaft, requires a long incision, and, when transferred around the subcutaneous border of the ulna, is conspicuous and may be objectionable in forearms with little subcutaneous coverage. This minor cosmetic problem, however, can be eliminated by resection of the flexor carpi ulnaris muscle distally. In the absence of significant wrist radial deviation, however, the flexor carpi ulnaris transfer to the extensor digitorum communis is acceptable for achieving digital extension.

To achieve full and independent thumb and digital extension, Boyes devised transfers using the flexor digitorum sublimis tendons of the middle and ring fingers. These transfers are more technically difficult, and adhesions may occur in the interosseous space through which the sublimis tendons are placed. His transfers include (1) pronator teres to extensor carpi radialis longus and extensor carpi radialis brevis, (2) flexor carpi radialis to extensor pollicis brevis and abductor pollicis longus, (3) middle flexor digitorum sublimis to extensor digitorum communis, and (4) ring flexor digitorum sublimis to extensor pollicis longus and extensor indicis proprius.

Brand suggested removing the insertion of the extensor carpi radialis longus and transferring it to a point between the extensor carpi radialis brevis and extensor carpi ulnaris to avoid radial deviation on extension of the wrist. Most surgeons attempt to balance the wrist and decrease the likelihood of radial deviation by transfer of the pronator teres into the more centrally located extensor carpi radialis brevis, rather than the extensor carpi radialis longus or extensor carpi radialis longus and brevis unit.

All procedures are done under general or axillary block anesthesia with the patient supine. All transfers are done at the same surgery, usually as outpatient procedures. A high arm tourniquet is used, and the hand, forearm, and elbow region are prepared for sterile draping. The most commonly performed series of transfers are described in Technique 8.17. In patients in whom the palmaris longus is not available for transfer, the sublimis of the long or ring finger generally is used (Table 8.2).

More recently, use of nerve transfers to restore radial nerve function has gained attention. Such transfers include (1) transfer of nerve branches of the flexor digitorum sublimus to the extensor carpi radialis brevis, (2) transfer of branches of the flexor carpi radialis and palmaris to the posterior interosseous nerve, and (3) transfer of branches of the flexor carpi ulnaris (ulnar nerve) to the posterior interosseous nerve. These transfers may offer both less morbidity with respect to scar formation and tendon gliding and also more physiologic function. However, nerve transfers take months rather than weeks to restore function and may sacrifice a potential tendon donor if the transfer fails.

TRANSFER OF PRONATOR TERES TO EXTENSOR CARPI RADIALIS BREVIS, FLEXOR CARPI RADIALIS TO EXTENSOR DIGITORUM COMMUNIS, AND PALMARIS LONGUS TO EXTENSOR POLLICIS LONGUS

TECHNIQUE 8.17   FIGURE 8.30

- Make a gently curved incision in the middle third of the dorsal forearm to expose the extensor pollicis longus and common extensor tendons and extensor indicis proprius proximal to the extensor retinaculum (Fig. 8.30A). Flex the fingers fully and hold the wrist in extension. Sequentially secure the extensor digitorum communis and extensor indicis proprius tendons together under equal tension proximal to the extensor retinaculum using 2.0 nonabsorbable braided sutures such that the suture site does not impinge on the extensor retinaculum proximal edge, thus limiting finger flexion with the wrist flexed.
- Place the wrist in neutral and evaluate synchronous metacarpophalangeal joint extension by placing traction on the extensor digitorum communis and extensor indicis proprius tendon composite. Additional extensor tendon balancing may need to be done by adjusting tension with additional mattress sutures between the individual tendons. Inclusion of the small finger proprius tendon may be necessary.
- Make a gently curved volar incision, extending from the junction of the proximal–middle third of the forearm to 4 cm proximal to the distal wrist flexion crease to expose the

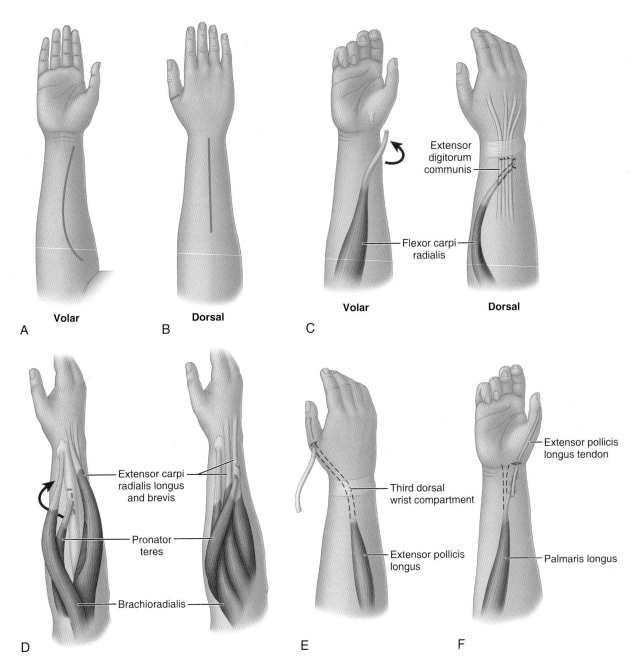

Volar **Dorsal**

A   B

Volar **Dorsal**

C

Extensor digitorum communis

Flexor carpi radialis

Extensor carpi radialis longus and brevis

Pronator teres

Brachioradialis

D

Third dorsal wrist compartment

Extensor pollicis longus

E

Extensor pollicis longus tendon

Palmaris longus

F

FIGURE 8.30 Transfer of pronator teres (PT) to extensor carpi radialis brevis (ECRB), transfer of flexor carpi radialis (FCR) to extensor digitorum communis (EDC), and transfer of palmaris longus (PL) to rerouted extensor pollicis longus (EPL). **A** and **B,** Volar and dorsal incisions used in combination of transfers. Note short transverse incisions over thumb metacarpal joint dorsally and wrist volarly used in rerouting EPL. **C,** FCR transfer to EDC. FCR motor tendon attachment at 45-degree angle into recipient tendon. **D,** Transfer of PT into more centralized ECRB. PT insertion is harvested with 2- to 3-cm periosteal extension strip. **E** and **F,** Transfer of PL to rerouted EPL. By rerouting EPL out of its third extensor compartment, combination of thumb abduction and extension can be achieved. **SEE TECHNIQUE 8.17.**

pronator teres, flexor carpi radialis, and palmaris longus musculotendinous units (Fig. 8.30B).
- Locate the interval between the brachioradialis and pronator teres and trace the pronator teres to its insertion. Sharply free the pronator teres from the radial shaft and remove as much periosteal extension as possible in continuity with the pronator teres tendinous insertion.

- Trace the flexor carpi radialis distally, and with the wrist flexed transect it at the distal wrist crease level.
- Verify the presence of the palmaris longus and trace its tendon distally, dividing it at the distal wrist flexion crease.
- Elevate and dissect these three motor units of their fascial attachments proximally to position them in line with their intended insertions.

- Transect the extensor pollicis longus at its musculotendinous junction and make a 2-cm incision dorsally just proximal to the thumb metacarpophalangeal joint. Release fascial attachments as necessary to deliver the extensor pollicis longus to this wound.
- Make another 2-cm transverse incision in the distal wrist flexion crease at the base of the thenar eminence. Make a tunnel to pass the extensor pollicis longus volar and radial to the thumb carpometacarpal joint so that the rerouted extensor pollicis longus will provide interphalangeal joint extension and palmar abduction.
- Likewise, tunnel the extensor pollicis longus tendon to the volar wound. Free extensor pollicis longus passage and effortless excursion is achieved by releasing again any fascial attachments (see Fig. 8.30E). Assess the desired thumb radial abduction and interphalangeal joint extension by placing traction on the free rerouted extensor pollicis longus tendon in line with the palmaris longus toward the medial epicondyle. Wrap the tendon in a moist 4 × 4–inch sponge.
- Develop subcutaneous tunnels from proximal volar to distal dorsal, keeping a straight-line approach to the destined tendon attachment sites for the pronator teres and flexor carpi radialis motors. Route the tendons dorsally around the radial shaft to avoid compressing the radial artery or superficial sensory nerves.
- Place the flexor carpi radialis tendon through the extensor digitorum communis and extensor indicis proprius tendon composite in a proximal-radial to distal-ulnar direction (Fig. 8.30C). Adjust the tension so that with full passive wrist flexion the metacarpophalangeal joints extend fully, and with full wrist extension the fingers can be passively flexed. A Pulvertaft-type weave is impossible; however, multiple horizontal mattress sutures should be used to anchor the flexor carpi radialis tendon to each individual tendon in the extensor digitorum communis and extensor indicis proprius composite.
- Weave the pronator teres tendon and its periosteal slip through the extensor carpi radialis brevis tendon (Fig. 8.30D). The pronator teres and extensor carpi radialis brevis tendons can be joined by several passages of the pronator teres tendon and its periosteal extension through the recipient extensor carpi radialis brevis tendon. Using multiple 2-0 braided nonabsorbable sutures in horizontal mattress fashion, secure the tendon weave with the wrist held in 40 degrees of extension with the pronator teres under near-maximal tension.
- Weave and suture together the extensor pollicis longus and palmaris longus tendons (Fig. 8.30E and F). Place traction on the tendon in line with the palmaris longus and check for the desired thumb palmar abduction and interphalangeal joint extension. The tension should be such as to permit passive flexion of the thumb across the palm with the wrist in neutral position.
- Achieve hemostasis after tourniquet deflation and close the wounds in routine fashion.
- When the flexor carpi ulnaris instead of the flexor carpi radialis is used for digital extension, a volar forearm incision should extend to the distal wrist flexion crease. The flexor carpi ulnaris tendon is detached near the pisiform. The procedure is analogous to that described for the flexor carpi radialis motor except for the details concerning proximal dissection of the flexor carpi ulnaris muscle and passing the tendon around the ulnar shaft. The flexor carpi ulnaris is muscular throughout, and in thin arms removal of the middle and distal muscle portion may make this motor less visible.

POSTOPERATIVE CARE　Although the sutures can be removed 10 to 14 days postoperatively, the wrist is kept in 40 degrees of extension, the metacarpophalangeal joints in full extension, and the thumb radially abducted and extended for 3 weeks. Supervised physical therapy is begun at this time. A removable custom-molded splint keeping the wrist, fingers, and thumb in the postoperative position is worn at night and between therapy sessions for approximately 3 months postoperatively.

TRANSFER OF PRONATOR TERES TO EXTENSOR CARPI RADIALIS LONGUS AND EXTENSOR CARPI RADIALIS BREVIS, FLEXOR CARPI RADIALIS TO EXTENSOR POLLICIS BREVIS AND ABDUCTOR POLLICIS LONGUS, FLEXOR DIGITORUM SUBLIMIS MIDDLE TO EXTENSOR DIGITORUM COMMUNIS, AND FLEXOR DIGITORUM SUBLIMIS RING TO EXTENSOR POLLICIS LONGUS AND EXTENSOR INDICIS PROPRIUS

TECHNIQUE 8.18

(BOYES)
- Make a long longitudinal incision on the volar side of the radial aspect of the forearm and free the insertion of the pronator teres with its strip of periosteum.
- Perforate the extensor carpi radialis longus and brevis tendons and pass the insertion of the pronator teres through these tendons.
- Expose the middle and ring finger sublimis tendons through a single incision in the distal palm over the metacarpal heads or through separate incisions at their insertions on the middle phalanges; divide each so that the free end of its distal segment lies within its sheath. Withdraw the proximal segments of the tendons through the forearm incision.
- Make a dorsal transverse incision on the wrist, extending from the radial styloid toward the ulnar styloid and curving it proximally. Expose the common digital extensors proximal to the dorsal carpal ligament, and incise the deep fascia.
- Make a 2-cm opening in the interosseous membrane at the proximal edge of the pronator quadratus muscle. Pass

the sublimis of the middle finger between the profundus muscle mass and the flexor pollicis longus muscle mass and through the interosseous membrane. Attach the donor tendon to the common digital extensors.

- Make another opening in the interosseous membrane. Pass the sublimis of the ring finger to the ulnar side of the profundus muscle mass and through the opening and attach it to the extensor pollicis longus and extensor indicis proprius. The sublimis tendons of the long and ring fingers must be separated proximally and not crossed over to prevent a scissors-type compression of the median nerve.
- Divide the flexor carpi radialis at the wrist and suture it to the extensor pollicis brevis and abductor pollicis longus at this level.
- Before the transferred tendons are sutured in place, remove the tourniquet and check the interosseous artery for bleeding.

POSTOPERATIVE CARE Immobilization should be implemented for 6 weeks. Usually a cast is maintained on the arm for 4 weeks, followed by a spring-loaded extension splint for the wrist and fingers for another week. During the cast immobilization, the metacarpophalangeal joints should not be completely extended but should be held in about 40 degrees of flexion. The wrist should be fully extended, however, with the thumb in abduction and extension. The interphalangeal joints of the fingers should be in "comfortable" flexion.

LOW ULNAR NERVE PALSY

The functional deficits caused by low ulnar nerve palsy are: (1) weakness of pinch resulting from paralysis of the adductor pollicis and first dorsal interosseous, (2) weakness of grip produced by paralysis of most of the finger intrinsics, and (3) clawing of the ring and little fingers associated with paralysis of all of their intrinsics.

Paralysis of the adductor pollicis results in a major functional loss that should be restored if possible by appropriate tendon transfer (see section on restoration of adduction of the thumb). Normal tightness of the metacarpophalangeal joints of the ring and little fingers may limit clawing of these fingers and enable the long extensors to extend their interphalangeal joints; in this instance, no treatment is indicated for clawing, but weakness of grip is still present. If clawing of these fingers is troublesome, however, function of their intrinsics should be restored by transferring the extensor indicis proprius tendon; it is split into two slips, passed volar to the deep transverse metacarpal ligament, and attached to the radial side of the extensor aponeurosis of each finger as in the Riordan transfer (see Fig. 8.21). Other dynamic transfers, such as that of Bunnell (see Technique 8.12) or Brand (see Technique 8.13), may be useful. As an alternative to tendon transfer, clawing of the ring and little fingers can be corrected by Zancolli capsulodesis. The utility of the Zancolli capsulodesis can be confirmed by performing Bouvier's test (Fig. 8.31). This is done by preventing metacarpophalangeal joint hyperextension. If the extensors can extend the proximal interphalangeal joints with the metacarpophalangeal joints flexed to or less than 40 degrees, a static procedure may be all that is required.

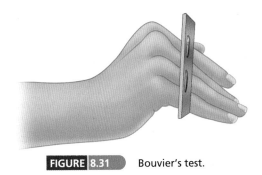

FIGURE 8.31 Bouvier's test.

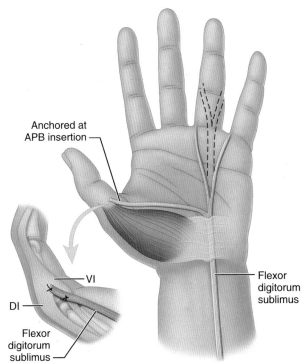

FIGURE 8.32 Single transfer of flexor digitorum sublimis tendon is used to correct clawing and to strengthen thumb-index pinch in isolated ulnar nerve palsy. *APB*, Adductor pollicis brevis; *DI*, dorsal interossei; *VI*, volar interossei. (Redrawn from Omer GE Jr: Tendon transfers in combined nerve lesions, *Orthop Clin North Am* 5:377, 1974.)

However, if a proximal interphalangeal joint extensor is not present, a dynamic procedure may yield a better result (see Technique 8.13). According to Hastings and McCollam, this technique is very successful in correcting claw deformity and increasing synchronous movement of the ring and small fingers; however, improvement in grip strength should not be expected with the Zancolli capsulodesis.

For low ulnar nerve palsy, Omer suggested the following procedure be done in one stage (Fig. 8.32). The metacarpophalangeal joint of the thumb is arthrodesed. The insertion of the flexor digitorum sublimis of the ring finger is freed, and the tendon is split into two slips. One slip is carried across the palm parallel to the fibers of the adductor pollicis and is anchored to the insertion of that muscle. The other slip is split into two tails; one is carried through the appropriate lumbrical canal and is anchored to the radial side of the extensor aponeurosis of the ring finger, and the other is transferred in a similar manner to the little finger. Instead of the procedure just described, Omer sometimes transferred the brachioradialis tendon, prolonged with a free graft, through the third interosseous space to restore adduction of the thumb (see section on restoration of adduction of the thumb); to restore abduction of the index finger, he freed the radial half of the insertion of the extensor indicis proprius, split the tendon, and anchored the freed half of the tendon to the insertion of the first dorsal interosseous.

Burkhalter suggested several tendon transfers and noted that insertion directly into the proximal phalanx diaphysis of the involved fingers resulted in a more secure attachment and has the advantage of a greater lever arm beyond the metacarpophalangeal joint. For motors, he used the brachioradialis or the extensor carpi radialis longus extended by free grafts, both of which are brought dorsally and passed through the intermetacarpal area volar to the transverse metacarpal ligament and then attached to bone (Fig. 8.33). Burkhalter also used the same bony attachment in transferring a split sublimis of the ring finger as a modification of the Stiles-Bunnell transfer. In addition, there should be a transfer to provide adduction of the thumb.

Brown suggested several transfers for thumb adduction. One uses the ring finger sublimis brought deep to the finger flexors, and another uses the extensor indicis proprius brought into the palm around the third metacarpal and then transversely across the palm, paralleling the paralyzed adductor muscle, to attach to the metacarpophalangeal joint area of the thumb. Occasionally, arthrodesis of the distal thumb joint is advised to increase the power of pinch; this is accompanied sometimes by advancing the pulley at the metacarpophalangeal joint by sectioning it proximally to provide a greater angle of approach of the flexor pollicis longus.

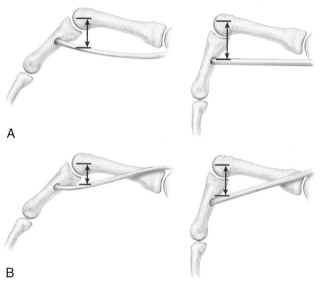

A

B

FIGURE 8.33 **A,** Burkhalter modification of Stiles-Bunnell transfer increases distance of moment arm with increased flexion of metacarpophalangeal joint. Force applied distally varies with square of distance. **B,** With intermetacarpal route for this transfer, moment arm also increases with increasing flexion of metacarpophalangeal joint. (Redrawn from Burkhalter WE: Restoration of power grip in ulnar nerve paralysis, *Orthop Clin North Am* 2:289, 1974.)

HIGH ULNAR NERVE PALSY

The functional deficits caused by high ulnar nerve palsy are the same as those described for low ulnar nerve palsy except that functions of the flexor digitorum profundus of the ring and little fingers and of the flexor carpi ulnaris also are lost. The transfers described for low ulnar nerve palsy can be used except that the sublimis of the ring finger must not be transferred because the profundus of this finger is paralyzed. Flexion of the distal interphalangeal joints of the ring and little fingers can be restored by suturing the profundus tendons of these fingers to that of the long finger. If further power is needed, transfer of the extensor carpi radialis longus into the profundus tendons of the long, ring, and little fingers also can be done. The innervation of the profundus of the long finger may be totally ulnar at times and frequently only partially ulnar.

The anterior interosseous nerve to ulnar motor nerve transfer can be used to restore intrinsic function. In contrast to radial nerve transfers, this transfer does not sacrifice potential tendon donors should it fail.

LOW MEDIAN NERVE PALSY

The important functional deficits caused by low median nerve palsy are loss of opposition of the thumb and loss of sensibility over the sensory distribution of the nerve; paralysis of the two radial lumbrical muscles is of little consequence when the ulnar nerve is intact. Restoration of thumb opposition is discussed in the section on restoration of thumb opposition. Restoration of sensibility by a neurovascular island graft is discussed in chapter 5.

HIGH MEDIAN NERVE PALSY

The important functional deficits caused by high median nerve palsy are loss of pronation of the forearm, flexion of the wrist, flexion of the index and long fingers, flexion of the thumb, opposition of the thumb, and median nerve sensation.

Function can be restored partially as follows. The paralyzed ulnar-innervated ring and small finger flexor digitorum profundus can be attached by side-to-side suture without sectioning of any of the nonparalyzed median nerve–innervated index and long finger flexor digitorum profundus tendons (Fig. 8.34). In addition, greater power can be achieved by transferring the extensor carpi radialis longus into the profundus tendons of the index and middle fingers. Thumb flexion can be restored by brachioradialis transfer to the long thumb flexor at the wrist level. Other options for restoration of the interphalangeal joint flexion include extensor carpi radialis longus transfer or extensor carpi ulnaris transfer to the flexor pollicis longus. Thumb opposition can be restored by using the extensor indicis proprius as a transfer, bringing it around the ulnar side of the wrist so that construction of a pulley is not needed (see Technique 8.3). The restoration of sensibility by a neurovascular island graft is discussed in chapter 5.

COMBINED LOW MEDIAN AND ULNAR NERVE PALSY (AT THE WRIST)

Combined median and ulnar nerve lesions at the wrist result in: (1) complete anesthesia of the palm, (2) loss of function of all intrinsics of the fingers, and (3) loss of opposition of the thumb (see the introduction to this section). If these lesions are not treated, skin and joint contractures develop and a fixed clawhand results.

Despite the palmar anesthesia, it is possible to restore some useful function after this severe paralysis. The success of treatment depends on several factors. Often the flexor tendons have been severely injured by the same trauma that caused the paralysis; in this event, the condition of the tendons is important in planning transfers. In Hansen disease, the paralysis is not accompanied by tendon injury but sometimes by deformity of the skin, fingernails, and bone. For tendon transfers to be successful, any contracture of the skin or joints must be corrected first because the transfers alone cannot accomplish this. Passive extension of the interphalangeal joints and flexion of the metacarpophalangeal joints must be possible. An attempt is made to mobilize the joints by splinting; if this fails, arthrodesis of the proximal interphalangeal joints must be considered. Any thumb web contracture, which is frequent after combined median and ulnar nerve palsy, also must be corrected (see the section on restoration of adduction of the thumb).

Function of the finger intrinsics can be restored by the Brand transfer, in which the extensor carpi radialis brevis is extended by tendon graft (see Technique 8.13). Opposition of the thumb can be restored by the Riordan transfer (see Technique 8.1), unless the sublimis tendon of the ring finger or the palmaris longus tendon has been injured by direct trauma.

For clawing, Brown suggested a transfer of the extensor carpi radialis longus tendon extended by a four-tailed graft to restore metacarpophalangeal flexion, as Brand described. For thumb adduction, he suggested using the extensor indicis proprius tendon passed through the third intermetacarpal

space and over the paralyzed adductor muscle, and attached to the adductor tendon insertion at the metacarpophalangeal joint of the thumb.

Thumb adduction also can be restored by transferring the ring flexor digitorum sublimis through the distal palmar fascia, using the vertical septum as a pulley, and passing it across the palm superficial to the fascia and attaching it to the radial side of the metacarpophalangeal joint of the thumb.

Omer suggested several possibilities. To restore digital balance, he used the middle finger flexor digitorum sublimis tendon split into four tails or the extensor carpi radialis longus tendon extended by a graft. The other two possibilities are the extensor indicis proprius tendon or the extensor digiti quinti proprius tendon, each split into two tails and attached to the second and third digits and fourth and fifth digits. For thumb adduction, the middle flexor digitorum sublimis tendon or the extensor carpi radialis longus tendon is brought through the third intermetacarpal space and extended by a graft to attach to the thumb adductor area. For opposition, he suggested using the extensor carpi ulnaris tendon extended by the extensor pollicis brevis tendon or a graft from the palmaris longus. Fusion also is suggested for increasing stability of the thumb.

COMBINED HIGH MEDIAN AND ULNAR NERVE PALSY (ABOVE THE ELBOW)

In combined high median and ulnar nerve palsy, the entire hand is anesthetic except for the dorsal surface, and the only muscles available for transfer are muscles innervated by the radial nerve—the brachioradialis, the extensor carpi radialis brevis, the extensor carpi radialis longus, the extensor carpi ulnaris, and the extensor indicis proprius. Recommended treatment of this palsy includes arthrodesis of the thumb metacarpophalangeal joint; Zancolli capsulodesis of the metacarpophalangeal joints of all fingers (see Technique 8.15) and release of the flexor tendon sheaths at the same time; transfer of the extensor carpi radialis longus around the radial side of the wrist to the flexor digitorum profundus; transfer of the brachioradialis to the flexor pollicis longus; and transfer of the extensor carpi ulnaris, extended with a free graft, around the ulnar border of the forearm to the extensor pollicis brevis. Amputating the index finger and its metacarpal and folding the radially innervated dorsal flap into the palm has been suggested.

SEVERE PARALYSIS FROM DAMAGE TO THE CERVICAL SPINAL CORD OR OTHER CAUSES
TETRAPLEGIA

Improved acute management and subsequent long-term care of victims of motor vehicle accidents and sports injuries have placed increased emphasis on rehabilitation of patients with tetraplegia. Most patients who survive cervical spinal cord injuries are young men with 25 to 30 years of life remaining, and nearly two thirds of survivors of cervical cord–level injury have C6 root level function remaining. Subjectively, most patients consider their lives considerably improved by upper-limb surgery. Three-fourths of young tetraplegic patients consider the use of the hands and upper extremities to be the function that they would like most to be restored. This is considered

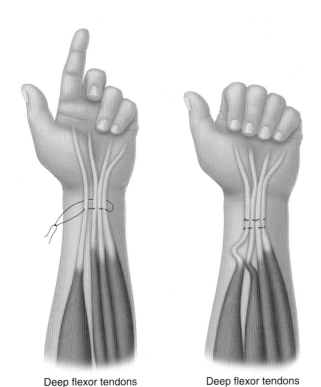

Deep flexor tendons   Deep flexor tendons
of fingers   of fingers

FIGURE 8.34 In high median nerve palsy, distal segments of profundus tendons of index and middle fingers are tightened and tendons are sutured to profundus tendons of ring and little fingers (see text). This tendon mass can be strengthened further by transfer of extensor carpi radialis longus to insert as additional motor. (Redrawn from Omer GE Jr: Evaluation and reconstruction of the forearm and hand after acute traumatic peripheral nerve injuries, *J Bone Joint Surg* 50A:1454, 1968.)

TABLE 8.3

International Classification for Surgery of the Hand in Tetraplegia

SENSIBILITY O OR CU GROUP*	MOTOR CHARACTERISTICS	DESCRIPTION/FUNCTION
0	No muscle below elbow suitable for transfer	Elbow flexion and forearm supination
1	BR	
2	ECRL	Extension of the wrist (weak or strong)
3[†]	ECRB	Extension of the wrist
4	PT	Wrist extension and forearm pronation
5	FCR	Flexion of the wrist
6	Finger extensors	Extrinsic extension of the fingers (partial or complete)
7	Thumb extensor	Extrinsic extension of the thumb
8	Partial digital flexors	Extrinsic flexion of the fingers (weak)
9	Lacks only intrinsic	Extrinsic flexion of the fingers
10	Exceptions	

Edinburgh, 1978; modified, Giens, France, 1984. *O, ocular; Cu, cutaneous.
[†]It is impossible to determine strength of ECRB without surgical exposure.
BR, Brachioradialis; ECRB, extensor carpi radialis brevis; ECRL, extensor carpi radialis longus; FCR, flexor carpi radialis; PT, pronator teres.
From McDowell CL, Moberg EA, House JH: The second international conference on surgical rehabilitation of the upper limb in tetraplegia (quadriplegia), J Hand Surg 11A:604, 1986.

by these patients to be more important than use of the legs, bladder or bowel function, and use and feeling of their sexual organs. Long-term follow-up after surgery in tetraplegic patients has demonstrated high overall satisfaction and positive impact on ability to perform activities of daily living and increased level of independence. Although surgical management of tetraplegia can improve patient function and independence, there is evidence that the techniques are underutilized. Of the 65% to 75% of patients with tetraplegia who would potentially benefit from surgery, tendon transfer procedures are performed in only 14%.

■ CLASSIFICATION

A useful classification scheme for tetraplegia takes into account sensory and motor level function (Table 8.3). The sensory afferent is designated either O (ocular) or Cu (cutaneous) depending on whether visual cue or at least 10-mm two-point discrimination is preserved. The motor groupings fall into 10 categories (0 through 9) depending on the lowest level of grade 4 or better motor function remaining, according to the Medical Research Council grading scale. An additional group (X) is added to accommodate patients who do not fit into any of the 10 categories. This classification system helps to tailor surgical management and outcomes assessment. The motor examination would seem to follow a predictable root level pattern (Fig. 8.35), but this often is not true. Asymmetrical upper-extremity involvement and skip lesions occur in sensory and motor function.

■ PRINCIPLES OF MANAGEMENT

Careful analysis of the motor and sensory status is necessary to determine which surgical procedure is warranted, if any. Same-level cervical spine injuries may yield varied physical findings, and different procedures may be

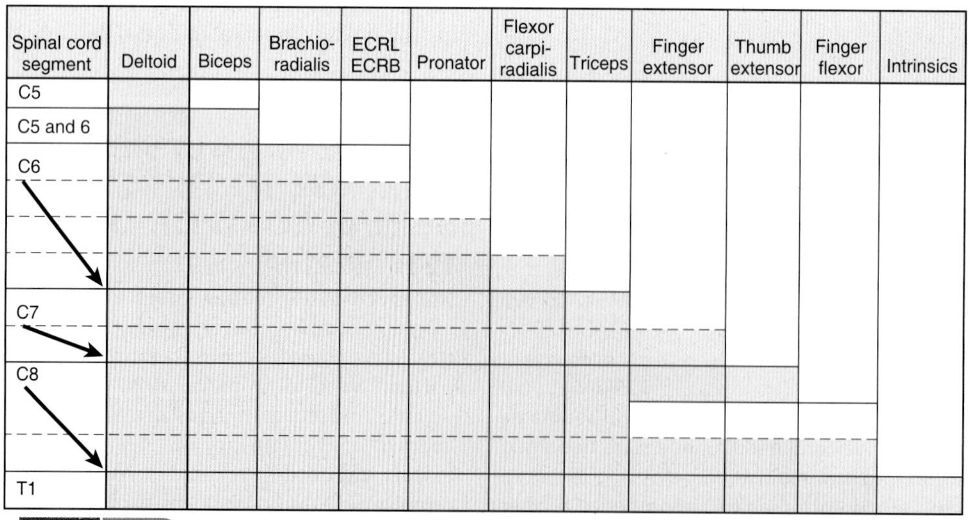

FIGURE 8.35 Normal spinal segmental level of muscles of upper limb. *Shaded areas* indicate main segmental muscle supply. *ECRB*, Extensor carpi radialis brevis; *ECRL*, extensor carpi radialis longus. (Modified from Lamb DW: *The paralysed hand: the hand and upper limb*, vol 2, Edinburgh, 1987, Churchill Livingstone.)

BOX 8.1

Protocol for Management of Tetraplegia

Acute Phase

- The spine is stabilized to preserve the remaining neurologic function and to allow early mobilization.
- Associated body system problems are managed.
- Associated upper extremity injuries are managed aggressively.
- An occupational therapy program is begun to prevent joint contracture and to maintain joint mobility.

Subacute Phase

- An aggressive rehabilitation program is begun.
- An occupational therapy maintenance program is instituted.
- Associated problems (e.g., decubitus ulcers, bladder) are treated.
- Psychologic problems are resolved.
- A serial examination is performed by the reconstructive surgeon at 3-month intervals; neurologic recovery is allowed to plateau.

Reconstructive Phase: Upper Extremity Reconstruction

- The patient is stable and psychologically well adjusted, and the neurologic recovery has plateaued. Generally, allow at least 12 months after injury.
- Reconstruction is begun on the side with the most intact function.
- If the sides are equal in function, reconstruction is begun on the dominant extremity.
- If cutaneous sensibility is absent (only ocular sensibility is present), reconstruction is limited to only one extremity to allow for visual control.
- The treatment plan is kept simple.
- Restoration of active elbow extension by the Moberg deltoid-to-triceps technique precedes other upper extremity reconstruction.
- Key grip is restored.
- The reconstruction plan is modified to fit the individual's needs.

Modified from Murphy CP, Chuinard RG: Management of the upper extremity in traumatic tetraplegia, *Hand Clin* 4:201, 1988.

Cutaneous sensation is measured by the two-point discrimination test with a paper clip (Moberg). If sensibility is not present, visual feedback is necessary for extremity control. In such an instance, only one upper extremity should undergo surgery.

After injury, it is essential to maintain mobility of the finger, wrist, elbow, and shoulder joints because contractures frequently develop, especially with spasticity. Elbow flexion, supination, and metacarpophalangeal extension contractures should be prevented through appropriate therapeutic techniques. Passive motion exercises and upper-extremity splinting are necessary preoperative measures in the postinjury period. Murphy and Chuinard developed a helpful protocol for the management of tetraplegia; they described acute, subacute, and reconstructive phases (Box 8.1).

McDowell, Moberg, and House summarized additional principles regarding surgical management in tetraplegia as follows:

1. Neurologic recovery should have ceased and at least 12 months should have passed before surgical reconstruction.
2. Uncontrolled spasticity of a muscle, despite good strength, precludes its use in transfer.
3. Painful paresthesias in a hand prohibit that hand from being reconstructed.
4. Wrist mobility and the natural tenodesis effect should be maintained.

For most authors, the goal of treatment usually has been to obtain key grip or key pinch. Key pinch posture provides a stronger, broader gripping surface, is cosmetically preferable, and is more easily achieved than the "chuckjaw," or three-fingered, pinch. Grasping with all fingers is desirable, but this cannot be accomplished without availability of more muscles. The surgical objective in tetraplegia is not to provide complex function through complex surgery. A simple surgical procedure for a given function should be planned whenever possible to provide some degree of freedom in patients who are severely handicapped.

Reconstructive surgery in tetraplegia can be simply a composite of methods necessary to provide control of a joint or a series of joints. Insufficient motor units around a joint often require arthrodesis of the joint, especially of the thumb carpometacarpal, metacarpophalangeal, and interphalangeal joints. Static and dynamic tenodeses (e.g., Moberg flexor pollicis longus tenodesis to the distal radius in group 1 tetraplegia) are versatile, frequently used procedures. For lower-level tetraplegia, a variety of tendon transfers are available, often supplemented by arthrodeses and tenodeses. Continued interest in tetraplegia has led to refinements in older techniques and new concepts as well, including possible use of nerve transfers in combination with tendon transfers.

Despite a slightly different approach to tendon transfers in patients with spinal cord injuries compared with patients with peripheral nerve injuries, the basic checklist of prerequisites for surgery must not be overlooked (Box 8.2). In addition, efforts to restore sensation should follow tendon transfers because cortical interpretation of sensation (localization and stereognosis) seems to be enhanced by movement of the part.

High-level tetraplegia without available motors for transfer has prompted the use of implanted electrical stimulation. Intact neuromuscular units lacking cortical efferent control

indicated in the upper extremities of an individual. Many patients are extremely hesitant to have any surgical procedure done for fear of losing what little function remains. The examiner not only must check for muscle function and grade its power but also should observe the patient in his or her daily activities and try to determine what additional function would best promote greater independence. If there is no muscle power, not even a flicker, immediately after injury and again nothing in 1 month, no function can be expected from this muscle. As a rule, however, surgery is begun after months of observation, usually after 1 year or longer. In partial or incomplete quadriplegia, spasticity usually becomes a consideration because it may jeopardize the end results of surgery. The better hand should be operated on first because rehabilitation is easier.

Patient Evaluation and Muscle Selection Guidelines for Tendon Transfers

Prerequisite Checks for Transfers
Sensibility
Stability
  Bone
  Neurologic
  Psychologic
  Soft tissue
Site adequacy
  Adequate soft-tissue bed
  Supple joints

Muscle Selection
Strength
  Tendon fraction
  Mass fraction
Excursion
Alignment
Synergy
Integrity
Expendability
  Staging
  Rehabilitation

are stimulated by impulses directed along the intact neural pathways. Combinations of stimuli to different neuromuscular units allow for programming of concerted activity.

ELBOW EXTENSION

Elbow extension is lost in approximately 70% of tetraplegics. Regaining elbow extension should be the function achieved first or in conjunction with other procedures. Elbow extension is crucial for overhead activities, weight shifting, and transfers. Several surgical techniques have been described for triceps substitution in patients with grade 3 or less muscle power.

The posterior deltoid-to-triceps transfer as described by Moberg has historically been the most commonly performed procedure to establish elbow extension. The Moberg procedure often incorporates a graft, usually autologous, and requires a long period of immobilization. Excellent results have been reported after such a transfer using the anterior tibial tendon as a donor. Direct deltoid-to-triceps transfer—simple attachment of the deltoid to the triceps aponeurosis—also has been recommended.

Transfer of the distal biceps to triceps tendon is a viable option if no elbow flexion contracture is present. Active supination and brachialis function are prerequisites to biceps-to-triceps transfer. In a prospective randomized study, Mulcahey et al. demonstrated superior results with biceps-to-triceps transfers compared with transfer of the posterior deltoid. Further investigation has shown satisfactory restoration of elbow function in a larger patient cohort. Hutchinson et al. also confirmed that the biceps achieves phasic reversal after transfer.

Nerve transfers of fascicles of the axillary or musculocutaneous nerve to motor branches of the radial nerve to the triceps also have been used.

DISTAL BICEPS-TO-TRICEPS TRANSFER

TECHNIQUE 8.19

- Make a 3-cm anterior transverse incision across the antecubital fossa (Fig. 8.36A) and a 7-cm longitudinal incision along the medial intermuscular septum (Fig. 8.36B).
- Mobilize or ligate large antecubital veins.
- Identify the musculocutaneous nerve just lateral to the biceps tendon and carefully protect it throughout the procedure (Fig. 8.36C).
- While protecting underlying neurovascular structures, incise the lacertus fibrosis.
- Perform blunt dissection carefully along the biceps tendon to its insertion into the radial tuberosity with the elbow in flexion and the forearm in supination (Fig. 8.36D).
- Release the biceps tendon from its attachment and place a large nonabsorbable grasping suture through the tendon.
- Through the previously performed medial incision, release the intermuscular septum and identify the ulnar nerve (Fig. 8.36E).
- Take care to carefully release the biceps tendon and muscle from surrounding fascial attachments to enhance excursion and line of pull.
- Continue the dissection until adequate excursion for transfer of the biceps to the olecranon is achieved.
- Make a third 7-cm posterior incision over the distal third of the triceps and carry it around the olecranon.
- Sharply split the triceps over the tip of the olecranon (Fig. 8.36F).
- Prepare the olecranon by placing a unicortical hole into the intramedullary canal and sequentially enlarge it to accommodate the distal biceps tendon (Fig. 8.36G).
- Transfer the biceps tendon from the anterior incision to the medial incision, superficial to the ulnar nerve into the posterior incision (Fig. 8.36H).
- Pass the biceps tendon obliquely through the medial portion of the triceps into the previously placed split in the triceps tendon (Fig. 8.36I).
- Drill two small holes into the opposite posterior cortex of the olecranon (i.e., inside-out technique) (Fig. 8.36J).
- With the elbow in full extension, dock the distal biceps into the unicortical hole in the olecranon and secure the sutures over the bone tunnel (an interference screw can also be used) (Fig. 8.36K).
- Subsequently augment the transfer with additional nonabsorbable sutures.
- After appropriate hemostasis and wound closure, apply a long arm splint incorporating the wrist with the elbow in full extension.

POSTOPERATIVE CARE The elbow is maintained in full extension for 4 weeks, after which time the patient is fitted with a fabricated nighttime extension brace. For daytime use, a controlled motion brace is used with a flexion block at 15 degrees. The brace is

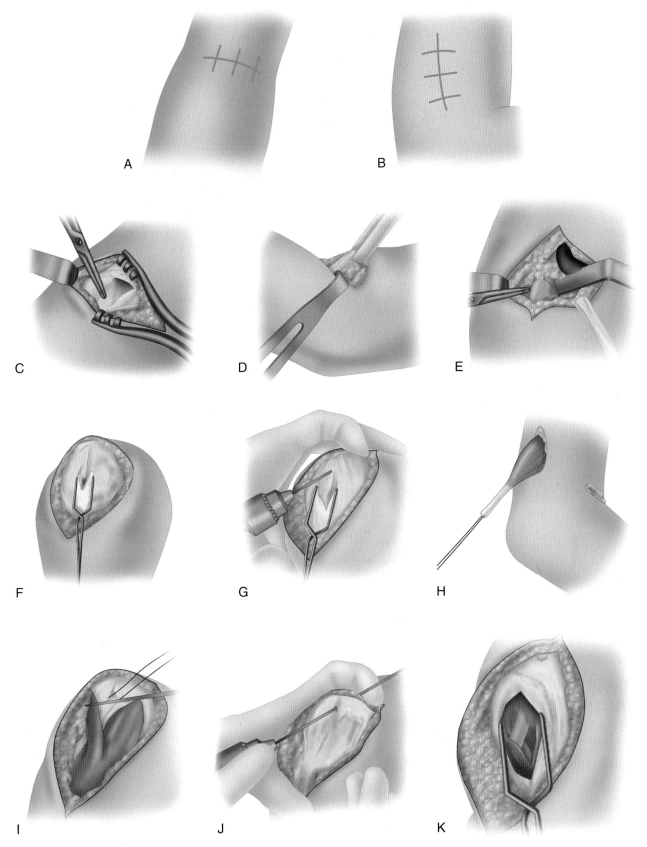

FIGURE 8.36 Biceps-to-triceps transfer. **A,** Transverse incision across antecubital fossa. **B,** Longitudinal incision along medial inter-muscular septum. **C,** Musculocutaneous nerve adjacent to biceps tendon. **D,** Elbow flexion and forearm supination to facilitate dissection of biceps tendon to insertion. **E,** Ulnar nerve identified through a medial incision. **F,** Triceps split over tip of olecranon and a self-retaining retractor between the incised tendon. **G,** Unicortical hole drilled from tip of olecranon to posterior or posterolateral cortex. **H,** Biceps tendon passed from anterior incision to medial incision. **I,** Biceps tendon passed obliquely through medial portion of triceps tendon using a tendon braider. **J,** Two small holes are drilled through opposite posterior cortex through the unicortical hole to accept the suture passer. **K,** Elbow extended and biceps tendon advanced into unicortical tunnel. **SEE TECHNIQUE 8.19.**

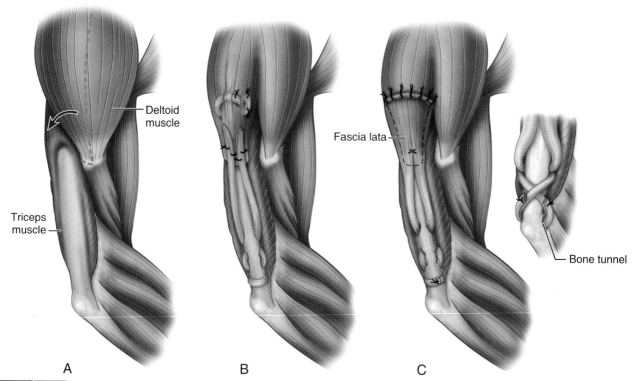

FIGURE 8.37   Deltoid-to-triceps transfer (Moberg). **A,** Posterior border of muscle belly is isolated, preserving as much of tendinous insertion as possible. **B,** Tendon grafts are laced into distal end of posterior deltoid muscle belly and triceps aponeurosis. **C,** Fascia lata can be used, as is done here, instead of tendon grafts. Direct insertion into olecranon through bone tunnel also can be done with either type of graft. **SEE TECHNIQUE 8.20.**

adjusted weekly to allow for additional flexion in 15-degree increments. Therapy is initiated with functional activities of daily living incorporated as elbow flexion increases. The controlled motion brace is discontinued when 90 degrees of elbow flexion is achieved without extension lag. Nighttime bracing is maintained for 12 weeks postoperatively, and strengthening is initiated at 3 months.

POSTERIOR DELTOID-TO-TRICEPS TRANSFER

TECHNIQUE 8.20

(MOBERG, MODIFIED)
- Place the patient in the lateral decubitus position and make a 10- to 13-cm incision along the posterior border of the deltoid muscle down to the insertion of the muscle. Raise flaps over the fascia of the deltoid and identify its humeral insertion.
- Using a periosteal elevator and sharp dissection, elevate the posterior third to half of the tendon with a strip of the periosteal insertion (Fig. 8.37A).
- Place this portion of the deltoid under slight tension and gently split the muscle fibers in a distal-to-proximal direc-

tion, taking care to palpate and inspect for the axillary nerve and posterior circumflex humeral vessels entering the muscle on its deep surface posteriorly. End the proximal dissection when this level is identified. The triceps generally is atrophied, and the posterior deltoid edge is easily palpable.
- Through a separate curved longitudinal incision, expose the distal triceps and its insertion on the olecranon distal to the musculotendinous junction. If there is adequate overlap of the tendinous portions of the deltoid insertion and the proximal portion of the triceps, the transfer can be accomplished without an interposition graft (Hentz et al.). If the overlap does not provide adequate weave fixation, however, a free tendon graft may be necessary (Fig. 8.37B). Moberg used great toe extensors, Lacey et al. used the anterior tibial tendon, and Hentz et al. used fascia lata; use of other graft sources also has been reported (Fig. 8.37C).
- Adjust the tension of the attachment so that full elbow flexion can be passively obtained. Stainless steel sutures can be placed on either side of the transfer site to radiographically follow the integrity of the attachment.

POSTOPERATIVE CARE The arm is splinted in 0 to 30 degrees of elbow flexion with the arm adducted. At 4 to 6 weeks, the elbow is gradually flexed at a rate of 10 to 15 degrees per week. Active and active-assisted range-of-

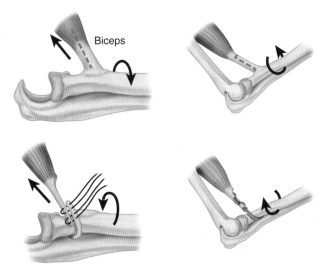

FIGURE 8.38 Rerouting of distal end of biceps and release of interosseous membrane for fixed supination deformity. (Redrawn from Zancolli EA: *Structural and dynamic bases of hand surgery,* Philadelphia, 1978, Lippincott.)

> motion exercises are then begun, with a progressive range of motion. The elbow is maintained in an elbow extension splint at night for 3 months. The patient should refrain from wheelchair push-ups and transfers for 3 months.

■ FOREARM PRONATION

Patients with group 3 function (transferable brachioradialis, extensor carpi radialis longus and brevis) or lower lack active forearm pronation. Resultant fixed or dynamic supination deformities prohibit the hand from being placed in a position necessary for a variety of functions. This deformity should be corrected before rehabilitation of the hand. Rerouting the biceps tendon around the lateral aspect of the proximal radius converts the biceps muscle into a pronator. Zancolli also recommended release of the interosseous membrane when the supination deformities are fixed (Fig. 8.38).

■ WRIST EXTENSION

In group 1 patients (transferable brachioradialis only), wrist extension can be accomplished by transferring the brachioradialis into the extensor carpi radialis brevis tendon. Transfer into the extensor carpi radialis longus produces more radial deviation. Transfer into the extensor carpi ulnaris is not advised because this muscle acts as a wrist extensor only when the wrist is in supination. Elbow extension must be present or reconstructed to stabilize the elbow against the significant flexion moment of the brachioradialis, or the transfer power would be reduced significantly. Procedures for wrist extension commonly are combined with other procedures, such as elbow extension and tenodesis procedures for key pinch. Only when the brachioradialis muscle has grade 4 power can it be transferred to provide wrist extension. The power of the brachioradialis can be graded by palpation over the muscle mass against resisted elbow flexion with the forearm in neutral.

Another option for restoration of wrist extension is nerve transfer. Transfer of the brachialis motor nerve to the extensor carpi radialis longus motor nerve in combination with

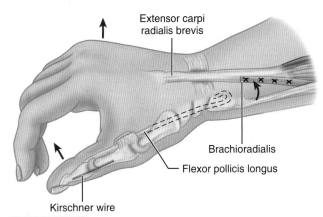

FIGURE 8.39 Restoration of wrist extension and key pinch when brachioradialis is only remaining functioning muscle unit, as recommended by Moberg. **SEE TECHNIQUE 8.21.**

tenodesis of the flexor pollicis longus to the distal radius can be done to restore tenodesis pinch.

TRANSFER OF THE BRACHIORADIALIS TO THE EXTENSOR CARPI RADIALIS BREVIS

TECHNIQUE 8.21

- Make a longitudinal incision 8 to 10 cm long dorsally along the radial aspect of the forearm.
- Carefully identify the dorsal sensory branch of the radial nerve and protect it during the mobilization of the brachioradialis. Proximal mobilization of the brachioradialis enhances the excursion and is safe because the nerve supply is proximal.
- Identify the extensor carpi radialis brevis tendon insertion into the third metacarpal base and pass the tendon of the brachioradialis through this tendon several times.
- Place tension on the tendon and temporarily suture it to check for full wrist flexion without undue tension or laxity of the transferred unit (Fig. 8.39). Suture the brachioradialis into place using nonabsorbable braided suture.

POSTOPERATIVE CARE A plaster splint is worn for 4 weeks, and then active range-of-motion exercises are begun. Splinting is continued between exercises and at night for 8 to 12 months.

■ KEY PINCH

Key, or lateral, pinch is more desirable and easier to achieve than chuckjaw pinch (three-fingered palmar pinch). Key pinch should be restored in all tetraplegic patients who have grade 4 or better wrist extensor motor power; at least 75% of all tetraplegic patients may be candidates for a key pinch procedure. Other prerequisites for the transfer include sufficient sensibility and thumb mobility. If ocular input is relied on, only one hand should be restored; however, if two-point discrimination is less than 12 to 15 mm, both hands should be reconstructed.

If no motors are expendable for active transfer, several well-designed tenodeses are available for accomplishing key pinch. The Moberg key grip procedure is the precursor of and the simplest of all thumb flexion tenodesis procedures. The flexor pollicis longus tendon is tenodesed to the distal radius so that on wrist extension the volar pulp of the thumb strongly contacts the radial side of the index finger. This may require stabilization procedures of the thumb interphalangeal and metacarpophalangeal joints. Moberg released the A1 pulley to increase the torque at the metacarpophalangeal joint by the subluxed flexor pollicis longus tendon.

Brand modified the Moberg key grip procedure by leaving the A1 pulley of the thumb metacarpophalangeal joint intact and routing the tendon across the palm, beneath the flexor tendons, and through the Guyon canal before tenodesing it to the distal radius. The line of pull is better with this technique, and bowstringing of the tendon is prevented (Fig. 8.40). A "winch" tenodesis for thumb flexion was described based on preservation of active forearm supination. The flexor pollicis longus tendon is routed around the distal ulna and is anchored to its dorsal aspect through a drill hole. During supination, the anchored tendon flexes the thumb (Fig. 8.41).

MOBERG KEY GRIP TENODESIS

TECHNIQUE 8.22

- Expose the musculotendinous junction of the flexor pollicis longus through a volar approach and divide the tendon at this level. Expose the distal end of the radius by subperiosteal dissection of the pronator quadratus in a radial-to-ulnar direction.
- Drill two holes in the volar cortex of the distal radius transverse to its longitudinal axis. The holes should be large enough to allow passage of the free flexor pollicis longus tendon.

- Connect the drill holes with a curved curet or power burr. Carefully round the edges of the cortical bone to prevent tendon attrition.
- Make a 2-cm incision over the A1 pulley and, after protecting the digital nerves, release the pulley.
- Deliver the flexor pollicis longus tendon into the wound. Stabilize the thumb interphalangeal joint in neutral position with a Kirschner wire (see Fig. 8.40).
- Make a 6-cm dorsal longitudinal incision centered over the thumb metacarpophalangeal joint. Open the hood of the dorsal apparatus in the line of the skin incision. After subperiosteal exposure, make several pairs of holes in the dorsal cortex of the thumb metacarpal. Tenodese the dorsal hood with sutures passed through them with the metacarpophalangeal joint in approximately 20 degrees of flexion.
- Adjust tension so that during full passive wrist extension the thumb firmly contacts the side of the index finger. When the proper tension has been obtained, secure the flexor pollicis longus tendon with multiple interrupted, nonabsorbable sutures.

POSTOPERATIVE CARE The transfer is protected with a splint for 4 weeks in neutral position with the thumb tip under the index finger middle phalanx. Splint protection is continued for 8 more weeks. When transfer of the brachioradialis to the extensor carpi radialis brevis is combined with this procedure, the wrist is kept in slight extension to lessen the tension on the active transfer.

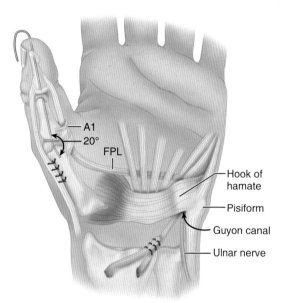

FIGURE 8.40 Modification of Moberg operation to create "simple hand grip" (see text). *FPL*, Flexor pollicis longus. **SEE TECHNIQUE 8.22.**

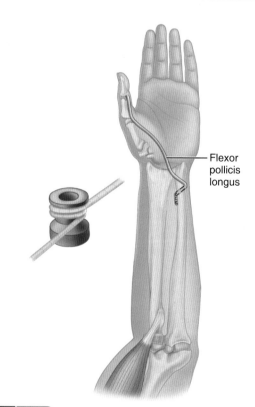

FIGURE 8.41 Brummer "winch" operation: temporary arthrodesis of interphalangeal joint and tenodesis of flexor pollicis longus against dorsal aspect of ulna. (Redrawn from Ejeskär A: Upper limb surgical rehabilitation in high-level tetraplegia, *Hand Clin* 4:585, 1988.)

Retained active wrist extension, as in group 2 or better patients, provides active transfer potential for thumb flexion and perhaps grasp. Increased pinch force of about 4 pounds has been reported, roughly equivalent to that obtained with the Dorrance prosthetic hook, as well as excellent excursion of the brachioradialis muscle, strength, and voluntary activation. An electromyographic study demonstrated that the brachioradialis muscle assumes the electrical synchrony of the paralyzed flexor pollicis longus after transfer. In normal subjects, the brachioradialis is electrically silent during lateral pinch and the triceps and flexor pollicis longus have synergistic activity. Patients who had a posterior deltoid-to-triceps transfer, in addition to brachioradialis-to-flexor pollicis longus transfer, showed a pattern of synergistic electrical activity similar to that of normal subjects with similar tasks of thumb flexion and elbow extension. If wrist extensor torque is good (>10 foot-lb), the brachioradialis transfer for thumb flexion is preferred; if wrist torque is less, wrist extension should be augmented by the brachioradialis and thumb flexion should be augmented by tenodesis.

House et al. reported a one-stage key pinch and release procedure in 18 patients (21 hands) with an average follow-up of 42 months. This procedure included carpometacarpal joint fusion, extensor pollicis longus tenodesis to the distal radius, and transfer of the brachioradialis to the flexor pollicis longus. Key pinch, which was nonmeasurable before surgery, increased to 3.3 kg and improved the activities of daily living (Fig. 8.42).

Patients in groups 4 and 5 constitute a large percentage of patients undergoing reconstructive efforts, and systematic programs have been developed to treat these patients. The two most popular reconstructions are the House two-stage procedure and the Zancolli two-step procedure. These procedures aim to restore grasp, key pinch, and release. They differ in that the Zancolli technique actively restores finger extension and the House procedure adds an adduction-opposition transfer to the thumb.

TWO-STAGE RECONSTRUCTION TO RESTORE DIGITAL FLEXION AND KEY PINCH

House et al. described a two-stage procedure for reconstruction of digital flexion and key pinch in patients who have at least strong wrist extension and a functioning pronator teres (group 4 or better function). The procedure is divided into flexor and extensor phases; the extensor phase is performed first. Digital flexion is accomplished by transferring the extensor carpi radialis longus to the flexor digitorum profundus. Adduction and opposition of the thumb are obtained by transfer of the brachioradialis to the thumb where the flexor digitorum sublimis of the ring finger is used as an in situ graft. Key pinch and grasp strength can be enhanced by an active transfer into the flexor pollicis longus using the pronator teres, the extensor or flexor carpi ulnaris, or the brachioradialis. The release phase of the reconstruction consists of intrinsic and extrinsic extensor tenodeses; however, if sufficient motors are available, active extension of the thumb and fingers is possible. The thumb carpometacarpal joint is stabilized by either fusion of that joint or tenodesis of the abductor pollicis longus.

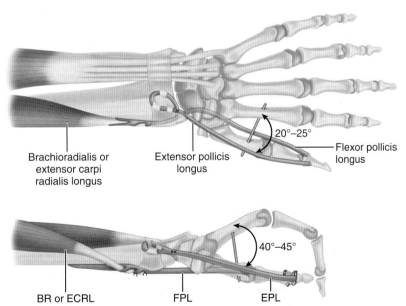

FIGURE 8.42 One-stage key pinch and release procedure (dorsal and lateral views). Thumb is prepositioned for lateral pinch by arthrodesis of trapezium–first metacarpophalangeal joint in 20 to 25 degrees of extension, 40 to 45 degrees of abduction, and slight pronation. Extensor pollicis longus (EPL) is fixed to Lister tubercle of distal radius by tenodesis. Brachioradialis (BR) or extensor carpi radialis longus (ECRL) is mobilized into proximal forearm and transferred to flexor pollicis longus (FPL) distally. (Redrawn from House JH, Comadoll J, Dahl AL: One-stage key pinch and release with thumb carpometacarpal fusion in tetraplegia, *J Hand Surg* 17A:530, 1992.)

House and Shannon compared the results of two modifications of this reconstruction. The procedures differed in the method of thumb control, intrinsic balance, and whether active extension was used. Qualitative differences between the two methods indicated that thumb carpometacarpal fusion allowed the hand better fine motor control, whereas the thumb adduction-opposition method afforded the ability to grasp larger objects. Both methods achieved good grasp and lateral pinch. Thumb adduction-opposition transfer produced slightly greater lateral pinch, and the thumb carpometacarpal arthrodesis provided slightly stronger grasp. Patients were pleased with having each hand reconstructed differently because they were able to use them for different tasks.

TECHNIQUE 8.23

STAGE 1—EXTENSOR PHASE

- Make an 8-cm incision along the dorsal aspect of the distal forearm beginning just distal to the Lister tubercle. Curve the incision gently to the radial side of the forearm if an active transfer is chosen; otherwise, make a straight incision for the tenodesis.
- Carefully protect the dorsal sensory branch of the radial nerve emerging beneath the brachioradialis radially and identify the extensor pollicis longus tendon ulnar and distal to the tubercle of Lister and the tendons of the extensor digitorum communis in the fourth dorsal compartment.
- Perform an extensor tenodesis by anchoring the tendons of the abductor pollicis longus, the extensor pollicis longus, and the extensor digitorum communis to the dorsum of the distal radius through two well-rounded holes. The holes should be several centimeters proximal to the radiocarpal joint for the extensor digitorum communis tendons and 2 cm proximal for the abductor pollicis longus and extensor pollicis longus tendons. Make tunnels into the proximal radius with a curet to accommodate the free ends of the tendons to be tenodesed.
- Make two suture holes proximal to the previously prepared holes with a 0.035-inch Kirschner wire (Fig. 8.43A). Remove the abductor pollicis longus and extensor pollicis longus tendons from the first dorsal compartment, and transpose them ulnarward.
- Suture the extensor digitorum communis tendons together under tension so that retraction of the single sutured tendon permits synchronous extension of the fingers.
- Likewise, suture the abductor pollicis longus and extensor pollicis longus tendons together to form a single tendon unit to be fixed to the distal radius.
- With the wrist in approximately 40 degrees of flexion, place tension on the proximal end of the divided extensor digitorum communis tendon so that the metacarpophalangeal joints are in full extension. Weave a heavy nonabsorbable suture into the tendon and deliver the free suture ends through the suture holes. Pull the sutures firmly and check the tenodesis; full metacarpophalangeal extension should be achieved when the wrist is flexed to 40 degrees, and full passive flexion of the fingers should be obtained when the wrist is extended 40 degrees.

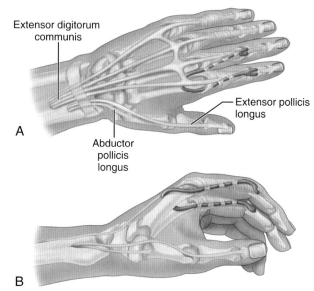

FIGURE 8.43 House two-stage technique for reconstruction of digital flexion and key pinch. **A,** Stage 1 (extensor phase). **B,** Stage 2 (flexor phase). (Redrawn from House JH, Comadoll J, Dahl AL: One-stage key pinch and release with thumb carpometacarpal fusion in tetraplegia, *J Hand Surg* 17A:530, 1992.) **SEE TECHNIQUE 8.23.**

- In the same fashion, fix the rerouted abductor pollicis longus and extensor pollicis longus tendons so that with 40 degrees of wrist flexion the thumb interphalangeal joint is extended to 0 degrees and the thumb metacarpal is in the plane of the hand and radially abducted 30 to 40 degrees.
- After checking the tenodesis, ensure that with wrist extension the thumb has acceptable passive motion for the second stage of the transfer.
- Intrinsic tenodesis can be achieved by transfer into either the A2 pulley or the dorsal apparatus. House et al. described a procedure in which a free tendon graft is sutured into the central slip and lateral tendon of the extensor apparatus and is taken through the lumbrical canals and around the dorsum of the metacarpal necks of the index and middle fingers. This forms in effect an "oblique retinacular ligament" so that when the proximal interphalangeal joint is flexed there is concomitant metacarpophalangeal flexion. It also prevents metacarpophalangeal hyperextension (Fig. 8.43B).

POSTOPERATIVE CARE The wrist is held in 40 to 45 degrees of extension, the thumb and the metacarpophalangeal joints in 40 degrees of flexion, and the interphalangeal joints in extension for 4 weeks; then active and passive motion is begun. If a thumb carpometacarpal joint arthrodesis was performed, the thumb is protected until fusion is obtained.

TECHNIQUE 8.24

STAGE 2—FLEXOR PHASE

- The flexor phase of reconstruction (Fig. 8.44) is performed 2 to 6 months after the extensor phase. Access

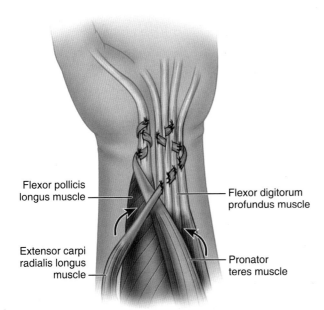

Flexor pollicis longus muscle

Flexor digitorum profundus muscle

Extensor carpi radialis longus muscle

Pronator teres muscle

FIGURE 8.44 House two-stage technique for reconstruction of digital flexion and key pinch-stage 2 (flexor phase). Extensor carpi radialis longus is transferred to flexor digitorum profundus, and pronator teres is transferred to flexor pollicis longus. **SEE TECHNIQUE 8.24.**

to the extensor carpi radialis longus and pronator teres for transfer into the flexor digitorum profundus and flexor pollicis longus requires three incisions.

- Make a volar longitudinal incision extending from the proximal wrist flexion crease just radial to the flexor carpi radialis tendon to the midshaft of the radius. Isolate the flexor pollicis longus, the pronator teres, and the flexor digitorum profundus tendons proximal to their musculotendinous junctions.
- Divide the extensor carpi radialis longus at its insertion into the base of the second metacarpal through a short transverse incision. Withdraw this tendon proximal to the abductor pollicis longus tendon in the midthird of the forearm using the proximal limb of the incision from the extensor phase of the reconstruction.
- Free the extensor carpi radialis longus tendon from its attachments so that free excursion is possible.
- Remove the pronator teres tendon from the shaft of the radius with a strip of its periosteal attachment.
- Weave the transfers together with the pronator teres to the flexor pollicis longus and the extensor carpi radialis longus to the flexor digitorum profundus.
- Adjust tension so that the thumb rests against the side of the index finger when the wrist is in 30 degrees of extension. The extensor carpi radialis longus–flexor digitorum profundus tension should allow reasonable synchronous finger flexion when the wrist is in 40 degrees of extension.
- The brachioradialis can be used as an opponens adductorplasty if it was not used in the extensor phase. This procedure is essentially the same as the Royle-Thompson transfer (see Technique 8.9).
- Harvest the ring finger sublimis tendon as for the Zancolli lasso procedure (see Fig. 8.48). Bring the sublimis tendon

out through a small incision at the distal-ulnar margin of the transverse carpal ligament.
- Tunnel the flexor digitorum sublimis tendon with its two slips across the palm to the metacarpophalangeal region of the thumb. Suture one slip into the extensor pollicis longus distal to the metacarpophalangeal joint and the other into the adductor tendon. Weave the free end of the brachioradialis into the intact ring flexor digitorum sublimis so that when the wrist is in neutral position, the thumb rests against the side of the index finger.

POSTOPERATIVE CARE The wrist is immobilized in 25 degrees of extension; the metacarpophalangeal joints, in flexion; and the interphalangeal joints, in extension. At 3 weeks, active and passive range-of-motion exercises and muscle reeducation are begun. The transfers should be protected for 3 months.

ZANCOLLI RECONSTRUCTION

Zancolli described a two-step technique for reconstruction in patients with C6 level function. The first step provides finger and thumb extension, and the second provides grasp. An accessory radial wrist extensor should be sought in the first step of the reconstruction because it may be helpful in the second step. In the first step, the thumb is stabilized by arthrodesis of the carpometacarpal joint or capsuloplasty of the metacarpophalangeal joint. The brachioradialis is transferred to the extensor digitorum communis and extensor pollicis longus. If the metacarpophalangeal joints tend to hyperextend, this is corrected by the Zancolli lasso procedure (see Fig. 8.48). If the flexor carpi radialis is nonfunctioning, the pronator teres is transferred to obtain wrist flexion.

TECHNIQUE 8.25

FIRST STEP
- Fuse the carpometacarpal joint in 45 degrees of palmar abduction and 20 degrees of radial abduction. Fix the fusion with two crossed Kirschner wires and with a third wire fix the relationship between the first and second metacarpals (Fig. 8.45B).
- If the metacarpophalangeal joint hyperextends, perform a volar plate capsuloplasty by suturing the volar plate and its radial sesamoid to the neck of the metacarpal (Fig. 8.45C).
- Transfer the brachioradialis into the extensor pollicis longus and extensor digitorum communis through a long curved radial incision (Fig. 8.45A). Adhesions at the graft site can be minimized by excising a portion of the proximal aspect of the dorsal carpal ligament and by placing the sutures as far proximal as possible.
- Keep the elbow at 60 degrees of flexion and use slightly more tension on the extensor digitorum communis than on

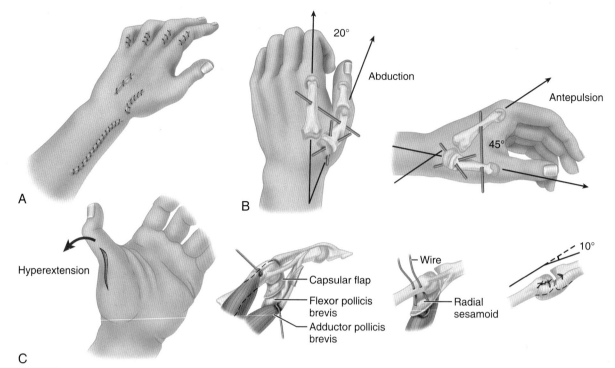

A

B

C

Hyperextension

20°

Abduction

Antepulsion

45°

Wire

Capsular flap

Flexor pollicis brevis

Adductor pollicis brevis

Radial sesamoid

10°

FIGURE 8.45 Zancolli two-step technique for reconstruction in patients with C6 level function (see text). **A,** Incisions required. **B,** Thumb fusion is fixed with three Kirschner wires. **C,** For hyperextension, volar plate capsuloplasty is performed. (Redrawn from Zancolli EA: Surgery for the quadriplegic hand with active, strong wrist extension preserved: a study of 97 cases, *Clin Orthop Relat Res* 112:101, 1975.) **SEE TECHNIQUE 8.25.**

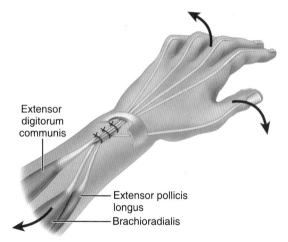

Extensor digitorum communis

Extensor pollicis longus

Brachioradialis

FIGURE 8.46 More tension is applied to extensor digitorum communis than to extensor pollicis longus because elbow extension reduces tension on extensor digitorum communis. (Redrawn from Zancolli EA: Surgery for the quadriplegic hand with active, strong wrist extension preserved: a study of 97 cases, *Clin Orthop Relat Res* 112:101, 1975.) **SEE TECHNIQUE 8.25.**

the extensor pollicis longus (Fig. 8.46). The tension is correct when full passive finger flexion can be obtained with maximal wrist extension and the elbow at 60 degrees of flexion. Passive wrist flexion should fully extend the metacarpophalangeal joints and the interphalangeal joint of the thumb. The intrinsic tenodesis can be performed at this stage, but it is often combined with the second step.

POSTOPERATIVE CARE The hand and elbow are immobilized for 4 weeks, after which the thumb fusion is protected with a splint for another 4 weeks. Muscle reeducation is begun by encouraging active metacarpophalangeal extension by elbow flexion. Passive finger flexion is necessary to prevent extension contractures (see Fig. 8.45).

Four to six months after the first step, the hand is ready for the second step of the reconstruction. This step provides finger flexion and active thumb flexion.

TECHNIQUE 8.26

SECOND STEP

- Transfer the extensor carpi radialis longus into the flexor digitorum profundus with slightly more tension applied to the more ulnar digits. The details are the same as in the House reconstruction (see Technique 8.23).
- The flexor pollicis longus can be activated by one of several methods. Zancolli's choice is the supernumerary radial wrist extensor (extensor carpi radialis tertius), which should be sought in the first step of the reconstruction. This is a synergistic transfer and allows independent control of thumb flexion (Fig. 8.47A).
- If this muscle is absent, side-to-side suturing of the extensor carpi radialis brevis with the flexor pollicis longus can be done. Thumb flexion occurs with wrist extension, and, conversely, thumb extension occurs with wrist flexion (Fig. 8.47B and C).

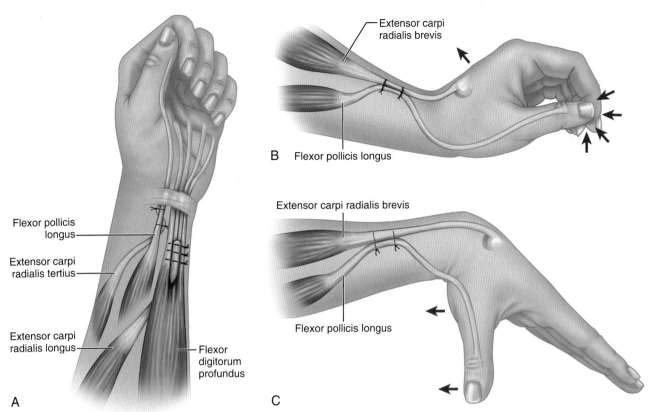

FIGURE 8.47 **A,** When both radial wrist extensors are active, extensor carpi radialis longus can be used to help provide finger flexion; thumb flexion may benefit from transfer of active extensor carpi radialis tertius when present (see text). **B,** Key pinch is obtained with wrist extension by active extensor carpi radialis brevis with tenodesis to flexor pollicis longus. To achieve correct tension, with wrist in complete passive extension, flexor pollicis longus tendon is sutured to extensor carpi radialis when pinching is produced. **C,** With passive wrist flexion, pinch is released. (Redrawn from Zancolli EA: Surgery for the quadriplegic hand with active, strong wrist extension preserved: a study of 97 cases, *Clin Orthop Relat Res* 112:101, 1975.) **SEE TECHNIQUE 8.26.**

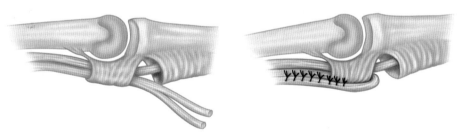

FIGURE 8.48 Zancolli lasso operation. Sublimis tendon is cut distally and turned proximally and sutured to itself and to A1 ligament with tension to prevent hyperextension of metacarpophalangeal joint. (Redrawn from Ejeskär A: Upper limb surgical rehabilitation in high-level tetraplegia, *Hand Clin* 4:585, 1988.) **SEE TECHNIQUE 8.26.**

Tension is set so that with complete passive wrist extension the thumb firmly rests against the index finger.
- A third option is passive tenodesis to the volar aspect of the distal radius, as in the Moberg key grip technique (see Technique 8.22).
- The Zancolli lasso procedure for intrinsic tenodesis can be added at this step. Tenodese the paralyzed sublimis tendons through a transverse incision in the palm just proximal to the metacarpophalangeal joint flexion crease. Expose the flexor digitorum sublimis tendons and the A1 and proximal A2 pulleys. Retract the flexor

digitorum sublimis tendons into the wound with the proximal interphalangeal joints in maximal flexion and divide them as far distally as possible. Take the two slips of each sublimis tendon out through the distal margins of the A1 pulleys and suture them back to themselves (Fig. 8.48). Adjust tension so that with the wrist in 40 degrees of flexion the metacarpophalangeal joints extend to 0 degrees.

POSTOPERATIVE CARE The arm is immobilized for 4 weeks in a long arm splint, as in step 1, but with the wrist

TABLE 8.4

Summary of Surgical Reconstruction Options in Tetraplegia According to the International Classification Scheme

GROUP	LOWEST MUSCLE GRADE 4 OR BETTER BELOW ELBOW	SURGICAL RECONSTRUCTION OPTIONS
0	0	Elbow extension (Moberg)
1	BR	Elbow extension, key grip
2	ECRL	Elbow extension, key grip
3	ECRB	Zancolli two-stage
		Key grip
		BR-thumb adductor
		ECRL-FDP
4	Pronator teres	Zancolli two-stage
5	Flexor carpi radialis	Zancolli two-stage
6	Finger extensors	Modified House (suture EPL to EDC side-to-side for thumb extension)
7	Thumb extensor	House two-stage
8	Partial finger flexors	Zancolli two-stage
9	Lacks only intrinsic	Opponens transfer
10	Exceptions	

BR, Brachioradialis; *ECRB,* extensor carpi radialis brevis; *ECRL,* extensor carpi radialis longus; *EDC,* extensor digitorum communis; *EPL,* extensor pollicis longus; *FDP,* flexor digitorum profundus.

in neutral, the thumb between the index and middle fingers, and the fingers gently flexed. Active and passive exercises are begun with muscle reeducation. The transfers are protected from heavy use for 3 months.

Surgery in tetraplegic patients in higher groups is easier because more function is retained. The previously outlined procedures can be incorporated into the management of these patients. Table 8.4 summarizes the classification scheme, with the surgical procedures of choice according to McDowell et al. Some patients do not fall neatly into groups 0 through 9 and a surgical plan must be tailored for them.

REFERENCES

Akinleye SD, Culbertson MD, Cappelleti G, et al.: The relative contribution to small finger abduction of the ulnar versus radial slip of the EDM: implications for tendon transfers, *Hand* 13(6):678, 2018.

Al-Qattan MH, Bednar MS: Tendon transfers for tetraplegia, *Hand Clin* 32:389, 2016.

Anderson GA, Thomas BP, Pallapati SC: Flexor carpi ulnaris tendon transfer to the split brachioradialis tendon to restore supination in paralytic forearms, *J Bone Joint Surg* 92B:230, 2010.

Bednar MS: Tendon transfers for tetraplegia, *Hand Clin* 32(3):389, 2016.

Bednar MS, Woodside JC: Management of upper extremities in tetraplegia: current concepts, *J Am Acad Orthop Surg* 26:e333, 2018.

Brown JM, Tung TH, Mackinnon SE: Medial to radial nerve transfer to restore wrist and finger extension: technical nuances, *Neurosurgery* 66(3 Suppl Operative):75, 2010.

Bumbasirevic M, Palibrk T, Lesic A, Atkinson HDE: Radial nerve plasty, *EFFORT Open Rev* 1:286, 2016.

Chadderdon RC, Gaston RG: Low median nerve transfers (opponensplasty), *Hand Clin* 32:349, 2016.

Chea AE, Etcheson J, Yao J: Radial nerve tendon transfers, *Hand Clin* 32:323, 2016.

Choo J, Wilhelmi BJ, Kasdan ML: Iatrogenic injury to the median nerve during palmaris longs harvest: an overview of safe harvesting techniques, *Hand* 12(1):NP6, 2017.

Cook S, Gaston G, Lourie GM: Ulnar nerve tendon transfers for pinch, *Hand Clin* 32:369, 2016.

Compton J, Owens J, Day M, Caldwell L: Systematic review of tendon transfer versus nerve transfer for the restoration of wrist extension in isolated traumatic radial nerve palsy, *JAAOS Glob Res Rev* 2:e001, 2018.

Coulet B: Principles of tendon transfers, *Hand Surg Rehabil* 35:68, 2016.

Coulet B, Waitzenegger T, Teissier J, et al.: Arthrodesis versus carpometacarpal preservation in key-grip procedures in tetraplegic patients: a comparative study of 40 cases, *J Hand Surg Am* 43:e2, 2018.

Dabas V, Suri T, Surapuraju PK, et al.: Functional restoration after early tendon transfer in high radial nerve paralysis, *J Hand Surg* 36:135, 2011.

DeSai MJ, Mithani SK, Lodha SJ, et al.: Major peripheral nerve injuries after elbow arthroscopy, *Arthroscopy* 32(6):999, 2016.

de Roode CP, James MA, Van Heest AE: Tendon transfers and releases for the forearm, wrist, and hand in spastic hemiplegic cerebral palsy, *Tech Hand Surg* 14:129, 2010.

Diaz-Garcia RJ, Chung KC: A comprehensive guide on restoring grasp using tendon transfer procedures for ulnar nerve palsy, *Hand Clin* 32:361, 2016.

Gangata H, Ndou R, Louw G: The contribution of the palmaris longus muscle to the strength of thumb abduction, *Clin Anat* 23:431, 2010.

Dunn JA, Sinnott KA, Rothwell AG, et al.: Tendon transfer surgery for people with tetraplegia: an overview, *Arch Phys Med Rehabil* 97(6 Suppl 2):S75, 2016.

Fox IK, Davidge KM, Novak CB, et al.: Use of peripheral nerve transfers in tetraplegia: evaluation of feasibility and morbidity, *Hand* 10:60, 2015.

Fridén J, Gohritz A: Tetraplegia management update, *J Hand Surg Am* 40(12):2489, 2015.

Giuffre JL, Bishop AT, Spinner RJ, Shin AY: The best of tendon and nerve transfers in the upper extremity, *Plast Reconstr Surg* 135:617e, 2015.

Gohritz A, Fridén J: Management of spinal cord injury-induced upper extremity spasticity, *Hand Clin* 34:555, 2018.

Gregersen H, Lybaek M, Lauge Johannesen I, et al.: Satisfaction with upper extremity surgery in individuals with tetraplegia, *J Spinal Cord Med* 38:161, 2015.

Gupta V, Consul A, Swamy MKS: Zancolli lasso procedure for correction of paralytic claw hands, *J Orthop Surg* 23(1):15, 2015.

Harris CA, Shauver MJ, Nasser JS, Chung KC: The golden year: how functional recovery sets the stage for tendon transfer surgery among patients with tetraplegia—a qualitative analysis, *Surgery* 165(365), 2019.

Isaacs J, Ugwu-Oju O: High median nerve injuries, *Hand Clin* 32:339, 2016.

Jaspers Focks-Feenstra JH, Snoek GJ, Bongers-Janssen HM, Nene AV: Long-term patient satisfaction after reconstructive upper extremity surgery to improve arm-hand function in tetraplegia, *Spinal Cord* 48:903, 2011.

Koch-Borner S, Dunn JA, Fridén J, Wangdell J: Rehabilitation after posterior deltoid to triceps transfer in tetraplegia, *Arch Phys Med Rehabil* 97(6 (Suppl 2)):S126, 2016.

Kozin SH, D'Addesi L, Chafetz RS, et al.: Biceps-to-triceps transfer for elbow extension in persons with tetraplegia, *J Hand Surg Am* 35:968, 2010.

Lalonde DH: Wide-awake extensor indicis proprius to extensor pollicis longus tendon transfer, *J Hand Surg Am* 39(11):2297, 2014.

Laravine J, Cambon-Binder A, Belkheyar Z: A new rerouting technique for the extensor pollicis longus in palliative treatment for wrist and finger extension paralysis resulting from radial nerve and C5C6C7 root injury, *Tech Hand Surg* 20:32, 2016.

Latheef L, Bhardwaj P, Sankaran A, Sabapathy SR: An objective functional evaluation of the flexor carpi ulnaris set of triple tendon transfer in radial nerve palsy, *J Hand Surg Eur* 42(2):170, 2017.

Laulan J: High radial nerve palsy, *Hand Surg Rehabil* 38:2, 2019.

Lee SK, Wisser JR: Restoration of pinch in intrinsic muscles of the hand, *Hand Clin* 28:45, 2012.

Livermore A, Tueting JL: Biomechanics of tendon transfers, *Hand Clin* 32:291, 2016.

Lucich EA, Fahrenkopf MP, Kelpin JP, et al.: Extensor tendon transfers for radial nerve palsy secondary to humeral shaft fracture, 21. Interesting Case, 2018. www.ePlasty.com.

Makarewich CA, Hutchinson DT: Tendon transfers for combined peripheral nerve injuries, *Hand Clin* 32:377, 2016.

Matter-Parrat V, Prunieres G, Collon S, et al.: Active extensor indicis proprius extension strength after its use as a tendon transfer: 19 cases, *Hand Surg Rehabil* 36:36, 2017.

Netscher DT, Sandvall BK: Surgical technique: posterior deltoid-to-triceps transfer in tetraplegic patients, *J Hand Surg* 36A:711, 2011.

Peljovich A, Ratner JA, Marino J: Update of the physiology and biomechanics of tendon transfer surgery, *J Hand Surg* 35A:1365, 2010.

Ratner JA, Peljovich A, Kozin SH: Update on tendon transfers for peripheral nerve injuries, *J Hand Surg* 35A:1371, 2010.

Rivlin M, Eberlin KR, Kachooei AR, et al.: Side-to-side versus Pulvertaft extensor tenorrhaphy-a biomedical study, *J Hand Surg Am* 41(11):e393, 2016.

Sapienza A, Green S: Correction of the claw hand, *Hand Clin* 28:53, 2012.

Sankaran A, Thora A, Arora S, Dhal A: Single tendon transfer of the flexor carpi ulnaris for high radial nerve injury, *J Orthop Surg* 23(3):345, 2015.

Seiler 3rd JG, Desai MJ, Payne SH: Tendon transfers for radial, median, and ulnar nerve palsy, *J Am Acad Orthop Surg* 21:675, 2013.

Tang JB: Wide-awake primary flexor tendon repair, tenolysis, and tendon transfer, *Clin Orthop Surg* 7(3):275, 2015.

Trehan SK, Little KJ: Technical pearls of tendon transfers for upper extremity spasticity, *Hand Clin* 34:529, 2018.

Titolo P, Fusini F, Arrigoni C, et al.: Combining nerve and tendon transfers in tetraplegia: a proposal of a new surgical strategy based on literature review, *Eur J Orthop Surg Traumatol* 29:521, 2019.

Waljee JF, Chung KC: Surgical management of spasticity of the thumb and fingers, *Hand Clin* 34:473, 2018.

Wangdell J, Reinholdt C, Fridén J: Activity gains after upper limb surgery for spasticity in patients with spinal cord injury, *J Hand Surg* 0:1, 2018.

Wilbur D, Hammert WC: Principles of tendon transfer, *Hand Clin* 32:283, 2016.

Woodside JC, Bondra RR: Rerouting extensor pollicis longus tendon transfer, *J Hand Surg Am* 40(4):822, 2015.

Zhang L, Dong Z, Zhang CL, Gu YD: Surgical anatomy of the radial nerve at the elbow and in the forearm: anatomical basis for intraplexus nerve transfer to reconstruct thumb and finger extension in C7-T1 brachial plexus palsy, *J Reconstr Microsurg* 32(9):670, 2016.

Zlotolow DA: The role of the upper extremity surgeon in the management of tetraplegia, *J Hand Surg Am* 36:929, 2011.

The complete list of references is available online at expertconsult.inkling.com.

CHAPTER 9

CEREBRAL PALSY OF THE HAND

Benjamin M. Mauck

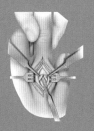

Cerebral palsy is a nonprogressive, nonhereditary encephalopathy that occurs in the prenatal or perinatal period and is characterized by altered motor, sensory, and, often, intellectual function. Cerebral palsy occurs in the industrialized world with an approximate annual frequency of 2 per 1000 live births. The most common motor disability of childhood, cerebral palsy can be caused by fetal stroke, anoxia, infection, teratogens, central nervous system malformations, metabolic diseases, and prematurity. Epidemiologic studies suggest that cerebral palsy is predominantly metabolic and not caused by neonatal ischemia. Approximately 75% of cases occur in utero, 5% during delivery, and 15% to 20% after delivery. Multiple-gestation pregnancies and intrauterine infections are other common risk factors. It can be classified as pyramidal, which includes spastic hemiplegia, diplegia, paraplegia, and quadriplegia, or as extrapyramidal, which includes athetoid and ataxic patterns. A mixed variety also occurs with spasticity and athetosis. Hand function is impaired to some extent in all types except possibly spastic paraplegia, with the most common deformities being shoulder adduction, internal rotation, elbow flexion, forearm pronation, wrist and finger flexion, thumb-in-palm, and swan-neck deformities (Fig. 9.1). Many surgical procedures have been performed in an attempt to correct these deformities. Earlier results were unpredictable and disappointing, primarily because of inappropriate patient selection. The extensive works of Green, Goldner, Swanson, Zancolli et al., and Hoffer et al. have proved certain principles in the evaluation and management of the cerebral palsied hand.

PATIENT EVALUATION

Most patients with cerebral palsy exhibit full passive range of motion at birth, but joint stiffness and contractures develop gradually, leading to variability at the time of presentation that depends on severity, location, and extent of brain injury, associated neurologic disorders, and baseline cognitive motor function. Careful repeated evaluations, often over a considerable length of time, are required before surgery can be advised or discouraged. Important information includes any birth or perinatal medical problems, achievement of developmental milestones, and especially the degree with which the child has previously used the hand. If the hand is completely ignored by the child, it is doubtful that function would be restored or improved with surgery. The early development of handedness may be especially helpful because it is uncommon before the age of 3 years and may represent some degree of particular weakness or incoordination in the less preferred extremity. The particular cerebral lesion should be identified and characterized as pyramidal with associated spasticity or extrapyramidal, because children with athetoid patterns are not surgical candidates. The persistence of any infantile postural reflexes should be documented. Deformities should be classified as static contractures (deformities that do not correct with compensatory positioning of muscle or joint) or dynamic deformities that are spastic and slowly correctable. Volkmann angle for finger flexor tightness (Fig. 9.2) should be assessed and documented. This is done by bringing the wrist from maximum palmar flexion into extension with the digits extended. The angle at which the digits move into a flexed posture is the Volkmann angle. Most children show dynamic deformities early in life; if left untreated, these deformities may progress to static contractures.

Muscle examination should determine the degree of spasticity, strength, and coordination of each major muscle, with special attention given to the child's ability to pinch, grasp, and release objects. The patient also should have sufficient proximal control of the extremity to place the hand voluntarily on top of the head and then on the opposite knee within 5 to 10 seconds. If a child does not show this degree of control, it is doubtful that he or she would use the extremity enough to justify reconstruction.

The sensibility pattern of the hand should be determined. Although most patients have intact epicritic sensation (the ability to discern pinprick, heat, and cold), about half have impaired sensibility, with diminished two-point discrimination, stereognosis, and proprioception. Because sensibility in the hand is so important in determining the prognosis after surgery, its status should be evaluated as accurately as possible before surgery. An indication may be gained by observing whether the hand is used or ignored; unless motor coordination is extremely poor, an ignored hand probably indicates the absence of sensibility. Further evaluation requires communication with the child, and this usually is impossible before 4 years of age. A cursory examination can be done by asking a blindfolded child to differentiate between a sphere and a cube or to indicate the position of the hand when the palm has been placed by the examiner facing upward or downward. A more detailed examination testing recognition of blunt and sharp points, of familiar objects such as coins, and of differences in temperature also is valuable. Examination of the contralateral extremity has been shown to be an important part of patient evaluation. Dexterity of the contralateral extremity also can be affected in patients with hemiplegia and may require intervention to improve overall function.

Further evaluation using dynamic electromyography may be helpful in determining which muscles are in phase with the function to be augmented and allow for appropriate donor muscle selection. After evaluation, the child's function and deformity can be described according to several available classification systems, including the House functional classification and the Manual Ability Classification System (MACS) (Tables 9.1 and 9.2). MACS level appears to be a strong predictor of contracture development. Patients with MACS level V have a 17 times greater risk of contracture than patients with MACS level I. Passive range of motion diminishes with age, with contractures occurring in one third of children overall. Neuromuscular blocking agents, such as 1% lidocaine, 0.25% bupivacaine, and 45% ethanol, are helpful in assessing weaker muscle groups without the overbearing effect of antagonist muscles and can assist in predicting surgical outcome after tendon lengthening or tenotomy. The classic presentation of established spastic hemiplegia is adduction, internal rotation of the shoulder, elbow flexion, forearm pronation, wrist and finger flexion, thumb-in-palm deformity, and swan-neck deformity of the fingers.

NONOPERATIVE MANAGEMENT

Traditionally, early splinting has been used to prevent fixed contractures of the muscles and joints; however, many surgeons have now abandoned this method because fixed contractures rarely occur in young children and because during sleep the upper extremity often is relaxed and supple, obviating the need for night splinting. Daytime splinting is cumbersome and often is rejected by an active child. If splinting is necessary, a well-formed splint without pressure points should hold the wrist in as much extension as tolerated with the fingers in almost complete extension and the thumb out of the palm (Fig. 9.3). A functional orthosis that provides wrist extension and thumb abduction has been found to improve measured hand function.

Hand therapy, although rarely successful in training a child to relax spastic muscles, strengthens weakened muscles and controls exaggerated reflexes. Therapy also is invaluable in providing support to the patient and family in dealing with the disorder, in evaluating patients for surgical procedures, and in postoperative recovery of functional activities.

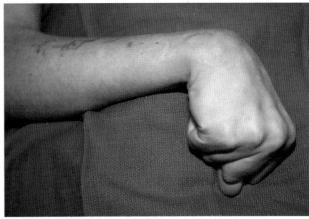

FIGURE 9.1 Typical upper extremity deformities in cerebral palsy: elbow flexion, forearm pronation, and wrist and finger flexion.

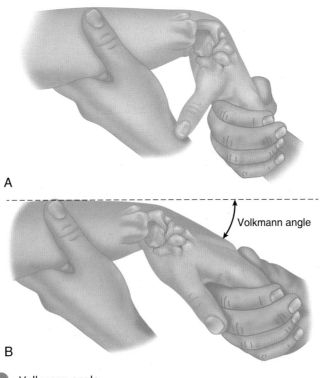

Volkmann angle

FIGURE 9.2 Volkmann angle.

TABLE 9.1

Functional Classification of House et al.

LEVEL	CATEGORY	DESCRIPTION
0	Does not use	Does not use
1	Poor passive assist	Uses as stabilizing weight only
2	Fair passive assist	Can hold object placed in hand
3	Good passive assist	Can hold object and stabilize it for use by other hand
4	Poor active assist	Can actively grasp object and hold it weakly
5	Fair active use	Can actively grasp object and stabilize it well
6	Good active assist	Can actively grasp object and manipulate it
7	Spontaneous use, partial	Can perform bimanual activities and occasionally uses the hand spontaneously
8	Spontaneous use, complete	Uses hand completely independently without reference to the other hand

From Van Heest AE, House JH, Cariello C: Upper extremity surgical treatment of cerebral palsy, *J Hand Surg* 24A:323, 1999.

TABLE 9.2

Summary of Manual Ability Classification System

MACS LEVEL	DESCRIPTION
I	Handles most objects easily and successfully
II	Handles most objects with somewhat reduced quality or speed of achievement
III	Handles objects with difficulty; needs help to prepare or modify activities
IV	Handles a limited selection of easily managed objects in adapted situations
V	Does not handle objects and has severely limited ability to perform even simple actions

MACS, Manual Ability Classification System.
From Arner M, Eliasson AC, Nicklasson S, et al: Hand function in cerebral palsy: report of 367 children in a population-based longitudinal health care program, *J Hand Surg* 33A:1337, 2008.

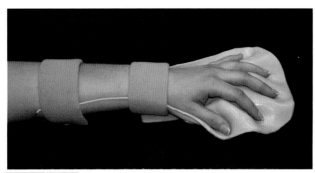

FIGURE 9.3 Splint for spastic hand.

Electrical stimulation aimed at strengthening nonspastic but weak extensor compartment muscles may have a role in nonoperative management. Previous reports have yielded conflicting results. Improvement has been reported with electrical stimulation and dynamic splinting; however, a lifelong application of the program is necessary.

Interest in the use of botulinum type A toxin in the treatment of cerebral palsy has increased. Decreasing spasticity should help to improve control of movement patterns through a combination of lengthening muscle groups, improving posture, and strengthening antagonistic muscles. Several studies have shown promising short-term results. In a randomized double-blind placebo-controlled study, Koman et al. demonstrated that children receiving multiple botulinum toxin A (BoNT-A) injections developed significant short-term improvements in upper extremity function without complications. In one 20-year study involving patients with MACS IV and V, Andersson et al. demonstrated that adjunctive Botox, movement training, and orthoses helped prevent significant loss of passive range of motion when started at an early age. Other long-term follow-up studies need to be conducted, however, to determine if there is any long-term functional improvement, or any possible resistance or allergic complications. Dramatic improvement has been shown but results are temporary (6 to 9 months). The most common reasons for failure are fixed joint contractures, absence of selective motor control in antagonist muscles, sensory impairment, and learned nonuse. In a smaller randomized controlled study, patients treated with BoNT-A injections in combination with occupational therapy showed improved function when compared with occupational therapy alone.

OPERATIVE MANAGEMENT
GOALS
The goals of operative treatment in a child with cerebral palsy should be specific and should be aimed at providing useful grasp and release and acceptable hygiene (Fig. 9.4). Sometimes improving the appearance of the hand by correcting an unsightly contracture may be a modest goal as well. Fine manipulation rarely is improved by surgery, and normal hand function is an unrealistic goal. Grasp and release are possible only in children who have at least sufficient sensibility to allow an awareness of the extremity. Stereognosis has been shown to improve with postoperative gains in motor function and functional use of the upper extremity. Undercorrection

rather than overcorrection of the deformity or dysfunction is always preferred.

PRINCIPLES
The ideal candidate for surgery is a spastic hemiplegic who is cooperative, intelligent, motivated to participate with postoperative rehabilitation protocol, and who has a pattern of grasp and release so functional that the hand is already useful to some extent; the hand should be reasonably sensitive, and the patient should be between 5 and 25 years old. In contrast, a poor candidate for surgery is a patient who is severely mentally delayed or disabled and who has definite athetosis in the extremity, a hand that has developed joint contractures and is insensitive, a wrist that passively cannot be brought to neutral, and fingers that cannot be extended even when the wrist is flexed. Children with spastic diplegia rarely have sufficient upper extremity spasticity to warrant surgery, and children with spastic quadriplegia or total body involvement have too little voluntary control to benefit from surgery aimed at improving grasp and release; however, they may benefit from surgery that improves hygiene.

Surgical options include myotomy, tenotomy, tendon lengthening, tendon transfer, tenodesis, capsulotomy, excisional arthroplasty, and arthrodesis. Tendon lengthening

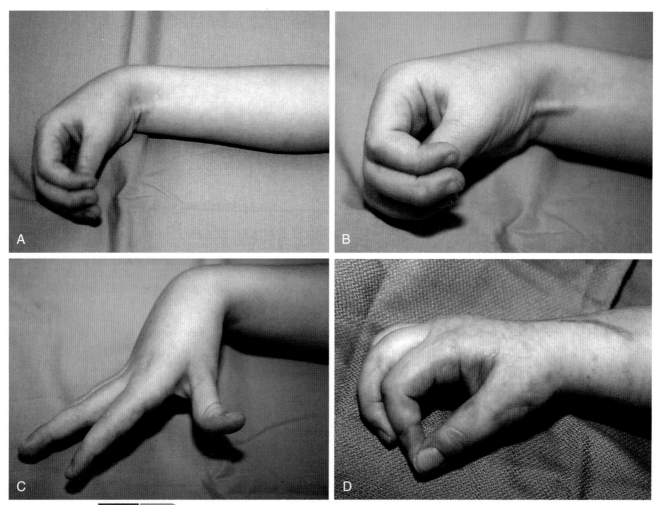

FIGURE 9.4 **A** to **C,** Preoperative flexion and pronation contracture. Thumb-in-palm deformity and weak wrist extension. **D,** After fractional lengthening, flexor carpi ulnaris-to-extensor carpi radialis longus transfer, and thumb-in-palm reconstruction, wrist extension and pinch are possible.

requires no particular compliance and can be performed in spastic and athetoid patients. It weakens the muscle and diminishes its excursion and stretch reflex, which subsequently diminishes spasticity, allowing antagonistic muscles to influence function to a greater extent. Tendon transfers require some postoperative compliance, should be synergistic, cannot overcome fixed deformity, and are not reliable in athetoid patients. Arthrodesis is useful in stabilizing the thumb metacarpophalangeal joint during reconstruction of a thumb-in-palm deformity and in correcting fixed flexion deformities of the wrist when sacrifice of its "windlass" effect is believed justifiable.

As to when the various types of operations may be indicated, myotomies are likely to be effective at the earliest age, tendon transfers later, and arthrodeses even later. Soft-tissue operations to correct flexion deformity of the wrist and pronation deformity of the forearm are probably indicated earliest. As a rule, indicated surgery usually is carried out at 4 to 8 years of age and ideally before significant contractures develop.

One study found that patients who had poor voluntary motor control had less improvement after surgery than patients with fair-to-good voluntary control. This was the only prediction of outcome after surgical intervention. Some literature would suggest that although surgical intervention can improve function, it may not provide improved ability to perform activities of daily living. Appropriate patient selection is of upmost importance, and a multidisciplinary approach is optimal. Using careful assessment for surgical eligibility and a multiple disciplinary approach, clinically relevant functional and cosmetic goals can be achieved (Table 9.3).

PRONATION CONTRACTURE OF THE FOREARM

Pronation deformity of the forearm is common and disabling in children with cerebral palsy and is caused by spasticity of the pronator teres and, at times, of the pronator quadratus. It can be aggravated by lengthening of the biceps tendon for elbow flexion contracture, and it can be improved by simple tenotomy of the insertion of the pronator teres. If the patient lacks supination just short of neutral and the pronator is contracted and fires out of phase with supination, then a simple pronator teres tenotomy is ideal. A pronation contracture also may be aggravated by a contracted biceps aponeurosis, and division of this structure may improve supination. Supination also can be improved by transfer of the flexor carpi ulnaris around the ulnar side of the forearm during augmentation of the extensor digitorum communis or the extensor carpi radialis brevis. However, overcorrection with supination contracture can occur postoperatively if the procedure is combined with a pronator teres release or transfer. Sakellarides et al. devised an operation principally to correct pronation contracture of the forearm. According to them, transferring the pronator teres tendon produces better correction than any other transfer. This method corrects one deforming force while providing a force for supination. The tendon is released, rerouted around the radius, and inserted into the bone. In their series of 22 patients so treated, 82% gained an average of 46 degrees of active supination. Bunata found similar improvement in 31 patients, with the average active supination improving 65 degrees and the average dynamic positioning changing from 26 to 7 degrees. The indication for surgery

was a pronation positioning of 25 degrees or greater because this prevented the child from grasping a cup full of water. Ozkan et al. described a brachioradialis rerouting procedure in combination with a pronator teres and quadratus release in a small series of patients with an average gain of 81 degrees of supination and no overcorrection. However, Čobeljić et al. did not find benefit to pronator quadratus release at 17.5-year follow-up. Gschwind and Tonkin classified pronation deformities into four groups to help guide surgical recommendations (Table 9.4). One should also note that transfer of the flexor carpi ulnaris to extensor carpi radialis will add to the supination moment and should be taken into consideration when contemplating pronator teres release versus rerouting.

TRANSFER OF THE PRONATOR TERES

TECHNIQUE 9.1

- Make a zigzag, curvilinear, or straight longitudinal incision over the anterior and radial aspects of the midforearm centered over the insertion of the pronator teres (Fig. 9.5A).
- Protect the lateral cutaneous nerve of the forearm and the superficial radial nerve.
- Identify and develop the interval between the brachioradialis and extensor carpi radialis longus.
- Identify the oblique fibers that insert into bone at the musculotendinous insertion of the pronator teres (Fig. 9.5B). Use sharp dissection to detach the insertion of the pronator teres, along with an attached strip of periosteum (Fig. 9.5C). Mobilize the muscle extraperiosteally, well proximal in the forearm.
- Free the interosseous membrane from the radius as far as necessary to gain maximal passive supination.
- Pass a right-angle clamp from the dorsolateral aspect of the radius through the interosseous membrane and use it to transfer the pronator teres through the interosseous membrane in a volar-to-dorsolateral direction.
- At the same level as the previous muscle insertion, drill an anchoring hole on the anterolateral aspect of the radial cortex (Fig. 9.5D). Drill a smaller hole through the posteromedial part of the radius using a 1.6-mm Kirschner wire. Enlarge the hole in the anterolateral cortex to 2.8 mm.
- Pass a suture with the tendon attached through the two holes from anteromedial to posterolateral (Fig. 9.5E). In this manner, the tendon is introduced into the larger hole on the anterolateral cortex and is secured (Fig. 9.5F,G). Apply further stay sutures through the tendon as indicated.
- Hold the forearm in approximately 45 degrees of supination and snug the tendon up to hold this position. Allow the brachioradialis to fall into place and close the incision.
- Apply a long arm cast, maintaining the elbow in 45 degrees of flexion and the forearm in 60 degrees of supination. Elevate the arm immediately after surgery.

TABLE 9.3

Surgical Procedures for Upper Limb Deformities

	ELBOW FLEXION	FOREARM PRONATION	WRIST FLEXION/ ULNAR DEVIATION	THUMB-IN-PALM	FINGER DEFORMITIES
Tendon releases	Lacertus fibrosus release BR release Biceps lengthening Brachialis lengthening	PT release	Flexor pronator slide FCR tenotomy or lengthening FCU tenotomy or lengthening	Adductor release FPB release FPL lengthening	FDS lengthening FDP lengthening Flexor pronator Slide
Tendon transfers		PT rerouting	FCU to ECRB FCU to EDC BR to ECRB ECU centralization	PL to AbPL, EPB, or EPL BR to AbPL, EPB, or EPL FCR to AbPL, EPB, or EPL AbPL tenodesis EPL rerouting	Lateral band rerouting (swan neck) FDS tenodesis (swan neck) STP transfer
Joint stabilization			Wrist fusion PRC	MCP fusion MCP capsulodesis IP fusion	PIP fusion (rare)

AbPL, Abductor pollicis longus; *BR,* brachioradialis; *ECRB,* extensor carpi radialis brevis; *ECU,* extensor carpi ulnaris; *EDC,* extensor digitorum communis; *EPB,* extensor pollicis brevis; *EPL,* extensor pollicis longus; *FCR,* flexor carpi radialis; *FCU,* flexor carpi ulnaris; *FDP,* flexor digitorum profundus; *FDS,* flexor digitorum superficialis; *FPB,* flexor pollicis brevis; *FPL,* flexor pollicis longus; *IP,* interphalangeal; *MCP,* metacarpophalangeal; *PIP,* proximal interphalangeal; *PL,* palmaris longus; *PRC,* proximal row carpectomy; *PT,* pronator teres; *STP,* superficialis-to-profundus.
From Waters PM, Bae DS: *Pediatric hand and upper limb surgery. A practical guide,* Philadelphia, 2012, Lippincott Williams and Wilkins, Table 22.1, pp 219–236.

TABLE 9.4

Gschwind Classification of Pronation Deformities as a Guide to Surgical Recommendations

CLASSIFICATION (GROUP)	PRONATION DEFORMITY	SURGICAL RECOMMENDATION
1	Active supination beyond neutral	No specific surgery
2	Active supination to or less than neutral	Pronator quadratus release with or without a flexor aponeurotic release
3	No active supination, yet free passive supination	Pronator teres rerouting procedure
4	No active supination and only limited passive supination	Pronator quadratus release and a flexor aponeurotic release*

*If after release no active supination is possible, a pronator teres rerouting may be added. Gschwind and Tonkin caution against performing a pronator teres transfer at the same time as a pronator quadratus release because an undesirable supination deformity may ensue.

POSTOPERATIVE CARE The sutures are removed at 2 weeks, and a new long arm cast that maintains forearm supination is applied and is worn for another 4 weeks. Supination splinting at night is continued for 6 months.

BRACHIORADIALIS REROUTING

TECHNIQUE 9.2

(OZKAN ET AL.)
■ Make a longitudinal incision on the radial aspect of the forearm to provide access to the brachioradialis, pronator teres, and pronator quadratus muscles. If additional procedures, such as flexor tendon lengthening, are also being performed, make a curvilinear incision on the palmar surface of the forearm.
■ Develop the skin flaps and retract.
■ Using monopolar diathermy, release the pronator quadratus muscle from its radial attachment by cutting through its muscle belly.
■ Isolate the pronator teres tendon and divide in a Z fashion for lengthening.
■ Suture the tendon ends with the forearm in neutral position and without any tension within the tendon. It is crucial not to overlengthen this tendon so as to preserve pronator function and prevent supination deformity.
■ Identify the superficial branch of the radial nerve and artery and retract in the distal forearm.

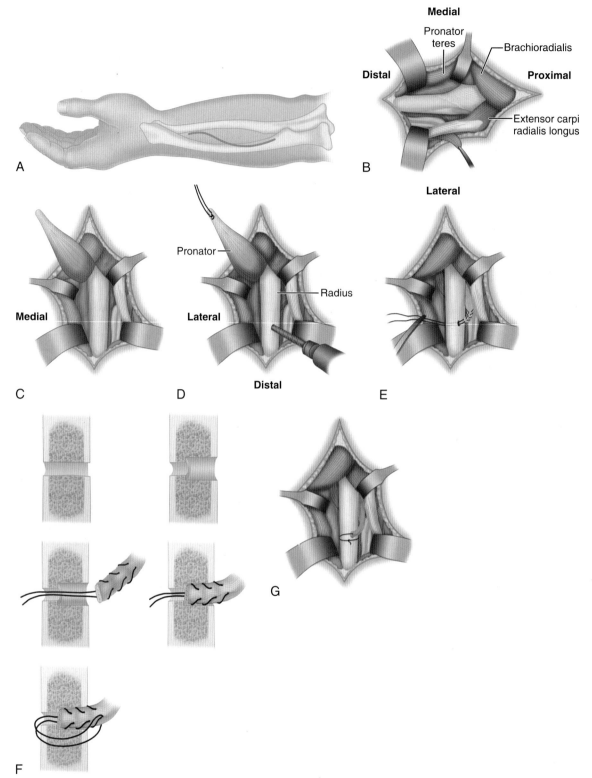

FIGURE 9.5 Transfer of pronator teres for pronation contracture of forearm. **A,** Incision along radial aspect of forearm centered over insertion of pronator teres. **B,** Exposure of pronator teres insertion on radius. **C,** Elevation of pronator teres insertion with strip of periosteum from radius. **D,** Anchoring hole drilled in anterolateral part of radial cortex, with smaller hole drilled through posteromedial part. **E–G,** Pronator teres tendon rerouted posteriorly through interosseous membrane, passed from lateral to medial through hole drilled in radius, and sutured. **SEE TECHNIQUE 9.1.**

- Prepare the brachioradialis tendon and muscle for transfer, preserving its distal attachment. It is important that the muscle is completely freed from all its fascial attachments because otherwise muscle excursion will be insufficient.
- Preserving the neurovascular structures of the muscle, the brachioradialis tendon is divided with a long Z-plasty to provide sufficient tendon length for rerouting (Fig. 9.6A).
- Pass the distal tendon end of the brachioradialis through a window created in the interosseous space, volar to dorsal, ulnar to radial direction, just proximal to the pronator quadratus muscle (Fig. 9.6B).
- Retract the radial artery and pass the tendon deep to this to avoid compression.
- Suture the proximal and distal tendons to each other with a Pulvertaft weave with the elbow at 90 degrees of flexion.
- Keep the forearm in neutral during reattachment without any tension on the tendon ends.
- Close the skin with absorbable sutures and apply an above-elbow plaster cast with the elbow in 90 degrees flexion and the forearm in neutral. Cast the wrist and fingers as necessary if additional procedures have been performed.

POSTOPERATIVE CARE The hand is elevated for 48 hours. Peripheral circulation should be closely monitored. The cast is worn for 4 weeks, after which time it is replaced with a splint that can be removed periodically for physical therapy. The splint is discontinued during the day after another 8 weeks but is applied at night for 4 additional weeks. Subsequently, the patient is encouraged to use the extremity in activities of daily living.

FLEXION DEFORMITIES OF THE WRIST AND FINGERS

The most frequent deformities in the upper extremity in spastic paralysis are those of flexion of the wrist and fingers. These deformities usually are accompanied by pronation of the forearm, flexion of the elbow, and the thumb-in-palm deformity. Zancolli et al. classified spastic flexion deformities of the wrist and hand into three patterns (Table 9.5):

Pattern 1. The fingers can be actively extended with the wrist in less than 20 degrees of flexion. This is a fairly mild deformity in which grasp and release are possible. Extension of the wrist is impossible with the fingers in full extension. Consideration may be given to flexor carpi ulnaris tenotomy combined with lengthening of the finger flexors, preferably by tenotomy at the musculotendinous junction, allowing for selective fractional lengthening as required. A flexor slide also can be selected.

Pattern 2. Active finger extension is possible only with the wrist in more than 20 degrees of flexion. This pattern is divided further into two subgroups. In pattern 2a, the patient has voluntary wrist extension with the fingers in flexion, indicating that the wrist extensors are active and the finger flexors are not severely spastic. In pattern 2b, the patient is unable to extend the wrist with the fingers in flexion, indicating that the wrist extensors are paralyzed and require augmentation to improve function. In pattern 2, lengthening of the finger flexors, combined with a tendon transfer to augment finger or wrist extension, should be considered. The classic transfer is of the flexor carpi ulnaris to the extensor carpi radialis brevis, which improves supination, wrist extension, and finger flexion (grasp). If weakness in finger extension (release) is considerable, transfer into the extensor digitorum communis is preferred. Preoperative electromyography may be useful to determine in which phase the donor muscle is active: grasp or release. Another

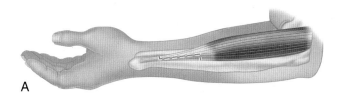

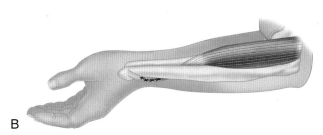

FIGURE 9.6 Ozkan brachioradialis rerouting technique. **A,** Tendon is cut in Z fashion. **B,** Distal tendon is passed between radius and ulna in dorsal to palmar direction and is sutured back to proximal brachioradialis tendon. **SEE TECHNIQUE 9.2.**

TABLE 9.5	
Classification of Flexion Deformities of Wrist and Fingers	
CLASSIFICATION (GROUP)	**DEFORMITY**
1	Active finger extension with <20 degrees of wrist flexion
2	Active finger extension with >20 degrees of wrist flexion
2a	Active wrist extension with fingers flexed
2b	No active wrist extension with fingers flexed
3	Wrist and finger extension absent even with full wrist flexion

From Van Heest AE: Surgical management of wrist and finger deformity, *Hand Clin* 19:657, 2003.

alternative is to fractionally lengthen the flexor carpi ulnaris and flexor carpi radialis and transfer the extensor carpi ulnaris into the extensor carpi radialis brevis to improve wrist extension power.

Pattern 3. The patient has severe flexion deformities and is unable to extend the fingers or wrist actively even when starting from a position of maximal flexion. Hand sensibility usually is poor. Surgery would not improve function but may improve hygiene. Tenotomy of the wrist flexors and sublimis-to-profundus transfers as described by Braun and Vice may be considered. Wrist arthrodesis and carpectomy may improve appearance in these severe deformities.

FRACTIONAL LENGTHENING OF THE FLEXOR CARPI RADIALIS MUSCLE AND FINGER FLEXORS

TECHNIQUE 9.3

- Begin a curved volar incision over the forearm about 3 cm proximal to the volar wrist crease and continue it proximally for 6 cm.
- Identify the flexor carpi radialis muscle and follow it proximally to the musculotendinous junction and farther proximally until the muscle belly is identified. The distal portion of the muscle belly is surrounded by an aponeurosis that thickens distally and forms the tendon of the muscle.
- Lengthen the muscle-tendon unit and leave it in continuity by making transverse cuts in the aponeurosis proximal to the musculotendinous junction. Completely identify the muscle circumferentially and make a transverse cut through the aponeurosis but not through the muscle (Fig. 9.7). Divide the aponeurosis transversely and do not leave any of the tendon intact; otherwise, the muscle-tendon unit does not lengthen.
- After the cut in the aponeurosis is made, place the wrist in dorsiflexion. The transverse cut in the aponeurosis widens as the muscle lengthens, but the entire muscle-tendon unit remains intact. A second cut for recession can be made if necessary.
- Other musculotendinous units may be contracted in addition to the flexor carpi radialis muscle. Frequently, the palmaris longus muscle also is spastic and contracted and may require lengthening in the same manner.
- Through this same incision, the finger flexors can be lengthened in a similar manner. First lengthen the flexor digitorum sublimis muscles and then the flexor digitorum profundus if they contribute to the contracture.

POSTOPERATIVE CARE A palmar (volar) short arm splint with the wrist in neutral position or slightly extended is worn for 3 to 4 weeks. Then mobilization of the wrist is begun, and a removable splint is used for protection. A volar short arm night splint is used for an additional 4 to 6 months.

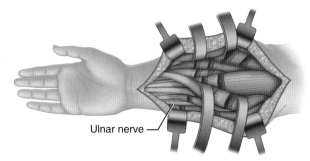

FIGURE 9.7 Fractional lengthening of flexor carpi radialis muscle and finger flexors. **SEE TECHNIQUE 9.3.**

RELEASE OF THE FLEXOR-PRONATOR ORIGIN

Release of the flexor-pronator origin may improve appearance and function of a hand with severe flexion deformities of the wrist and fingers. It is not indicated in hands that can be corrected passively but assume a flexed position during grasp; for these, less extensive operations, such as transfer of the flexor carpi ulnaris to a wrist extensor, are more useful. Release of the flexor-pronator origin was first described by Page in 1923 and later by Inglis and Cooper and by Williams and Haddad. Ezaki recommended a flexor-pronator slide if more than 45 degrees of wrist flexion is required to extend the fingers.

TECHNIQUE 9.4

(INGLIS AND COOPER)

- Make an incision over the anterior part of the medial epicondyle of the humerus beginning 5 cm proximal to the epicondyle and continuing distally to the midpoint of the forearm over the ulna (Fig. 9.8A). The medial antebrachial cutaneous nerve often is seen in the distal part of the incision, and the medial brachial cutaneous nerve can be seen posterior to the medial part of the epicondyle.
- Identify the ulnar nerve proximal to the epicondyle, dissect and elevate it from its groove behind the epicondyle, and carefully free it distally (Fig. 9.8B). Identify, free, and protect the branches of the ulnar nerve to the flexor carpi ulnaris and to the two ulnar heads of the flexor digitorum profundus.
- To release the origins of the flexor carpi ulnaris and flexor digitorum profundus, begin distally at about the middle of the ulna and elevate both muscles from the bone at the subcutaneous border; the interosseous membrane is seen around the volar surface of the bone. Continue proximally along the ulna as far as the ulnar groove at the epicondyle. During this dissection, the interosseous membrane and the fascia of the brachialis muscle are seen in the depths of the wound.
- Replace the ulnar nerve in its groove and divide the entire flexor-pronator muscle mass at its origin from the medial part of the epicondyle. At this point, the median nerve can be seen as it passes through the pronator teres.
- Continue the dissection anteriorly over the flexor aspect of the elbow, dividing the lacertus fibrosus (Fig. 9.8C) and any remaining parts of the flexor muscle origin.
- If a flexion contracture of the elbow persists, incise the fascia of the brachialis muscle. Then transplant the ulnar

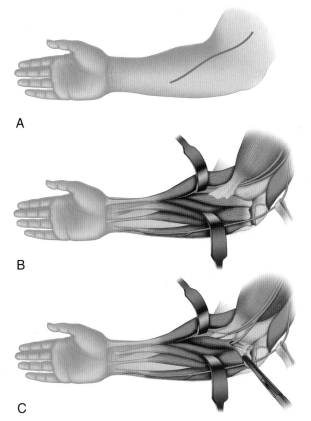

A

B

C

FIGURE 9.8 Flexor slide (Inglis and Cooper). **A,** Incision on medial aspect of volar side of arm, beginning approximately 5 cm proximal to medial epicondyle and continuing distally to midpoint of forearm over ulna. **B,** Ulnar nerve is identified, protected, and released from cubital tunnel. Tendinous origins of muscles on medial epicondyle are cut, and flexor carpi ulnaris and flexor digitorum profundus muscles are completely released from medial epicondyle and ulna. **C,** Lacertus fibrosus is divided, along with any remaining portions of flexor muscle origin, and ulnar nerve is transposed anteriorly. **SEE TECHNIQUE 9.4.**

nerve anterior to the epicondyle. Now the muscle mass has been displaced 3 to 4 cm distal to its original location.
- Close the wound and apply a cast or plaster splints to hold the forearm in supination and the wrist and fingers in neutral positions.

POSTOPERATIVE CARE At 3 weeks, the cast or splints and the sutures are removed. An extension hand splint is applied, which is worn constantly for 3 months and then only at night for 3 more months or, in children, until growth is complete.

EXTENSIVE RELEASE OF THE FLEXOR PRONATOR ORIGIN

Williams and Haddad recommended a similar but more extensive release of the flexor-pronator origin than that just described. It frees completely the origins of the flexor mass almost to the wrist.

TECHNIQUE 9.5

(WILLIAMS AND HADDAD)
- Make an incision over the medial aspect of the arm and forearm anterior to the medial epicondyle of the humerus, beginning 5 cm proximal to the elbow and extending distally to about 5 cm proximal to the wrist (Fig. 9.9A).
- Protecting the medial antebrachial cutaneous nerve and the basilic vein, anteriorly dissect a flap of skin and subcutaneous tissue to expose the lacertus fibrosus and the antecubital fossa (Fig. 9.9B). Expose the ulnar nerve as it passes between the two heads of origin of the flexor carpi ulnaris.
- Avoiding the ulnar collateral ligament and capsule of the elbow joint, divide the common tendon of origin of the superficial group of muscles just distal to the epicondyle (Fig. 9.9C).
- Protecting the median nerve and its motor branches to the superficial group of muscles, free the ulnar origin of the pronator teres. Extend the dissection along the lateral border of the pronator teres to its insertion on the radius, but avoid injuring the radial artery. At this level, divide the aponeurotic radial origin of the flexor digitorum sublimis.
- Retract anteriorly the ulnar nerve and the stump of the common flexor tendon and free the origin of the flexor carpi ulnaris from the medial border of the olecranon. During this dissection, ligate and divide the posterior ulnar recurrent artery. Avoiding the periosteum of the ulna, release the aponeurotic origin of the flexor carpi ulnaris and flexor digitorum profundus from the ulna throughout its entire length (Fig. 9.9D).
- Identify the common interosseous artery, its volar branch, and the anterior interosseous nerve, and release from the volar aspect of the ulna and adjacent interosseous membrane the origin of the flexor digitorum profundus as far distally as the pronator quadratus (Fig. 9.9E).
- Release from the radius the origin of the flexor digitorum profundus to the index finger.
- Release from the medial side of the coronoid process the remaining origin of the flexor digitorum sublimis proximal to the common interosseous artery (Fig. 9.9F).
- Extend the wrist and fingers and identify and release any remaining tight bands. If there is any tension on the ulnar nerve, transplant it anteriorly into the brachialis (Fig. 9.9G); and if any elbow contracture persists, divide the brachialis tendon.
- If necessary, divide or lengthen the tendon of the flexor pollicis longus through a separate incision proximal to the wrist.
- Splint the extremity with the wrist and fingers extended and the elbow flexed.

POSTOPERATIVE CARE At 3 weeks, the splint and sutures are removed and another splint is applied that keeps the wrist and fingers extended and the thumb abducted. This splint is worn for 3 months except when it is removed for exercises of the wrist and fingers. It is then worn only at night for 6 weeks. Both occupational and physical therapy are continued as necessary.

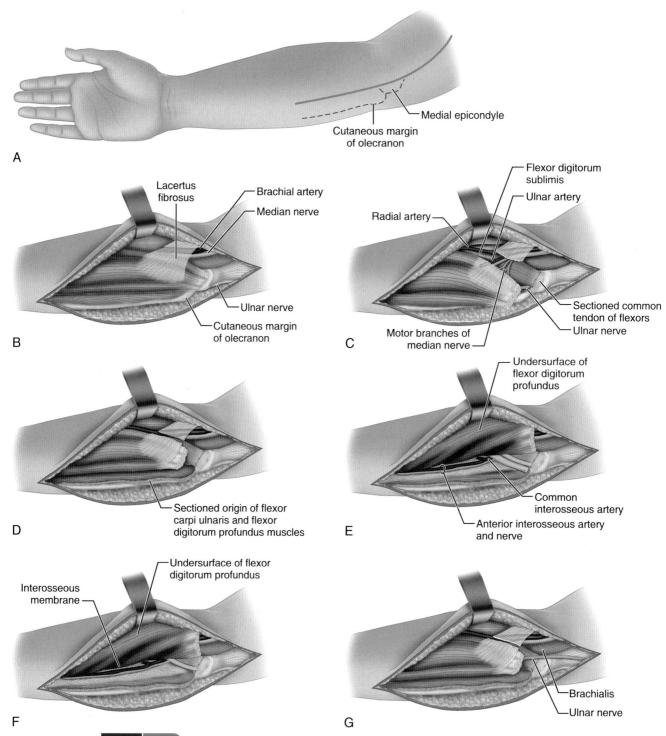

A

B
Lacertus fibrosus
Brachial artery
Median nerve
Ulnar nerve
Cutaneous margin of olecranon

Medial epicondyle
Cutaneous margin of olecranon

C
Flexor digitorum sublimis
Ulnar artery
Radial artery
Sectioned common tendon of flexors
Ulnar nerve
Motor branches of median nerve

D
Sectioned origin of flexor carpi ulnaris and flexor digitorum profundus muscles

E
Undersurface of flexor digitorum profundus
Common interosseous artery
Anterior interosseous artery and nerve

F
Undersurface of flexor digitorum profundus
Interosseous membrane

G
Brachialis
Ulnar nerve

FIGURE 9.9   Williams and Haddad technique for releasing flexor-pronator origin. **A,** Incision. **B,** Structures anteriorly and medially at elbow have been exposed (see text). **C,** Lacertus fibrosus has been divided, origin of superficial flexors has been released from medial epicondyle, and origin of flexor digitorum sublimis has been released from radius (see text). **D,** Origin of flexor carpi ulnaris has been released from olecranon, and common origin of flexor carpi ulnaris and flexor digitorum profundus has been released from ulna (see text). **E,** Origin of flexor digitorum profundus has been released from volar aspect of ulna and interosseous membrane (see text). **F,** Origin of flexor digitorum profundus to index finger has been released from radius, and remaining origin of flexor digitorum sublimis has been released from coronoid process (see text). **G,** Ulnar nerve has been transplanted anteriorly into brachialis muscle (see text). **SEE TECHNIQUE 9.5.**

TRANSFER OF THE FLEXOR CARPI ULNARIS

Transfer of the flexor carpi ulnaris dorsally to a radial wrist extensor removes a deforming force that pulls the hand into ulnar deviation and flexion and provides a force that promotes supination of the forearm and extension of the wrist. For this operation to be effective there must be active finger extension, passive flexibility of the hand, wrist, and forearm, and a favorable diagnostic profile. Any fixed deformity should be corrected before surgery by successive casts or by any operations as indicated. If active supination is possible before surgery, the muscle can be carried through the interosseous membrane instead of around the ulnar side of the forearm and can be prevented from acting as a supinator. This procedure should not be performed in conjunction with a release or lengthening of the flexor carpi radialis because it may cause a hyperextension deformity of the wrist. A normal patient has synergistic wrist and finger motion, that is, wrist extension is synergistic with finger flexion and wrist flexion with finger extension. A wrist flexion deformity may be accompanied by a primary weakness of the finger extensors; a child is able to release objects only by flexing the wrist. In this situation, transfer of the flexor carpi ulnaris to wrist extensors may only strengthen grasp, making it difficult for the child to release objects. With significant finger extensor weakness, flexor carpi ulnaris transfer to extensor digitorum communis is recommended. Van Heest et al. demonstrated in seven patients that flexor carpi ulnaris activation was most common during grasp, and relaxation was present during release. This phasic activation did not appear to change after transfer and proved beneficial during grasp and release. Wolf et al. improved function and cosmesis, with an average final wrist resting position of 9 degrees extension with transfer of the flexor carpi ulnaris to the extensor carpi radialis longus. Some authors have reported late extension deformity in patients younger than 13 years in whom tendon transfer was performed.

TECHNIQUE 9.6

(GREEN AND BANKS)
- Make an anterior longitudinal incision (Fig. 9.10A) extending from the flexor crease of the wrist proximally for about 3 cm to expose the insertion of the flexor carpi ulnaris on the pisiform bone.
- Detach the tendon from the bone and dissect it proximally (Fig. 9.10B).
- The attachment of the muscle to the ulna often extends almost the full length of the tendon; free it by sharp dissection from the ulna, leaving the periosteum in place. The ulnar nerve now may be seen in a sheath posterior to the tendon.
- Introduce a nylon suture into the distal end of the tendon and, by pulling on it gently, outline the course of the muscle proximally.

- Beginning about 5 cm distal to the medial epicondyle of the humerus, make a second incision 7 to 10 cm long over the belly of the muscle. Define the lateral margin of the muscle and make an incision there through the deep fascia to expose this margin and the deep surface of the muscle.
- When the muscle belly has been defined, dissect it from its origin on the deep surface of the deep fascia and from the ulna distally.
- Pull the tendon into the proximal incision and free the muscle further until it passes straight from its origin across the border of the ulna to the dorsal aspect of the wrist. Locate and preserve branches of the ulnar nerve to the muscle because they limit the dissection proximally.
- At a suitable level at the medial margin of the ulna, excise the intermuscular septum separating the volar and dorsal compartments of the forearm for 4 to 5 cm and expose the dorsal compartment.
- Starting just proximal to the transverse skin crease on the dorsum of the wrist and extending proximally, make a third incision (Fig. 9.10C) about 3 cm long over the extensor carpi radialis brevis and longus tendons and expose these tendons.
- Choose the extensor carpi radialis brevis or longus tendon for insertion of the transferred tendon; the extensor carpi radialis brevis gives a more central action in extension of the wrist, whereas the extensor carpi radialis longus gives a better pull for supination of the forearm and radial deviation of the wrist.
- Using a tendon passer (Fig. 9.10D), direct the free end of the flexor carpi ulnaris from the proximal incision into the dorsal compartment along the path of the extensor tendons to the chosen extensor radialis tendon.
- Make a buttonhole (Fig. 9.10E) in the chosen tendon and pass through it the flexor carpi ulnaris tendon; suture the flexor carpi ulnaris tendon (Fig. 9.10F) there under tension with the forearm in full supination and the wrist in at least 45 degrees of extension. Manske prefers to tension the transfer by placing the wrist in slight flexion (15 degrees) to avoid a hyperextension deformity. We have not encountered this complication, provided that the flexor carpi radialis is not overlengthened.
- If the flexor carpi ulnaris is to be transferred into the extensor digitorum communis tendons, suture it under tension, so that when the wrist is in the neutral position the metacarpophalangeal joints are hyperextended.
- Close the wounds and apply a cast extending from near the axilla to the tips of the fingers, holding the wrist in extension, the forearm in supination, the fingers in almost complete extension, and the thumb in abduction and opposition.

POSTOPERATIVE CARE The sutures are removed at 2 weeks, and a new cast is applied and worn for 4 weeks. Hand therapy is begun at 6 weeks after surgery. Night splints are used intermittently for several months as necessary to keep the hand in a corrected position.

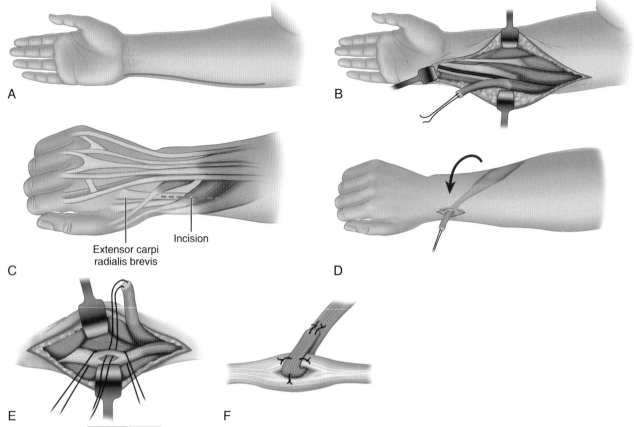

A

B

C

Extensor carpi
radialis brevis

Incision

D

E

F

FIGURE 9.10 Transfer of flexor carpi ulnaris. **A,** Anterior longitudinal incision over flexor carpi ulnaris. This may be divided into two separate incisions as described in the text. **B,** Flexor carpi ulnaris tendon is detached from pisiform insertion, and muscle is dissected proximally off ulna. **C,** Small longitudinal incision on dorsum of wrist over extensor carpi radialis brevis just proximal to first extensor compartment. **D,** Flexor carpi ulnaris tendon is passed subcutaneously around ulnar border of forearm using a tendon passer. **E,** Buttonhole is made in extensor carpi radialis brevis tendon. **F,** Flexor carpi ulnaris is passed through buttonhole and sutured to itself under appropriate tension. **SEE TECHNIQUE 9.6.**

WRIST ARTHRODESIS

Wrist arthrodesis is useful in a patient with a severe wrist flexion contracture and a nonfunctional hand. It is used primarily to control position and improve hygiene in a hand with poor motor control and sensibility. A proximal row carpectomy is typically incorporated with the fusion to improve the flexion contracture and to provide a bone graft. Complete release of wrist flexors (palmaris longus, flexor carpi ulnaris, and flexor carpi radialis) is accomplished first. Because the epiphysis of the distal radius is damaged, a standard wrist fusion must be delayed until the patient is at least 12 years old. For skeletally immature patients, an epiphyseal arthrodesis can be done that allows for continued distal radial growth. The wrist ideally should be fused in neutral flexion and ulnar deviation; however, a mild degree of flexion is well tolerated.

TECHNIQUE 9.7

- After lengthening or releasing the flexor tendons as necessary, make a dorsal longitudinal incision over the wrist.

- Excise the proximal carpal row as necessary to achieve correction. Denude all remaining cartilage from the radiocarpal and intercarpal joints and from the second and third carpometacarpal joints.
- Use corticocancellous portions of the excised carpal bones or iliac crest grafts to supplement the fusion.
- Transfix the carpus with two Steinmann pins measuring 7/64 to 9/64 of an inch (Fig. 9.11) or 3.5 mm dorsal plate.
- Apply a long arm cast with the elbow at 90 degrees of flexion and the forearm in neutral pronation and supination. If the finger flexors have been lengthened, extend the cast to include the fingers in the extended position.

POSTOPERATIVE CARE At 4 weeks, the long arm cast can be converted to a short arm cast and finger flexion and extension are encouraged. The wrist is protected until fusion is apparent, usually at 10 to 12 weeks. The pins may be removed when the arthrodesis is solid.

CARPECTOMY

Omer and Capen reported proximal row carpectomies to improve appearance in eight patients with cerebral palsy. At the same time, transfers of the flexor carpi ulnaris tendon around the ulna to the extensor carpi radialis brevis were done to strengthen wrist extension and increase supination. Omer and Capen warn that this does not improve function. All their patients were older than 11 years of age. They emphasized prolonged postoperative splinting because the procedure increases the relative length of all flexor muscle-tendon units that cross the wrist and increases wrist extension and forearm supination; they further emphasized that only the proximal half of the carpal scaphoid is taken.

TECHNIQUE 9.8

(OMER AND CAPEN)
- Make a longitudinal incision over the dorsum of the wrist. Identify the distal edge of the dorsal carpal ligament and retract the common digital extensor tendons ulnarward. Make a T-shaped incision in the dorsal capsule to expose the carpal bones.
- Excise the lunate and the proximal half of the scaphoid. Leave the distal half of the scaphoid with its capsular attachments.
- Excise the triquetrum, but leave the pisiform bone.
- Make a longitudinal incision over the volar aspect of the wrist, beginning at the pisiform and extending proximally over the flexor carpi ulnaris tendon.
- Protect the neurovascular bundle and free the flexor carpi ulnaris from the intermuscular septum.
- Divide the muscle near its insertion and pass its tendon through a window in the interosseous membrane. (If more supination is needed, pass the transfer around the ulna.)
- Insert the flexor carpi ulnaris into the extensor carpi radialis brevis and anchor it with nonabsorbable monofilament sutures.
- Place the wrist in maximal passive dorsiflexion and imbricate the dorsal capsule of the wrist.

POSTOPERATIVE CARE The arm is placed in a bulky dressing and a volar plaster splint that holds the fingers and wrist in extension. On or about postoperative day 5, a circular long arm cast is applied, holding the elbow flexed, the forearm supinated, and the wrist and fingers extended. This position is maintained for 6 weeks. Then a circular short arm cast, incorporating outriggers for extension of the fingers, is applied. Splinting is continued for 4 months and subsequently used only at night for an indefinite time.

THUMB-IN-PALM DEFORMITY

The second most frequent and important deformity of the hand in cerebral palsy is the thumb-in-palm, adducted thumb, or clutched thumb deformity. This deformity blocks entry of objects into the palm and prevents the thumb from assisting fingers in grasp or pinch. Contributing to thumb-in-palm

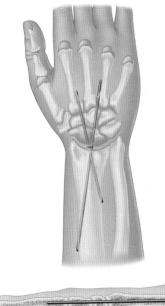

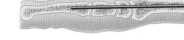

FIGURE 9.11 Wrist arthrodesis using two Steinmann pins. **SEE TECHNIQUE 9.7.**

deformity are spasticity of the flexor pollicis longus, flexor pollicis brevis, adductor pollicis, and first dorsal interosseous, as well as weakness of the extensor pollicis longus, extensor pollicis brevis, and abductor pollicis longus muscles. Spasticity in the extensor pollicis longus muscle also may contribute to an adduction deformity of the thumb during the release phase (Fig. 9.12). House, Gwathney, and Fidler classified thumb-in-palm deformities into four major types based on the clinical appearance of the thumb. A type I deformity consists of a simple metacarpal adduction contracture and is the most common pattern. A type II deformity consists of a metacarpal adduction contracture combined with a metacarpophalangeal flexion deformity. A type III deformity consists of a metacarpal adduction contracture combined with a metacarpophalangeal hyperextension deformity or instability; this is the second most common pattern. A type IV deformity consists of a metacarpal adduction contracture combined with metacarpophalangeal and interphalangeal flexion deformities; this is believed to be the most severe deformity, being caused by spasticity in the flexor pollicis longus and in the intrinsic muscles in the thumb. Tonkin et al. divided thumb-in-palm deformities into three types: type 1, a flexed metacarpophalangeal joint and an extended interphalangeal joint; type 2, flexed metacarpophalangeal and interphalangeal joints; and type 3, a flexed metacarpophalangeal and interphalangeal joint with an adduction contracture as well (Table 9.6).

Although thumb-in-palm deformity can be caused principally by spasticity of the flexor pollicis longus muscle, it is not caused solely by this muscle. The flexor pollicis longus flexes the interphalangeal joint, the metacarpophalangeal joint, and the carpometacarpal joint and acts as an adductor of the thumb. To be certain that it is a principal deforming force, the patient should be able to decrease the flexion of these joints by flexing the wrist. Conversely, extending the wrist causes an increase in deformity. The

TABLE 9.6

Classification of Thumb Deformity

TYPE OF DEFORMITY	DEFORMING FORCES	THUMB POSITION
1—intrinsic	Adductor pollicis First dorsal interosseous Flexor pollicis brevis	Metacarpal adduction MCP joint flexion IP joint extension
2—extrinsic	Flexor pollicis longus	MCP joint flexion IP joint flexion Metacarpal adduction less marked
3—combined	Adductor pollicis First dorsal interosseous Flexor pollicis brevis Flexor pollicis longus	Metacarpal adduction MCP joint flexion IP joint flexion (true "thumb-in-palm" deformity)

IP, Interphalangeal; *MCP*, metacarpophalangeal.

From Tonkin MA, Hatrick NC, Eckersley JRT, et al: Surgery for cerebral palsy, part 3: classification and operative procedures for thumb deformity, *J Hand Surg* 26B:465, 2001.

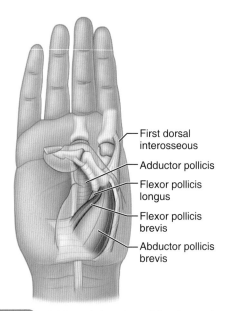

- First dorsal interosseous
- Adductor pollicis
- Flexor pollicis longus
- Flexor pollicis brevis
- Abductor pollicis brevis

FIGURE 9.12　Adducted thumb position in cerebral palsy is result of forces exerted by powerful muscles.

examiner should determine whether an accompanying severe adduction deformity, caused by contracture of muscle or other structures, is present. A weak adductor pollicis may be overpowered by a tendon transfer; active adduction of the thumb by the adductor pollicis should be checked with the wrist palmar flexed to determine the strength of the muscle. Surgical correction of thumb-in-palm deformity has demonstrated both high clinical success rates and overall patient satisfaction in the short and long term. Although clinical correction was shown to diminish over time, there appeared to be minimal effect on patient satisfaction.

■ TREATMENT

Treatment of thumb-in-palm deformity must be individualized after careful, repeated assessments of the overall hand function and function of the specific muscles contributing to the deformity. Currently, a dynamic approach is used in the surgical correction of this deformity, as

described by House et al. This involves release of contractures, augmentation of weak muscles, and skeletal stabilization (Table 9.7), especially of the metacarpophalangeal joint when necessary. A myotomy of the adductor pollicis may be done through a palmar incision, as described by Matev, or through a Z-plasty incision placed in the first web if a skin contracture is present. Preoperative electromyography of the adductor pollicis has been found to be useful in determining whether a partial or complete release of this muscle was necessary. If the adductor is active during grasp, the patients are said to have selective control, and release of the transverse head of the muscle only should be considered because pinch may be weak if complete myotomy is performed. Release of the origin of the first dorsal interosseous muscle also may be required. In long-standing type II deformities, the origin of the adductor and the flexor pollicis brevis may require release, as described by Matev. In type IV deformities, the flexor pollicis longus may require lengthening proximal to the wrist. Augmentation of a weak abductor pollicis longus may be necessary. The most common muscles used for this augmentation are the palmaris longus, the brachioradialis, and the flexor carpi radialis. Fusion of the thumb metacarpophalangeal joint is especially useful if a hyperextension deformity of that joint is present. Arthrodesis may be performed without damage to the physis if only articular cartilage is removed, and a smooth Kirschner wire is used for fixation. Alternatively, if instability of the thumb metacarpophalangeal extension is present, a sesamoid metacarpal synostosis may be used, as described by Zancolli et al. In this procedure, the radial sesamoid with the volar plate is advanced proximally and fused to the thumb metacarpal neck.

Smith proposed transfer of the flexor pollicis longus tendon to the radial side of the thumb combined with tenodesis of the distal joint. He recommended the operation for patients who have some use of the affected hand, in addition to passive extension of the metacarpophalangeal joint and abduction of the carpometacarpal joint with the wrist in flexion.

If the extensor pollicis longus contributes to the thumb deformity, it may be rerouted from the Lister tubercle, as recommended by Manske. Significant improvement in

TABLE 9.7	
Surgical Options	
Surgical options for releases or lengthening of contracted or spastic muscles	Adductor release in palm Adductor tenotomy First interosseous release Flexor pollicis brevis (thenar) release FPL lengthening Thumb web Z-plasty w/ fascial release
Surgical options for tendon transfers	EPL rerouting To augment abductor pollicis longus, EPL, or extensor pollicis brevis Flexor digitorum superficialis Brachioradialis Palmaris longus Flexor carpi radialis Extensor carpi radialis longus
Surgical options for joint stabilization	CMC arthrodesis MCP arthrodesis MCP joint volar capsulodesis IP joint arthrodesis

CMC, Carpometacarpal; *EPL,* extensor pollicis longus; *FPL,* flexor pollicis longus; *IP,* interphalangeal; *MCP,* metacarpophalangeal.
From Van Heest AE: Surgical technique for thumb-in-palm deformity in cerebral palsy, *J Hand Surg* 36A:1526, 2011.

functional activities was noted in 90% of his patients treated with this technique. Long-term satisfaction of surgical correction in patients remains high despite deterioration of position in up to 30% of patients at 5 years.

MYOTOMY

TECHNIQUE 9.9

- Make an incision bordering the thenar crease in the palm but avoid damaging the recurrent branch of the median nerve or the innervation of the adductor pollicis.
- Retract the long flexors of the fingers and strip from the third metacarpal the origin of the adductor pollicis.
- Cut from the deep transverse carpal ligament about two thirds of the origin of the abductor pollicis brevis and all of the origins of the flexor pollicis brevis and opponens pollicis (Fig. 9.13).
- Strip from the first metacarpal the origin of the first dorsal interosseous.
- If necessary, do a capsulorrhaphy of the metacarpophalangeal joint.

POSTOPERATIVE CARE A pressure dressing and a cast are applied holding the first metacarpal (not the phalanges) in wide abduction and opposition. At 3 weeks, the cast and sutures are removed and a splint is applied to hold the thumb in this same position. If tendon transfers have been necessary, the cast is retained for 6 weeks. Splinting at night may be necessary for a long time if the deformity tends to recur.

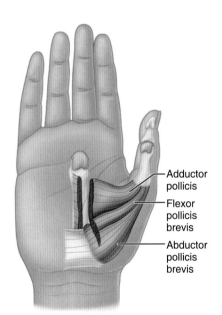

FIGURE 9.13 Myotomies of intrinsic muscles of thumb for thumb-in-palm deformity. **SEE TECHNIQUE 9.9.**

Labels: Adductor pollicis; Flexor pollicis brevis; Abductor pollicis brevis

RELEASE OF CONTRACTURES, AUGMENTATION OF WEAK MUSCLES, AND SKELETAL STABILIZATION

TECHNIQUE 9.10

(HOUSE ET AL.)

STEP 1: RELEASE OF CONTRACTURES

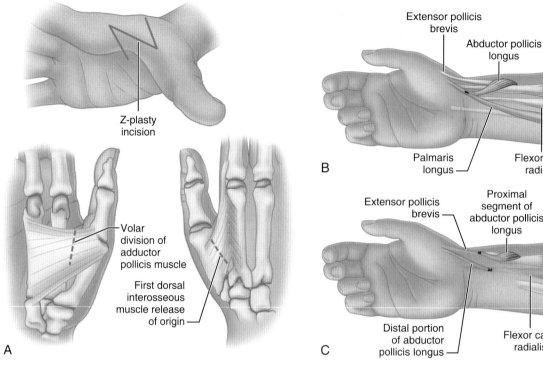

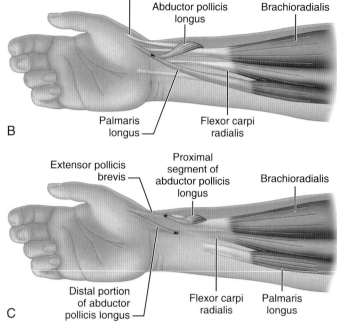

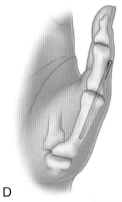

FIGURE 9.14   Dynamic approach to thumb-in-palm deformity. **A,** Release of adduction contracture through Z-plasty first web incision (see text). **B,** Transfer of palmaris longus to intact abductor pollicis longus, which has been released from first dorsal compartment. **C,** Transfer of distal portion of tendon of abductor pollicis longus to flexor carpi radialis, so-called dynamic tenodesis, and transfer of proximal segment of abductor pollicis longus into extensor pollicis brevis. **D,** Chondrodesis of thumb metacarpophalangeal joint for hyperextension deformity. **SEE TECHNIQUE 9.10.**

- Through a Z-plasty incision located along the first web space, release the origin of the first dorsal interosseous muscle from the thumb metacarpal (Fig. 9.14A).
- Expose the intramuscular portion of the tendon of the adductor pollicis and divide it obliquely to allow a relative lengthening of the tendon while preserving bridging muscle fibers. If a long-standing type II deformity exists with a flexion deformity of the metacarpophalangeal joint, release the origin of the adductor and the flexor pollicis brevis if necessary. For a type IV deformity with spasticity of the flexor pollicis longus muscle and interphalangeal flexion deformity, lengthen the tendon of the flexor pollicis longus proximal to the wrist.

STEP 2: AUGMENTATION OF WEAK MUSCLES
- If adduction of the thumb at the carpometacarpal joint is considerable, with weakness of the abductor pollicis

longus, release the abductor pollicis longus tendon from the first extensor compartment and allow the tendon to subluxate volarly.
- Divide the palmaris longus tendon at the level of the wrist and suture it into the abductor pollicis longus tendon in an end-to-side fashion (Fig. 9.14B). The brachioradialis and the flexor carpi radialis can be used instead of the palmaris longus if desired.
- If there is no suitable donor for active transfer, divide the abductor pollicis longus tendon and reroute its distal portion volarly, attaching it in an end-to-side fashion to the flexor carpi radialis tendon under sufficient tension to maintain metacarpal abduction Fig. 9.14C). This provides a dynamic abductor tenodesis.
- If the flexion deformity at the metacarpophalangeal joint is significant but joint stability is normal, a similar tenodesis

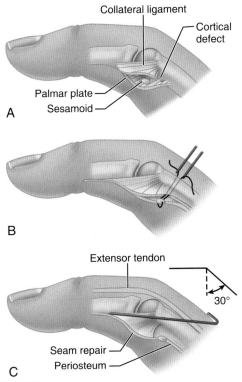

Collateral ligament

Cortical defect

Palmar plate

Sesamoid

A

B

Extensor tendon

30°

Seam repair

Periosteum

C

FIGURE 9.15 Sesamoid arthrodesis. **A,** Palmar plate is mobilized by dividing accessory collateral ligament at its insertion into palmar plate. Articular surface of sesamoid is denuded of cartilage. Cortical defect is created at head-neck junction of metacarpal. **B,** Two straight needles (with Kirschner wire driver) are used to pass polypropylene (Prolene) suture through sesamoid-palmar plate complex and metacarpal neck to secure sesamoid into cortical defect created. **C,** Intraosseous suture is tied over metacarpal under extensor tendons as permanent suture. Kirschner wire is placed across metacarpophalangeal joint to maintain joint in approximately 30 degrees of flexion. Seam in collateral ligament is repaired, and proximal radial edge of palmar plate is sutured to metacarpal periosteum and aponeurotic fibers of abductor pollicis brevis. **SEE TECHNIQUE 9.10.**

of the extensor pollicis brevis tendon may be performed. Care must be taken not to create a disabling hyperextension deformity at this joint.

STEP 3: SKELETAL STABILIZATION

- If there is a hyperextension deformity of the metacarpophalangeal joint (type III deformity), carefully remove the articular cartilage of the metacarpophalangeal joint without damaging the physis.
- Position the thumb and secure it with one centrally placed 1-mm Kirschner wire (Fig. 9.14D).
- Alternatively, if thumb metacarpophalangeal extension instability is present, advance the sesamoid with the palmar plate as described by Zancolli et al., and Lawson, and Tonkin (Fig. 9.15). Approach the metacarpophalangeal joint through a dorsoradial incision.
- Divide the accessory collateral ligament insertion and mobilize the palmar plate.
- Denude the sesamoid of cartilage.
- Create a cortical defect at the head-neck junction of the metacarpal.
- Fix the sesamoid in the defect created at the head-neck junction of the metacarpal with the thumb in 30 degrees of

flexion. Pass two intraosseous sutures across the sesamoid and tie them over the dorsal surface of the metacarpal.
- Stabilize the joint with a Kirschner wire. (The wire is removed at 5 weeks.)

POSTOPERATIVE CARE The forearm and hand are immobilized for 4 weeks with the thumb held in abduction and extension by a volar plaster splint. Then active and assisted exercises of the wrist, thumb, and fingers are started. A long opponens splint modified by the addition of a C-bar or molded plastic orthosis is worn between exercise periods for the next few weeks, after which splinting is continued at night, only until growth is completed or dynamic balance is attained and stabilized.

FLEXOR POLLICIS LONGUS ABDUCTORPLASTY

TECHNIQUE 9.11

(SMITH)

- Make a radial midlateral incision from the middle of the distal phalanx of the thumb to the neck of the first metacarpal (Fig. 9.16A).
- Elevate a volar skin flap and transect the flexor pollicis longus tendon opposite the proximal phalanx (Fig. 9.16B).
- Tenodese the flexor pollicis longus stump to the proximal phalanx, or arthrodese the distal joint in 15 degrees of flexion (Fig. 9.16C-E).
- Make a longitudinal incision in the forearm just radial to the tendon of the flexor carpi radialis, curving its distal portion ulnarward. Identify the flexor pollicis longus tendon and draw it out through this incision.
- Tunnel subcutaneously by blunt dissection on the radial side of the thumb to the lateral side of the metacarpophalangeal joint and pass the flexor pollicis longus tendon through this tunnel.
- With the wrist in neutral position and the thumb at 50 degrees of abduction, suture the tendon to the dorsoradial aspect of the metacarpophalangeal joint with tension (Fig. 9.16F).

POSTOPERATIVE CARE The hand is immobilized for 6 weeks with the thumb in abduction and the wrist in 30 degrees of flexion. The thumb is splinted with a C-bar in the web for an additional 6 weeks.

REDIRECTION OF EXTENSOR POLLICIS LONGUS

TECHNIQUE 9.12

(MANSKE)

- Through a palmar incision, release the adductor pollicis and the deep head of the flexor pollicis brevis, as described by Matev and by Swanson.

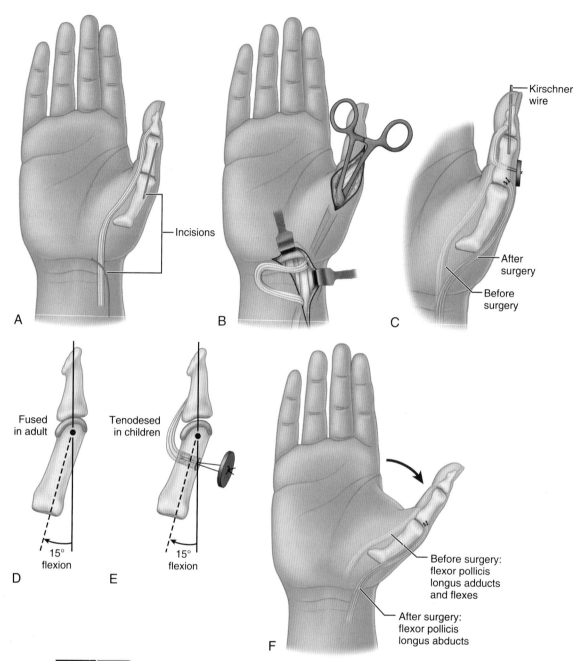

FIGURE 9.16   Flexor pollicis longus abductorplasty. **A,** Incision to radial side of thumb exposes insertion of flexor pollicis longus, interphalangeal joint, and base of proximal phalanx. Second curved incision to radial side of wrist exposes flexor pollicis longus near its musculotendinous juncture and permits tendon to be withdrawn from carpal canal. **B,** Flexor pollicis longus is transected at its insertion and withdrawn from carpal canal through wrist incision. It is passed subcutaneously to radial side of base of proximal phalanx. **C** to **E,** Interphalangeal joint of thumb is arthrodesed in about 15 degrees of flexion in adult. In child with open physis, distal joint may be tenodesed in about 15 degrees of flexion. **F,** Transfer of flexor pollicis longus to radial side of proximal phalanx reduces adduction-flexion deformity and augments thumb abduction by transferred position of flexor pollicis longus. Interphalangeal arthrodesis improves metacarpophalangeal joint extension by increasing lever arm of extensor pollicis longus on metacarpophalangeal joint. **SEE TECHNIQUE 9.11.**

- Release the first dorsal interosseous muscle at its origin from the first metacarpal through a longitudinal incision on the dorsum of the thumb.
- Extend the incision on the dorsum of the thumb distally to the proximal phalanx, exposing the extensor aponeurotic hood (Fig. 9.17A).
- Identify the extensor pollicis longus at the metacarpophalangeal joint and dissect it out from the extensor aponeurosis for a distance of 10 mm distal to the joint. This leaves a longitudinal defect 4 mm wide in the extensor hood. Preserve the margins of the aponeurosis sufficiently for subsequent closure.
- Identify the extensor pollicis longus through a longitudinal incision at the distal radius and withdraw it into the forearm (Fig. 9.17B).
- Redirect the extensor pollicis longus tendon along the radial aspect of the wrist, using the first extensor retinacular compartment as a pulley to maintain its position by passing a curved hemostat or tendon passer from the dorsal incision on the thumb along the course of the extensor pollicis brevis tendon through the first extensor compartment.
- Grasp the extensor pollicis longus tendon with the hemostat and retract it distally through the first extensor compartment (Fig. 9.17C). If redirecting the tendon through this compartment is difficult, the extensor pollicis longus can be routed around the extensor pollicis brevis and abductor pollicis longus tendons just proximal to the compartment and into the dorsal incision on the thumb.
- Pass the extensor pollicis longus tendon through a transverse tunnel made in the capsule of the metacarpophalangeal joint and suture it under sufficient tension to advance it 1 to 2 cm from its original position (Fig. 9.17D). If the metacarpophalangeal joint is hyperextensible, this tunnel should be placed proximal to the articular surface to prevent further hyperextension. In this situation, a temporary Kirschner wire should be inserted across the slightly flexed metacarpophalangeal joint.
- Suture the distal portion of the extensor pollicis longus tendon into the extensor aponeurosis to close the longitudinal defect and prevent flexion deformity at the interphalangeal joint (Fig. 9.17E).
- Close the incisions in routine fashion.

POSTOPERATIVE CARE The thumb is immobilized in abduction and extension in a short arm–thumb spica cast for 4 weeks. If a Kirschner wire has been inserted in the metacarpophalangeal joint, it should be removed at 4 weeks. A removable thumb spica splint is worn for 2 weeks; this splint is removed three to four times daily for controlled active motion.

SWAN-NECK DEFORMITY

Compared with other deformities of the upper extremity in cerebral palsy, swan-neck deformities of the fingers are infrequent; however, they can be quite disabling. They are secondary to hand intrinsic muscle spasticity or extrinsic overpull, which causes intrinsic spasticity and by secondary ligamentous and capsular relaxation at the proximal interphalangeal joints, allowing these joints to hyperextend. In general, only a swan-neck deformity greater than 20 degrees should be considered for surgical treatment. In the involved finger, the middle extensor band is relatively short compared with the lateral bands because of tension exerted on the middle band by the long extensor and the intrinsic muscle. In this deformity, the Curtis sublimis tenodesis of the proximal interphalangeal joint may improve function. Lateral band translocation originally described by Zancolli, and later by Tonkin, Hughes, and Smith, in which the radial lateral band is translocated volarly beneath a soft-tissue sling created by suturing the accessory collateral ligament to the radial slip of the sublimis, also may be useful. The reported results by Tonkin, Hughes, and Smith in 12 patients were excellent; however, the follow-up was less than 1 year in most patients. More recently, de Bruin reported long-term results of lateral band translocation for swan-neck deformity in patients with cerebral palsy and found that the success rate decreased from 84% at 1 year to 60% at 5 years. We have not used this technique.

SUBLIMIS TENODESIS OF THE PROXIMAL INTERPHALANGEAL JOINT

TECHNIQUE 9.13

(CURTIS)
- The Curtis technique employs one slip of the flexor digitorum sublimis that is left at its insertion on the bone and cut free at the bifurcation.
- Bring the tendon slip to the opposite side of the joint under the remaining tendons and insert it into the lateral aspect of the proximal phalanx with a pull-out wire suture (Fig. 9.18).
- Hold the proximal interphalangeal joint in flexion with a traversing Kirschner wire for 6 weeks.

INTRINSIC LENGTHENING

Other surgical options include intrinsic lengthening or central slip tenotomy, depending on the defining force. This can be differentiated by the position of the metacarpophalangeal joint during active digital extension. Intrinsic spasticity will cause metacarpophalangeal joint flexion and hyperextension of the proximal interphalangeal joints. Patients with full metacarpophalangeal joint extension with active finger extension develop swan-neck deformity secondary to extensor digitorum communis spasticity. A Bunnell test can confirm intrinsic spasticity.

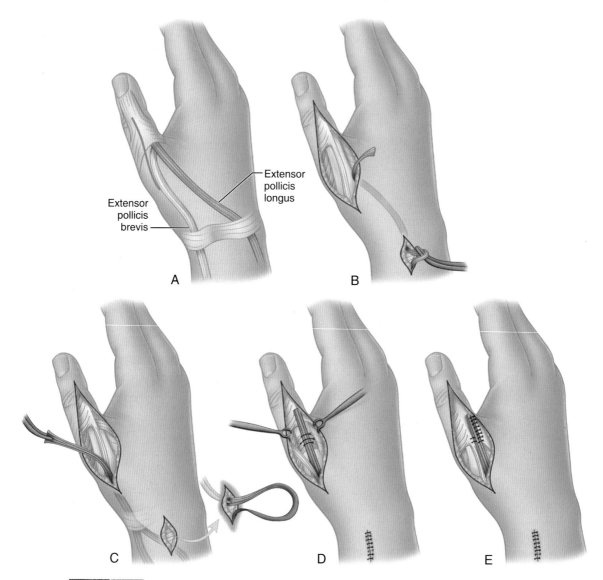

Extensor pollicis longus

Extensor pollicis brevis

A

B

C

D

E

FIGURE 9.17   **A** to **E,** Manske technique for redirecting extensor pollicis longus tendon to correct thumb-in-palm deformity. **SEE TECHNIQUE 9.12.**

TECHNIQUE 9.14

Figure 9.19

(MATSUO ET AL. AND CARLSON ET AL.)

- Make a single transverse incision in the palm over the affected digits at the level of the distal palmar crease.
- Expose the intermetacarpal area. Identify and protect the neurovascular structures.
- Identify the lumbricals and perform fractional lengthening with two tenotomies at the musculotendinous junction.
- Similarly perform fractional lengthening for the dorsal interossei.
- Confirm intrinsic release by gentle Bunnell testing.
- Do not overlengthen by flexing the proximal interphalangeal joint greater than 70 degrees with the metacarpophalangeal joint extended.
- Avoid lengthening the first dorsal interossei because this will weaken pinch.

- Apply a soft dressing.

POSTOPERATIVE CARE Patients are encouraged to perform early range of motion as soon as possible after surgery with or without assisted therapy.

LATERAL BAND TRANSLOCATION

TECHNIQUE 9.15

(TONKIN, HUGHES, AND SMITH)

- Make a midlateral incision on the radial side of the finger.
- Mobilize the lateral band of the extensor mechanism from the midpoint of the proximal phalanx to the midpoint of the middle phalanx by separating it from the central

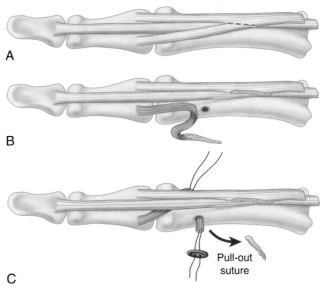

FIGURE 9.18 Curtis technique for correcting recurrent hyperextension and locking of proximal interphalangeal joint. **A,** Palmar view of flexor tendons. **B,** One half of flexor digitorum sublimis tendon has been divided at bifurcation of tendon. Hole has been drilled in proximal phalanx. **C,** Freed half of tendon has been carried deep to flexor digitorum profundus tendon to opposite side of proximal phalanx, threaded through hole in bone, and anchored with pull-out suture under enough tension to cause slight flexion contracture of proximal interphalangeal joint. **SEE TECHNIQUE 9.13.**

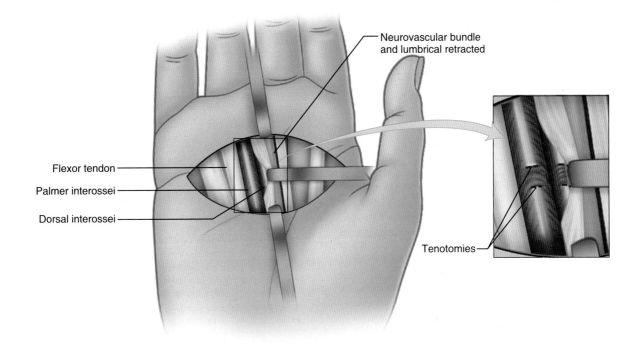

FIGURE 9.19 Intrinsic lengthening. **SEE TECHNIQUE 9.14.**

tendon mechanism dorsally and by dividing the transverse retinaculum ligament of Landsmeer on the palmar aspect of the lateral band.

- Divide the accessory collateral ligament at its insertion into the palmar plate, displaying the free lateral margin of that structure. The insertion of the palmar plate into the base of the middle phalanx and its origin from the proximal phalanx remain intact. A synovectomy of the proximal interphalangeal joint may be done if needed.

- Open the flexor tendon sheath between the A2 and A4 pulleys and identify the radial slip of the superficialis insertion.
- Translocate palmarward the mobilized lateral band below the proximal interphalangeal joint axis. Create a sling, using two 4-0 sutures placed at the distal edge of the proximal interphalangeal joint, between the free margin of the palmar plate and the radial slip of the superficial tendon to maintain the position of the lateral band.

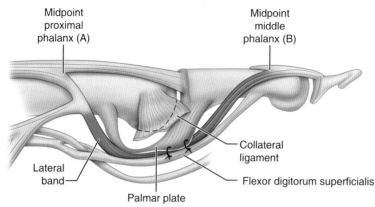

Midpoint proximal phalanx (A)

Midpoint middle phalanx (B)

Collateral ligament

Flexor digitorum superficialis

Lateral band

Palmar plate

FIGURE 9.20 Tonkin et al. lateral band translocation technique. Separation of the lateral band from the midpoint of the proximal phalanx to the midpoint of the middle phalanx. Release of accessory collateral ligament. Suture of palmar plate to flexor digitorum superficialis tendon to create retaining sling. **SEE TECHNIQUE 9.15.**

- Check the tension of the translocated tendon so that the proximal interphalangeal joint does not extend beyond 5 degrees of flexion when the finger is supported at the finger pulp alone. The tension can be adjusted by changing the position of the proximal point of dissection of the lateral band from the central tendon mechanism. To loosen tension, dissect farther proximally. To tighten the translocated band, resuture it to the central slip. To prevent subsequent splitting of the translocated tendon from the central tendon, place a single suture at the point of proximal and distal separation (Fig. 9.20).
- If an extension lag remains at the distal interphalangeal joint, place a temporary Kirschner wire to maintain this joint in extension for 4 weeks. Alternatively, a distal interphalangeal joint arthrodesis may be considered.
- After hemostasis is obtained, suture the skin and place the forearm and hand in a palmar resting splint with the metacarpophalangeal joints flexed and the interphalangeal joints in the position obtained after the procedure.

POSTOPERATIVE CARE

The dressings are reduced at 48 hours. Gentle, active mobilization should be started. A dorsal splint should be worn to protect the joint from hyperextension for 2 weeks.

REFERENCES

Alewijnse JV, Smeulders MJ, Kreulen M: Short-term and long-term clinical results of the surgical correction of thumb-in-palm deformity in patients with cerebral palsy, *J Pediatr Orthop* 35:825, 2015.

Andersson G, Renström B, Blaszczyk I, Domellöf E: Upper-extremity spasticity-reducing treatment in adjunct to movement training and orthoses in children with cerebral palsy at gross motor function and manual ability classification system levels IV-V: a descriptive study, *Dev Neurorehabil* 1–10, 2019, E-pub ahead of print.

Barroso PN, Vecchio SD, Xavier YR, et al.: Improvement of hand function in children with cerebral palsy via an orthosis that provides wrist extension and thumb abduction, *Clin Biomech* 26:937, 2011.

Carlson EJ, Carlson MG: Treatment of swan neck deformity in cerebral palsy, *J Hand Surg Am* 39:768, 2014.

Čobeljić G, Rajković S, Bajin Z, et al.: The results of surgical treatment for pronation deformities of the forearm in cerebral palsy after a mean follow-up of 17.5 years, *J Orthop Surg Res* 10:106, 2015.

de Bruin M, van Vliet DC, Smeulders MJ, Kreulen M: Long-term results of lateral band translocation for the correction of swan neck deformity in cerebral palsy, *J Pediatr Orthop* 30:67, 2010.

de Roode CP, James MA, Van Heest AE: Tendon transfers and releases for the forearm, wrist, and hand in spastic hemiplegic cerebral palsy, *Tech Hand Up Extrem Surg* 14:129, 2010.

Gong HS, Chung CY, Park MS, et al.: Functional outcomes after upper extremity surgery for cerebral palsy: comparison of high and low manual ability classification system levels, *J Hand Surg Am* 35A:277, 2010.

Hedberg-Graf J, Granström F, Arner M, Krumlinde-Sundholm L: Upper-limb contracture development in children with cerebral palsy: a population-based study, *Dev Med Child Neurol* 61(2):204, 2019.

Koman LA, Smith BP, Williams R, et al.: Upper extremity spasticity in children with cerebral palsy: a randomized, double-blind, placebo-controlled study of the short-term outcomes of treatment with botulinum A toxin, *J Hand Surg Am* 38:435, 2013.

Lidman G, Nachemson A, Peny-Deahlstrand M, Himmelmann K: Botulinum toxin A injections and occupational therapy in children with unilateral spastic cerebral palsy: a randomized controlled trial, *Dev Med Child Neurol* 57:754, 2015.

Lin H, Hou C, Chen A, Xu Z: Long term outcome of division of the C8 nerve root for spasticity of the hand in cerebral palsy, *J Hand Surg Am* 35E:558, 2010.

Lomita C, Ezaki M, Oishi S: Upper extremity surgery in children with cerebral palsy, *J Am Acad Orthop Surg* 18:160, 2010.

Patterson JM, Wang AA, Hutchinson DT: Late deformities following the transfer of the flexor carpi ulnaris to the extensor carpi radialis brevis in children with cerebral palsy, *J Hand Surg Am* 35:1774, 2010.

Tomhave WA, Van Heest AE, Bagley A, James MA: Affected and contralateral hand strength and dexterity measures in children with hemiplegic cerebral palsy, *J Hand Surg Am* 40:900, 2015.

Van Heest AE: Surgical technique for thumb-in-palm deformity in cerebral palsy, *J Hand Surg Am* 36A:1526, 2011.

Van Heest A, Stout J, Wervey R, Garcia L: Follow-up motion laboratory analysis for patients with spastic hemiplegia due to cerebral palsy: analysis of the flexor carpi ulnaris firing pattern before and after tendon transfer surgery, *J Hand Surg Am* 35(2):284, 2010.

The complete list of references is available online at ExpertConsult.com.

SUPPLEMENTAL REFERENCES

Arner M, Eliasson A-C, Nicklasson S, et al.: Hand function in cerebral palsy: report of 367 children in a population-based longitudinal health care program, *J Hand Surg Am* 33A:1337, 2008.

Atwater SW, Tatarka ME, Kathrein JE, et al.: Electromyography-triggered electrical muscle stimulation for children with cerebral palsy: a pilot study, *Pediatr Phys Ther* 3:190, 1991.

Braun RM, Vice BT: Sublimis to profundus transfers in the hemiplegic upper extremity, *J Bone Joint Surg* 55A:873, 1973.

Bunata RE: Pronator teres rerouting in children with cerebral palsy, *J Hand Surg Am* 31A:474, 2006, e1–474.e11.

Carlson MG, Athwal GS, Bueno RE: Treatment of the wrist and hand in cerebral palsy, *J Hand Surg Am* 31A:483–490, 2006.

Carlson MG, Gallegher K, Spirtos M: Surgical treatment of swan-neck deformity in hemiplegic cerebral palsy, *J Hand Surg Am* 32A:1418, 2007.

Carlson MG, Spincola LJ, Lewin J, McDermott E: Impact of video review on surgical procedure determination for patients with cerebral palsy, *J Hand Surg Am* 34A:1225, 2009.

Carmick J: Use of neuromuscular electrical stimulation and a dorsal wrist splint to improve the hand function of a child with spastic hemiparesis, *Phys Ther* 77:661, 1997.

Chait LA, Kaplan I, Stewart-Lord B, et al.: Early surgical correction in the cerebral palsied hand, *J Hand Surg Am* 5A 122, 1980.

Chin TYP, Duncan JA, Johnstone BR, Graham HK: Management of the upper limb in cerebral palsy, *J Pediatr Orthop B* 14:389, 2005.

Chin TYP, Graham HK: Botulinum toxin A in the management of upper limb spasticity in cerebral palsy, *Hand Clin* 19:591, 2003.

Corry IS, Cosgrove AP, Walsh EG, et al.: Botulinum toxin A in the hemiplegic upper limb: a double-blind trial, *Dev Med Child Neurol* 39:185, 1997.

Curtis RM: Treatment of injuries of proximal interphalangeal joints of fingers. In Adams JP, editor: *Current practice in orthopaedic surgery*, vol. 2. St. Louis, 1964, Mosby.

Dahlin LB, Komoto-Tufvesson Y, Salgeback S: Surgery of the spastic hand in cerebral palsy: improvement in stereognosis and hand function after surgery, *J Hand Surg Am* 23B:334, 1998.

Davids JR, Sebesan VJ, Ortmann F, et al.: Surgical management of thumb deformity in children with hemiplegic-type cerebral palsy, *J Pediatr Orthop* 29:504, 2009.

Denislic M, Meh D: Botulinum toxin in the treatment of cerebral palsy, *Neuropediatrics* 26:249, 1995.

El-Said NS: Selective release of the flexor origin with transfer of the flexor carpi ulnaris in cerebral palsy, *J Bone Joint Surg* 83B:259, 2001.

Fehlings D, Rang M, Glazier J, et al.: An evaluation of the botulinum-A toxin injections to improve upper extremity function in children with hemiplegic cerebral palsy, *J Pediatr* 137:321, 2000.

Goldner JL: Surgical reconstruction of the upper extremity in cerebral palsy, *Instr Course Lect* 36:207, 1987.

Goldner JL: Surgical reconstruction of the upper extremity in cerebral palsy, *Hand Clin* 4:223, 1988.

Goldner JL, Koman LA, Gelberman R, et al.: Arthrodesis of the metacarpophalangeal joint of the thumb in children and adults, *Clin Orthop Relat Res* 253:75, 1990.

Green NE: Cerebral palsy. In Canale ST, Beaty JH, editors: *Operative pediatric orthopaedics*, St. Louis, 1991, Mosby.

Green WT, Banks HH: Flexor carpi ulnaris transplant and its use in cerebral palsy, *J Bone Joint Surg* 44A:1343, 1962.

Gschwind CR: Surgical management of forearm pronation, *Hand Clin* 19:649, 2003.

Gschwind C, Tonkin M: Surgery for cerebral palsy, part 1: classification and operative procedures for pronation deformity, *J Hand Surg Am* 17B:391, 1992.

Hargreaves DG, Warwick DJ, Tonkin MA: Changes in hand function following wrist arthrodesis in cerebral palsy, *J Hand Surg Am* 25B:193, 2000.

Hoffer MM, Leham M, Mitani M: Long-term follow-up on tendon transfers to the extensors of the wrist and fingers in patients with cerebral palsy, *J Hand Surg Am* 11A 836, 1986.

Hoffer MM, Lehman M, Mitani M: Surgical indications in children with cerebral palsy, *Hand Clin* 5:69, 1989.

Hoffer MM, Perry J, Garcia M, et al.: Adduction contracture of the thumb in cerebral palsy: a preoperative electromyographic study, *J Bone Joint Surg* 65A:755, 1983.

Hoffer MM, Perry J, Melkonian GJ: Dynamic electromyography and decision-making for surgery in the upper extremity of patients with cerebral palsy, *J Hand Surg Am* 4A:424, 1979.

Hoffer MM, Zeitzew S: Wrist fusion in cerebral palsy, *J Hand Surg Am 13A* 667, 1988.

House JH, Gwathney FW, Fidler MO: A dynamic approach to the thumb-in-palm deformity in cerebral palsy: evaluation and results in fifty-six patients, *J Bone Joint Surg* 63A:216, 1981.

House JH, Shannon MA: Restoration of strong grasp and lateral pinch in tetraplegia: a comparison of two methods of thumb control in each patient, *J Hand Surg Am* 10A:21, 1985.

Hurvitz EA, Conti GE, Flansburg EL, et al.: Motor control testing of upper limb function after botulinum toxin injection: a case study, *Arch Phys Med Rehabil* 81:1408, 2000.

Inglis AE, Cooper W: Release of the flexor-pronator origin for flexion deformities of the hand and wrist in spastic paralysis: a study of eighteen cases, *J Bone Joint Surg* 48A:847, 1966.

Inglis AE, Cooper W, Bruton W: Surgical correction of thumb deformities in spastic paralysis, *J Bone Joint Surg* 52A:253, 1970.

Koman LA, Gelberman RH, Toby EB, et al.: Cerebral palsy: management of the upper extremity, *Clin Orthop Relat Res* 253:62, 1990.

Kreulen M, Smeulders MJC, Veeger HEJ, et al.: Three-dimensional video analysis of forearm rotation before and after combined pronator teres rerouting and flexor carpi ulnaris tendon transfer surgery in patients with cerebral palsy, *J Hand Surg Am* 29B:55, 2004.

Lawson RD, Tonkin MA: Surgical management of the thumb in cerebral palsy, *Hand Clin* 19:667, 2003.

Manske PR: Redirection of extensor pollicis longus in the treatment of spastic thumb-in-palm deformity, *J Hand Surg Am 10A* 553, 1985.

Manske PR: Cerebral palsy of the upper extremity, *Hand Clin* 6:697, 1990.

Matev IB: Surgical treatment of spastic "thumb-in-palm" deformity, *J Bone Joint Surg* 45B:703, 1963.

Matev IB: Surgical treatment of flexion-adduction contracture of the thumb in cerebral palsy, *Acta Orthop Scand* 41:439, 1970.

Matev IB: Thumb reconstruction through metacarpal bone lengthening, *J Hand Surg Am* 5:482, 1980.

Matsuo T, Matsuo A, Hajime T, et al.: Release of flexors and intrinsic muscles for finger spasticity in cerebral palsy, *Clin Orthop Relat Res* 384:162, 2001.

Mital MA, Sakellarides HT: Surgery of the upper extremity in the retarded individual with spastic cerebral palsy, *Orthop Clin North Am* 12:127, 1981.

Mowery CA, Gelberman RH, Rhoades CE: Upper extremity tendon transfers in cerebral palsy: electromyographic and functional analysis, *J Pediatr Orthop* 5:69, 1985.

Nossaman BC, Rayan GM: Extensor tendon dislocation in cerebral palsy, *J Hand Surg Am* 24B:233, 1999.

Omer GE, Capen DA: Proximal row carpectomy with muscle transfers for spastic paralysis, *J Hand Surg Am* 1A:197, 1976.

Ozkan T, Aydin A, Ozer K, et al.: A surgical technique for pediatric forearm pronation: brachioradialis rerouting with interosseous membrane release, *J Hand Surg Am* 29A:22, 2004.

Ozkan T, Tuncer S, Aydin A, et al.: Brachioradialis rerouting for the restoration of active supination and correction of forearm pronation deformity in cerebral palsy, *J Hand Surg Am* 29B:265, 2004.

Page CM: An operation for the relief of flexion-contracture in the forearm, *J Bone Joint Surg* 21:233, 1923.

Rayan GM, Young BT: Arthrodesis of the spastic wrist, *J Hand Surg Am* 24A:944, 1999.

Sakellarides HT, Mital MA, Lenzi WD: Treatment of pronation contractures of the forearm in cerebral palsy, *J Bone Joint Surg* 63A:645, 1981.

Sakellarides HT, Mital MA, Lenzi WD: Treatment of pronation contractures of the forearm in cerebral palsy by changing the insertion of the pronator radii teres, *J Bone Joint Surg* 63A:645, 1982.

Scheker LR, Ozer K: Electrical stimulation in the management of spastic deformity, *Hand Clin* 19:601, 2003.

Sherk HH: Treatment of severe rigid contractures of cerebral palsied upper limbs, *Clin Orthop Relat Res* 125:151, 1977.

Skoff H, Woodbury DF: Current concepts review: management of the upper extremity in cerebral palsy, *J Bone Joint Surg* 67A:500, 1985.

Smeulders MJ, Kreulen CA, Surgical treatment for the thumb-in-palm deformity in patients with cerebral palsy [review]: *The Cochrane Collaboration*, John Wiley & Sons Ltd, 20092009. www.thecochranelibrary.com.

Smith RJ: Flexor pollicis longus abductor-plasty for spastic thumb-in-palm deformity, *J Hand Surg Am* 7A:327, 1982.

Strecker WB, Emanuel JP, Dailey L, et al.: Comparison of pronator tenotomy and pronator rerouting in children with spastic cerebral palsy, *J Hand Surg Am* 13A:540, 1988.

Swanson AB: Surgery of the hand in cerebral palsy and the swan-neck deformity, *J Bone Joint Surg* 42A:951, 1960.

Swanson AB: Surgery of the hand in cerebral palsy, *Surg Clin North Am* 44:1061, 1964.

Swanson AB: Treatment of the swan-neck deformity in the cerebral palsied hand, *Clin Orthop Relat Res* 48:167, 1966.

Swanson AB: Surgery of the hand in cerebral palsy and muscle origin release procedures, *Surg Clin North Am* 48:1129, 1968.

Tonkin M, Freitas A, Leclercq C, et al.: *The surgical management of thumb deformity in cerebral palsy. IFSSH cerebral palsy Committee report*, 2007. http://sagepub.com. .

Tonkin MA, Hatrick NC, Eckersley JRT, et al.: Surgery for cerebral palsy, part 3: classification and operative procedures for thumb deformity, *J Hand Surg Am* 26B:465, 2001.

Tonkin MA, Hughes J, Smith KL: Lateral band translocation for swan-neck deformity, *J Hand Surg Am* 17A:260, 1992.

Van Heest AE: Surgical management of wrist and finger deformity, *Hand Clin* 19:657, 2003.

Van Heest AE, House JA, Cariello C: Upper extremity surgical treatment of cerebral palsy, *J Hand Surg Am* 24A:323, 1999.

Van Heest AE, Ramachandran V, Stout J, et al.: Quantitative and qualitative functional evaluation of upper extremity tendon transfers in spastic hemiplegia caused by cerebral palsy, *J Pediatr Orthop* 28:679, 2008.

Van Munster JC, Maathuis KGB, Haga N, et al.: Does surgical management of the hand in children with spastic unilateral cerebral palsy affect functional outcome? *Dev Med Child Neurol* 49:385, 2007.

Wenner SM, Johnson KA: Transfer of the flexor carpi ulnaris to the radial wrist extensors in cerebral palsy, *J Hand Surg Am* 13A:231, 1988.

Westdock KA, Kott K, Sharps C: Pre- and postsurgical evaluation of hand function in hemiplegic cerebral palsy: exemplar cases, *J Hand Surg Am* 21:386, 2008.

Williams R, Haddad RJ: Release of flexor origin for spastic deformities of the wrist and hand, *South Med J* 60:1033, 1967.

Wolf TM, Clinkscales CM, Hamlin C: Flexor carpi ulnaris tendon transfers in cerebral palsy, *J Hand Surg Am* 23B:340, 1998.

Wright PA, Granat MH: Improvement in hand function and wrist range of motion following electrical stimulation of wrist extensor muscles in an adult with cerebral palsy, *Clin Rehabil* 14:244, 2000.

Wright PA, Granat MH: Therapeutic effects of functional electrical stimulation of the upper limb of eight children with cerebral palsy, *Dev Med Child Neurol* 42:724, 2000.

Zancolli EA, Goldner LJ, Swanson AB: Surgery of the spastic hand in cerebral palsy: report of the Committee on Spastic Hand Evaluation, *J Hand Surg Am* 8A:766, 1983.-->

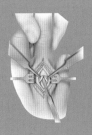

CHAPTER 10

ARTHRITIC HAND

James H. Calandruccio

RHEUMATOID ARTHRITIS

Rheumatoid arthritis is the most common idiopathic inflammatory arthritis, affecting approximately 0.8% of the population, and it is two to four times more common in women than in men. The disease is characterized by hypertrophic synovitis that leads to joint laxity from soft-tissue attenuation, which may lead to joint subluxation and dislocation. Joint cartilage destruction usually ensues and may lead to attritional tendon rupture. However, isolated nodular tendon involvement may exist independent of overt joint pathology, leading to joint motion limitation, such as triggering or locking of flexor tendons. Similarly, extensor tendon nodularity may limit wrist extension from impingement on the extensor retinaculum. Despite preservation of function, socialization sometimes is altered by disfiguring deformities, especially of the hands.

At various times in the disease course, treatment of patients with rheumatoid arthritis involves a management team, including a rheumatologist, internist, other medical specialists, surgeon, therapist, and counselor. Operative treatment should be considered a part of the general disease management.

Since the introduction of medical therapies, such as disease modifying antirheumatic drugs in the mid-1990s and biologics in the early 2000s, there has been an 83% reduction in rheumatoid hand surgery in the United Kingdom. This indicates that medical treatments and strategies have been successful at preventing disease progression. Patients with rheumatologic diseases, however, may present initially to a hand surgeon with varied symptoms and signs without a specific diagnosis. When the history, physical examination, and radiographs suggest a rheumatologic condition, nonsurgical management may be more appropriate.

Rheumatoid arthritis patients may be treated with one or more medications, such as nonsteroidal antiinflammatory drugs (NSAIDs), corticosteroids, and disease-modifying antirheumatic drugs, which may have significant side effects. Because of their effect on platelets, salicylates usually are discontinued 1 to 2 weeks before surgery; NSAIDs should be discontinued 2 to 5 days before surgery. Patients who have taken corticosteroids for more than a 3-week period in the previous 12 months should receive supplemental corticosteroid therapy before, during, and after surgery. Side effects of patient prescription and nonprescription medications, including those used for their arthritic condition, should be considered before surgery. In some cases, perioperative medical management by an internist is warranted.

If a general anesthetic is to be used during an operation on a patient with rheumatoid arthritis, the alignment and stability of the cervical spine should be investigated before surgery. If the disease has been generalized and prolonged, radiographs of the cervical spine are indicated to discover any subluxations. The degree of cervical spine instability alerts the anesthesiologist to the possibility of spinal cord injury that may result from hyperextension or hyperflexion of the neck during intubation or while maintaining a free airway. Extensive involvement of the temporomandibular joint also may influence the approach to endotracheal intubation.

Procedures usually considered for patients with rheumatoid arthritis include tenosynovectomy, tendon repair or realignment, synovectomy, arthroplasty, and arthrodesis. The goals of surgery are to relieve pain, restore function, correct or prevent deformity, and inhibit disease progression. If pain is not the primary consideration, the surgeon should have a reasonable level of confidence that the selected procedure can restore enough function to justify the surgery. Conversely, if pain can be significantly relieved by a surgical procedure, it is worthwhile when adequate medical treatment has failed to do so. Although patients may complain principally of pain, cosmesis is an important consideration for some, if not most. Hand appearance and pain relief are highly correlated with patient satisfaction. If rheumatoid synovitis or tenosynovitis persists despite good medical treatment and supervision, synovectomy and tenosynovectomy are worthwhile prophylactic procedures that may help delay further distention of the joint capsule and ligament, as well as prevent tendon rupture.

Before surgery, the patient is advised of the details of the anticipated procedure. This usually includes information about (1) the location of incisions, (2) anticipated implants required for the surgical procedure(s), (3) the expected appearance after surgery, (4) the type of anesthesia, (5) the alternatives to and risks of surgery, (6) the postoperative care and the rehabilitation period, and especially (7) the expected benefit from the operation. Patients with severe deformities may have developed substitution patterns that enable them to perform their daily tasks; these should not be interrupted without careful analysis of the pathologic anatomy

and functional patterns. This is especially true in older, retired individuals who have no pain. The patient should be advised emphatically that surgery neither cures the disease nor restores the hand to normal. It is helpful for the patient to understand that although many deformities are correctable, the local progression of the disease may not be altered by surgical procedures.

Rheumatoid hand deformities usually are bilateral and symmetric. Each deformity must be analyzed in detail before surgery is considered. Although combinations of deformities occur, involvement of the fingers, thumb, and wrist is typical. The metacarpophalangeal joints and the wrist are affected early in rheumatoid arthritis, whereas the distal joints usually are affected later. The metacarpophalangeal is the most important joint affecting finger function in rheumatoid disease. Finger ulnar deviation with metacarpophalangeal palmar subluxation or dislocation typifies the rheumatoid hand deformity. Ligamentous, osteochondral, and intraarticular damage and the forces applied through the intrinsic and extrinsic muscles at the metacarpophalangeal joint affect the metacarpophalangeal joint deformities and at the proximal and distal interphalangeal joints. The disease extent and wrist deformity affect finger joint deformities. In addition to the typical metacarpophalangeal deformities, the proximal interphalangeal joints may develop boutonniere or swanneck deformities, and the distal interphalangeal joints, when affected, usually develop a mallet or hyperflexed deformity, depending on the extent of capsular disruption (Fig. 10.1).

Thumb involvement can cause a variety of deformities, depending on the joint in which synovitis begins. Synovitis beginning in the thumb metacarpophalangeal joint frequently leads to a boutonniere deformity of the thumb, with palmar subluxation of the proximal phalanx and subsequent metacarpophalangeal joint flexion, and interphalangeal joint hyperextension (Fig. 10.2). When synovitis begins in the thumb

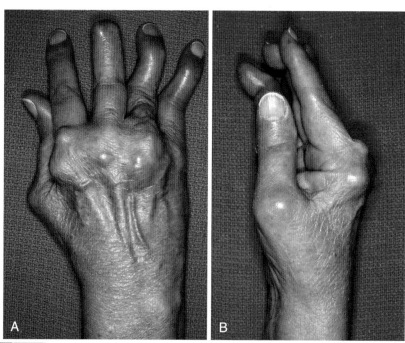

FIGURE 10.1   A and **B,** Rheumatoid swan-neck deformities of varying severity in all fingers. Metacarpophalangeal synovitis and subluxation and flexion contractures also are present.

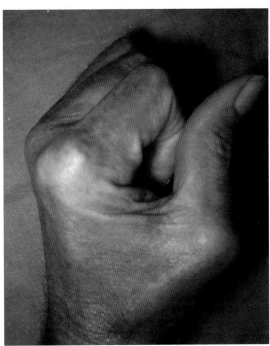

Thumb with fixed rheumatoid boutonniere deformity with metacarpophalangeal flexion and interphalangeal hyperextension (type I deformity).

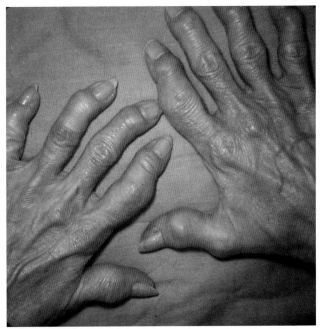

Osteoarthritic hands with Heberden (distal interphalangeal) and Bouchard (proximal interphalangeal) nodes on both index fingers and thumbs. Note angular changes at distal joints as result of loss of joint cartilage and instability.

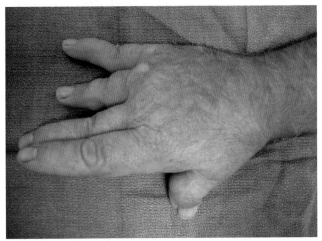

"Main en lorgnette" (opera glass hand). Late changes in progressive rheumatoid arthritis.

carpometacarpal (CMC) joint, the deformity includes dorsal subluxation of the metacarpal base and hyperextension of the metacarpophalangeal joint (swan-neck deformity). Another thumb deformity caused by synovitic destruction of the capsuloligamentous supports on the ulnar side of the metacarpophalangeal joint is the gamekeeper thumb, which results from laxity of the ulnar collateral ligament of the thumb metacarpophalangeal joint. Involvement of the metacarpophalangeal joint also can result in laxity of the capsuloligamentous structures in the volar plate, leading to hyperextension of the metacarpophalangeal joint and interphalangeal hyperflexion, but with a stable CMC joint. Other, more severe deformities of the fingers and thumb can be caused by an erosive rheumatoid disease, leading to the "main en lorgnette" (opera-glass hand; Fig. 10.3).

Significant flexor and extensor tendon tenosynovitis in the digits, palm, and over the wrist flexor and extensor surfaces can lead to erosive and attritional changes and tendon ruptures. Rheumatoid wrist deformities have a significant effect on hand function, especially the metacarpophalangeal joint finger position. Rheumatoid synovitis can result in intercarpal ligament disruption, especially the radioscaphocapitate ligament, leading to rotatory instability of the carpal scaphoid and subsequent destructive changes throughout the entire wrist. The distal radioulnar joint stabilizing ligaments are destroyed in a similar fashion, leading to ulnar head dorsal dislocation and subluxation of the extensor carpi ulnaris tendon with secondary ulnar translocation of the carpus.

OSTEOARTHRITIS

Osteoarthritis is the most common arthritic hand disorder. The condition may be unilateral but occurs as frequently in the nondominant hand as in the dominant one. Although it can be associated with tendon ruptures and triggering of fingers, these are not seen as frequently in osteoarthritis as in rheumatoid arthritis. It frequently is seen at the trapeziometacarpal joint, more often in women, and sometimes as a single joint involvement. Osteophytes that form at the distal interphalangeal joint are known as *Heberden nodes*. Mucoid cysts may form at the joint margins. At the proximal interphalangeal joint, such osteophytes are known as *Bouchard nodes* (Fig. 10.4). Spur formation, cartilage fragmentation, and limited motion without dislocation are common. During the active phase, pain is severe and the joints and overlying skin may be inflamed; direct trauma to an inflamed joint is especially painful. Osteoarthritis may be the natural consequence of longevity; however, the etiology of early onset of osteoarthritis and its prevention remain elusive. Moreover, osteoarthritic

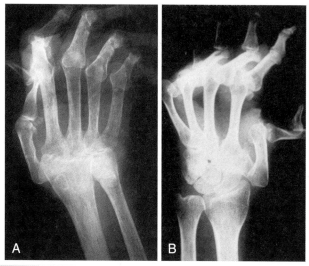

radiographic signs often do not correlate with symptoms or the severity of patient's pain complaints. Asymptomatic scapholunate advanced collapse wrist deformities are common, as are thumb basal and finger joint degeneration, and explanations and effective initial treatments must be individualized.

SYSTEMIC LUPUS ERYTHEMATOSUS

Systemic lupus erythematosus, one of the diffuse connective tissue diseases, can affect many organ systems. Pericarditis, pleuritis, and renal disease represent involvement of major organ systems. Cutaneous involvement is present in 85% of patients with this condition. Musculoskeletal involvement is characterized by stiffness, swelling, tenderness, and pain, with tendons, joint capsules, and ligaments particularly involved. Joint surface destruction can occur late in the disease process. Hand involvement may be among the earliest manifestations. Usually the metacarpophalangeal and proximal interphalangeal joints are involved, as first manifested by ligamentous laxity. Raynaud phenomenon, with tissue necrosis, ulceration, and cold intolerance, also is seen. Although the hand deformities of systemic lupus erythematosus are similar to rheumatoid hand deformities, they result primarily from soft-tissue abnormalities unrelated to proliferative synovitis, and the articular cartilage is well preserved (Fig. 10.5). Soft-tissue procedures (capsulodesis, tenodesis, tendon realignment), bone procedures (arthrodesis, arthroplasty), and digital sympathectomy for relief of the digital ischemia of Raynaud phenomenon may be necessary in patients with systemic lupus erythematosus.

PSORIATIC ARTHRITIS

An estimated 25% of patients with psoriatic arthritis have polyarthritis similar to rheumatoid arthritis; 5% to 10% have distal interphalangeal joint involvement. About 15% to

20% develop the typical psoriatic rash after they develop the arthritis. Almost 95% of patients with psoriatic arthritis have asymmetric peripheral joint involvement. Fusiform swelling of the entire digit may occur. Uniquely, the nails may separate from the nail bed and have a white, flaking discoloration near their distal borders; they also may be ridged. Fingernail changes, the most common of which is pitting, are reported to be present in about 15% of patients with joint involvement (Fig. 10.6). Radiographic changes in psoriatic arthritis of the hand include erosion of terminal phalangeal tufts (acroosteolysis), tapering of the phalanges and metacarpals, cupping of the proximal ends of phalanges and metacarpals ("pencil-in-cup" deformity), severe destruction or ankylosis of isolated small joints, and a predilection for the interphalangeal joints with sparing of the metacarpophalangeal joints. Contractures of the proximal interphalangeal joints most often require surgical treatment, usually arthrodesis. Patients with psoriatic arthritis can, in general, be placed into three groups, depending on the timing of the onset of the arthritis and the skin lesions. Patients with type 1 disease have early onset of joint involvement with late development of skin lesions. Those with type 2 disease have late joint involvement and early skin changes. In type 3, there is almost simultaneous onset of joint and skin involvement. In patients with type 1, the arthritic involvement is mild, whereas in type 2 the arthritis is more severe. In patients with type 3, the severity of arthritic involvement is unpredictable. Although fusion or arthroplasty may improve hand function, infection may occur more frequently after implant arthroplasty in these patients than in patients with rheumatoid disease. Scheduling surgical procedures during summer months has been recommended, because the skin lesions tend to be smaller and may be less likely to pose a significant risk of infection.

REITER SYNDROME

Reiter syndrome is described as a triad of conjunctivitis, urethritis, and synovitis. The synovitis usually involves asymmetrically four or fewer joints. Heel pain, back pain, and nail deformities may occur in this syndrome, sometimes making it difficult to distinguish it from psoriatic arthritis. It affects the lower extremity more often than the upper, and 90% of patients have remission of symptoms after several weeks; in about 10%, the disease may become chronic. It is typically found in young men. Surgery rarely is indicated.

GOUT

Gout usually causes an erythematous, painful joint in men. The attack often is sudden with severe pain around a single joint. The joint is swollen, hot, and tender, suggesting a severe cellulitis or abscess. In chronic gout, massive deposits of monosodium urate crystals can be found around the joints and tendon sheaths, causing nerve compression, such as carpal tunnel syndrome. Intratendinous monosodium urate crystal deposition can lead to tendon rupture. The skin may be ulcerated by pressure from within (Fig. 10.7). Amputation may be necessary because of the extreme bony disruption resulting from gout. The deposits may be visible on radiographs. Women rarely have gouty arthritis until after menopause; however, the typical patient with tophaceous gout is an elderly woman. The presence of hyperuricemia alone

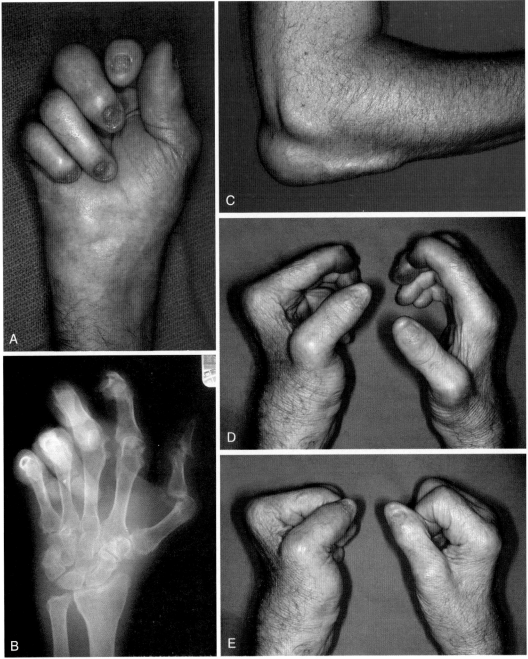

FIGURE 10.6 Common findings of psoriatic arthritis. **A,** Pitted nail deformities. **B,** Metacarpophalangeal joint dislocations and thumb interphalangeal joint destruction. **C,** Typical psoriatic elbow lesion. **D** and **E,** Right-hand limited finger flexion and extension after metacarpal arthroplasty.

does not establish the diagnosis of gout; the uric acid level may be elevated, and an acute attack of gout may never occur. Conversely, during an acute attack of gout, the uric acid level may be normal. Joint aspiration provides the only definitive diagnosis of gout, and polarized microscopy usually shows negatively birefringent crystals in the joint fluid. Surgery for tophaceous deposits rarely is indicated, unless an important structure is compressed or if the patient cannot tolerate uric acid–lowering measures. In addition to tophus excision and debridement, other procedures that may benefit a patient with gout include tenosynovectomy, tendon repair, or transfer for

tendon ruptures, carpal tunnel release, and appropriate management of destroyed gouty arthritic joints.

Pseudogout, also known as calcium pyrophosphate dihydrate crystal deposition disease, although more common in the knee, may involve the hands and can mimic septic arthritis. Clinically, it is characterized by intermittent acute attacks resembling acute gouty arthritis. It may be associated with a flexor tenosynovitis, leading to carpal tunnel syndrome. Calcium pyrophosphate crystal deposition may be visible on routine radiographs as opaque areas in the articular cartilage or the fibrocartilaginous disc of the distal radioulnar

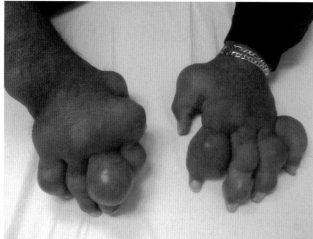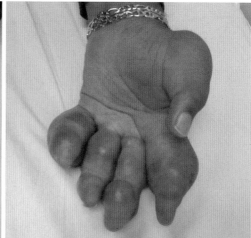

FIGURE 10.7 Severe gout in multiple joints of the hand of a 54-year-old man. Heavy calcium urate deposits have caused severe deformities of all fingers.

joint, and definitive diagnosis is made by the identification of calcium pyrophosphate crystals in the joint aspirate. As with gout, initial management is medical.

SCLERODERMA (PROGRESSIVE SYSTEMIC SCLEROSIS)

Two types of scleroderma are recognized: progressive systemic sclerosis and CREST (calcinosis, Raynaud phenomenon, esophageal dysmotility, sclerodactyly, and telangiectasia) syndrome. Diffuse scleroderma, or progressive systemic sclerosis, is usually more severe and affects the extremities and the trunk. The disease may involve not only the skin but also the gastrointestinal tract, especially the esophagus, heart, lungs, and kidneys. Telangiectasia also may be seen. The hand surgeon may see these patients because of calcinosis of the fingertips, ulcerations, or Raynaud phenomenon. The age at onset usually is older than 40 years.

Arthritic involvement usually causes finger contractures, but synovial thickening is minimal. Involvement of hand tendons and tendon sheaths can cause a palpable tendon friction rub or a leathery crepitus, as distinguished from the coarse, gritty crepitus palpable in osteoarthritis. Extensor tendons may rupture at the interphalangeal joint as they become attenuated, the overlying skin breaks down, and the joint may be exposed. Changes at the distal interphalangeal joint include skin ulceration, joint contracture, gangrene, and osteomyelitis. The usual surgical choices for these changes at the distal joint are amputation and arthrodesis.

At the proximal interphalangeal joint, scleroderma changes lead to the previously mentioned flexion contractures. Because the severe contracture of all structures limits the potential for movement, arthrodesis is usually the best choice for the proximal interphalangeal joint.

Metacarpophalangeal joint flexion or hyperextension deformities may occur. Resection arthroplasty has been found to be an effective method to preserve joint motion. If there is a flexion deformity, the metacarpophalangeal joint is approached through a dorsal incision. If the metacarpophalangeal joint is hyperextended with proximal interphalangeal joint flexion, Nalebuff recommended approaching the metacarpophalangeal joint through a palmar incision to perform the metacarpal head resection, followed by proximal interphalangeal joint fusion.

Thumb web adduction contractures may require adductor pollicis muscle release with trapezial excision. Thumb metacarpophalangeal and interphalangeal joint fusions may be required.

Fingertip ulceration from vascular impairment is best treated by an extremely conservative approach, including waiting for the tips to amputate spontaneously, because this retains digital length. Surgical sympathectomies and intra-arterial injection of vasodilating drugs have been effective in improving digital circulation. Although recurrence of ischemic changes may follow procedures on the vessels, the short-term result can be beneficial for wound healing and pain relief. Calcification around the eroded fingertip pulps may be excised through a lateral incision, or they may be curetted, but healing may be slow.

NONOPERATIVE TREATMENT OF SYNOVITIS AND TENOSYNOVITIS

Persistent tenosynovitis or arthritis with obvious swelling that persists for several weeks even when treated with antiinflammatory drugs can be treated by local injections of a steroid preparation and a local anesthetic. In many instances, pain may be relieved and surgery delayed by this technique.

This treatment is especially applicable to trigger fingers, carpal tunnel syndrome, and trapeziometacarpal joint osteoarthritis. Osteoarthritis of the distal interphalangeal joints and rheumatoid arthritis of the proximal interphalangeal joints also respond favorably to injections for several weeks; however, after repeated injections, the response may be less dramatic. If synovitis and tenosynovitis persist after 4 to 6 months of adequate medical therapy, consideration should be given to synovectomy or tenosynovectomy.

RHEUMATOID NODULES

Rheumatoid subcutaneous nodules occur on the dorsum of the hand, palmar surface of the fingers and thumb,

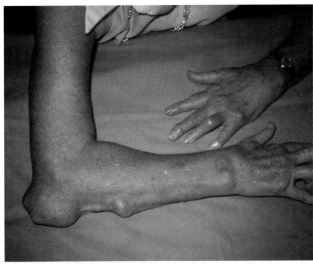

FIGURE 10.8 Rheumatoid nodules in olecranon bursa and on subcutaneous surface of ulna.

subcutaneous border of the ulna, and in the olecranon bursa (Fig. 10.8). They may interfere with finger motion because of their size; they may be uncomfortable and are at risk for ulceration. If the nodules cause sufficient symptoms, they can be removed. Care should be taken to avoid injuring neurovascular structures, which may be adherent to the larger masses.

STAGING OF OPERATIONS

When considering operative procedures for patients with rheumatoid arthritis, all aspects of the musculoskeletal involvement should be considered. The extent to which pain limits function is given high priority. Patients who function well despite significant deformity may be less inclined to have a surgical procedure than patients whose activities are limited by pain. Souter recommended starting with a procedure that is likely to succeed, beginning with the least involved hand. He grouped hand procedures from the most effective (group I) to the least effective (group V) (Table 10.1). In addition, Souter advocated correcting significant disease and deformity in the elbow and shoulder before correcting hand deformities. Surgical priorities are, in descending order of importance, the spine, foot, hip, knee, wrist, shoulder, thumb, elbow, and fingers. Each patient should be considered individually, and the patient's requirements and the forces and demands on the extremity should be considered.

When several operations are indicated on a single hand, their order of priority must be considered. Persistent tenosynovitis, tendon rupture, and nerve compression are high-priority problems. In general, when wrist arthroplasty or arthrodesis is indicated, it should be done first because the position of the wrist determines the balance of the digital flexor and extensor tendons. At the time of wrist surgery, an additional procedure, such as arthrodesis of the metacarpophalangeal joint of the thumb, can be done. Other, more extensive surgery usually is best delayed.

When multiple small joint procedures, such as metacarpophalangeal arthroplasties or proximal interphalangeal joint fusions, are to be performed, they can be done at the same time. Frequently, a patient with rheumatoid arthritis requires surgery not only on the opposite hand but also on the feet,

TABLE 10.1

Grading of Surgical Procedures for Rheumatoid Arthritis (Souter)

GROUP	PROCEDURE
I	Fusion of thumb MCP joint
	Extensor synovectomy and Darrach procedure
II	Flexor synovectomy
	MCP joint arthroplasty
III	PIP joint fusion
	Wrist stabilization
IV	Swan-neck correction
	MCP, PIP joint synovectomy
	Thumb IP joint fusion
V	PIP joint arthroplasty
	Boutonniere correction

IP, Interphalangeal; *MCP*, metacarpophalangeal; *PIP*, proximal interphalangeal.
From Souter WA: Planning treatment of the rheumatoid hand, *Hand* 11:3, 1979.

the hips, and other joints. Usually, surgery is performed on only one hand at a given time because of the requirements for daily independent living and personal hygiene. If the lower extremities require external support, a platform or forearm crutch should be provided.

FINGER DEFORMITIES CAUSED BY RHEUMATOID ARTHRITIS

Finger deformities can be caused by the normal forces applied to damaged joints by the extrinsic flexors and extensors, tightness of the intrinsic muscles, displacement of the lateral bands of the extensor hood, central slip rupture, or rupture of the long extensor or long flexor tendons. Abnormal forces also act on joints already weakened by the disease. In addition, flexor tenosynovitis may produce limitation of interphalangeal joint motion, so the range of active flexion of these joints is significantly less than passive flexion.

INTRINSIC PLUS DEFORMITY

The intrinsic plus deformity is caused by excessive intrinsic muscle tension, in which the proximal interphalangeal joint cannot be flexed fully when the metacarpophalangeal joint is fully extended. Often, the deformity develops in combination with volar subluxation of the metacarpophalangeal joints and ulnar deviation of the fingers. The Bunnell test is a test for intrinsic tightness; the degree of passive proximal interphalangeal joint flexion is compared with the metacarpophalangeal joint in full extension (intrinsic muscles stretched) and full flexion (intrinsic muscles relaxed). Variable degrees of passive proximal interphalangeal joint flexion loss with the metacarpophalangeal joint in extension indicates intrinsic tightness (Fig. 10.9). With ulnar drift of the fingers, this intrinsic tightness may be present only on the ulnar side. To test this accurately, axial alignment of the finger with the metacarpal should be maintained in checking intrinsic tightness. Any ulnar deviation at the metacarpophalangeal joint during the test slackens the intrinsics on the ulnar side of the finger and may confuse the findings. A tight first volar interosseous

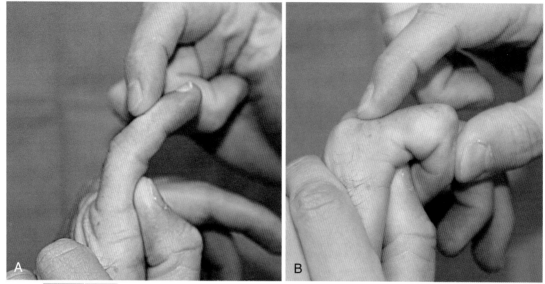

FIGURE **10.9**   Test for intrinsic tightness. **A,** Proximal interphalangeal (PIP) joint passive flexion is limited with the metacarpophalangeal (MP) joint in full extension. **B,** Full PIP joint flexion possible from intrinsic relaxation when the MP joint is fully flexed.

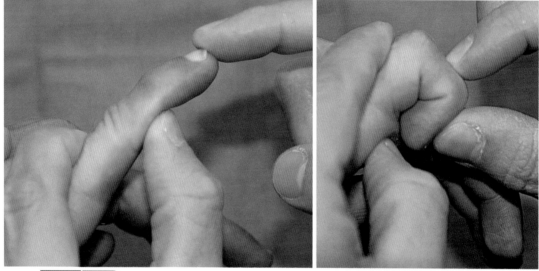

FIGURE **10.10**   Test for tightness of oblique retinacular ligament. Proximal interphalangeal joint held in maximal extension by examiner. Resistance to passive flexion of distal interphalangeal joint is evaluated.

muscle pulls the extended index finger ulnarward, but if the finger is held in line with the second metacarpal during the test, then tightness of this muscle can be shown.

Tightness in the oblique retinacular ligament can be shown by maintaining the proximal interphalangeal joint in extension while testing the distal interphalangeal joint resistance to passive flexion (Fig. 10.10). This can be helpful when evaluating a digit with a boutonniere deformity.

When indicated, intrinsic tightness can be released in conjunction with synovectomy by lateral band mobilization. When degeneration of the metacarpophalangeal joints requires arthroplasty, there may be sufficient resection of

bone to relax the intrinsic mechanism; however, it must be determined specifically at the time of surgery when a release is necessary. A specific tendon release of the intrinsics may be indicated (see Technique 10.5).

SWAN-NECK DEFORMITY

Swan-neck deformity is characterized by a flexion posture of the distal interphalangeal joint and hyperextension posture of the proximal interphalangeal joint (Fig. 10.11). It is caused by muscle imbalance and may be passively correctable, depending on the original and secondary deformities (Fig. 10.12). Although usually associated with rheumatoid arthritis,

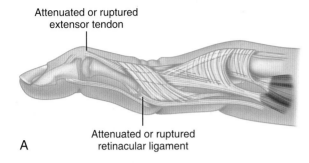

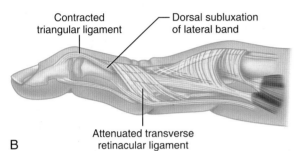

FIGURE 10.11 Swan-neck deformity. **A,** Terminal tendon rupture may be associated with synovitis of distal interphalangeal joint, leading to distal interphalangeal joint flexion and subsequent proximal interphalangeal joint hyperextension. Rupture of flexor digitorum superficialis tendon can be caused by infiltrative synovitis, which can lead to decreased volar support of proximal interphalangeal joint and subsequent hyperextension deformity. **B,** Lateral-band subluxation dorsal to axis of rotation of proximal interphalangeal joint. Contraction of triangular ligament and attenuation of transverse retinacular ligament are depicted. (Copyright 1999 by Jesse B. Jupiter, MD.)

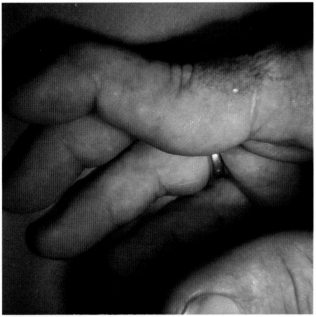

FIGURE 10.12 Fixed rheumatoid swan-neck deformity, with proximal interphalangeal joint hyperextension and distal interphalangeal joint flexion.

swan-neck deformity may occur in patients with volar plate laxity and in patients with conditions such as Ehlers-Danlos syndrome.

This deformity may begin as a mallet deformity associated with extensor tendon disruption at the distal joint with secondary overpull of the central slip, causing secondary proximal interphalangeal joint hyperextension This deformity also may begin at the proximal interphalangeal joint because synovitis causes capsular disruption, tightening of the lateral bands and central tendon, and eventual adherence of the lateral bands in a fixed dorsal position, so they can no longer slide over the condyles when the proximal interphalangeal joint is flexed, thereby limiting proximal interphalangeal flexion. The dorsally and centrally displaced lateral bands become relatively slack and may be ineffective in extending the distal interphalangeal joint, which may secondarily assume a mallet deformity. This mallet deformity usually is not as severe, however, as that produced by terminal slip tendon rupture. A swan-neck deformity may require proximal interphalangeal joint synovectomy, mobilization of the lateral bands, and release of the skin distal to the proximal interphalangeal joint. Wrinkles and normal laxity of the skin are lost at the proximal interphalangeal joint level after several weeks. Nalebuff, Feldon, and Millender categorized swan-neck deformities into four types and recommended treatment for each type. Type I deformities are flexible and require dermodesis, flexor tenodesis of the proximal interphalangeal joint, fusion of the distal interphalangeal joint, and reconstruction of the retinacular ligament. Type II deformities are caused by intrinsic muscle tightness and require intrinsic release in addition to one or more of the aforementioned procedures. Type III deformities are stiff and do not allow satisfactory flexion but do not have significant joint destruction radiographically. These deformities require joint manipulation, mobilization of the lateral bands, and dorsal skin release. Type IV deformities have radiographic evidence of destruction of the joint surface and stiff proximal interphalangeal joints, which usually can be best treated with arthrodesis of the proximal interphalangeal joint or, in the ring and small fingers, possibly proximal interphalangeal joint arthroplasty if the metacarpophalangeal joints are well preserved. Proximal interphalangeal capsulotomy and lateral band mobilization may improve interphalangeal flexion by changing the arc of motion of the proximal interphalangeal joint.

Flexor tenosynovitis results in ineffective support by the flexor digitorum sublimis tendon and may be an important factor in initiating the development of swan-neck deformity in the rheumatoid hand. The overpull of the central tendon slip, combined with synovitis of the proximal interphalangeal joint, stretches the surrounding tissue, resulting in a swan-neck deformity. A tenodesis can be created across the proximal interphalangeal joint, using one half of the flexor sublimis tendon. If there is marked proximal interphalangeal joint hyperextension and a normal radiographic joint space appearance, tenodesis with the flexor sublimis tendon can be combined with release of the lateral bands and the distal skin. Either the Curtis technique of sublimis tenodesis (see Technique 9.13) or the technique described by Beckenbaugh (Technique 10.1; Fig. 10.13) can be used.

Temporary pinning of the proximal interphalangeal joint may be indicated for most reconstructions; however, postoperative immobilization of the joint may be unnecessary

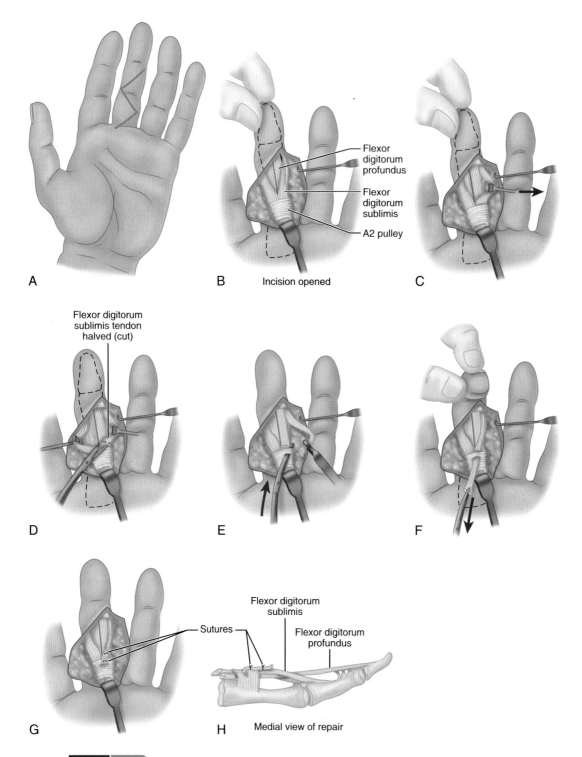

Flexor
digitorum
profundus

Flexor
digitorum
sublimis

A2 pulley

A

B   Incision opened

C

Flexor digitorum
sublimis tendon
halved (cut)

D

E

F

Sutures

Flexor digitorum
sublimis

Flexor digitorum
profundus

G

H   Medial view of repair

FIGURE 10.13   **A-H,** Beckenbaugh technique for correcting hyperextension deformity of proximal interphalangeal joint. (Copyright Mayo Clinic, Rochester, MN.) **SEE TECHNIQUE 10.1.**

at times, allowing immediate movement of the joint without protective splinting. A complication of this technique is flexion contracture of the proximal interphalangeal joint, which may exceed 30 degrees. If there is marked proximal interphalangeal joint extension associated with joint destruction on radiographs, arthrodesis may be best if metacarpophalangeal joint arthroplasty is anticipated. Numerous fixation techniques have been described to obtain successful proximal

interphalangeal joint arthrodesis in arthritic joints, including a single Kirschner wire, crossed Kirschner wires, intraosseous or tension band wiring, bone pegs, miniplates, compression plates, and subchondral screws.

■ INTRINSIC RELEASE

For intrinsic release, see chapter 11 (Fig. 11.11 and Technique 11.7).

CORRECTION OF PROXIMAL INTERPHALANGEAL JOINT HYPEREXTENSION DEFORMITY

TECHNIQUE 10.1

(BECKENBAUGH)

- Make a zigzag incision over the proximal interphalangeal joint (Fig. 10.13A). Avoid damaging the digital nerves that may adhere to the pulley system volar to the hyperextended proximal interphalangeal joint.
- Expose the pulley system over the proximal and middle phalanges by elevating the neurovascular bundles medially and laterally.
- Expose the A2 pulley (Fig. 10.13B).
- Incise the first cruciate pulley between the distal end of the A2 and proximal end of the A4 pulleys and expose the flexor tendons.
- Retract the profundus tendon and release any adhesions; expose the sublimis tendon and its adhesions and perform a synovectomy (Fig. 10.13C).
- Pull the sublimis tendon distally and incise the decussation, splitting the tendon into two slips.
- Pull the divided sublimis tendon distally and incise the ulnar slip, leaving a 5-cm slip of tendon attached to the ulnar side of the middle phalanx (Fig. 10.13D). Pull the slip firmly to ensure that its insertion is not weakened by synovitis. In the little finger, both slips are incised because a single slip usually is too small.
- Puncture the A2 pulley 3 to 4 mm from its distal border (Fig. 10.13E).
- Pass a small curved hemostat through the hole distally into the sheath and clamp the tip of the sublimis tendon slip and pull it proximally through the A2 pulley (Fig. 10.13F).
- Bring the slip of tendon distally and suture it to itself with nonabsorbable 4-0 sutures (Fig. 10.13G and H).

- Adjust the tension so that the proximal interphalangeal joint is held at only 5 degrees of flexion. A tenodesis is accomplished with this slip of tendon fixed across the joint.
- Repair the cruciate pulley if feasible.
- Several fingers can be operated on at one sitting.
- If the distal interphalangeal joints are fixed in a flexed position, they can be manipulated and pinned in extension for 3 weeks.
- Close the skin over a small drain. Apply a bandage, supported by a dorsal splint to prevent proximal interphalangeal joint hyperextension.

POSTOPERATIVE CARE Motion is begun on day 3 after removal of the dressing. A static splint is worn at night for 6 weeks to hold the metacarpophalangeal joints in extension and the proximal interphalangeal joints in slight flexion.

LATERAL BAND MOBILIZATION AND SKIN RELEASE

TECHNIQUE 10.2

(NALEBUFF AND MILLENDER)

- Begin a slightly curved dorsal incision at the midportion of the proximal phalanx, continue it distally from this point over the dorsolateral aspect of the proximal interphalangeal joint and over the middle of the middle phalanx, and traverse obliquely dorsally (Fig. 10.14A).
- Elevate the skin carefully, taking with it the veins.
- Make a longitudinal incision between each lateral band and the central tendon, releasing them from their fixed dorsal position (Fig. 10.14B and C).

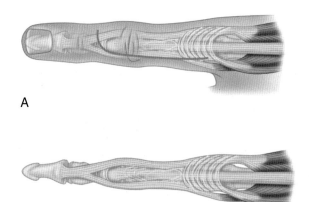

A

C

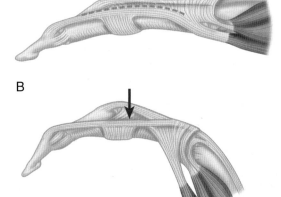

B

D

FIGURE 10.14 Nalebuff and Millender technique for correction of swan-neck deformity. **A,** Skin incision is shown curved to permit release of contracted skin. Incision should not be completely sutured. **B,** Lateral view of skin incision. Medial view incision not shown. **C** and **D,** Lateral tendons are mobilized by two longitudinal releasing incisions, and joint is flexed. **SEE TECHNIQUE 10.2.**

- Passively flex the proximal interphalangeal joint to observe that the lateral bands now slip volarward, sliding over the condyles of the joint (Fig. 10.14D).
- A synovectomy can now be done, and good passive motion usually is established.
- Suture the skin incision proximally. Distally, suturing may not be possible; the distal incision, being placed obliquely across the middle phalanx, gapes open and releases skin tension. The open portion of the incision usually heals without a graft in about 2 weeks.
- Ensure in the preoperative evaluation that active motion can be established by evaluating active flexion of the joint by the profundus and sublimis tendons. When active flexor function is not confirmed, check the tendons by making an incision in the palm and pulling on the tendons through the palm to see that they are not stuck and are not held by rheumatoid nodules.
- Pass a Kirschner wire across the proximal interphalangeal joint to maintain this joint in flexion postoperatively for approximately 3 weeks.

BOUTONNIERE DEFORMITY

A finger with the so-called boutonniere deformity has a flexed proximal interphalangeal joint, with a hyperextended distal interphalangeal joint. It is commonly seen in patients with rheumatoid arthritis, although this tendon imbalance is not unique to rheumatoid disease. In a patient with rheumatoid arthritis, it is thought to be caused by synovitis of the proximal interphalangeal joint with a stretching out of the central slip, allowing the lateral bands to begin subluxating volarward. As the deformity progresses, the lateral bands are forced farther over the proximal interphalangeal joint condyles. They finally become fixed in a subluxated position volar to the joint rotation axis and act as proximal interphalangeal joint flexors. This tightening causes a secondary hyperextension deformity of the distal interphalangeal joint. The flexion deformity of the proximal interphalangeal joint is compensated for by an extension of the metacarpophalangeal joint (Fig. 10.15). The metacarpophalangeal joint deformity does not become fixed, as do the distal two joints. Nalebuff and Millender categorized boutonniere deformities on the basis of the radiographic appearance of the joint surface and the amount of active and passive motion. The mildest deformities, with satisfactory motion and normal-appearing radiographs, can be treated with repositioning the lateral bands, proximal interphalangeal joint synovectomy, and extensor tenotomy over the middle phalanx (Dolphin-Fowler procedure). For moderate deformities with a passively correctable proximal interphalangeal joint, normal flexor tendon function, and satisfactory preservation of joint space radiographically, a soft-tissue procedure with central slip reconstruction using the lateral band or a tendon graft is an option. For severe deformities with stiff joints, the long, ring, and little fingers can be treated with extensor reconstruction and possible implant

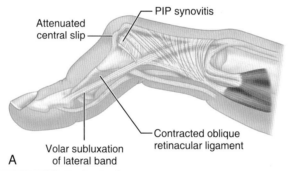

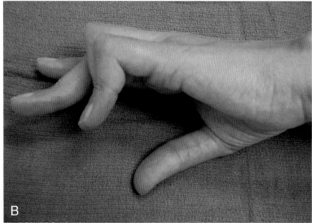

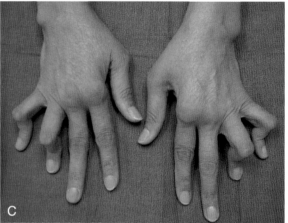

FIGURE **10.15** Boutonniere deformity. **A,** Primary synovitis of proximal interphalangeal *(PIP)* joint can lead to attenuation of overlying central slip and dorsal capsule and increased flexion at PIP joint. Lateral band subluxation volar to axis of rotation of PIP joint can lead in time to hyperextension. Contraction of oblique retinacular ligament, which originates from flexor sheath and inserts into dorsal base of distal phalanx, can lead to extension contracture of distal interphalangeal joint. **B and C,** Clinical photographs illustrate flexion posture of PIP joint and hyperextension posture of distal interphalangeal joint in boutonniere deformity.

arthroplasty; in the index finger, arthrodesis of the proximal interphalangeal joint may be a more durable procedure.

In mild boutonniere deformities, there is a flexion deformity at the proximal interphalangeal joint with lessened ability to flex the distal joint fully, but the joint is not fixed in hyperextension. The flexion deformity at the proximal interphalangeal joint is passively correctable from a position of approximately 15 degrees of flexion. In these deformities, treatment may consist of releasing the lateral tendons near their insertion into the distal phalanx.

A moderate boutonniere deformity has an approximately 40-degree proximal interphalangeal joint flexion contracture, most of which is passively correctable, and the distal interphalangeal joint is hyperextended. The lateral bands are fixed in their subluxated position volarward by virtue of the contracted transverse retinacular ligament. To correct this deformity, there must be functional restoration of the central slip and correction of the lateral band subluxation. Radiographs of these joints should show no severe joint destruction. If the proximal interphalangeal joint is destroyed and fixed, but the distal interphalangeal joint is preserved, this deformity can be treated with proximal interphalangeal joint arthroplasty or fusion.

A fixed boutonniere deformity usually has joint changes on radiographs and a passively uncorrectable proximal interphalangeal joint flexion contracture. Kiefhaber and Strickland found central extensor tendon reconstruction for rheumatoid boutonniere deformities unpredictable and recommended arthrodesis for severe boutonniere deformities.

CORRECTION OF MILD BOUTONNIERE DEFORMITY BY EXTENSOR TENOTOMY

TECHNIQUE 10.3

- Make a dorsal transverse or oblique incision over the distal third of the middle phalanx and expose the extensor tendon.
- Divide this tendon obliquely to enable it to lengthen and remain partially in apposition after the distal interphalangeal joint is flexed.
- Carefully stretch the distal interphalangeal joint into flexion. This uncommonly may become overstretched and develop a mallet deformity that requires splinting.
- Do not suture the extensor tendon.
- Close the wound and begin motion in the next several days, ensuring that active motion is carried out by the patient. Splint only if there is a mallet deformity.

CORRECTION OF MODERATE BOUTONNIERE DEFORMITY

TECHNIQUE 10.4

- Make a curved, dorsal, longitudinal incision over the proximal interphalangeal joint and extend it distally to the distal interphalangeal joint.

- Mobilize the lateral bands by incising the transverse retinacular ligament longitudinally and dissecting underneath the displaced lateral slips.
- Tenotomize the terminal slips of the two lateral tendons just proximal to the distal interphalangeal joint.
- When the central tendon appears to be stretched, shorten it by suture after tenotomy, taking care not to create a proximal interphalangeal joint extension contracture.
- Align the lateral bands with the central slip at the middle phalanx base.
- Be certain of 80 degrees of proximal interphalangeal joint passive flexion to ensure that an extension contracture is not being created. Tendon balance is crucial in this operation.
- Perform a synovectomy after mobilizing the lateral bands.
- Pass a small-caliber transfixing Kirschner wire obliquely through the joint to hold it in extension.
- After 3 to 4 weeks, remove the wire and place the joint in a dynamic extension splint if it is indicated. Active motion should be initiated promptly to achieve and maintain active joint flexion.

CORRECTION OF SEVERE BOUTONNIERE DEFORMITY

TECHNIQUE 10.5

- When proximal interphalangeal joint arthrodesis is indicated, release the distal interphalangeal joint by oblique tenotomy of the lateral tendons just proximal to the joint and use the technique of arthrodesis described in Technique 10.15.
- The resection arthroplasty and implant technique can be used as an option if the flexion contracture is not so severe that it requires extreme bone shortening to accommodate the implant.

◼ INTERPHALANGEAL JOINT ARTHROPLASTY

Proximal interphalangeal joint arthroplasties can be done when metacarpophalangeal joints are reasonably well preserved. Some surgeons consider the central two digits more suitable for proximal interphalangeal arthroplasty because lateral stability can be supported by digits on either side. We have found proximal interphalangeal joint arthroplasty satisfactory in the middle, ring, and small fingers. Distal interphalangeal joint or thumb interphalangeal joint arthroplasty rarely is necessary because arthroplasty of these joints results in limited motion and because function after arthrodesis is quite satisfactory and predictable. Metacarpophalangeal joint and proximal interphalangeal joint arthroplasties of the same finger rarely are indicated.

Lin, Wyrick, and Stern reported 69 proximal interphalangeal silicone arthroplasties and found that (1) an anterior approach (Schneider) preserved the extensor central slip, allowing earlier motion; (2) pain relief was achieved in 67 of 69 patients; (3) coronal plane deformities were not easily corrected; and (4) total motion was not improved.

Alternative arthroplasty implants continue to evolve with variable success. The surface replacement arthroplasty devices are, in general, two-piece constructs designed to replace the normal joint anatomy. Features common to these devices include minimal bone resection, motion center recreation, and soft-tissue preservation. Despite these intuitive advantages, categorically these have not proven superior to flexible implant arthroplasty. Dislocations, implant squeaking, loosening, and high revision rates are not uncommon, especially when used in the index proximal interphalangeal joint. Pelligrini and Burton compared the results of arthroplasty and arthrodesis in 43 proximal interphalangeal joints. All cemented arthroplasty devices failed at an average of 2.25 years after surgery. None of the flexible silicone interposition arthroplasties in ulnar digits required revision, but progressive bone resorption was evident radiographically adjacent to the implant. They concluded that no currently available cemented articulated device provides adequate lateral stability in the radial proximal interphalangeal joints; arthrodesis remains their procedure of choice for the index and occasionally the long finger proximal interphalangeal joints with arthritic involvement that interferes with lateral pinch.

Results of pyrolytic carbon surface replacement arthroplasty have been mixed. In a consecutive series of 170 patients, Wagner et al. found that one in five patients will require revision within 5 years and one in three will require more than one operation. Moreover, high rates of radiolucent loosening and subsidence make this implant choice a concern in younger patients with posttraumatic arthritis. In an earlier series, Wagner et al. found a second revision necessary in 25% of 75 pyrolytic carbon revision arthroplasties. Revision to silicone arthroplasty produced superior results.

The proximal interphalangeal joint volar plate may be used as an interposition arthroplasty in selected individuals. Although technically demanding, this procedure may benefit patients who wish to retain motion but have contraindications to or wish not to have a nonbiologic arthroplasty. Small patient series with proximal interphalangeal joint volar plate arthroplasty have reported pain reduction and maintenance of the preoperative strength and motion.

PROXIMAL INTERPHALANGEAL JOINT VOLAR PLATE INTERPOSITION ARTHROPLASTY

TECHNIQUE 10.6

- Approach the proximal interphalangeal joint through a volar incision and detach the volar plate from the middle phalanx base (Fig. 10.16A).
- Debride the irregular surfaces of the proximal phalanx head and contour them to allow enough space for the interposition.
- Use a Kirschner wire to make two parallel 1.2-mm holes perpendicular to the middle phalanx base for passing sutures. Attach nonabsorbable sutures to the free distal end of the volar plate (Fig. 10.16B). Use fine needles to draw the sutures from dorsal to volar through the bone tunnels

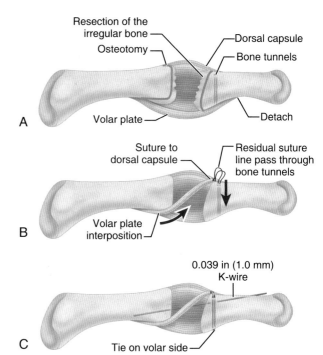

FIGURE 10.16 Proximal interphalangeal joint volar plate interposition arthroplasty. **A,** Through proximal interphalangeal joint volar approach, volar plate is detached from middle phalangeal base. Two holes are drilled perpendicular to middle phalangeal base for passing sutures. **B,** Sutures are attached to volar plate and drawn dorsal to volar through bone tunnels and tied on the volar side of middle phalangeal base. **C,** A 1-mm Kirschner wire is used to fix joint in 20 degrees of flexion. (Redrawn from Lin SY, Chuo CY, Lin GT, et al: Volar plate interposition arthroplasty for posttraumatic arthritis of the finger joints, *J Hand Surg* 33A:35, 2008.) **SEE TECHNIQUE 10.6.**

and tie the sutures on the volar side of the middle phalanx base.
- Obtain hemostasis and close the wound.
- Use a 1-mm Kirschner wire to fix the joint in 20 degrees of flexion and apply a well-molded dorsal splint (Fig. 10.16C).

POSTOPERATIVE CARE

The splint and sutures are removed at 2 weeks, and a proximal interphalangeal joint extension block splint is applied. Progressive range-of-motion exercises are begun with interval splinting.

Both flexible implant and surface replacement metacarpophalangeal joint arthroplasties have had better outcomes than proximal interphalangeal joint arthroplasty. When the metacarpophalangeal joints are stable, surface replacement arthroplasties may offer some advantages compared with the one-piece silicone implants, which, despite high fracture rates, still result in satisfactory outcomes. All surgical techniques, regardless of the device chosen, should preserve the joint soft-tissue restraints, especially with two-piece surface replacement arthroplasties (see Technique 10.7). We still tend to favor the flexible implant devices, especially in rheumatoid arthritis patients, but the metacarpophalangeal joint surface replacement devices may yield some improvement in strength and motion and do not appear to have the same concerns as in the proximal interphalangeal joint.

Metacarpophalangeal joint volar plate arthroplasty also can be done as a biologic alternative to implant arthroplasty. Again, small patient series indicate reasonable outcomes with resurfacing of either the proximal phalanx base or the metacarpal head (see Technique 10.6).

PROXIMAL INTERPHALANGEAL JOINT IMPLANT ARTHROPLASTY

If the index and middle finger proximal interphalangeal joints are involved, index finger proximal interphalangeal joint arthrodesis and middle finger proximal interphalangeal joint arthroplasty may be indicated. This procedure gives a more stable index finger for pinch and permits middle finger flexion for grasp. Vitale et al. found 4.3 times more complications with arthroplasty than with arthrodesis in 79 posttraumatic proximal interphalangeal joints. Ring and little finger arthroplasty also can be done when indicated. If the joint contracture is so tight that extensive bone resection is required for satisfactory implant placement, arthrodesis should be considered.

Joint stiffness and angular and rotational instability may compromise outcomes when interposition arthroplasty is done for osteoarthritis or traumatic arthritis. Silicone arthroplasty for traumatic arthritis of the proximal interphalangeal joint has been shown to work satisfactorily. Proximal interphalangeal joint silicone arthroplasty has been shown to provide pain relief without significant improvement in motion. Proximal interphalangeal silicone arthroplasty generally produces better results in patients with traumatic arthritis than in patients with rheumatoid arthritis. High fracture rates have been reported with proximal interphalangeal joint silicone spacers despite reasonable clinical outcomes. Patients should be clearly informed that all arthroplasty procedures are done for pain reduction or elimination and not for improvement in motion or strength. Moreover, joint motion may be decreased after the procedure, and some patients may elect to endure the pain rather than risk motion loss, especially of the dominant hand ring finger when loss of motion may significantly alter activities such as handwriting.

PROXIMAL INTERPHALANGEAL JOINT ARTHROPLASTY THROUGH A DORSAL APPROACH

TECHNIQUE 10.7

(SWANSON)
- Make a dorsal, longitudinal, slightly curved incision over the joint. Incise the central tendon longitudinally, preserving the insertion at the middle phalanx. Maintain the collateral ligament insertions as much as possible.
- Resect the proximal phalangeal head sufficiently to accommodate the implant.
- Accurately determine the central canal axis of the proximal phalanx with the awl (sometimes fluoroscopy is helpful in this step). Ream and broach the medullary canal with the provided instruments to accommodate the largest implant possible.
- Enter the middle phalangeal base with the awl or small power burr. The articular surface usually is not resected; however, sometimes bony distortion requires recontouring to remove osteophytes and make the base perpendicular to the long axis of the middle phalanx. Ream and broach to accommodate the largest implant possible in accordance with the proximal phalangeal canal preparation.
- With gentle traction and the joint in full extension, check that the distance between the prepared bone ends will accommodate the waist portion of the implant. Place a prosthetic implant trial in the newly created joint space by folding the implant and placing both stems in their respective canals simultaneously with the proximal interphalangeal joint flexed. The proximal and distal implant stems should be fully seated in the medullary canals and the waist not compressed with the joint in full extension. In flexion, the cortices of the phalanges should not abut.
- Reattach the central tendon, if necessary, through a hole drilled at the dorsal cortex of the proximal phalanx.
- In a swan-neck deformity (Fig. 10.17), a release of the triangular ligament and a release of the lateral tendon from the central tendon and elongation of the central tendon may be necessary.
- In a boutonniere deformity (Fig. 10.18), release and imbrication of the triangular ligament are necessary to permit proximal interphalangeal joint extension. The central tendon may have to be advanced and reinserted at the dorsum of the middle phalanx.
- Collateral ligaments may require release or excision to permit satisfactory joint alignment. Fluoroscopic imaging may be helpful, especially in joints distorted by the arthritic process.

PROXIMAL INTERPHALANGEAL JOINT ARTHROPLASTY THROUGH AN ANTERIOR (VOLAR) APPROACH

TECHNIQUE 10.8

(LIN, WYRICK, AND STERN; SCHNEIDER)
- Select an appropriate anesthetic; Lin et al. used an intermetacarpal block with intravenous sedation to allow assessment of proximal interphalangeal active motion. A sterile wrist tourniquet also can be used.
- Approach the joint through a V-shaped or similar incision, centered at the proximal interphalangeal joint crease (Fig. 10.19A).
- Incise the A3 pulley of the flexor sheath on the side with the apex of the skin flap.
- Retract both flexor tendons and detach the volar plate proximally (Fig. 10.19B).
- Release the collateral ligaments partially or completely from the proximal phalanx, allowing nearly 180 degrees of joint extension (Fig. 10.19C).

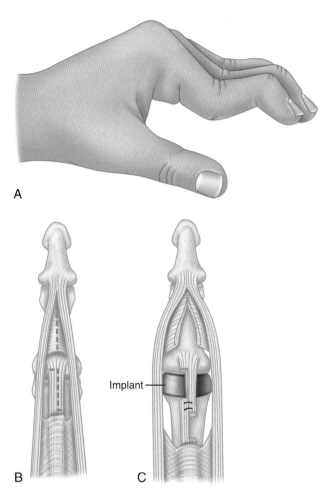

FIGURE 10.17 Technique for swan-neck deformity. **A,** Swan-neck deformity of fingers. **B,** Central tendon is separated from lateral tendons by dividing connecting fibers. Central tendon is step-cut transversely and dissected proximally, lengthening it. **C,** Lateral tendons are relocated palmarward. After insertion of implant, cut ends of central tendon are approximated with interrupted sutures. Knots are buried. (Adapted from an original painting by Frank H. Netter, MD, from Clinical Symposia, copyright Elsevier.) **SEE TECHNIQUE 10.7.**

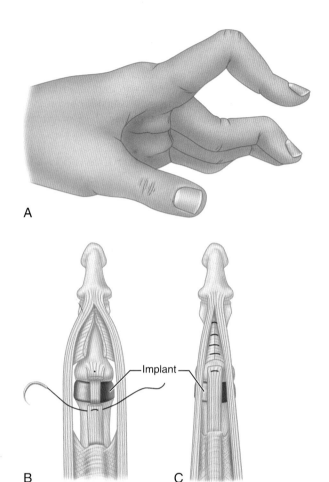

FIGURE 10.18 Technique for boutonniere deformity. **A,** Boutonniere deformity of index finger with swan-neck deformity of other fingers. **B and C,** Lengthened central tendon is advanced, and lateral tendons are released and relocated dorsally by suturing their connecting fibers. (Adapted from an original painting by Frank H. Netter, MD, from Clinical Symposia, copyright Elsevier.) **SEE TECHNIQUE 10.7.**

- Cut through the neck of the proximal phalanx with an oscillating saw (Fig. 10.19D). Do not resect the base of the middle phalanx to preserve digital length.
- Prepare the medullary canals with square broaches to prevent malrotation (Fig. 10.19E).
- Insert provisional "sizing" implants (Fig. 10.19F). Insert the permanent implant without the metal grommets.
- If possible, reattach the collateral ligaments to the proximal phalanx through drill holes.
- Split the volar plate longitudinally to reinforce the collateral ligaments (Fig. 10.19G).
- Close the skin and apply a nonadherent gauze bandage, supported by a splint.

POSTOPERATIVE CARE The dressing is removed within the first week. A dynamic proximal interphalangeal dorsal outrigger extension splint with a middle phalangeal block is used for 4 weeks. Active flexion against rubber bands allows graduated strengthening. Active and passive exercises are begun, and blocking techniques and resting extension splints to prevent flexion deformity are used. The dynamic extension splint is discontinued after 4 to 6 weeks. Side-to-side "buddy" taping for 3 months is encouraged.

Volar plate interposition into the proximal interphalangeal joint remains an alternative to implant arthroplasty (see Technique 10.6). Although the procedure is technically more difficult than implant arthroplasty, reports suggest that this technique can provide durable clinical results.

DISTAL INTERPHALANGEAL JOINT DEFORMITIES

The rheumatoid deformities at the distal joint include a mallet, hyperflexed distal interphalangeal joint, which may occur in conjunction with a swan-neck deformity or as a result of attenuation of the terminal slip, and a hyperextensible distal interphalangeal joint, which also may be related to attenuation of capsuloligamentous structures or to flexor tendon

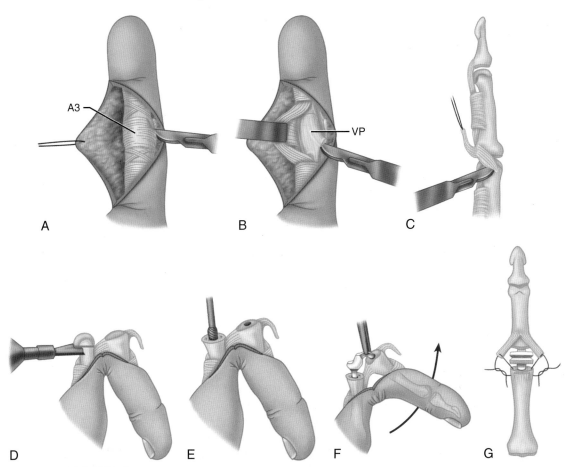

FIGURE 10.19 Anterior approach for proximal interphalangeal joint arthroplasty. **A,** V-shaped incision allows exposure of flexor tendon sheath and division of A3 pulley. **B,** Flexor tendons retracted to allow proximal detachment of volar plate. **C,** Collateral ligament origins completely released. **D,** Proximal interphalangeal joint hyperextended to expose articular surfaces. Head of proximal phalanx removed with oscillating saw. **E,** Medullary canals prepared with properly sized burrs. **F,** Provisional implants are sized, and trial of active motion is shown. Permanent implant is then inserted. **G,** Volar plate can be split and used to reconstruct collateral ligaments. *VP,* Volar plate. **SEE TECHNIQUE 10.8.**

rupture. Usually either of these deformities can be treated with distal interphalangeal joint arthrodesis. In a patient who has had a proximal interphalangeal joint arthrodesis, the distal interphalangeal joint mallet deformity might be left untreated because the small amount of mobility remaining in the distal interphalangeal joint can contribute significantly to fingertip function.

■ ULNAR DRIFT OR DEVIATION OF THE FINGERS

Ulnar drift or deviation of the fingers (Fig. 10.20) is found in conditions other than rheumatoid arthritis. In the normal hand, predisposing factors include (1) metacarpophalangeal joint ulnar deviation, especially of the index finger; (2) smaller and sloping ulnar condyles of asymmetric metacarpal heads, especially those of the index and middle fingers; (3) the approach of the long flexor and extensor tendons from the ulnar side of the metacarpophalangeal joints; (4) greater ulnar deviation than radial deviation of the digits permitted by the radial collateral ligaments when the metacarpophalangeal joints are flexed; and (5) greater strength of the abductor digiti quinti and flexor digiti quinti than the third volar interosseous. Pathologic

changes in the rheumatoid hand accentuating ulnar deviation and drift include (1) metacarpophalangeal joint synovitis that weakens the dorsoradial capsular restraints; (2) stretching of the metacarpophalangeal joint collateral ligaments by the volarly directed forces of the flexor tendons, permitting volar displacement of the proximal phalanges; (3) stretching of the accessory collateral ligaments that permits ulnar displacement of the flexor tendons within their tunnels; (4) stretching of the flexor tunnels that permits even more ulnar displacement of the long flexor tendons; (5) interosseous muscle contracture that causes ulnar deviation and proximal interphalangeal joint hyperextension, as well as metacarpophalangeal joint flexion and eventually subluxation; (6) attenuated radial sagittal bands that allow long extensor tendon ulnar displacement; and (7) long extensor tendon rupture at the wrist level that increases the possibility of metacarpophalangeal joint dislocations.

■ MILD-TO-MODERATE ULNAR DRIFT

In the surgical treatment of mild-to-moderate ulnar drift, reasonable success is possible only when the major deforming forces have been properly evaluated. This type of ulnar drift

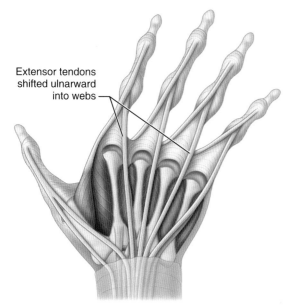

Extensor tendons shifted ulnarward into webs

FIGURE **10.20** Ulnar deviation of fingers in rheumatoid arthritis.

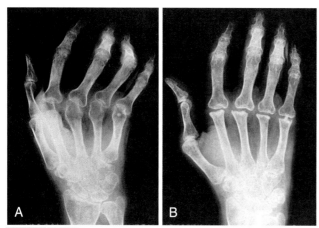

FIGURE **10.21** **A,** Subluxation of metacarpophalangeal joints in severe rheumatoid arthritis. **B,** Subluxations have been treated by resecting metacarpal heads because intrinsic release provides insufficient correction.

implies the absence of severely diseased articular surfaces of dislocated joints (Fig. 10.21). Often, however, the flexor and extensor tendons are displaced ulnarward, the intrinsic muscles are imbalanced, and the joints are swollen. Surgical procedures that may be indicated are intrinsic release or transfer for balance, extensor tendon realignment, and metacarpophalangeal joint synovectomy. No operation has been devised to realign easily the ulnarly displaced flexor tendons and their sheaths.

Extensor tendon realignment procedures ideally are performed under local anesthesia so that the effectiveness of the construct can be verified. The presumed tension on the realigned tendon often requires adjustment for proper tendon tracking over the metacarpophalangeal joint. Release of the tightened sagittal band and transfer of this into the radial collateral ligament or use of a distally based portion of the extensor tendon or juncture around the lumbrical tendon or collateral ligament are common extensor tendon realignment techniques.

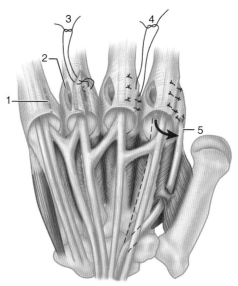

FIGURE **10.22** Correction of mild to moderate ulnar drift. *(1)* Joint is entered through incision in radial side of hood. *(2)* Relaxing incision is made in ulnar side of hood to permit repositioning of extensor tendon. *(3)* and *(4)* Incision in radial side of hood is closed after its edges are overlapped. *(5)* Extensor indicis proprius tendon is transferred to first dorsal interosseous muscle to reinforce it. **SEE TECHNIQUE 10.9.**

EXTENSOR TENDON REALIGNMENT AND INTRINSIC REBALANCING

TECHNIQUE 10.9

- Make a transverse dorsal incision over the metacarpal heads or longitudinal incisions between the metacarpophalangeal joints. If multiple common extensor tendons are to be realigned and longitudinal incisions are preferred, incisions between the index and middle and ring and small metacarpophalangeal joints will allow access to all four metacarpophalangeal joints. Identify and preserve the dorsal veins.
- Enter each metacarpophalangeal joint through a longitudinal incision on the ulnar side of the extensor hood (radial if the tendons are subluxing radially).
- Dissect the extensor hood from the underlying capsule to release the ulnarly displaced extensor mechanism.
- Preserve the joint capsule as possible, and remove the synovium, especially that herniating out through the capsule and over the dorsal neck of the metacarpal.
- Reposition the displaced extensor mechanism.
- Realign the extensor tendon over the metacarpophalangeal joint by taking a distally based portion of the extensor tendon and passing it around the radial lumbrical tendon or collateral ligament with nonabsorbable sutures.
- When the index finger is markedly deviated, a transfer of the extensor indicis proprius tendon to its radial side may be beneficial (Fig. 10.22). In addition, the intrinsic ten-

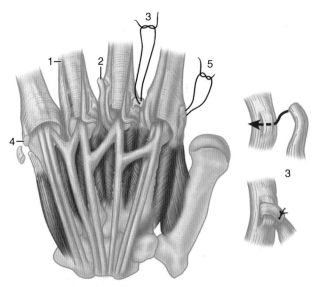

FIGURE 10.23 Flatt transfer of released ulnar intrinsics to radial side of digits for ulnar drift. *(1)* Incision is made on ulnar side of central tendon, releasing ulnar intrinsic insertion. *(2)* Ulnar intrinsic insertion is free. *(3)* Insertion is sutured to capsule on radial side of metacarpophalangeal joint of adjacent finger. *(4)* Segment of abductor digiti quinti tendon is excised to relieve ulnar pull of muscle on little finger. *(5)* First dorsal interosseous tendon is shortened to increase radial pull of muscle on index finger. **SEE TECHNIQUE 10.9.**

dons can be transferred from the ulnar side of the digits to the radial side of the adjacent joint, as shown in Figure 10.23.

■ Have the patient actively flex and extend the finger to ensure that the common extensor tendon remains over the metacarpophalangeal joint.

POSTOPERATIVE CARE At 2 weeks, the sutures are removed and the hand is continually supported in a splint to avoid recurrence of ulnar deviation for another week. Supervised therapy is then begun with intermittent splint wear and progressive metacarpophalangeal joint flexion. The splint is worn for another 3 to 4 weeks.

SEVERE ULNAR DRIFT AND METACARPOPHALANGEAL DISLOCATION

In severe ulnar drift, often one or more metacarpophalangeal joints have dislocated; consequently, this type of drift and dislocation of these joints are discussed together. Metacarpophalangeal joint dislocations in effect release the soft-tissue tension across the joint and thus decrease tension more distally and protect, at least partially, the proximal interphalangeal joint. Conversely, the proximal interphalangeal joints may dislocate first. It should be emphasized, however, that the long flexor tendons are a major deforming force that drifts ulnarward, either within or without their sheaths, exerting an ulnar and palmarly directed force leading to metacarpophalangeal joint dislocation. For this type of ulnar drift, surgery is done mainly on the metacarpal head and its surrounding ligaments and tendons.

Function of a dislocated and arthritic metacarpophalangeal joint may be improved by arthroplasty. Many different designs of metacarpophalangeal joint interposition arthroplasty implants are available. We have had more experience with the Swanson implant than any other. An average expected range of motion at the metacarpophalangeal joint is about 55 degrees, and usually this occurs in the functional range. Complications include an infection rate between 0% and 3%, a breakage rate between 2% and 82%, a subluxation rate of 20%, and a dislocation rate of 5%. Although obvious fractures of the prosthesis may occur, the function of the joint usually is not impaired because it is not only the prosthesis but also the encapsulating scar that provides joint stability. Metal sleeves or grommets, which have been added to diminish abrasion at the bone-prosthesis interface, do not seem to make a significant difference in the fracture rate. The prostheses are easily removed when necessary. Of the many alternative designs for metacarpophalangeal implant arthroplasty, the pyrolytic carbon design has shown promising results.

Pyrolytic carbon metacarpophalangeal joint arthroplasties have fared better than their proximal interphalangeal joint counterparts. Wall and Stern found satisfactory outcomes in pyrolytic carbon metacarpophalangeal arthroplasties at an average 4-year follow-up, with improved joint motion, good pain relief and patient satisfaction, and few complications. Radiographic outcomes revealed a consistent asymptomatic surrounding lucency with no evidence of implant failure or migration. Dickson et al. reported a mean arc of motion of 54 degrees (20 to 80 degrees) in 35 index and 16 middle metacarpophalangeal arthroplasties at an average follow-up of 103 months (range, 60 to 72 months). Good pain relief, a functional range of motion, and high satisfaction were seen in most patients, with an 88% survival rate at 10 years and average subsidence of 2 mm in the proximal and 1 mm in the distal component.

Metacarpophalangeal joint arthroplasty reliably relieves pain, maintains stability and alignment, and permits acceptable motion (Fig. 10.24). Results deteriorate over time, however, and the patient should be advised that revision may be necessary. The presence of active infection is a contraindication to implant arthroplasty. Loss of bone stock, skin changes that prohibit good closure, and irreparable tendon damage also compromise the outcome of implant arthroplasty.

METACARPOPHALANGEAL JOINT ARTHROPLASTY

TECHNIQUE 10.10

(SWANSON)

■ Make a transverse incision on the dorsum of the hand, beginning on the radial aspect of the second metacarpophalangeal joint, and extend it ulnarward to the ulnar aspect of the fifth metacarpophalangeal joint. (Alternatively, two longitudinal incisions can be used for the metacarpophalangeal joint exposure, one between the index and middle and one between the ring and small fingers.) Preserve all sensory nerves and carefully observe

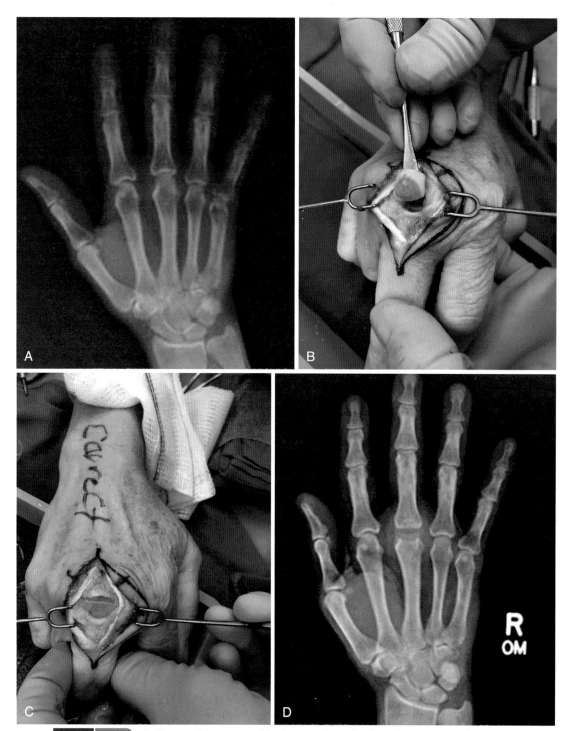

FIGURE 10.24 A 60-year-old woman with rheumatoid arthritis and persistent pain in right middle finger metacarpophalangeal joint despite no signs of significant joint degeneration on plain radiographs **(A)**. **B,** Appearance of metacarpal head with significant cartilage loss. **C,** Silicone spacer before capsular and extensor tendon closure. **D,** Radiograph after metacarpophalangeal joint arthroplasty.

the pattern of the superficial veins; preserve them as well when possible.

- This transverse incision permits a flap that can be dissected proximally and folded back, exposing the heads of the metacarpals. Through this, incise the shroud ligament of the extensor mechanism on the radial aspect of each joint

and, if necessary, on the ulnar aspect also. This permits entry into the joint capsule, which already may be ruptured dorsally with herniation of hypertrophied synovium.

- Incise and preserve when possible the capsule longitudinally, and perform a synovectomy with small rongeurs before and after metacarpal head resection.

- With a thin osteotome or an oscillating saw, resect each metacarpal head to shorten the bone sufficiently to permit easy reduction of the volarly dislocated proximal phalangeal base. This may require resection proximal to the collateral ligaments origin, necessitating radial collateral ligament repair or reconstruction.
- After synovectomy, introduce into the metacarpal medullary canal an awl or, if necessary, a reamer to provide space for the prosthesis stem. The metacarpal head-neck region should be cut carefully so that it is at a 90-degree angle with the axis of the metacarpal shaft.
- Do not resect the proximal phalangeal base, although deformity from the arthritic process may require recontouring to make the base perpendicular to the phalangeal shaft. Soft-tissue dissection from the proximal phalangeal base should be sufficient to ensure that the entry point in the phalangeal canal is appropriate, centered from medial to lateral and more dorsal than volar to prevent volar cortex perforation. Prepare the base to accept the distal stem of the prosthesis by appropriate drilling, reaming, and broaching.
- Select the largest implant that can be inserted comfortably.
- Place gentle traction on the finger with the metacarpophalangeal joint in full extension and examine the distance between the metacarpal head and the phalangeal base. This should be sufficient to accommodate the implant midsection. Moreover, bone resection should be sufficient to prevent prosthesis buckling and volar abutment with joint flexion.
- To help correct or avoid index finger pronation, Swanson recommended that a radial slip of the proximal phalangeal volar plate be split off proximally and reattached to the radial aspect of the metacarpal neck (Fig. 10.25).
- Remove the prosthesis from the package after a trial prosthesis has been inserted and the desired size determined. Handle the prosthesis with instruments without sharp edges to avoid scoring or other damage.

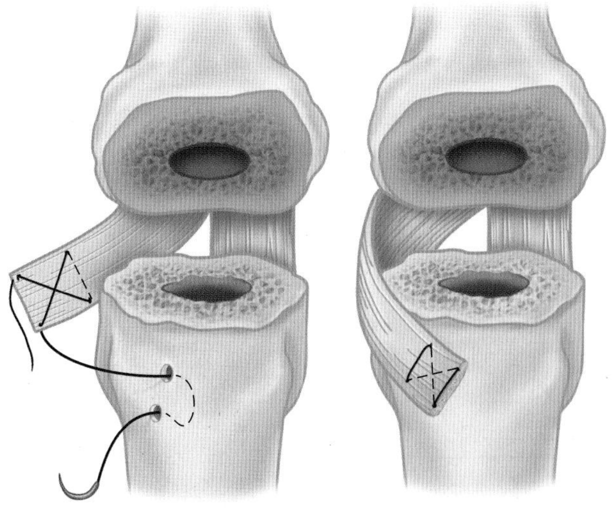

- Insert the prosthesis and check that metacarpophalangeal joint passive motion is from full extension to almost 90 degrees of flexion.
- Check all fingers carefully for alignment and for rotary deformity.
- Close any remaining capsule over the prosthesis and centralize the extensor tendon over the metacarpophalangeal joint. Check finally for the need for further intrinsic release by placing the metacarpophalangeal joint in full extension and passively flexing the proximal interphalangeal joint. Note that ulnar intrinsic release is commonly required in rheumatoid arthritis patients, especially for the ring and small fingers.
- Insert a drain, close the wound, and apply a supportive dressing to splint the fingers in slight radial deviation.

POSTOPERATIVE CARE The splint is removed, and the dressing is changed at 5 to 7 days after surgery. The fingers are held in extension and deviated radially in the postoperative splint for 7 to 10 days until sutures are removed at about 10 days or longer, depending on wound healing. After suture removal, a program of passive and active motion is begun under the supervision of a therapist. Dynamic splinting is used to assist metacarpophalangeal extension and radial deviation during the day and is combined with static volar wrist, metacarpophalangeal, and proximal interphalangeal extension splinting at night. The daytime static splint is discontinued at 6 to 8 weeks, and supervised therapy with static splinting at night is continued for at least 3 months.

Surface replacement arthroplasty is reserved for patients with stable metacarpal joints. Most rheumatoid arthritis patients, however, are not candidates for this technique because joint instability and joint dislocations are contraindications to this procedure. Thus surface replacement arthroplasty is more ideally suited for patients with osteoarthritis or posttraumatic disorders with intact and stable metacarpal joint collateral ligaments and volar plates.

METACARPAL JOINT SURFACE ARTHROPLASTY

TECHNIQUE 10.11

(BECKENBAUGH)
- If a single joint is to be replaced, make a curved longitudinal incision centered over the metacarpal joint dorsally; if multiple joints are involved, make a transverse incision across the metacarpal joints dorsally or longitudinal incisions between the joints to be addressed.
- Incise the extensor hood on the radial side of the central tendon or through its center if no dislocation or subluxation of the tendon is present.
- Dissect the extensor tendon free from the joint capsule when possible and split it longitudinally to expose the joint

FIGURE 10.25 Swanson technique for reconstruction of radial collateral ligament of index metacarpophalangeal joint by using slip of volar plate. **SEE TECHNIQUE 10.10.**

so that the proximal phalangeal dorsal base and the metacarpal head with the collateral ligament origins are visible. Preserve the capsule as much as possible for later repair.

- Use an awl to puncture the metacarpal head in its dorsal third, centered in the width of the head and aligned with the long axis of the metacarpal medullary canal.
- Attach the alignment guide and insert the alignment awl through the puncture and advance it into the medullary canal one half to two thirds the length of the metacarpal. The alignment guide should be parallel to the dorsal surface of the metacarpal shaft and in line with the long axis of the bone.
- Begin a partial metacarpal osteotomy using the proximal osteotomy guide mounted on the alignment awl and complete it free hand by following the previously established osteotomy plane. Attach the proximal osteotomy guide (Fig. 10.26A) on the alignment awl and advance it until the cutting plane of the guide is positioned 1 to 2 mm distal to the dorsal attachments of the collateral ligaments. Keep the volar surface of the guide parallel to the dorsal metacarpal surface to maintain proper rotational alignment. Remove the alignment awl and complete the

osteotomy by following the plane established by the guided cut.

- Puncture the proximal phalangeal base volar to the dorsal surface of the proximal phalanx a distance one third of the sagittal height and centered across the base in line with the phalangeal medullary canal.
- Advance the alignment guide one half to two thirds the length of the phalangeal medullary canal and attach the distal osteotomy guide. Advance until the cutting plane of the guide is positioned 0.5 to 1.0 mm distal to the dorsal edge of the proximal phalanx. Keep the volar surface of the guide parallel to the phalanx dorsal surface.
- Make the phalangeal cut with a small sagittal saw through the blade slot of the osteotomy guide (Fig. 10.26B). Make the dorsal portion of the osteotomy, remove the alignment awl, and complete the osteotomy free hand.
- Open the phalangeal opening with the starter awl and distally broach along the previously established medullary axis. Keep the dorsal surface of the broach parallel to the dorsal surface of the phalangeal bone. A side-cutting burr may be necessary to assist in proper seating of the broaches. Continue broaching until the seating plane of

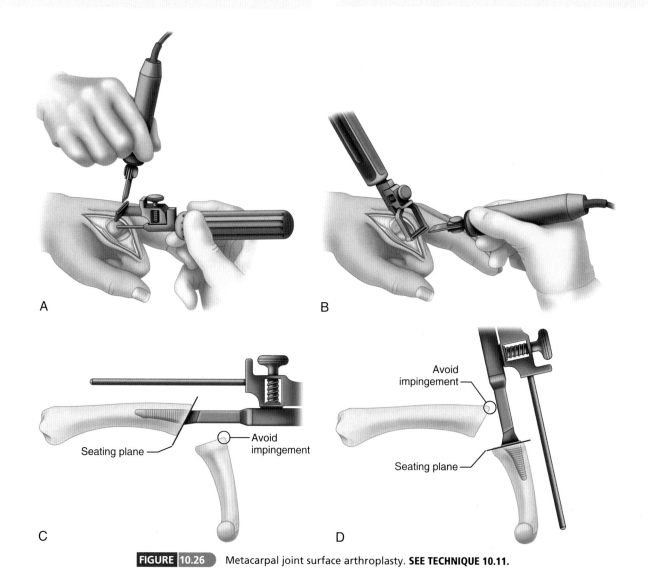

A

B

C

D

FIGURE **10.26** Metacarpal joint surface arthroplasty. **SEE TECHNIQUE 10.11.**

the broach is flush to 1 mm deeper than the osteotomy (Fig. 10.26C, D). During broaching, evaluate fit and movement resistance. Repeat the broaching process with the next larger size broach until the largest size possible can be inserted and properly seated.

- Broach the metacarpal beginning with the size 10 proximal broach working up to the broach determined from the phalangeal broaching process. Continue broaching until the seating plane of the broach is 1 mm deeper than the osteotomy. Do not mismatch proximal and distal component sizes.
- Assess range of motion with trial components. Tightness in extension can be relieved by further impaction or removal of more bone. Insert and impact the appropriate size distal component until the component collar is flush with the proximal phalangeal base.
- Insert and impact the matching metacarpal component and assess stability and range of motion.
- Repair the capsule, centralize the common extensor tendon, and perform intrinsic releases and transfers when indicated.
- Apply a volar splint with the wrist in 10 to 15 degrees of extension, the metacarpal joints in full extension, and the proximal interphalangeal joints in slight flexion.

POSTOPERATIVE CARE Active and passive range-of-motion exercises are begun under the supervision of a therapist within the first week following the procedure. The sutures are removed at 10 to 14 days after surgery. Supervised physical therapy is continued until satisfactory motion has been achieved and the patient understands various exercises sufficiently to perform them independently.

EXTENSOR TENOSYNOVITIS

Wrist and digital extensor tenosynovitis causes visible swelling yet is usually relatively painless. This condition is more common at the wrist level, and mobile masses associated with the extensor tendons distinguish this from dorsal capsular synovitis and ganglion cysts. These extensor tendon nodules may impinge on the distal edge of the extensor retinaculum, producing discomfort and limiting concomitant wrist and finger extension. One or all extensor tendons may be affected, and significant tendon involvement may lead to tendon rupture. In the absence of extensor tendon rupture, splinting and medical treatment should be used initially and may lead to symptom resolution. Corticosteroid injections have limited use because of the possibility of extensor tendon rupture, and an extensor tenosynovectomy usually is recommended if there has been no improvement in the tenosynovitis with nonoperative treatment.

EXTENSOR TENDON RUPTURE

Rheumatoid tenosynovitis is a common cause of tendon rupture and a major cause of deformity and disability. Distal ulna, dorsal subluxation contributes to extensor tendon rupture because the extensor tendons usually glide between the arthritic distal ulnar head and the tight, intact dorsal carpal ligament. The small finger usually is involved first and subsequently the ring (Vaughn-Jackson syndrome) and then

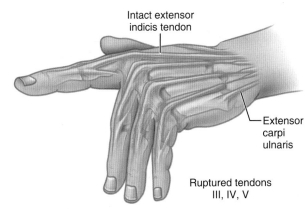

Intact extensor indicis tendon

Extensor carpi ulnaris

Ruptured tendons III, IV, V

FIGURE 10.27 Rupture of extensor tendons at level of extensor retinaculum in rheumatoid arthritis. Most ruptures of common finger extensors occur at an abrasive point created by dorsally dislocated distal ulna.

sequentially more radial digital extensors (Fig. 10.27). The long extensor tendon of the thumb, because of its tortuous course, frequently ruptures at Lister's tubercle, where it angles through the third extensor compartment. At surgery, white strips of pseudotendon connective tissue may be seen between the more normal proximal and distal tendon ends, and although these are not true tendons, they may be responsible for some remaining limited metacarpophalangeal joint extension and clinically suggest less extensive tendon disruption.

A ruptured extensor tendon can be repaired by direct suture if found within a few days and if the remaining tendon is adequate. If surgery must be delayed for several days, it is well to splint the wrist in extension to relieve the constant tension on the remaining intact tendons. If the ruptured tendon is diagnosed after several weeks, a segmental tendon graft may be possible between the proximal and distal segments of the ruptured tendon to an adjoining intact tendon. Although attachment of the ruptured distal tendons to an intact tendon is possible (Fig. 10.28), tendon transfers, such as extensor indicis proprius to power the ulnar ruptured tendons, are more often required. A synovectomy is always indicated in the region of the rupture and the repair.

If the tendon of the ring finger or little finger alone is ruptured, repair of the ring finger tendon may be possible by suturing its distal and proximal segments to the intact middle finger extensor tendon under appropriate tension. The extensor indicis proprius might be transferred for use as a motor to the little finger. Transfer of the extensor pollicis brevis is an alternative, unless there is an extension deficit of the thumb metacarpometacarpal joint. When three extensor tendons, those of the middle, ring, and little fingers, have been ruptured for an extended period, the transfer of a motor usually is indicated. An acceptable source for this motor is the sublimis of the ring finger. This tendon has enough excursion and might be even more effective because of the tenodesis effect when the wrist is flexed. Extensor pollicis longus tendon rupture can be repaired by transfer of the extensor indicis proprius, a common and useful transfer when the extensor pollicis ruptures from other causes.

As mentioned, the clinical examination usually underestimates the amount of tendon attenuation and rupture, and reconstruction may be more complex than anticipated. Moreover, surgery may be done as an attempt to identify and

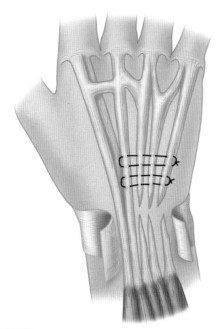

FIGURE 10.28 Extensor tendon rupture under extensor retinaculum. Repair can be accomplished by side-to-side repair to adjacent intact tendon.

eliminate the source of tendon degeneration to limit further loss of metacarpophalangeal joint extension.

FLEXOR TENDON RUPTURE

Flexor tendon rupture in rheumatoid patients is not as common as extensor tendon rupture but is much more difficult to treat surgically. Rupture may occur within the digit as a result of infiltrative tenosynovitis or at wrist level, especially of the flexor pollicis longus tendon, because of bony prominences about the carpal tunnel.

Triggering of the fingers commonly comes from tendon nodularity within the zone II flexor sheath but may also be secondary to a sublimis slip rupture. Infiltration, weakening, and eventual rupture of the profundus tendons may likewise occur and are more obvious and disabling clinically. The location of either sublimis or profundus ruptures is variable and indeterminate on physical examination, and either may result in secondary joint stiffness. Grafting of ruptured rheumatoid finger flexor tendons almost always fails. The exception is at the wrist, where a segmental graft occasionally can be used as a treatment for a ruptured flexor pollicis longus tendon. Another approach to flexor pollicis longus rupture is distal joint arthrodesis if hyperextension of the interphalangeal joint compromises thumb function. If the flexor profundus and superficialis are ruptured in the digit, proximal and distal interphalangeal joint stabilization by arthrodesis may be preferred.

PERSISTENT PROXIMAL INTERPHALANGEAL JOINT SYNOVITIS

Synovectomy is a useful operation for persistent proximal interphalangeal joint synovitis and can be performed on all four fingers of one hand at the same time and in conjunction with other synovectomies. Since the advent of disease-modifying antirheumatic drugs, the need for synovectomies has declined significantly.

SYNOVECTOMY

TECHNIQUE 10.12

- A curved dorsal incision centered over the proximal interphalangeal joint provides a more extensile approach and is preferred, especially when extensor tendon rebalancing procedures are needed; however, midlateral incisions can also be incorporated to perform this procedure.
- Locate the transverse retinacular ligament(s), sever the attachments, and elevate the extensor hood.
- Under the hood, identify the collateral ligament. Enter the joint dorsal to this ligament and lateral to the central tendon, explore the joint, and excise as much synovium as possible.
- Remove the synovium from the area behind the volar plate and the area inferior to the collateral ligament, dividing, if necessary, the accessory collateral ligament.
- Relocate the lateral tendon and transverse retinacular ligament.
- Close the incisions. Apply a dressing and a volar splint.

POSTOPERATIVE CARE The sutures are removed at 10 to 14 days after surgery. Active and passive range-of-motion exercises are begun under the supervision of a therapist at the time of suture removal. The supervised physical therapy is continued until satisfactory motion has been achieved and the patient understands various exercises sufficiently to perform them independently.

FLEXOR TENOSYNOVITIS

Although flexor tenosynovitis at the wrist may not be as apparent as that seen on the extensor surface, the bulk of the tenosynovium interferes with finger motion, compresses the median nerve in the carpal tunnel, and leads to tendon rupture. Erosion of the volar capsule and ligaments over radial osteophytes contribute to flexor pollicis longus rupture in the carpal tunnel (Mannerfelt lesion). In the digits, flexor tenosynovitis may lead to triggering in the flexor sheath. The triggering may be caused by localized tenosynovitis or tendon nodules catching within the fibroosseous sheath. Rarely, the flexor profundus may trigger through the sublimis decussation.

Tenosynovitis occurs most often on the volar surface of the wrist and fingers and the wrist dorsal surface. Often there is a progressive fusiform swelling of one or more flexor tendon sheaths extending from the middle of the palm to the distal interphalangeal joint. The swelling is typically painful and causes a gradual decrease in finger flexion. On palpation, the synovium is thickened and nodules can be felt along the tendon sheath with tendon excursion; crepitus and grating usually are present. Tenosynovectomies seem to have a lasting effect, and flexor sublimis ulnar slip removal has been suggested to reduce the recurrence. Although tenosynovectomy and joint synovectomy usually can be expected to relieve pain, a concomitant improvement in joint motion may not be seen.

FLEXOR TENDON SHEATH SYNOVECTOMY

TECHNIQUE 10.13

- Make a long zigzag incision (Fig. 10.29) on the palmar surface of each involved finger.
- Expose the flexor tendon sheath by raising skin flaps and protect the anterolaterally oriented neurovascular bundles.
- Excise portions of the sheath, leaving as much of the annular pulley system intact as possible, especially the A2 and A4 pulleys over the middle of the proximal and middle phalanges.
- Excise as much synovium as possible, taking care to remove it from behind the slips of the sublimis and between the profundus and sublimis.
- Traction on the tendons individually proximal to the A1 pulley will assist in identifying the source of triggering if present. If triggering persists after a careful synovectomy and flexor tendon nodule debridement, excise the ulnar flexor digitorum sublimis slip. An A1 annular pulley release should rarely be required.
- Close the incision with interrupted sutures, apply a compression dressing, support the wrist with a volar plaster splint, and elevate the hand. Motion of the fingers is started as soon as tolerated.

POSTOPERATIVE CARE The sutures are removed at 10 to 14 days after surgery. Active and passive range-of-motion exercises are begun under the supervision of a therapist at the time of suture removal. Supervised physi-cal therapy is continued until satisfactory motion has been achieved and the patient understands various exercises sufficiently to perform them independently.

■ FINGER JOINT ARTHRODESIS

Thumb or finger joint arthrodeses may be indicated when arthroplasty cannot reliably restore stability and motion. Ligamentous instability and angular and rotational deformities, especially those of the index and thumb, are more reliably treated by arthrodesis because the stress from pinch and grasp may further the deformity. Occasionally, a joint must be arthrodesed because the muscles that control the digit are not strong enough to stabilize and move all joints. When the metacarpophalangeal joint is destroyed, if good muscle strength is present, arthroplasty is indicated more often than arthrodesis.

The following are the preferred positions for arthrodesis of the various joints. In the fingers, the metacarpophalangeal joint should be fixed in 20 to 30 degrees of flexion. The proximal interphalangeal joints should be fixed from 25 degrees of flexion in the index finger to almost 40 degrees in the small finger (less flexion in the radial fingers than in the ulnar fingers). The distal interphalangeal joints are fixed in 0 to 20 degrees of flexion depending on the patient's preference and the method of fixation. Techniques for arthrodesis with internal fixation include Kirschner wires, screws, and bone grafting techniques. Tension band wiring can provide reliable fixation for proximal interphalangeal and metacarpophalangeal joint arthrodesis (Figs. 10.30 and 10.31). Kirschner wire fixation is rapid and simple and allows control of the fusion position in flexion, angulation, and rotation before fixation. It preserves maximal length, it allows early motion, and rapid union is achieved (Figs. 10.32 and 10.33).

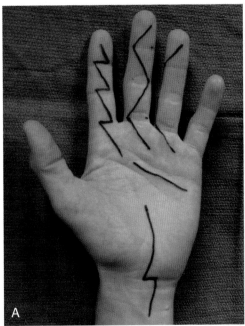
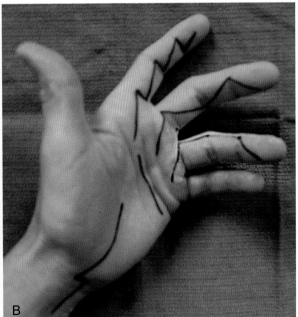

FIGURE 10.29 Discontinuous, extensile incision used in extended approach. Similar incisions for ring and little fingers are made as needed. **SEE TECHNIQUE 10.13.**

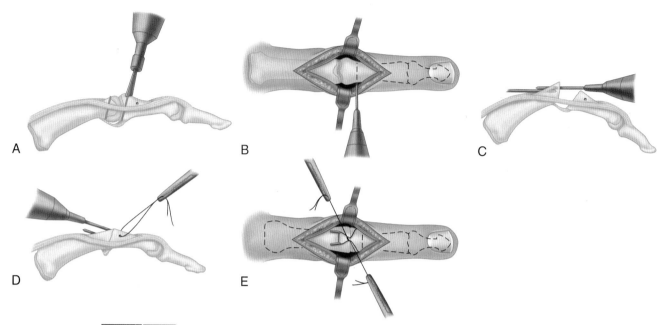

FIGURE 10.30 Tension band arthrodesis. **A,** Phalangeal osteotomy. Cuts are made parallel at desired angle with oscillating saw. **B,** Hole for 25-gauge or 26-gauge stainless steel wire made through middle phalangeal base dorsal to midaxial line. **C,** Retrograde insertion of 0.028-inch or 0.035-inch Kirschner wire into proximal phalanx. **D,** Kirschner wire driven into anterior cortex of middle phalanx. **E,** Figure-of-eight tension band created and tightened. **SEE TECHNIQUE 10.14.**

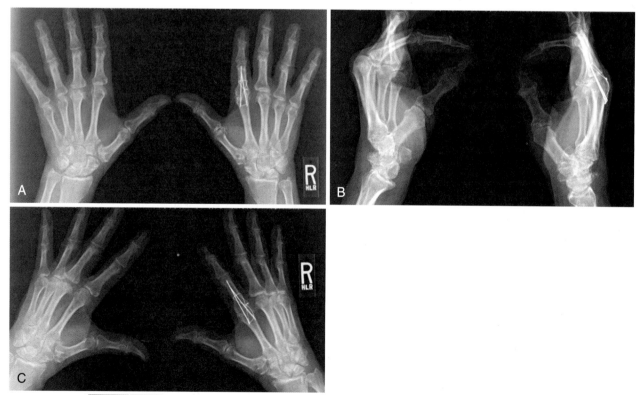

FIGURE 10.31 Anteroposterior **(A)**, lateral **(B)**, and oblique **(C)** radiographs of a 64-year-old right-handed surgeon with right index finger osteoarthritis treated with a tension band fusion. Note prior thumb arthroplasties and left middle finger treated with a silicone arthroplasty.

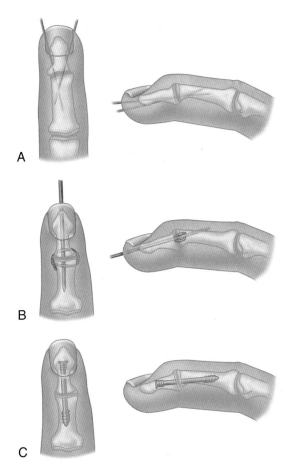

FIGURE 10.32 **A,** Anteroposterior and lateral views of crossed Kirschner wires. **B,** Anteroposterior and lateral views of interfragmentary wire and longitudinal Kirschner wire. **C,** Anteroposterior and lateral views of an intramedullary screw.

METACARPOPHALANGEAL JOINT ARTHRODESIS

TECHNIQUE 10.14

(STERN ET AL.; SEGMÜLLER, MODIFIED)
- Make a dorsal incision over the metacarpophalangeal joint to be fused.
- Split the extensor hood and joint capsule longitudinally in the center of the central extensor tendon.
- Remove sufficient capsule to gain exposure of the joint.
- Release the collateral ligaments to allow full flexion of the joint, exposing the joint surfaces proximally and distally.
- Remove any remaining articular cartilage from the destroyed joint and remove subchondral bone down to cancellous bone. Resect the joint surfaces with an osteotome or oscillating saw to achieve the desired angle (20 to 30 degrees), or remove the metacarpal head and proximal phalangeal base to make a cup-and-cone or ball-and-socket fit.
- With a 0.028-inch Kirschner wire, drill a transverse hole 5 to 10 mm distal to the fusion site slightly dorsal to the midaxial line.

- Thread a 25-gauge or 26-gauge stainless steel wire through this hole.
- Drive two 0.028-inch or 0.035-inch Kirschner wires retrograde into the metacarpal to exit dorsally 10 to 15 mm proximal to the fusion site.
- Compress the cut bone surfaces; avoid malrotation.
- Drive the Kirschner wires antegrade into the proximal phalanx, seating them either into the palmar cortex without penetrating it or distally in the medullary canal. Verify the fusion position and implant alignment fluoroscopically before definitive fixation.
- Loop the steel wire around the Kirschner wires in a figure-of-eight manner. Twist the ends of the steel wire together with a needle holder. Bend the ends of the Kirschner wires over the steel wire loops and cut the Kirschner wires close to bone (see Fig. 10.30).
- Close the remaining capsule over the wires and the extensor mechanism.
- Close the skin and apply a dressing and a splint, usually a dorsal splint to block extension.

POSTOPERATIVE CARE The splint is removed in 3 to 5 days, and active motion exercises are begun for mobile joints. Skin sutures are removed in 10 to 14 days. Interval splinting is appropriate for compliant patients. Internal fixation usually is not removed. Periodic radiographs are obtained to assess healing, and several months may pass before solid bone union is apparent radiographically.

PROXIMAL INTERPHALANGEAL JOINT ARTHRODESIS

TECHNIQUE 10.15

- Open the joint through a curved dorsal midline incision centered over the proximal interphalangeal joint. Incise the extensor tendon and capsule longitudinally.
- Release the extensor central tendon from the middle phalanx.
- Release and excise the collateral ligaments as required to flex and fully access the joint surfaces.
- Shape the joint surfaces either by making flat surfaces with an oscillating saw or by making a ball-and-socket shape so that the surfaces can be closely apposed at the proper angle (25 to 45 degrees progressively from the index to small finger proximal interphalangeal joint).
- Fusion fixation may be by Kirschner wires, tension band technique, or screws.
- The techniques of tendon repair, skin closure, and splint application and postoperative care are the same as for the metacarpophalangeal joint described previously.

■ DISTAL INTERPHALANGEAL JOINT ARTHRODESIS

Distal interphalangeal joint arthrodesis can be performed as described for the proximal interphalangeal joint. A number of dorsal approaches allow adequate distal interphalangeal

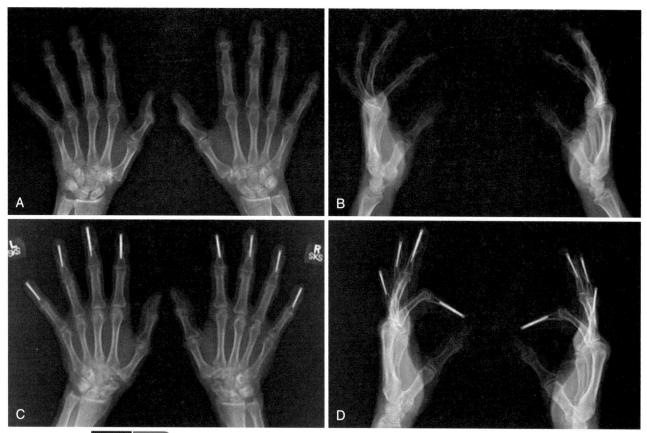

FIGURE 10.33 A 58-year-old female with persistent pain in distal interphalangeal joints of index through small fingers of both hands. **A** and **B,** Anteroposterior and lateral views of hands showing osteoarthritic deformities of distal interphalangeal joints. **C** and **D,** Anteroposterior and lateral views showing successful fusion of using fusion screws. Also note thumb arthroplasties done at same time as the fusions.

joint exposure, including longitudinal, V-shaped, and transverse curved incisions on contralateral limbs. A transverse incision centered over the thumb interphalangeal or finger distal interphalangeal joint with proximal and distal extensions at right angles on contralateral sides of the transverse limb heals with almost imperceptible scars (Fig. 10.34). Skin over the distal joint usually is insufficient to allow elaborate internal fixation. Because of ease of insertion, a buried headless screw or Kirschner wires are preferred. Union rates are similar. In compliant patients, interval splinting may be permitted until fusion is achieved, usually 6 to 8 weeks.

DEFORMITIES OF THE THUMB
CLASSIFICATION

Rheumatoid thumb deformities frequently are complex and can involve the joints individually or in combination. The classification of rheumatoid thumb deformities proposed by Nalebuff is helpful in understanding the problems and developing a plan for treatment. He described four types of rheumatoid thumb deformities.

Type I, the most common, is a boutonniere deformity; type II, which is rare, includes metacarpophalangeal joint flexion, interphalangeal joint hyperextension, and trapeziometacarpal

joint subluxation or dislocation; type III, the second most common, is a swan-neck deformity; and type IV, which is unusual, results from ulnar collateral ligament laxity and includes abduction of the proximal phalanx with metacarpal adduction. Type I (boutonniere) deformity results from synovitis that begins at the metacarpophalangeal joint and stretches out the dorsal capsule and extensor hood, with attenuation of the extensor pollicis brevis insertion. The extensor pollicis longus migrates medially. The deformities that eventually develop are metacarpophalangeal joint flexion, palmar subluxation of the proximal phalanx on the metacarpal, and interphalangeal joint hyperextension. As the deformity begins to develop, the joints usually can be passively corrected; with progression, the deformities become fixed.

■ TYPE I

Treatment of type I thumb deformities depends on the passive correctability of the joints and the extent of joint destruction. If the metacarpophalangeal subluxation and interphalangeal joint hyperextension are correctable, and radiographically the joints are normal, metacarpophalangeal synovectomy and extensor reconstruction may suffice. If the metacarpophalangeal contracture is fixed and the interphalangeal joint is correctable, but joint destruction is radiographically significant, then metacarpophalangeal arthrodesis is indicated. In

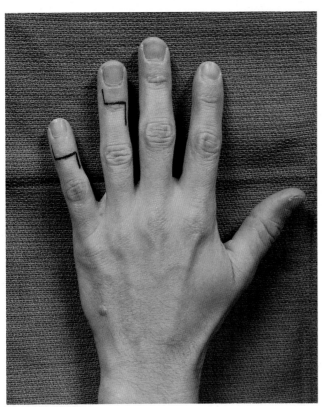

FIGURE 10.34 Incision for distal interphalangeal joint arthrodesis.

the presence of joint destruction at the interphalangeal and trapeziometacarpal joints, metacarpophalangeal arthroplasty may be more satisfactory, especially in older patients with fewer demands on their hands. If the deformities at the metacarpophalangeal and interphalangeal joints are fixed, with a satisfactory trapeziometacarpal joint but interphalangeal and metacarpophalangeal joint damage, metacarpophalangeal motion may be preserved with arthroplasty and interphalangeal arthrodesis may provide a satisfactory thumb for patients with low demands. Metacarpophalangeal and interphalangeal arthrodeses usually provide a stable opposable thumb when both joints are severely damaged radiographically.

TYPE II

Type II thumb deformities include metacarpophalangeal joint flexion, interphalangeal joint hyperextension, and dislocation or subluxation of the trapeziometacarpal joint. By using combinations of interphalangeal fusion and metacarpophalangeal and trapeziometacarpal arthroplasty, type II deformities can be treated similar to type I and type III deformities.

TYPE III

Type III (swan-neck) thumb deformities generally are believed to begin with synovitis at the trapeziometacarpal joint. Eventually the trapeziometacarpal joint subluxates laterally because of joint destruction and capsular attenuation. An adduction contracture of the metacarpal develops, and the metacarpophalangeal joint hyperextends as a result of the metacarpophalangeal joint extension forces and volar plate laxity. The treatment of type III deformities depends on the extent of metacarpophalangeal joint destruction, pain, the passive correctability of the metacarpophalangeal joint deformity and trapeziometacarpal subluxation, metacarpal adduction contractures, and metacarpophalangeal joint hyperextension. For mild type III deformities, if conservative treatment fails and pain persists, trapeziometacarpal arthroplasty, without total excision of the trapezium, provides a satisfactory basal joint. If the metacarpophalangeal deformity is mild, trapeziometacarpal implant hemiarthroplasty or resection arthroplasty can provide a satisfactory joint. If the deformity and metacarpophalangeal joint destruction are advanced, however, metacarpophalangeal joint fusion can be added to the trapeziometacarpal hemiarthroplasty or resection arthroplasty. In advanced metacarpophalangeal deformity with trapeziometacarpal dislocation, a fixed thumb metacarpal adduction contracture, and a fixed hyperextension of the metacarpophalangeal joint, better results can be obtained with trapeziometacarpal hemiarthroplasty or resection arthroplasty, combined with metacarpophalangeal joint fusion. This usually relieves the thumb metacarpal adduction posture without release of the first dorsal interosseous or first web space.

TYPE IV

Type IV (gamekeeper) thumb deformity includes a thumb proximal phalanx abduction deformity and an adducted metacarpal caused by stretching of the ulnar collateral ligament and attenuation of the capsuloligamentous structures by chronic rheumatoid synovitis. Metacarpophalangeal synovectomy, ligament reconstruction, and adductor release may be sufficient for milder deformities. For more advanced deformities, metacarpophalangeal arthroplasty or arthrodesis may be required to stabilize the joint. Additional adduction deformity of the thumb metacarpal usually is avoided after metacarpophalangeal stabilization.

Although the pathomechanics may be different for rheumatoid and osteoarthritic patients, techniques for treating the thumb, including soft-tissue procedures, arthrodesis, and arthroplasty, are similar in both diseases.

OSTEOARTHRITIS

The thumb joints affected by osteoarthritis are, in descending order of frequency, the trapeziometacarpal, metacarpophalangeal, and distal interphalangeal joints. The trapeziometacarpal joint is most often affected by primary osteoarthritis or posttraumatic arthritis. Trapeziometacarpal osteoarthritis is a consequence of a progressive volar trapezial articular surface eburnation, which is greater than that on the metacarpal beak articular surface, supporting the concept of trapeziometacarpal translational instability as a major factor in trapeziometacarpal joint osteoarthritis. The metacarpophalangeal joint is most often disabled by ligament instability, usually of the ulnar collateral ligament.

CORRECTION OF ARTHRITIC THUMB DEFORMITIES

The operative techniques available for the treatment of arthritic thumb deformities include synovectomy, soft-tissue reconstructions, osteotomy, arthroplasty, and arthrodesis. The following techniques can be used for rheumatoid arthritis and osteoarthritis. Although most of the soft-tissue procedures are used more frequently for rheumatoid arthritis, the bony procedures, including osteotomy, arthroplasty, and arthrodesis, are used in the treatment of osteoarthritis as well.

SYNOVECTOMY

Synovectomy may prevent rheumatoid capsular distention and capsuloligamentous destruction and attenuation and is effective especially in the absence of significant radiographic changes or joint instability. Synovectomy is done more commonly for interphalangeal and metacarpophalangeal involvement and less often for trapeziometacarpal involvement.

THUMB INTERPHALANGEAL JOINT SYNOVECTOMY

TECHNIQUE 10.16

- Approach the thumb interphalangeal joint using a straight dorsal, longitudinal curved, or dual flap incision as for the fingers.
- Carefully examine the radial and ulnar sides of the joint and perform synovectomy on either side of the extensor tendon as needed.
- If the radial collateral ligament is released, reattach the collateral ligament to bone with a pull-out wire or suture anchor and fix the joint with a Kirschner wire for temporary stabilization.
- Close the wound and apply a splint with the interphalangeal joint in extension.

POSTOPERATIVE CARE The sutures and Kirschner wire are removed at 10 to 14 days, and active movement is begun. The finger is splinted in extension except for exercise periods for another 10 to 14 days.

THUMB METACARPOPHALANGEAL JOINT SYNOVECTOMY

TECHNIQUE 10.17

- Approach the metacarpophalangeal joint through a dorsal curved incision.
- Expose the dorsal joint capsule between the extensor pollicis brevis and extensor pollicis longus tendons, retracting them to either side of the joint. (Splitting the extensor pollicis brevis provides the same exposure and may result in better soft tissue for closure.)
- Open the capsule dorsally and clean the joint using a rongeur and curet.
- Apply traction to the proximal phalanx to open the joint and flex the joint to allow access to the more volar recesses.
- Close the capsule, extensor mechanism, and skin. Apply a splint to maintain the metacarpophalangeal joint in extension.

POSTOPERATIVE CARE The splint and sutures are removed at 10 to 14 days, and exercises are begun. Splinting of the joint is continued for another 2 weeks except for exercise periods.

THUMB TRAPEZIOMETACARPAL JOINT SYNOVECTOMY

TECHNIQUE 10.18

- Approach the thumb trapeziometacarpal joint through either a straight dorsal incision curving toward the palm over the trapeziometacarpal joint or an extended Wagner approach between the glabrous and nonglabrous skin.
- Retract the skin, avoiding injury to the cutaneous nerve branches.
- Open the capsule and clean the joint as much as possible with a rongeur and curet.
- Close the capsule and skin and splint the thumb in extension and abduction.
- If extensive ligamentous laxity is noted, reconstruction of the trapeziometacarpal capsuloligamentous structures may be required.

SOFT-TISSUE RECONSTRUCTION

Soft-tissue reconstruction may be required for thumb interphalangeal, metacarpophalangeal, and trapeziometacarpal joint instability, whether related to osteoarthritic or rheumatoid deformities, especially at the metacarpophalangeal and trapeziometacarpal joints.

INTERPHALANGEAL SOFT-TISSUE RECONSTRUCTION

TECHNIQUE 10.19

- If the interphalangeal joint is passively correctable and there are no significant radiographic changes, release of this joint may be effective in restoring some of its flexion.
- Expose the joint; if there is a severe extension contracture deformity, convert the incision to a Z-plasty as the wound is closed.
- Perform an extensor tenolysis and release the dorsal capsule by retracting the extensor tendon to the side and incising the dorsal part of the metacarpophalangeal joint capsule along with the dorsal portions of the collateral ligaments.
- Flex the joint 20 to 30 degrees and pin it with a Kirschner wire.
- Secondary intention healing is suitable for wounds that cannot be closed, especially distally.
- Apply a thumb spica splint.

POSTOPERATIVE CARE The splint and Kirschner wire and sutures are removed at 10 to 14 days, and gentle exercises are begun. The thumb is splinted for another 2 to 3 weeks, except for periods of exercise. If an incomplete extension (extensor lag) develops, splinting is continued for another 2 to 3 weeks. Normal motion rarely is regained.

Soft-tissue reconstructions are effective for mild, easily correctable rheumatoid metacarpophalangeal joint deformities without significant radiographic changes. Metacarpophalangeal synovectomy and extensor tendon reconstruction usually restore metacarpophalangeal joint extension. Nalebuff and Inglis et al. described effective procedures for improving function in the rheumatoid thumb. In patients with long-standing posttraumatic ulnar collateral ligament laxity or ligament laxity related to osteoarthritis, ulnar collateral ligament reconstruction may be required to stabilize the joint if there is no significant radiographic joint destruction.

METACARPOPHALANGEAL SYNOVECTOMY WITH EXTENSOR TENDON RECONSTRUCTION

TECHNIQUE 10.20

- Determine the passive correctability of metacarpophalangeal joint flexion.
- Make either a straight or a curved incision over the dorsum of the metacarpophalangeal joint, and retract skin flaps, avoiding injury to cutaneous nerves.
- Identify the extensor pollicis brevis and longus tendons, which may be displaced medially, and make an incision between them.
- Incise along each side of the extensor pollicis longus to free it of its intrinsic muscle attachment.
- Transect the extensor pollicis longus over the distal third of the proximal phalanx.
- Dissect and release the extensor pollicis brevis from the base of the proximal phalanx and detach it from the extensor mechanism.
- Make a transverse incision in the capsule and mobilize a flap of capsule based distally at its attachment to the base of the proximal phalanx.
- Make a transverse slit incision in the base of the capsule to allow passage of the extensor pollicis longus.
- Remove the synovium from the joint with a rongeur and curet.
- Pass the extensor pollicis longus through the transverse slit incision in the capsule and reflect it over itself.
- Hold the joint in full extension and suture the extensor pollicis longus tendon to itself under tension.
- Apply traction to the extensor pollicis brevis distally and suture it into the side of the extensor pollicis longus.
- Ensure that the intrinsic tendon insertions into the extensor mechanism are properly positioned to maintain active extension of the distal phalanx and that the intrinsic tendons do not subluxate toward the palm.
- Tighten the transverse fibers of the extensor tendons over the dorsal aspect of the distal phalanx if needed. Insert a Kirschner wire across the metacarpophalangeal joint to maintain it in extension.
- Apply a splint to maintain interphalangeal extension.

POSTOPERATIVE CARE The splint and sutures are removed at 10 to 14 days, and the splint is reapplied. The Kirschner wire across the metacarpophalangeal joint is removed at 4 weeks, and splinting of the metacarpophalangeal joint in extension is continued for another 2 weeks. Interphalangeal joint flexion and extension are maintained from the early postoperative period throughout recovery.

THUMB METACARPOPHALANGEAL JOINT RECONSTRUCTION FOR RHEUMATOID ARTHRITIS

TECHNIQUE 10.21

(INGLIS ET AL.)
- Make a longitudinal incision over the dorsum of the metacarpophalangeal joint from the middle of the proximal phalanx to the midshaft of the first metacarpal.
- Observe the extensor pollicis brevis to determine if it has become detached and retracted proximally (Fig. 10.35A).
- Split the extensor hood longitudinally between the extensor pollicis longus and extensor pollicis brevis.
- Detach the abductor pollicis brevis from the extensor hood on the radial side and the adductor pollicis from the ulnar side (Fig. 10.35B).
- Retract the remaining tendon structures laterally to expose the capsule and the synovium.
- Preserve the collateral ligaments, but excise all the synovium within the joint (Fig. 10.35C); this may be facilitated by flexing the joint.
- Attach the extensor pollicis brevis (or extensor indicis proprius if indicated) to the proximal phalanx base dorsally.
- Attach the extensor pollicis brevis with sufficient tension to maintain extension of the metacarpophalangeal joint, and attach the abductor pollicis brevis and adductor pollicis dorsally to preserve the balance of this joint (Fig. 10.35D).
- Maintain the metacarpophalangeal joint in extension by transfixing Kirschner wires for 4 weeks.
- Apply a splint to maintain the thumb in the desired position.

POSTOPERATIVE CARE The splint and sutures are removed at about 2 weeks, and the splint is reapplied. The Kirschner wires are removed at about 4 weeks, and splinting is continued except for exercise periods for another 2 to 3 weeks.

ARTHROPLASTY

Arthroplasty may be preferable to an attempt to maintain metacarpophalangeal joint motion if the interphalangeal joint is sufficiently damaged to require arthrodesis. Sufficient bone stock should be present to allow stable arthroplasty, and it should be possible to obtain reasonable joint stability with restoration or preservation of capsuloligamentous structures (Fig. 10.36). If restoration of joint stability is doubtful, arthrodesis is more predictable. Normal motion is not expected after metacarpophalangeal arthroplasty. Silicone implant arthroplasty can provide a satisfactorily functioning joint, despite implant breakage, dislocation, and particulate synovitis.

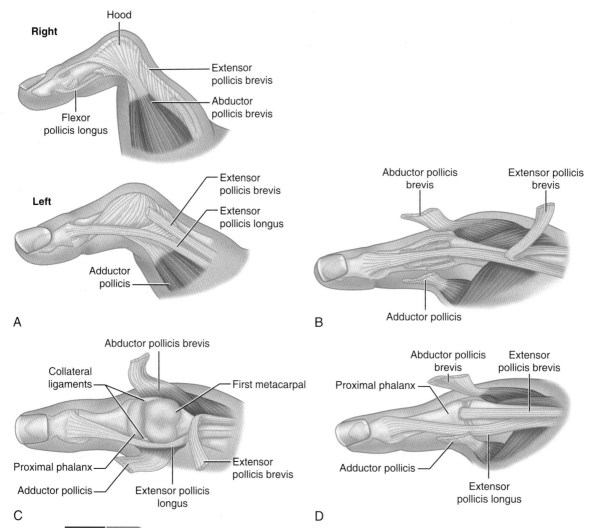

FIGURE 10.35 Reconstruction of metacarpophalangeal joint of thumb in rheumatoid arthritis. **A,** Metacarpophalangeal joint of thumb with extensive tendon damage. After rupture of insertion of extensor pollicis brevis tendon proximal retraction, extensor hood becomes attenuated and allows abductor pollicis brevis and extensor pollicis longus to migrate volarward below center of rotation of metacarpophalangeal joint. **B,** Extensor pollicis brevis and adductor pollicis insertions are dissected free from remaining attenuated extensor tendon hood. **C,** Synovectomy is facilitated by joint flexion. Collateral ligaments are preserved. **D,** Attachment of extensor pollicis brevis tendon into base of proximal phalanx. When extensor pollicis brevis cannot be advanced, extensor indicis proprius can be transferred from index finger and inserted into base of proximal phalanx. (Redrawn from Inglis AE, Hamlin C, Sengelmann RP, et al: Reconstruction of the metacarpophalangeal joint of the thumb in rheumatoid arthritis, *J Bone Joint Surg* 54A:704, 1972.) **SEE TECHNIQUE 10.21.**

METACARPOPHALANGEAL ARTHROPLASTY

TECHNIQUE 10.22

- Expose the metacarpophalangeal joint extensor mechanism through a longitudinal dorsal oblique skin incision.
- Enter the metacarpophalangeal joint by longitudinally splitting the extensor pollicis brevis and the radial extensor expansion distally. Note that the extensor pollicis

brevis typically does not have a phalangeal bony insertion. If the extensor pollicis longus is translocated ulnarward, then release the extensor expansion along the extensor pollicis longus ulnarly to centralize this tendon.

- Resect the metacarpal head perpendicular to the shaft, leaving the metaphyseal flare of the metacarpal. Preserve the collateral ligaments.
- If a flexion contracture persists, partially release the collateral ligament proximally.
- Leave the base of the proximal phalanx, unless additional space is required for the prosthesis, in which case remove a portion of the cartilage and subchondral bone.

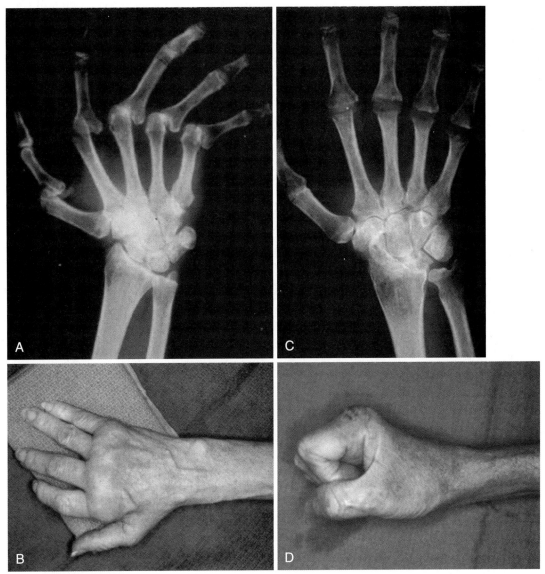

FIGURE 10.36   **A** and **B,** Type I thumb, fixed finger metacarpophalangeal joint subluxations with degenerative changes and ulnar translocation of wrist with relatively preserved midcarpal joint. **C** and **D,** Appearance after radioscapholunate fusion, metacarpophalangeal implant arthroplasty, and thumb metacarpophalangeal joint fusion. **SEE TECHNIQUE 10.22.**

- Ream the medullary canal of the metacarpal and the proximal phalanx using the temporary trial prostheses to determine the largest size that the metacarpal shaft will accept.
- Drill small holes in the dorsal base of the proximal phalanx to allow attachment of the extensor pollicis brevis.
- Pass a suture through these holes so that it is in place for reattachment of the extensor pollicis brevis after the prosthesis has been inserted.
- Reattach the extensor pollicis brevis under sufficient tension to allow proximal phalangeal extension.
- Repair the extensor expansion over the insertion of the extensor pollicis brevis tendon.

- Advance and repair the extensor pollicis longus tendon centered over the extensor expansion.
- Close the skin and apply a splint to immobilize the hand and thumb with the metacarpophalangeal joint held in extension.
- Pin the distal joint if needed.

POSTOPERATIVE CARE The sutures are removed at 10 to 14 days and a splint is applied to keep the metacarpophalangeal joint in extension. Interphalangeal joint motion is encouraged. The metacarpophalangeal joint is splinted in extension for 3 to 4 weeks. Forceful, strenuous activities are avoided for at least 6 to 8 weeks.

▌TRAPEZIOMETACARPAL LIGAMENT RECONSTRUCTION

Trapeziometacarpal soft-tissue reconstruction is used for posttraumatic ligamentous laxity related to recurrent dislocation. It rarely is indicated for laxity related to rheumatoid changes because arthroplasty and arthrodesis usually are better options. Reconstruction of the trapeziometacarpal volar ligament in patients with hypermobile prearthritic joints may provide significant pain relief and reduce the chance of future progression of trapeziometacarpal arthritis.

Although suture techniques may provide adequate stabilization, we prefer to use this as an adjunct to biologic reconstruction.

TRAPEZIOMETACARPAL LIGAMENT RECONSTRUCTION

TECHNIQUE 10.23

(EATON AND LITTLER)

- Expose the thumb CMC joint through an incision along the radial border of the metacarpal, curving ulnarly in the distal wrist flexion crease as far as the flexor carpi radialis tendon. Three special structures should be protected: the superficial branch of the radial nerve, the superficial branch of the radial artery, and any sensory branches, especially the palmar cutaneous branch of the median nerve (Fig. 10.37A).
- Reflect the thenar muscles extraperiosteally from the metacarpal and volar aspects of the trapezium ulnarward.
- Deep dissection at the proximal border of the trapezium exposes a sheet of transverse fascial fibers that form a roof over the separate fibrous flexor carpi radialis tunnel. This tunnel is separated from the carpal tunnel by a septum parallel to and between the flexor carpi radialis and the flexor pollicis longus.
- A reflection of the transverse carpal ligament forms a roof over this fibroosseous tunnel (Fig. 10.37B). Incise this layer longitudinally, exposing the flexor carpi radialis tendon course, which disappears distally beneath a horizontal trapezial ridge projection.
- Free the tendon approximately 0.5 cm distal to this point by sharp release of the overlying muscle origins and the transverse carpal ligament, exposing the volar and radial aspect of the CMC joint.
- Perform an arthrotomy of the radial capsule to allow debridement of synovium and marginal osteophytes and inspection of the articular cartilage.
- Remove as much diseased synovium as possible.
- Create an extraarticular tunnel from the metacarpal dorsum to the metacarpal volar beak apex, in a plane perpendicular to the thumb nail. Start the tunnel just distal to the dorsal base of the metacarpal between the extensor pollicis brevis and extensor pollicis longus tendons (Fig. 10.37C).
- Obtain a strip of the distally based flexor carpi radialis by making two transverse incisions 3 and 6 cm proximal to the distal wrist flexion crease.

- Split a strip of half its width away radially and tunnel beneath skin bridges to emerge beyond the wrist crease, remaining in continuity distally (Fig. 10.37D).
- Continue the split distal to the crest of the trapezium, at which point the free end is redirected across the crest to enter the volar portion of the previously created intramedullary channel at the thumb metacarpal beak.
- Draw the tendon dorsally using a previously placed wire suture (Fig. 10.37E). The distal portion of the new ligament reconstruction should remain in continuity with the intact flexor carpi radialis tendon.
- At this point, accurately reduce the joint under direct vision and hold it in extension-abduction, seating the metacarpal against the deep facet of the trapezium.
- Insert a Kirschner wire from the dorsum of the metacarpal into the trapezium to maintain the reduction. Do not impale the intramedullary portion of the tendon strip.
- With the reduction stabilized, draw the tendon strip taut. Ensure that it courses directly between its point of emergence from the flexor radialis tunnel to the beak of the metacarpal.
- Securely suture this tendon to the dorsal periosteum of the metacarpal and route the remainder proximally to pass across the dorsal basal joint capsule and beneath the extensor pollicis brevis and abductor pollicis longus (APL) insertion. Suture this tendon strip under tension to the APL bony insertion.
- Pass the remainder of the flexor carpi radialis tendon strip beneath or through a short split in the remaining flexor carpi radialis tendon just proximal to the trapezium and back across the radial margin of the joint to insert into the metacarpal periosteum, suturing at each point where its direction is changed (Fig. 10.37F).
- Apply a short arm thumb spica splint.

▌TRAPEZIOMETACARPAL ARTHROPLASTY

Many surgical techniques have been described for thumb trapeziometacarpal joint arthritic deformity, including ligament reconstruction, open or arthroscopic partial or complete trapezial resection arthroplasty with or without interposition, metacarpal osteotomy, implant arthroplasty, and fusion. Although patients with rheumatoid arthritis involving the trapeziometacarpal joint seem to benefit more from resection arthroplasty, with or without tendon interposition or ligament reconstruction, or from hemiarthroplasty, this seems to be related to joint laxity, destruction, and osteoporosis. More treatment options are available for osteoarthritic trapeziometacarpal deformities, including procedures mentioned previously for rheumatoid arthritis and trapeziometacarpal arthrodesis in younger patients with heavy demands on their joints.

Efforts to simplify the surgical techniques, lessen the potential complications, and shorten the usually prolonged recovery period continue to evolve. The observation that failed attempts to achieve a CMC arthrodesis usually resulted in a painless pseudarthrosis led Rubino et al. to a procedure designed to specifically achieve this result (Fig. 10.38). Between 1 and 2 mm of the opposing CMC joint surfaces are resected, and crossed Kirschner wires are removed at approximately 4 weeks. In a retrospective review of 248 consecutive patients treated for Eaton stages II and III osteoarthritis,

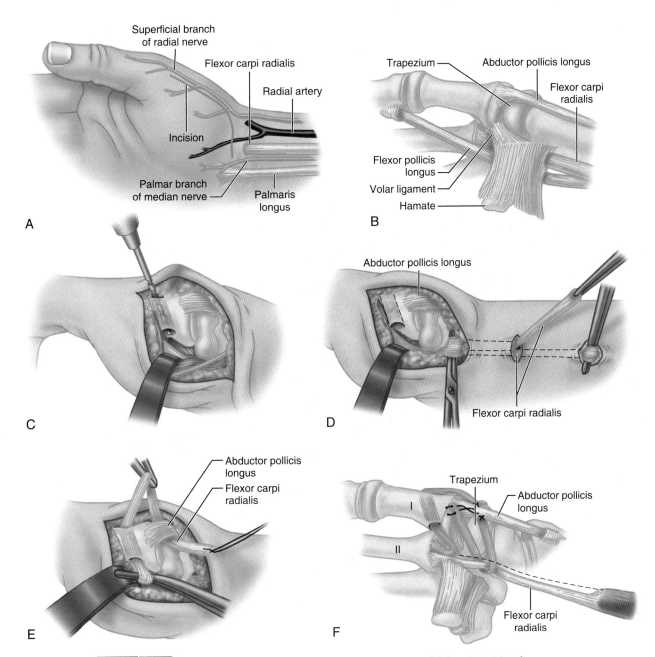

FIGURE 10.37 Reconstruction for painful thumb carpometacarpal joint. **A,** Incision for exposure. **B,** Schema of ligament support. The volar ligament is reflection of transverse carpal ligament after insertion into crest of trapezium. Note flexor radialis passing directly beneath this ligament. **C,** Gouge track created in sagittal diameter of metacarpal, emerging at its volar beak. Small branch of radial nerve retracted volarly. **D,** A 6-cm to 8-cm strip, representing half width of flexor radialis tendon split away and remaining in continuity distally. Split continues 5 mm distal to crest of trapezium. **E,** Scissor point indicates path of flexor radialis strip rerouted to enter channel at metacarpal beak. Emerging dorsally, flexor carpi radialis is passed deep to extensor pollicis brevis and under insertion of abductor pollicis longus, also reinforcing dorsal capsule. **F,** Schema of volar and radial ligament reconstruction. Course of tendon strip creates reinforcement in volar, dorsal, and radial aspect of joint. (Redrawn from Eaton RG, Littler JW: Ligament reconstruction for the painful thumb carpometacarpal joint, *J Bone Joint Surg* 55A:1665, 1973.) **SEE TECHNIQUE 10.23.**

these authors observed a statistically significant improvement in mean appositional and oppositional pinch strength, mean disabilities of the arm, shoulder, and hand (DASH) score (63.8 preoperatively to 10.5 at final follow-up), and the mean pain score (8.3 to 0.2). No revisions were required. They concluded

that trapeziometacarpal limited excision arthroplasty is a simple and reliable alternative to existing surgical techniques for treating stage II or III thumb CMC joint arthritis.

Resection arthroplasty involving total trapeziectomy may relieve pain in patients with rheumatoid arthritis, but patients

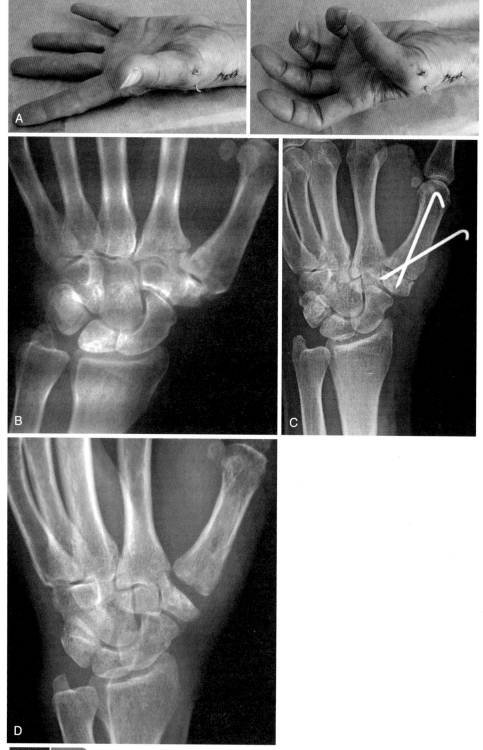

FIGURE 10.38 Trapeziometacarpal pseudarthrosis. **A,** Percutaneous Kirschner wires allow pain-free mobilization of thumb. **B,** Dorso-palmar radiograph showing advanced degenerative changes in carpometacarpal joint. **C,** After surgery, before removal of Kirschner wires. **D,** Dorso-palmar radiograph 3 years after surgery; note maintenance of trapeziometacarpal joint line. (From Rubino M, Civani A, Pagani D, Sansone V: Trapeziometacarpal narrow pseudarthrosis: a new surgical technique to treat thumb carpometacarpal joint arthritis, *J Hand Surg Eur* 38:844, 2013.)

with extreme ligamentous laxity may not have as good results. Patients with advanced osteoarthritic changes may obtain satisfactory results. Resection arthroplasty allows early thumb mobilization and is technically easier than other arthroplasty methods.

Gangopadhyay et al. compared simple trapeziectomy, trapeziectomy with palmaris longus interposition, and trapeziectomy with ligament reconstruction and tendon interposition using 50% of the flexor carpi radialis tendon in a group of 153 thumbs at a minimum follow-up of 5 years (5 to 18 years). All thumbs were temporarily pinned for 4 weeks and had similar postoperative treatment protocols. Subjective and objective assessments of thumb pain, function, and strength in this randomized prospective study found no differences among the three treatment groups. Good results were achieved in 78% of patients, and pain relief was maintained in the long term, regardless of the type of surgery. The authors concluded that there appears to be no benefit to tendon interposition or ligament reconstruction in the longer term. The common step in all three groups, however, is temporary Kirschner wire fixation that requires a second surgery for wire removal. Taking this into consideration, as well as factors specific to surgeon preference, most surgeons prefer reconstructions not requiring secondary procedures.

Burton and Eaton and Littler proposed classification systems of thumb trapeziometacarpal arthrosis (Table 10.2). The deformities are divided into four stages based on joint involvement, trapeziometacarpal joint subluxation, and joint debris. At best these systems quantify the radiographic disease state; however, they do not reliably correlate with a patient's symptoms or necessarily help select the best surgical procedure for a given condition. Nevertheless, more significant joint destruction, including pantrapezial arthritis, intermetacarpal osteophyte formation, and adduction deformities, are end-stage findings usually best treated by complete trapezium techniques.

DISTRACTION ARTHROPLASTY

TECHNIQUE 10.24

- Make an incision parallel to the APL tendon and extend it into the web space as far as necessary to release the soft tissue.
- Divide the superficial fascia and release the fascia over the abductor, the adductor insertion, and the part of the adductor origin on the third metacarpal.
- Reflect dorsally the dorsal branch of the radial artery and the sensory branch of the radial nerve and identify the first metacarpal base.
- Remove the periosteum and capsule to expose the first trapeziometacarpal joint and then the scaphotrapezial joint.
- With a small osteotome, split the trapezium into segments and remove it.
- Maintain the intermetacarpal ligament so that the thumb metacarpal base retains its attachments to the index finger metacarpal.
- Remove osteophytes from the thumb metacarpal base and, if necessary, resect a part of the base of the index (second) metacarpal.
- Perform a tenolysis of the extensor pollicis longus and APL if needed.

TABLE 10.2

Classification Systems of Thumb Carpometacarpal Arthrosis

EATON	BURTON	DELL
STAGE I		
No joint destruction Joint space widened if effusion present Less than one third subluxation	Ligamentous laxity, pain, positive grind test Dorsoradial metacarpal subluxation	Symptoms with heavy use, positive grind test Narrowed joint space, subchondral sclerosis
STAGE II		
Slight decrease in joint space Marginal osteophytes <2 mm May be one third subluxation	Crepitus, instability, chronic subluxation Degenerative changes on radiograph	Pain with normal use, crepitus Ulnar osteophyte, less than one third subluxation
STAGE III		
Significant joint destruction with cysts and sclerosis Osteophytes >2 mm Greater than one third subluxation	Pantrapezial degenerative changes	CMC adduction deformity, MCP joint hyperextension May have pantrapezial arthritis and one third subluxation
STAGE IV		
Involvement of multiple joint surfaces	Stage II or III with arthritis at the MCP joint	Cystic changes and total loss of joint space CMC joint may be totally immobile

CMC, Carpometacarpal; *MCP,* metacarpophalangeal.
From Wolock BS, Moore JR, Weiland AJ: Arthritis of the basal joint of the thumb: a critical analysis of treatment options, *J Arthroplasty* 4:65, 1989.

- Hold the thumb and index metacarpals with a Kirschner wire, maintaining the thumb in a rotated, abducted position.
- Thumb web space contractures may require skin grafting, rotation or pedicle flaps, or Z-plasties.
- Close the skin and apply a compression dressing combined with a plaster splint to maintain thumb abduction and rotation.

POSTOPERATIVE CARE The splint or cast and sutures are removed at 2 weeks. The Kirschner wire is removed at 4 to 6 weeks, and exercises are begun; the thumb is splinted between exercise sessions.

After complete trapezial excision, surprising longitudinal stability is sometimes retained as demonstrated by axial loading of the thumb metacarpal shaft. However, more commonly, once the trapezium has been excised, the thumb tends to shorten as the distance between the metacarpal base and distal scaphoid lessens. The Gothic arch relationship between the thumb and index metacarpals can be maintained in ways other than Kirschner wire fixation, as in Technique 10.24. Another option is to suspend the thumb metacarpal by a suture and button technique (Fig. 10.39). According to Yao and Song, 21 patients with a minimum 2-year follow-up had satisfactory results with this technique, although there was a 25% loss of trapezial height. Because biologic stabilization is not required for this method, earlier rehabilitation may be possible.

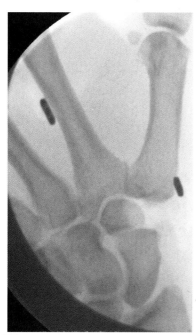

FIGURE 10.39 Suture-button suspensionplasty for thumb carpometacarpal arthritis. One button lies on dorsoradial base of thumb metacarpal and other on ulnar border of second metacarpal. A suture between two buttons provides suspension of thumb metacarpal (because the suture is radiolucent, it is not visible on radiograph). (From Yao J, Song Y: Suture-button suspensionplasty for thumb carpometacarpal arthritis: a minimum 2-year follow-up, *J Hand Surg* 38A:1161, 2013.)

TENDON INTERPOSITION ARTHROPLASTY WITH LIGAMENT RECONSTRUCTION

Biologic interposition materials used for resection arthroplasty have included fascia lata, hematoma, Gelfoam, and the flexor carpi radialis or palmaris longus and the APL tendons. Ligament reconstructions have included free grafts and strips of the flexor carpi radialis tendon, APL tendon, and extensor carpi radialis longus tendon and APL tendon shortening. Ligament reconstruction alone seems to be suitable for posttraumatic or early osteoarthritic changes at the trapeziometacarpal joint.

This section on trapeziometacarpal arthroplasties presents the procedures in current use that incorporate available biologic structures. The following techniques have similarities, can be used for rheumatoid arthritis or osteoarthritis, can provide predictable and reliable stability of the thumb metacarpal base, can provide pain relief, may be used with complete or partial trapezial excision, and have produced satisfactory results according to the reports of their proponents.

TECHNIQUE 10.25

(BURTON AND PELLEGRINI)

- With the patient under satisfactory anesthesia and a pneumatic tourniquet inflated, expose the trapeziometacarpal joint with a dorsoradial incision in line with the thumb metacarpal, extending proximally across the trapeziometacarpal joint and medially toward the palm.
- Elevate the thenar muscles extraperiosteally and expose the trapezium by opening the capsule of the trapeziometacarpal joint.
- Reflect the APL palmarward.
- If preoperative radiographs reveal only trapeziometacarpal arthrosis, a hemitrapeziectomy procedure can be performed.
- If there is pantrapezial involvement, or if there is a severe thumb-web contracture, excise the entire trapezium. Avoid damage to the flexor carpi radialis tendon during trapezial excision.
- Excise only the articular surface of the thumb metacarpal perpendicular to its long axis.
- Make the hole in the base of the radial cortex of the thumb metacarpal with a 6-mm gouge perpendicular to the plane of the thumbnail.
- Split the flexor carpi radialis longitudinally and release a 10- to 12-cm portion of the radial half of the flexor carpi radialis, leaving it attached distally.
- Harvest the flexor carpi radialis either through a series of short transverse incisions or through a single longitudinal incision.
- Split the flexor carpi radialis tendon to its insertion on the index metacarpal base and pass it into the dorsoradial wound through the trapezium fossa. Avoid transecting the flexor carpi radialis at its insertion.
- Place two nonabsorbable sutures in the deep capsule for later use.
- Seat the metacarpal in a medial direction toward the index metacarpal and stabilize it in the abducted position with a longitudinal Kirschner wire.

- Apply traction to the metacarpal and slide it on the Kirschner wire to preserve the arthroplasty space in the trapezium fossa.
- Pass the free end of the flexor carpi radialis from its distal insertion proximally to the base of the metacarpal cortex, into the medullary canal, and out the hole in the radial metacarpal cortex.
- Pull the tendon slip tight and suture it to the lateral periosteum and soft tissues around the metacarpal, then back onto itself to resurface the base of the metacarpal.
- Fold the remainder of the tendon to act as a spacer in the trapezium fossa and suture it to itself and the deep palmar capsule with one of the previously placed sutures.
- Use the second capsular suture to complete a two-layered lateral capsular closure over and including the tendon arthroplasty spacer.
- The distal orientation of the flexor carpi radialis tendon slip from the base of the thumb metacarpal to its insertion on the base of the index metacarpal is important because this is the ligament reconstruction that supports the thumb metacarpal, preventing proximal migration and radial subluxation of the thumb.
- Transfer the extensor pollicis brevis proximally and insert it on the metacarpal shaft to augment the metacarpal abduction and remove the hyperextension-deforming force in the proximal phalanx at the metacarpophalangeal joint.
- Apply a short arm thumb spica splint.

Following are modifications to this technique that are helpful in expediting the procedure and that do not seem to affect the outcome.

- We do not find it necessary to always use a Kirschner wire to stabilize the thumb, as a secure intermetacarpal ligament reconstruction and a thumb spica splint accurately maintain thumb position.
- In most cases, the entire trapezium has to be removed to aid in mobilization of the flexor carpi radialis. Based on preoperative radiographs and intraoperative evaluations of the proximal trapezoid, if arthrosis is identified, the proximal portion of the trapezoid can be resected to alleviate this contact point known to affect the outcome. Moreover, a wrist that shows signs of a midcarpal instability pattern with the lunate tilted dorsally before the thumb arthroplasty would seem to be at further risk of collapse from disengagement of the scaphoid distal pole.
- Rather than harvesting a longitudinal strip of the flexor carpi radialis through multiple transverse incisions, the entire flexor carpi radialis tendon can be used and harvested through a single transverse incision at the musculoskeletal junction. The flexor carpi radialis tendon is delivered to the base of the thumb by traction, and the sequence of ligament reconstruction and tendon interposition is carried out in routine fashion.
- Instead of removing the entire articular surface of the base of the thumb metacarpal, fashion a tunnel in the base of the thumb metacarpal using gradually larger drill points, entering the dorsum of the base of the thumb metacarpal about 1 cm distal to the articular margin. Orient the tunnel obliquely, medially, and proximally, allowing the drill point to exit through the joint surface at the medial (ulnar) side of the joint. Gradually enlarge the tunnel in the thumb metacarpal with drill points or curets. A number 1 curet usually makes a tunnel that is 4 to 5 mm

in diameter, which is sufficient for passage of the entire tendon. Avoid disrupting the bone bridge between the tunnel and the joint surface. Pass the tendon through the tunnel, securing the tendon to itself with nonabsorbable mattress sutures. Fold and attach the remainder of the tendon to the capsule deep in the trapezial defect with nonabsorbable sutures. Fold and suture the remaining half of the tendon to the deep capsule in a similar fashion. The folded tendon slips also can be secured to the trapezoid and the distal pole of the scaphoid.

See Video 10.1

POSTOPERATIVE CARE The sutures are removed in about 10 to 14 days. A splint is worn for an additional 3 to 4 weeks, at which time the Kirschner wire (if used) is removed and a removable thumb spica splint is applied. Range-of-motion exercises are begun at about the end of the first month. Initially, range-of-motion exercises are focused on metacarpal abduction and extension, avoiding flexion and adduction. Splinting is continued except for hand exercises and bathing for 2 to 4 weeks after the start of exercises. At about 6 weeks, thenar strengthening is begun and is continued for 4 to 6 months. Pinch and grip strengthening exercises are begun at about 12 weeks after surgery. Splinting is discontinued when range of motion and thenar strength are improved to a functional level, usually at 8 to 12 weeks. Recovery periods vary, and full recovery to pain-free use with good strength requires a minimum of 4 to 6 months.

TECHNIQUE 10.26

(KLEINMAN AND ECKENRODE)
- Use a regional or general anesthetic with a pneumatic tourniquet on the well-padded arm.
- Make a palmar curvilinear basilar thumb incision to extend proximally in a sufficient zigzag to allow access to the flexor carpi radialis and the tendons of the first extensor compartment (APL, extensor pollicis brevis) (Fig. 10.40A).
- If present, transect the palmar slip of the APL at the level of the trapeziometacarpal capsule and reflect the thenar muscles distally to expose the capsule of the trapeziometacarpal joint.
- Elevate a U-shaped, distally based flap of capsule, exposing the entire trapezium.
- Use an osteotome to fragment the trapezium carefully and remove the trapezium piecemeal, including all medial osteophytes (Fig. 10.40B).
- Dissect the flexor carpi radialis distally to its insertion on the second metacarpal. Develop a distally based 8-cm slip of 50% of the flexor carpi radialis tendon (split longitudinally).
- Pass the slip of tendon through the trapezial space, around the APL, and back around the intact 50% of flexor carpi radialis in a figure-of-eight pattern.
- Repeat this maneuver, completing a double figure-of-eight. Suture the tendon in place with several nonabsorbable sutures (Fig. 10.40C).

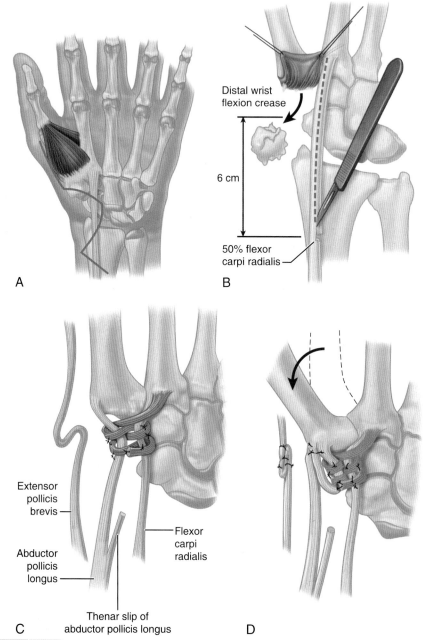

A

B

Distal wrist
flexion crease

6 cm

50% flexor
carpi radialis

C

Extensor
pollicis
brevis

Flexor
carpi
radialis

Abductor
pollicis
longus

Thenar slip of
abductor pollicis longus

D

FIGURE 10.40 Tendon interposition arthroplasty with ligament reconstruction. **A,** Incision. **B,** Distally based flap is raised over trapezium, and entire bone is removed piecemeal. **C,** Double figure-of-eight sling, using one half of flexor carpi radialis. **D,** Distal advancement of abductor pollicis longus onto periosteum of proximal portion of first metacarpal. **SEE TECHNIQUE 10.26.**

- Advance the APL tendon from a point proximal to the suspension sling to the proximal metacarpal periosteum. Suture the tendon securely just distal to its usual insertion at the base of the thumb metacarpal (Fig. 10.40D).
- Repair the capsule, the thenar muscle mass, and the previously transected thenar slip of the APL. Repair the latter by shortening with a weave. Imbricate the extensor pollicis brevis to take up any "slack."

- Close the skin and apply a bulky dressing supported by a short arm thumb spica splint.

POSTOPERATIVE CARE The dressing is replaced in about 10 to 14 days with a short arm thumb spica cast, which is worn another 3 weeks. Active-assisted and passive range-of-motion exercises are begun at 5 weeks. As the healing progresses, strengthening exercises are added.

TECHNIQUE MODIFICATION (CALANDRUCCIO)

- Carefully protect all sensory nerves through an extended Wagner incision and reflect ulnarly the thenar musculature. Isolate and protect the flexor carpi radialis tendon and the APL insertion.
- Subperiosteally expose and excise the trapezium.
- Remove loose bodies and redundant synovium from the thumb index recess and contour the metacarpal beak to cancellous bone by removing osteophytes.
- Use a 4-mm rough bur to make holes through the thumb metacarpal base proximally and radially, leaving a 1.0 cm bridge between them (Fig. 10.41A). Connect these holes with a series of curets, usually up to a No. 1, taking great care not to fracture the bony bridge.
- Pass the flexor carpi radialis tendon through the bone tunnel and hold it perpendicular to the index metacarpal shaft. Passage of the entire tendon can be aided by using a running locking 2-0 nonabsorbable suture to pull the tubulized, tapered end of the tendon.
- Approximate the index and thumb metacarpal bases by slight ulnarly directed pressure while the flexor carpi radialis tendon is firmly secured to the APL bony insertion with 2-0 braided nonabsorbable sutures (Fig. 10.41B).
- Next draw the flexor carpi radialis tendon between the thumb and index intermetacarpal ligament reconstruction and secure it to itself with the same suture (Fig. 10.41C and D).
- Weave the remaining portion of the suture still attached to the deep intermetacarpal ligament through the remaining flexor carpi radialis tendon so that it can be slid down the suture to form a firm accordion-like interposition mass (Fig. 10.41E and F).
- Secure the flexor carpi radialis mass to the volar radial capsular tissue and distal scaphotrapezial ligament so that this interposition is between the distal scaphoid pole and metacarpal base (Fig. 10.41G).
- Approximate the thenar muscles to the APL tendon with a buried suture. After wound closure, apply a thumb spica splint with the interphalangeal joint free.

POSTOPERATIVE CARE The sutures are removed at 10 to 14 days and either a thumb spica splint or cast is applied and worn for another 3 to 4 weeks. Secure constructs in reliable patients may be treated with a custom-fit removable thumb spica splint. At 6 weeks, range-of-motion exercises are initiated and tight grip and pinch are not allowed until 3 months postoperatively. Formal physical therapy rarely is indicated.

When the flexor carpi radialis is absent, structurally weakened by attrition, or ruptured, alternate tendons are available for a biologic suspension arthroplasty. A slip of the APL has been shown to be suitable (Fig. 10.42A) when a proximally detached section of the tendon is passed through drill holes in the thumb and index metacarpal bases (Fig. 10.42B-E). Temporary pinning can be used for 8 weeks, and a stable, pain-free thumb with excellent strength and motion has been reported at an average of 5.5 years after the procedure.

ARTHROSCOPIC THUMB CARPOMETACARPAL ARTHROPLASTY

Although more equipment-intensive and technically challenging, arthroscopic techniques have been developed for treatment of peritrapezial thumb basal joint arthritis. Both early stage disease with thumb CMC debridement and late stage disease with arthroscopic resection of both the CMC and scaphotrapeziotrapezoidal joints have favorable patient outcomes. Moreover, materials interposed following resection do not appear to offer any additional benefit, but do increase the cost of the procedure, potentially increase the difficulty of the procedure, and introduce other sources of complications. Cobb et al. concluded from their findings in 144 arthroscopic resection arthroplasties with or without interposition materials (52 and 73 patients at 7.4- and 5.6-year follow-up, respectively) that interposition was unnecessary. Changes in pinch and grip and postoperative mean satisfaction, in addition to complications, were similar in both groups. Similarly, Edwards and Ramsey found that the average DASH score improved from 61 to 10 and pain scores decreased from 8.3 to 1.5 at 3 months after arthroscopic hemitrapeziectomy. Grip and key pinch strength improved 6.8 and 1.9 kg, respectively, and wrist and digital motion were unchanged. Proximal migration of the first metacarpal averaged 3 mm, and translation decreased from 30% to 10%. Nineteen of 23 patients were pleased with their overall outcomes, and patient satisfaction, radiographic subsidence, and translation remained unchanged for a minimum of 4 years. Similar to other reports, hemitrapeziectomy and thermal capsular modification were found to offer patients with Eaton stage III arthritis a minimally invasive alternative that can provide increased function and decreased pain by 3 months after surgery. These results are comparable to those reported for open techniques involving trapeziectomy.

Arthroscopic staging has been devised to direct treatment regimens. Stage I is characterized by diffuse synovitis without significant cartilage loss, and ligamentous laxity of the volar capsule is frequently present; simple synovectomy with or without electrothermal shrinkage is the preferred treatment. Stage II is present when there is focal wear of the central to dorsal articular surface of the trapezium. Although an osteotomy of the metacarpal base to place the thumb in a more extended and abducted position usually is recommended, this stage can also be treated arthroscopically. Stage III has diffuse articular cartilage loss on the trapezium with or without metacarpal base articular cartilage loss. This stage can also be treated with arthroscopic hemiresection of the trapezium.

TECHNIQUE 10.27

(SLUTSKY)

- Position the patient supine on the operating table with the involved extremity supported on a hand table and the thumb suspended by Chinese finger traps with 10 to 15 pounds (4.5 to 6.8 kg) of countertraction, which forces the wrist into ulnar deviation.

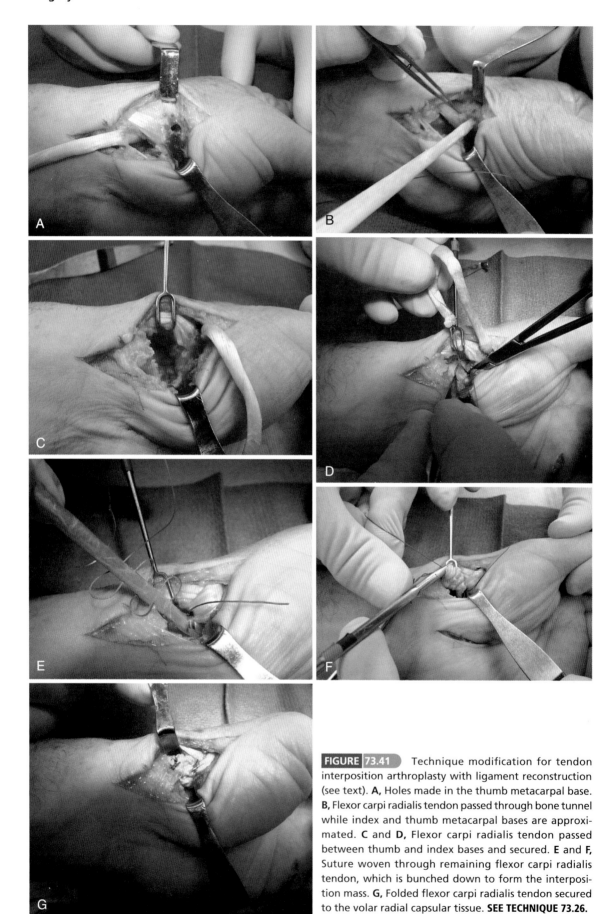

FIGURE 73.41 Technique modification for tendon interposition arthroplasty with ligament reconstruction (see text). **A,** Holes made in the thumb metacarpal base. **B,** Flexor carpi radialis tendon passed through bone tunnel while index and thumb metacarpal bases are approximated. **C** and **D,** Flexor carpi radialis tendon passed between thumb and index bases and secured. **E** and **F,** Suture woven through remaining flexor carpi radialis tendon, which is bunched down to form the interposition mass. **G,** Folded flexor carpi radialis tendon secured to the volar radial capsular tissue. **SEE TECHNIQUE 73.26.**

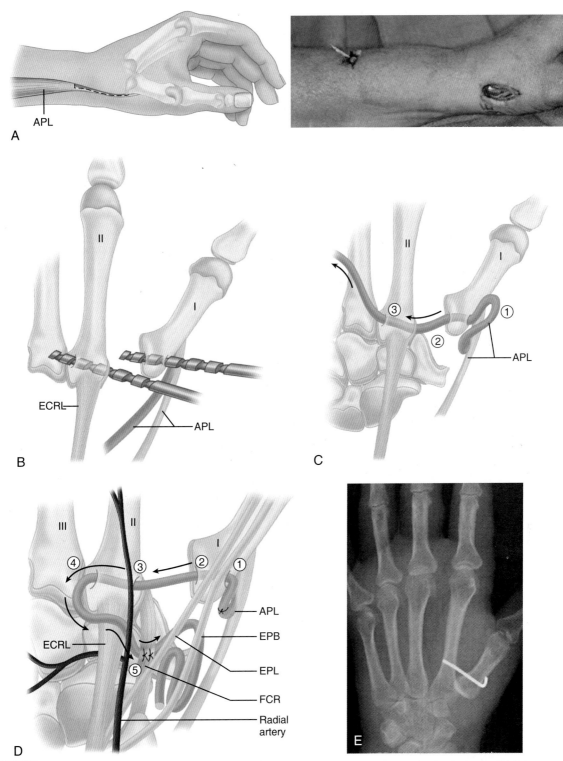

FIGURE 10.42 Thumb arthroplasty using the abductor pollicis longus *(APL)* tendon. **A,** One leash of APL tendon is harvested. Second incision is made over tendon at distal third of forearm; one leash of tendon is divided at muscle junction and passed beneath fascia distally into incision. **B,** A 3.5-mm hole is drilled at base of the thumb metacarpal from point 1 cm distal to base, through bone in dorsal-to-volar fashion. A second 3.5-mm hole is drilled at base of index metacarpal, 1 cm distal to its base in radiovolar-to-ulnodorsal fashion. **C,** APL tendon is passed through holes in index and thumb metacarpals and then pulled snugly outside wrist to remove slack in tendon. **D,** APL graft is passed back inside wrist above extensor carpi radialis longus *(ECRL)* and volar to dorsal radial artery (radial a), flexor carpi radialis *(FCR)*, extensor pollicis longus *(EPL)*, and extensor pollicis brevis *(EPB)* tendons. Numbers indicate sequence of construction. **E,** Thumb metacarpal is distracted to maintain carpometacarpal joint space while 1.6-mm (0.062 inch) Kirschner wire is inserted percutaneously 1 cm distal to thumb metacarpal and advanced through the index metacarpal. *APL,* abductor pollicis longus; *ECRL,* extensor carpi radialis longus; *EPB,* extensor pollicis brevis; *EPL,* extensor pollicis longus; *FCR,* flexor carpi radialis. (From Kochevar AJ, Adham CN, Adham MN, et al: Thumb basal joint arthroplasty using abductor pollicis longus tendon: an average 5.5-year follow-up, *J Hand Surg* 36A:1326, 2011.)

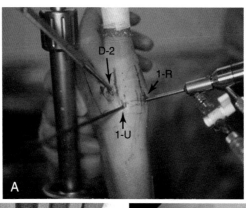

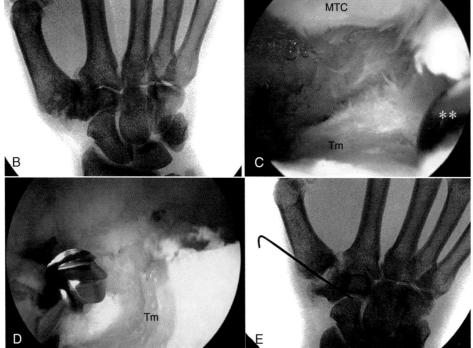

FIGURE 10.43 Arthroscopic thumb carpometacarpal arthroplasty. **A,** Surface landmarks for D-2 portal. **B,** Anteroposterior view showing advanced trapeziometacarpal osteoarthritis. **C,** Arthroscopic view of right thumb from 1-U portal shows the resection *(asterisks)* in 1-R portal. **D,** Partial resection of trapezium *(Tm)*. **E,** Completed hemitrapeziectomy. (From Slutsky DJ: The role of arthroscopy in trapeziometacarpal arthritis, *Clin Orthop Relat Res* 472:1173, 2014; with permission of David J. Slutsky.) **SEE TECHNIQUE 10.27.**

- Outline the relevant landmarks, including the proximal and dorsal edge of the thumb metacarpal base, the tendons of the APL and the extensor pollicis longus, and the radial artery in the snuff box (Fig. 10.43A).
- Inflate a tourniquet to 250 mm Hg and establish saline inflow irrigation through the arthroscope and a small joint pump or pressure bag.
- To establish the 1-R portal, palpate the thumb metacarpal base and identify the joint with a 22-gauge needle just radial to the APL, followed by injection of 2 mL of saline. This step may be facilitated by fluoroscopy. Make a small skin incision and spread the wound with tenotomy scissors.
- Pierce the capsule and insert a cannula and blunt trocar, followed by the arthroscope.

- Use an identical procedure to establish the 1-U portal, just ulnar to the extensor pollicis brevis tendon, followed by insertion of a 3-mm hook probe. The portals are used interchangeably to systematically inspect the joint, which is facilitated by expedient use of a 2.0-mm synovial resector.
- The D-2 portal is used to facilitate resection of the medial osteophytes (see Fig. 10.43A). To establish the D-2 portal, identify the intersection of the base of the index and thumb metacarpal just distal and ulnar to the extensor pollicis longus tendon. Insert a 22-gauge needle 1 cm distal to this juncture and angle it in a proximal, radial, and palmar direction, hugging the thumb metacarpal while viewing from either the 1-R or 1-U portal (see Fig. 10.43A).

- Make a small skin incision and use tenotomy scissors to spread the soft tissue and pierce the joint capsule. Then insert a blunt trocar and cannula, followed by the arthroscope or a hook probe, motorized shaver, or 2.9-mm burr.

ARTHROSCOPIC DEBRIDEMENT AND CAPSULAR SHRINKAGE

- The essence of arthroscopic capsular relies on thermal heating of the collagenous fibers in the surrounding ligaments and capsule, followed by a period of joint immobilization in a reduced position.
- Use a motorized shaver to debride any synovitis and to expose the capsular ligaments.
- Then use a diathermy probe to "paint" the anterior oblique ligament and surrounding capsule, taking care to leave bands of tissue in between. Be sure to keep the probe away from the joint surfaces to prevent cartilage necrosis. In light of the meager joint volume, the outflow fluid temperature can be monitored to prevent overheating. Use an 18-gauge needle in an accessory portal to enhance fluid circulation, which minimizes this risk.

ARTHROSCOPIC PARTIAL OR COMPLETE TRAPEZIECTOMY WITHOUT TENDON INTERPOSITION

- After joint debridement, use a 2.9-mm burr in a to-and-fro manner to resect 3 to 4 mm of the distal trapezium. The diameter of the burr along with fluoroscopy provides a gauge as to the amount of bony resection. A larger 3.5-mm burr can be substituted as the space between the metacarpal base and distal trapezium enlarges.
- After the bony resection is complete, fix the thumb in a pronated and abducted position with a Kirschner wire (Fig. 10.43B-E).
- If there is lateral subluxation of the metacarpal base, thermal shrinkage of the anterior oblique ligament can be done at this time.

┃ IMPLANT ARTHROPLASTY

Trapeziometacarpal implant arthroplasty may be indicated when pain from rheumatoid arthritis or osteoarthritis has not responded to conservative treatment. Several techniques are available that may provide stability and pain relief yet preserve some mobility and strength of pinch. The ligaments and capsule around this prosthesis must be reconstructed carefully, and the position of the prosthesis must be immobilized in a cast for 6 weeks to prevent subluxation. This technique is generally used in patients with a subluxated trapeziometacarpal joint with synovitis, joint narrowing, osteophytes, and a positive grind test. Complications include implant subluxation (5% to 20%) or dislocation (0% to 19%) and silicone synovitis (50%). Relief of pain has been excellent in most instances. Some motion and pinch power may be lost with various degrees of subluxation. Although various modifications of the flexible silicone implant have been devised and their results satisfactory, the outcomes do not appear to differ significantly enough to recommend any particular device. Currently we favor nonimplant arthroplasty techniques, regardless of the arthritic condition, and find that these soft-tissue techniques are quite reliable.

▓ ARTHRODESIS OF THUMB JOINTS

Arthrodesis may be required for thumb joint deformities caused by rheumatoid arthritis or osteoarthritic processes. Patients with rheumatoid arthritis often have soft and insufficient bone that may limit the choice of internal fixation to small Kirschner wires and, in addition, may require bone grafting. If adequate bone is present, fixation can be obtained with Kirschner wires, plate, screws, or a tension band technique. The more stable and rigid the fixation, the shorter the time for immobilization. Arthrodesis is indicated most often for the metacarpophalangeal joint, which greatly relieves pain and improves strength by rigid stabilization. Although the union and complication rates of tension band and headless compression screw fixation are similar, the need for removal of symptomatic implants appears to be greater with the tension band technique (Fig. 10.44).

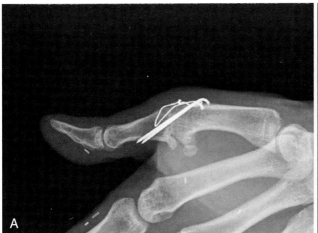
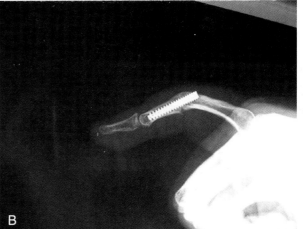

FIGURE 10.44   Proximal interphalangeal arthrodesis with **(A)** tension-band and **(B)** compression-screw fixation. (From Breyer JM, Vergas P, Parra L, et al: Metacarpophalangeal and interphalangeal arthrodesis: a comparative study between tension band and compression screw fixation, *J Hand Surg Eur* 40:374, 2015.)

Interphalangeal joint arthrodesis is indicated mainly for painful deformed joints, and repositioning extremely deviated joints may require soft-tissue release or bone resection. Intramedullary screws placed retrograde and buried in the distal phalanx work well, although bone quality may dictate simple Kirschner wire fixation. The fusion position of the interphalangeal joint can be varied; however, fusion in 0 to 15 degrees of flexion does not seem to compromise thumb function.

CMC joint arthrodesis can give very satisfactory outcomes if distal metacarpophalangeal and interphalangeal joint mobility is satisfactory. Placing the thumb so that it overlies the fully flexed fingers (fist position) will adequately position the CMC joint fusion.

INTERPHALANGEAL ARTHRODESIS OF THE THUMB

TECHNIQUE 10.28

- Approach the interphalangeal joint through a dorsal incision.
- Divide the extensor tendon, release and excise the collateral ligaments, and flex open the joint.
- Remove the articular surface and just enough subchondral bone from the distal and proximal phalanges for cancellous bone contact. Make sure to excise the soft tissue so that it does not become interposed into the joint.
- Position the interphalangeal joint in 0 to 15 degrees of flexion and fix it with small Kirschner wires driven out through the distal phalanx distally and then proximally into the proximal phalanx after the interphalangeal joint has been appropriately positioned.
- Alternatively, headless screws can be used for fixation if the medullary canal allows; the medullary canal of the thumb proximal phalanx may be too large in some instances for an interference fit of some intramedullary screws. Moreover, screw fixation requires the interphalangeal joint to be in full extension.
- After the interphalangeal joint has been stabilized with the internal fixation, evaluate the thumb for appropriate position and length. If the thumb is shortened excessively, as may be seen in patients with arthritis mutilans, obtain a small corticocancellous iliac crest bone graft to restore length and transfix it with Kirschner wires.

METACARPOPHALANGEAL ARTHRODESIS OF THE THUMB

TECHNIQUE 10.29

- With an osteotome, oscillating saw, burr, or rongeurs, cut across the articular surface of the proximal phalanx in a straight line at 90 degrees to its long axis to expose the cancellous bone. The articular surfaces also can be removed in a "cup-and-cone" configuration.

- After the articular surface is resected, place the phalanx at an angle of 15 degrees of flexion with the metacarpal. There is a tendency to osteotomize the distal metacarpal head also at 90 degrees; rather, make the osteotomy so that the metacarpophalangeal joint is flexed 15 degrees. This requires removing more bone toward the palmar aspect. The two raw surfaces should fit flush.
- When this joint is subluxated, shortening of the bone may be required.
- Remove any protruding small edges of bone.
- The arthrodesis can be accomplished with Kirschner wires inserted longitudinally. Insert them first through the metacarpal and advance them through the phalanx. Ensure that the wires do not pierce the flexor tendon or the distal joint and cut them off under the skin. Pack small fragments of bone into any spaces around the joint margins.
- Approximate the tendons with a small absorbable suture.
- Close the wound and place the hand in a small splint to be replaced later by a cast if indicated.
- Ensure that the thumb is in appropriate pronation so that the pulp of the thumb can be placed against the other digit.

POSTOPERATIVE CARE The splint and sutures are removed at 10 to 14 days. The thumb is protected in a short arm thumb spica cast for another 4 weeks or until union occurs. The Kirschner wires may be removed at about 6 weeks, and a splint is worn another 3 to 4 weeks. Active use of the thumb is resumed gradually. Sometimes despite the radiographic nonunion the joints are stable and pain free, allowing unprotected thumb use and resumption of daily activities.

TENSION BAND ARTHRODESIS OF THE THUMB METACARPOPHALANGEAL JOINT

TECHNIQUE 10.30

- Make a curved dorsal incision to allow safe dissection of sensory nerves from underlying extensor apparatus (Fig. 10.45A).
- Make a longitudinal incision through the extensor pollicis brevis tendon and radial aponeurotic fibers to expose the dorsal capsule (Fig. 10.45B).
- Split the capsule longitudinally to expose the metacarpal head and proximal phalanx base and excise osteophytes, collateral ligaments, and synovitic tissue (Fig. 10.45C).
- With rongeurs, a coarse-tooth oscillating saw, or congruent reamers, prepare the subchondral bone such that a 20-degree flexion angle is achieved with full contact of the raw cancellous metacarpal and proximal phalangeal surfaces (Fig. 10.45D).
- Make a transverse hole with a 0.045-inch Kirschner wire in the distal proximal phalangeal shaft to allow a 22-gauge spool wire to pass through this hole (Fig. 10.45E).

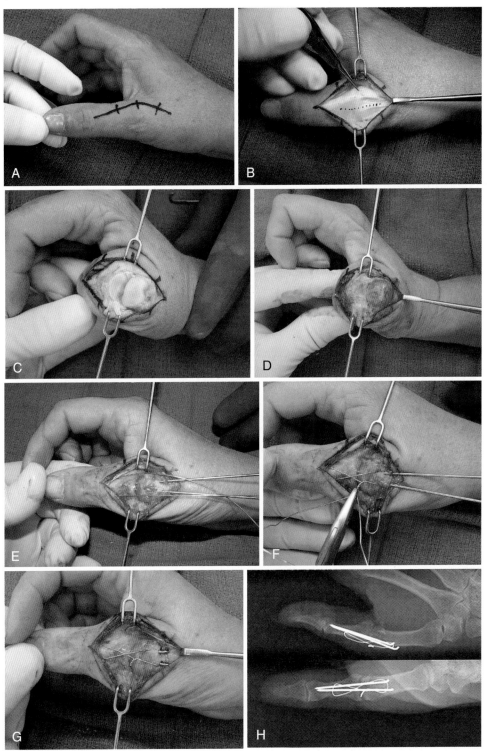

FIGURE 10.45 Tension band technique for thumb metacarpophalangeal joint arthrodesis. **A,** Curved dorsal incision. **B,** Incision through extensor pollicis brevis tendon and radial aponeurotic fibers exposing dorsal capsule. **C,** Capsule split longitudinally to expose metacarpal head and proximal phalanx base and excise osteophytes, collateral ligaments, and synovitic tissue. **D,** Exposure of subchondral bone to obtain full contact of raw cancellous metacarpal and proximal phalangeal surfaces. **E,** Placement of Kirschner wire in distal third of proximal phalangeal neck completing tension band construct. **F,** Wire twisted and ends buried about fusion site. **G,** Ends of wires cut and tamped into metacarpal over low-profile construct. **H,** Postoperative radiographic appearance. **SEE TECHNIQUE 10.30.**

- Hold the metacarpophalangeal joint in the desired position and pass two 0.045-inch Kirschner wires longitudinally across the fusion site and into the proximal phalangeal medullary canal, verifying their position on fluoroscopy before completing the tension band construct.
- Cross the 22-gauge wire and place one limb beneath the Kirschner wires projecting from the metacarpal neck.
- Take the slack out of the 22-gauge wire before twisting the wire and burying the end about the fusion site (Fig. 10.45F).
- Hold the Kirschner wires and bend the ends with a neuro-tip sucker so that the hooked ends can be cut and tamped into the metacarpal neck (Fig. 10.45G).
- Close the extensor pollicis brevis with a 4-0 nonabsorbable braided suture after the capsule has been closed over the low-profile construct (Fig. 10.45H).

POSTOPERATIVE CARE A thumb spica splint or cast is worn until signs of radiographic union. The interphalangeal joint is left free for range-of-motion exercises.

THUMB METACARPOPHALANGEAL JOINT ARTHRODESIS WITH INTRAMEDULLARY SCREW FIXATION

TECHNIQUE 10.31   *Figure 10.46*

- Make the skin and capsular exposures as described in Technique 10.30.
- With rongeurs, a coarse-tooth oscillating saw, or congruent reamers, prepare the subchondral bone such that a 20-degree flexion angle is achieved with full contact of the raw cancellous metacarpal and proximal phalangeal surfaces.
- Position the metacarpophalangeal joint at the desired angle with the cancellous surfaces in maximal contact. Verify the guidewire position with fluoroscopy.
- Perform reaming according to the screw diameter.
- Seat the screw(s) just beneath the metacarpal neck cortex and evaluate the stability of the construct (Fig. 10.46B).
- Obtain fluoroscopic images to verify position of the arthrodesis before routine wound closure.

   Thumb metacarpophalangeal joint arthrodesis can be accomplished using miniplate fixation (see Fig. 10.47D), and this may be preferable when other methods have failed or when intercalary bone grafting is required. In some situations, supplementary fixation is required for rigid fixation during the fusion period.

◼ TRAPEZIOMETACARPAL ARTHRODESIS

Although trapeziometacarpal joint arthroplasty usually provides stability and strength in most cases, arthrodesis may be recommended for joints affected by traumatic arthritis and osteoarthritis in younger patients.

Arthrodesis can be expected to relieve pain and to provide a stable and strong joint at the expense of thumb mobility. It traditionally has been used for patients who require a strong, powerful, stable, and painless thumb. It also is useful in stabilizing the joint for congenital and paralytic deformities and in hands impaired by cerebral palsy.

Careful consideration should be given to other causes of pain in and around the trapeziometacarpal area. Pain on passive thumb adduction and wrist ulnar deviation (Finkelstein test) suggests first extensor compartment tenosynovitis (de Quervain). Typical symptoms and signs of median nerve compression (carpal tunnel syndrome), tenderness of the flexor carpi radialis at its fibro-osseous tunnel (flexor carpi radialis tunnel syndrome), and radiographic evidence of arthritis in adjacent joints suggest other potential sources of pain, whereas pain on passive rotation of the thumb metacarpal with trapeziometacarpal compression ("grind test") reasonably localizes the problem to the trapeziometacarpal joint. For any trapeziometacarpal arthrodesis technique, the thumb metacarpal position should permit pulp opposition to fingers.

The "cone and cup," sliding graft, and fixation techniques using Kirschner wires, screws, plates, and staples are effective in achieving a fusion rate greater than 90%. Increased nonunion rates have been reported when screws alone have been used to attempt fusion.

TRAPEZIOMETACARPAL ARTHRODESIS

TECHNIQUE 10.32   *Figure 10.47*

(STARK ET AL.)
- Expose the trapeziometacarpal joint through a curved volar incision at the thumb base at the level of the APL tendon insertion, avoiding branches of the superficial radial, lateral antebrachial cutaneous, and palmar cutaneous nerves.
- Divide this tendon and the origin of the opponens muscle at the first metacarpal base; open the joint capsule through a transverse incision.
- Remove all the articular cartilage and the subchondral cortical bone on both joint surfaces with instruments of choice.
- Compress the bony surfaces in the position desired and maintain this by two or three small Kirschner wires. Cannulated screws and blade plates also may provide satisfactory fixation.
- If more bony contact is needed, additional bone graft may be required.
- Repair the capsule and the APL tendon and suture the skin.

POSTOPERATIVE CARE The thumb is maintained in a thumb spica cast for 2 weeks, after which the skin sutures are removed. The thumb spica cast is reapplied, and radiographs are used periodically to check healing until fusion is obtained, usually at 12 weeks.

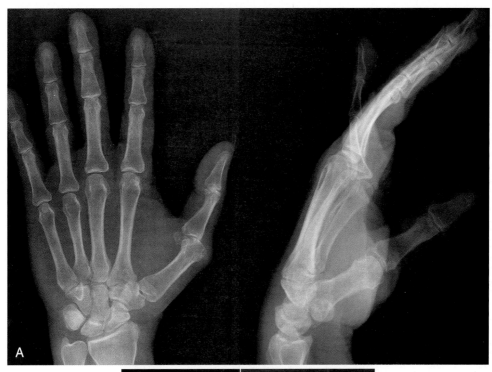

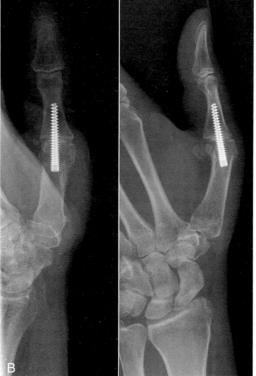

FIGURE 10.46 Thumb metacarpophalangeal arthrodesis with intramedullary screw fixation. **A,** Preoperative radiograph showing severe involvement of thumb metacarpophalangeal joint. **B,** After arthrodesis with intramedullary screw fixation. **SEE TECHNIQUE 10.31.**

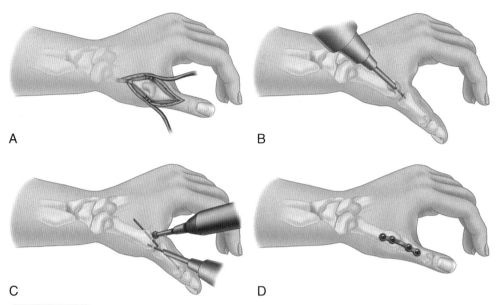

A

B

C

D

FIGURE 10.47 Trapeziometacarpal arthrodesis. **A,** Incision. **B,** Air-driven burr used to remove articular surfaces town to cancellous bone. **C,** Osteotome used to make multiple small cuts into opposing articular surfaces. **D,** Fixation with plate and screws. (Redrawn from Doyle JR: Sliding bone graft technique for arthrodesis of the trapeziometacarpal joint of the thumb, *J Hand Surg* 16A:363, 1991). **SEE TECHNIQUES 10.32 AND 10.33.**

TRAPEZIOMETACARPAL ARTHRODESIS

TECHNIQUE 10.33   *see Figure 10.47*

(DOYLE)
- With the patient supine and the hand supinated on the hand table, use a pneumatic tourniquet.
- Make a curved incision exposing the proximal two thirds of the thumb metacarpal and the dorsal and palmar sides of the trapeziometacarpal joint.
- Identify and protect the branches of the superficial radial nerve and the extensor pollicis brevis tendon.
- Detach the APL tendons with a portion of the joint capsule for later reattachment.
- Reflect the thenar muscles distally; incise the dorsal and palmar capsule and expose the joint.
- Use an air-driven burr to remove the articular cartilage and the subchondral bone down to cancellous bone.
- Slightly round the base of the thumb metacarpal and make a matching shallow concavity in the trapezium. Preserve the overall shape of the joint to avoid undue shortening of the thumb.
- Use a small osteotome to make small, shallow cuts in the bone surface.
- Insert crossed Kirschner wires to hold the joint firmly in 30 to 40 degrees of palmar abduction and 30 to 35 degrees of radial abduction ("clenched fist").
- Using a small drill point or a Kirschner wire, make drill holes to outline a rectangular corticocancellous graft on the dorsum of the thumb metacarpal.

- Connect the drill holes with a small osteotome to mobilize the corticocancellous "sliding graft."
- Make a rectangular recess in the dorsum of the trapezium to receive the graft.
- Move the graft proximally into the trapezial recess and impact the graft.
- Stabilize the graft with an additional Kirschner wire or screws to avoid graft displacement.
- Reattach the APL tendon and close the skin. Over a nonadhering dressing, apply cast padding and a thumb spica splint.

POSTOPERATIVE CARE At 10 days, the splint and skin sutures are removed, if wound healing permits. A thumb spica cast is applied. The cast and Kirschner wires are removed at 8 weeks after the operation. Arthrodesis is monitored with serial radiographs. Motion and strengthening exercises are begun after successful arthrodesis and pin removal.

THUMB CARPOMETACARPAL ARTHRODESIS WITH KIRSCHNER WIRE OR BLADE-PLATE FIXATION

TECHNIQUE 10.34

(GOLDFARB AND STERN)
- Make a longitudinal incision from the midpoint of the dorsal surface of the first metacarpal to the proximal aspect of the radial styloid.

- Identify and protect the superficial branches of the radial sensory nerve and the lateral antebrachial cutaneous nerve.
- Identify the APL and extensor pollicis brevis and develop the interval between them to access the joint.
- Reflect the thumb CMC joint capsule and soft-tissue attachments sharply in a circumferential fashion from both the trapezium and metacarpal, and deliver the metacarpal base into the wound with two small Hohmann retractors (Fig. 10.48A).
- Remove the remaining articular cartilage and dense subchondral bone from the base of the metacarpal with a rongeur, forming a cone-shaped surface of cancellous bone.
- Use a rongeur, curet, and small osteotome to shape the trapezium into a cup configuration of matching radius of curvature, and appose the prepared bone surfaces (see Fig. 10.48A).
- Place the thumb at approximately 45 degrees to the coronal and sagittal planes of the hand. Slight prona-

tion of the thumb may improve digital opposition. In the ideal position, the thumb will overlie the dorsum of the index finger middle phalanx when the hand is held in a fist.
- Temporarily stabilize the joint with a 1.6-mm Kirschner wire and confirm bony apposition with fluoroscopy (Fig. 10.48B).
- Once satisfactory joint positioning is confirmed, evaluate the quality of the bony apposition. If areas of suboptimal contact are present, supplemental bone graft can be harvested from the distal radius by extending the incision proximally. Protect the sensory nerves and release the first dorsal compartment. Mobilize the APL and extensor pollicis brevis tendons and make a 5 × 5-mm cortical window in the radius to harvest the cancellous bone graft; pack the graft into any fusion defects.
- With the provisional Kirschner wire in place, position a 2.4-mm T-plate or 2.0-mm/2.4-mm minicondylar blade plate (Synthes USA, Paoli, PA) and insert the screws (Fig. 10.48C). Take care to use image intensification in multiple

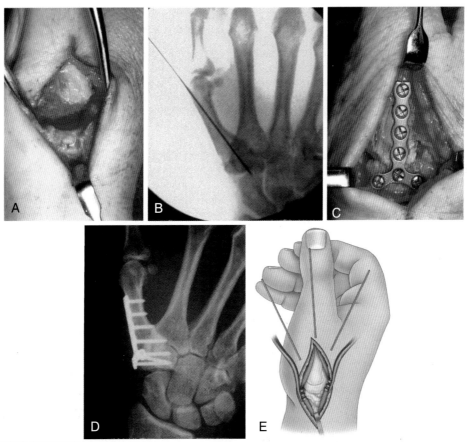

FIGURE 10.48 Thumb carpometacarpal joint arthrodesis with plate fixation. **A,** Prepared surfaces of metacarpal and trapezium in cup-and-cone configuration. **B,** Radiographic confirmation of positioning with temporary Kirschner wire; note bony apposition. **C,** Application of 2-mm T-plate. **D,** Radiographic appearance after arthrodesis. **E,** Placement of Kirschner wires for arthrodesis. (**A-D** from Doyle JR: Sliding bone graft technique for arthrodesis of the trapeziometacarpal joint of the thumb, *J Hand Surg* 16A:383, 1991; **E** redrawn from Goldfarb CA, Stren PJ: Indications and techniques for thumb carpometacarpal arthrodesis, *Tech Hand Upper Extremity Surg* 6:178, 2001.) **SEE TECHNIQUE 10.34.**

planes to ensure that the screws or blades do not penetrate adjacent joints (Fig. 10.48D).

- If Kirschner wire fixation is chosen, drive three 1.1-mm wires retrograde from the metacarpal into the trapezium. The first pin follows the planned axis of the bone fusion, and the other two pins diverge 10 to 20 degrees from this axis (Fig. 10.48E). Take care to avoid pin penetration of the scaphotrapeziotrapezoid joint. Leave the pins outside the skin for later removal.
- Close the skin in routine fashion and apply a short arm thumb spica cast, leaving the interphalangeal joint free.

RHEUMATOID DEFORMITIES OF THE WRIST

SYNOVITIS OF THE WRIST

Painful dorsal wrist swelling may be the presenting symptom in rheumatoid arthritis. The tenosynovial swelling may contribute to de Quervain disease, trigger finger, or carpal tunnel syndrome, whereas rheumatoid arthritis as the underlying cause may not be suspected. The swelling may begin as a small soft mass at the distal end of the ulna; radiographs may reveal a small pit at the base of the ulnar styloid as the first radiographic evidence of the disease. The synovitis can spread and cause massive swelling in the shape of an hourglass, its middle being constricted by the extensor retinaculum. Eventually, destruction of joints may contribute to dorsal subluxation of the distal ulna, ulnar shifting of the carpal bones, radial angulation of the metacarpals, and ulnar deviation of the fingers. Finally, the wrist may subluxate volarly. Tendons, especially those of the three ulnar finger extensors, may rupture.

If the synovitis is only moderate, and if changes in the bones are absent, but pain is significant, dorsal synovectomy of the wrist may be of lasting benefit. Persistent swelling at the dorsum of the wrist that continues for 6 weeks or longer despite adequate medical treatment may be an indication for a dorsal synovectomy. This may be considered a prophylactic measure to avoid extensor tendon rupture. Rupture of these tendons is quite disabling, and function can never be restored completely. Any tendons ruptured at the wrist level can be repaired or reconstructed at the time of synovectomy. Options include distal side-to-side suture of the ruptured to intact tendon, free tendon graft, and tendon transfers to bridge a defect in a tendon. If synovitis involves the wrist and the metacarpophalangeal joints, synovectomy often can be done at both levels during the same operation, usually only on one limb at a time.

Hypertrophy of the volar wrist synovium even though undetectable clinically can cause median nerve compression and symptoms of carpal tunnel syndrome. Compression of the nerve in rheumatoid arthritis should be relieved surgically if conservative treatment with splinting and corticosteroid injections has been unsuccessful. If hypertrophy of the tenosynovium on the volar aspect of the wrist is obvious clinically with or without symptoms of compression of the median nerve, a palmar (flexor) tenosynovectomy may be useful in relieving pain and in preventing rupture of tendons. The carpal tunnel is a frequent site of rupture of flexor tendons. Distal radius or scaphoid bony prominences in the floor of the carpal tunnel can cause fraying and eventual rupture of

the thumb (Mannerfelt syndrome) and other finger flexor tendons. More commonly, the flexor pollicis longus or index profundus is involved. Synovitis within the carpal articulations themselves and in the surrounding tendon sheaths is also common in rheumatoid arthritis.

The various options for surgical treatment depend on the pathologic process involved and the severity of the disease. As already mentioned, synovectomy of the dorsal compartment is a worthwhile procedure when indicated (Fig. 10.49). Capsuloligamentous repairs may be required to stabilize joints. Repair of the extensor tendons is best done, if possible, by repair to an adjoining tendon rather than by segmental grafting. Wrist level flexor tendon rupture is best repaired by suture to adjoining tendons or by segmental grafts; however, in the thumb an arthrodesis of the distal joint may be a more preferred procedure if the interphalangeal joint is unstable or degenerative. However, if the thumb interphalangeal joint is not arthritic and is stable, a ring flexor digitorum superficialis transfer can be considered.

DORSAL SYNOVECTOMY

TECHNIQUE 10.35

- Make a dorsal longitudinal incision curved only slightly ulnarward and long enough to expose the distal ulna and the extensor retinaculum; avoid curving it sharply because the flap circulation may be impaired. Preserve the larger veins and all identifiable sensory nerves.
- Raise a laterally based retinacular flap.
- Make transverse incisions at the proximal and distal ends of the retinaculum.
- At the proximal end, make the transverse incision so that a band 5 to 10 mm wide is preserved proximally.
- Connect the transverse, parallel retinacular incisions with a longitudinal incision over the extensor carpi ulnaris.
- Raise the flap from medial to lateral, dividing the septa between the compartments. Avoid injury to the extensor tendons, especially the extensor pollicis longus.
- Detach from the radial side and reflect as a sheet the extensor retinaculum.
- Carefully excise the synovium from around the finger and radial wrist extensor tendons. Excise any hypertrophied synovium from the distal ulna and the distal radioulnar joint.
- If the attachments of the distal ulna to the radius and carpus seem to be intact, do not disturb them, but if the distal ulna is found subluxated, excise about 1 cm of it, smooth off the remaining end, and cover the end with periosteum and surrounding soft tissues.
- Incise the sheath of the extensor carpi ulnaris tendon near its attachment to the base of the fifth metacarpal.
- If the sheath is disintegrated and the tendon is dislocated palmarward, it has become a flexor, causing palmar flexion and ulnar deviation of the wrist. In this case, remove the tendon from the sheath as needed and return it to the dorsum of the wrist by creation of a pulley with a strip of the extensor retinaculum.

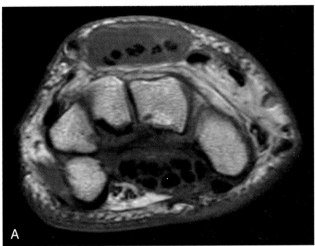
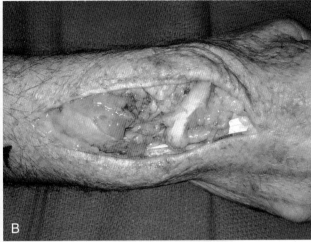
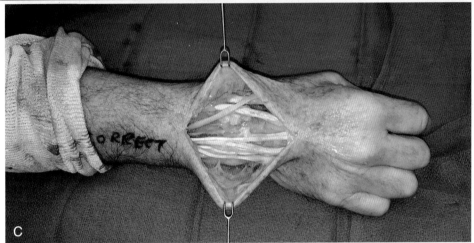

FIGURE 10.49 Extensor tenosynovectomy in a 69-year-old, right-hand-dominant male with negative rheumatologic work up and persistent extensor tenosynovitis: **A,** MRI showing isolated 4th extensor compartment involvement. **B,** Midline dorsal approach exposing proliferative extensor tenosynovitis. **C,** Wrist after tenosynovectomy. Note that rheumatologic studies, histopathology, and cultures were inconclusive as to etiology of extensor tenosynovitis, which is not uncommon with such conditions.

- If before surgery the wrist is radially deviated, transfer the insertion of the extensor carpi radialis longus to the extensor carpi ulnaris tendon.
- While an assistant applies traction to the hand, remove the synovium from among the carpal bones. Pass the extensor retinacular flap deep to the long extensor tendons and suture its detached end in place medially.
- Elevate the hand and control bleeding.
- Close the skin with interrupted sutures over a drain.
- Apply a compression dressing and a volar plaster splint to hold the wrist in neutral position.

POSTOPERATIVE CARE Active motion of the finger joints is encouraged early. The drain is removed at 24 to 48 hours, and the wound is inspected. Hematomas compromising the skin are evacuated. At 10 to 14 days, the sutures are removed; at 3 weeks, the splint is removed.

VOLAR SYNOVECTOMY

TECHNIQUE 10.36   *Figure 10.50*

- Make a volar longitudinal incision beginning distally at the middle of the palm and proceeding proximally to the wrist, and then curving slightly ulnarward, and ending about 7.5 cm proximal to the wrist.
- Open the deep fascia proximally and identify the median nerve. It is safer to stay on the ulnar side of the median nerve, beginning proximally in the forearm and carefully freeing the nerve distally.
- Divide completely the transverse carpal ligament to expose the flexor tendons; its distal border is more distal in the palm than is usually realized.
- Beginning proximally and proceeding distally, and keeping constantly in mind the location of the median nerve,

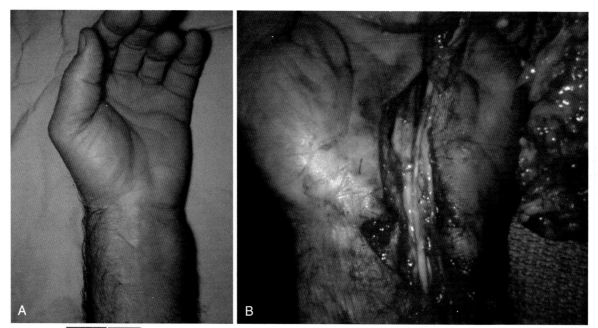

FIGURE 10.50   **A,** Flexor surface, left hand and wrist with rheumatoid tenosynovium bulging to palmar and ulnar (medial) side of distal forearm. **B,** At flexor tenosynovectomy. Note extension of incision distally into palm and proximally into forearm. Excised tenosynovial mass lies to medial side of hand. **SEE TECHNIQUE 10.36.**

dissect the synovium from each flexor tendon. Evaluate the flexor tendons for ruptures and erosions.

■ Inspect the volar capsule and ligaments over the carpal bones for osteophytes, especially those from the distal radial rim and the scaphoid. Remove osteophytes with a rongeur and close the capsule-ligament layer over the carpal bones. Do not close the deep transverse carpal ligament.

■ Release the tourniquet, obtain hemostasis, insert a drain, and close the wound.

■ Apply a compression dressing and a volar plaster splint from the proximal forearm to the distal palmar crease.

■ Keep the wrist extended for a minimum of 3 weeks.

POSTOPERATIVE CARE Postoperative care is the same as for dorsal synovectomy. Immediate finger range-of-motion exercises are begun the day of surgery as motion restriction in both flexion and extension often accompany such procedures.

WRIST ARTHRODESIS AND ARTHROPLASTY

The reconstructive procedures available for an arthritic wrist joint include partial arthrodesis, total wrist arthrodesis, and arthroplasty. If bilateral wrist bony procedures are necessary, arthroplasty on at least one side should be considered. In some cases, arthroplasty may be indicated initially because eventual collapse of the opposite wrist may require reconstruction. Several types of arthroplasties are available. Resection of the distal radius to form a shelf in cases of palmar dislocation maintains some stability, increases motion, and relieves pain without the insertion of foreign material; however, resection arthroplasty does not produce a stable joint.

Implant arthroplasties historically include silicone (Swanson) arthroplasties and plastic and metal arthroplasties (Fig. 10.51). Swanson wrist arthroplasty does not require fixation and entails minimal bone resection, but it is associated with a prosthetic fracture rate of 10% to 52% and an overall revision rate of 14% to 41%. This implant has fallen out of favor as other designs have proven more reliable and without the reactive synovitis issues.

Although total joint arthroplasty has the advantages of preserving motion, providing a fixed fulcrum, and obtaining stable fixation, problems such as distal component loosening compromise the results in 50% of patients. Complications lead to an overall revision rate of 9% to 35% for metal and plastic total wrist implants. Constrained designs, such as the Meuli and Volz wrist implants, allow excessive forces to be transmitted to the prosthesis, resulting in displacement of the distal portion of the prosthesis and leading to median nerve compression and flexor tendon abrasion. Although Meuli and Fernandez found excellent results in 24 of 50 wrists treated for rheumatoid or traumatic arthritis with a Meuli III wrist prosthesis, loosening occurred in eight wrists. Adequate muscle balance and correctable wrist contractures are important requirements for this implant to be successful. Beckenbaugh and Linscheid reported satisfactory preliminary results with a semiconstrained "biaxial" wrist implant. It is porous coated to improve cement fixation or to eliminate the need for cement. Rettig and Beckenbaugh evaluated 13 failed total wrist arthroplasties, salvaged with the biaxial total wrist implant. Although improvement was achieved, loosening was a persistent problem, especially in patients with rheumatoid disease. Takwale et al. found that of 66 biaxial wrist replacements

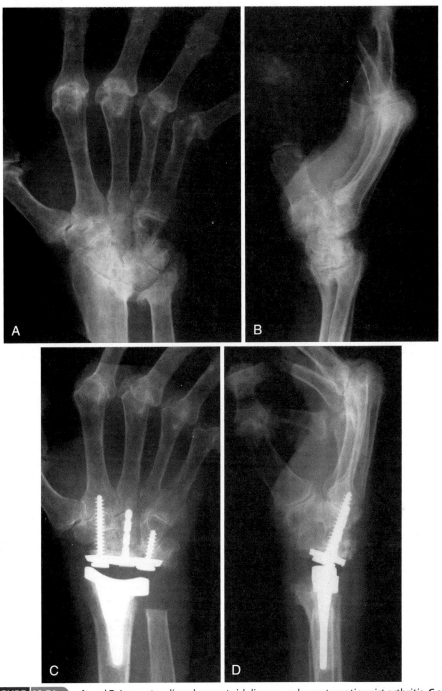

FIGURE 10.51   **A** and **B,** Long-standing rheumatoid disease and symptomatic wrist arthritis. **C** and **D,** Two years after total wrist arthroplasty. (From Divelbiss BJ, Sollerman C, Adams BD: Original communications: early results of the universal total wrist arthroplasty in rheumatoid arthritis, *J Hand Surg* 27A:195, 2002.)

reviewed at an average of 52 months, five required revisions. An 8-year survivorship probability of 83% was seen. Menon and Divelbiss, Sollerman, and Adams reported that the Universal total wrist implant was promising in the early groups of patients with rheumatoid arthritis. Despite implant modifications, careful patient selection, close attention to meticulous surgical technique, and thoughtful consideration of salvage options are important considerations when implant arthroplasty is considered for a patient with incapacitating wrist arthritis. According to Carlson and Simmons, contraindications to total wrist arthroplasty include chronic

subluxation, poor bone, prior infection, impaired motor or neurologic function, use of a walker or cane, and impaired wrist extensor tendons.

Whether wrist arthrodesis or arthroplasty is best in rheumatoid arthritis is controversial. Wrist arthroplasty usually has a higher percentage of late complications than does arthrodesis; however, arthrodesis provides a painless and stable wrist after fusion has occurred. Most authors consider it the procedure of choice for marked flexion deformity of the wrist and fingers, for carpal dislocation, or for a painful wrist associated with multiple ruptures of tendons. This

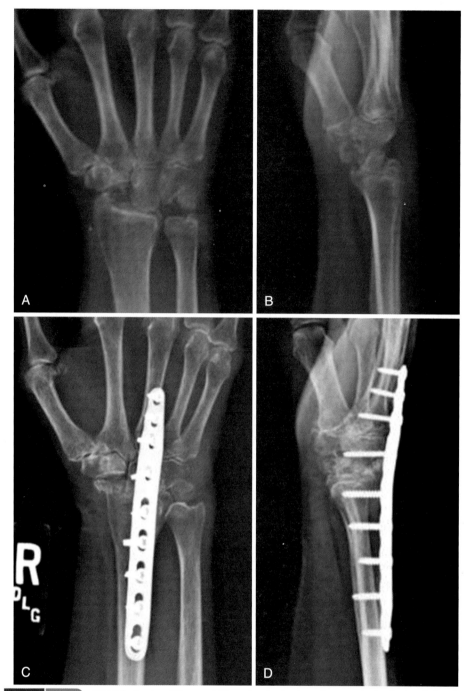

FIGURE 10.52   Wrist fusion in a 65-year-old female who had persistent pain for 2 years following proximal row carpectomy. Anteroposterior **(A)** and lateral **(B)** views of wrist indicating radiocapitate joint space narrowing. Anteroposterior **(C)** and lateral **(D)** views of successful total wrist fusion with Synthes wrist fusion plate.

is especially true for ruptures of the extensor carpi radialis longus and brevis because they are necessary for wrist balance. Also, when wrist deformities are bilateral and require major procedures on both sides, one wrist can be arthrodesed to provide stability, especially when the use of crutches may be necessary; an arthroplasty can be performed on the other wrist. Successful wrist arthrodesis reliably relieves pain, corrects deformity, and maintains stability (Fig. 10.52).

The position in which to fuse for maximal function also is controversial; recommended positions include 10 to 30 degrees of extension. In bilateral fusions, some authors prefer to place one wrist in extension and the other in flexion. Usually, both wrists should not be fused in extension because this would make it difficult for personal hygiene. Several satisfactory techniques are available for arthrodesis. Most require some type of internal fixation, including a pin inserted between the second and third metacarpal shafts, through the carpus, and then through the medullary canal of the radius, with a supplementary staple to prevent rotation; an intramedullary Steinmann pin and bone grafting of the dorsum of the wrist; and a Steinmann pin down the shaft of the third metacarpal with additional fixation by a staple or oblique pin, which permits operations to be done on the metacarpophalangeal joints at the same time. Because these procedures for fusion of the rheumatoid wrist are similar, the procedure of Millender and Nalebuff is described here. Radiocarpal fusions (radioscaphoid, radiolunate, radioscapholunate) are useful to preserve motion in relatively uninvolved midcarpal joints and to stabilize the radiocarpal joint against ulnar translation. Motomiya et al. used a half-slip of the extensor carpi ulnaris tendon to stabilize the distal ulnar stump (Fig. 10.53) and reported fusion in all 22 wrists with radiolunate fusions. Moreover, at mean follow-up of 7 years, the average motion arc was just beyond 70 degrees, and there was no progression in arthritis stage (Fig. 10.54). Similarly, Raven et al. found radioulnar fusion useful for both rheumatoid and psoriatic patients with painful ulnar translation and preserved midcarpal joints, despite slight progression in Larsen stage at just over 11 years' mean follow-up.

ARTHRODESIS OF THE WRIST

TECHNIQUE 10.37

(MILLENDER AND NALEBUFF)

- Make a dorsal, straight longitudinal incision and protect the wrist and finger extensor tendons.
- Curet away the remaining cartilage and remove the sclerotic bone from the carpus and radius down to cancellous bone. Varying amounts of bone may require resection for reduction of a dislocated wrist.

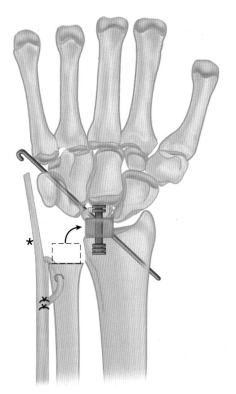

FIGURE 10.53   Radiolunate fusion. A half-slip of extensor carpi ulnaris tendon *(asterisk)* is used to stabilize the distal ulnar stump. Kirschner wire used to transfix triquetrum, bone graft, and radius is removed 6 weeks after surgery. (From Motomiya M, Iwasaki N, Minami A, et al: Clinical and radiological results of radiolunate arthrodesis for rheumatoid arthritis: 22 wrists followed for an average of 7 years, *J Hand Surg* 38A:1484, 2013.)

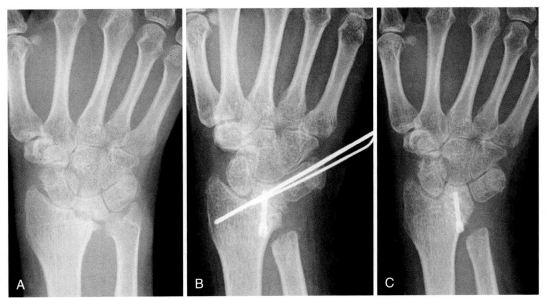

FIGURE 10.54   **A,** Larsen grade III involvement in 36-year-old woman improved to grade II immediately after radiolunate arthrodesis **(B). C,** Approximately 8 years after surgery, there is continued good condition of preserved joints. (From Motomiya M, Iwasaki N, Minami A, et al: Clinical and radiological results of radiolunate arthrodesis for rheumatoid arthritis: 22 wrists followed for an average of 7 years, *J Hand Surg* 38A:1484, 2013.)

- Drill a Steinmann pin of appropriate size into the carpus and out distally between the second and third metacarpals. Then drill it proximally into the medullary canal of the radius and cut off its end beneath the skin.
- As an alternative, resect the third metacarpal head for later insertion of a joint prosthesis.
- Insert the Steinmann pin through the medullary canal of the third metacarpal, through the carpus, and finally into the radius, leaving sufficient room distally in the metacarpal to allow insertion of the proximal stem of a metacarpophalangeal prosthesis. This places the wrist in neutral position.
- To avoid rotational deformities, drive a staple across the radiocarpal joint or insert an oblique Kirschner wire.
- Close the wound loosely to permit ample drainage.
- Proceed with any other operations necessary on the digits.

POSTOPERATIVE CARE For the first 2 weeks, a splint is preferred to avoid complications from swelling. The wrist is protected with a cast or splint until bony union has occurred. The extent and type of splinting depend on the activities and needs of the patient.

■ DISTAL RADIOULNAR JOINT ARTHROPLASTY

Instability and degenerative arthritic deformities isolated to the distal radioulnar joint can be managed by a number of techniques (see chapter 6, Wrist Disorders). When these conditions warrant surgical intervention, the use of a number of implants may prove beneficial (Fig. 10.55). The details specific to each implant are best outlined in the manufacturers' surgical guides. Both instability and arthritis may be treated with the Aptis-Scheker implant (Fig. 10.56). The most common complication associated with this implant was extensor carpi ulnaris tendonitis, for which an adipose fascial flap was designed to minimize this issue. The functional outcomes of a challenging group of patients (including those with Madelung deformity and Ehlers-Danlos syndrome) were reported by Rampazzo et al. Their retrospective analysis of 46 Aptis-Scheker implants placed in patients under 40 years

of age (18 to 39 years) found a 5-year survival rate of 96%. Although extensor carpi ulnaris tendinitis was satisfactorily treated by the adipofascial flap, other reasons for revision in this group included replacement of the polyethylene ball (2), ulnar stem exchange (2), radial plate repositioning, partial lunate excision, and posterior interosseous neuroma excision. Radial plate loosening is a potential concern in the long term because fixation to the radial shaft is not by ingrowth.

Ulnar head prosthetic implants of various designs have been devised to alleviate the pain following distal radioulnar joint degenerative and instability conditions (Fig. 10.57). Although survival rates seem satisfactory at midterm follow-up, concerns remain because stem lucencies and other factors make revision not uncommon. At a 56-month median follow-up (16 to 126 months), Kakar et al. reported an 83% survival of 47 implants followed over a 10-year period. Although 92% of patients reported feeling better after the surgery, 30% required revision; the most common reasons for revision were soft-tissue stabilization and implant loosening. These authors noted that, although pain reduction and functional improvement can be expected with distal ulnar replacement arthroplasty for instability, arthrosis, or both, patients should be counseled about the need for revision surgery.

■ TOTAL WRIST ARTHROPLASTY

Total wrist arthroplasty designs continue to evolve, and functional results and survivorship remain variable. The soft tissues must be released adequately, the bones must be aligned correctly, and the musculotendinous units must be balanced to prevent recurrence of deformity. Newer designs rely on shorter screw fixation in the carpals and osseous integration to reduce distal component loosening. Complication rates remain high, and surface replacement arthroplasties must be used with caution especially in patients with rheumatoid arthritis. Ward et al. reported a 50% failure rate in a 5-year minimum follow-up study on a group of 20 rheumatoid wrists undergoing replacement. Yeoh and Tourret reported much higher survivorship in a literature review on fourth-generation wrist implants. The results of 405 prostheses from eight articles were available, including seven different manufacturers (Table 10.3). The mean follow-up

TABLE 10.3				
Implant Survival				
PROSTHESIS	AUTHOR	NUMBER	LOSS TO FOLLOW-UP/DEATHS	SURVIVAL
Universal	Ward et al., 2011	24	5	75% at 5 years
Universal 2	Morapudi et al., 2012 Ferreres et al., 2011	21	3	100% at 3–5 years
Remotion	Boeckstyns et al., 2013	65	8	90% at 6 years
Biaxial	Krukhaug et al., 2011 Harlingen et al., 2011	90 40	NA 1	85% at 5 years 81% at 7 years
Motec	Krukhaug et al., 2011 Reigstad et al., 2012	76 30	NA 1	77% at 4 years 93.3% at 6 years
Elos	Krukhaug et al., 2011	23	NA	57% at 5 years (Krukhaug)
Maestro	Nydick et al., 2012	23	0	95.7% at 2.3 years
All prosthesis				57%–100% at 5 years

From Yeoh D, Tourret L: Total wrist arthroplasty: a systematic review of the evidence from the last 5 years, *J Hand Surg Eur* 40:458, 2015.

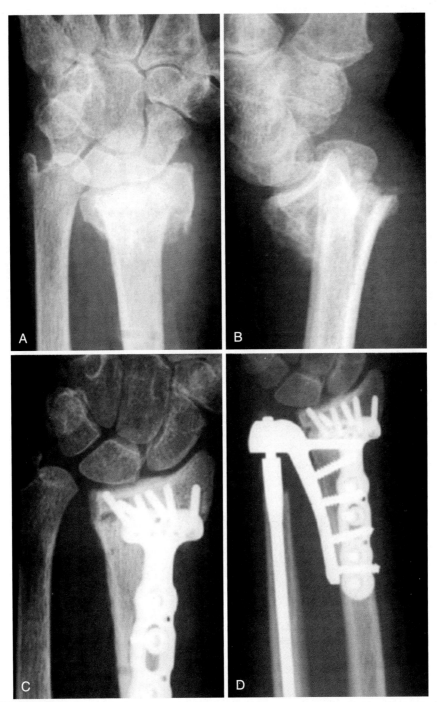

FIGURE 10.55 A 55-year-old man who had corrective osteotomy for distal radial malunion, followed by total distal radioulnar joint arthroplasty for residual instability and pain. **A** and **B,** Preoperative radiographs showing an apex-volar malunion of distal radius with marked ulnar-positive variance. **C,** Two months after corrective osteotomy, the apex-volar malunion was corrected but distal radioulnar joint dysfunction persisted, with wide diastasis at sigmoid notch and ulnar-positive variance. **D,** One month after total distal radioulnar joint arthroplasty, which resulted in resolution of pain and restoration of grip and lifting strength. There were no clinical or radiographic indications of loosening at more than 3 years of follow-up. (From Faucher GK, Zimmerman RM, Zimmerman NB: Instability and arthritis of the distal radioulnar joint: a critical analysis review, *JBJS Rev* 4(12):pii: 01874474-201612000-00001, 2016.)

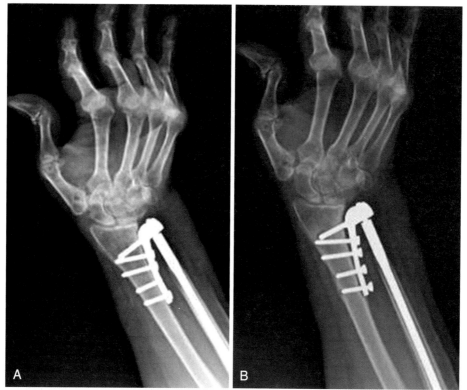

FIGURE 10.56 Arthroplasty with an Aptis-Scheker implant in 65-year-old female with lupus in whom fascial interposition failed to relieve symptoms. **A,** Early postoperative radiograph. **B,** At 2-year follow-up with recent onset of wrist pain, swelling, and mechanical symptoms.

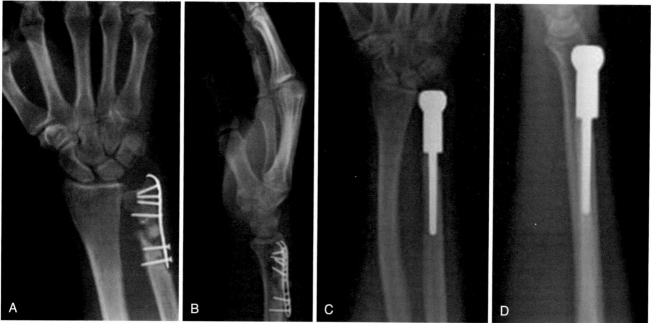

FIGURE 10.57 Ulnar head replacement in 50-year-old female package handler. **A** and **B,** Anteroposterior and lateral views of wrist after revision bone grafting, which subsequently united after nonunion of an ulnar-shortening osteotomy for degenerative impaction syndrome. **C** and **D,** Anteroposterior and lateral views after ulnar head replacement. Moderate degree of clinical improvement was achieved.

ranged from 2.3 to 7.3 years, and average patient age from 52 to 63 years. Rheumatoid arthritis was the indication in 42% of patients. Motec (Swemac, LinKöping, Sweden) demonstrated the best postoperative DASH scores. Only Maestro (Biomet Orthopedics, Warsaw, IN) achieved a defined functional range of motion postoperatively. Universal 2 (Integra, Cincinnati, OH) displayed the highest survival rates (100% at 3 to 5 years), whereas Elos (Elos Medtech, Gorlose, Denmark) had the lowest (57% at 5 years). Biaxial had the highest complication rate (68.7%), whereas Re-Motion (Small Bone Innovations Inc., Morrisville, PA) had the lowest (11%). Functional scores improved and were maintained over the mid- to long-term. A single-center study of 189 consecutive patients (219 wrist arthroplasties) found high satisfaction rates among all implants studied at an average follow-up of 7 years (2 to 13 years). This group consisted of 33 male and 186 female patients (34 with osteoarthritis and 185 with rheumatoid arthritis), with an average age of 60 years (25 to 88 years). Cumulative implant survivorship at 8 years was 81% for the Biax (DePuy Orthopaedics Inc, Warsaw, IN), 94% for the Re-Motion, and 95% for the Maestro, with radiographic evidence of loosening in 26%, 18%, and 2%, respectively.

Complication rates were higher than for wrist fusion, with reports of radiographic loosening and osteolysis. The evidence does not support the widespread use of arthroplasty over arthrodesis, and careful patient selection is essential.

REFERENCES

GENERAL ARTHRITIS

Bernstein RA: Arthritis of the thumb and digits: current concepts, *Instr Course Lect* 64:281, 2015.

Cavaliere CM, Chung KC: A cost-utility analysis of nonsurgical management, total wrist arthroplasty, and total wrist arthrodesis in rheumatoid arthritis, *J Hand Surg* 35A:379, 2010.

Chung KC, Kotsis SV: Outcomes of hand surgery in the patient with rheumatoid arthritis, *Curr Opin Rheumatol* 22:336, 2010.

Chung KC, Pushman AG: Current concepts in the management of the rheumatoid hand, *J Hand Surg* 36A:736, 2011.

Farr S, Girsch W: The hand and wrist in juvenile rheumatoid arthritis, *J Hand Surg Am* 40:2289, 2015.

Gogna R, Cheung G, Arundell M, et al.: Rheumatoid hand surgery: is there a decline? a 22-year population-based study, *Hand* 10:272, 2015.

Kahlenberg JM, Fox DA: Advances in the medical treatment of rheumatoid arthritis, *Hand Clin* 27:11, 2011.

Murray PM: Current concepts in the treatment of rheumatoid arthritis of the distal radioulnar joint, *Hand Clin* 27:49, 2011.

Pegoli L, Pozzi A, Pivato G, et al.: Arthroscopic resection of distal pole of the scaphoid for scaphotrapeziotrapezoid joint arthritis: comparison between and simple resection and implant interposition, *J Wrist Surg* 5:227, 2016.

Riches PL, Elherik FK, Dolan S, et al.: Patient rated outcomes study into the surgical interventions available for the rheumatoid hand and wrist, *Arch Orthop Trauma* 136:563, 2016.

Rizzo M, Cooney 3rd WP: Current concepts and treatment for the rheumatoid wrist, *Hand Clin* 27:57, 2011.

Sebastin SJ, Chung KC: Reconstruction of digital deformities in rheumatoid arthritis, *Hand Clin* 27:87, 2011.

Watt AJ, Shin AY, Vedder NB, Chang J: Joint arthritis and soft-tissue problems of the hand, *Plast Reconstr Surg* 126:288e, 2010.

Wilczynski MC, Gelberman RH, Adams A, Goldfarb CA: Arthroscopic findings in gout of the wrist, *J Hand Surg* 34A:244, 2009.

ARTHRITIS SOFT-TISSUE PROCEDURES

Chung CS, Yen CH, Yip MR, et al.: Arthroscopic synovectomy for rheumatoid wrists and elbows, *J Orthop Surg* 20:219, 2012.

Gehrmann SV, Tang J, Li ZM, et al.: Motion deficit of the thumb in CMC joint arthritis, *J Hand Surg* 35A:1449, 2010.

Ishikawa H, Abe A, Kojima T, et al.: Overall benefits provided by orthopedic surgical intervention in patients with rheumatoid arthritis, *Mod Rheumatol* 1–9, 2018, https://doi.org/10.1080/14397595.2018.1457468, [Epub ahead of print].

To P, Watson JT: Boutonniere deformity, *J Hand Surg* 36A:139, 2011.

Ursum J, Horsten NC, Hoeksma AF, et al.: Predictors of stenosing tenosynovitis in the hand and hand-related activity limitations in patients with rheumatoid arthritis, *Arch Phys Med Rehabil* 92:96, 2011.

THUMB METACARPOPHALANGEAL JOINT ARTHRITIS

Abzug JM, Osteroman AL: Arthroscopic hemiresection for stage II-III trapeziometacaral osteoarthritis, *Hand Clin* 27:347, 2011.

Adams JE, Steinmann SP, Culp RW: Bone-preserving arthrosopic options for treatment of thumb basilar joint arthritis, *Hand Clin* 27:355, 2011.

Avisar E, Elvey M, Tzang C, Sorene E: Trapeziectomy with a tendon tie-in implant for osteoarthritis of the trapeziometacarpal joint, *J Hand Surg* 40:1292, 2015.

Bachoura A, Yakish EJ, Lubahn JD: Survival and long-term outcomes of thumb metacarpal extension osteotomy for symptomatic carpometacarpal laxity and early basal joint arthritis, *J Hand Surg Am* 43:772, 2018.

Barrerra-Ochoa S, Vidal-Tarrason N, Correa-Vazquez E, et al.: Pyrocarbon interposition (PyroDisk) implant for trapeziometacarpal osteoarthritis: minimum 5-year follow-up, *J Hand Surg Am* 39:2150, 2014.

Berger AJ, Meals RA: Management of osteoarthritis of the thumb joints, *J Hand Surg Am* 40:843, 2015.

Bodin ND, Spangler R, Thoder JJ: Interposition arthroplasty options for carpometacarpal arthritis of the thumb, *Hand Clin* 26:339, 2010.

Bozentka DJ: Implant arthroplasty of the carpometacarpal joint of the thumb, *Hand Clin* 26:327, 2010.

Braun RM, Rechnic M, Shah KN: Salvage reconstruction of failed interposition arthroplasty at the base of the thumb, *Tech Hand Surg* 16:230, 2012.

Brogan DM, Kakar S: Metacarpophalangeal joint hyperextension and the treatment of thumb basilar joint arthritis, *J Hand Surg* 37A:837, 2012.

Cebrian-Gomez R, Lizaur-Utrilla A, Sebastia-Forcada E, et al.: Outcomes of cementless joint prosthesis versus tendon interposition for trapeziometacarpal osteoarthritis: a prospective study, *J Hand Surg Eur* 2018, 1753193418787151, https://doi.org/10.1177/1753193418787151. [Epub ahead of print].

Cheema T, Salas C, Morrell N, et al.: Opening wedge trapezial osteotomy as possible treatment for early trapeziometacarpal osteoarthritis: a biomechanical investigation of radial subluxation, contact area, and contact pressure, *J Hand Surg* 37A:699, 2012.

Chou FH, Irrgang JJ, Goitz RJ: Long-term follow-up of first metacarpal extension osteotomy for early CMC arthritis, *Hand* 9:478, 2014.

Chug M, Williams N, Benn D, Brindley S: Outcome of uncemented trapeziometacarpal prosthesis for treatment of carpometacarpal arthritis, *Indian J Orthop* 48:394, 2014.

Cobb TK, Walden AL, Cao Y: Long-term outcome of arthroscopic resection arthroplasty with or without interposition for thumb basal joint arthritis, *J Hand Surg Am* 40:1844, 2015.

De Smet L, Vandenberghe L, Didden K, Degreef I: Outcome of simultaneous treatment of hyperextension of metacarpophalangeal and basal joint osteoarthritis of the thumb, *Acta Orthop Belg* 79:514, 2013.

Dickson DR, Badge R, Nuttall D, et al.: Pyrocarbon metacarpophalangeal joint arthroplasty in noninflammatory arthritis: minimum 5-year follow-up, *J Hand Surg* 40:1956, 2015.

Escott BG, Ronald K, Judd MG, Bogoch ER: NuFlex and Swanson metacarpophalangeal implants for rheumatoid arthritis: prospective randomized, controlled clinical trial, *J Hand Surg* 35A:44, 2010.

Frizziero A, Maffulli N, Masiero S, Frizziero L: Six-months pain relief and functional recovery after intra-articular injections with hyaluronic acid (ms 500-730 KDa) in trapeziometacarpal osteoarthritis, *Muscles Ligaments Tendons J* 4:256, 2014.

Gangopadhyay S, McKenna H, Burke FD, Davis TRC: Five- to 18-year follow-up for treatment of trapeziometacarpal osteoarthritis: a prospective comparison of excision, tendon interposition, and ligament reconstruction and tendon interposition, *J Hand Surg* 37A:411, 2012.

Givissis P, Sachinis NP, Akritopouos P, et al.: The "pillow technique for thumb carpometacarpal joint arthritis: cohort study with 10- to 15-year follow-up, *J Hand Surg Am* 41:775, 2016.

Goubau JF, Gooren CK, Van Hoonacker P, et al.: Clinical and radiological outcomes of the Ivory arthroplasty for trapeziometacarpal joint arthritis with a minimum of 5 years of follow-up: a prospective single-centre cohort study, *J Hand Surg Eur* 38E:866, 2013.

Hattori Y, Doi K, Dormitorio B, et al.: Arthrodesis for primary osteoarthritis of the trapeziometacarpal joint in elderly patients, *J Hand Surg Am* 41:753, 2016.

Hentz VR: Surgical treatment of trapeziometacarpal joint arthritis. a historical perspective, *Clin Orthop Relat Res* 472:1183, 2014.

Hess DE, Crace P, Franco MJ, et al.: Failed thumb carpometacarpal arthroplasty: common etiologies and surgical options for revision, *J Hand Surg AM* 43:844, 2018.

Hippensteel KJ, Calfee R, Dardas AZ, et al.: Functional outcomes of thumb trapeziometacarpal arthrodesis with a locked plate versus ligament reconstruction and tendon interposition, *J Hand Surg Am* 42:685, 2017.

Kapoutsis DV, Dardas A, Day CS: Carpometacarpal and scaphotrapeziotrapezoid arthritis: arthroscopy, arthroplasty, and arthrodesis, *J Hand Surg* 36A:354, 2011.

Kochevar AJ, Adham CN, Adham MN, et al.: Thumb basal joint arthroplasty using abductor pollicis longus tendon: an average 5.5-year follow-up, *J Hand Surg* 36A:1326, 2011.

Landes G, Gaspar MP, Goljan P, et al.: Arthroscopic trapeziectomy with suture button suspensionplasty: a retrospective review of 153 cases, *Hand* 11:232, 2016.

Logli AL, Twu J, Bear BJ, et al.: Arthroscopic partial trapeziectomy with soft tissue interposition for symptomatic trapeziometacarpal arthritis: 6-month and 5-year minimum follow-up, *J Hand Surg Am* 43:384.e1, 2018.

Marks M, Hensler S, Wehrli M, et al.: Trapeziectomy with suspension-interposition arthroplasty for thumb carpometacarpal osteoarthritis: a randomized controlled trial comparing the use of allograft versus flexor carpi radialis tendon, *J Hand Sur Am* 42:978, 2017.

Martin-Ferrero M: Ten-year long-term results of total joint arthroplasties with ARPE® implant in the treatment of trapeziometacarpal osteoarthritis, *J Hand Surg Eur* 39E:826, 2014.

Moneim MS, Morrell NT, Mercer DM: Partial trapeziectomy with capsular interposition arthroplasty (PTCI): a novel technique for thumb basal joint arthritis, *Tech Hand Surg* 18:116, 2014.

Noland SS, Saber S, Endress R, Hentz VR: The scaphotrapezial joint after partial trapeziectomy for trapeziometacarpal joint arthritis: long-term follow-up, *J Hand Surg* 37A:1125, 2012.

Park MJ, Lee AT, Yao J: Treatment of thumb carpometacarpal arthritis with arthroscopic hemitrapeziectomy and interposition arthroplasty, *Orthopedics* 35:e1759, 2012.

Pegoli L, Pozzi A: Arthroscopic management of scaphoid-trapezium-trapezoid joint arthritis, *Hand Clin* 33:813, 2017.

Qadir R, Duncan SFM, Smith AA, et al.: Volar capsulodesis of the thumb metacarpophalangeal joint at the time of basal joint arthroplasty: a surgical technique using suture anchors, *J Hand Surg Am* 39:1999, 2014.

Raskolnikov D, White NJ, Swart E, et al.: Volar plate capsulodesis for metacarpophalangeal hyperextension with basal joint arthritis, *Am J Orthop (Belle Mead NJ)* 43:354, 2014.

Reissner L, Marks M, Schindele S, et al.: Comparison of clinical outcome with radiological findings after trapeziectomy with ligament reconstruction and tendon interposition, *J Hand Surg Eur* 41:335, 2016.

Robles-Molina MJ, Lopez-Caba F, Gómez-Sánchez RC, et al.: Trapeziectomy with ligament reconstruction and tendon interposition versus a trapeziometacarpal prosthesis for the treatment of thumb basal joint osteoarthritis, *Orthopedics* 40:e681, 2017.

Roman PB, Linnell JD, Moore JB: Trapeziectomy arthroplasty with suture suspension: short- to medium-term outcomes from a single-surgeon experience, *J Hand Surg Am* 41:34, 2016.

Rubino M, Cavagnaro L, Sansone V: A new surgical technique for the treatment of scaphotrapezial arthritis associated with trapeziometacarpal arthritis: the narrow pseudoarthrosis, *J Hand Surg Eur* 41:710, 2016.

Shuler MS, Luria S, Trumble TE: Basal joint arthritis of the thumb, *J Am Acad Orthop Surg* 16:418, 2008.

Slutsky DJ: The role of arthroscopy in trapeziometacarpal arthritis, *Clin Orthop Relat Res* 472:1173, 2014.

Spaans AJ, van Minnen P, Kon M, et al.: Conservative treatment of thumb base osteoarthritis: a systematic review, *J Hand Surg Am* 40:16, 2015.

Spekreijse KR, Selles RW, Kediloglu MA, et al.: Trapeziometacarpal arthrodesis or trapeziectomy with ligament reconstruction in primary trapeziometacarpal osteoarthritis: a 5-year follow-up, *J Hand Surg Am* 41:910, 2016.

Spekreijse KR, Vermeulen GM, Kedilioglu MA, et al.: The effect of a bone tunnel during ligament reconstruction for trapeziometacarpal osteoarthritis: a 5-year follow-up, *J Hand Surg Am* 40:2214, 2015.

Toffoli A, Teissier J: MAÏA trapeziometacarpal joint arthroplasty: clinical and radiological outcomes of 80 patients with more than 6 years of follow-up, *J Hand Surg Am* 42:838, 2017.

Vermeulen GM, Brink SM, Slijper H, et al.: Trapeziometacarpal arthrodesis or trapeziectomy with ligament reconstruction in primary trapeziometacarpal osteoarthritis. A randomized controlled trial, *J Bone Joint Surg* 96:726, 2014.

Wajon A, Vinycomb T, Carr E, et al.: Surgery for thumb (trapeziometacarpal joint) osteoarthritis, *Cochrane Database Syst Rev* 2:CD004631, 2015.

Waljee JF, Chung KC: Objective functional outcomes and patient satisfaction after silicone metacarpophalangeal arthroplasty for rheumatoid arthritis, *J Hand Surg* 37A:47, 2012.

Wall LB, Stern PJ: Clinical and radiographic outcomes of metacarpophalangeal joint pyrolytic carbon arthroplasty for osteoarthritis, *J Hand Surg* 38A:537, 2013.

Wysocki RW, Cohen MS, Shott S, Fernandez JJ: Thumb carpometacarpal suspension arthroplasty using interference screw fixation: surgical technique and clinical results, *J Hand Surg Am* 35:913, 2010.

Yao J, Song Y: Suture-button suspensionplasty for thumb carpometacarpal arthritis: a minimum 2-year follow-up, *J Hand Surg* 38A:1161, 2013.

Zancolli 3rd ER, Andrés BG: The modified Zancolli arthroplasty for basal thumb arthritis, *Tech Hand Up Extrem Surg* 14:248, 2010.

DISTAL RADIOULNAR JOINT

Faucher GK, Zimmerman RM, Zimmerman NB: Instability and arthritis of the distal radioulnar joint: a critical analysis review, *JBJS Rev* 4:pii: 01874474-201612000-00001, 2016.

Jain A, Ball C, Freidin AJ, Nanchahal J: Effects of extensor synovectomy and excision of the distal ulnar in rheumatoid arthritis on long-term function, *J Hand Surg* 35A:1442, 2010.

Kakar S, Fox T, Wagner E, et al.: Linked distal radioulnara joint arthroplasty: an analysis of the APTIS prosthesis, *J Hand Surg Eur* 39:739, 2014.

Kakar S, Swann P, Perry KI, et al.: Functional and radiographic outcomes following distal ulna implant arthroplasty, *J Hand Surg* 37A:1364, 2012.

Motomiya M, Iwasaki N, Minami A, et al.: Clinical and radiological results of radiolunate arthrodesis for rheumatoid arthritis: 22 wrists followed for an average of 7 years, *J Hand Surg* 38A:1484, 2013.

Rampazzo A, Gharb BB, Brock G, et al.: Functional outcomes of the Aptis-Scheker distal radioulnar joint replacement in patients under 40 years old, *J Hand Surg Am* 40:1397, 2015.

Raven EE, Ottink KD, Doets KC: Radiolunate and radioscapholunate arthrodeses as treatments for rheumatoid and psoriatic arthritis: long-term follow-up, 37(1):55, 2012.

WRIST ARTHRODESIS/ARTHROPLASTY

Adams BD, Kleinhenz BP, Guan JJ: Wrist arthrodesis for failed total wrist arthroplasty, *J Hand Surg Am* 41:673, 2016.

Bedford B, Yang SS: High fusion rates with circular plate fixation for four-corner arthrodesis of the wrist, *Clin Orthop Relat Res* 468:163, 2010.

Bhamra J, Bhamra K, Hindocha S, et al.: The role of wrist fusion and wrist arthroplasty in rheumatoid arthritis, *Curr Rheumatol Rev* 13:23, 2017.

Delattre O, Goulon G, Vogels J, et al.: Three-corner arthrodesis with scaphoid and triquetrum excision for wrist arthritis, *J Hand Surg Am* 40:2176, 2015.

Ferreres A, Lluch A, del Valle M: Universal total wrist arthroplasty: midterm follow-up study, *J Hand Surg* 36A:967, 2011.

Gaspar MP, Lou J, Kane PM, et al: Complications following partial and total wrist arthroplasty: a single-center retrospective review, J Hand Surg Am 41:47, 20156.

Reigstad O, Holm-Glad T, Bolstad B, et al.: Five to 10-year prospective follow-up of wrist arthroplasty in 56 nonrheumatoid patients, *J Hand Surg Am* 42:788, 2017.

Sagerfors M, Gupta A, Brus O, Pettersson K: Total wrist arthrolasty: a single-center study of 219 caes with 5-year follow-up, *J Hand Surg Am* 40:2380, 2015.

Ward CM, Kuhl T, Adams BD: Five to ten-year outcomes of the Universal total wrist arthroplasty in patients with rheumatoid arthritis, *J Bone Joint Surg* 93:914, 2011.

Wysocki RW, Cohen MS: Complications of limited and total wrist arthrodesis, *Hand Clin* 26:221, 2010.

Yeoh D, Tourret L: Total wrist arthroplasty: a systematic review of the evidence from the last 5 years, *J Hand Surg Eur* 40E:458, 2015.

INTERPHALANGEAL ARTHROPLASTY AND ARTHRODESIS

Beldner S, Polatsch DB: Arthrodesis of the metacarpophalangeal and interphalangeal joints of the hand: current concepts, *J Am Acad Orthop Surg* 24:290, 2016.

Breyer JM, Vergas P, Parra L, et al.: Metacarpphalangeal and interphalangeal arthrodesis: a comparative study between tension band and compression screw fixation, *J Hand Surg Eur* 40:374, 2015.

Dickson DR, Nuttall D, Watts AC, et al.: Pyrocarbon proximal interphalangeal joint arthroplasty: minimum five-year follow-up, *J Hand Surg Am* 40:2142, 2015.

Edwards SG, Ramsey PN: Prospective outcomes of stage III thumb carpometacarpal arthritis treated with arthroscopic hemitrapeziectomy and thermal capsular modification without interposition, *J Hand Surg* 35(4):566, 2010.

Heers G, Springorum JR, Baier C, et al.: Proximal interphalangeal joint replacement with an unconstrained pyrocarbon prosthesis (Ascension®): a long-term follow-up, *J Hand Surg Eur* Vol. 38E:680, 2012.

Herren DB, Keuchel T, Marks M, Schindele S: Revision arthroplasty for failed silicone proximal interphalangeal joint arthroplasty: indications and 8-year results, *J Hand Surg Am* 39:462, 2014.

Jacobs BJ, Verbruggen G, Kaufmann RA: Proximal interphalangeal joint arthritis, *J Hand Surg* 35A:2107, 2010.

Jennings CD, Livingstone DP: Surface replacement arthroplasty of the proximal interphalangeal joint using the SR PIP implant: long-term results, *J Hand Surg Am* 40:469, 2015.

Lin EA, Papatheodorou LK, Sotereanos DG, et al.: Cheilectomy for treatment of symptomatic distal interphalangeal joint osteoarthritis: a review of 78 patients, *J Hand Surg Am* 42:889, 2017.

Luther C, Germann G, Sauerbier M: Proximal interphalangeal joint replacement with surface replacement arthroplasty (SR-PIP): functional results and complications, *Hand (N Y)* 5:233, 2010.

McGuire DT, Whilte CD, Carter SL, Solomons NW: Pyrocarbon proximal interphalangeal joint arthroplasty: outcomes of a cohort study, *J Hand Surg Eur* 37E:490, 2011.

Mikolyzk DK, Stern PJ: Steinmann pin arthrodesis for salvage of failed small joint arthroplasty, *J Hand Surg* 36A:1383, 2011.

Pettersson K, Amilon A, Rizzo M: Pyrolytic carbon hemiarthroplasty in the management of proximal interphalangeal joint arthritis, *J Hand Surg Am* 40:462, 2015.

Srnec JJ, Wagner ER, Rizzo M: Implant arthroplasty for proximal interphalangeal, metacarpophalangeal, and trapeziometacarpal joint degeneration, *J Hand Surg Am* 42:817, 2017.

Van Nuffel M, Degreef I, Willems S, De Smet L: Proximal interphalangeal joint replacement: resurfacing pyrocarbon versus silicone arthroplasty, *Acta Orthop Belg* 80:190, 2014.

Vitale MA, Fruth KM, Rizzo M, et al.: Prosthetic arthroplasty versus arthrodesis for osteoarthritis and posttraumatic arthritis of the index finger proximal interphalangeal joint, *J Hand Surg* 40:1937, 2015.

Wagner ER, Luo TD, Houdek MT, et al.: Revision proximal interphalangeal arthroplasty: an outcome analysis of 75 consecutive cases, *J Hand Surg Am* 40:1949, 2015.

Wagner ER, Van Denmark 3rd R, Kor DJ, et al.: Intraoperative periprosthetic fractures in proximal interphalangeal joint arthroplasty, *J Hand Surg Am* 409:2149, 2015.

Wagner ER, Weston JT, Houdek MT, et al.: Medium-term outcomes with pyrocarbon proximal interphalangeal arthroplasty: a study of 170 consecutive arthroplasties, *J Hand Surg Am* 43:979, 2018.

Watts AC, Heranden AJ, Trail IA, et al.: Pyrocarbon proximal interphalangeal joint arthroplasty: minimum two-year follow-up, *J Hand Surg* 37A:882, 2012.

The complete list of references is available online at Expert Consult.com.

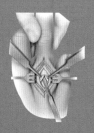
COMPARTMENT SYNDROMES AND VOLKMANN CONTRACTURE

Norfleet B. Thompson

DEFINITION AND HISTORY

Compartment syndrome is a condition in which the circulation within a closed compartment is compromised by an increase in pressure within the compartment, causing necrosis of muscles, nerves, and eventually the skin because of excessive swelling. Volkmann ischemic contracture is a sequela of untreated or inadequately treated compartment syndrome in which necrotic muscle and nerve tissue have been replaced with fibrous tissue.

In the upper extremity, compartment syndrome is most common in the forearm. The intrinsic muscle compartments of the hand also may be involved, and compartment syndrome of the upper arm has been reported.

In 1881, Volkmann stated in his classic paper that the paralytic contractures that could develop only a few hours after injury were caused by arterial insufficiency or ischemia of the muscles. He suggested that tight bandages were the cause of vascular insufficiency. This concept of extrinsic pressure as the primary cause of paralytic contracture persisted for some time in the English literature. In 1909, Thomas studied 107 paralytic contractures and found that some developed following severe contusions of the forearm in the absence of fractures, splints, or bandages. The idea was established that extrinsic pressure was not the sole cause of the ischemia. In 1914, Murphy reported that hemorrhage and effusion into the muscles could cause internal pressures to increase within the unyielding deep fascial compartments of the forearm, with subsequent obstruction of the venous return. In 1928, Jones concluded that Volkmann contracture could be caused by pressure from within, from without, or from both. Eichler and Lipscomb outlined the early technique of fasciotomy as the primary surgical treatment.

ANATOMY

Four interconnected compartments of the forearm are recognized (Fig. 11.1): (1) the superficial volar compartment, (2) the deep volar compartment, (3) the dorsal compartment, and (4) the compartment containing the mobile wad of Henry (brachioradialis and extensor carpi radialis longus and brevis). The volar compartments are most commonly involved, but the dorsal and mobile wad compartments can be involved alone or in addition to the volar compartments. It is usually difficult to clinically differentiate between isolated or combined involvement of the deep and superficial volar compartments; however, the deep volar compartment (flexor digitorum profundus, flexor pollicis longus, and pronator quadratus) may be solely involved.

In the hand, three palmar and four dorsal interosseous muscles are each surrounded by a tough, investing fascial layer, creating individual compartments, as shown by the injection dissections of Halpern and Mochizuki. The adductor pollicis, thenar, and hypothenar muscles also form three separate compartments (Fig. 11.2). The neurovascular bundles of each digit also are compartmentalized by fascial layers, making them vulnerable to excessive swelling (Fig. 11.3).

ETIOLOGY

Numerous injuries have been shown to result in compartment syndrome, including crush injuries, prolonged external compression, internal bleeding (especially after injury in patients with hemophilia), fractures, excessive exercise, burns, snake bites, and intraarterial injections of drugs or sclerosing agents. Infections also have been noted to increase pressures within compartments.

Elliott and Johnstone found that 18% of forearm compartment syndromes were caused by fractures, and 23% were caused by soft-tissue injuries without fractures. Although isolated distal radial fractures rarely were associated with compartment syndrome (0.3%), an ipsilateral elbow injury resulted in forearm compartment syndrome in 15% of patients. Historically, supracondylar humeral fractures were most frequently associated with forearm compartment syndrome in children; however, Grottkau et al. found that forearm fractures were actually more commonly associated (74% vs. 15%). In children, supracondylar humeral fractures with an associated neurovascular or floating elbow injury significantly increase the risk of compartment syndrome.

Acute compartment syndrome of the intrinsic muscles of the hand, resulting in contracture or necrosis of the muscle bellies such as those in the larger muscles in the forearm, can occur after compression injuries of the hand without fracture. Compartment syndrome has been noted in neonates following intrauterine malposition or strangulation of the extremity by the umbilical cord.

Direct trauma, crushing of the upper arm, shoulder dislocation, avulsion of the triceps muscle, pneumatic tourniquet use, and arteriography have all been reported as causes of compartment syndrome. Intravenous regional anesthesia has also been implicated as a cause when hypertonic saline is used to dilute an anesthetic.

Although more common in the lower extremity, chronic exertional compartment syndrome (CECS) may also involve the upper extremity. CECS most commonly affects the volar forearm compartment and the first dorsal interosseous muscle in the hand. It is most frequently diagnosed in competitive off-road motorcyclists. It has also been reported in kayakers and elite rowers and may occur in adolescents after puberty.

Any situation that causes a decrease in compartment size, an increase in compartment pressure, or a decrease in soft-tissue compliance can initiate compartment syndrome. As the intracompartmental pressure increases, capillary blood perfusion is reduced to a level that cannot maintain tissue viability. The increase in interstitial pressure overcomes the intravascular pressure of the small vessels and capillaries, which causes the walls to collapse and impedes local blood flow. In a canine model, muscle necrosis was shown to occur with a rise in pressure to within 20 mm Hg below the diastolic pressure. Local tissue ischemia leads to local edema, which increases the intracompartmental pressure. This cycle of increasing muscle ischemia was depicted by Eaton and Green, as shown in Figure 11.4.

The tolerance of tissue to prolonged ischemia varies according to the type of tissue. Functional impairment in muscles has been demonstrated after 2 to 4 hours of ischemia, and irreversible functional loss occurs after 4 to 12 hours. Nerve tissue shows abnormal function after 30 minutes of ischemia, with irreversible functional loss after 12 to 24 hours.

DIAGNOSIS

A crush injury or fracture of the forearm or elbow, especially in the supracondylar area of the humerus, should raise suspicion that a forearm compartment syndrome may develop.

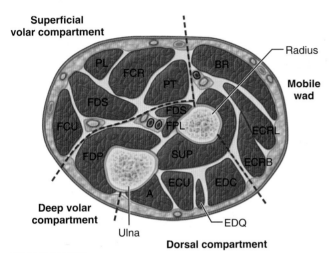

FIGURE 11.1 Cross-section through upper third of forearm. *A,* Anconeus muscle; *BR,* brachioradialis; *ECRB,* extensor carpi radialis brevis; *ECRL,* extensor carpi radialis longus; *ECU,* extensor carpi ulnaris; *EDC,* extensor digitorum communis; *EDQ,* extensor digiti quinti; *FCR,* flexor carpi radialis; *FCU,* flexor carpi ulnaris; *FDP,* flexor digitorum profundus; *FDS,* flexor digitorum sublimis; *FPL,* flexor pollicis longus; *PL,* palmaris longus; *PT,* pronator teres; *SUP,* supinator.

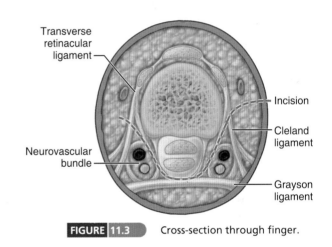

FIGURE 11.3 Cross-section through finger.

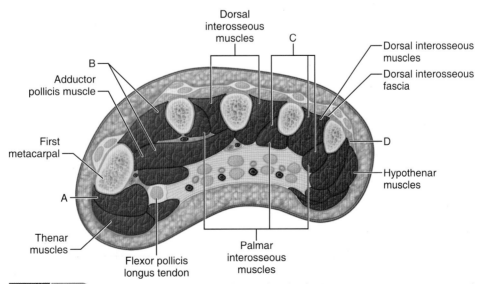

FIGURE 11.2 Cross-section through hand. Dorsal and volar interosseous compartments and adductor compartment to thumb *(B and C)*; thenar and hypothenar compartments *(A and D)*.

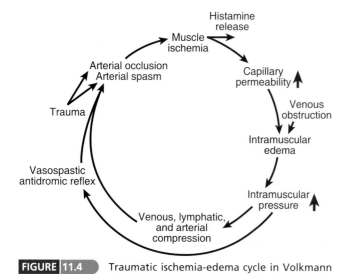

FIGURE 11.4   Traumatic ischemia-edema cycle in Volkmann contracture.

Early diagnosis of impending ischemia is essential because irreversible damage can occur quickly. Commonly described characteristics of compartment syndrome in adults include the five "P's": pain with passive stretch of the involved compartment (or pain out of proportion to examination), paresthesias, pallor, paralysis, and pulselessness. Increasing pain that is out of proportion to the injury and worsens with passive stretching of the involved muscles is an early indication that a compartment syndrome is developing. The volar and/or dorsal forearm is tender and tense with swelling, and sensibility of the fingertips may be diminished. Two-point discrimination and 256-cycle vibratory testing can be helpful in determining nerve ischemia. Paralysis of involved muscle function and loss of the radial and/or ulnar pulse present as late findings unless there is direct arterial injury.

Diagnosis of compartment syndrome in an individual interosseous muscle can be difficult. The hand is swollen and tense, and the fingers are held almost rigid in a partially flexed position with the wrist in neutral. Any passive movement of the fingers that causes metacarpophalangeal joint extension usually causes considerable pain. The adductor compartment of the thumb can be tested by pulling the thumb into palmar abduction and stretching the adductor muscle. The thenar muscles rarely are involved. Diagnosis in obtunded and pediatric patients is more difficult. In children, the five "P's" are considered less reliable. Bae et al. advocated using the three "A's" (increasing analgesic requirements, unremitting agitation, and anxiety) as more reliable indicators of developing pediatric compartment syndrome. Compartment syndrome in a neonate may manifest as a sentinel bullous or ulcerative skin lesion, usually over the dorsum of the forearm, wrist, or hand. Unilateral aplasia cutis congenita also must be considered in this setting.

When compartment syndrome is suspected and the necessary equipment is available, compartment pressures should be obtained to confirm the diagnosis. Compartment pressures over 30 mm Hg or within 30 mm Hg of the diastolic pressure (delta P) are indicative of compartment syndrome. The delta P value compares the compartment pressure to the diastolic blood pressure and thus controls for variation in a patient's blood pressure. All involved compartments should be measured, and the results should be interpreted with regard to the overall clinical picture. Forearm measurements can be obtained from the superficial and deep volar compartments, and the mobile wad and dorsal compartments. The location for pressure monitoring using a needle manometer is commonly the middle third of the forearm for both flexor compartments and for the dorsal extensor compartment. The deep flexor compartment is measured just anterior to the ulna. The mobile wad of Henry may be entered in the midline of its bulk. Hand measurements may be obtained from the thenar, hypothenar, adductor pollicis, and interosseous muscles. Digital pressures are not routinely obtained.

In 1975, Whitesides et al. described a technique for measuring compartment pressures using an 18-gauge needle, saline syringe, three-way stopcock, and a mercury manometer; however, a handheld pressure monitoring device or an arterial line monitoring system, connected to either a straight needle, a side-port needle, or slit catheter, is currently preferred. Boody and Wongworawat compared the intracompartmental pressure monitoring system, an arterial line manometer, and the Whitesides apparatus, each with a straight needle, a side-port needle, and a slit catheter, and found that the arterial line manometer with a slit catheter was the most accurate technique. The handheld pressure monitoring system also was found to be accurate. Side-port needles and slit catheters were more accurate, whereas straight needles tended to overestimate the pressure. We most commonly use the Stryker handheld pressure monitoring device to determine intracompartmental pressures. The arterial line monitoring system is useful if continuous monitoring is desired.

To use the handheld pressure monitoring device (Stryker), the needle is placed firmly onto the chamber stem, a prefilled syringe is placed into the remaining chamber stem, and the chamber is firmly seated into the device. The needle is held at 45 degrees from horizontal and the system is purged of excess air. When the unit is turned on, the display should read 0 to 9 mm Hg. To calibrate the system, the zero button should be pressed and the display should read 00. The needle is then inserted into the desired compartment, and no more than 0.3 mL of solution is injected. The device then displays the pressure of the compartment. In an experimental model, Doro et al. showed that measurement of intramuscular glucose levels can identify compartment syndrome with high sensitivity and specificity.

MEASURING COMPARTMENT PRESSURES IN THE FOREARM AND HAND USING A HANDHELD MONITORING DEVICE

TECHNIQUE 11.1

(LIPSCHITZ AND LIFCHEZ)

MEASURING FOREARM COMPARTMENT PRESSURE
- Place the compartment to be measured at heart level.
- Use adequate local analgesia infiltrated into the skin only, taking care to avoid the underlying muscle and fascia, to control discomfort and pressure spikes.

- To measure the volar compartment pressure, insert the needle just ulnar to the palmaris longus, through the superficial fascia to a depth of 1 cm. Confirm proper needle depth by observing a rise in pressure during external compression of the volar forearm or passive extension of fingers. The deep volar compartment may be measured just anterior to the ulna on the flexor side of the forearm, taking care to avoid the neurovascular bundle.
- To measure the dorsal compartment, insert the needle just radial to the border of the ulna to a depth of 1 to 2 cm. Confirm placement by external compression of the dorsal compartment with passive flexion of the wrist.
- To test the mobile wad, identify the radialmost portion of the forearm and insert the needle perpendicular to the skin to a depth of 1 to 1.5 cm. A rise in pressure is identified by external pressure or passive flexion of the wrist.

MEASURING HAND COMPARTMENT PRESSURE

- Insert the needle perpendicular to the skin.
- Evaluate the compartments individually. Pressure measurements are not obtained from the digits, but at the site of maximal swelling of the thenar, hypothenar, and interosseous compartments.
- If a single compartment pressure is elevated, release all compartments and the carpal tunnel.
- To measure the dorsal interosseous compartment pressure, insert the needle through the dorsal hand 1 cm proximal to the metacarpal head until it rests in the muscle belly. To judge the depth, it is helpful to place identifiable marks on the needle at depths of 1.0, 1.5, and 2.0 cm.
- To measure the adductor pollicis compartment pressure, insert the needle on the radial side of the second metacarpal in the substance of the thumb-index web space.
- To measure the thenar and hypothenar spaces, insert the needle at the junction of the glabrous and nonglabrous skin over the maximal bulk of the muscle compartment. Advance the needle at least 5 mm below the enveloping fascia for pressure assessment.

MANAGEMENT

ACUTE COMPARTMENT SYNDROME OF THE FOREARM

Impending tissue ischemia may be considered when the tissue pressure reaches between 30 and 20 mm Hg below the diastolic blood pressure. A higher pressure is a strong indication that fasciotomy should be recommended. In a hypotensive patient, the acceptable pressure is lower. Fasciotomy should be performed in (1) normotensive patients with positive clinical findings and compartment pressures of greater than 30 mm Hg, and when the duration of the increased pressure is unknown or thought to be longer than 8 hours; (2) uncooperative or unconscious patients with compartment pressures of greater than 30 mm Hg; (3) patients with low blood pressure and compartment pressures of greater than 20 mm Hg; and (4) patients with a delta P value of less than 30 mm Hg. As a general rule, when in doubt, the compartment should be released. If it proves later to have been unnecessary, only a scar will result. However, if a fasciotomy should have been

done but was not, loss of muscle and nerve tissue carries a high risk for a poor functional outcome. In one study, a delay in diagnosis was the most important determining factor for poor outcome. Compartment pressure should be monitored in young patients with injury to the forearm diaphysis or distal radius, or in patients with significant soft-tissue injury and a bleeding diathesis. Normal function was regained in 68% of patients in one study when fasciotomy was performed within 12 hours of the onset of compartment syndrome. When performing a volar fasciotomy, a volar curvilinear incision is used; this allows release of the lacertus fibrosus proximally and the carpal tunnel distally. The interval between the flexor carpi ulnaris and the flexor digitorum sublimis is used for release of deep and superficial compartments. The dorsal forearm fascia is released through the interval between the extensor carpi radialis brevis and the extensor digitorum communis. The mobile wad of Henry can be released through this same incision.

FOREARM FASCIOTOMY AND ARTERIAL EXPLORATION

TECHNIQUE 11.2

- For the volar fasciotomy (Fig. 11.5B), make an anterior curvilinear skin incision medial to the biceps tendon, crossing the elbow flexion crease at an angle. Carry the incision distally and radially over the brachioradialis, then distally and ulnarward, eventually coursing medial to the palmaris longus. Cross the wrist flexion crease at an angle and continue in the midline of the palm to allow for a carpal tunnel release. Curving the incision at the wrist ulnarly will decrease the risk of injury to the palmar cutaneous branch of the median nerve. The underlying subcutaneous tissues should be spread longitudinally, protecting the lateral and medial antebrachial cutaneous nerves and the palmar cutaneous branch of the median nerve.

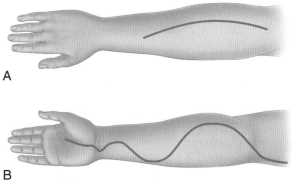

FIGURE 11.5 Incisions used in forearm for severe Volkmann contracture. **A,** Extensive opening of fascia of the forearm dorsum in dorsal compartment syndromes. **B,** Incision used for anterior forearm compartment syndromes in which skin and underlying fascia are released completely throughout. **SEE TECHNIQUES 11.2, 11.5, AND 11.6.**

- Divide the lacertus fibrosus proximally and evacuate any hematoma.
- In patients with suspected brachial artery injury, expose the brachial artery and determine if there is free blood flow. If the flow is unsatisfactory, remove the adventitia to expose any underlying clot, spasm, or intimal tear. Resect the adventitia, if necessary, and anastomose or graft the artery.
- Release the superficial volar compartment throughout its length with open scissors, freeing the fascia over the superficial compartment muscles.
- Identify the flexor carpi ulnaris and retract it with its underlying ulnar neurovascular bundle medially, and then retract the flexor digitorum superficialis and median nerve laterally to expose the flexor digitorum profundus in its deep compartment. Check to see if the overlying fascia or epimysium is tight and incise it longitudinally.
- If the muscle is gray or dusky, the prognosis for recovery may be poor; however, the muscle may still be viable and should be allowed to perfuse.
- Continue the dissection distally by incising the transverse carpal ligament along the ulnar border of the palmaris longus tendon and median nerve.
- In cases of median nerve palsy or paresthesia, observe the median nerve along the entire zone of injury to ensure that it is not severed, contused, or entrapped between the ulnar and humeral heads of the pronator teres. If it is, a partial pronator tenotomy is necessary.
- In a patient with a supracondylar fracture, reduce the fracture, pin it with Kirschner wires, and control the bleeding.
- Do not close the skin at this time; anticipate secondary closure later.
- If the median nerve is exposed within the distal forearm, suture the distal, radial-based forearm flap loosely over the nerve.
- Check the dorsal compartments clinically or repeat the pressure measurements. Usually, the volar fasciotomy decompresses the dorsal musculature sufficiently, but if involvement of the dorsal compartments is still suspected, release them also.
- Make the incision distal to the lateral epicondyle between the extensor digitorum communis and extensor carpi radialis brevis, extending approximately 10 cm distally. Gently undermine the subcutaneous tissue and release the fascia overlying the mobile wad of Henry and the extensor retinaculum.
- Apply a sterile moist dressing and a long-arm splint. The elbow should not be allowed to flex beyond 90 degrees.

POSTOPERATIVE CARE The arm is elevated for 24-48 hours after surgery. If closure is not possible within 5 days, a split-thickness skin graft should be applied. Alternatively, closure of fasciotomy wounds can be accomplished gradually, using vessel loops that are progressively tightened postoperatively during dressing changes. Wound closure using this method usually can be accomplished in 2 weeks (Fig. 11.6). A vacuum-assisted wound closure system may be used to assist in wound management. The splint is worn until the sutures are removed, or as determined by fracture care requirements.

HAND FASCIOTOMIES

TECHNIQUE 11.3

- Make two dorsal parallel incisions through the skin overlying the second and fourth metacarpals, beginning at the level of the metacarpophalangeal joints and extending just distal to the wrist (Fig. 11.7A). Make each incision down to the musculofascial area.
- Incise the fascia and release the compression of the distended muscles by allowing them to extrude into the wound if necessary. Through the two dorsal incisions, all four dorsal interosseous compartments, all three palmar interosseous compartments, and the adductor compartment can be released.
- Identify each muscle individually to ensure that a complete release is achieved. Passively flex the metacarpophalangeal joints and extend the proximal interphalangeal joints to stretch the muscles, ensuring that all are adequately released.
- Release the thenar and hypothenar compartments by making additional palmar radial and palmar ulnar incisions along the glabrous and nonglabrous intervals to allow for their separate decompression.
- Release the carpal tunnel through a palmar midline incision.
- Do not attempt to debride the interosseous muscles at this point. If the fingers are tensely swollen and capillary refill is delayed, continue with digital fasciotomies through midlateral incisions along the radial border of the ring and small fingers and the ulnar border of the index and long fingers (Fig. 11.7B).
- In general, it is prudent to release all compartments, including the carpal tunnel if any of the hand compartments are involved.
- Do not attempt to close the wounds at this time. They may be permitted to granulate and heal, or after the swelling has decreased, they can be closed secondarily. A vacuum-assisted wound closure system may be used to assist in wound management.

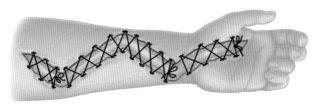

FIGURE 11.6   Vessel loop shoelace technique for fasciotomy closure. **SEE TECHNIQUE 11.2.**

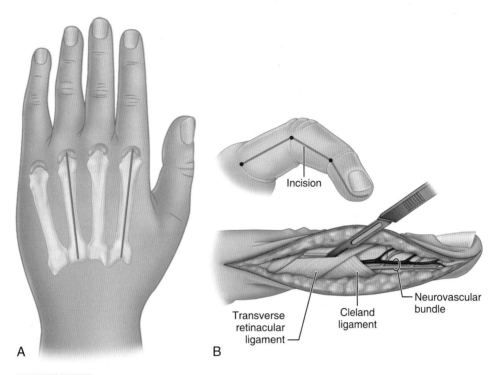

FIGURE 11.7 **A,** Longitudinal incisions over second and third metacarpals. **B,** Midaxial incision of finger. **SEE TECHNIQUE 11.3**.

CHRONIC EXERTIONAL COMPARTMENT SYNDROME OF THE FOREARM

Because CECS of the forearm is rare, statements regarding diagnosis and management are inherently provisional. Most experience with the condition involves competitive motocross riders who develop symptoms described as "arm pump," which includes severe pain, tightness, weakness, and difficulty controlling bike handles. Cessation of activity typically leads to symptom resolution within 20 to 30 minutes. The diagnosis is made primarily by history and confirmed with compartment pressure measurements after the activity. Pedowitz et al. proposed diagnostic pressure measurements for CECS as a resting compartment pressure of greater than 15 mm Hg, a compartment pressure of 30 mm Hg or greater 1 minute after exercise, or greater than 20 mm Hg at 5 minutes after exercise. A recent study has proposed a T_{Rest} (or time to return from peak measurement to the patient's own baseline compartment pressure) of 14.5 minutes as another potential screening tool. Management of CECS initially consists of rest and adjustments to the racing technique and bike setup. If nonoperative treatment fails after a trial of at least 3 months, fasciotomy has been shown to allow a return to the sport in most patients. Fasciotomy may be performed through multiple techniques, including open, mini-open, and endoscopic. It seems that all techniques produce adequate results, allowing surgeon preference to guide the choice of technique. Mini-open and endoscopic techniques may allow quicker recovery and improved cosmesis, but open methods improve exposure and allow formal nerve decompression if needed. The deep flexor compartment is not released in the endoscopic approaches.

MINI-OPEN FOREARM FASCIOTOMY

TECHNIQUE 11.4

(HARRISON ET AL.)
- With the patient supine and the arm abducted on an arm table, exsanguinate the limb and apply a tourniquet.

EXTENSOR COMPARTMENT RELEASE
- Mark a line between the lateral epicondyle and Lister's tubercle and measure it at the junction of the middle and distal thirds.
- Make a skin incision from 5 cm distal to the epicondyle to 5 cm proximal of the two thirds mark (Fig. 11.8A); the incision usually is about 8 cm long.
- Perform a fasciotomy along the septum between the mobile wad and the extensor digitorum communis to release both extensor compartments.
- Once all structures have been identified, extend the fascial incisions proximally and distally to fully release from the epicondyle to the musculotendinous junction.

FLEXOR COMPARTMENT RELEASE
- Draw a line between the medial epicondyle to the junction of the palmaris longus at the distal wrist crease and mark it at two thirds of its length for extensor compartment release.

- Make a skin incision from 5 cm distal to the epicondyle to 5 cm short of the two thirds mark (Fig. 11.8B).
- Split the fascia in line with the incision to release the superficial flexor compartment.
- Develop the interval between the flexor digitorum superficialis and flexor carpi ulnaris down to the deep fascia.
- Identify the ulnar nerve and release the deep fascia over the flexor digitorum profundus, taking care to protect the nerve and its branches.
- Extend the fascial releases proximally from the epicondyle and distally to the musculotendinous junction.

ESTABLISHED VOLKMANN CONTRACTURE OF THE FOREARM

If compartment syndrome is untreated or inadequately treated, compartment pressures continue to increase until irreversible tissue ischemia occurs. Volkmann ischemic contracture is the result of several different degrees of tissue injury; however, the earliest changes usually involve the flexor digitorum profundus muscles in the middle third of the forearm (Fig. 11.9). The typical clinical picture of established Volkmann contracture includes elbow flexion, forearm pronation, wrist flexion, thumb adduction, metacarpophalangeal joint extension, and finger flexion.

A mild contracture, also termed *localized Volkmann contracture*, results from partial ischemia of the profundus mass, with flexion contractures usually involving only two or three fingers. Sensory changes usually are mild or absent. Intrinsic muscle contractures and joint contractures are absent. During the early stages of a mild contracture, dynamic splinting to prevent wrist contracture, functional training, and active use of the muscles may be helpful. After

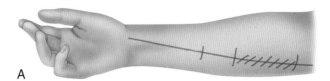

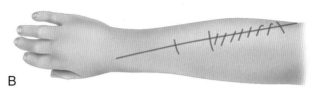

FIGURE 11.8 Incision for mini-open release of extensor compartment **(A)** and flexor compartment **(B).** (Redrawn from Harrison JWK, Thomas P, Aster A, et al: Chronic exertional compartment syndrome of the forearm in elite rowers: a technique for mini-open fasciotomy and a report of six cases, Hand 8:450, 2013.) **SEE TECHNIQUE 11.4**.

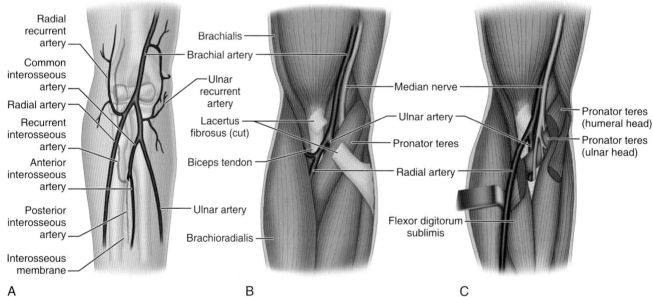

FIGURE 11.9 Anatomy of Volkmann ischemia. **A,** "Collateral circulation" of elbow does not communicate with vessels within flexor compartment. These elbow collaterals join radial and ulnar arteries proximal to pronator teres, the proximal guardian of flexor compartment. **B,** Brachial artery and median nerve enter forearm through tight opening formed by biceps tendon insertion laterally and pronator teres muscle medially and are tightly covered by lacertus fibrosus. Proximal angulation, hematoma, or muscle swelling within this cruciate tendon-muscle portal is capable of major compression of neurovascular bundle. **C,** Radial artery, arising from brachial artery, passes distally superficial to pronator teres and all flexor muscles. It is not crossed by any structure along this route. Ulnar artery passes beneath pronator teres and lies in deepest portions of compartment. Median nerve usually passes between humeral and ulnar heads of fleshy pronator teres, and, emerging, it becomes compressed against firm arcuate band of flexor sublimis origin (see text).

3 months, the involved muscle-tendon units can be released and lengthened. When multiple tendon units are involved, however, a muscle sliding operation is preferable to lengthening of multiple tendons, wrist resection, or other possible procedures. If involved, the pronator teres may require excision.

A moderate contracture usually involves not only the long finger flexors, but also the flexor pollicis longus and possibly the wrist flexors. Median and ulnar nerve sensory changes and intrinsic minus deformities are present. In this instance, the muscle sliding operation, careful neurolysis of the median and ulnar nerves without injuring their branches, and the excision of any fibrotic muscle mass encountered can be done. When no useful movement of the finger flexors has been retained, volar transfers of dorsal wrist extensors, such as the brachioradialis and extensor carpi radialis longus, and a complete release of the wrist and finger flexors may be required.

A severe contracture involves the flexors and extensors of the forearm. Fractures of the forearm bones and scars on the skin also may be present. Sensory feedback is usually impaired because the nerves are strangulated by the contracted and scarred muscles surrounding them. The preferred treatment in these instances is early excision of all necrotic muscles, combined with complete median and ulnar neurolysis to restore sensibility and possibly intrinsic function. Although one author recommended this be done no sooner than 3 months but no later than 1 year after the ischemic event, others have recommended surgical intervention within 3 weeks to prevent additional contractures from developing. Tendon transfers to restore function should be performed as a secondary procedure. These may include transfer of the brachioradialis to the flexor pollicis longus and the extensor carpi radialis longus to the flexor digitorum profundus tendons. If motors to restore finger flexion are unavailable, a free innervated muscle transfer using the gracilis muscle may be considered. In one long-term study (32 years), substantial improvement was noted with excision of fibrotic muscle, neurolysis, and tendon or free gracilis transfers; however, tendon lengthening alone was rarely satisfactory. For severe Volkmann ischemic contracture, Oishi and Ezaki recommended a two-stage procedure with initial muscle debridement and neurolysis, followed by a free-functioning gracilis transfer after return of sensation and intrinsic function to the hand. Satisfactory results have also been reported using a free medial gastrocnemius myocutaneous flap for reconstruction in patients with established Volkmann contracture.

■ MUSCLE SLIDING OPERATION OF FLEXORS FOR ESTABLISHED VOLKMANN CONTRACTURE

The muscle sliding operation was first described by Page in 1923 and was endorsed by Scaglietti in 1957. It has been used for Volkmann and other contractures caused by conditions such as brain damage and burns. In cases of Volkmann contracture, usually the muscle is fibrotic and noncontractile, and a muscle sliding operation alone is rarely indicated.

EXCISION OF NECROTIC MUSCLES COMBINED WITH NEUROLYSIS OF MEDIAN AND ULNAR NERVES FOR SEVERE CONTRACTURE

This is a salvage procedure that may result in only modest improvement. If the contracture is diffuse but incomplete throughout all digital and wrist flexors, the muscle sliding technique may be considered (see chapter 9).

TECHNIQUE 11.5

- Make an extensive volar forearm incision (Fig. 11.5) and excise all avascular masses of the flexor profundus and sublimis muscles, leaving any muscle that might survive or appears viable.
- Perform a neurolysis of the median and ulnar nerves. The median nerve usually is affected and may have an hourglass deformity in the midforearm. Neuroma excision and secondary nerve grafting may be necessary.
- Correct finger and wrist flexion deformities by dividing the involved flexor tendons at the musculotendinous junctions and excising the fibrotic muscle. At this time, at least the functional position of the hand will have been restored.
- At a second-stage procedure, any viable extensor muscles can be transferred to the finger flexors. At least one wrist extensor must be retained, however. Otherwise, any wrist flexor or extensor muscle can be transferred to power the profundus and flexor pollicis longus tendons. Most commonly, the brachioradialis is transferred to the flexor pollicis longus and the extensor carpi radialis longus to the flexor digitorum profundus of all four fingers.

TWO-STAGED FREE GRACILIS TRANSFER

TECHNIQUE 11.6

(OISHI AND EZAKI)

FIRST STAGE

- Widely expose the volar forearm compartment from the elbow to the wrist (see Fig. 11.5B) and elevate the skin flaps.
- Identify and mobilize the ulnar nerve at the elbow. After isolating and protecting the median nerve and brachial artery at the antecubital fossa, dissect the median and ulnar nerves and vascular structures all the way from the elbow to the wrist to free adherences to fibrotic necrotic muscle.
- Debride all the involved muscle, including the deep layers. Sometimes the only structures remaining after debridement are the median and ulnar nerves, the vascular structures, and the tendon ends.

- Perform any necessary nerve grafting or vascular reconstruction at this point.
- Keep the proximal ends of the flexor tendon as long as possible (it is helpful to suture the proximal ends of the flexor digitorum profundus and the flexor pollicis longus together for later identification). In young or small children, suture these ends to an area proximal to the carpal tunnel to prevent retraction into the carpal tunnel.
- Close the skin and immobilize the arm in a cast for 3 weeks to allow the wound to heal. After removal of the cast, begin passive range-of-motion exercises to the fingers and wrist. The patient is observed over the ensuing 6 months for muscle and sensory recovery.

SECOND STAGE

For the second-stage procedure, a two-person team approach is used; one is responsible for exposing the forearm, including the neurovascular structures and tendinous ends, and the other for harvesting the gracilis muscle.

- Identify the brachial artery in the forearm and follow it distally to determine its suitability or that of any of its branches. Also identify a vein for anastomosis because the venae comitantes or subcutaneous veins may not be suitable.
- Identify the anterior interosseous branch, and in the distal forearm, identify and prepare the ends of the flexor digitorum profundus and flexor pollicis longus tendons.
- In the lower extremity, expose the gracilis muscle with or without an accompanying skin paddle. If a skin paddle is necessary, use only the proximal two thirds of overlying skin because the blood supply to the distal third of skin overlying the muscle is unreliable.
- Tag the anterior surface of the gracilis muscle with sutures at 2-cm intervals to correctly identify the resting tension of the muscle.
- Identify the neurovascular bundle and dissect it. Careful dissection is mandatory because the anterior branch of the obturator nerve runs superiorly from the muscle.
- When the forearm recipient site has been prepared, release the origin and divide the neurovascular bundle.
- If a vein graft is deemed necessary, microvascular anastomosis of the vein graft to the gracilis artery can be done on a back table using an operating microscope.
- Suture the proximal gracilis to the medial epicondyle using nonabsorbable suture. Note the location of the ulnar nerve before carrying out this step. Also, take care to position the muscle so as not to cause undue tension on the upcoming microvascular work.
- Using an operating microscope, perform anastomoses of the artery, vein(s), and nerve. Examine the anterior interosseous nerve under the operating microscope and cut it back until good fascicles are seen. The closer the nerve coaptation is to the muscle, the shorter the distance necessary for reinnervation.
- Place an implantable Doppler probe around the artery for postoperative monitoring. After assessment of adequate flow, suture the flexor digitorum profundus ends to each other and to the gracilis muscle at its resting tension (marked earlier).
- Suture the flexor pollicis longus tendon to a separate portion of the gracilis muscle with the wrist in 10-20 degrees of extension and slight overcorrection of the normal finger cascade.
- Flex the wrist to ensure that the tenodesis allows the fingers to extend appropriately.
- Close the skin flaps and immobilize and elevate the upper extremity. Failure to elevate the extremity could jeopardize flap viability.

POSTOPERATIVE CARE The patient is placed in a warm room and started on one low-dose (81 mg) aspirin per day. The dressing is changed, and the Doppler device is removed at 6-7 days with the patient under anesthesia. The upper extremity is immobilized for 4 weeks, and then range-of-motion exercises are begun. Protective splinting is used for the first few months. Muscle function may take up to 6 months to return.

ESTABLISHED INTRINSIC MUSCLE CONTRACTURES OF THE HAND

Proper surgical release of established intrinsic muscle contractures depends on the severity of the contractures. When the contractures are mild (Fig. 11.10), the metacarpophalangeal joints can be passively extended completely, but while they are held extended, the proximal interphalangeal joints cannot be flexed (positive intrinsic tightness test); in these instances, the distal intrinsic release of Littler may be indicated (Fig. 11.11).

In contractures that are more severe, the interosseous muscles are viable but contracted, and the intrinsic tightness test is positive. Active spreading of the fingers may be possible. In these instances, the contracted muscles may be released from the metacarpal shafts by a muscle sliding operation (Fig. 11.12A).

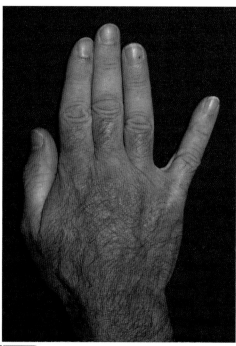

FIGURE 11.10 Abduction contracture of fifth finger in patient who developed fibrosis in abductor digiti quinti, probably secondary to ischemic myositis from compressive bandage.

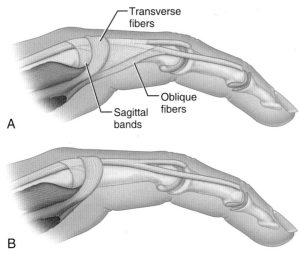

FIGURE 11.11 Littler release of intrinsic contracture. **A,** Extensor aponeurosis at level of metacarpophalangeal joint consists of long extensor tendon, transverse fibers (which flex the metacarpophalangeal joint), and oblique fibers (which extend the interphalangeal joint). Crosshatched part is resected from each side of hood. **B,** Appearance of aponeurosis after release. **SEE TECHNIQUE 11.7.**

In the most severe contractures, the intrinsic muscles not only may be contracted, but also necrotic and fibrosed, so any useful muscle excursion is absent. In these instances, the tendon of each muscle must be divided to release the contractures (Fig. 11.12B). Other procedures, such as capsulotomies and tendon transfers, also may be necessary.

RELEASE OF ESTABLISHED INTRINSIC MUSCLE CONTRACTURES OF THE HAND

TECHNIQUE 11.7

(LITTLER)
- The same procedure is done on any finger as needed.
- Make a single midline incision on the dorsum of the proximal phalanx, extending from the metacarpophalangeal joint to the proximal interphalangeal joint to allow good exposure of both sides of the extensor aponeurosis. Incise the insertion of the oblique fibers of the extensor aponeurosis into the extensor tendon; make the incision parallel with the tendon (Fig. 11.11A).
- Preserve the transverse fibers to avoid hyperextension of the metacarpophalangeal joint with its resultant clawhand deformity and limitation of extension of the interphalangeal joints.
- After adequate excision of the oblique fibers, the proximal interphalangeal joint should have full passive flexion with the metacarpophalangeal joints in neutral (Fig. 11.11B).
- Close the incision.
- Apply a volar plaster splint from the elbow to the middle of the proximal phalanges, immobilizing the metacarpophalangeal joints in extension and permitting full motion of the interphalangeal joints.

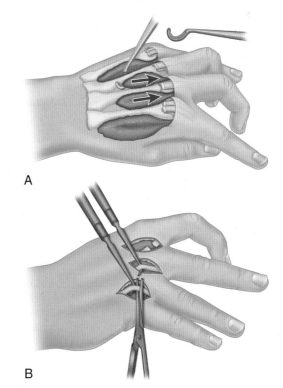

FIGURE 11.12 **A,** Method of stripping and advancing interosseous muscles to slacken them, allowing proximal finger joints to extend and distal two to flex. Interosseous muscles of two clefts have been stripped. Stripping of interossei is done only when muscles still retain considerable function. Nerve supply should be spared. **B,** Complete intrinsic tenotomy for severe intrinsic contractures in which nonfunctioning interosseous muscle remains.

POSTOPERATIVE CARE Active motion of the interphalangeal joints is begun the day after surgery, and the splint and sutures are removed at 10-14 days.

RELEASE OF SEVERE INTRINSIC CONTRACTURES WITH MUSCLE FIBROSIS

TECHNIQUE 11.8

(SMITH)
- Make a dorsal transverse incision just proximal to the metacarpophalangeal joints.
- Resect the lateral tendons of all the interossei and the abductor digiti quinti at the level of the metacarpophalangeal joints. If these joints remain flexed, retract the sagittal bands distally, and divide each accessory collateral ligament at its insertion into the volar plate.
- Free the volar plate from its attachments to the base of the proximal phalanx, and with a blunt probe, separate any adhesions between the volar plate and the metacarpal head.

- If maintaining extension of the proximal phalanx is difficult after soft-tissue release, insert a Kirschner wire obliquely through the metacarpophalangeal joint with the joint in maximal extension. When the phalanx is extended, ensure that its base articulates properly with the metacarpal head before inserting the wire.
- If passive flexion of the proximal interphalangeal joints is incomplete with the metacarpophalangeal joints extended, resect the lateral bands at the distal half of the proximal phalanges through separate dorsal incisions.

POSTOPERATIVE CARE Passive and active flexion exercises of the proximal interphalangeal joints are begun within 1 day of surgery. The Kirschner wires are removed at about 3 weeks.

ADDUCTED THUMB

Only complete loss of the thumb causes more disability in the hand than a fixed severe adduction of the thumb (web contracture). The thumb is the only digit with the ability to bring its terminal sensory pad over the entire surface of any chosen finger or over the distal palmar eminence. The saddlelike first carpometacarpal joint provides the circumductive movement of the thumb necessary for pinch or grasp functions. The intrinsic muscles of the thumb and the extrinsic flexors and extensors all are important in the balanced control required to perform these functions effectively. The short abductor muscle positions and stabilizes the thumb metacarpal for pinch; the adductor muscle supplies the power for pinch by acting on the proximal phalanx; the long extrinsic flexor muscle positions the distal phalanx in varying degrees of flexion and consequently controls the type of pinch, whether it be fingernail-to-fingernail opposition or pulp-to-pulp opposition with another digit. The thumb web must be supple if these important movements of the thumb are to be possible. Any contracture of the thumb web causes limited opposition of varying degrees. In severe contracture, the thumb is in a position of adduction and external rotation.

The thumb web consists of skin, subcutaneous tissue, muscle, fascia, and joint capsule. Contracture of any one of these tissues can cause a secondary contracture of the others; rarely is there contracture of only one. Causes of some injuries include scarring of the skin, burns, infection, crush injuries, congenital webbing, paralysis, Dupuytren contracture, and faulty immobilization.

The proper treatment of a contracted web is determined by which structures of the web are involved; little is accomplished by releasing the skin alone when deeper structures, such as muscle, fascia, or joint capsule, also are contracted. When the skin alone is contracted from a hypertrophic scar after a surgical incision or a laceration along the border of the web, it sometimes can be released by a Z-plasty or a local flap. The four-flap Z-plasty is a commonly utilized technique to expand the first web space when the predominant causative factor involves the skin. It is described in chapter 1.

Crushing injuries, infections, or deep burns result in extensive fibrosis within the thumb web that cannot be treated by release of the skin alone; rather, the scarred components of the contracted skin, muscle, fascia, and capsule must be excised with care to avoid damaging the radial artery near the carpometacarpal joint. This excision produces a deep fissure that must be filled with skin and subcutaneous fat to provide an elastic functioning web. This may be accomplished by dorsal rotation or a sliding flap with supplemental skin grafting (Figs. 11.13 and 11.14).

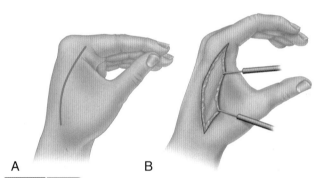

A   B

FIGURE 11.13 One method of releasing dorsal skin of adducted thumb (see text) (Brand and Milford). **A,** Skin incision. **B,** Skin grafting covers defect after release has been accomplished by undermining dissection.

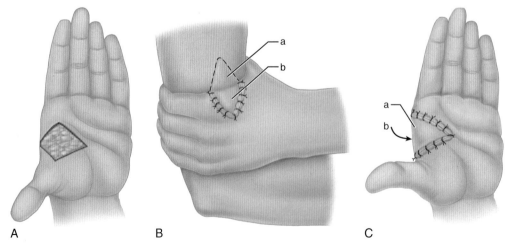

A   B   C

FIGURE 11.14 Cross-arm flap coverage of deepened thumb web. **A,** Web space deepening after skin division and muscle recession. **B,** Position of hand with triangular distal flap *(b)* sutured into dorsal thumb web defect. Outline of proximal triangular flap *(a)* that will be used for palmar web coverage. **C,** Web space reconstruction after transfer of palmar flap at second-stage operation 3 weeks later.

If the adjacent tissue is unsuitable for transfer, several other options are available to treat moderate-to-severe first web space contractures. Rotational axial pattern flaps include reverse posterior interosseous artery flap, reverse radial forearm flap, or a groin flap (described in chapter 2). A free lateral arm flap may also be used. The cross-arm flap has been described as well. It is fashioned as a double triangle, one on the dorsal surface and one on the volar surface of the web, to eliminate any line of scar paralleling the border of the web. The first and second metacarpals are fixed in the desired position with Kirschner wires. When motion in the carpometacarpal joint can be restored, any necessary tendon transfers for apposition can be done later, but if motion cannot be restored the carpometacarpal joint must be arthrodesed to maintain the new position of the thumb permanently.

Paralysis of the muscles of apposition can result in secondary contracture of the skin and joint capsule, and in contracture of the thumb web, requiring release by a Z-plasty or using a local flap and a skin graft as described by Brand and Milford (see Fig. 11.13). Contracted fascia and bands of muscle must be released, and capsulotomy of the carpometacarpal joint must be done at the same time.

Occasionally, a useless index finger may provide a filleted pedicle with which a satisfactory thumb web can be constructed in one stage. This procedure not only widens the web, in that the index metacarpal is excised, but also provides skin that can be repositioned over a nearby defect or scar (see discussion of filleted graft in chapter 2).

REFERENCES

COMPARTMENT SYNDROME AND VOLKMANN CONTRACTURE

Auld TS, Hwang JS, Stekas N, et al.: The correlation between the OTA/AO classification system and compartment syndrome in both bone forearm fractures, *J Orthop Trauma* 31(11):606, 2017.

Barrera-Ochoa, Correa-Vazquez E, Gallardo-Calero I, et al.: TR$_{est}$ as a new diagnostic variable for chronic exertional compartment syndrome of the forearm: a prospective cohort analysis of 124 athletes, *Clin J Sport Med* 28(6):516, 2018.

Barrera-Ochoa S, Haddad S, Correa-Vázquez E, et al.: Surgical decompression of exertional compartment syndrome of the forearm in professional motorcycling racers: comparative long-term results of wide-open versus mini-open fasciotomy, *Clin J Sport Med* 26(2):108, 2016.

Benamran L, Masquelet AC: A cadaver study into the number of fasciotomies required to decompress the anterior compartment in forearm compartment syndrome, *Surg Radiol Anat* 40(3):281, 2018.

Beniwal RK, Bansal A: Osteofascial compartment pressure measurement in closed limb injuries – Whitesides' technique revisited, *J Clin Orthop Trauma* 7(4):225, 2016.

Blackman AJ, Wall LB, Keeler KA, et al.: Acute compartment syndrome after intramedullary nailing of isolated radius and ulna fractures in children, *J Pediatr Orthop* 34:50, 2014.

Capo JT, Renard RL, Moulton MJ, et al.: How is forearm compliance affected by various circumferential dressings? *Clin Orthop Relat Res* 472:3228, 2014.

Davies J, Fallon V, Kyaw Tun J: Ultrasound-guided percutaneous compartment release: a novel technique, proof of concept, and clinical relevance, *Skeletal Radiol* 48(6):959, 2019.

Diesselhorst MM, Deck JW, Davey JP: Compartment syndrome of the upper arm after closed reduction and percutaneous pinning of a supracondylar humerus fracture, *J Pediatr Orthop* 34:e1, 2014.

Doro CJ, Sitzman TJ, O'Toole RV: Can intramuscular glucose levels diagnose compartment syndrome? *J Trauma Acute Care Surg* 76:474, 2014.

Garcia-Mata S: Chronic exertional compartment syndrome of the forearm in adolescents, *J Pediatr Orthop* 33:832, 2013.

Gondolini G, Shiavi P, Pogliacomi F, et al.: Long-term outcome of mini-open surgical decompression for chronic exertional compartment syndrome of the forearm in professional motorcycling riders, *Clin J Sport Med* 2017, [Epub ahead of print].

Gottlieb M, Adams S, Landas T: Current approach to the evaluation and management of acute compartment syndrome in pediatric patients, *Pediatr Emerg Care* 35(6):432, 2019.

Griffart A, Gautheir E, Vaiss L, et al.: Functional and socioprofessional outcome of surgery for Volkmann's contracture, *Orthop Traumatol Surg Res* 105(3):423, 2019.

Harrison JW, Thomas P, Aster A, et al.: Chronic exertional compartment syndrome of the forearm in elite rowers: a technique for mini-open fasciotomy and a report of six cases, *Hand (N Y)* 8:450, 2013.

Hashimoto K, Kuniyoshi K, Suzuki T, et al.: Biomecanical study of the digital flexor tendon sliding lengthening technique, *J Hand Surg Am* 40(10):1981, 2015.

Hosseinzadeh P, Hayes CB: Compartment syndrome in children, *Orthop Clin North Am* 47(3):579, 2016.

Hosseinzadeh P, Talwalkar VR: Compartment syndrome in children: diagnosis and management, *Am J Orthop (Belle Mead NJ)* 45(1):19, 2016.

Humpherys J, Lum Z, Cohen J: Diagnosis and treatment of chronic exertional compartment syndrome of the forearm in motorcross riders, *JBJS Rev* 6(1):e3, 2018.

Kalyani BS, Fisher BE, Roberts CS, Giannoudis PV: Compartment syndrome of the forearm: a systematic review, *J Hand Surg [Am]* 36A:535, 2011.

Kenny EM, Egro FM, Russavage JM, et al.: Primary closure of wide fasciotomy and surgical wounds using rubber band-assisted external tissue expansion: a simple, safe, and cost-effective technique, *Ann Plast Surg* 81(3):344, 2018.

Kistler JM, Ilyas AM, Thoder JJ: Forearm compartment syndrome: evaluation and management, *Hand Clin* 34(1):53, 2018.

Lipschitz AH, Lifchez SD: Measurement of compartment pressures in the hand and forearm, *J Hand Surg [Am]* 35A:1893, 2010.

Liu B, Barrazueta G, Ruchelsman DE: Chronic exertional compartment syndrome in athletes, *J Hand Surg Am* 42(11):917, 2017.

Meena DK, Thalanki S, Patni P, et al.: Results of neurolysis in established upper limb Volkmann's ischemic contracture, *Indian J Orthop* 50(6):602, 2016.

Mehta SK, Dale WW, Dedwylder MD, et al.: Rates of neurovascular injury, compartment syndrome, and early infection in operatively treated civilian ballistic forearm fractures, *Injury* 49(12):2244, 2018.

Miller EA, Cobb AL, Cobb TK: Endoscopic fascia release for forearm chronic exertional compartment syndrome: case report and surgical technique, *Hand (NY)* 12(5):NP58, 2017.

Neri I, Magnano M, Pini A, et al.: Congenital Volkmann syndrome and aplasia cutis of the forearm: a challenging differential diagnosis, *JAMA Dermatol* 150:978, 2014.

O'heireamhoin S, Baker JF, Neligan M: Chronic exertional compartment syndrome of the forearm in an elite rower, *Case Rep Orthop* 2011:497854, 2011.

Oishi SN, Ezaki M: Free gracilis transfer to restore finger flexion in Volkmann ischemic contracture, *Tech Hand Up Extrem Surg* 14:104, 2010.

Pegoli L, Pozzi A, Pivato G: Endoscopic single approach forearm fasciotomy for chronic exertional compartment syndrome: long term follow-up, *J Hand Surg Asian Pac* 21(1):8, 2016.

Pozzi A, Pivato G, Kask K, et al.: Single portal endoscopic treatment for chronic exertional compartment syndrome of the forearm, *Tech Hand Up Extrem Surg* 18(3):153, 2014.

Raveendran S, Rajendra Benny K, Monica S, et al.: Multiple stab incisions and evacuation technique for contrast extravasation of the hand and forearm, *J Hand Surg Amd* 44: (1), 71.e1, 2019.

Reichman EF: Compartment syndrome of the hand: a little thought about diagnosis, *Case Rep Emerg Med* 2016: 2907067, 2016.

Robertson AK, snow E, Browne TS, et al.: Who gets compartment syndrome?: a retrospective analysis of the national and local incidence of compartment syndrome in patients with supracondylar humerus fracture, *J Pediatr Orthop* 38(5):e252, 2018.

Turkula SC, Fuller DA: Extensile fasciotomy for compartment syndrome of the forearm and hand, *J Orthop Trauma* 31(Suppl 3):S50, 2017.

Winkes MB, EJT L, van Zoest WJF, et al.: Long-term results of surgical decompression of chronic exertional compartment syndrome of the forearm in motocross racers, *Am J Sports Med* 40:452, 2012.

Zuchelli D, Divaris N, McCormack JE, et al.: Extremity compartment syndrome following blunt trauma: a level I trauma center's 5-year experience, *J Surg Res* 217:131, 2017.

The complete list of references is available online at Expert Consult.com.

DUPUYTREN CONTRACTURE

James H. Calandruccio

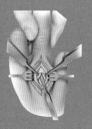

Dupuytren disease is a proliferation of previously normal subcutaneous palmar and digital tissues that may manifest as nodules and cords that may compromise hand function by the resultant finger and thumb joint flexion contractures. Other secondary changes include thinning of the overlying subcutaneous fat and subsequent adhesion to and later pitting or dimpling of the skin. The lesion activity and the ensuing deformity rate vary considerably. Occasionally, a finger may become markedly flexed within a few weeks or months, but development of severe deformity usually requires several years.

Ectopic Dupuytren disease deposits may occur in a variety of areas (Fig. 12.1). Approximately 5% of patients with Dupuytren contractures have similar lesions in the medial plantar fascia of one or both feet (Ledderhose disease), 3% of patients have plastic penile induration (Peyronie disease), and "knuckle pads" (Garrod nodules) may present over the proximal interphalangeal (PIP) joints dorsally. Patients with these associated findings are considered to have a Dupuytren diathesis and are prone to a more progressive and recurrent form of this disease.

Commonly occurring in adults in their 40s to 60s, Dupuytren contracture occurs 6 to 10 times more frequently in men than in women. According to McFarlane, the disease occurs significantly earlier in men (33 to 63 years old) than in women (46 to 70 years old). It is most common in white northern European individuals, although it has been reported occasionally in blacks and rarely in Asians. The lesion has been reported to be more frequent and severe in individuals with diabetes mellitus or with epilepsy (42%), and conflicting reports exist concerning the disease in individuals with alcoholism. The involvement, although often bilateral (45%), rarely is symmetric (Fig. 12.2). Mikkelsen et al. found that mortality may be increased in men who develop the disease before age 60.

Although the causes of this disease are unknown, hand trauma and the type of manual labor performed by an individual may be contributing factors. The presence of hemosiderin in these lesions suggests hemorrhage from tears; however, the nondominant hand is affected as often as the dominant one, making trauma alone an unlikely cause. Occasionally a single injury may precipitate the onset of the disease in genetically susceptible individuals. Likewise, surgical trauma, even release of a trigger finger in susceptible patients, may precipitate significant pretendinous cords, palmar thickening, and subsequent troublesome contractures. Accordingly, minor palmar surgical procedures should be approached with

caution when pretendinous cords are present. Similarly, excision of an isolated Dupuytren nodule, especially in younger patients, is rarely warranted as it is more likely than not a more significant lesion will ensue.

According to McFarlane, a causal relationship may be assumed if consistent histologic changes occur within 2 years after a focal injury in women younger than 50 years of age and men younger than 40 without a strong diathesis for Dupuytren disease. In patients with bilateral disease, the disease usually develops in the uninjured hand after age 40 years in men and 50 years in women.

Evidence also points to heredity as a predisposing factor in Dupuytren disease. The lesion seems to occur earlier and more frequently in some families, with a variable penetrance autosomal dominant pattern. Vascular insufficiency and cigarette smoking have been linked to Dupuytren disease as possible causative factors.

The lesion usually begins on the ulnar side of the hand at the distal palmar crease and progresses to involve the ring and little fingers, these being affected more frequently than all other digits combined. Metacarpophalangeal (MP) and PIP joint flexion contractures gradually develop; their severity depends on the extent and maturity of the fibroplasia. The lesions are more commonly painless, although some patients may complain of itching or minor discomfort. However, these nodules have been shown histologically to have neural entrapment, the reason some individuals present with pain primarily.

PATHOGENESIS

The cause of Dupuytren disease is unknown; however, the cellular and connective tissue changes that occur with this disorder have some similarity to malignant tumors despite being a benign process. Dupuytren contracture begins with increased fibroblast proliferation followed by type III collagen deposition resulting in uncontrolled palmar fascia growth ultimately causing flexion contractures. Dupuytren disease has been compared with wound healing in that myofibroblasts, which produce type III collagen, are dominant in both granulation tissue and Dupuytren tissue. In addition, growth factors and their receptors have been shown to have increased expression in diseased fascia, especially transforming growth factor-β and basic fibroblast growth factor. Transforming growth factor-β has been shown to induce differentiation of fibroblasts into myofibroblasts. An increase in glycosaminoglycans, matrix metalloproteinase activity, the presence of fibrofatty tissue between

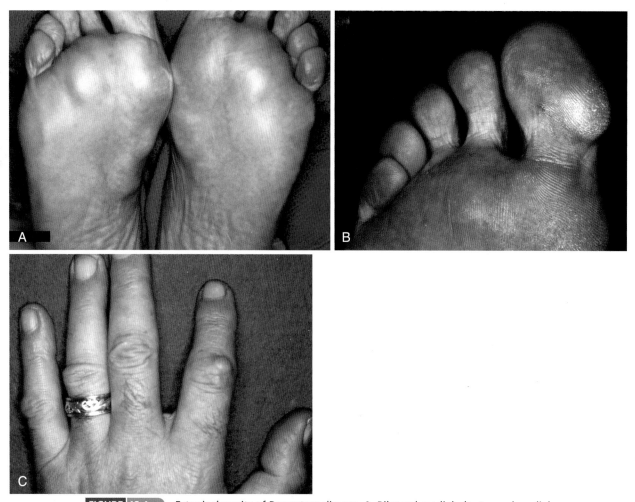

FIGURE 12.1 Ectopic deposits of Dupuytren disease. **A,** Bilateral medial plantar and medial great toe involvement. **B,** Right foot involvement (Ledderhose disease). **C,** Dorsal proximal interphalangeal joint nodules (Garrod nodules).

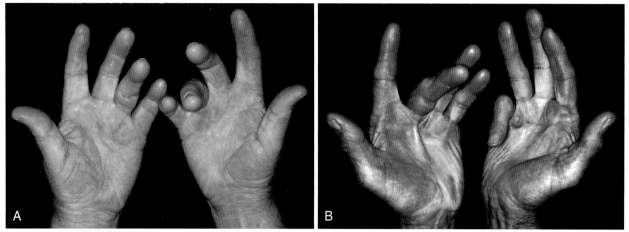

FIGURE 12.2 Asymmetric hand involvement. **A,** Mild bilateral ulnar hand disease. **B,** More diffuse bilateral disease with severe contracture of interphalangeal joint of right small finger.

the skin and fascia, trauma, and microtrauma caused by free radicals also have been theorized as playing a role in the development of Dupuytren contracture.

Dupuytren disease progresses through several stages: proliferative, involutional, and residual. In the proliferative stage, nodules, composed of type III collagen and fibroblasts, develop and expand to displace the subcutaneous tissue and fuse to the skin. The nodules typically appear at the distal palmar crease over the MP joints and distally over the PIP joints but not over the distal interphalangeal joints. They eventually stop growing

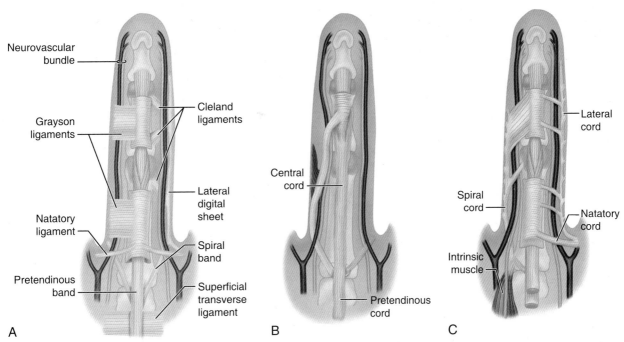

FIGURE 12.3 **A,** Normal palmar and digital fascia. **B,** Diseased fascia in continuity with the pretendinous cord. **C,** Other common fascial disease patterns.

and begin to contract in the involutional stage. Stress alignment of the fibroblasts occurs, and more collagen is produced. Myofibroblasts then replace the fibroblasts as the predominant cell type, producing type III collagen and causing contraction. Nodule expansion places tension on the normal fascia proximally, producing fascial hypertrophy and nodule-cord units. In the residual phase, the nodules decrease in size and may become acellular fibrous cords. Contractures of the MP and PIP joints and displacement of digital neurovascular bundles result from predictable patterns of fascial cord involvement.

The fascial structures that may become involved in the fibroproliferative process have been clearly outlined by McFarlane (Fig. 12.3). Thomine described a longitudinally oriented fascia located dorsal to the neurovascular bundle, which he termed the *retrovascular cord*. This structure often is involved in the disease and may be implicated as a cause for recurrent PIP contractures. The Cleland ligament generally is believed to be spared. The pretendinous cord nearly always is responsible for primary contracture of the MP joint. It may attach to the distal palmar crease skin, base of the proximal phalanx, or the tendon sheath at this level, or it may extend to attach to the flexor tendon sheath over the middle phalanx or the skin in this area. A spiral cord occurs when four normally existing structures (pretendinous band, spiral band, lateral digital sheet, and Grayson ligament) become diseased. The spiral cord runs dorsal to the neurovascular bundle proximally and volar to it distally. When the spiral cord is contracted, the neurovascular bundle is drawn superficially and toward the midline of the finger (Fig. 12.4). Neurovascular displacement is found most commonly on the ulnar aspect of the little and ring fingers, and tedious dissection is required to prevent digital nerve injury.

The lateral digital cord may extend distally and contribute to a flexion contracture of the distal interphalangeal joint. The plane between this cord and the overlying skin is minimal and must be developed sharply. The retrovascular cord is not believed to contribute significantly to flexion contracture of

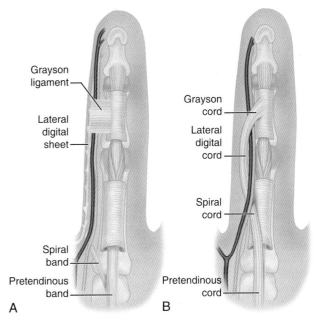

FIGURE 12.4 **A,** Normal parts of fascia that produce spiral cord: pretendinous band, spiral band, lateral digital sheet, and Grayson ligament. **B,** Spiral cord showing medial displacement of neurovascular bundle. (Diseased spiral band is not synonymous with spiral cord.)

the PIP joint; however, it may be responsible for some residual flexion contracture or recurrence if not excised.

MP and distal interphalangeal (DIP) joint contractures seem to result from pretendinous and lateral cord development. PIP joint contractures may develop from isolated digital cords in addition to central, spiral, or retrovascular cords (Figs. 12.5 and 12.6). The diseased tissue in this unusual form of Dupuytren contracture most commonly affects the small

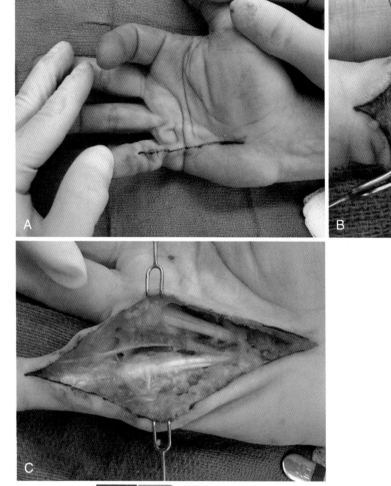

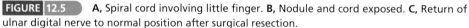

FIGURE 12.5   **A,** Spiral cord involving little finger. **B,** Nodule and cord exposed. **C,** Return of ulnar digital nerve to normal position after surgical resection.

finger; however, any digit may be involved. The cord originates from the periosteum of the proximal phalanx and fascia overlying the intrinsic muscles and distally courses dorsal to the neurovascular bundles, inserting into the middle phalanx or the overlying flexor tendon sheath volar to the neurovascular bundles. This digital cord frequently displaces the neurovascular bundle superficially and to the midline of the finger, similar to a spiral cord.

Skoog suggested that, of the palmar fascia components, only the longitudinal pretendinous bands are involved and that the superficial transverse palmar ligaments are always spared. We agree with McFarlane that the superficial transverse ligaments, in addition to natatory cord prominence, may be involved and require excision especially in symptomatic thumb web space contractures.

PROGNOSIS

The prognosis in Dupuytren contracture seems to depend on the following factors, which may determine the appropriate intervention:

1. *Heredity.* A family history of the disease indicates that the lesion is likely to progress more rapidly than usual, especially if the onset is early.

2. *Sex.* The lesion usually begins later and progresses more slowly in women, who often accommodate better to the resulting deformity; however, long-term results after operation are worse in women than in men, with postoperative flare reaction being twice as likely.

3. *Epilepsy.* Despite earlier statements positively associating Dupuytren contracture with epilepsy, Geoghegan et al. concluded that neither epilepsy nor antiepileptic medications were associated with the disease.

4. *Diabetes mellitus.* Diabetes mellitus is a risk factor for Dupuytren disease, especially in patients requiring medical management compared with patients with diet-controlled diabetes mellitus. According to Geoghegan et al., patients taking insulin were more likely to have Dupuytren disease than patients taking metformin or sulfonylureas.

5. *Alcoholism or smoking.* The lesions are more severe, progress more rapidly, and recur more frequently when associated with these conditions. Godtfredsen et al. found a dose-dependent relationship to alcohol intake and smoking and concluded that the combination of these two factors conveys a high risk for the development of Dupuytren disease.

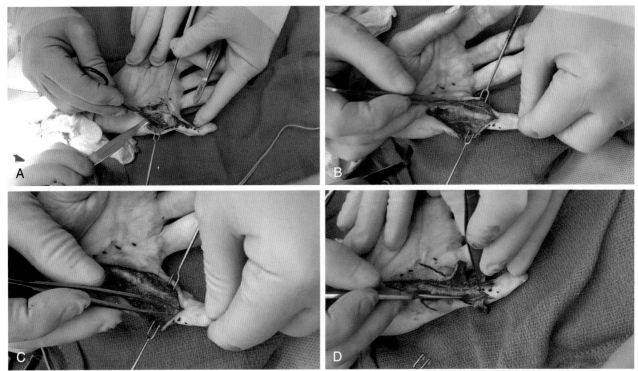

FIGURE 12.6 Retrovascular cord. **A** and **B,** 50-year-old right-handed woman with diabetes mellitus and previous isolated Dupuytren nodule excision from small finger with resultant proximal interphalangeal and distal interphalangeal joint contractures. **C,** Retrovascular cord responsible for DIP contracture. **D,** Clearer view of the retrovascular cord before excision with Z-plasty flap incision.

6. *Location and extent of disease.* When the disease is bilateral and especially when it is associated with knuckle pads and nodules in the plantar fascia, progression is more rapid and recurrence is more frequent. Progression is more rapid on the ulnar side of the hand.

7. *Behavior of disease.* How the disease has behaved in the past, whether treated or not, is an indication of its probable behavior in the future.

Patients need to know that Dupuytren disease is not a curable disorder and that interventions are designed to manage functional deficits resulting from the nodules and cords. Contracture management usually focuses on isolated deformities; however, recurrence in the areas treated is common and more widespread disease may follow (disease extension) and be a cause for patient concern. Hence, counseling patients regarding disease recurrence and extension is important prior to engaging various treatment regimens (Fig. 12.7).

NONOPERATIVE TREATMENT

Various nonoperative treatment regimens for Dupuytren disease continue to focus on the fundamental disease histopathology (Box 12.1).

EXTERNAL BEAM RADIATION

Management of early stage Dupuytren disease by external beam radiation has been reported to regress the disease in up to 45% and stop progression in up to 80% of patients. Low-dose radiation (less than 30 Gy) using various protocols have been published, and no protocol has reported any malignant transformation in up to 13 years after treatment. Chronic side effects reported to persist more than 4 weeks after treatment were dryness of the skin (20%), skin atrophy (3%), lack of sweating (4%), telangiectasia (3%), desquamation (2%), and sensory alteration (2%). We have no experience with this treatment method.

Nodule-derived fibroblast contractile properties were shown by Bisson et al. to be greater than those of cord-derived fibroblasts, and both of these fibroblast lines had significantly greater force generation than carpal tunnel ligament fibroblasts. Ketchum and Donahue found that after an average of 3.2 injections per nodule of triamcinolone acetonide, 97% of 75 hands had softening or flattening of the nodules. Although complete resolution of the disease was rare, only half of the patients had nodule reactivation within 3 years after the injections.

COLLAGENASE INJECTIONS

Clinical trials evaluating clostridial collagenase histolyticum (CCH) injections as a nonoperative treatment have indicated prompt and impressive MP and PIP joint contracture release. Badalamente et al. reported on the safety and efficacy of this enzymatic degradation in studies, including a randomized placebo-controlled study in which Hurst et al. reported contracture reduction to 0 to 5 degrees in 77% of MP joint and 40% of PIP joint contractures in 204 joints receiving collagenase injections. Despite these results being significantly better

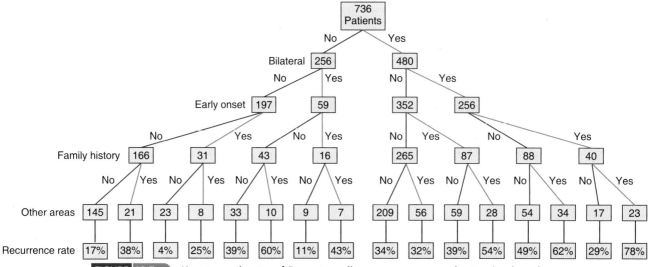

FIGURE 12.7 Hueston estimates of Dupuytren disease recurrence and extension based on bilateral disease presence, age of onset, family history, and ectopic deposits. (From McFarlane RM: Some observations on the etiology of Dupuytren's disease. In Hueston JT, Tubiana R, editors: *Dupuytren's Disease*, London, 1985, Churchill Livingstone, p 123.)

BOX 12.1

Treatment of Dupuytren Disease

Nonoperative
- External beam radiation
- Steroid injection
- Collagenase

Operative
- Subcutaneous fasciotomy
  - Scalpel
  - Needle
- Partial (selective) fasciectomy
- Complete fasciectomy
- Fasciectomy with skin grafting
- Staged external fixation
- Arthrodesis
- Amputation

---

than in the 104 joint placebo group, the 30-day outcome did not allow the authors to comment in regard to recurrence. In a previous 2-month follow-up study, similar results were achieved compared with placebo and only 5 of 62 joints had recurrence. Transient side effects included localized swelling, pain, bruising, pruritus, regional lymph node enlargement, and tenderness; however, permanent adverse serious side effects were rare, aside from two flexor tendon ruptures in the prior study. Our experience with collagenase injections has been limited but favorable. Best results are obtained in patients with a well-defined palpable cord that is located away from the flexor tendon. Collagenase injection may be contraindicated in patients who are on anticoagulation or who have lymphedema, lymph node surgery, or implants.

Publications involving CCH safety, tolerability, and efficacy continue to document the reliability of management of MP contractures and the difficulty with PIP joint contractures. Peimer et al. collected data on 463 patients (78% males with an average age of 65 years) and found that 1.08 CCH injections were used per treated joint, compared with a mean of 1.7 injections in registration trials. Ninety-three percent of joints received only one injection, and 67% of first injections resulted in full correction compared with the clinical trial rate of 39%. Atroshi et al., however, reported skin tears in 66 hands (40%) of 164 treated with collagenase injections; only 14 were larger than 1 cm, and all healed without complications. Although original labeling of CCH included a restriction that only one affected joint be treated at a time, Gaston et al., in a study of 714 patients (724 joint pairs), reported that CCH injections can be used to effectively treat two affected joints concurrently without increasing the risk of adverse events. The US Food and Drug Administration (FDA) recently approved the use of CCH to treat two affected joints concurrently and to perform finger manipulations 1 to 3 days after the injections.

COLLAGENASE INJECTIONS

TECHNIQUE 12.1

(HENTZ)
- Use a 1-mL syringe and a 0.5-in, 27-gauge needle. Local anesthesia is not recommended at the time of injection because of distortion of the soft-tissue anatomy and the potential for deactivation of the drug.
- Use the nondominant hand to apply gentle extension to the finger undergoing injection, displacing the cord superficially from the underlying flexor tendon mechanism.
- Insert the needle perpendicularly through the skin into the underlying cord. The tissue should be firm and resist easy passage of the needle.
- Use passive manipulation of the proximal or distal interphalangeal joint to ensure that the needle has not been improperly positioned within the underlying flexor tendon.

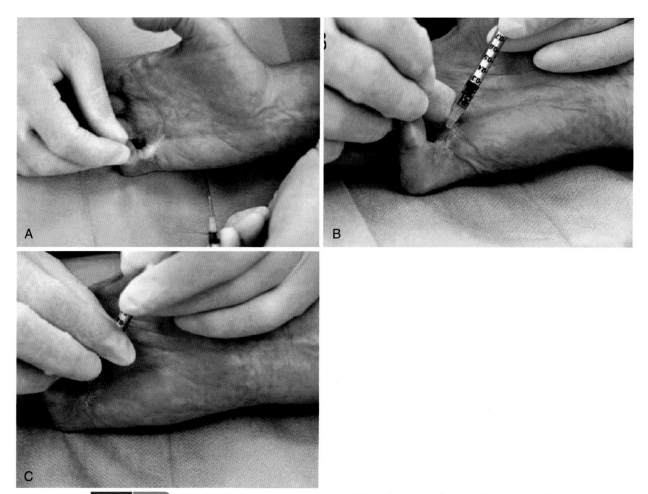

FIGURE 12.8 Two-handed clostridial collagenase histolyticum injection technique. **A,** Cord is delineated by palpation. **B,** Needle is inserted into cord while tension is applied to cord. **C,** Both hands are used to support syringe while the plunger is pressed. (From Hentz VR, Watt AJ, Desai SS: Advances in the management of Dupuytren's disease: collagenase, *Hand Clin* 28:552, 2012.) **SEE TECHNIQUE 12.1.**

- Inject one third of the volume. Resistance to fluid flow indicates that the needle is within the cord.
- Withdraw the needle slightly, incline it distally, and reinsert it into the cord approximately 3 mm from the site of the first insertion. Confirm proper positioning, and inject one third of the dose.
- Reposition the needle 2 to 3 mm proximal to the initial injection site and administer the final one third of the dose (Figs. 12.8 and 12.9).

POSTOPERATIVE CARE The hand is wrapped in a soft dressing, and the patient is instructed to avoid hand-intensive activity for the next few hours. They can resume a normal schedule that evening but should be cautioned that this is not always possible.

MANIPULATION

Although current FDA guidelines stipulate that finger manipulation is done the day following injection, studies have shown that a delay in manipulation for up to 7 days does not increase adverse events or result in loss of efficacy.

Finger extension without local anesthesia can be extremely painful; a midpalm (proximal to the area of swelling and ecchymosis), intermetacarpal, or wrist block can be used for anesthesia. Care should be taken during rupture of the cord because skin splitting can occur. Most skin tears are of the palmar skin with a contracture of more than 45 degrees, heavily calloused skin, or marked ecchymosis at the injection site. Tearing can be minimized by not pulling vigorously in the area of blood blisters and following a four-step protocol described by Meals and Hentz:

1. Flex the PIP joint while extending the MP joint.
2. Flex the MP joint while extending the PIP joint.
3. Extend both joints together.
4. While keeping the finger extended under moderate tension, continue to extend the MP and PIP joints and disrupt any residual intact cord fibers.

If necessary, these four steps can be repeated at 5- to 10-minute intervals while observing carefully for skin tears; however, no more than three attempts are recommended. If a skin tear begins, manipulation should be stopped and the patient instructed to begin gentle progressive passive extension. After manipulation, the patient is fitted with a splint and instructed to use it at bedtime for up to 4 months to maintain finger extension. The patient also is instructed to perform finger

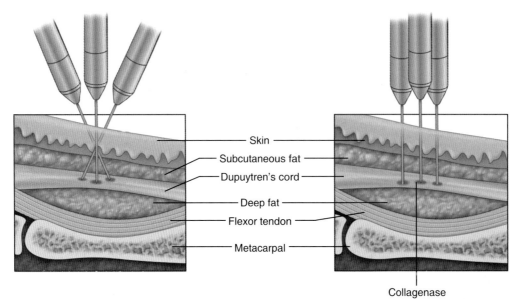

Skin
Subcutaneous fat
Dupuytren's cord
Deep fat
Flexor tendon
Metacarpal
Collagenase

FIGURE 12.9   Two injection techniques; goal is to inject total volume into cord over a distance of 5 to 6 mm. (Redrawn from Hentz VR, Watt AJ, Desai SS: Advances in the management of Dupuytren's disease: collagenase, *Hand Clin* 28:552, 2012.) **SEE TECHNIQUE 12.1.**

extension and flexion exercises several times a day for several months.

Coleman et al. and Verheyden reported success with CCH injections of multiple cords at the same time. Coleman et al. treated 60 patients with 2 concurrent injections; 88% were satisfied with their results, and 92% reported being very much or much improved. Adverse events (pruritus, lymphadenopathy, blood blister, skin laceration) were more frequent than after single injections. Verheyden treated 144 patients with the entire bottle of enzyme, approximately 0.78 mg compared with 0.58 mg in other reports, using a novel slow intracord multicord technique. He found that the technique safely allowed injection of multiple Dupuytren contracture cords at one setting. Correction at the MP and PIP joints, taken individually, was comparable with the collagenase option for the reduction of Dupuytren contractures (43 degrees and 33 degrees, respectively). With multicord injections, Verheyden achieved 94 degrees average immediate and 76 degrees average final combined MP and PIP joint contracture releases per bottle of enzyme. This may result in significant health care savings when CCH is the chosen treatment. However, the cost-benefit ratio has been questioned in a level 1 study by Strömberg et al. comparing CCH and percutaneous needle aponeurotomy (PNA). After evaluation of 156 randomized patients evaluated by a blinded observer over 2 years, they concluded that PNA achieved results equivalent to or slightly better than CCH (79% vs. 76% straight fingers), with CCH being nearly three times more expensive. A smaller prospective study by Skov et al. reached similar conclusions, with better clinical results with PNA and higher complication rates with CCH.

PERCUTANEOUS NEEDLE APONEUROTOMY

PNA has had a resurgence of interest since first being described by Lermusiaux and Debeyre in 1980. A 25-gauge needle mounted on a 10-mL syringe is used to divide the contractile cords after infiltration with 1.0 mL or less of 1% lidocaine with 1:100,000 epinephrine. Multiple contractile cord areas can be sectioned in the palm and fingers with special care to avoid sensory nerves. No splint or physiotherapy is used. PNA has been reported to give satisfactory short-term results in a group of 74 releases at 33-month follow-up, with an 88% MP joint and 46% PIP joint contracture reduction. However, in this group the recurrence rate was 65%, where recurrence was defined as loss of 30 degrees or more from the immediate postoperative correction. Although sensory disturbance was noted in only two fingers, digital nerve stretch injury and needle trauma remain concerns. This may be an office procedure and repeated as necessary to gain extension. It appears to be effective for those who are elderly, patients who desire minimally invasive procedures, and those knowing additional releases may be required in the near future. Several studies have shown PNA to be a cost-effective alternative to fasciectomy, as noted by Strömberg et al., Skov et al., and Leafblade et al., who reported results equivalent or superior to CCH at much lower medical expense.

Hovius et al. described combining PNA with lipofilling (injection of a lipoaspirate containing adipose-derived stem cells) to restore the subdermal fat deficiency present in Dupuytren disease. Adipose-derived stem cells also have been shown in laboratory studies to inhibit the contractile myofibroblast in Dupuytren disease. In their technique, multiple nicks are made with a 19-gauge needle from proximal to distal in the palpable cord, and a hooked needle is used to release the skin from the underlying tissue; when the cord is fully released, the lipoaspirate is diffusely injected through 2 or 3 needle entry sites in the palm and digit. Suggested advantages of this technique include the ability to treat multiple digits, shorter recovery time, restoration of deficient subcutaneous fat, and supple skin without scars. In a series of 91 patients (99 hands), 94% returned to normal use of the hand within 2 to 4 weeks, and 95% were very satisfied with their results.

OPERATIVE TREATMENT

Operative treatment is technically easier when joint contractures are less severe; however, minor contractures are encountered more often early in the disease progression.

Where ill-defined planes between normal and abnormal tissue are encountered, the cellular process is more active, and recurrence is more likely. Ideally, patients are operated on when their diseased tissues are more mature and the tendency for surgical trauma to accelerate the disease process is less. Nonetheless, PIP joint and MP joint contractures of 15 degrees and 30 degrees or more, respectively, may be disabling and warrant surgical intervention. Stiffening and increase in flexion contractures may occur when surgical intervention occurs in the proliferative stage. Indications for and timing of surgery should also take into account the disability of the joint contracture, presence of degenerative joint disease, and other predisposing factors for poor outcomes, rather than merely the degree of contracture.

Operative procedures commonly used in treating Dupuytren contracture are (1) subcutaneous fasciotomy, (2) partial (selective) fasciectomy, (3) complete fasciectomy, (4) fasciectomy with skin grafting, (5) staged resection preceded by external fixation, (6) joint resection and arthrodesis, and (7) amputation. The appropriate procedure depends on the degree of contracture; nutritional status of the palmar skin; the presence or absence of bony deformities; and the patient's age, occupation, and general health. Generally, more severe involvement requires more extensive surgery, done in stages if necessary, and preceded perhaps by a subcutaneous fasciotomy and joint extension therapy.

The least extensive procedure, subcutaneous fasciotomy, is commonly used for elderly patients who are not concerned with the appearance of the disease or in patients who have poor general health. The results of this procedure are better in the residual phase when dense, mature cords are present than when the lesions are more immature and diffuse. However, many require repeat surgery. In subcutaneous tenotomy, the pretendinous cords are simply divided in an attempt to correct MP joint contractures; however, some PIP joint contractures may be lessened immediately from dynamic MP joint contractures and others eventually from cord and nodule regression. We have found percutaneous fasciotomy to be an effective treatment for Dupuytren contracture, and we investigated the effectiveness of an office-based percutaneous fasciotomy both objectively and subjectively. Thirty-two patients (36 digits) were followed to determine active and passive MP joint correction and patient-perceived effects after percutaneous release. Patient-reported outcome measures (QuickDASH, Work Module Score [WMS], Sports Module Score [SMS]) were collected preoperatively and postoperatively at 6 weeks, 3 months, and 1 year. At 1 year, the rate of recurrence was 33%. The average MP joint correction was active extension of 39.6 to 9.3 degrees and passive 25.4 to 3.6 degrees of hyperextension. The improvement in patient-reported outcomes (WMS and SMS) was correlated at 6 weeks and 1 year with active extension improvement. On average, the wound closed within 7 days, with pain resolution by 2 days. No patient sustained a sensory deficit. Patients had a statistically significant contracture reduction after release, sustained at 1 year in most. The increase in extension deficit correlated with improvement in patient-reported outcomes at 1 year; 82% of patients were satisfied with the procedure, and 87% thought the procedure was worth having done.

Partial (selective) fasciectomy is the procedure most commonly performed, results in the greatest reduction in extension deficit, has the best long-term results of any

procedure to date, and is indicated when contractures compromise hand function. Although the ulnar digits are most commonly involved, all fingers and the thumb may require surgical management at the same setting. This operation is used more frequently because postoperative morbidity is less and complications are fewer than after complete fasciectomy. Although the rate of recurrence after partial fasciectomy is 50%, the need for another surgical procedure is only 15%. In this operation, only the mature deforming tissue is excised and, although all the visible diseased tissue typically is removed, biochemically or microscopically involved fascia may not be clinically apparent and not excised during an operation. Various incisions can be used to expose the pathologic tissue (Fig. 12.10). When the PIP contracture is not significant, a zigzag or Bruner incision may be sufficient (Fig. 12.10B) or a variant of it because adequate exposure and removal of the pathologic tissue usually is possible. The incision chosen should be fashioned to fit the needs of the individual patient. When tightness of the palmar skin limits extension of a finger or when there is a significant PIP joint contracture, a straight midline incision converted to appropriate Z-plasties is indicated (Fig. 12.10A). Multiple transverse incisions can be used when the diseased tissue can be safely dissected free from the neurovascular bundles; however, following and excising diseased cords through discontinuous incisions is more difficult. Patients suitable for this surgical exposure usually have well-defined disease and minor PIP joint contractures. Successful disease removal from this exposure may result in a faster recovery and acceptable cosmetic results. Regardless of the incision, dissection is made easier by loupe magnification, and great care must be taken to avoid damage to neurovascular structures.

Sometimes after fasciectomy, extension of the PIP joint is incomplete, which may result from incomplete excision of less obvious diseased tissue, skin tightness, joint capsular contractures, flexor tendon pathology, or joint incongruity. Projections of isolated cords passing volar to the rotation axis of the PIP joint are common causes of residual joint flexion deformity. These problematic cords often insert onto the flexor tendon sheath laterally or the middle phalanx. Dissection of faintly detectable deforming cords intimately associated with the skin and skin Z-plasty may be required for sufficient correction of PIP joint contracture. Significant residual PIP joint flexion contractures may require volar joint capsulotomies. PIP joint flexion contractures of more than 60 degrees are in general correctable to about 50% of the existing contracture, regardless of a concomitant PIP joint capsulotomy, according to Weinzweig et al. These authors found an average 16-degree loss of preoperative flexion in the capsulotomy group compared with an 8-degree loss in the noncapsulotomy group.

More severe PIP joint contractures may benefit from a staged procedure in which an external fixator is used to gradually correct the flexion contracture before the definitive surgical excision. Success with this method has been reported by Agee and Goss and White et al. White et al. treated 38 fingers in 27 patients with PIP joint contractures of more than 70 degrees with a staged technique. The first stage involved applying a mini-external fixator across the PIP joint for continuous extension over 6 weeks (Fig. 12.11). The tension of the elastic band across the minifixator was increased twice weekly, allowing full active flexion of the PIP joint against the elastic

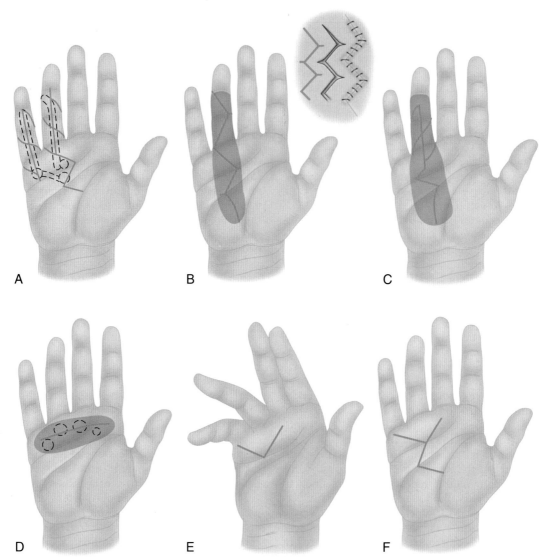

FIGURE 12.10 **A,** Multiple Z-plasties can be used to provide exposure and convert longitudinal skin contractures to zigzag closures. Only one extension typically needs to be made into palm because wide palmar exposure usually allows excision of adjacent diseased tissue. **B,** When joint or skin contracture is not a major problem, zigzag pattern can be used for exposure, with extended corners as shown to make use of redundant skin. **C,** Extent of possible undermining of skin is shown in *shaded area.* **D,** When only the palm is involved, transverse incisions can be used. **E** and **F,** V-Y plasty method of Mukerjea.

band. The second stage involved an open palm fasciectomy for the contracted cords restricting MCP joint movement and dermofasciectomy with full-thickness skin grafting over the proximal phalanx for bands restricting PIP joint movement. The external fixator was used to maintain active extension force until the graft healed; it generally was removed in the outpatient clinic under ring block 2 weeks after the second-stage procedure. At a mean follow-up of 20.6 (6 to 48) months, the mean preoperative PIP joint of 75 degrees had improved to 37 degrees. Despite complications including pin site infection, pin loosening, and complex regional pain syndrome, the authors concluded that the staged procedure is a valid alternative in the management of severe Dupuytren PIP joint contracture.

Skoog described a partial or selective fasciectomy in which only the pretendinous fibers of the palmar fascia are excised. According to Skoog, there is a definite plane between the pretendinous longitudinal fibers of the palmar fascia and the transverse palmar ligament that is limited to the midpalmar area. The pretendinous fibers may seem to be attached to the ligament. He suggested that the interdigital or natatory ligaments do become involved in Dupuytren contracture and prevent the fingers from spreading normally and are distinguishable from the transverse palmar ligament by their more distal location. Adduction and MP joint flexion contractures can be addressed through a transverse palmar incision and wounds left to heal by secondary intention.

Complete fasciectomy rarely, if ever, is indicated because it frequently is associated with complications of hematoma, joint stiffness, and delayed healing, and it does not completely prevent recurrence of the disease.

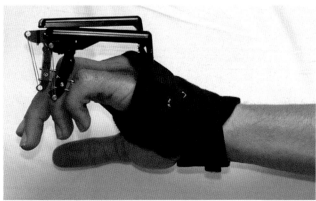

FIGURE 12.11 Mini-external fixator applied on patient with proximal interphalangeal joint contractures from Dupuytren disease. (From Agee JM, Goss BC: The use of skeletal tension torque in reversing Dupuytren contractures of the proximal interphalangeal joint, *J Hand Surg* 37A:1467, 2012.)

Fasciectomy with skin grafting may be indicated for young people in whom the prognosis is poor because of such factors as epilepsy, alcoholism, the presence of the disease elsewhere in the body, and recurrence of the lesion after excision. The skin and underlying abnormal fascia are excised, and a full-thickness or split-thickness skin graft is applied. Recurrence has not been reported in areas of the palm treated in this manner.

Amputation, although rarely necessary, may be indicated if flexion contracture of the PIP joint, especially of the little finger, is severe and cannot be corrected enough to make the finger useful. A 40-degree flexion contracture usually is tolerated fairly well. The skin from the involved finger can be used to cover a palmar skin defect; the finger is filleted, and the skin is folded into the palm as a pedicle with its neurovascular bundles.

Another alternative for a severely contracted PIP joint is joint resection and arthrodesis. This procedure results in a shortened finger but avoids the potential for recurrent PIP joint contracture and a potential amputation neuroma.

The scope of procedures for recurrent Dupuytren disease is essentially the same as for the initial intervention, which includes subcutaneous fasciotomy (scalpel, needle, or enzymatic release), fasciectomy (limited, selective, or complete), nodule fasciectomy and skin grafting, arthrodesis, or amputation. The procedure chosen for reoperation may not necessarily be similar to that chosen for the first procedure. Disease extension in regions remote from that previously excised may need to be treated and require a much more extensive approach, multiple incisions, and possibly a combination of procedures.

Regardless of the treatment method, the most significant injury following cord management is digital nerve injury. Surface landmarks provide a good reference to the underlying proper digital nerves to the ulnar side of the small finger and radial side of the index finger. Great care should be taken in isolation of the pertinent digital nerves associated with a particular cord. In general, cord excision should be preceded by nerve protection, and nerve dissection and isolation should proceed from areas where the nerve is easily identified and free of disease (Fig. 12.12).

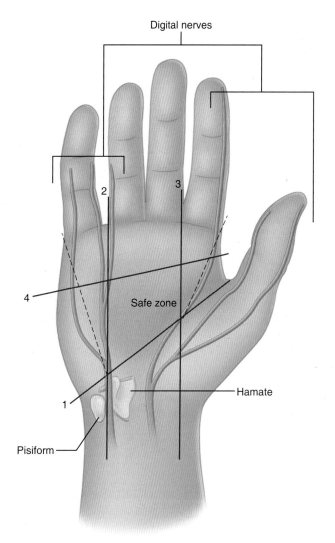

FIGURE 12.12 Correlation of digital nerves to skin surface creases. Small finger ulnar digital nerve courses obliquely across hand under line drawn from small finger ulnar palmar crease (4) to intersection point of Kaplan cardinal line (1) and one parallel to the ulnar border of ring finger (2). Similarly, index radial digital nerve courses obliquely across hand under line drawn from index finger radial palmar digital crease (4) to intersection point of Kaplan cardinal line (1) and one parallel to radial border of middle finger (3). (Redrawn from Calandruccio JH, Hecox SE: Reoperative Dupuytren's contracture. In Duncan SFM, editor: *Reoperative hand surgery*, New York, 2012, Springer Science+Business Media LLC.)

SUBCUTANEOUS FASCIOTOMY

TECHNIQUE 12.2

(LUCK)

- Using a pointed scalpel, make skin puncture wounds on the ulnar side of the diseased palmar fascia at the following levels: (1) just distal to the apex of the palmar fascia between the thenar and hypothenar eminences, (2) at or near the level of the proximal palmar crease, and (3) at the level of the distal palmar crease. Digital nerves are more likely to be injured at the distal palm where they may become more superficial and may be intertwined with the diseased tissue.

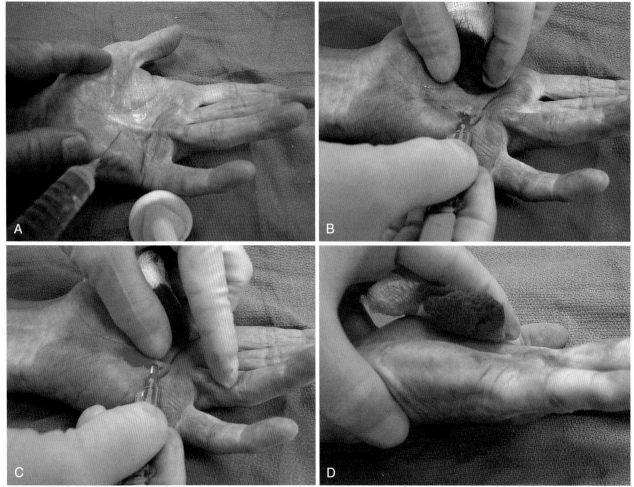

FIGURE 12.13 Subcutaneous Dupuytren cordotomy. **A,** Well-defined pretendinous cord in ring finger with a 60-degree MP joint contracture. **B,** No. 15 scalpel blade inserted between skin and pretendinous cord. **C,** Forceful extension effectively delivers more superficially abnormal cord onto scalpel blade held at 90 degrees to tight cord. **D,** Resultant MP joint extension achieved. **SEE TECHNIQUE 12.2.**

- Insert a small tenotomy knife or a fasciotome (Luck) that resembles a myringotome, with its blade parallel with the palm, through each of the puncture wounds. A 15- or 11-blade works satisfactorily for this purpose. Pass the cutting instrument across the palm beneath the skin but superficial to the fascia (Figs. 12.13 and 12.14).
- Turn the edge of the blade dorsally toward the palmar fascia and extend the fingers to tighten the involved tissue. Carefully divide the fascial cords by pressing the blade onto the tense cords with gentle pressure over the blade or at most a gentle rocking motion; never use a sawing motion. Whenever a cord is divided, the sense of the gritty, firm resistance disappears, indicating that the blade has passed completely through the diseased fascial cord.
- Keep the blade in a plane parallel with the skin and free the skin from the underlying fascia. The corrugated skin, although very thin at times, can be safely undermined and released as necessary with little fear of skin necrosis.
- In the fingers, subcutaneous fasciotomy is safe only for a fascial cord located in the midline. Insert the blade through a puncture wound adjacent to the cord and divide it obliquely.

- For a laterally placed cord, use a short longitudinal incision, and excise or divide the diseased segment under direct vision. Also enucleate larger nodules in both fingers and palm under direct vision.

POSTOPERATIVE CARE A pressure dressing is used for 24 hours; then a smaller dressing is applied, and active range of motion of the hand and fingers is encouraged. A night splint that conforms to the contracture correction is worn for 3 months, and progressive extension splinting and a formal physical therapy program often enhance the final result.

PARTIAL (SELECTIVE) FASCIECTOMY

TECHNIQUE 12.3

- Outline the proposed incision with a marking pen before inflation of the tourniquet (Figs. 12.15A–C and 12.16A–C). Take into consideration the pits and other areas of skin

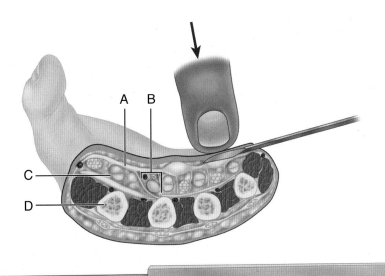

FIGURE 12.14 Luck subcutaneous fasciotomy. *Top,* Cross section of hand to show relations of palmar fascia and technique of subcutaneous fasciotomy. Palmar fascia *(A),* neurovascular bundle *(B),* flexor tendons *(C),* and metacarpal *(D).* Fasciotome is being pressed *(arrow)* through fascial cord. *Bottom,* Fasciotome (note that a No. 15 blade scalpel can be used for this purpose). **SEE TECHNIQUE 12.2.**

with diminished vascularity by making an incision over or near these areas, avoiding their presence at the base of a flap. These areas sometimes can be excised when the final rotation of the skin takes place in closure.

- Make a zigzag or longitudinal incision over the deforming pathologic structure. Because zigzag incisions tend to straighten out, causing tension lines at the creases, we often prefer incorporating longitudinal incisions, which are converted to Z-plasties at closure (Fig. 12.17). Design the Z-plasty flaps so that a transverse segment is within or near each joint crease. Continue the incision proximally into the palm, avoiding crossing the palmar creases at right angles.
- Elevate the skin and underlying normal subcutaneous tissue from the pathologic fascia from proximal to distal (Figs. 12.15D and 12.16D). Create the Z-plasty flaps when the wound is ready for closure (Figs. 12.15E and 12.16E).
- Excise the pathologic fascia proximal to distal, taking great care to isolate and protect the neurovascular bundles of each finger. Carefully cauterize small vessels as necessary. Excision of superficial transverse palmar fascial fibers may be unnecessary. Avoid entering tendon sheaths if possible because bleeding into the flexor tendon sheaths may cause adhesions.
- Carefully excise the pathologic fascia by sharp dissection. Avoid cutting displaced digital nerves by locating each nerve in the fatty pad at the level of the MP joint and following it distally.
- Excise the natatory ligament if it prevents separation from its adjacent digit.
- Follow all the contracted fascial cords to their distal insertions. Insertions may be into tendon sheaths, bone, and skin; occasionally, they are dorsolateral to the proximal interphalangeal joint.
- When excision of the diseased tissue has been completed, all joints should permit full passive extension unless capsular contractures exist.
- Fashion the skin flaps. If there is any extra skin, the pitted or thinned areas can be excised (Figs. 12.15F and G and 12.16F).

- Before closing, elevate the hand, compress the wound, release the tourniquet, hold for 10 minutes, and check for and control bleeding.
- Using skin hooks and with minimal handling of the flaps, suture them in place with 4-0 or 5-0 monofilament nylon.
- Close the palmar wound loosely to allow necessary drainage. A red rubber drain can be placed in the palm or, alternatively, a closed suction drainage system can be constructed with the use of butterfly catheters and Vacutainer tubes (Fig. 12.18). One catheter tube for each operated finger provides adequate and efficient drainage. The likelihood of a flare reaction occurring 4 to 6 weeks postoperatively may be decreased by infusing 15 to 20 mg of betamethasone (Celestone) into the catheters before connecting the Vacutainer tubes. This also seems to decrease the amount of postoperative discomfort, decreasing the need for narcotic analgesics in many patients even after complex fasciectomies.
- Apply a layer of nonadherent gauze and a moist dressing compressed gently against the wound to conform to the contours of the palm and fingers. Apply a compression dressing over this and use a volar plaster splint to maintain the fingers in the degree of extension achieved at surgery.

POSTOPERATIVE CARE Drains usually are removed within 24 to 48 hours after surgery. The hand is kept elevated for a minimum of 48 hours. Early proximal interphalangeal motion is encouraged. The shoulder is moved actively at intervals during this period to avoid cramping. If there is undue pain in the hand or fever after 48 hours, the wound should be inspected. If a hematoma is found elevating the skin, it should be expressed manually and the involved area of the wound be left open. Otherwise, the first dressing change is done 3 to 5 days after surgery, and range-of-motion exercises are begun. A resting pan splint is fitted with the fingers in maximal extension to be worn at night.

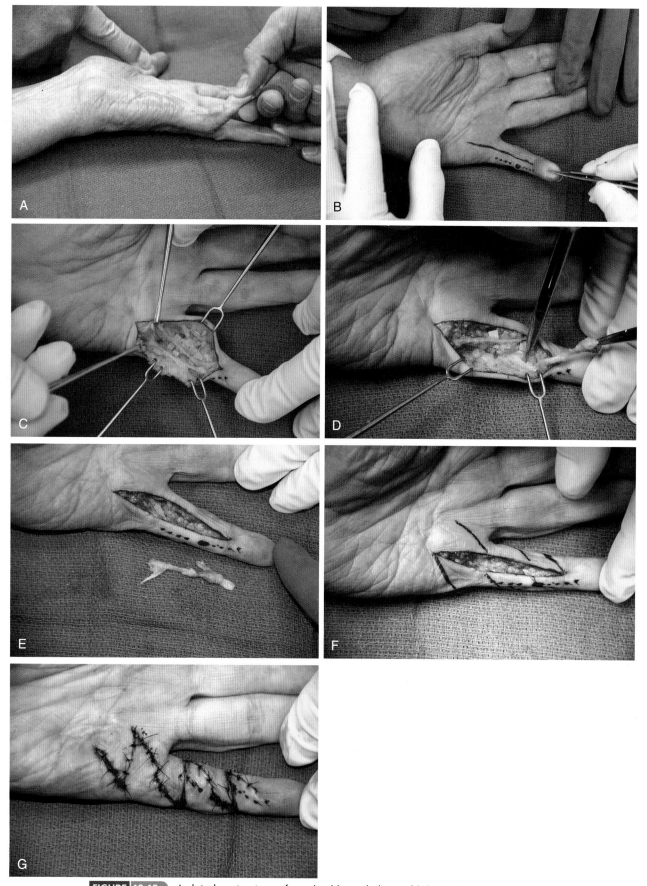

FIGURE 12.15 Isolated contracture of proximal interphalangeal joint in 71-year-old woman.
A, Maximal passive proximal interphalangeal joint extension of 55 degrees. **B,** Palpable diseased
cord and nodule denoted with planned longitudinal incision. **C,** Cord and digital nerve underlaid
with blue plastic markers. **D,** Distal retraction of digital cord depicting underlying diseased Cleland
ligament. **E,** Pathology pattern. **F** and **G,** Z-plasty skin flap design and closure. **SEE TECHNIQUE 12.3.**

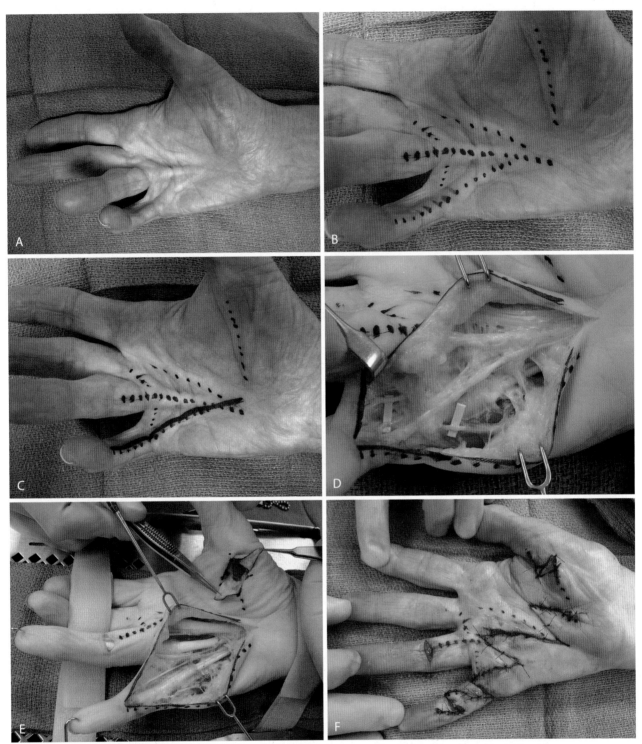

FIGURE 12.16   More complex selective fasciectomy. **A,** Disease involving thumb, middle, ring, and small fingers. **B,** Cords to be released are dotted with skin-marking pen. **C,** Planned incisions are solidly outlined before tourniquet inflation. **D,** Palmar and digital cords are exposed through the longitudinal incision. **E,** Exposure after cord excisions. Note the additional transverse incision required to excise ring finger central cord and additional thumb cord incision. **F,** After meticulous hemostasis, Z-plasty wounds are closed. **SEE TECHNIQUE 12.3.**

At 2 weeks, the sutures are removed and the hand is left free of all dressings. The patient is warned not to place the hand in a dependent position for rest and not to soak the hand in hot water. Active exercise in warm water is permissible, but no passive stretching is allowed. Moderate use of the hand is permitted at 3 weeks; however, several months of

rehabilitation may be necessary before unrestricted activities can comfortably be performed. The resting pan splint is worn for 3 months after surgery. Silicone putty may be a valuable adjunct to an exercise program.

Chronic PIP joint contractures of more than 60 degrees may have central slip attenuation. If a tenodesis test is positive

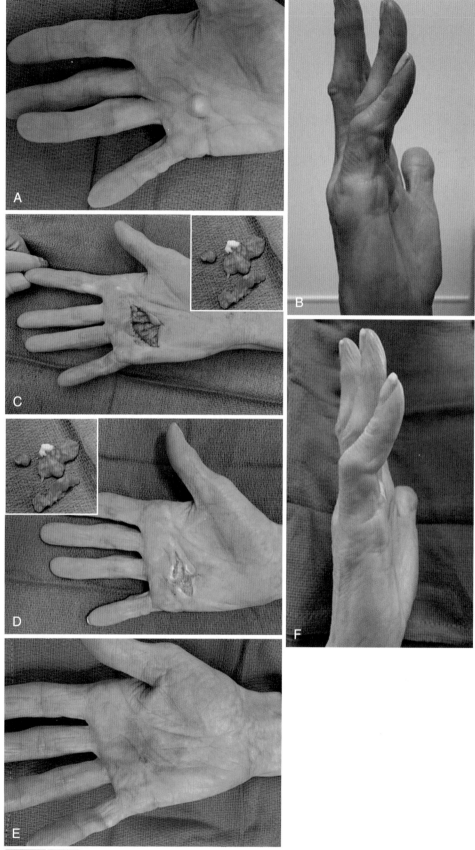

FIGURE 12.17 Open palm (McCash) technique in 53-year-old right-handed female with previous PNA and collagenase treatment. **A** and **B,** Preoperative appearance. **C** and **D,** Intraoperative images after cordectomies and excision of incidental inclusion cyst *(inset).* **E** and **F,** Secondary wound healing images at 12 and 38 days after surgery.

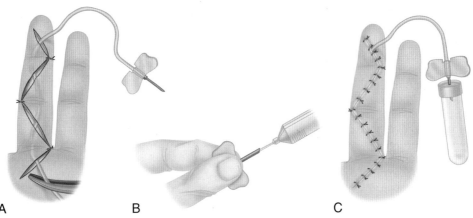

FIGURE 12.18 Closed suction drainage system for individual fingers and palm can be constructed from 21-gauge sterile catheters and Vacutainer tubes. **A,** Multiple tubing holes are made with scissors, and catheter is placed under skin flaps. **B,** After wound closure, 25-gauge needle can be used to instill steroid preparation through 21-gauge catheter needle. **C,** Vacutainer tube attached after dressing is applied and tourniquet is deflated.

(failure of the PIP joint to extend fully with full wrist and MP joint in full passive flexion), PIP joint splinting for 3 weeks postoperatively may be indicated. During these 3 weeks, distal interphalangeal joint exercises are performed to mobilize the lateral bands dorsally.

The Jacobsen flap technique has been described as a safe, simple alternative to open-palm procedures in the treatment of advanced Dupuytren disease of the little finger. Rather than a zigzag incision, the procedure creates an L-shaped full-thickness flap with two linear incisions, one in the transverse crease of the palm and the other in the midlateral line of the little finger to the distal interphalangeal joint (Fig. 12.19). After contracture release, full extension of the finger moves the flap distally, and the longitudinal arm of the L-shaped incision is closed, leaving a 15-mm skin defect open in the palm, which is left open to heal by secondary intention within 4 to 6 weeks. When the palmar wound is healed, a dynamic extension splint is worn for 10 weeks. Suggested advantages of this technique are reduction of hematoma and edema, avoidance of skin grafting and donor site scars, and immediate active mobilization of the hand. Disadvantages include the need for 10 weeks of splint wear and extensive potential prolonged physical therapy. The palm wound must be carefully monitored to avoid infections and delayed healing. Tripoli et al. reported only two complications in 15 patients in whom the Jacobsen flap was used: chronic regional pain syndrome in one patient and delayed wound healing in another.

In summary, patients with Dupuytren disease can be simply treated by education about their condition, especially those with new-onset disease and minor nodules and cords; however, rather significant degrees of contractures frequently are well tolerated by many individuals. In contrast, some patients' functions will be compromised by thumb and finger flexion, as well as varying degrees of adduction contractures. For patients in whom surgical intervention is contemplated, an informed discussion regarding the anticipated outcome, especially the likelihood of recurrence and disease extension, is indicated. Factors including family history, ectopic deposits, age of onset, and the presence of bilateral disease should be taken into consideration, in addition to

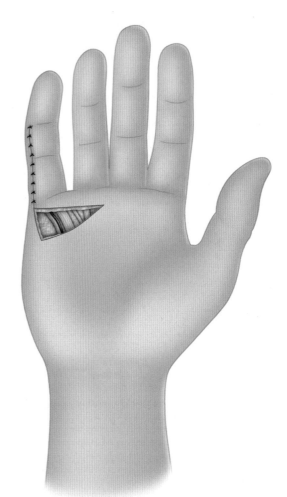

FIGURE 12.19 Jacobsen flap. The L-shaped full-thickness flap is created by making two linear incisions: the first in the transverse crease of the palm, the second in the midlateral line of the little finger to the distal interphalangeal joint. (Redrawn from Tripoli M, Cordova A, Moschella F: The "Jacobsen flap" technique: a safe, simple surgical procedure to treat Dupuytren disease of the little finger in advanced stage, *Tech Hand Up Extrem Surg* 14:172, 2010.)

other confounding variables related to patient health status, such as but not limited to smoking, diabetes mellitus, and other metabolic issues.

Surgical interventions we use include minimally invasive cordotomy techniques and selective fasciectomies. Needle or scalpel releases are reserved for patients with well-defined cords causing moderate degrees of MP and PIP contractures and in whom the resultant skin tears usually are minor and of little consequence. Recurrence is common (33% or higher) and does not preclude repeat needle or scalpel aponeurotomy, nor does it appear to complicate selective fasciectomy procedures. Selective fasciectomy remains the most durable technique resulting in the best long-standing contracture correction. We prefer designing incisions tailored to each patient, which provide clear visualization to excise as much of the cords and nodules as possible with subsequent skin rearrangement. Sometimes skin deficiency results in open wounds that can be left open to heal by secondary intention. Permanent and full correction of all joint contractures is rare; approximately 50% of the pre-existing PIP joint contracture correction is to be expected, and perhaps 15% of previously operated patients may require another surgical intervention.

REFERENCES

Agee JM, Goss BC: Dupuytren contractures of the proximal interphalangeal joint, *J Hand Surg Am* 37A:1467, 2012.

Akhavani MA, McMurtie A, Webb M, et al.: A review of the classification of Dupuytren's disease, *J Hand Surg Eur* 40E:155, 2015.

Atroshi I, Nordenskjold J, Lauritzson A, et al.: Collagenase treatment of Dupuytren's contracture using a modified injection method: a prospective cohort study of skin tears in 164 hands, including short-term outcome, *Acta Orthop* 86:310, 2015.

Ball C, Izadi D, Verjee LS, et al.: Systematic review of non-surgical treatments for early dupuytren's disease, *BMC Musculoskel Dis* 17:345, 2016.

Bogdanov I, Payne CR: Dupuytren contracture as a sign of systemic disease, *Clin Dermatol* 37:675, 2019.

Calandruccio JH, Hecox SE: Reoperative dupuytren contracture. In Duncan SFM, editor: *Reoperative hand surgery*, New York, 2012, Springer Science+Business Media.

Coleman S, Gilpin D, Kaplan FT, et al.: Efficacy and safety of concurrent collagenase clostridium histolyticum injections for multiple Dupuytren contractures, *J Hand Surg Am* 39:57, 2014.

Dolmans GH, de Bock GH, Werker PM: Dupuytren diathesis and genetic risk, *J Hand Surg Am* 37A:2106, 2012.

Eaton C: Percutaneous fasciotomy for Dupuytren's contracture, *J Hand Surg Am* 36A:910, 2011.

Eckerdal D, Nivestam A, Dahlin LB: Surgical treatment of Dupuytren's disease—outcome and health economy in relationship to smoking and diabetes, *BMC Musculoskelet Disord* 15:117, 2014.

Gajendran VK, Hentz V, Kenney D, Curtin CM: Multiple collagenase injections are safe for treatment of Dupuytren's contractures, *Orthopedics* 37:e657, 2014.

Gaston RG, Larsen SE, Pess GM, et al.: The efficacy and safety of concurrent collagenase clostridium histolyticum injections for 2 Dupuytren contractures in the same hand: a prospective multicenter study, *Hand Surg Am* 40:193, 2015.

Hentz VR: Collagenase injections for treatment of Dupuytren disease, *Hand Clin* 30:25, 2014.

Herrera FA, Benhaim P, Suliman A, et al.: Cost comparison of open fasciectomy versus percutaneous needle aponeurotomy for treatment of Dupuytren contracture, *Ann Plast Surg* 70:454, 2013.

Hovius SER, Kan HJ, Smit X, et al.: Extensive percutaneous aponeurotomy and lipografting: a new treatment for Dupuytren disease, *Plast Reconstr Surg* 128:221, 2011.

Hovius SER, Kan JH, Verhoekx JSN, Khouri RK: Percutaneous aponeurotomy and lipofilling (PALF). A regenerative approach to Dupuytren contracture, *Clin Plast Surg* 42:375, 2015.

Izadpanah A, Viezel-Mathieu A, Izadpanah A, Luc M: Dupuytren contracture in the pediatric population: a systematic review, *Eur J Pediatr Surg* 25:151, 2015.

Kaplan FT, Badalamente MA, Hurst LC, et al.: Delayed manipulation after collagenase clostridium histolyticum injection for Dupuytren contracture, *Hand (N Y)* 10:578, 2015.

Kirkpatrick K: New treatment for Dupuytren contracture, *AAOS Now* October 11–12, 2010.

Leafblad ND, Wagner E, Wanderman ER, et al.: Outcomes and direct costs of needle aponeurotomy, collagenase injection, and fasciectomy in the treatment of Dupuytren constracture, *J Hand Surg Am* 44:919, 2019.

Lilly SI Stern PJ: Simultaneous carpal tunnel release and Dupuytren's fasciectomy, *J Hand Surg Am* 35A:754, 2010.

McMillan C, Binhammer P: Steroid injection and needle aponeurotomy for Dupuytren contracture: a randomized, controlled trial, *J Hand Surg Am* 37A:1307, 2012.

Meals RA, Hentz VR: Technical tips for collagenase injection for Dupuytren contracture, *J Hand Surg Am* 39:1195, 2014.

Muppavarapu RC, Waters MJ, Leibman MI, et al.: Clinical outcomes following collagenase injections compared to fasciectomy in the treatment of Dupuytren's contracture, *Hand* 10:260, 2015.

Peimer CA, Skodny P, Mackowiak JI: Collagenase clostridium histolyticum for Dupuytren contracture: patterns of use and effectiveness in clinical practice, *J Hand Surg Am* 38:2370, 2013.

Rizzo M, Stern PJ, Benhaim P, Hurst LC: Contemporary management of Dupuytren contracture, *Instr Course Lect* 63:131, 2014.

Sanjuan-Cerveró R, Carrera-Hueso FJ, Ferreiro P, et al.: Efficacy and adverse effects of collagenase use in the treatment of Dupuytren's disease: a meta-analysis, *Bone Joint Lett J* 100-B:73, 2018.

Satish L, Gallo PH, Baratz ME, et al.: Reversal of TGF- ß1 stimulation of α-smooth muscled actin and extracellular matrix components by cyclic AMP in Dupuytren's-derived fibroblasts, *BMC Musculoskelet Disord* 12:133, 2011.

Scherman P, Jenmalm P, Dahlin LB: Three-year recurrence of Dupuytren's contracture after needle fasciotomy and collagenase injection: a two-centre randomized controlled trial, *J Hand Surg Eur* 43:836, 2018.

Shewring DJ: Rethnam U: Cleland's ligaments and Dupuytren's disease, *J Hand Surg Eur* 39:477, 2014.

Skov ST, Bisgaard T, Søndergaard P, et al.: Injectable collagenase versus percutaneous needle fasciotomy for Dupuytren contracture in proximal interphalangeal joints: a randomized controlled trial, *J Hand Surg Am* 42:321, 2017.

Soreide E, Murad MH, Denbeigh JM, et al.: Treatment of Dupuytren's constracture: a systematic review, *Bone Joint Lett J* 100-B:1138, 2018.

Steenbeck LM, Dreise MM, Werker PMN: Durability of collagenase treatment for Dupuytren disease of the thumb and first web after at least 2 years' follow-up, *J Hand Surg Am* 44:694, 2019.

Strömberg J, Sörensen AI, Fridén J: Percutaneous needle fasciotomy versus collagenase treatment for Dupuytren contracture. A randomized controlled trial with a two-year follow-up, *J Bone Joint Surg Am* 100:1079, 2018.

Tripoli M, Cordova A, Moschella F: The "Jacobsen flap" technique: a safe, simple surgical procedure to treat Dupuytren disease of the little finger in advanced stage, *Tech Hand Up Extrem Surg* 14:172, 2010.

Verheyden JR: Early outcomes of a sequential series of 144 patients with Dupuytren's contracture treated by collagenase injection using an increased dose, multi-cord technique, *J Hand Surg Eur* 40E:133, 2015.

von Campe A, Mende K, Omaren H, Meuli-Simmen C: Painful nodules and cords in Dupuytren disease, *J Hand Surg Am* 37A:1313, 2012.

White JW, Kang SN, Nancoo T: Management of severe Dupuytren's contracture of the proximal interphalangeal joint with use of a central slip facilitation device, *J Hand Surg Eur* 37E:728, 2012.

Zhou C, Hovius ER, Slijper HP, et al.: Predictors of patient satisfaction with hand function after fasciectomy for Dupuytren's contracture, *Plast Reconstr Surg* 138:649, 2016.

Zyluk A, Debniak T, Puchalski P: Common variants of the *ALDH2* and *DHDH* genes and the risk of Dupuytren's disease, *J Hand Surg Eur* 38E:430, 2013.

The complete list of references is available online at ExpertConsult.com.

CHAPTER 13

STENOSING TENOSYNOVITIS OF THE WRIST AND HAND

William J. Weller

STENOSING TENOSYNOVITIS

Stenosing tenosynovitis in the hand and wrist are common conditions resulting in significant functional impairment for which treatments usually are straightforward; symptom resolution usually is complete with appropriate management. When the extensor pollicis brevis (EPB) and the abductor pollicis longus (APL) tendons in the first dorsal compartment are affected, the condition is named after the Swiss physician Fritz de Quervain, who described this malady in 1895. A peritendinitis also may affect these tendons proximal to the extensor retinaculum, causing pain, swelling, and crepitus in some patients. Cysts attached to the first dorsal compartment retinaculum and tendon triggering may also occur.

The long flexor tendons to the thumb and fingers may develop focal areas of swelling resulting in mechanical symptoms at various tendon pulley interfaces. Less often, the extensor pollicis longus may be affected at the level of Lister tubercle. Any of the other tendons that pass beneath the dorsal wrist retinaculum also may be involved. The tenosynovitis that precedes the stenosis may result from an otherwise subclinical collagen disease or recurrent mild trauma, such as that experienced by carpenters and wait staff. Some case histories indicate that acute trauma may initiate the pathologic condition; however, most commonly these conditions develop gradually with no known cause. The stenosis occurs at a point where the direction of a tendon changes, for here a fibrous sheath acts as a pulley and friction is maximal. Although the tenosynovium lubricates the sheath, friction can cause a reaction when the repetition of a particular movement is necessary.

Many cases of tenosynovitis in various locations, even stenosing tenosynovitis, respond favorably to nonoperative intervention such as rest, antiinflammatory medications, and corticosteroid injections. Pain may increase temporarily during the initial 24 hours after loss of the local anesthetic effect; the patient should be warned about this possibility. It may be 3 to 7 days before the steroid becomes effective, but surgery is avoided in many instances. Before injection, it should be determined that the tenosynovitis is not caused by other conditions, such as gout or infection, which could be worsened by steroid injections. Patients with diabetes mellitus should be counseled about the potential rise in blood sugars for days following injection; patients with prior unfavorable response or brittle bone disease are not candidates for this treatment.

Most often, triggering digits are from flexor tendon-pulley pathology; however, it is important to evaluate for metacarpophalangeal joint arthritis and extensor tendon subluxation. Middle finger osteoarthritis may mimic middle trigger finger, and dorsal metacarpophalangeal joint swelling and joint space narrowing on radiographic examination usually clarify the distinction between these two entities. Oddly, trigger finger in conjunction with osteoarthritis is rare, and symptoms are unlikely to resolve with treatment of the trigger finger alone. Similarly, extensor tendon subluxation may be mistaken for simple trigger finger conditions. A sudden radial or ulnar shift of the finger associated with snapping or triggering of the finger should alert the examiner to check the dorsum of the hand for extensor tendon instability over the metacarpophalangeal joint. Similarly, coexistent trigger finger with extensor tendon subluxation is rare, and management of the extensor tendon alone usually is warranted.

DE QUERVAIN DISEASE

Stenosing tenosynovitis of the APL and EPB tendons typically occurs in adults 30 to 50 years old; however, in women of childbearing age radial-sided wrist pain is commonly related to de Quervain tenosynovitis from repetitive ulnar deviation required in newborn care. Women are affected 6 to 10 times more frequently than men. The cause is almost always related to overuse, either in the home or at work, or is associated with rheumatoid arthritis. The presenting symptoms usually are pain and tenderness at the radial styloid. Sometimes a thickening of the fibrous sheath is palpable. The Finkelstein test usually is positive: "on grasping the patient's thumb and quickly abducting the hand ulnarward, the pain over the styloid tip is excruciating." Although Finkelstein stated that this test is "probably the most pathognomonic objective sign," it is not diagnostic; the patient's history and occupation, the radiographs, and other physical findings also must be considered. Similar symptoms also can be caused by arthritis in the trapeziometacarpal, scaphotrapeziotrapezoid, and radiocarpal joints; superficial radial nerve entrapment or neuroma; and tenosynovitis at the crossing of the EPB and APL over the extensor carpi radialis longus and brevis (intersection syndrome).

Conservative treatment consisting of splint wear and the injection of a steroid preparation (Fig. 13.1) may be successful early after onset. Initial treatment with steroid injections may yield complete pain relief in over 70% of patients. When pain persists, surgery is the treatment of choice.

Anatomic variations are common in the first dorsal compartment, and separate compartments have been noted in 21% of anatomic specimens. Reports of separate compartments found at surgery vary from 20% to 58%. More than half of patients may have "aberrant" or duplicated tendons

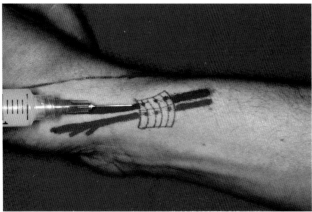

FIGURE 13.1 Injection for de Quervain tenosynovitis. Regardless of whether injection is given distal-to-proximal or proximal-to-distal, care should be made not to direct the needle past radial styloid toward radial artery.

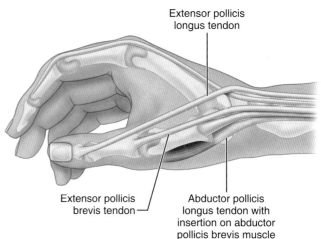

FIGURE 13.3 In rare cases, abductor pollicis longus inserts onto trapezium.

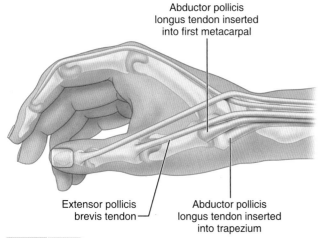

FIGURE 13.2 During surgery for de Quervain disease, at least one aberrant tendon often is found. Abductor pollicis longus routinely inserts on first metacarpal base and commonly has thenar fascial slip.

(usually the APL). These tendons sometimes insert more proximally and medially than usual, into the trapezium (Fig. 13.2), the abductor pollicis brevis muscle (Fig. 13.3), the opponens pollicis muscle, or the muscle fascia. The EPB is considered a "late" tendon phylogenetically and is absent in about 5% of wrists. The presence of these variations and failure to deal with them at the time of surgery may account for any persistence of pain.

SURGICAL TREATMENT OF DE QUERVAIN DISEASE

TECHNIQUE 13.1

- Use a local anesthetic and a tourniquet.
- Infiltrate the skin well proximal to the area of the first dorsal compartment with sufficient local anesthetic before skin preparation and draping. An Esmarch bandage on the proximal forearm usually suffices as a tourniquet.
- Make an incision carefully through the skin only. An oblique incision coursing along the extensor brevis tendon is preferred; however, a transverse, oblique, or longitudinal incision is also perfectly satisfactory (Fig. 13.4). The longitudinal incision advocated by some surgeons creates a longer area in which skin scar may make cutaneous nerves more subject to scar adherence.
- Carry sharp dissection just through the dermis and not into the subcutaneous fat, avoiding the sensory branches (lateral antebrachial cutaneous nerve above the cephalic vein and superficial radial nerve branches more deeply).
- After retracting the skin edges, use blunt dissection in the subcutaneous fat to clearly expose the retinaculum over the first dorsal compartment tendons.
- Identify the first dorsal compartment tendons proximal to the stenosing dorsal ligament and sheath and open the first dorsal compartment on its dorsoulnar side. The EPB tendon is most dorsal and can be identified by its distally oriented muscle fibers; the APL tendon has no muscular fibers in this area.
- With the thumb abducted and the wrist flexed, lift the APL and the EPB tendons from their groove. If they cannot be easily retracted from the radial styloid, look for additional "aberrant" tendons and separate compartments. Releasing the EPB tendon first and then the APL usually reveals the presence or absence of a septum. If there is no EPB present, inspect the floor of the compartment for the footprint of the brachioradialis tendon. This has a Y-shaped tendinous insertion; if this is clearly seen, release of this compartment is assured. Sometimes the septum is quite pronounced, and its resection is warranted, ensuring not to injure the underlying radial artery coursing dorsally just beyond the radial styloid.
- Make sure that the volarly based retinacular flap remains over the released tendons to prevent volar tendon subluxation.
- Close the skin incision only and apply a small pressure dressing.

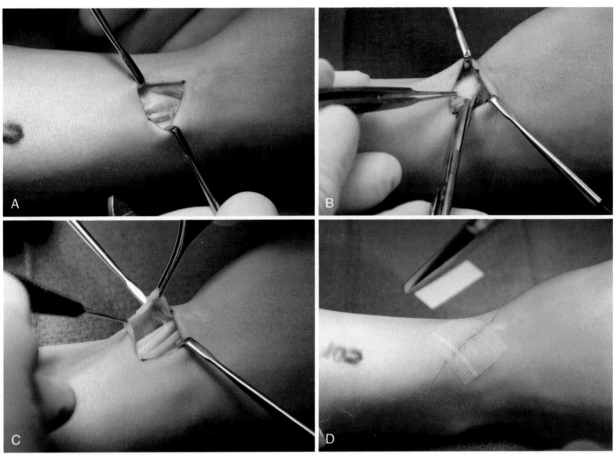

FIGURE 13.4 Surgical treatment of de Quervain disease. **A**, Skin incision. **B**, Dorsal carpal ligament has been exposed. **C**, First dorsal compartment has been opened on its ulnar side. **D**, Occasionally, separate compartments are found for extensor pollicis brevis and abductor pollicis longus tendons **SEE TECHNIQUE 13.1.**

POSTOPERATIVE CARE The small pressure dressing is removed after 48 hours; an additional dressing can be applied if needed. Thumb and hand motion is immediately encouraged and is increased as tolerated, except for forceful wrist flexion, which may predispose the tendons toward subluxation during the first 2 weeks after surgery.

Failure to obtain complete relief after surgery may result from (1) neural adhesions or neuroma formation, (2) volar tendon subluxation, (3) failure to find and release a separate aberrant tendon within a separate compartment, (4) scar hypertrophy, or (5) incorrect diagnosis such as a bone lesion in the distal radius, intersection syndrome, localized arthritic deformities, or more proximal nerve compression syndromes. For recurrent subluxation of the EPB and APL tendons, a distally based brachioradialis tendon slip can be used to reconstruct a nonstenosing compartment to house the first dorsal compartment tendons. Ramesh and Britton used the extensor retinaculum to prevent subluxation (Fig. 13.5). Littler et al. also described a reconstruction for the first compartment in which the septum dividing the first extensor compartment is removed, the EPB is removed from the compartment, and

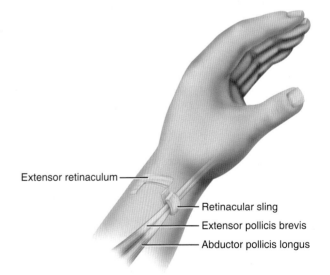

Extensor retinaculum

Retinacular sling

Extensor pollicis brevis

Abductor pollicis longus

FIGURE 13.5 Part of extensor retinaculum is used to create U-shaped sling to retain tendons of extensor pollicis brevis and abductor pollicis longus.

the retinacular sheath is reapproximated loosely over the APL tendon to prevent tendon subluxation.

TRIGGER FINGER AND THUMB

Trigger thumb in adults is a distinctly separate entity from "congenital" trigger thumb. Stenosing tenosynovitis, leading to inability to extend the flexed digit or flex the extended digit often produces a palpable "triggering" and usually is seen in individuals older than 45 years of age. When associated with a collagen disease, several fingers may be involved (most often the long and ring fingers). Patients may note a lump or knot in the palm. The lump may be the thickened area in the first annular pulley or a nodule or fusiform swelling of the flexor tendon just distal to it. The nodule can be palpated by the examiner's fingertip and moves with the tendon. The tendon nodule usually is just proximal to the anulus at the metacarpophalangeal joint level; however, in a rheumatoid patient, a nodule distal to this point may cause triggering. Patients may experience triggering after operative release because of catching of the tendon on the palmar aponeurosis transverse fibers, which usually resolves with time. Occasionally, a partially lacerated flexor tendon at this level heals with a nodule sufficiently large to cause triggering. Local tenderness may be present but is not a prominent complaint. Pressure accentuates the apparent snapping or triggering of the more distal joints. Patients frequently state that the problem is in the proximal interphalangeal joint with trigger finger or in the interphalangeal joint with trigger thumb. Other conditions, such as intraarticular disorders (e.g., loose bodies, degenerative joint disease, and fractures) and common extensor tendon subluxation, can cause similar symptoms and must be considered to determine effective treatment for idiopathic trigger finger.

Initial treatment of trigger digits usually is nonoperative, especially in uncomplicated conditions in patients with a short duration of symptoms. Nonoperative methods include stretching, night splinting, and combinations of heat and ice. Corticosteroid injection is effective, with 60% achieving success after one injection. In their study of 292 corticosteroid injections for trigger digits, Dardas et al. found that repeat injections provided symptomatic relief for a year or more in 50% of patients; they recommended consideration of repeat injections in patients who prefer nonoperative management.

Patients with diabetes mellitus may be more refractory to nonoperative management; however, corticosteroid injections may elevate serum glucose levels for 5 days or more, and patients with unstable diabetes may be better treated without injection. Database review (153,479 injections and 70,290 releases) found that preoperative hypoglycemia increased infection risk after both procedures. In a cost analysis study, immediate surgical release in the clinic was identified as the most cost-effective treatment strategy for trigger finger in diabetic patients.

Surgical release reliably relieves the problem for most patients: approximately 97% of patients have complete resolution after operative treatment. Persistence of triggering is more common than recurrence. Trigger release should be done with a local block so that the cessation of triggering of a particular finger can be evaluated. Some adjacent finger triggering may become obvious only after a given finger is released; both can be released at the same surgical setting.

The safety and effectiveness of percutaneous trigger finger release using a needle or a push knife have literature support.

Incomplete pulley release and damage to the flexor tendons and digital nerves, especially in the index finger and thumb, remain of some concern, especially with limited exposure techniques.

SURGICAL RELEASE OF TRIGGER FINGER

TECHNIQUE 13.2

- Local anesthetic infiltration in the palm proximal to the incision site is preferred (Fig. 13.6). The use of a pneumatic arm tourniquet may be helpful, although a high forearm Esmarch wrap usually is sufficient.
- Make a transverse incision about 2 cm long several millimeters distal to the distal palmar crease for middle, ring, and small trigger finger releases and several millimeters distal to the proximal palmar crease for index trigger finger releases (Fig. 13.7A). Trigger thumb releases can be done through incisions either distal or proximal to the metacarpophalangeal joint flexion crease (Fig. 13.8). Alternative incisions for the fingers can be made obliquely or longitudinally between the metacarpophalangeal and distal palmar creases and obliquely across the thumb metacarpophalangeal flexion crease.
- Avoid the digital nerves, which on the thumb are more palmar and closer to the flexor sheath than might be anticipated. The thumb radial digital nerve is especially vulnerable.

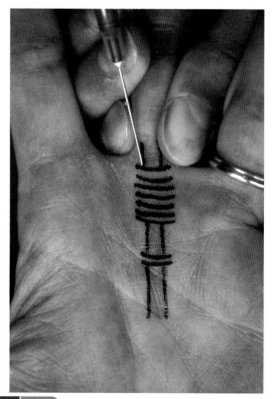

FIGURE 13.6   Local anesthetic for trigger finger release **SEE TECHNIQUE 13.2.**

- Spread the subcutaneous tissues away from the underlying annular pulley system and make sure the digital nerves are safely protected. Trigger thumbs require release of only the A1 pulley, whereas trigger digits require division of the A1 and A0, or proximal palmar pulley.
- Pulley division usually is accomplished with an initial opening of the pulley with a No. 15 knife blade and a pair of tenotomy scissors. For trigger thumb release, avoid cutting too far distally and disrupting the oblique pulley (Fig. 13.7B). Incise the sheath from proximal to distal, approximately 1 cm, and reassess for triggering.
- Have the patient actively flex and extend the digit; persistent triggering implies that either the A1 and palmar pulleys are incompletely released or an alternate site of triggering is present. The distinction between the A1 and A2 pulleys may not be apparent; however, when the distal A1 pulley edge is released, the divided pulley leaves are parallel rather than ending in a V-shaped pattern.
- After the tendon sheath has been released, encourage the patient to actively flex and extend the digit to ensure that the release is complete. Sometimes other fingers can be found to trigger at the same surgical setting and can be managed at the same time. Close the skin and apply a small, dry compression dressing.

POSTOPERATIVE CARE The compression dressing is removed after 48 hours. Sutures are removed at 10 to 14 days. Normal use of the finger or thumb is encouraged.

PERCUTANEOUS RELEASE OF TRIGGER FINGER

TECHNIQUE 13.3   *Figure 13.8*

- Before attempting the percutaneous release, it is helpful to have the patient understand that the procedure might fail and that subsequent open release may be necessary.
- Inject local anesthetic into the palmar skin and more deeply proximal to the intended release site (between the proximal and distal palmar creases for the middle, ring, and small fingers and proximal to the proximal palmar crease for the index finger). Maintain an orientation along the flexor tendon sheaths in the midline of the digit being released.
- Although specialized instruments have been devised for trigger release, an 18- or 19-gauge needle may suffice.
- Turn the palm up, resting the hand on a folded towel to permit slight hyperextension of the metacarpophalangeal joint.
- Insert the needle onto the A1 pulley and orient the bevel of the needle so that it is longitudinally aligned parallel to the flexor tendons.
- Move the needle proximally and distally along the A1 pulley, pressing firmly proximally and distally. Feel for a scraping or grating sensation as the sheath is incised.
- When the grating is eliminated, remove the needle and check for triggering as the patient flexes and extends the digit. Additional needle passes might be needed.
- Injection of corticosteroid is optional.

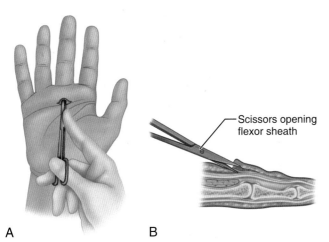

FIGURE 13.7   **A,** Surgical treatment of trigger finger. **B,** One blade of scissors has been placed beneath proximal edge of tendon sheath **SEE TECHNIQUE 13.2.**

Scissors opening flexor sheath

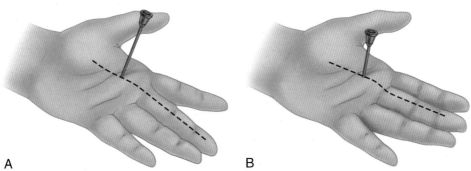

FIGURE 13.8   **A,** Percutaneous release of long finger A1 pulley. Metacarpophalangeal joint hyperextended and 19-gauge needle inserted just distal to flexor crease. Bevel of needle oriented longitudinally with tendon. Skin markings indicate path of flexor tendons. **B,** Needle stabilized and pulley released from proximal to distal. Loss of grating sensation as pulley is cut indicates completion of release **SEE TECHNIQUE 13.2.**

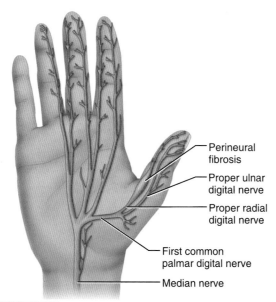

FIGURE 13.9 Bowler's thumb. Distal sensory branches of median nerve in hand and location of perineural fibrosis of proper ulnar digital nerve of thumb are shown.

POSTOPERATIVE CARE The needle entry site is covered with an adhesive bandage or light nonrestrictive dressing, and active hand and finger use is encouraged with stretching exercises.

Normal use of the finger or thumb is encouraged.

BOWLER'S THUMB

Bowler's thumb is a perineural fibrosis caused by repetitious compression of the ulnar digital nerve of the thumb while grasping a bowling ball (Fig. 13.9). Bowlers with this condition usually are those who bowl several times a week. Tingling and hyperesthesia around the pulp accompany this condition. A palpable lump that is exceedingly tender and at times accompanied by distal skin atrophy usually is present. Early awareness of the cause can lead to protection of the thumb by a shield or splint and rest from bowling to help reduce the symptoms and to prevent the condition from becoming chronic. Occasionally, neurolysis and dorsal transfer of the nerve become necessary.

REFERENCES

DE QUERVAIN DISEASE
Adams JE, Habbu R: Tendinopathies of the hand and wrist, *J Am Acad Orthop Surg* 23:741, 2015.
Earp BE, Han CH, Floyd WE, et al.: De Quervain tendinopathy: survivorship and prognostic indicators of recurrence following a single corticosteroid injection, *J Hand Surg Am* 40:1161, 2015.
Goubau JF, Goubau L, Van Tongel A, et al.: The wrist hyperflexion and abduction of the thumb (WHAT) test: a more specific and sensitive test to diagnose de Quervain tenosynovitis than the Eichoff's test, *J Hand Surg Eur* 39:286, 2014.
Kazmers NH, Liu TC, Gordon JA, et al.: Patient- and disease-specific factors associated with operative management of de Quervain tendinopathy, *J Hand Surg Am* 42:931, 2017.

Lee HJ, Kim PT, Aminata IW, et al.: Surgical release of the first extensor compartment for refractory de Quervain's tenosynovitis: surgical findings and functional evaluation using DASH scores, *Clin Orthop Surg* 6:405, 2014.
Leversedge FJ, Cotterell IH, Nickel BT, et al.: Ultrasonography-guided de Quervain injection: accuracy and anatomic considerations in a cadaver model, *J Am Acad Orthop Surg* 24:399, 2016.
Luther GA, Murthy P, Blazar PE: Cost of immediate surgery versus non-operative treatment for trigger finger in diabetic patients, *J Hand Surg Am* 41:1056, 2016.
Mardani-Kivi M, Karimi Mobarakeh M, Bahrami F, et al.: Corticosteroid injection with or without thumb spica cast for de Quervain tenosynovitis, *J Hand Surg Am* 39:37, 2014.
Nam YS, Doh G, Hong KY, et al.: Anatomical study of the first dorsal extensor compartment for the treatment of de Quervain's disease, *Ann Anat* 218:250, 2018.
Pagonis T, Ditsios K, Toli P, et al.: Improved corticosteroid treatment of recalcitrant de Quervain tenosynovitis with a novel 4-point injection technique, *Am J Sports Med* 339:398, 2011.
Pensak MJ, Bayron J, Wolf JM: Current treatment of de Quervain tendinopathy, *J Hand Surg Am* 38:2247, 2013.
van der Wijk J, Goubau JF, Mermuys K, et al.: Pulley reconstruction as part of the surgical treatment for de Quervain disease: surgical technique with medium-term results, *J Wrist Surg* 4:300, 2015.

TRIGGER THUMB AND TRIGGER FINGER
Abe Y: Clinical results of a percutaneous technique for trigger digit release using a 25-gauge hypodermic needle with corticosteroid infiltration, *J Plast Reconstr Aesthet Surg* 69:270, 2016.
Adams JE, Habbu R: Tendinopathies of the hand and wrist, *J Am Acad Orthop Surg* 23:741, 2015.
Amirfeyz R, McNich R, Watts A, et al.: Evidence-based management of adult trigger digits, *J Hand Surg Eur* 42:473, 2017.
Becker SJ, Braun Y, Janssen SJ, et al.: Early patient satisfaction with different treatment pathways for trigger finger and thumb, *J Hand Microsurg* 7:283, 2015.
Brito JL, Rozental TD: Corticosteroid injection for idiopathic trigger finger, *J Hand Surg* 35A:831, 2010.
Bruijnzeel H, Neuhaus V, Fostvedt S, et al.: Adverse events of open A1 pulley release for idiopathic trigger finger, *J Hand Surg Am* 37:1650, 2012.
Buchanan PJ, Law T, Rosas S, et al.: Preoperative hypoglycemia increases infection risk after trigger finger injection and release, *Ann Plast Surg* Oct 15. 2018, [Epub ahead of print].
Cakmak F, Wolf MB, Bruckner T, et al.: Follow-up investigation of open trigger digit release, *Arch Orthop Trauma Surg* 132:685, 2012.
Calleja H, Tanchuling A, Alagar D, et al.: Anatomic outcome of percutaneous release among patients with trigger finger, *J Hand Surg* 35A:1671, 2010.
Castellanos J, Munoz-Mahamud E, Dominguez E, et al.: Long-term effectiveness of corticosteroid injections for trigger finger and thumb, *J Hand Surg Am* 40:121, 2015.
Chang EY, Chen KC, Chung CB: MR imaging findings of trigger thumb, *Skeletal Radiol* 44:1201, 2015.
Choudhury MM, Tay SC: Prospective study on the management of trigger finger, *Hand Surg* 19:393, 2014.
Dala-Ali BM, Nakhdjevani A, Lloyd MA, Schreuder RB: The efficacy of steroid injection in the treatment of trigger finger, *Clin Orthop Surg* 4:263, 2012.
Dardas AZ, VandenBerg J, Shen T, et al.: Long-term effectiveness of repeat corticosteroid injections for trigger finger, *J Hand Surg Am* 42:227, 2017.
Döring AC, Hageman MG, Mulder FJ, et al.: Trigger finger: assessment of surgeon and patient preferences and priorities for decision making, *J Hand Surg Am* 39:2208, 2014.
Everding NG, Bishop GB, Belyea CM, Soong MC: Risk factors for complications of open trigger finger release, *Hand (N Y)* 10:297, 2015.
Hansen RL, Søndergaard M, Lange J: Open surgery versus ultrasound-guided corticosteroid injection for trigger finger: a randomized controlled trial with 1-year follow-up, *J Hand Surg Am* 42:359, 2017.
Huang HK, Wang JP, Lin CJ, et al.: Short-term versus long-term outcomes after open or percutaneous release for trigger thumb, *Orthopaedics* 41:e131, 2017.

Giugale JM, Fowler JR: Trigger finger: adult and pediatric treatment strategies, *Orthop Clin North Am* 46:561, 2015.

Gulabi D, Cecen GS, Bekler HI, et al.: A study of 60 patients with percutaneous trigger finger releases: clinical and ultrasonographic findings, *J Hand Surg Eur* 39:699, 2014.

Hoang D, Lin AC, Essilfie A, et al.: Evaluation of percutaneous first annular pulley release: efficacy and complications in a perfused cadaveric study, *J Hand Surg Am* 2016. [Epub ahead of print].

Huang HK, Wang JP, Wang ST, et al.: Outcomes and complications after percutaneous release for trigger digits in diabetic and non-diabetic patients, *J Hand Surg Eur* 40:735, 2015.

Kloeters O, Ulrich DJ, Bloemsma C, van Houdt CI: Comparison of three different incision techniques in A1 pulley release on scar tissue formation and postoperative rehabilitation, *Arch Orthop Trauma Surg* 136:731, 2016.

Miyamoto H, Miura T, Isayama H, et al.: Stiffness of the first annular pulley in normal and trigger fingers, *J Hand Surg* 36A:1486, 2011.

Ng KY, Olmscheid N, Worhacz K, et al.: Steroid injection and open trigger finger release outcomes: a retrospective review of 999 digits, *Hand (N Y)* Sep 21, 2018. [Epub ahead of print].

Patel RM, Chilelli BJ, Ivy AD, Kalainov DM: Hand surface landmarks and measurements in the treatment of trigger thumb, *J Hand Surg Am* 38:1166, 2013.

Potulsak-Chromik A, Lipowska M, Gawel M, et al.: Carpal tunnel syndrome in children, *J Child Neurol* 29:227, 2014.

Schubert C, Hui-Chou HG, See AP, Deune EG: Corticosteroid injection therapy for trigger finger or thumb: a retrospective review of 577 digits, *Hand (N Y)* 8:439, 2013.

Shah AS, Bae DS: Management of pediatric trigger thumb and trigger finger, *J Am Acad Orthop Surg* 20:206, 2012.

Shakeel H, Ahmad TS: Steroid injection versus NSAID injection for trigger finger: a comparative study of early outcomes, *J Hand Surg Am* 37:1319, 2012.

Shiozawa R, Uchiyama S, Sugimoto Y, et al.: Comparison of splinting versus nonsplinting in the treatment of pediatric trigger finger, *J Hand Surg Am* 37:1211, 2012.

Wang J, Zhao JG, Liang CC: Percutaneous release, open surgery, or corticosteroid injection, which is the best treatment method for trigger digits? *Clin Orthop Relat Res* 471:1879, 2013.

Will R, Lubahn J: Complications of open trigger finger release, *J Hand Surg* 35A:594, 2010.

Wojahn RD, Feoger NC, Gelberman RH, Calfee RP: Long-term outcomes following a single corticosteroid injection for trigger finger, *J Bone Joint Surg* 96A:1849, 2014.

Ztluk A, Jagielski G: Percutaneous A1 pulley release vs steroid injection for trigger digit: the results of a prospective, randomized trial, *J Hand Surg Eur* 36(53), 2011.

BOWLER'S THUMB

Halsey JN, Therattil PJ, Viviano SL, et al.: Bowler's thumb: case report and review of the literature, *Eplasty* 15:e47, 2015.

Showalter MF, Flemming DJ, Bernard SA: MRI manifestataions of bowler's thumb, *Radiol Case Rep* 6:458, 2015.

Terence T, Khoo YP: Friction neuropathy of the ulnar digital nerve in a writer's thumb which was successfully treated with corticosteroid injection, *J Hand Surg Eur* 36:711, 2011.

Wajid H, LeBlanc J, Shapiro DB, et al.: Bowler's thumb: ultrasound diagnosis of a neuroma of the ulnar digital nerve of the thumb, *Skeletal Radiol* 45:1589, 2016.

The complete list of references is available online at Expert Consult.com

CHAPTER 14

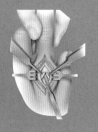

COMPRESSIVE NEUROPATHIES OF THE HAND, FOREARM, AND ELBOW

William J. Weller, James H. Calandruccio, Mark T. Jobe

CARPAL TUNNEL SYNDROME

Carpal tunnel syndrome, described by Paget in 1854, is the most common upper extremity compression neuropathy and results from median nerve compression within the carpal tunnel. The carpal tunnel is bound by the carpal bones arching dorsally; the hook of the hamate and the pisiform medially; and the scaphoid tubercle and trapezial ridge laterally. The palmar aspect, or "roof," of the carpal tunnel is formed by the flexor retinaculum, consisting of the deep forearm fascia proximally, the transverse carpal ligament (TCL) over the wrist, and the aponeurosis between the thenar and hypothenar muscles distally. The most palmar structure in the carpal tunnel is the median nerve. Lying dorsal (deep) to the median nerve in the carpal tunnel are the nine long finger and thumb flexor tendons.

Carpal tunnel syndrome is primarily a clinical diagnosis, with symptoms of tingling and numbness in the typical median nerve distribution (thumb, index, long, and radial side of ring fingers). Pain, described as deep, aching, or throbbing, occurs diffusely in the hand and may radiate up the forearm. Thenar muscle atrophy usually is seen in late-stage nerve compression. It occurs most often in patients 30 to 60 years old and is two to three times more common in women than in men. Carpal tunnel syndrome may affect 1% to 10% of the U.S. population. Older, overweight, and physically inactive individuals are more likely to develop carpal tunnel syndrome, and female sex, obesity, cigarette smoking, and vibrations associated with job tasks have been identified as carpal tunnel risk factors in industrial workers.

Elevation of carpal tunnel pressures of more than 20 to 30 mm Hg impedes epineurial blood flow, and nerve function is impaired. Reduction in cross-sectional area along the length of the carpal tunnel may result from various conditions such as malaligned Colles fractures, edema from infection or trauma, tumors or tumorous conditions, and other space-occupying lesions. Distal radial fracture immobilization with the wrist in marked flexion and ulnar deviation can cause acute median nerve compression immediately after reduction. Systemic conditions, such as obesity, diabetes mellitus, thyroid dysfunction,

amyloidosis, rheumatoid arthritis, and Raynaud disease, sometimes are associated with the syndrome. Occasionally, a patient has carpal tunnel syndrome symptoms caused by a habitual sleeping posture in which the wrist is kept acutely flexed. Trauma caused by repetitive hand motions has been identified as a possible aggravating factor, especially in patients whose work requires repeated forceful finger and wrist flexion and extension. Laborers using vibrating machinery also are at risk. The causative effect of light, repetitive activities experienced by office workers is controversial and unresolved. Many factors are implicated in the causation and aggravation of carpal tunnel syndrome (Box 14.1).

When carpal tunnel syndrome occurs in pregnant women, the symptoms usually resolve after delivery. Aberrant muscles of the forearm and thrombosis of the median artery also may contribute to median nerve compression. The cause, however, in most patients is idiopathic, its direct association with work is difficult to substantiate, and involvement of the nondominant hand is frequent.

In children, carpal tunnel syndrome is unusual. Macrodactyly, lysosomal storage diseases, and a strong family history of carpal tunnel syndrome may be predisposing factors in children. Symptoms in children may be confusing and include decreased dexterity and diffuse pain. Findings such as thenar muscle atrophy and weakness suggest that the condition is severe by the time of presentation. The Phalen test and Tinel sign may be absent if the nerve compression has been present for a long time. Carpal tunnel syndrome frequently is associated with nonspecific tenosynovial edema and rheumatoid tenosynovitis, as are trigger finger and de Quervain disease. Flexor tendon synovium biopsy specimens from patients with idiopathic carpal tunnel syndrome show benign fibrous tissue without inflammatory changes. The tenosynovium in patients with carpal tunnel disease shows increased fibroblast density, collagen fiber size, vascular proliferation, and more type III collagen fibers than controls.

DIAGNOSIS

Patients with carpal tunnel syndrome usually have symptoms of numbness, pain, or paresthesia in the median nerve distribution.

Factors Involved in the Pathogenesis of Carpal Tunnel Syndrome

Anatomy
Decrease in Size of Carpal Tunnel
- Bony abnormalities of the carpal bones
- Acromegaly
- Flexion or extension of wrist

Increase in Contents of Canal
- Forearm and wrist fractures (Colles fracture, scaphoid fracture)
- Dislocations and subluxations (scaphoid rotary subluxation, lunate volar dislocation)
- Posttraumatic arthritis (osteophytes)
- Musculotendinous variants
- Aberrant muscles (lumbrical, palmaris longus, palmaris profundus)
- Local tumors (neuroma, lipoma, multiple myeloma, ganglion cysts)
- Persistent medial artery (thrombosed or patent)
- Hypertrophic synovium
- Hematoma (hemophilia, anticoagulation therapy, trauma)

Physiology
Neuropathic Conditions
- Diabetes mellitus
- Alcoholism
- Double-crush syndrome
- Exposure to industrial solvents

Inflammatory Conditions
- Rheumatoid arthritis
- Gout
- Nonspecific tenosynovitis
- Infection

Alterations of Fluid Balance
- Pregnancy
- Menopause
- Eclampsia
- Thyroid disorders (especially hypothyroidism)
- Renal failure
- Long-term hemodialysis
- Raynaud disease
- Obesity
- Lupus erythematosus
- Scleroderma
- Amyloidosis
- Paget disease

External Forces
- Vibration
- Direct pressure

From Kerwin G, Williams CS, Seiler JG: The pathophysiology of carpal tunnel syndrome, *Hand Clin* 12:243–251, 1996.

Paresthesia in the median nerve sensory distribution is the most frequent symptom, often awakening patients with burning and numbness of the hand that is relieved by exercise. The Tinel sign also may be shown in most patients by percussing the median nerve at the wrist. Atrophy to some degree of the median-innervated thenar muscles has been reported in about half of patients treated by operation. Acute flexion of the wrist for 60 seconds (Phalen test) or strenuous use of the hand increases the paresthesia in some but not all patients.

Evaluation of the clinical usefulness of several commonly used provocative tests, including wrist flexion, nerve percussion, and the tourniquet test, found the most sensitive test to be the wrist flexion test, whereas nerve percussion was the most specific and the least sensitive. Gellman et al. found that with the wrist in neutral position, the mean pressure within the carpal tunnel in patients with carpal tunnel syndrome was 32 mm Hg. This pressure increased to 99 mm Hg with 90 degrees of wrist flexion and to 110 mm Hg with the wrist at 90 degrees of extension. The pressures in the control subjects were 25 mm Hg with the wrist in neutral position, 31 mm Hg with the wrist in flexion, and 30 mm Hg with the wrist in extension.

A carpal compression test (Durkan test), in which direct compression is applied to the median nerve for 30 seconds with the thumbs or an atomizer bulb attached to a manometer, was found to be more specific (90%) and more sensitive (87%) than either the Tinel or Phalen test. Szabo et al. evaluated the validity of tests for carpal tunnel syndrome, including Phalen wrist flexion, Tinel nerve percussion, Durkan compression, and Semmes-Weinstein monofilaments. Grip and pinch strength, a hand diagram, and patient symptoms were assessed. Durkan nerve compression, the hand diagram score, night pain, and Semmes-Weinstein testing after a Phalen test had the highest sensitivity. The most specific tests were the hand diagram and Tinel sign. These authors concluded that a patient with an abnormal hand diagram, a positive Durkan test, abnormal Semmes-Weinstein sensibility testing, and night pain had a very high probability of having carpal tunnel syndrome. Conversely, they found that if all four of the just-mentioned examinations were normal, the probability of the patient having carpal tunnel syndrome was very low.

Sensibility testing in peripheral nerve compression syndromes found that threshold tests of sensibility correlated accurately with symptoms of nerve compression and electrodiagnostic studies. Semmes-Weinstein monofilament pressure testing was the most accurate in determining early nerve compression. A combination of the Semmes-Weinstein monofilament test with the wrist flexion test for a "quantitative provocational" diagnostic test was reported to have 82% sensitivity and 86% specificity.

According to some authors, electrodiagnostic studies including nerve conduction velocities and electromyography (EMG) are reliable confirmatory tests. A distal motor latency of more than 4.5 milliseconds (ms) and a sensory latency of more than 3.5 ms are considered abnormal. EMG may show increased insertional activity, positive sharp waves, fibrillations at rest, decreased motor recruitment, and complex repetitive discharges indicative of nerve damage. These studies are occasionally normal, however, even in patients with classic clinical signs and symptoms of carpal tunnel syndrome are present. Similarly, electrodiagnostic tests may be abnormal in asymptomatic patients. Nerve conduction studies are reported to be 90% sensitive and 60% specific for the diagnosis of carpal tunnel syndrome. They also are helpful in evaluating the upper extremity for nerve compression at the elbow, axilla, and cervical spine and for showing changes of peripheral neuropathy. Studies have shown, however, that electrodiagnostic testing provides no significant data for prediction of functional recovery or reemployment after carpal tunnel release, nor does it increase the diagnostic value of the four commonly used tests (i.e., abnormal hand diagram, abnormal Semmes-Weinstein testing, positive Durkan compression, and night pain). These findings, combined with reported false-negative rates of 10%, limit the usefulness of this type of testing to determine treatment. Postoperative electrodiagnostic testing may be helpful in assessing recurrent symptoms. The various tests for nerve compression in the carpal tunnel are summarized in Table 14.1.

Reports of MRI in carpal tunnel syndrome are promising, especially with newer techniques such as diffusion tensor imaging, but MRI is not routinely used for diagnosis. A major advantage of MRI is its high soft-tissue contrast, which gives detailed images of bones and soft tissues. Ultrasound sensitivity for carpal tunnel syndrome has been reported to be over 97% when the median nerve diameter is greater than 10 mm^2 at the level of the pisiform and is suggested to be a useful diagnostic technique by some authors. In patients with negative electrodiagnostic studies but a clinical diagnosis of carpal tunnel syndrome, high-resolution ultrasonography has been used to diagnose carpal tunnel, with a sensitivity of 73% if the cutoff of 9.4 mm^2 at the inlet of the carpal tunnel is used. Nonetheless, the diagnosis of carpal tunnel syndrome should be based on clinical acumen and physical examination in the vast majority of patients, and ancillary tests should be reserved for patients without clear presentations.

TREATMENT

If mild symptoms have been present and there is no thenar muscle atrophy, the use of night splints and injection of cortisone preparations into the carpal tunnel may provide temporary relief, but long-term benefit is obtained in only about 10% of patients treated with corticosteroid injection and splinting. The response to injection treatment has been reported to be faster in men and in patients older than 40 years old. Care should be taken not to inject directly into the nerve. Injection also can be used as a diagnostic tool in patients without osteophytes or tumors in the canal. Most of these cases are probably caused by a nonspecific synovial edema, and these seem to respond more favorably to injection. Injection also helps to eliminate the possibility of other syndromes, especially cervical disc or thoracic outlet syndrome. Some patients prefer to receive injections two or three times before a surgical procedure is done. If the symptoms and physical findings improve, and there is no muscle atrophy, conservative treatment with splinting and injection is reasonable.

In a study of 331 patients with carpal tunnel syndrome, Kaplan, Glickel, and Eaton identified five important factors in determining the success of nonoperative treatment: (1) age older than 50 years, (2) duration longer than 10 months, (3) constant paresthesia, (4) stenosing flexor tenosynovitis, and (5) a positive Phalen test result in less than 30 seconds. Two thirds of patients were cured by medical treatment when none of these factors was present; 59.6% were cured when one factor was present; and 83.3% when two factors were noted. Of patients with three factors, 93.2% did not experience any improvement. No patient with four or five factors was cured by medical management.

Patients with intermediate and advanced (chronic) syndromes probably are better treated with early carpal tunnel release. Extensive neurolysis has not been shown to have any significant effect. Internal neurolysis does not improve the motor or sensory outcome of carpal tunnel release. Moreover, epineurotomy offers no clinical benefit to carpal tunnel release. Treatment of acute carpal tunnel syndrome should be individualized, depending on its cause. For carpal tunnel syndrome caused by an acute increase in carpal tunnel pressure (e.g., after a Colles fracture treated with flexed wrist immobilization), relief may be obtained by a change in wrist position without surgical release of the tunnel.

Patients with florid tenosynovitis caused by rheumatoid arthritis or other inflammatory conditions are managed by tenosynovectomy at the time of carpal tunnel release. The palmaris longus opponensplasty (Camitz) may be beneficial, particularly in an elderly patient with thenar muscle wasting, weakness, and poor opposition. Trapeziometacarpal arthroplasty and carpal tunnel release can be done safely through two incisions.

Idiopathic carpal tunnel syndrome in the pediatric population is uncommon; however, night pain, hand clumsiness, and thenar atrophy may be the initial findings as these patients rarely present with complaints of sensory disturbance. Congenital bone abnormalities, hypothyroidism, lysosomal storage disease, and myopathic contractures account for some of the predisposing etiologies in this age group.

If signs and symptoms are persistent and progressive, especially if they include thenar atrophy, then a carpal tunnel release should be performed. The results of surgery are good in most instances, and benefits seem to last in most patients. Maximal improvement is seen in the first 6 months after carpal tunnel release. After 6 months, there is no significant improvement in the Tinel and Phalen tests, pinch strength, motor latency, symptom severity, or functional scoring. Although thenar atrophy may disappear, it resolves slowly, if at all. Surgical release might not achieve complete relief of all symptoms for patients older than 70 years or those with advanced nerve compression. When symptoms of median nerve compression develop during treatment of an acute distal radial fracture, the constricting bandages and cast should be loosened, and the wrist should be extended to neutral position. When median nerve symptoms persist after a distal radial fracture and have not improved after positional change, surgery usually is indicated.

Despite variable recovery periods, the results of carpal tunnel release in patients with idiopathic carpal tunnel syndrome with intermittent symptoms usually are uniformly successful; however, carpal tunnel release in diabetic and nondiabetic patients was shown to be similarly beneficial in a prospective study with a follow-up period of 6 months. When the same patients were followed for long-term (10 years), however, patients with diabetes had worse surgical outcomes compared with patients with idiopathic carpal tunnel syndrome when using the self-administered Boston Questionnaire to assess symptom severity and functional status. According to Roh et al., patients with a metabolic syndrome were found to have only a delay in the recovery process. Metabolic syndrome was defined by the presence of at least three of the five criteria: a clinical diagnosis of diabetes or hypertension or use of antihypertensive medication; elevated plasma triglyceride level (150 mg/dL or higher); decreased high-density lipoprotein cholesterol levels (less than 50 mg/dL for females or less than 40 mg/dL for males); increased waist size (greater than 80 cm for females or 90 cm for males); and body mass index of

TABLE 14.1

Tests for Nerve Compression

TEST	HOW PERFORMED	CONDITION TESTED	POSITIVE RESULT	INTERPRETATION OF POSITIVE RESULT
Phalen test	Elbows on table, forearms vertical, wrists flexed	Paresthesia in response to position	Numbness or tingling on radial digits within 60 s	Probable CTS (sensitivity 0.75, specificity 0.47)
Percussion test (Tinel sign)	Lightly tap along median nerve from proximal to distal	Site of nerve lesion	"Electric" tingling response in fingers	Probable CTS if positive at the wrist (sensitivity 0.60, specificity 0.67)
Carpal tunnel compression test (Durkan)	Direct compression of median nerve at carpal tunnel	Paresthesia in response to compression	Paresthesia within 30 s	Probable CTS (sensitivity 0.87, specificity 0.90)
Hand diagram	Patient marks site of pain or altered sensation on outlined hand diagram	Patient's perception of symptoms	Markings on palmar side of radial digits, without markings in palm	Probable CTS (sensitivity 0.96, specificity 0.73, negative predictive value 0.91)
Hand volume stress test	Hand volume measured by displacement, repeat after 7-min stress test and 10-min rest	Hand volume	Hand volume increased by ≥10 mL	Probable dynamic CTS
Direct measurement of carpal tunnel pressure	Wick or infusion catheter placed in carpal tunnel	Hydrostatic pressure in resting and provocative positioning	Resting pressure ≥25 mm Hg (variable and technique related)	Hydrostatic compression is probable cause of CTS
Static two-point discrimination	Determine minimal separation of two distinct points when applied to palmar fingertip	Innervation density of slow-adapting fibers	Failure to determine separation of at least 5 mm	Advanced nerve dysfunction
Moving two-point discrimination	As above, with movement of the points	Innervation density of fast-adapting fibers	Failure to determine separation at least 4 mm	Advanced nerve dysfunction
Vibrometry	Vibrometer placed on palmar side of digit, amplitude at 120 Hz, increased to threshold of perception; compare median and ulnar bilaterally	Threshold of fast-adapting fibers	Asymmetry compared with contralateral hand or median to ulnar in ipsilateral hand	Probable CTS (sensitivity 0.87)
Semmes-Weinstein monofilaments	Monofilaments of increasing diameter touched to palmar side of digit until patient can determine which digit is touched	Threshold of slowly adapting fibers	Value >2.83	Median nerve impairment (sensitivity 0.83)
Distal sensory latency and conduction velocity	Orthodromic stimulus and recording across wrist	Latency, conduction velocity of sensory fibers	Latency >3.5 ms or asymmetry of conduction velocity >0.5 m/s vs. opposite hand	Probable CTS
Distal motor latency and conduction velocity	Orthodromic stimulus and recording across wrist	Latency, conduction velocity of motor fibers of median nerve	Latency >4.5 ms or asymmetry of conduction velocity >1 m/s	Probable CTS
Electromyography	Needle electrodes placed in muscle	Denervation of thenar muscles	Fibrillation potentials, sharp waves, increased insertional activity	Advanced motor median nerve compression

CTS, Carpal tunnel syndrome; *ms,* milliseconds; *m/s,* millimeter per second.
From Abrams R, Meunier M: Carpal tunnel syndrome. In Trumble TE, editor: *Hand surgery update 3,* Rosemont, 2003, American Society for Surgery of the Hand.

more than 30. These authors found that metabolic syndrome was related to a more severe grade of carpal tunnel syndrome and was a risk factor for delayed functional recovery at up to 6 months' follow-up, yet significant improvements in symptom severity and hand function were similar in both groups after 12 months, except for pinch strength being higher in the control group. Similar findings were noted by Kronlage and Menendez when the results of carpal tunnel release were compared among moderate and severe electrophysiologic carpal tunnel syndrome patients. Patients with moderate disease (prolonged sensory and motor latencies) had nearly complete resolution of pain and paresthesias at 3 months after surgery, whereas those with severe disease (prolonged sensory or motor latencies plus either absent sensory or mixed nerve action potential or low amplitude or absent compound motor action potential), despite considerable improvement, had prolonged and incomplete symptom reduction at 1 year after carpal tunnel release.

Worker's compensation patients do well with carpal tunnel release overall; however, surgeon expectations for improvement similar to that in non–worker's compensation patients should be cautious. In addition, patients should be counseled that outcomes may be delayed or inferior compared with non–worker's compensation patient. Pallis et al. found that worker's compensation patients had three times the number of complications and nearly twice the rate of persistent pain. They also took 5 weeks longer to return to work and were 16% more likely to not return to preinjury vocation.

The surgical technique chosen for median nerve decompression should be tailored by the surgeon's expertise. Although minimally invasive techniques purport earlier return to work and less postoperative discomfort, the results suggest that outcomes are similar at 6 months. In a meta-analysis of high-level evidence (randomized controlled trials), Sayegh and Strauch found that endoscopic release allows earlier return to work and improved strength during the early postoperative period. Results at 6 months or later were similar according to current data except that patients with endoscopic release are at greater risk of nerve injury and lower risk of scar tenderness compared with open release. The authors concluded that, although endoscopic release may appeal to patients who require an early return to work and activities, surgeons should be cognizant of its elevated incidence of transient nerve injury amid its similar overall efficacy to open carpal tunnel release. Seiler et al. showed that since the introduction of endoscopic carpal tunnel release the frequency of vascular injuries has decreased; however, nerve injuries have not declined, and this should be taken into consideration when determining treatment options.

Publications have described ultra-minimally invasive techniques, such as ultrasound- guided carpal tunnel release and looped-thread carpal tunnel release. We have limited experience with these treatment options. A single study by Lytie et al. of 159 hands treated with a modified looped-thread technique showed improved short- and long-term Boston Carpal Tunnel Syndrome Questionnaire responses compared with the available data for open or endoscopic carpal tunnel release. Apard and Candelier reviewed ultrasound-guided carpal tunnel release and made several recommendations: the practitioner attempting these techniques (1) must be able to identify all structures clearly, (2) must be aware of all the possible intraoperative and postoperative complications, and (3) must be able to treat the complications appropriately.

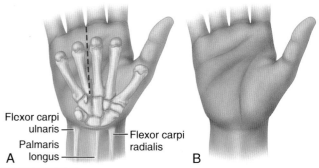

FIGURE 14.1 Two approaches for open carpal tunnel release. **A,** Transverse incision proximal to anterior wrist crease between flexor carpi ulnaris and flexor carpi radialis tendons. Distal longitudinal incision made between proximal palmar crease and 1 cm distal to hamate hook in line with radial border of ring finger. **B,** Incision used for minimal-incision approach.

■ **SURGICAL RELEASE**

Limited approaches, such as the "double incision" of Wilson (Fig. 14.1A) and the "minimal incision" of Bromley (Fig. 14.1B), may offer rapid recovery as ascribed to the endoscopic techniques. Similarly, the use of the "carpal tunnel tome" through a small palmar incision is a technical modification that may minimize the soft-tissue trauma of the traditional open technique and provides adequate exposure in most cases. Regardless of the technique selected, all structures to be incised should be seen and identified and safety of the median nerve verified before carpal tunnel release (Fig. 14.2).

"MINI-PALM" OPEN CARPAL TUNNEL RELEASE

TECHNIQUE 14.1

- Mark the planned surgical incision with a skin pen so that the longitudinal incision begins just distal to the distal wrist flexion crease and slightly ulnar to the midline of the wrist (center dot reference point) and extends distally approximately 2.0 to 3.0 cm in line with the third web space (Fig. 14.3A). (Note: only rarely is it necessary to extend the incision into the distal forearm.)
- Exposure of the transverse carpal ligament (TCL) requires splitting of the parallel palmar fascia fibers and ulnar retraction of the hypothenar fat (Fig. 14.3B). Frequently, intrinsic muscles obscure the midline of the TCL and can be released from their origin and reflected away from the underlying TCL.
- Carefully open the carpel tunnel by division of the TCL with a no. 15 blade. The TCL division should be such that 3 to 4 mm of it is left attached to the hamate hook to avoid flexor tendon ulnar subluxation. Make sure the contents of the carpal tunnel are not adherent to the undersurface of the TCL by gently spreading with a blunt instrument such as a mosquito hemostat the remaining portions of the distal and proximal portions of the undi-

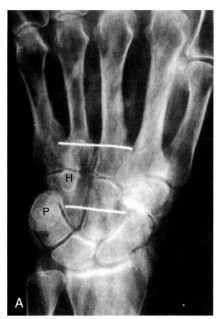
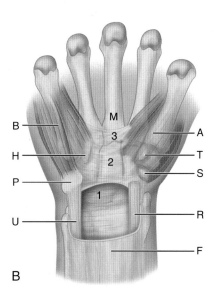

FIGURE 14.2 **A,** Anteroposterior radiograph of dissected right hand. Wires mark proximal and distal extents of classic flexor retinaculum, which includes middle portion of flexor retinaculum (transverse carpal ligament) and distal portion of flexor retinaculum. Note proximal limit is at distal aspect of pisiform *(P)* and distal limit is distal to hook of hamate *(H)*. **B,** Three portions of flexor retinaculum *(1 to 3)* consist of thick aponeurosis between thenar *(A)* and hypothenar *(B)* muscles. Thenar muscles attach to radial half of classic flexor retinaculum, composed of distal portion of flexor retinaculum *(3)*; trapezial ridge *(T)* and scaphoid tubercle *(S)* also are shown. Proximal portion of flexor retinaculum *(1)* courses deep to flexor carpi ulnaris *(U)* and flexor carpi radialis *(R)*. Flexor carpi radialis tendon is shown as it pierces flexor retinaculum at junction of proximal and middle portions to enter its fibroosseous canal. *F,* Antebrachial fascia; *M,* third metacarpal. (**A** from and **B** redrawn from Cobb TK, Dalley BK, Posteraro R, et al: Anatomy of the flexor retinaculum, *J Hand Surg Am* 18A:91–99, 1993.)

vided TCL and antebrachial fascia. The distal 2.0 cm of the antebrachial fascia can then be safely divided with blunt-tipped Metzenbaum or Mayo scissors (Fig. 14.3C).
- If the median nerve is adherent to the divided radial TCL leaf (Fig. 14.3D), external neurolysis may be needed.
- Close the incision in routine fashion (Fig. 14.3E) and apply a compressive dressing (Fig. 14.3F to H).

EXTENDED OPEN CARPAL TUNNEL RELEASE

TECHNIQUE 14.2

- The thenar crease takes a variable course, and palmar incisions should be well ulnar to it to avoid the median nerve palmar cutaneous branch. A curved incision ulnar and parallel to the thenar crease is not advisable because the palmar cutaneous branch of the median nerve proximally may be more at risk of injury. We prefer to use the incision described for the mini-palm technique (see Technique 14.1).
- Extend the incision proximally to the flexor crease of the wrist, where it can be continued farther proximally

if necessary. Angle the incision toward the ulnar side of the wrist to avoid crossing the flexor creases at a right angle, but especially to avoid cutting the palmar cutaneous sensory branch, which lies in the interval between the palmaris longus and the flexor carpi radialis tendons (Fig. 14.4). Maintain longitudinal orientation so that the incision is generally to the ulnar side of the long finger axis or radial border of the ring fourth ray. When severed, the palmar sensory branch frequently causes a painful neuroma that may later require excision from the scar. Should this nerve be severed, we do not attempt to repair it but section it more proximally to be covered by the middle finger sublimis muscle.
- Incise and reflect the skin and subcutaneous tissue.
- Identify the palmar fascia from the wrist flexion crease distally and the distal forearm antebrachial fascia proximally by subcutaneous blunt dissection. Split the palmar fascia, and expose the underlying transverse carpal ligament (TCL), avoiding the median nerve beneath it.
- Identify the TCL, and carefully divide it and avoid damage to the median nerve and its recurrent branch, which may perforate the ligament and leave the median nerve on the volar side (Fig. 14.5). Fibers of the TCL can extend distally farther than expected (Fig. 14.6).
- The flexor retinaculum includes the distal deep fascia of the forearm proximally, the TCL, and the aponeurosis between the thenar and hypothenar muscles. A successful

carpal tunnel release usually requires division of all these components.

- Be aware of potential anomalies: connections between the flexor pollicis longus and the index flexor digitorum profundus tendons; anomalous flexor digitorum superficialis; palmaris longus, hypothenar, lumbrical muscle bellies; and median and ulnar nerve branches and interconnections.
- Avoid injury to the superficial palmar arterial arch, which is 5 to 8 mm distal to the distal margin of the TCL.
- Inspect the flexor tenosynovium. Tenosynovectomy occasionally may be indicated, especially in patients with rheumatoid arthritis.
- Close only the skin and drain the wound as needed.

POSTOPERATIVE CARE A light compression dressing and a volar splint may be applied. The hand is actively used as soon as possible after surgery, but the dependent position is avoided. Usually the dressing can be removed by the patient at home 2 or 3 days after the surgery, and then gentle washing and showering of the hand is permitted. Gradual resumption of normal hand use is encouraged. The sutures are removed after 10 to 14 days. A splint may be continued for comfort as needed for 14 to 21 days.

ENDOSCOPIC RELEASE

Advocates of endoscopic carpal tunnel release cite less palmar scarring and ulnar "pillar" pain, rapid and complete return of strength, and return to work and activities at least 2 weeks sooner than for open release. Some studies comparing open and endoscopic carpal tunnel release found no significant differences in function. The advantages of the endoscopic technique in grip strength and pain relief are realized within the first 12 weeks and seem to benefit those patients not involved in compensable injuries. Anecdotal reports of intraoperative injury to flexor tendons; to median, ulnar, and digital nerves; and to the superficial palmar arterial arch emphasize

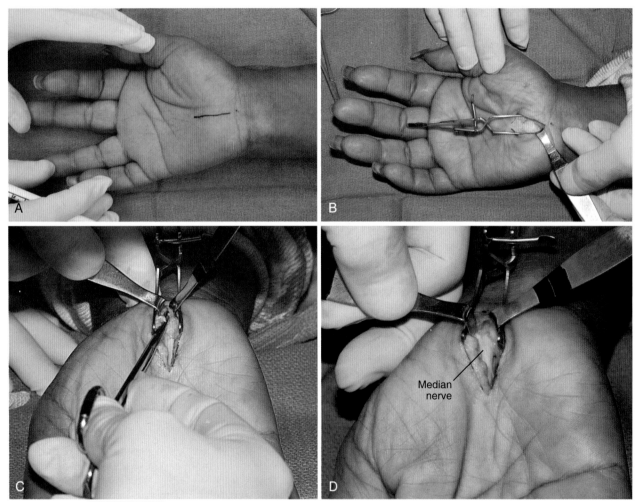

FIGURE 14.3   Mini-palm open release technique (see text). **A,** Incision is marked with skin pen (only rarely is it necessary to extend the incision into the distal forearm). **B,** Exposure of transverse carpal ligament (TCL) with parallel palmar fascia fibers and hypothenar fat retraction. **C,** After division of TCL, distal 2.0 cm of antebrachial fascia is divided with Metzenbaum scissors. **D,** In this patient, median nerve is adherent to divided radial TCL leaf and was subsequently externally neurolyzed.

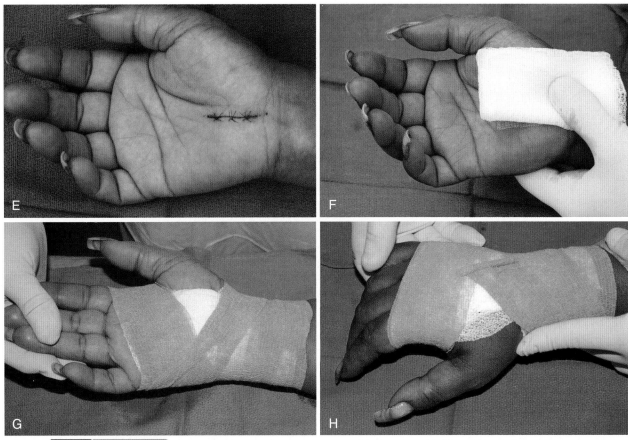

FIGURE 14.3, Cont'd **E**, Incision is closed and compressive dressing is applied (**F to H**). **SEE TECHNIQUE 14.1.**

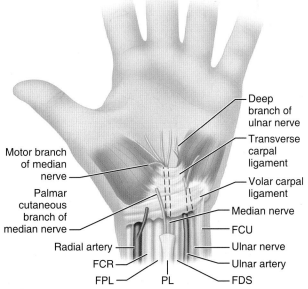

FIGURE 14.4 Care should be taken in any wrist incision to avoid cutting palmar cutaneous branch of median nerve. *FCR,* Flexor carpi radialis; *FCU,* flexor carpi ulnaris; *FDS,* flexor digitorum superficialis; *FPL,* flexor pollicis longus; *PL,* palmaris longus. **SEE TECHNIQUE 14.2.**

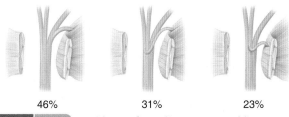

46%   31%   23%

FIGURE 14.5 Incidence of extraligamentous, subligamentous, and transligamentous course of thenar branch. **SEE TECHNIQUE 14.2.**

the need to exercise great care and caution when performing the endoscopic procedure. Cadaver studies have shown the close proximity of the median and ulnar nerves, superficial palmar arterial arch, and flexor tendons to the endoscopic instruments. Problems related to endoscopic carpal tunnel release include (1) a technically demanding procedure; (2) a limited visual field that prevents inspection of other structures; (3) the vulnerability of the median nerve, flexor tendons, and superficial palmar arterial arch; (4) the inability to control bleeding easily; and (5) the limitations imposed by mechanical failure. Agee, McCarroll, and North developed the following 10 guidelines for the single-incision endoscopic technique to prevent injury to the carpal tunnel structures:

1. Know the anatomy.
2. Never overcommit to the procedure.
3. Ascertain that the equipment is working properly.

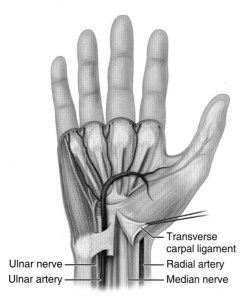

Transverse carpal ligament
Ulnar nerve
Radial artery
Ulnar artery
Median nerve

FIGURE 14.6 Anatomic relationships of deep transverse carpal ligament. **SEE TECHNIQUE 14.2.**

4. If scope insertion is obstructed, abort the procedure.
5. Ascertain that the blade assembly is in the carpal tunnel and not in Guyon's canal.
6. If a clear view cannot be obtained, abort the procedure.
7. Do not explore the carpal canal with the scope.
8. If the view is not normal, abort the procedure.
9. Stay in line with the ring finger.
10. "When in doubt, get out."

Although this technique has proved to be effective, it may not be applicable to every patient with carpal tunnel syndrome. If an endoscopic release cannot be accomplished safely, the procedure should be converted to an open technique.

There are various equipment manufacturers, but the two methods can be divided into single-portal (Chow) and two-portal (Agee) techniques. According to Chow, contraindications to endoscopic carpal tunnel release include the following: (1) the patient requires neurolysis, tenosynovectomy, Z-plasty of the TCL, or decompression of Guyon's canal; (2) the surgeon suspects a space-occupying lesion or other severe abnormality of the muscles, tendons, or vessels in the carpal tunnel; and (3) the patient has localized infection or severe hand edema, or the vascular status of the upper extremities is tenuous. Fischer and Hastings added the following contraindications to the use of endoscopic technique: (1) revision surgery for unresolved or recurrent carpal tunnel syndrome; (2) anatomic variation in the median nerve, suggested by clinical findings of wasting in the abductor pollicis brevis without significant median sensory changes; and (3) previous tendon surgery or flexor injury that would cause scarring in the carpal tunnel, preventing the safe placement of the instruments for endoscopic carpal tunnel release. Additionally, limitation of wrist extension is another contraindication to an endoscopic procedure because the endoscopic instruments cannot be introduced into the carpal tunnel and remain juxtaposed to the dorsal surface of the TCL. The general scheme of the techniques is shown in Figures 14.7 and 14.8. Before any surgeon attempts endoscopic carpal tunnel release, thorough familiarization with the technique through participation in "hands-on" laboratory practice sessions is recommended.

Endoscopic carpal tunnel release often has been performed with sedation or even general anesthesia. More recently, however, Tulipan et al. compared endoscopic carpal tunnel release using local anesthesia alone with the same procedure with local anesthesia and sedation. They found equal satisfaction and outcomes, indicating that the endoscopic technique can be done in a procedure room.

ENDOSCOPIC CARPAL TUNNEL RELEASE THROUGH A SINGLE INCISION

TECHNIQUE 14.3

(AGEE)
- Ascertain that the operating room setup is satisfactory. Ensure there is an unobstructed view of the patient's hand and the television monitor.
- Use general or regional anesthesia. Although the procedure can be done safely using local anesthesia, the increase in tissue fluid can compromise endoscopic viewing.
- Exsanguinate the limb with an elastic wrap and inflate a pneumatic tourniquet applied over adequate padding. Leave the arm exposed distal to the tourniquet.
- In a patient with two or more wrist flexion creases, make the incision in the more proximal crease between the tendons of the flexor carpi radialis and flexor carpi ulnaris (Fig. 14.7A).
- Use longitudinal blunt dissection to protect the subcutaneous nerves and expose the forearm fascia.
- Incise and elevate a U-shaped, distally based flap of forearm fascia (Fig. 14.7B), and retract it palmarward to facilitate dissection of the synovium from the deep surface of the ligament, creating a mouth-like opening at the proximal end of the carpal tunnel.
- When using the tunneling tools and the endoscopic blade assembly, keep them aligned with the ring finger, hug the hook of the hamate, and keep the tools snugly apposed to the deep surface of the transverse carpal ligament (TCL), maintaining a path between the median and ulnar nerves for the instruments.
- Use the synovium elevator to scrape the synovium from the deep surface of the TCL. Extend the wrist slightly; insert the blade assembly to the carpal tunnel, pressing the viewing window snugly against the deep surface of the TCL (Fig. 14.7C). While advancing the blade assembly distally, maintain alignment with the ring finger and hug the hook of the hamate, staying to the ulnar side. Make several proximal-to-distal passes to define the distal edge of the TCL with the fat overlying it.
- Define the distal edge of the TCL by viewing the video picture, ballottement, and light transilluminated through the skin. Correctly position the blade assembly and touch the distal end of the ligament with the partially elevated blade to judge its entry point for ligament division. Elevate the blade and withdraw the device, incising the ligament.
- Fat from the proximal palm may compromise endoscopic viewing by protruding through the divided proximal half

of the ligament, leaving an oil layer on the lens. Avoid this by first releasing only the distal one half to two thirds of the ligament (Fig. 14.7D).

- Using the unobstructed path for reinsertion of the instrument, accurately complete the distal ligament division with good viewing. Complete proximal ligament division with a final proximal pass of the elevated blade.
- Assess the completeness of ligament division using the following endoscopic observations.
- Through the endoscope, note that the partially divided ligament separates on the deep surface, creating a V-shaped defect (Fig. 14.7E).
- Make subsequent cuts viewing the trapezoidal defect created by complete division as the two halves of the ligament spring apart. Through this defect, observe the longitudinal palmar fascia fibers intermingled with fat and muscle. Force these structures to protrude by pressing on the palmar skin.
- Confirm complete division by rotating the blade assembly in radial and ulnar directions, noting that the edges of the

ligament abruptly "flop" into the window, obstructing the view.
- Palpate the palmar skin over the blade assembly window, observing motion between the divided TCL and the more superficial palmar fascia, fat, and muscle.
- Ensure complete median nerve decompression by releasing the forearm fascia with tenotomy scissors (Fig. 14.7F).
- Use small right-angle retractors to view the fascia directly, avoiding nerve and tendon injury.
- Close the incision with subcuticular or simple stitches.
- Apply a nonadhering dressing. Apply a well-padded volar splint, or, in selected patients, leave the wrist unsplinted.

POSTOPERATIVE CARE The splint and sutures may be removed early or at 10 to 14 days. Active finger motion is allowed early in the postoperative period. Forceful pulling with wrist flexion is discouraged for 4 to 6 weeks to allow maturation of soft-tissue healing. Progression of light activities of daily living is allowed at 2 to 3 weeks, and more strenuous activities are gradually added in the next 4 to 6 weeks.

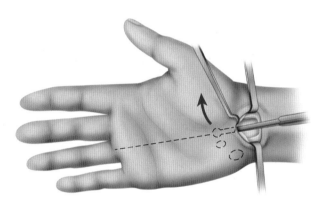

A

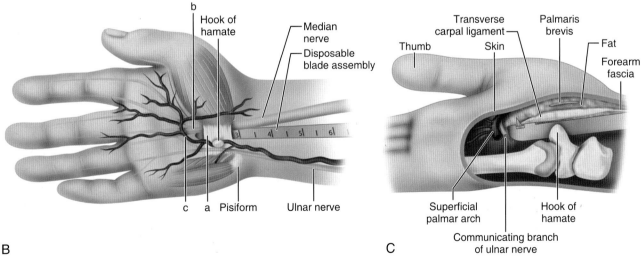

B

C

FIGURE 14.7 Agee technique. **A,** U-shaped flap elevated in palmar direction. Synovium elevator prepares wrist for optimal endoscopic view by separating synovium from deep side of ligament. **B,** Safe zone of blade elevation is triangle defined by ulnar half of distal edge of transverse carpal ligament *(a)* ulnar border of median nerve, *(b)* median nerve common digital branch to long/ring web space, and *(c)* superficial palmar arch. **C,** Longitudinal cross section through carpal tunnel depicts blade elevation in triangular safe zone.

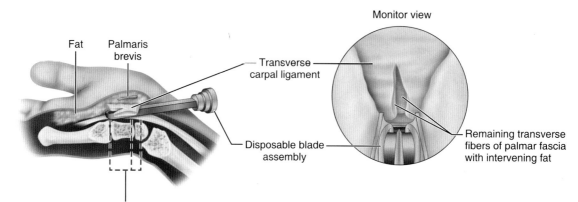

Fat   Palmaris brevis

Monitor view

Transverse carpal ligament

Disposable blade assembly

Remaining transverse fibers of palmar fascia with intervening fat

One half to two thirds of distal transverse carpal ligament is released completely before final pass to release remainder of ligament. This prevents fat located superficial to proximal portion of ligament from dropping into wound and compromising surgeon's endoscopic view of extent of ligament division.

D

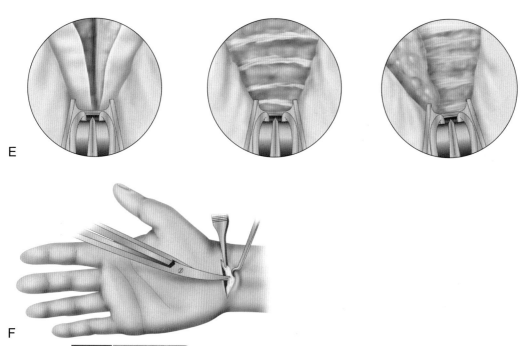

E

F

FIGURE 14.7, Cont'd   **D,** Initial release facilitates accurate viewing and division of ligament. **E,** Inspection of incised transverse carpal ligament in which left view depicts incomplete release as V-shaped defect, with superficial fibers of transverse carpal ligament remaining intact. Center view depicts complete release of ligament after reinsertion of blade assembly. Fat and transverse fibers of palmar fascia that remain palmar to divided ligament can be noted. View on right shows that rotating blade assembly approximately 20 degrees in either direction causes separated cut edges of ligament to fall into window. **F,** Tenotomy scissors used to release forearm fascia proximal to skin incision. (Redrawn from Agee JM, McCarroll HR, North ER: Endoscopic carpal tunnel release using the single proximal incision technique, *Hand Clin* 10:647–659, 1994.) **SEE TECHNIQUE 14.3.**

TWO-PORTAL ENDOSCOPIC CARPAL TUNNEL RELEASE

TECHNIQUE 14.4

(CHOW)

■ Perform the procedure using anesthesia believed most appropriate by the patient, surgeon, and anesthesiologist. Local anesthetic infiltration supplemented with intravenous sedation is commonly used, although regional block or even general anesthesia may be more suitable in some situations.

■ With the patient supine, place the hand and wrist on a hand table. The surgeon usually sits on the axillary side, and an assistant should be on the cephalad side of the upper extremity; however, the endoscopic dissection is proximal to distal and the surgeon may elect to be on the cephalad side depending on his or her hand dominance.

■ A well-padded pneumatic upper arm or forearm Esmarch tourniquet can be used.

■ At least one television monitor should be placed on the extremity side opposite the surgeon (toward the head of

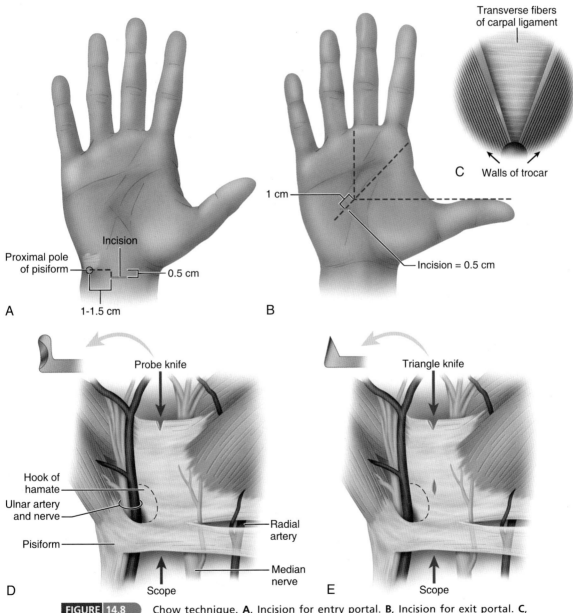

FIGURE 14.8 Chow technique. **A,** Incision for entry portal. **B,** Incision for exit portal. **C,** Following proximal portal dissection and placement of slotted cannula, transverse fibers of transverse carpal ligament are identified in its entirety, by camera placement in slotted cannula. **D,** First cut is made with probe knife, cutting distal to proximal, to release distal edge of carpal ligament. **E,** Second cut made with triangle knife, with cut made in midsection of transverse carpal ligament.

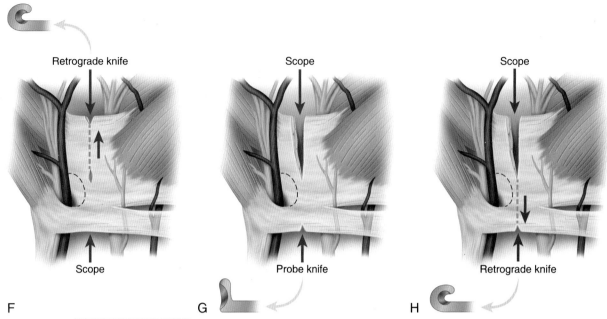

FIGURE 14.8, Cont'd **F,** Third cut made by placing retrograde knife in second cut and drawing it distally to join first cut. **G,** Proximal section of carpal ligament is identified, and proximal edge is released; probe knife is used to make fourth cut. **H,** Final cut is made by reinserting retrograde knife into midsection and drawing it proximally to complete release of carpal ligament. (Redrawn from Chow JCY: Endoscopic carpal tunnel release: two-portal technique, *Hand Clin* 10:637–646, 1994.)
SEE TECHNIQUE 14.4.

the table), or, as preferred by Chow, two monitors should be used, one for the surgeon and the other for the assistant.

- Define the entry and exit portals with a marking pen. Begin at the pisiform proximally and, depending on the size of the hand, draw a line extending 1.0 to 1.5 cm radially. From the end of this line, extend a second line 0.5 cm proximally. From the end of the second line, draw a third line extending about 1.0 cm radially. The third line is the entry portal (Fig. 14.8A). Passively, fully abduct the thumb. Draw a line along the distal border of the fully abducted thumb across the palm toward the ulnar border of the hand. Draw another line extending proximally from the web space between the long finger and the ring finger, intersecting the line drawn from the thumb. About 1.0 cm proximal to the intersection of these lines, draw a third line about 0.5 cm long transverse to the long axis of the hand (Fig. 14.8B).
- Make an incision in the previously marked entry portal just through the skin and bluntly dissect down to the transverse fibers of the forearm fascia. If a palmaris tendon is present, it should remain radial to the dissection field. Gently lift the forearm fascia and make a longitudinal incision through the fascia only. Only the distal 2.0 cm of forearm fascia typically needs to be released. Release the distal forearm fascia distally to the proximal edge of the transverse carpal ligament (TCL).
- Gently lift the distal edge of the entry portal incision with a small right-angle retractor, revealing the small space

between the TCL and the ulnar bursa. Bluntly dissect and develop the space between the TCL and the underlying bursa.
- Use the curved dissector obturator/slotted cannula assembly with the pointed side toward the TCL to enter the space and to push the bursal tissue free from the deep surface of the TCL.
- Use the curved dissector to feel the curved shape of the deep surface of the TCL. Move the dissector back and forth to feel the "washboard" effect of the transverse fibers of the TCL.
- Apply a lifting force to the dissector to test the tightness of the ligament and to ensure that the dissector is deep to the ligament, rather than in the tissues superficial to the ligament. Ensure that the dissector and trocar are oriented in the longitudinal axis of the forearm.
- Touch the hook of the hamate with the tip of the assembly; lift the patient's hand above the table, extending the wrist and fingers over the hand holder. Gently advance the slotted cannula assembly distally and direct it toward the exit portal. Palpate the tip of the assembly in the palm.
- Make a second small incision as marked for the exit portal in the palm. Pass the assembly through the exit portal, and secure the hand to the hand holder.
- Insert the endoscope at the proximal opening of the tube (Fig. 14.9).
- Examine the entire length of the slotted cannula opening to ensure that there is no other tissue between the slotted cannula and the TCL (Fig. 14.10A). If there is any doubt,

remove the tube and reevaluate for correct instrumentation placement.

- With the endoscope inserted from the proximal direction and remaining in the tube, insert a probe distally and identify the distal edge of the TCL (Figs. 14.8C and 14.10B).
- Use the probe knife to cut from distal to proximal to release the distal edge of the ligament (Fig. 14.8D).
- Insert the triangle knife to cut through the midsection of the TCL (Fig. 14.8E).
- Insert the retrograde knife and position it in the second cut. Draw the retrograde knife distally to join the first cut, completely releasing the distal half of the ligament (Fig. 14.8F).
- Remove the endoscope from the proximal opening of the open tube and insert the endoscope into the distal opening.
- Insert the instruments from the proximal opening.
- Identify the uncut proximal section of the ligament and use the probe knife to release the proximal edge (Fig. 14.8G). Draw the retrograde knife proximally to complete the release of the ligament (Fig. 14.8H).
- Choose the proper knife to make additional cuts to complete transection of the ligament as needed.

- Reinsert the trocar, and remove the slotted cannula from the hand.
- If a tourniquet is used, deflate it, and then ascertain hemostasis and that there is no pulsatile or excessive bleeding.
- Suture the incisions and apply a soft dressing.

POSTOPERATIVE CARE Active movement is encouraged immediately after surgery. The dressing usually is removed by the patient at home 2 to 3 days after the procedure, and sutures are removed at 10 to 14 days at the first postoperative visit. Direct pressure to the palm area and heavy lifting should be avoided for 2 to 3 weeks or until discomfort disappears.

UNRELIEVED OR RECURRENT CARPAL TUNNEL SYNDROME

The recurrence rate after primary carpal tunnel release is approximately 2%. Complications and failures are estimated to be 3% to 19%. Unrelieved symptoms may lead to repeat operation in 12% of patients. Because most patients obtain relief in the early postoperative period, it is difficult to attribute one anatomic cause to recurrent symptoms. Findings reported at reoperation include incomplete release of the TCL, re-formation of the flexor retinaculum, scarring in the carpal tunnel, median or palmar cutaneous neuroma, palmar cutaneous nerve entrapment, recurrent granulomatous or inflammatory tenosynovitis, and hypertrophic scar in the skin. Botte et al. categorized procedures for recurrent problems after carpal tunnel release as follows:

Incomplete ligament release: reexploration, rerelease of TCL, excision, release of re-formed retinaculum.

Fibrosis or painful scar: epineurolysis, local muscle flaps, local or remote free fat or radial forearm fascial grafts, excision, Z-plasty of painful scar, nerve wrapping or interposition materials.

Recurrent tenosynovitis: tenosynovectomy, appropriate medical management (appropriate antibiotics in patients with infectious granulomatous tenosynovitis from fungi or mycobacteria).

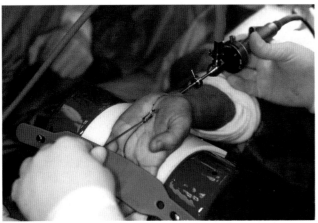

FIGURE 14.9 Intraoperative photo: Chow technique. **SEE TECHNIQUE 14.4.**

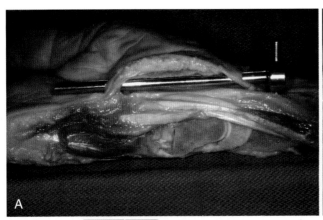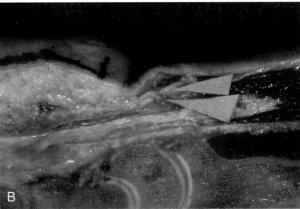

FIGURE 14.10 Cadaver photos: Chow technique. **A,** Longitudinal section showing slotted cannula beneath the transverse carpal ligament. **B,** Longitudinal wrist section showing two distinct layers of distal forearm fascia (*pink triangle* indicates superficial and *green triangle* indicates deep forearm fascia) which envelop palmaris longus when present.

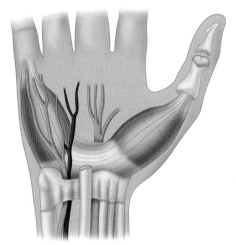

FIGURE **14.11** Anatomic relationships of structures within ulnar tunnel.

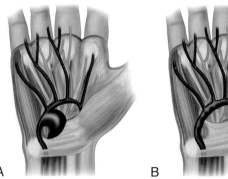
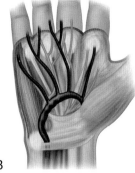

A   B

FIGURE **14.12**   Two types of traumatic aneurysms of ulnar artery in hand. **A,** Saccular "false" aneurysm arising from ulnar artery. **B,** "True" fusiform aneurysm of ulnar artery.

Patients with normal preoperative electrodiagnostic studies, patients who had filed for compensation, and patients with ulnar nerve symptoms have been reported to have results significantly worse than patients without these findings. Careful patient evaluation must be done when considering reoperation for recurrent symptoms and complications after initial carpal tunnel release. Temporary relief following a corticosteroid injection is a good prognostic sign when considering reoperation. Recurrent carpal tunnel syndrome was demonstrated more often in patients with diabetes by Zieske et al., and incomplete release of the flexor retinaculum and scarring of the median nerve were common intraoperative findings in all patients. Postoperative pinch strength, grip strength, and pain significantly improved from baseline, apart from strength measures in the recurrent group. Persistent symptoms and more than one prior carpal tunnel syndrome had higher odds of not changing or worsening postoperative pain. Higher preoperative pain, use of pain medication, and workers' compensation were significant predictors of higher postoperative average pain according to these authors. Our experience has been similar; however, we find the TCL that reforms indistinguishable from the native ligament and thus, determination of incomplete release is not possible. Moreover, neural adhesion lysis and early nerve gliding exercises are essential, and rarely do we find synovial or hypothenar fat pad flaps necessary in the management of these problematic cases.

ULNAR TUNNEL SYNDROME

Ulnar tunnel syndrome results from compression of the ulnar nerve within a tight triangular fibroosseous Guyon's tunnel or canal. The walls of the tunnel consist of the superficial TCL anteriorly, the deep TCL posteriorly, and the pisiform bone and pisohamate ligament medially (Fig. 14.11). Similar to the median nerve within the carpal tunnel, the ulnar nerve is subject to compression within this tunnel. Compared with carpal tunnel syndrome, ulnar tunnel syndrome is much less common because the space occupied by the ulnar nerve at the wrist is much more yielding. The more common location of ulnar nerve constriction is at the elbow. When both volar and dorsal sensory complaints are present, the ulnar nerve involvement usually is proximal to the dorsal sensory branch

division from the parent nerve, which is at least 8.0 cm proximal to the pisiform.

The exact level of compression determines whether symptoms are motor or sensory or both. Compression just distal to the tunnel affects the deep branch of the nerve that supplies most of the intrinsic muscles. A space-occupying lesion, such as a ganglion or tumor, can cause compression in this area. True or false aneurysm of the ulnar artery (Fig. 14.12), thrombosis of the ulnar artery, or fracture of the hamate with hemorrhage may be the cause of pressure on the ulnar nerve. Other reported causes are lipoma and aberrant muscles. Occasionally in rheumatoid disease, carpal tunnel and ulnar tunnel syndromes develop in the same hand. In the differential diagnosis, herniation of a cervical disc, thoracic outlet syndrome, and peripheral neuropathy must be considered. Treatment consists of exploration of the ulnar nerve at the wrist and removal of any cause of compression. Should the ulnar artery be occluded for several millimeters, Raynaud syndrome may be produced in the ulnar three digits because the sympathetic nerve fibers to these digits pass along the ulnar artery.

Segmental resection of the occluded section and replacement with a vein graft is the preferred procedure when it is feasible. Usually symptoms are relieved, and weakened or atrophic intrinsic muscles may recover in 3 to 12 months after surgery. For the technique of exploration, see the approach described for repair of the deep branch of the ulnar nerve (see chapter 5).

CUBITAL TUNNEL SYNDROME AND TARDY ULNAR NERVE PALSY

The prevalence of cubital tunnel syndrome in the United States population is between 1.8% and 5.9% according to the most recent population study. Treatment of refractory tardy ulnar nerve palsy may require removal of the nerve from its groove, neurolysis if necessary, and anterior transposition of the nerve to the flexor surface of the elbow. Conservative treatment for this syndrome should be attempted before surgical treatment. The severity of cubital tunnel syndrome was divided into three categories by McGowan and later revised by Dellon. *Mild dysfunction* implies intermittent paresthesias and subjective weakness; *moderate dysfunction* presents as intermittent paresthesias and measurable weakness; and *severe dysfunction* is characterized by persistent paresthesias and measurable weakness. In mild-to-moderate cubital tunnel syndrome, patients are instructed to avoid prolonged elbow flexion in the workplace and are given elbow extension splints for sleeping. The splint should not be fitted with the forearm held in pronation because this may aggravate the symptoms. Towels or pillows secured around the elbow may limit elbow flexion adequately during sleep. Conservative treatment usually is attempted for 3 months before surgical treatment is considered. Svernlöv reported improvement in 89.5% of patients with mild-to-moderate cubital tunnel syndrome who were treated conservatively with elbow extension splinting, patient education, and activity modification. Decompression is recommended for some moderate and severe involvement.

The demographics of patients who required operative release of the carpal tunnel or cubital tunnel were compared by Zhang et al. The two groups were found to be dissimilar, with the exception of those with diabetes. Patients with cubital tunnel release often had a history of trauma to the anatomic site of the cubital tunnel. Patients with carpal tunnel release were older and more often female, had higher body mass indexes, and had concomitant hand tendinopathies. The diabetic population was found to have both procedures more often. Other studies have shown male gender to be a risk factor for cubital tunnel syndrome.

Before surgical treatment, careful preoperative evaluation and EMG are recommended. The surgical treatment of cubital tunnel syndrome includes simple decompression (either open or endoscopically), medial epicondylectomy, and anterior transposition of the ulnar nerve into a subcutaneous, intramuscular, or submuscular bed. Taniguchi et al. reported good-to-excellent results in 14 of 17 patients treated with simple decompression through a small incision. Goldfarb et al. reported that only 7% of 56 patients had recurrent symptoms postoperatively.

More recently, prospective randomized studies have shown that in situ decompression of the ulnar nerve is as effective as anterior transposition. Staples et al., in a randomized level 2 prospective cohort study comparing early morbidity with in situ cubital tunnel release to that with anterior subcutaneous transposition of the ulnar nerve, found that prior to 8 weeks after surgery patients with transposed nerves had greater narcotic consumption, scar sensitivity, and poorer patient-rated elbow evaluation; however, the differences in morbidity between the two cohorts was not significant after 8 weeks, indicating only short-term morbidity for either procedure. The authors also found that in situ decompression had a 11% occurrence of postoperative hematoma, none of which required operative intervention. The transposition group had a 15% frequency of hematoma, only one of which required operative debridement. In contrast, a retrospective study comparing in situ release with transposition found a complication rate of 11% for transposition and a 2.5% rate for in situ release. The overall rate of secondary surgery for both in situ release and transposition of the ulnar nerve together was 6%.

The subluxated or "perched" ulnar nerve with elbow flexion after in situ release should be transposed to prevent symptomatic instability. This is required in 21% to 34% of in situ releases and most often in younger males. In a retrospective review of 67 in situ releases, Henn et al. found that 45% were unstable and required transposition. At 5 years after surgery patients with instability that required transposition were less likely to have persistent symptoms and more likely to have a lower Disabilities

of the Arm, Shoulder, and Hand (DASH) score than the stable cohort who had simple in situ release.

Good results of 45% to 93% have been reported after medial epicondylectomy, although persistent medial elbow pain has been reported in up to 45% of patients 6 months after surgery. In comparing minimal medial epicondylectomy with partial medial epicondylectomy, Amako et al. found no difference in improvement and recommended the minimal epicondylectomy technique. Good results also have been reported in ulnar neuropathies treated by anterior nerve transposition and construction of a fasciodermal sling from the antebrachial fascia overlying the flexor pronator muscles.

No significant differences in results have been reported after release of the cubital tunnel, subcutaneous anterior transposition, or submuscular anterior transposition. The current trend is to perform a simple or in situ decompression, taking care to release any and all constricting tissue, and perform transpositions only in patients who have subluxation or develop recurrent symptoms. Revision surgery after simple decompression is more common in patients with a previous elbow fracture or dislocation, younger patients (<50 years old), tobacco users, and patients having surgery for mild symptoms.

IN SITU DECOMPRESSION OF THE ULNAR NERVE

TECHNIQUE 14.5

- With the elbow flexed and the arm abducted and externally rotated, make a 3- to 5-cm incision along the course of the ulnar nerve between the medial epicondyle and the olecranon.
- Spread the subcutaneous tissues, and develop the avascular plane overlying the fascia. Take care to avoid damaging the medial antebrachial cutaneous nerve that lies along the fascia usually about 3 cm distal to the medial epicondyle. Use right-angle retractors to carefully elevate the subcutaneous tissue and elevate cutaneous nerves off the fascia.
- Identify the thickened fascia between the medial epicondyle and olecranon known as Osbourne's ligament, and incise the fascia overlying the ulnar nerve proximally for a distance of 8 to 9 cm and distally including the deep and superficial fascia between the two heads of the flexor carpi ulnaris. Leave the nerve undisturbed in its soft-tissue bed to avoid iatrogenic anterior subluxation.
- Dissect proximally to release the arcade of Struthers and the medial intermuscular septum, and pass a finger proximally along the nerve 5 to 8 cm to ensure no constricting bands. Protect the superior ulnar collateral artery with the nerve when dissecting proximally to limit the risk of nerve infarction.
- Reinspect carefully for any remaining areas of compression. Flex the elbow and make certain that the nerve does not subluxate across the medial epicondyle. If subluxation occurs, a formal anterior transposition is recommended.
- Obtain careful hemostasis and close the incision. A soft dressing is applied, and immediate elbow motion is allowed to prevent neural adhesions.

ENDOSCOPIC DECOMPRESSION OF THE ULNAR NERVE

Endoscopic decompression of the ulnar nerve at the elbow was first described by Tsai in 1995 and has since grown in popularity. Results have been comparable to open in situ decompression. The advantages reported are a smaller skin incision with less soft-tissue dissection, perhaps resulting in less chance of incisional tenderness and damage to the medial antebrachial cutaneous nerve. A nonrandomized level III study reported a 60% (9 of 15) patient satisfaction rate with the open in situ decompression compared with a 79% (15 of 19) rate in the endoscopic group. Dützmann et al. found no significant differences in long-term outcomes after open and retractor-endoscopic in situ decompression of the ulnar nerve in cubital tunnel syndrome. The short-term results were significantly better with endoscopic surgery. A double-blind, prospective randomized controlled study found equivalent outcomes at 2 years in endoscopic and "open" releases. Two meta-analysis, one by Buchanan et al. of 655 patients with endoscopic or situ decompression showed no significant differences in terms of outcomes (Bishop score) or visual analog scores between the two treatment groups. The second meta-analysis by Aldekhayel et al. also found no significant difference between the two treatments in terms of complications, outcomes and reoperation rates.

We have no experience with this technique.

ENDOSCOPIC CUBITAL TUNNEL RELEASE

TECHNIQUE 14.6

(COBB)
- Place the patient supine, with the shoulder abducted and externally rotated and the arm on an arm table. Place a tourniquet high on the brachium so as not to interfere with the surgical release. Elevate the arm off the table sufficiently to facilitate instrumentation of the cubital tunnel (Fig. 14.13A).
- After exsanguination and elevation of the tourniquet, make a 2-cm incision through the skin over the cubital tunnel, just posterior to the medial epicondyle. Carry the dissection down with scissors to the medial epicondyle, protecting the superficial nerves as they are encountered. Avoid violating the deep fascia during the initial exposure.
- Identify the medial epicondyle. With blunt scissors, dissect directly down to the deep fascia then develop the space between the deep adipose tissue and deep fascia. Dissect the adipose tissue and superficial nerves off the deep fascia both proximally and distally over the course of the ulnar nerve. During this portion of the exposure, do not develop multiple layers through the adipose tissue or expose the ulnar nerve.
- Identify the ulnar nerve by palpation directly posterior to the medial epicondyle, and make an incision through the roof of the canal for exposure. The opening in the cubital tunnel should be sufficient to allow instrumentation to be placed without binding. If the anconeus epitrochlearis muscle is encountered, incise it directly over the cubital tunnel.
- Insert a spatula into the space between the ulnar nerve and the roof of the canal proximally and distally to confirm the course of the ulnar nerve and that adipose tissue and superficial nerves have been sufficiently elevated (Fig. 14.13B).
- Insert a cannula/trocar into the canal and advance it proximally between the superficial ulnar nerve and the roof of the canal. The attached retractor slides on the external surface of the fascia, atraumatically elevating the superficial nerves (Fig. 14.13C). If resistance is encountered, remove the instrumentation and confirm that the superficial tissue is sufficiently elevated off the fascia.
- Once the cannula/trocar has been placed, remove the trocar and place the scope initially between the cannula and retractor to confirm that no superficial nerves are in the way. Place the scope into the cannula and turn it to view the inferior slots so the ulnar nerve can be identified throughout the entire course of the cannula (Fig. 14.13D).
- After the nerve has been clearly identified, divide the fascia (roof of the canal) with the blade along the superior slot of the cannula (Fig. 14.13E and inset). Check for completeness of the release by pulling the cannula back on the scope. If the release cannot be confirmed in this manner, place a narrow retractor, exposing the nerve, and hold the endoscope under the retractor to view the nerve.
- Next, place the cannula/trocar into the canal and advance it distally using the same technique as just described. The flexor pronator mass, which can be seen through the superior slot of the cannula, can be released; however, this is not necessary and results in unnecessary bleeding.
- Deflate the tourniquet and apply pressure. With the retractor in place, view the surgical field both proximally and distally with the endoscope to confirm complete release and hemostasis. Bipolar cautery can be used if necessary.
- Place a 20-gauge angiocatheter through the skin and into the wound and close the wound with subcuticular absorbable sutures. Infiltrate 15 to 20 mL of 0.5% bupivacaine and epinephrine and then remove the angiocatheter and apply a compressive dressing.

POSTOPERATIVE CARE Patients are instructed on gentle range of motion, with the expectation that full range of motion will be obtained within 5 to 7 days. They may debulk the dressing to facilitate full motion.

MEDIAL EPICONDYLECTOMY

TECHNIQUE 14.7

- Make an 8-cm skin incision along the course of the ulnar nerve centered over the posterior aspect of the medial epicondyle.

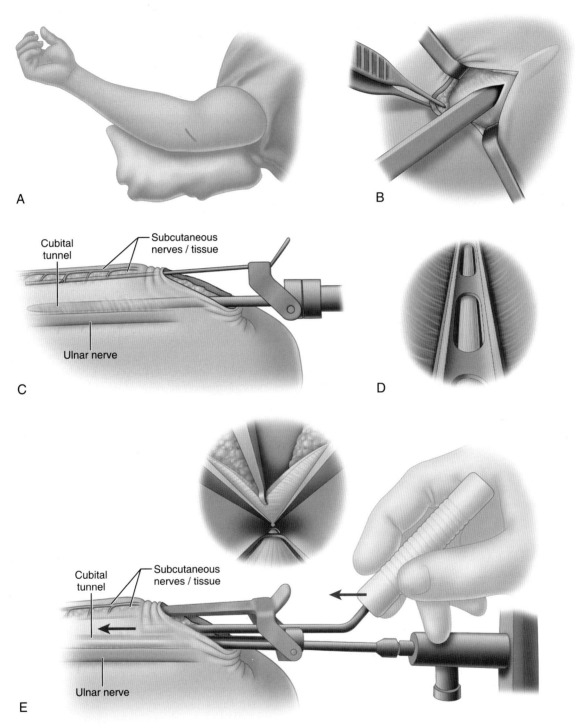

FIGURE 14.13 Endoscopic cubital tunnel release. **A,** Incision. **B,** Spatula used to open space between ulnar nerve and roof of canal (fascia). **C,** Trocar/cannula placed into canal. Attached retractor slides on external surface of fascia elevating superficial nerves. **D,** Ulnar nerve seen through inferior slots of cannula. **E,** Roof of canal (fascia) is divided with blade along superior slot of cannula. Inset shows arthroscopic view of ulnar nerve as fascia is being divided through superior slot. **SEE TECHNIQUE 14.6.**

- Carry the incision to the deep fascia, carefully protecting the medial brachial and antebrachial cutaneous nerves (Fig. 14.14A).
- Expose the medial epicondyle subperiosteally, incising the common flexor-pronator origin but protecting the ulnar collateral ligament.
- Identify and retract the ulnar nerve posteriorly during exposure of the medial epicondyle, taking care to protect the mesoneurium.
- With an osteotome or rongeur, remove the entire medial epicondyle and a portion of the supracondylar ridge to release the insertion of the medial intermuscular septum (Fig. 14.14B).
- Expose and excise the medial intermuscular septum proximally to the insertion of the coracobrachialis muscle, releasing the arcade of Struthers as a potential area of compression.
- Using a bone rasp, ensure that no bony ridges remain in the area of the osteotomy.
- Reattach the periosteum to the common flexor-pronator tendon to separate the raw cancellous surface from the ulnar nerve.

- Allow the ulnar nerve to seek its own position adjacent to the medial humeral condyle.
- Deflate the tourniquet to allow adequate hemostasis before routine closure of the subcutaneous tissues and skin.

POSTOPERATIVE CARE The wound is protected in a soft bulky dressing, and early range of motion is allowed as tolerated.

TRANSPOSITION OF THE ULNAR NERVE

TECHNIQUE 14.8

- With the arm abducted and externally rotated, make an incision on the posteromedial surface of the elbow beginning 7 cm proximal to the epicondyle, passing distally anterior to the epicondyle, and proceeding farther distally in line with the course of the nerve (Fig. 14.15A).
- Reflect the anterior skin flap to expose the common origin of the flexor muscles. Avoid damaging the medial antebrachial cutaneous nerve by keeping the dissection just superficial to the flexor-pronator fascia.
- Identify the ulnar nerve in its groove posterior to the medial epicondyle and free it of soft tissues. Free the flexor carpi ulnaris from its humeral origin on the epicondyle to expose the nerve further.
- Identify its branches to the flexor profundus and flexor carpi ulnaris, and carefully dissect them intraneurally up the nerve.

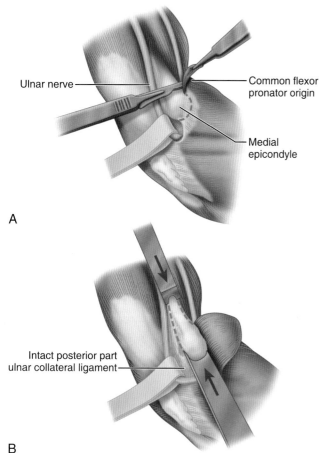

A

B

FIGURE 14.14   Technique of medial epicondylectomy for treatment of cubital tunnel syndrome (see text). **A,** Ulnar nerve is protected, and common flexor pronator origin is elevated from medial epicondyle. **B,** Guide for plane of osteotomy is medial border of trochlea; sharp posterior edge of osteotomy must be smoothed and rounded. **SEE TECHNIQUE 14.7.**

Ulnar nerve

Common flexor pronator origin

Medial epicondyle

Intact posterior part ulnar collateral ligament

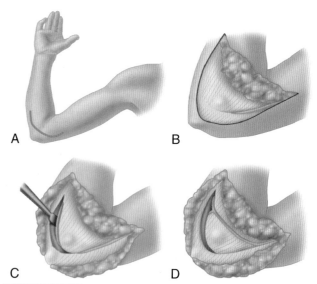

A   **B**

C   **D**

FIGURE 14.15   Technique of transposing ulnar nerve for tardy ulnar nerve palsy. **A,** Skin incision. **B** and **C,** Exposing and freeing of nerve. It is freed from scar tissue posterior to medial epicondyle and from beneath tendinous arch between humeral and ulnar heads of the flexor carpi ulnaris. **D,** Nerve has been transposed anteriorly. **SEE TECHNIQUE 14.8.**

- Dissect any fibrous tissue or callus from the area adjacent to the groove, and remove the nerve (Fig. 14.15B,C).
- Carry out a neurolysis or endoneurolysis as indicated if there is extensive scarring; keep the superior ulnar collateral artery with the nerve as far distal as possible. It often requires division at the level of just distal to the medial epicondyle.
- Draw the nerve over the epicondyle to the anterior surface of the elbow, and place it on the surface of the fascia of the flexor-pronator group beneath the thick fat in this region (Fig. 14.15D).
- Excise the medial intermuscular septum and any other tendinous bands that may constrict or otherwise injure the transposed nerve. Ensure that the intermuscular septum is excised as far proximally as the arcade of Struthers, where the ulnar nerve passes from the anterior to the posterior compartment. Obtain good hemostasis here as there are large veins anterior and piercing the septum in the supracondylar area.
- Place a few interrupted sutures through the fascia and subcutaneous fat medial to the nerve to keep the nerve from slipping back posterior to the epicondyle.
- The tourniquet should be deflated and hemostasis achieved before closure because postoperative hematoma may be significant in this area.
- If an anterior submuscular transfer is preferred, place a hemostat beneath the superficial head of the pronator teres, the flexor carpi radialis, the palmaris longus, and the superficial head of the flexor carpi ulnaris, being certain not to include the median nerve.
- Sharply divide the tendinous origin of the medial epicondyle, and retract the flexor mass distally, carefully protecting the small motor branches from the median and ulnar nerves (Fig. 14.16).
- After placing the ulnar nerve deep to the flexor mass, repair the tendinous origin to the medial epicondyle with a nonabsorbable suture.
- As an alternative, divide the medial epicondyle, transpose the ulnar nerve anterior to the elbow near the median nerve, and reattach the epicondyle.

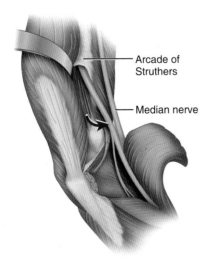

FIGURE 14.16 Anterior submuscular transposition of ulnar nerve. **SEE TECHNIQUE 14.8.**

Arcade of Struthers

Median nerve

POSTOPERATIVE CARE The elbow is immobilized at a 90-degree angle for 3 weeks. Physical therapy is started and continued to prevent secondary changes in the muscles of the hand. Appropriate splinting is continued until sufficient function has returned to allow the patient to be free of the brace or splint.

REVISION CUBITAL TUNNEL SURGERY

Revision surgery for cubital tunnel release spans a wide range of treatment. If the nerve was not transposed, then transposition is indicated; however, the literature is unclear as to whether a subcutaneous, submuscular, or intramuscular transposition is best. Verveld et al. described a pedicled adipofascial flap used to wrap the nerve and compared it to anterior transposition; both treatments had high (>95%) good-to-excellent outcome scores and symptom improvement. Aleem et al. compared primary with revision cubital tunnel release and found that at 2 years' follow-up, despite 79% of revision patients reporting symptomatic improvement, they also reported worse outcomes on all measured standardized questionnaires compared with primary patients. Additionally, 21% of patients with revision surgery had worsening of their McGowan grade. Complete symptomatic resolution after revision cubital tunnel release is unlikely, and this should be discussed with the patient before surgery.

PRONATOR SYNDROME AND ANTERIOR INTEROSSEOUS SYNDROME

Median nerve deficits, as seen in the pronator syndrome, may result from compression of the nerve at the pronator teres, the lacertus fibrosus, or the fibrous flexor digitorum sublimis arch or from anomalies including a hypertrophic pronator teres, a high origin of the pronator teres, fibrous bands within the pronator teres, the median nerve passing posterior to both heads of the pronator teres, or an accessory tendinous arch of the flexor carpi radialis arising from the ulna. The anterior interosseous nerve may be injured in fractures and lacerations or may be compressed or entrapped by any of the following: the tendinous origins of the flexor digitorum sublimis or the pronator teres, variant muscles such as the palmaris profundus and flexor carpi radialis brevis, accessory muscle slips and tendons from the flexor digitorum sublimis to the flexor pollicis longus, an accessory head of the flexor pollicis longus (Gantzer's muscle), an aberrant radial artery, thrombosis of the ulnar collateral vessels, enlargement of the bicipital bursa, or a Volkmann ischemic contracture. For detailed discussions of these particular nerve compressions, the reader is referred to the extensive reports by Spinner and to the references at the end of the chapter.

At the wrist, the median nerve may be injured by fractures of the distal radius and by fractures and dislocations of the carpal bones.

EXAMINATION

The muscles of the forearm and hand supplied by the median nerve that can be tested with relative accuracy are the pronator teres, flexor carpi radialis, flexor digitorum profundus (index), flexor pollicis longus, flexor digitorum sublimis, and abductor pollicis brevis. Substitution movements caused by action of intact muscles may cause confusion during the examination. The works of Sunderland provide an excellent review of these movements and the methods of recognizing and preventing them. Usually, if the forearm can be actively maintained in pronation against resistance, the pronator teres is intact. If the wrist can be actively maintained in flexion, and a contracting flexor carpi radialis is palpated, this muscle is intact. Similarly, if the interphalangeal joint of the thumb can be maintained in flexion against resistance with the wrist in the neutral position and the thumb adducted, the flexor pollicis longus is functioning. The flexor digitorum sublimis to each finger is examined separately, and the remaining fingers are held in full passive extension. Although opposition of the thumb can be difficult to confirm, if the thumb can be actively maintained in palmar abduction and a contracting abductor pollicis brevis is palpated, this muscle is functioning. The lumbricals cannot be discretely tested because they cannot be palpated and because their function may be confused with that of the interosseous muscles.

When examining a patient with suspected pronator teres syndrome, three resistive tests have been found helpful: (1) production of symptoms with pronation of the forearm against resistance with the elbow flexed and gradually extended localizes the lesion to the pronator teres, (2) independent flexion of the flexor sublimis of the long finger with reproduction of paresthesias or numbness in the radial three and a half fingers localizes the entrapment level at the fibrous arcade of the flexor sublimis, and (3) flexion-supination of the elbow against resistance shows the presence or absence of entrapment of the nerve by the lacertus fibrosus. To perform the pronator compression test, the examiner pushes with the thumb just proximal and lateral to the proximal edge of the pronator teres muscle. Pain and paresthesias in the median nerve distribution within 30 seconds are considered a positive test. Other findings suggesting pronator teres syndrome include tenderness, firmness, or apparent enlargement of the pronator teres; a positive Tinel sign on percussion of the proximal muscle mass; variable weakness in the median-innervated extrinsics and intrinsics; and, occasionally, a depression in the contour of the forearm superficial to the lacertus fibrosus. Nerve conduction studies often are found to be normal in pronator teres syndrome.

The anterior interosseous syndrome can cause various signs and symptoms. Typically, the patient has pain in the proximal forearm lasting for several hours and is found to have weakness or paralysis of the flexor pollicis longus, the flexor digitorum profundus to the index and long fingers, and the pronator quadratus. When the patient attempts to pinch, active flexion of the distal phalanx of the index finger is impossible. Variations from these signs and symptoms usually result from atypical patterns of innervation. If all of the flexor digitorum profundus muscles are supplied by the anterior interosseous nerve, all of these muscles are weak or paralyzed. Conversely, if innervation overlaps and the ulnar nerve supplies the flexor digitorum profundus to the long finger, this finger is spared. EMG, the ninhydrin print test, and clinical examination help to differentiate the syndromes. In well-established lesions, atrophy of the forearm flexor mass and of the thenar muscles may be seen.

TREATMENT

Surgical exploration and decompression of the median nerve for refractory pronator teres syndrome, as reported by Hartz

et al. and by Johnson, Spinner, and Shrewsbury, has been successful in relieving symptoms in 80% to 92% of patients. Some persistence of symptoms has been reported in 66% of patients. In patients who have symptoms of carpal tunnel syndrome and pronator teres syndrome, particular attention should be paid to the nerve conduction studies during preoperative planning. If the nerve conduction test is positive for carpal tunnel syndrome, we agree in recommending carpal tunnel release in anticipation that the proximal symptoms will resolve. If the nerve conduction test is negative for carpal tunnel syndrome, we recommend proximal median nerve exploration and proximal decompression as the initial procedure of choice. For the anterior interosseous syndrome, Spinner recommended the following plan. If the onset of paralysis has been spontaneous, the initial treatment is nonoperative. Surgical exploration is indicated in the absence of clinical or EMG improvement after 12 weeks. If an anterior interosseous nerve injury is caused by a penetrating wound, primary repair is recommended. In irreparable injury to the nerve, tendon transfers are indicated (see chapter 5).

APPROACH TO THE MEDIAN NERVE

TECHNIQUE 14.9

- To expose the median nerve, use the same approach as that for the ulnar nerve in the arm and at the elbow and avoid crossing the folds of the antecubital fossa (Fig. 14.17).
- To expose the median nerve in the forearm, continue the incision from the medial epicondyle onto the volar aspect of the forearm and distally over the course of the nerve. In approaching the wrist, curve it toward the radial side (or if exploration of the median and ulnar nerves is indicated, curve it toward the ulnar side). As the flexor creases of the wrist are reached, return the incision along one of them to the middle of the wrist. If the nerve is to be explored distal to the wrist, extend the incision down the thenar crease.
- Deepen the incision through the fascia along the course of the nerve. To accomplish this at the elbow, undermine the skin flap widely.

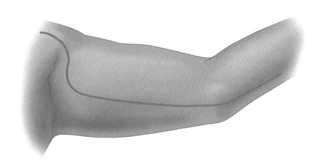

FIGURE 14.17 Skin incision for exploration of median and ulnar nerves in upper arm. **SEE TECHNIQUE 14.9.**

- In the arm, retract the brachial artery and vein medially to expose the nerve on the lateral aspect of the neurovascular bundle.
- At the junction of the middle and distal thirds of the arm, the nerve crosses to the medial side of the artery, usually coursing posteriorly, although occasionally anteriorly to it.
- The nerve enters the forearm beneath the lacertus fibrosus medial to the artery, and then courses between the two heads of the pronator teres and continues distally in the forearm beneath the flexor sublimis, lying on the flexor profundus. Approaching the wrist, the nerve becomes more superficial, lies beneath the tendon of the flexor carpi radialis, and is easily found if approached between this tendon and that of the palmaris longus.
- At the elbow, expose the nerve by incising the fibers of the lacertus fibrosus at its attachment to the fascia over the pronator-flexor group.
- Dissect the fascia radially from this group of muscles and incise it distally and radially along the proximal border of the pronator teres and then distally across this muscle and along the medial side of the flexor carpi radialis. The pronator teres may be widely mobilized and separated from the flexor carpi radialis, permitting easy exposure of the nerve and making closure easier later.
- Expose the nerve where it emerges from beneath the fibers of the flexor digitorum sublimis. Trace the nerve proximally by retracting the flexor carpi radialis laterally and the pronator proximally and by separating the fibers of the flexor digitorum sublimis. In this way, the nerve can be exposed over its entire course.
- As an alternative, cut the radial origin of the flexor digitorum sublimis in line with the nerve and sever the pronator teres by a Z-shaped incision near its insertion (Fig. 14.18).
- The median nerve gives off no branches in the upper arm.
- The branches to the pronator teres and flexor carpi radialis emerge as the nerve courses beneath the lacertus fibro-

sus. Usually, two branches go to the pronator: one to the superficial head and one to the deep head. Also, several branches go to the flexor carpi radialis and palmaris longus, one to the flexor sublimis, and one to the profundus.
- The anterior interosseous nerve emerges from the posteromedial side of the nerve after passing through the two heads of the pronator teres and supplies the flexor pollicis longus, the radial half of the flexor profundus, and the pronator quadratus. Farther distally, several more branches are given off to the flexor digitorum sublimis. No other significant branches are given off until the nerve enters the hand.
- When exposure of the anterior interosseous nerve deep to the pronator teres is required, or when anterior transposition of the median nerve is preferred, a method whereby the pronator teres insertion is released and is repaired by Z-plasty or a tongue-in-groove suture after the median nerve has been transposed is suitable.
- In decompressing the median nerve for pronator teres syndrome, explore and release all points of potential compression.
- If a ligament of Struthers is encountered, excise it from its origin on the supracondylar process to its insertion on the medial epicondyle.
- Divide the lacertus fibrosus and trace the median nerve through the two heads of the pronator teres.
- Release any intermuscular tendinous bands within or under the pronator and fascial constricting bands between the superficial and deep heads of the muscle.
- If necessary, divide the deep head of the pronator teres.
- Alternatively, the superficial head of the pronator teres can be excised from its radial insertion, although this rarely is necessary in our experience.
- Retract the superficial head of the pronator teres anteriorly, distally, and ulnarward to allow exploration of the nerve into the flexor digitorum sublimis.
- Divide the aponeurotic arch, which commonly is encountered as the median nerve enters the sublimis muscle.
- If Gantzer's muscle is encountered, resect any proximal fibrous bands that may be compressing the median nerve.

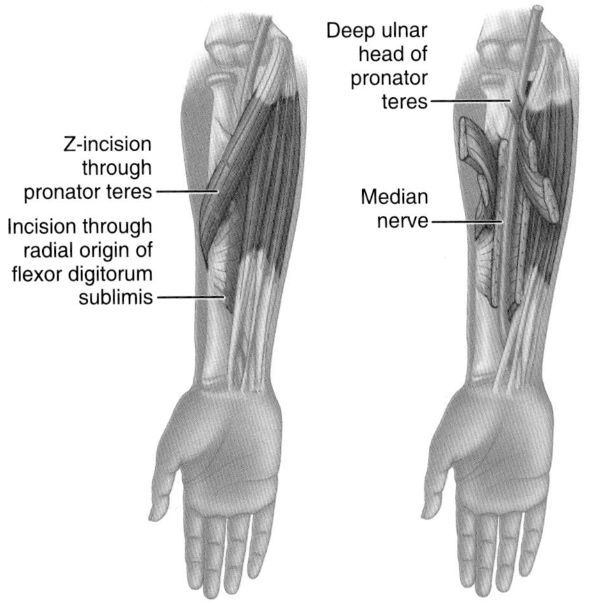

FIGURE 14.18 Alternative method of exposing median nerve throughout forearm (see text). **SEE TECHNIQUE 14.9.**

Labels: Z-incision through pronator teres; Incision through radial origin of flexor digitorum sublimis; Deep ulnar head of pronator teres; Median nerve

RADIAL TUNNEL SYNDROME

Entrapment syndromes of the radial nerve may develop when the nerve or one of its branches is compressed at some point along its course. Compression of the radial nerve in the arm may be caused by the fibrous arch of the lateral head of the triceps muscle. The posterior interosseous nerve may be compressed by the fibrous arcade of Frohse, fracture-dislocations or dislocations of the elbow, fractures of the forearm, Volkmann ischemic contracture, neoplasms, enlarged bursae, aneurysms, or rheumatoid synovitis of the elbow. According to Spinner, posterior interosseous nerve entrapment is of two types. In one type, all the muscles supplied by the nerve are completely paralyzed; these include the extensor digitorum communis, extensor indicis proprius, extensor digiti quinti, extensor carpi ulnaris, abductor pollicis longus, and extensor pollicis brevis. In the second type, only one or a few of these muscles are paralyzed. Entrapment of the posterior interosseous nerve can cause chronic and refractory tennis elbow. Such entrapment is called radial tunnel syndrome and can occur at four potentially compressive anatomic structures: (1) the origin of the extensor carpi radialis brevis, (2) adhesions around the radial head, (3) the radial recurrent arterial fan, and (4) the arcade of Frohse as the posterior interosseous nerve enters the supinator. Occasionally, compression occurs at the distal border of the supinator as the nerve exits. Pain in the region of the radial nerve beneath the extensor mass at and just distal to the radial head, pain on resistance to supination of the forearm, and electrodiagnostic measures aid in differentiating this particular type of tennis elbow. When symptoms and signs of radial nerve entrapment in the arm develop only after muscular effort, spontaneous recovery can be anticipated. Marchese et al. evaluated the usefulness of a single corticosteroid injection in those patients with radial tunnel syndrome. Thirty-five patients completed 1-year follow-up, and a minimal clinically important difference in quick DASH was achieved in 57% of subjects; however, 23% failed nonoperative treatment and required surgery. Corticosteroid injection thus is a potential option for conservative treatment of radial tunnel syndrome. When entrapment is caused by other space occupying conditions; however, especially in the forearm, surgical exploration and decompression of the nerve (Fig. 14.19) usually are beneficial.

Compression of the superficial radial nerve causes pain in the forearm and sensory impairment on the dorsum of the thumb. The nerve may be caught in scar tissue at the wrist after surgery or trauma. Constricting jewelry also has been cited as a potential cause of entrapment here.

After repair of the radial nerve, the prognosis for regeneration is more favorable than for any other major nerve in the upper extremity, primarily because it is predominantly a motor nerve and secondarily because the muscles innervated by it are not involved in the finer movements of the fingers and hand.

EXAMINATION

The following muscles supplied by the radial nerve can be tested accurately because their bellies or tendons or both can be palpated: the triceps brachii, brachioradialis, extensor carpi radialis, extensor digitorum communis, extensor carpi ulnaris, abductor pollicis longus, and extensor pollicis longus. Injury to this nerve results in inability to extend the elbow or supinate the forearm and in a typical wristdrop. An inexperienced examiner often may be misled by the patient's ability to extend the wrist merely by flexing the fingers. The examiner should be discriminating because analysis of movements often may result in error in evaluating the function of a nerve. The triceps is not seriously affected by injuries of the nerve at the level of the middle of the humerus or distally. In injuries of the nerve at its bifurcation into the deep and superficial branches, the brachioradialis and the extensor carpi radialis longus continue to function; the arm can be supinated, and the wrist can be extended. The nerve is especially susceptible to electrical stimulation in situ just proximal to the elbow; elsewhere this is difficult, and the results are uncertain.

Sensory examination is relatively unimportant, even when the nerve is divided in the axilla, because usually there is no autonomous zone. When present, the autonomous zone usually is over the first dorsal interosseous muscle, between the first and second metacarpals. It usually is too inconsistent to afford more than confirmatory evidence of complete interruption of the nerve proximal to its bifurcation at the elbow.

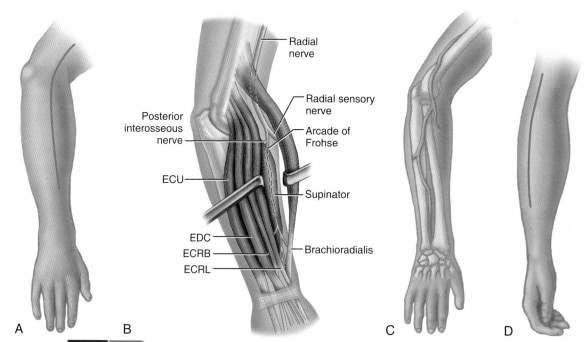

FIGURE 14.19 Exposure of posterior interosseous branch of the radial nerve for repair or decompression in radial tunnel syndrome. **A,** Line of incision, forearm prone, elbow flexed. **B,** Nerve exposed. **C,** Diagram of course of nerve with arm in position A. **D,** Line of incision, elbow extended. ECU, extensor carpi ulnaris; ECRB, extensor carpi radialis brevis; ECRL, extensor carpi radialis longus; EDC, extensor digitorum communis.

TREATMENT

APPROACH TO THE RADIAL NERVE

TECHNIQUE 14.10

- Expose the radial nerve in the axilla and proximal third of the arm by the usual incision for the distal part of the brachial plexus (Fig. 14.20) and carry this incision distally in the arm a little more posteriorly than is necessary for exposing the ulnar and median nerves.
- Incise the fascia over the neurovascular bundle and expose the bundle between the triceps posteriorly and the biceps, brachialis, and coracobrachialis anteriorly.
- Expose and retract laterally the more superficial structures of the bundle—the ulnar nerve, the brachial artery and vein, and the median nerve—exposing the radial nerve and one or two of its branches, first to the long head and then to the medial head of the triceps.
- Trace the nerve to the point where it winds around the humerus.
- To expose the nerve on the posterior and lateral aspects of the humeral shaft, begin the incision along the poste-

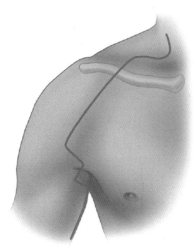

FIGURE 14.20   Incision for approach to brachial plexus (see text). **SEE TECHNIQUE 14.10.**

rior border of the distal third of the deltoid between the deltoid and the long head of the triceps. Curve it distalward along the lateral aspect of the arm, curving at first anteriorly along the medial aspect of the brachioradialis and then, if necessary, laterally at the elbow across the belly of this muscle and the extensor carpi radialis longus. Finally, if the deep radial nerve is to be explored, carry the incision distally on the dorsum of the forearm along the radial side of the extensor digitorum communis.

- In the incision proximal to the elbow it is wise to expose the nerve at its most superficial position by incising the fascia between the brachialis and brachioradialis and to identify the nerve at this point by retracting the brachioradialis laterally. The nerve can be exposed proximally by incising the fascia and retracting the lateral head of the triceps laterally to the point where the nerve winds around the humerus. This approach, with minor changes, is shown in Figure 14.21.
- The nerve can be carefully traced distally to the elbow; 5 or 6 cm proximal to the elbow it sends branches to the brachioradialis and a little more distally to the extensor carpi radialis longus and brevis. At the elbow, the nerve divides into the superficial and deep radial (posterior interosseous) nerves.
- The superficial radial nerve is entirely sensory but should be protected to avoid painful neuromas. The deep radial nerve often is injured, and such an injury is quite disabling.
- Expose this nerve through the distal part of the incision just described, beginning 8 to 10 cm proximal to the elbow and continuing to the middle of the dorsum of the forearm (see Fig. 14.19). Follow the nerve beneath the brachioradialis into the supinator muscle.
- If the injury is at this point or is more distal, expose the nerve distal to the supinator by incising the fascia between the extensor carpi radialis longus and brevis and the extensor digitorum communis and by developing this plane of cleavage.
- After exposing the nerve, follow it proximally to the distal border of the supinator where numerous branches are given off.
- After identifying these branches, incise the superficial part of the supinator at a right angle to the direction of its fibers to complete the exposure of the entire deep radial nerve.

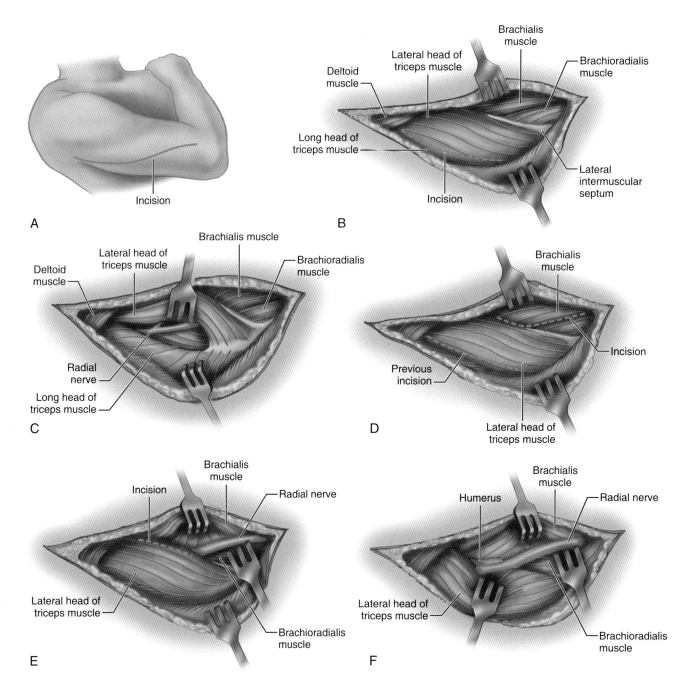

FIGURE 14.21 Exposure of radial nerve in middle and distal thirds of arm. **A,** Skin incision begins at posterior margin of deltoid muscle and extends distally in midline and laterally and anteriorly. It ends at interval between brachioradialis and brachialis. **B,** Posterior skin flap has been dissected and retracted; deep fascia is incised in line with skin incision. *Dotted line* indicates incision in triceps muscle between long and lateral heads. **C,** Radial nerve and accompanying vascular bundle have been exposed by retraction of these two heads of triceps muscle. Radial nerve has been dissected to point at which it passes beneath lateral head of triceps muscle. **D,** Arm is externally rotated a few degrees. Interval between proximal end of brachioradialis and brachialis is to be dissected, exposing radial nerve along anterolateral aspect of humerus. **E,** *Dotted line* indicates incision through which lateral head of triceps is mobilized from underlying bone, facilitating exposure of radial nerve deep to it. **F,** Exposure. **SEE TECHNIQUE 14.10.**

REFERENCES

CARPAL TUNNEL SYNDROME

Alter TH, Warrender WJ, Liss FE, et al.: A cost analysis of carpal tunnel release surgery performed wide awake versus under sedation, *Plast Reconstr Surg* 142:1532, 2018.

Apard T, Candelier G: Surgical ultrasound-guided carpal tunnel release, *Hand Surg Rehabil* 36:333, 2017.

Beck JD, Brothers JG, Maloney PJ, et al.: Predicting the outcome of revision carpal tunnel release, *J Hand Surg* 37A:282, 2012.

Beck JD, Deegan JH, Rhoades D, Klena JC: Results of endoscopic carpal tunnel release relative to surgeon experience with the Agee technique, *J Hand Surg* 36A:61, 2011.

Bland JD, Ashworth NL: Does prior local corticosteroid injection prejudice the outcome of subsequent carpal tunnel decompression? *J Hand Surg Eur* 41:130, 2016.

Blazar PE, Floyd 4th WE, Han CH, et al.: Prognostic indicators for recurrent symptoms after a single corticosteroid injection for carpal tunnel syndrome, *J Bone Joint Surg* 97A:1563, 2015.

Burnham R, Playfair L, Loh E, et al.: Evaluation of the effectiveness and safety of ultrasound-guided percutaneous carpal tunnel release: a cadaveric study, *Am J Phys Med Rehabil* 96:457, 2017.

Burton CL, Chesterton LS, Chen Y, van der Windt DA: Clinical course and prognostic factors in conservatively managed carpal tunnel syndrome: a systematic review, *Arch Phys Med Rehabil* 97:836, 2016.

Calandruccio JH, Thompson NB: Carpal tunnel syndrome: making evidence-based treatment decisions, *Orthop Clin North Am* 49:223, 2018.

Calleja H, Tsai TM, Kaufman C: Carpal tunnel release using the radial sided approach compared with the two-incision approach, *Hand Surg* 19:375, 2014.

Castillo TN, Yao J: Comparison of longitudinal open incision and two-incision techniques for carpal tunnel release, *J Hand Surg* 35A:1813, 2010.

Chen L, Duan X, Huang X, et al.: Effectiveness and safety of endoscopic versus open carpal tunnel decompression, *Arch Orthop Trauma Surg* 134:585, 2014.

Chen CH, Wu T, Sun JS, et al.: Unusual causes of carpal tunnel syndrome: space occupying lesions, *J Hand Surg Eur* 37:14, 2012.

Cho YI, Lee JH, Shin DJ, Park KH: Comparison of short wrist transverse open and limited open techniques for carpal tunnel release: a randomized controlled trial of two incisions, *J Hand Surg Eur* 41:143, 2016.

Conzen C, Conzen M, Rübsamen N, Mikolajczky R: Predictors of the patient-centered outcomes of surgical carpal tunnel release—a prospective cohort study, *BMC Musculoskelet Disrod* 17:190, 2016.

Deniz FE, Oksüz E, Sarikaya B, et al.: Electromography, ultrasonography, computed tomography, magnetic resonance imaging in idiopathic carpal tunnel syndrome determined by clinical findings, *Neurosurgery* 70:610, 2012.

Duckworth AD, Jenkins PJ, McEachan JE: Diagnosing carpal tunnel syndrome, *J Hand Surg Am* 39:1403, 2014.

Dunn JC, Kusnezov NA, Koehler LR,et al.: Outcomes following carpal tunnel release in patients receiving workers' compensation: a systematic review, Hand (NY) 13:137, 2018.

English JH, Gwynne-Jones DP: Incidence of carpal tunnel syndrome requiring surgical decompression: a 10.5-year review of 2,309 patients, *J Hand Surg Am* 40:2427, 2015.

Ettema AM, Amadio PC, Cha SS, et al.: Survery versus conservative therapy in carpal tunnel syndrome in people aged 70 years and older, *Plast Reconstr Surg* 118:947, 2006.

Fowler JR, Cipolli W, Hanson T: A comparison of three diagnostic tests for carpal tunnel syndrome using latent class analysis, *J Bone Joint Surg* 97A:2015, 1958.

Fowler JR, Munsch M, Huang Y, et al.: Pre-operative electrodiagnostic testing predicts time to resolution of symptoms after carpal tunnel release, *J Hand Surg Eur* 41:137, 2016.

Fowler JR, Munsch M, Tosti R, et al.: Comparison of ultrasound and electrodiagnostic testing for diagnosis of carpal tunnel syndrome: study using a validated clinical tool as the reference standard, *J Bone Joint Surg* 96A:e148, 2014.

Goldfarb CA: The clinical practice guideline on carpal tunnel syndrome and workers' compensation, *J Hand Surg Am* 41:723, 2016.

Gulabi D, Cecen G, Guclu B, Cecen A: Carpal tunnel release in patients with diabetes results in poor outcomes in long-term study, *Eur J Orthop Surg Traumatol* 24:1181, 2014.

Guo D, Guo D, Guo J, et al: A clinical study of the modified thread carpal tunnel release, *Hand (N Y)* 12:453, 2017.

Hattori Y, Koi K, Koide S, Sakamoto S: Endoscopic release for severe carpal tunnel syndrome in octogenarians, *J Hand Surg Am* 39:2448, 2014.

Jones NF, Ahn H, Eo S: Revision surgery for persistent and recurrent carpal tunnel syndrome and for failed carpal tunnel release, *Plast Reconstr Surg* 129:683, 2012.

Kang HJ, Koh IH, Lee TJ, Choi YR: Endoscopic carpal tunnel release is preferred over mini-open despite similar outcome: a randomized trial, *Clin Orthop Relat Res* 471:1548, 2013.

Kang JH, Koh IH, Lee WY, et al.: Does carpal tunnel release provide long-term relief in patients with hemodialysis-associated carpal tunnel syndrome? *Clin Orthop Relat Res* 470:2561, 2012.

Karl JW, Gancarczyk SM, Strauch RJ: Complications of carpal tunnel release, *Orthop Clin North Am* 47:425, 2016.

Kazmers NH, Presson AP, Xu Y, et al.: Cost implications of varying the surgical technique, surgical setting, and anesthesia for carpal tunnel release surgery, *J Hand Surg Am* 43:971, 2018.

Kikuchi K, Matsumoto K, Seo K, et al.: Risk factors for re-recurrent carpal tunnel syndrome in patients undergoing long-term hemodialysis, *Hand Surg* 18:63, 2013.

Kohanzadeh S, Herrera FA, Dobke M: Outcomes of open and endoscopic carpal tunnel release: a meta-analysis, *Hand (N Y)* 7:247, 2012.

Kronlage SC, Menendez ME: The benefit of carpal tunnel release in patients with electrophysiologically moderate and severe disease, *J Hand Surg Am* 40:438, 2015.

Larsen MB, Sørensen AI, Crone KL, et al.: Carpal tunnel release a randomized comparison of three surgical methods, *J Hand Surg Eur* 38:646, 2013.

Louie D, Earp B, Blazar P: Long-term outcomes of carpal tunnel release: a critical review of the literature, *Hand (N Y)* 7:242, 2012.

Mahmoud M, El Shafie S, Coppola EE, Elfar JC: Perforator-based radial forearm fascial flap for management of recurrent caral tunnel syndrome, *J Hand Surg Am* 38:2151, 2013.

McDonagh C, Alexander M, Kane D: The role of ultrasound in the diagnosis and management of carpal tunnel syndrome: a new paradigm, *Rheumatology (Oxford)* 54(9), 2015.

Means Jr KR, Dubin NH, Patel KM, Pletka JD: Long-term outcomes following single-portal endoscopic carpal tunnel release, *Hand (N Y)* 9:384, 2014.

Mosier BA, Hughes TB: Recurrent carpal tunnel syndrome, *Hand Clin* 29:427, 2013.

Nassar WAM, Atiyya AN: New technique for reducing fibrosis in recurrent cases of carpal tunnel syndrome, *Hand Surg* 19:381, 2014.

Neuhaus V, Christoforou D, Cheiryan T, Mudgal CS: Evaluation and treatment of failed carpal tunnel release, *Orthop Clin N Am* 43:439, 2012.

Pimentel BFR, Faloppa F, Tamaoki MJS, et al.: Effectiveness of ultrasonography and nerve conduction studies in the diagnosing of carpal tunnel syndrome: clinical trial on accuracy, *BMC Musculoskeletal Disord* 19:115, 2018.

Povlsen B, Bashir M, Wong F: Long-term result and patient reported outcome of wrist splint treatment for carpal tunnel syndrome, *J Plast Surg Hand Surg* 48:175, 2014.

Roghani RS, Holisaz MT, Norouzi AAS, et al.: Sensitivity of high-resolution ultrasonography in clinically diagnosed carpal tunnel syndrome patients with hand pain and normal nerve conduction studies, *J Pain Res* 11:1319, 2018.

Roh YH, Lee BK, Noh JH, et al.: Effects of metabolic syndrome on the outcome of carpal tunnel release: a matched case-control study, *J Hand Surg Am* 40:1303, 2015.

Sayegh ET, Strauch RJ: Open versus endoscopic carpal tunnel release: a meat-analysis of randomized controlled trials, *Clin Orthop Relat Res* 473:1120, 2015.

Sears ED, Swiatek PR, Hou H, Chung KC: Utilization of preoperative electrodiagnostic studies for carpal tunnel syndrome: an analysis of national practice patterns, *J Hand Surg Am* 41:665, 2016.

Shiri R: Arthritis as a risk factor for carpal tunnel syndrome: a meta-analysis, *Scand J Rheumatol* 45:339, 2016.

Staples JR, Calfee R: Cubital tunnel syndrome: current concepts. *J Am Acad Orthop Surg* 25:e215, 2017.

Staples R, London D, Dardas AZ, Goldfarb CA: Calfee RP: Comparative morbidity of cubital tunnel surgeries: a prospective cohort study, *J Hand Surg Am* 43:207, 2018.

Szabo RM: Perioperative antibiotics for carpal tunnel surgery, *J Hand Surg* 35A:122, 2010.

Tulipan JE, Kim N, Ilyas AM, et al.: Endoscopic carpal tunnel release with and without sedation, *Plast Reconstr Surg* 141:685, 2018.

Vasiliadis HS, Xenakis TA, Mitsionis G, et al.: Endoscopic versus open carpal tunnel release, *Arthroscopy* 26:26, 2010.

Wang CK, Jou IM, Huang HW, et al.: Carpal tunnel syndrome assessed with diffusion tensor imaging: comparison with electrophysiological studies of patients and healthy volunteers, *Eur J Radiol* 81:3378, 2012.

Wang WL, Buterbaugh K, Kadow TR, et al.: A prospective comparison of diagnostic tools for the diagnosis of carpal tunnel syndrome, *J Hand Surg Am* 43:833, 2018.

Zhang D, Collins JE, Earp BE, et al.: Surgical demographics of carpal tunnel and cubital tunnel syndrome over 5 years at a single institution, *J Hand Surg Am* 42:929, 2017.

Zhang X, Huang X, Wang X, et al.: A randomized comparison of double small, standard, and endoscopioc approaches for carpal tunnel release, *Plast Reconstr Surg* 138:641, 2016.

Zieske L, Ebersole GC, Davidge K, et al.: Revision carpal tunnel surgery: a 10-year review of intraoperative findings and outcomes, *J Hand Surg Am* 38:1530, 2013.

Zuo D, Zhou Z, Wang H, et al.: Endoscopic versus open carpal tunnel release for idiopathic carpal tunnel syndrome: a meta-analysis of randomized controlled trials, *J Orthop Surg Res* 10:12, 2015.

Zyluk A, Puchalski P: A comparison of outcomes of carpal tunnel release in diabetic and non-diabetic patients, *J Hand Surg Eur* 38:485, 2013.

ULNAR TUNNEL SYNDROME

Bachoura A, Jacoby SM: Ulnar tunnel syndrome, *Orthop Clin North Am* 43:467, 2012.

Calfee RP, Manske PR, Gelberman RH, et al.: Clinical assessment of the ulnar nerve at the elbow: reliability of instabiity testing and the association of hypermobility with clinical symptoms, *J Bone Joint Surg Am* 92:2801, 2010.

Chen SH, Tsai TM: Ulnar tunnel syndrome, *J Hand Surg Am* 39:571, 2014.

Maroukis BL, Ogawa T, Rehim SA, Chung KC: Guyon canale: the evolution of clinical anatomy, *J Hand Surg Am* 40:560, 2015.

CUBITAL TUNNEL SYNDROME

Aldekhayel S, Govshievich A, Lee J, et al.: Endoscopic versus open cubital tunnel release: a systematic review and meta-analysis, *Hand (N Y)* 11:36, 2016.

Aleem AW, Krogue JD, Calfee RP: Outcomes of revision surgery for cubital tunnel syndrome, *J Hand Surg Am* 39:2141, 2014.

An TW, Evanoff BA, Boyer MI, et al.: The prevalence of cubital tunnel syndrome: a cross-sectional study in a U.S. metropolitan cohort, *J Bone Joint Surg Am* 99:408, 2017.

Buchanan PJ, Chieng LO, Hubbard ZS, et al.: Endoscopic versus open in situ cubital tunnel release: a systematic review of the literature and meta-analysis of 655 patients, *Plast Reconstr Surg* 141:679, 2018.

Camp CL, Ryan B, Degen RM, et al.: Risk factors for revision surgery following isolated ulnar nerve release at the cubital tunnel: a study of 25,977 cases, *J Shoulder Elbow Surg* 26:710, 2017.

Choudhry IK, Bracey DN, Hutchinson ID, Li Z: Comparison of transposition techniques to reduce gap associated with high ulnar nerve lesions, *J Hand Surg Am* 39:2460, 2014.

Cobb TK: Endoscopic cubital tunnel release, *J Hand Surg Am* 35A:1690, 2010.

Dützmann S, Martin KD, Sobottka S, et al.: Open vs retractor-endoscopic in situ decompression of the ulnar nerve in cubital tunnel syndrome: a retrospective cohort study, *Neurosurgery* 72:604, 2013.

Gaspar MP, Kane PM, Putthiwara D, et al.: Predicting revision following in situ ulnar nerve decompression for patients with idiopathic cubital tunnel syndrome, *J Hand Surg Am* 41:427, 2016.

Henn CM, Ptel A, Wall LB, et al.: Outcomes following cubital tunnel surgery in young patients: the importance of nerve mobility, *J Hand Surg Am* 41:e1, 2016.

Kokkalis ZT, Efstathopoulos DG, Papanastassiou ID, et al.: Ulnar nerve injuries in Guyon Canal: a report of 32 cases, *Microsurgery* 32:296, 2012.

Krogue JD, Aleem AW, Osei DA, et al.: Predictors of surgical revision after in situ decompression of the ulnar nerves, *J Shoulder Elbow Surg* 24:634, 2015.

Matzon JL, Lutsky KF, Hoffler CE, et al.: Risk factors for ulnar nerve instability in transposition in patients with cubital tunnel syndrome, *J Hand Surg Am* 41:180, 2016.

Ochi K, Horiuchi Y, Tanabe A, et al.: Comparison of shoulder internal rotation test with the elbow flexion test in the diagnosis of cubital tunnel syndrome, *J Hand Surg Am* 36:782, 2011.

Palmer BA, Hughes TB: Cubital tunnel syndrome, *J Hand Surg Am* 35:153, 2010.

Said J, Frizzell K, Heimur J, et al.: Visualization during endoscopic versus open cubital tunnel decompression: a cadaveric study, *J Hand Surg Am* 2018 Nov 9. pii: S0363-5023(18)30190-30194. https://doi: 10.1016/j.jhsa.2018.10.004. [Epub ahead of print]

Schmidt S, Kleist-Welch-Guerra W, Matthes M, et al.: Endoscopic vs open decompression of the ulnar nerve in cubital tunnel syndrome: a prospective randomized double-blind study, *Neurosurgery* 77:960, 2015.

Staples R, London DA, Dardas AZ, et al.: Comparative morbidity of cubital tunnel surgeries: a prospective cohort study, *J Hand Surg Am* 43:207, 2018.

Uzunkulaoglu A, Ikbali A, Karatas M: Association between gender, body mass index, and ulnar nerve entrapment at the elbow: a retrospective study, *J Clin Neurophysiol* 33:545, 2016.

Verveld CJ, Daqnoff Jr , Lombardi JM, et al.: Adipose flap versus fascial sling for anterior subcutaneous transposition of the ulnar nerve, *Am J Orthop (Belle Mead NJ)* 45:89, 2016.

Zhang D, Collins JE, Earp BE, et al.: Surgical demographics of carpal tunnel and cubital tunnel syndrome over 5 years at a single institution, *J Hand Surg Am* 42:929, 2017.

Zhang D, Earp BE, Blazar P: Rates of complications an secondary surgeries after in situ cubital tunnel release compared with ulnar nerve transposition: a retrospective review, *J Hand Surg Am* 42:294, 2017.

PRONATOR SYNDROME AND ANTERIOR INTEROSSEOUS SYNDROME

Komaru Y, Inokuchi R: Anterior interosseous nerve syndrome, *QJM* 110:243, 2017.

Lee HJ, Kim I, Hong JT, et al.: Early surgical treatment of pronator teres syndrome, *J Korean Neurosurg Soc* 55:296, 2014.

Nzeako OJ, Tahmassebi R: Idiopathic anterior interosseous nerve dysfunction, *J Hand Surg Am* 40:2277, 2015.

Rodner CM, Tinsley BA, O'Malley MP: Pronator syndrome and anterior interosseos nerve syndrome, *J Am Acad Orthop Surg* 21:268, 2013.

Strohl AB, Zelouf DS: Ulnar tunnel syndrome, radial tunnel syndrome, anterior interosseous nerve syndrome, and pronator syndrome, *Instr Course Lect* 66:153, 2017.

RADIAL TUNNEL SYNDROME

Marchese I, Coyle K, Cote M, et al: Prospective evaluation of a single corticosteroid injection in radial tunnel syndrome, *Hand* 1558944718787282. https://doi: 10.1177/1558944718787282. [Epub ahead of print].

Moradi A, Ebrahimzadeh MH, Jupiter JB: Radial tunnel syndrome, diagnostic and treatment dilemma, *Arch Bone Jt Surg* 3:156, 2015.

Popinchalk SP, Schaffer AA: Physical examination of upper extremity compressive neuropathies, *Orthop Clin North Am* 43:417, 2012.

Strohl AB, Zelouf DS: Ulnar tunnel syndrome, radial tunnel syndrome, anterior interosseous nerve syndrome, and pronator syndrome, *Instr Course Lect* 66:153, 2017.

Ummel JR, Coury JG, Lum ZC, et al.: Transbrachioradialis approach to the radial tunnel: an anatomic study of 5 potential compression sites, *Hand (N Y)* 558944717750916, 2018, https://doi.org/10.1177/1558944717750916, [Epub ahead of print].

The complete list of references is available online at Expert Consult.com.

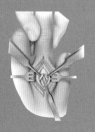

Hand masses may result from tumors and tumorous conditions, and although most of these masses are benign, they should be considered potentially problematic and managed with great diligence. Because the hand has limited free space and exquisite sensitivity, even small and histologically benign masses can cause pain and significantly impair function. However, most hand neoplasms develop insidiously without significant pain or tenderness (including those that are malignant) and thus cosmetic concerns may be the patient's only presenting complaint. Therefore, most hand and finger growths should be biopsied even when considered benign. Malignant lesions that arise primarily from tissues other than the skin are rare, and management of these tumors is derived mainly from small series and case reports. The hand may be the site of distant breast, lung, or kidney adenocarcinoma metastases, most of which occur in the distal phalanges.

CLASSIFICATION

Tumors involving the hand are classified in a manner similar to that for tumors involving the rest of the body. Benign tumors are classified as latent, active, or aggressive, according to their local biologic activity (Table 15.1). Benign latent tumors are those in which tumor growth has occurred during childhood or adolescence and has subsequently entered an inactive or healing phase. Solitary and unicameral bone cysts are examples of benign latent tumors. A benign active tumor continues to enlarge and although it is well encapsulated, may have an irregular or lumpy border. Most benign tumors of the hand fall into this category. Although a benign aggressive

tumor is nonmetastasizing and appears innocent on histologic sections, it is locally destructive and is surrounded by a thin, tenuous capsule that may not contain all the tumor cells. A giant cell tumor of bone often behaves in this aggressive manner. A wide margin is often necessary for complete eradication of benign aggressive tumors.

Malignant tumors are classified as low grade (I), high grade (II), or associated with metastasis (III) (Table 15.2). Most malignant tumors of the hand are low-grade tumors and are classified further, according to the degree of local extension, as either intracompartmental (A) or extracompartmental (B). In the hand, each ray forms a distinct compartment. The individual phalanges are not considered separate compartments but rather that they, along with their corresponding intrinsic muscles, are included in the ray compartment. The ray compartment includes the flexor tendon and sheath of each finger as far proximally as the midpalmar space and the extensor tendon as far as the metacarpophalangeal joint. Each metacarpal is a separate compartment. If a tumor involves the palmar space or the loose areolar tissue on the dorsum of the hand, it is considered extracompartmental because proximal spread is unobstructed. Tumors arising in the digits remain confined to that compartment for long periods and then extend into the palm.

DIAGNOSIS

A pertinent history, physical examination, and plain radiographs are frequently all that are necessary to determine the diagnosis and appropriate treatment of benign-appearing

---

TABLE 15.1

Classification of Benign Tumors

STAGE	TYPE
1	Latent
2	Active
3	Aggressive

Modified from Enneking WE: *Musculoskeletal tumor surgery*, New York, 1983, Churchill Livingstone.

TABLE 15.2

Classification of Malignant Tumors

STAGE	TYPE
IA	Low grade, intracompartmental
IB	Low grade, extracompartmental
IIA	High grade, intracompartmental
IIB	High grade, extracompartmental
III	Either grade with regional or distant metastasis

Modified from Enneking WF, Spanier SS, Goodman MA: The surgical staging of musculoskeletal sarcoma, *Clin Orthop Relat Res* 153:106, 1980.

TABLE 15.3

Classification of Surgical Margins

TYPE	PLANE OF DISSECTION
Intracapsular	Piecemeal, debulking, or curettage
Marginal	Shell out (en bloc) through pseudocapsule or reactive zone
Wide	Intracompartmental (en bloc) with cuff of normal tissue
Radical	Extracompartmental (en bloc) with entire compartment

Modified from Enneking WE: *Musculoskeletal tumor surgery*, New York, 1983, Churchill Livingstone.

---

hand and finger tumors. If a more aggressive process is present, causing considerable pain, inflammation, tumor enlargement, or bony destruction, further diagnostic and staging studies are warranted before biopsy or a definitive surgical procedure. Local imaging studies, including bone scans, angiograms, CT, and MRI, are helpful in surgical planning. A metastatic workup is indicated in most malignant lesions, and a chest CT is necessary for those tumors with a propensity for metastasizing to the lungs.

TREATMENT

Generally, hand and finger tumors are treated surgically. Incisional biopsy is rarely required in most benign tumors because marginal excision is usually definitive and curative. Incisional biopsy is advised if a malignant tumor is suspected, or if the morbidity of surgical excision outweighs the morbidity caused by the tumor itself, as may be true in some benign neural tumors. Incisions should be made directly over the mass for biopsy and should be oriented so as not to jeopardize hand function or interfere with complete removal of the tumor. The way in which a tumor is removed depends on its location, aggressiveness, potential for metastasizing, and, at times, sensitivity to adjuvant chemotherapy and radiation therapy. The various surgical margins are summarized in Table 15.3.

Benign soft-tissue tumors are treated by excisional biopsy (marginal excision). Benign tumors of bone are often treated by curettage (intracapsular) and, occasionally, bone grafting. Malignant tumors require a wide excision in which a 2 cm tumor-free cuff of tissue is removed with the tumor. Malignant tumors involving the distal phalanx can be treated with a transdiaphyseal amputation through the middle phalanx, and malignant tumors of the middle phalanx can be treated with a transdiaphyseal amputation through the proximal phalanx. If the malignant tumor involves the proximal phalanx, a ray amputation is usually required. Malignant tumors of the metacarpals, especially if large and extracompartmental, often require adjacent amputations to achieve adequate surgical margins. Grade IIB lesions involving the hand may require amputation through the distal third of the forearm at a level just proximal to the musculotendinous junctions. Reconstruction after wide or radical excisions for malignant tumors of the hand should be delayed until tumor-free margins have been documented.

BENIGN TUMORS (TABLE 15.4)
LIPOMA
Although lipomas are more common elsewhere in the body, they are also found in the hand and are common solid cellular hand tumors (Fig. 15.1). These lightly encapsulated tumors are composed of mature fatty tissue in which the central lipid droplet and peripherally located nucleus form the characteristic signet-ring cell. They arise from mesenchymal primordial fatty tissue cells. These tumors can be superficial, arising from the subcutaneous tissues and having the characteristic signs of a soft, bulging mass, or they can be nonpalpable, occurring deep in the palm, arising in Guyon's canal, the carpal tunnel, or the deep palmar space. Usually, a painless mass is present that impairs grasp. Lateral deviation of the fingers may also be present when the tumor is located between the metacarpophalangeal joints.

Median or ulnar nerve compression from these tumors can cause muscular weakness or diminished sensibility. Lipomas project through spaces of least resistance, and those deep palmar space lesions tend to present distally between the fingers and thumb because of the unyielding overlying palmar aponeurosis. Careful dissection is necessary for removal because the tumor often envelops digital nerves and is much larger than is clinically apparent. Recurrence after marginal excision is unlikely.

■ INFILTRATING LIPOMAS
Infiltrating lipomas are rare tumors that usually occur in adults. Two types, intermuscular and intramuscular, have been reported. Intermuscular lipomas grow between large muscles and arise from septa; intramuscular lipomas arise between muscle fibers. Despite tissue infiltration, no malignant transformation has been reported; however, these uncommon, nonencapsulated, benign tumors have a recurrence rate of 60%.

TABLE 15.4

Benign Tumors of the Hand

TUMOR	AGE AT ONSET M:F	LOCATION	IMAGING	TREATMENT	RECURRENCE	SPECIAL NOTES
Lipoma	Infiltrating lipoma occurs mostly in adults M=F	Palm	Radiograph: Bufalini sign MRI: well marginated	Marginal excision	Low: 60% for infiltrating lipoma	No malignant transformation
Lipoblastoma	<7 yr	Rare in hand		Surgical excision	14%	Absence of cellular atypia and mitosis necessary to differentiate from congenital liposarcoma
Intraneural lipofibromas	<30 yr	Median nerve with mass located in the palmar aspect of hand or wrist		Surgical decompression if extrinsic neural compression Intraneural excision may debulk tumor but may increase neural deficit En bloc excision with nerve grafting if digital nerve affected		Malignant transformation rare but intractable pain may warrant tumor excision
Giant cell tumor tendon sheath (xanthoma)	8-80 yr 2M:3F	Frequent in hand Flexor surface of fingers	Radiograph: possible bone erosion MRI: low-intensity T1- and T2-weighted images	Excision	13%	Most common primary hand tumor Histology like pigmented villonodular synovitis
Infantile digital fibromatosis	1/3 congenital within first 2 yr of life M=F	Dorsolateral fingers		Observation Marginal excision	Frequent (60%)	Dermal lesion often multiple Possible spontaneous resolution at 2-3 yr
Calcifying aponeurotic fibroma	First to fifth decades 2M:1F	Palms, fingers, plantar surfaces Not adherent to skin	Radiograph: stippled calcifications possible scalloping MRI: bands of low-signal intensity	Observation Excision	>50% Common locally	Intermediate aggressive behavior
Fibroma of tendon sheath	Third to fifth decades M>F	Thumb, index, middle fingers	MRI: heterogeneous, no enhancement	Excision	Rare	
Neurofibroma	Solitary form first decade; multiple form >30 yr M=F	Deeper nerves fusiform nerve	Radiograph: normal MRI: nerve fibers in tumor	Excision expendable nerves	Rare after excision	Common in neurofibromatosis (possible malignant degeneration 15%) Arise from nerve

Continued

TABLE 15.4—cont'd

Benign Tumors of the Hand

TUMOR	AGE AT ONSET M:F	LOCATION	IMAGING	TREATMENT	RECURRENCE	SPECIAL NOTES
Glomus tumor	Third to fifth decades M<F	Subungual mass	Radiograph: possible scalloping distal phalanx MRI: ±	Excision	1%-18% Rare at same site	Localized pain, bluish discoloration, cold intolerance Autosomal dominant 1% malignant Lesions >2 cm suggest malignancy When malignant, 25% are metastatic
Hemangioma	<4 wk M1:F3	Occasionally in hand	Radiograph: calcifications	Spontaneous resolution (70% at 7 yr) Complete excision for cavernous type with symptoms	Frequent recurrence in diffuse lesions	Rapid growth in first year
Lymphangioma	Tendency to occur in childhood	Rarely occur in the hand		Excisional biopsy for diagnostic confirmation and debulking	Tendency to recur after excision	No malignant potential Overly aggressive surgery to be avoided
Neurilemoma (schwannoma)	Fourth to sixth decades M=F	Small cutaneous nerves Eccentric in nerve Flexor surface of hand	Radiograph: normal MRI: isointense to skeletal muscle, possible capsule, no nerve fascicles in tumor	Excision	Rare	Most common benign nerve tumor Antoni A pattern (storiform tumor cells) Antoni B pattern (disorganized myxoid pattern) Arise from Schwann cells
Osteoid osteoma	<30 yr M2:F1	Most lesions in upper extremity occur in wrist or hand Proximal phalanx Carpus	Radiograph: sclerotic lesion with central nidus	Central nidus excision	Recurrence to be expected with incomplete excision	Night pain relieved by aspirin or NSAID
Enchondroma	First to second decades M=F	Phalanx Pathologic fracture common Histology worrisome	Radiograph: central well-circumscribed	Curettage ± bone graft CaPhos bone cement Amputation if digit dysfunctional	>10%	Possible malignant degeneration
Benign osteoblastoma	<30 yr M>F	Small bones of the handa/feet	Radiograph: similar to osteoid osteoma but more expansile Ground-glass appearance: intact cortical shell	Curettage and bone grafting Excision with interpositional bone grafting for locally aggressive	20%-30%	Histology, areas of mature bone, osteoid, and plump osteoblasts
Aneurysmal bone cyst	Second decade M=F	Metacarpals metaphyseal epiphyseal	Radiograph: central expansion MRI: fluid filled	Curettage and bone grafting	Tendency to recur	Locally aggressive

Continued

TUMOR	AGE AT ONSET M:F	LOCATION	IMAGING	TREATMENT	RECURRENCE	SPECIAL NOTES
Giant cell tumor of bone	Third to fourth decades M=F	Radius Metaphysis/epiphysis Carpus-hamate	Radiograph: expansile Chest CT: rule out pulmonary metastases	Resection of bone and reconstruction with cementation and allograft En bloc excision and allograft reconstruction for cortical invasion or recurrence Cryosurgery and adjunctive treatment	Local recurrence high after curettage alone	Benign but aggressive and has a tendency to metastasize Campanacci: I: well marginated II: thinned cortex III: soft tissue
Osteochondroma	First to third decades Earlier for hereditary multiple exostosis M>F	Rare in the hand Occasionally phalanx Metacarpal Carpus (scaphoid) Metaphyseal	Radiograph: bony erosion	Excision	Rare	Hereditary multiple exostosis (autosomal dominant) with malignant degeneration 1%-25%
Periosteal chondroma	Second to third decades M>F	Rare in hand Surface of long bones	Radiograph: central scalloping MRI: cartilage tumor	Resect underlying cortex	20%	
Parosteal osteochondromatous proliferation (Nora tumor)	Third to fourth decades M=F	Hands/feet Surface long bones	Radiograph: No cortical scalloping MRI: lesion separate from medullary canal	Resect underlying periosteum	High local recurrence rate	
Osteochondromatosis	Third to fifth decades M2:F4	Proximal interphalangeal joint Metacarpophalangeal joint Distal radioulnar joint	Radiograph: stippled calcification cortical scalloping MRI: low-intense bodies	Excision Synovectomy	Rare	Monarticular mechanical symptoms
Chondromyxoid fibroma	Second to third decades M2:F1	Rare in hand Metaphysis Eccentric	Radiograph: radiolucent lesion	Curettage and bone grafting	7%-25%	

CT, Computed tomography; MRI, magnetic resonance imaging; NSAID, nonsteroidal antiinflammatory drug.

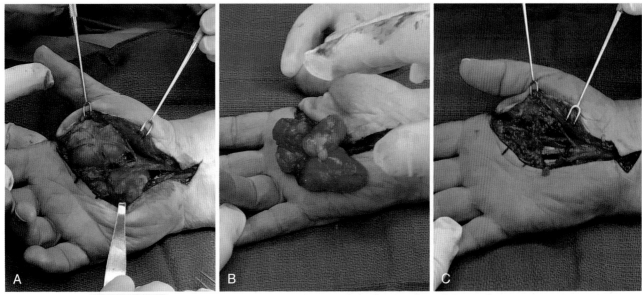

FIGURE 15.1   **A,** Palmar lipoma with significant palmar radial prominence causing interference with grasp (note sensory nerves draped across the tumor). **B,** Encapsulated lesion removed en bloc. **C,** Appearance of tumor bed prior to closure.

LIPOBLASTOMAS

Lipoblastomas are rare, benign tumors composed of immature, spindle-shaped cells that occur in children younger than 7 years old, with 90% occurring before age 3 years. They usually grow rapidly and are painless. Two forms of this tumor exist; one is a diffuse infiltrative form, which is deeply seated and poorly circumscribed, and the other is more superficial and well circumscribed. Absence of cellular atypia and mitosis is necessary to differentiate them from the exceptionally rare congenital liposarcomas. A cytogenic analysis may help to identify the lipoblastomas that have a characteristic chromosome abnormality found on the long arm of chromosome 8 (8q11-8q13). Surgical excision after MRI to assess the extension of the mass is usually necessary. A recurrence rate up to 22% after excision has been reported.

INTRANEURAL LIPOFIBROMAS

Intraneural lipofibromas or lipofibromatous hamartomas (LFHs) are rare benign tumors that usually involve the median nerve; one third of individuals also have macrodactyly. Males and females are equally afflicted, and nearly three fourths of LFH patients present within the first 3 decades of life with a mass located in the palmar aspect of the hand or wrist, possibly with altered median nerve function (Fig. 15.2). Microscopically, fibroadipose tissue is seen infiltrating the epineurium, separating and compressing the fascicles. A conservative approach should be taken in treating these tumors. Histologic examination is definitive for LFH tumors; however, biopsy is rarely necessary because T1- and T2-weighted MRI showing characteristic low-intensity serpentine nerve bundles embedded within abundant hyperintense adipose material, with fine, fibrous tissue septa coursing along the median nerve, is pathognomic (Fig. 15.3B and C). If extrinsic neural compression exists, surgical decompression should be performed by fasciotomy or carpal tunnel release (Fig. 15.3D and E). Intraneural excision may debulk the tumor, but this procedure is not recommended because intraneural fibrosis

can increase the neural deficit. Malignant transformation has not been reported; however, intractable pain and expanding tumor size or increased firmness may warrant tumor biopsy and excision. If a digital nerve is involved, en bloc excision with nerve grafting may be performed (Fig. 15.4).

GIANT CELL TUMOR OF THE TENDON SHEATH (XANTHOMA)

Giant cell tumors of tendon sheaths were first described by Targett in 1897, and some consider these to be the most common solid cellular hand tumors (Fig. 15.5). The reported age distribution is 8 to 80 years, although most present in middle-aged patients. These tumors may occur anywhere in the hand but more commonly present as firm lobulated masses on the lateral side of the hand (index and middle fingers more so than the thumb).

Giant cell tumors usually grow slowly and can remain the same size for many years. Pain and tenderness are rare. If these tumors occur at a joint (often the proximal interphalangeal joint), they can enlarge enough to interfere with joint motion. They may rarely erode bone. Grossly, the tumors appear as well-encapsulated yellow or tan lobular masses. Histologic sections reveal spindle cells, fibrous tissue, cholesterol-laden histiocytes, multinucleated giant cells similar to osteoclasts, and hemosiderin.

The lesions are benign, but recurrence is noted in up to 40% of patients (10% to 20% more commonly reported) even after meticulous excision of the friable fragments. Risk factors for recurrence or persistence include adjacent degenerative joint disease, location at the finger distal interphalangeal and thumb interphalangeal joint, bony invasion, multifocal disease, tendon involvement, and poor surgical technique. Excision often is difficult because the tumors may wind in and around the flexor tendons and their sheaths, the digital nerves, and even the extensor tendons, and may involve three fourths of the circumference of involved digits; however, this benign lesion is considered surgically curable. Extensile surgical approaches are frequently required, and gentle blunt

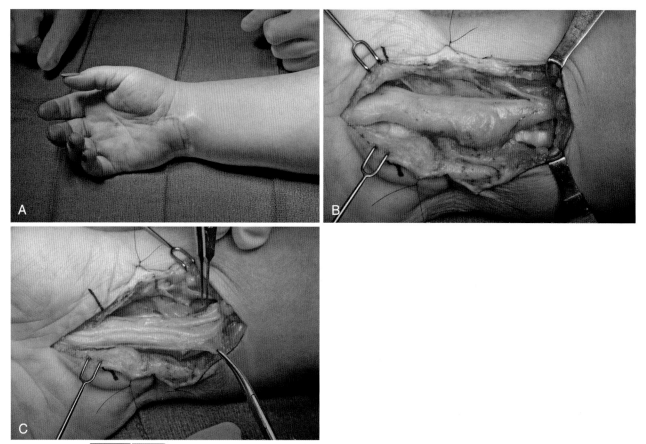

FIGURE 15.2   Median nerve lipofibroma. **A,** A 42-year-old woman with carpal tunnel syndrome recurrence 18 years postoperatively and incidental finding of median nerve enlargement. **B,** Segmental median nerve lipofibromatous enlargement. Note sparing of the palmar cutaneous branch. **C,** Epineurotomy demonstrating fascicular enlargement and expansion of connective tissue.

dissection should be performed to minimize fragmentation of the encapsulated tumor mass. Magnified vision is helpful to discover discolored synovial tumor, which should be removed during the marginal tumor resection.

BENIGN TUMORS OF FIBROUS ORIGIN

Fibrous tissue frequently proliferates in the hand as a response to local injury and is considered simple scar tissue; for this reason, the diagnosis of fibrous tumor must be made based on the appearance of the tumor, the age of the patient, the clinical behavior of the tumor, and its histologic appearance. All tumors of fibrous origin may involve the hand and although most are benign, they are frequently active or aggressive lesions with a tendency to recur after local excision. The differential diagnosis in benign fibrous tumors includes simple fibroma, recurring digital fibrous tumor of childhood, juvenile aponeurotic fibroma, Dupuytren contractures or nodules, fibromatosis or desmoid tumors, and pseudosarcomatous fasciitis. Fibromatosis or extraabdominal desmoid and pseudosarcomatous fasciitis are especially aggressive tumors that usually involve the more proximal portions of extremities.

▪ RECURRING DIGITAL FIBROUS TUMOR OF CHILDHOOD OR INFANTILE DIGITAL FIBROMATOSIS

In 1965, Reye described a benign fibrous tumor that develops in the fingers and toes of infants and young children. The

distinguishing feature of this tumor is the presence of intracytoplasmic inclusion bodies within proliferating fibroblasts. These inclusion bodies are invisible with routine hematoxylin and eosin staining. A viral causative factor has been suggested, although this is uncertain. These tumors tend to be multicentric, occurring on several digits. The dermis appears to be the site of involvement with sparing of the overlying epidermis. No malignant potential is present, and spontaneous regression has been reported. A marginal excision is recommended when function seems compromised or appearance is bothersome, especially if tendons, joints, or nails are involved. Local recurrence after marginal excision is common, occurring in 60% of patients.

▪ JUVENILE APONEUROTIC FIBROMA OR CALCIFYING APONEUROTIC FIBROMA

First described by Keasbey in 1953, juvenile aponeurotic fibroma is a benign fibrous tumor typically appearing in the hands or wrists of children and young adults. It has also been called *calcifying aponeurotic fibroma* because in older patients, calcification of the cartilaginous component may be present, a feature that distinguishes it from other benign tumors of fibrous origin. Clinically, it is a painless, solitary, and mobile mass less than 4 cm in diameter, usually involving the palm (Fig. 15.6). The tumor is usually on the volar side of the hand and is connected to peritendinous tissues and fascia. It has no gender predilection and no tendency to involve the ulnar side of the hand, as do Dupuytren nodules. Juvenile aponeurotic fibromas tend to develop close to

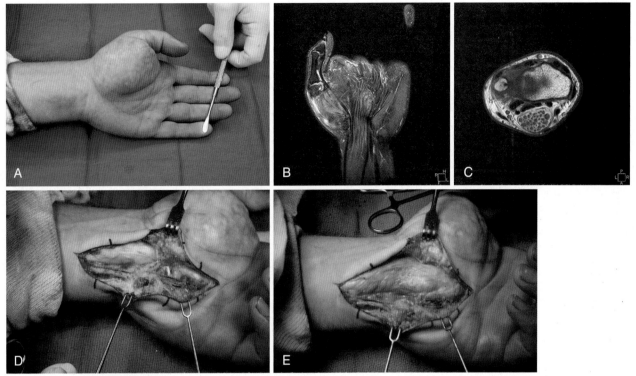

FIGURE 15.3 Lipofibroma hamartoma. **A,** A 21-year-old man with progressive neurologic symptoms with palmar and thumb hypertrophy since 5 years of age. **B** and **C,** MRI with classic findings of median nerve lipofibromatous hamartoma. **D** and **E,** Median nerve before and after division of transverse carpal ligament.

tendons and are able to infiltrate surrounding muscle and fat. On radiographs, calcifications can be seen within the soft-tissue mass. Because juvenile aponeurotic fibroma has a distinct tendency for local recurrence after marginal excision, especially in younger children (50%), a wide excision, preferably without sacrifice of function, is recommended.

■ FIBROMA

Fibromas are rare in the hand and can be deep, arising from a joint capsule, or superficial. They tend to occur early in life, grow for a limited time, and then subside. There are no calcifications, as seen in juvenile aponeurotic fibroma, unless they have been present for a long time. Clinically, these tumors are distinguishable from Dupuytren nodules because they occur earlier in life, tend not to multiply, have no predilection for the ulnar side of the hand, and are not associated with contractures. These tumors are well encapsulated and are easily dissected free from surrounding tissue by blunt dissection. They are firm, white, and composed of dense mature fibroblasts and fibrous tissue. Marginal extracapsular excision usually is curative.

DESMOID TUMOR

Extraabdominal desmoid tumors are benign, rare, aggressive, and infiltrative lesions that make surgical excision difficult and recurrence common. There is no sex predilection, and the tumors more commonly affect the forearm than the hand (Fig. 15.7). Tumor excision is the mainstay of treatment; however, disease-free margins may be difficult to obtain. Nonetheless, recurrence rates in the forearm and hand are 60% and 33%, respectively. Disease recurrence is more common in younger patients. Adjunctive radiation treatment does not appear to

decrease the recurrence rate but does increase the 5-year disease-free interval. Hence, radiation therapy may be reasonable for patients with incomplete excision or in whom tumor resection resulted in substantial morbidity.

NEUROFIBROMA

Neurofibromas rarely exist as solitary lesions, and most that occur as multiple lesions are associated with neurofibromatosis or von Recklinghausen disease. The solitary form usually occurs in the first decade of life, and the multiple form frequently manifests after 30 years of age. These lesions in the hand involve the more distal digital nerves (Fig. 15.8), where enlargement may produce grotesque finger angulation and gigantism. They are usually centrally located, nontender, more nodular, and nonencapsulated, and may involve the skin, making them less mobile than schwannomas. The lesion is not resectable without sacrificing nerve elements because the nerve fibers intersperse in the tumor mass. Often these involve cutaneous nerves where proximal, and distal to the lesion the nerve caliber appears normal. The solitary and multiple forms are histologically indistinguishable; both have a plexiform mass of irregular, thickened nerve fibers separated by increased endoneural matrix. Malignant transformation in neurofibromatosis has been reported to occur in 15% of patients, and complete excision is necessary for lesions that enlarge and become painful.

GLOMUS TUMOR

A glomus body is a specialized neuromyoarterial receptor composed of an afferent arteriole, an anastomotic Sucquet-Hoyer canal, an afferent venule, actin-containing glomus cells surrounding the canals, intraglomerular retinaculum, and capsule. The glomus body functions as a dermal shunt that normally

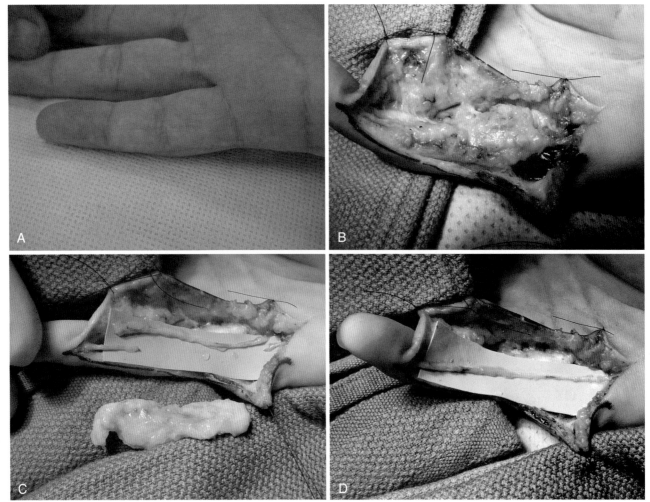

FIGURE 15.4 **A,** Recurrent intraneural lipofibroma of ulnar digital nerve to small finger. **B,** Surgical exposure showing 4 cm segment of involved ulnar digital nerve with normal-appearing proximal and distal segments. **C,** En bloc excision of digital nerve and tumor with nerve graft placed in proximity. **D,** Nerve graft sutured in place.

regulates skin temperature and blood pressure. Hyperplasia of one or more parts of the glomus body causes this tumor or a variant. Glomus cells are specialized perivascular muscle cells that are round or oval and have a dense, granular cytoplasm. The etiology for glomus tumors is unknown, but trauma and genetic mutations have been implicated. Nonmyelinated nerve fibers that are intermixed with thick-walled capillaries are postulated to be responsible for the lancinating pain.

Pain, cold sensitivity, and point tenderness are the characteristic of glomus tumors (described by Wood in 1812 and histologically clarified by Barre and Masson in 1924). Glomus tumors may be solitary or multiple. The lesions arise mainly in women (75%) and occur at an average age of 46 years (18 to 72 years). Seventy-five percent are subungual in location (Trehan et al.) (Fig. 15.9). Although they occur more often in the hand, up to 25% may be located elsewhere, and a diagnosis requires a high index of suspicion. Multiple lesions are associated with neurofibromatosis I and may be nontender, making their diagnosis sometimes elusive. Direct pressure on the tumor by a small, firm object causes excruciating pain (Love test), whereas pressure applied slightly to one side of it elicits no pain. Elimination of the pin-point tenderness with

tourniquet-induced ischemia (Hildredth test) is also characteristic of glomus tumors. Immersing the involved hand or digit in ice water also exacerbates the discomfort, and a red, opaque dot seen with transillumination of the finger pad may be a useful additional test for some glomus tumors.

Glomus tumors are usually less than 1 cm in diameter, often being only a few millimeters in diameter. High-Tesla MRI scans may prove helpful in diagnosing these rare tumors, with a cold T1 and bright T2 signal being classic but nondiagnostic. Moreover, smaller tumors, those with atypical pathology or location, and tumors not suspected clinically may produce a false-negative MRI study. Trehan et al. found that 33% of histologically proven glomus tumors had negative MRI studies.

Most of these tumors are benign; however, if the lesion exceeds 2.0 cm and histologic parameters suggest malignancy, then metastatic rates exceed 25%. Most of these tumors can be removed under local anesthesia and should be accurately localized by marking the lesion(s) just before surgery. Meticulous and complete excision of the usually well-encapsulated lesions is normally curative, although reoperation rates of 12% to 24% have been reported. Unrecognized synchronous satellite lesions may explain tumors developing in new sites; however,

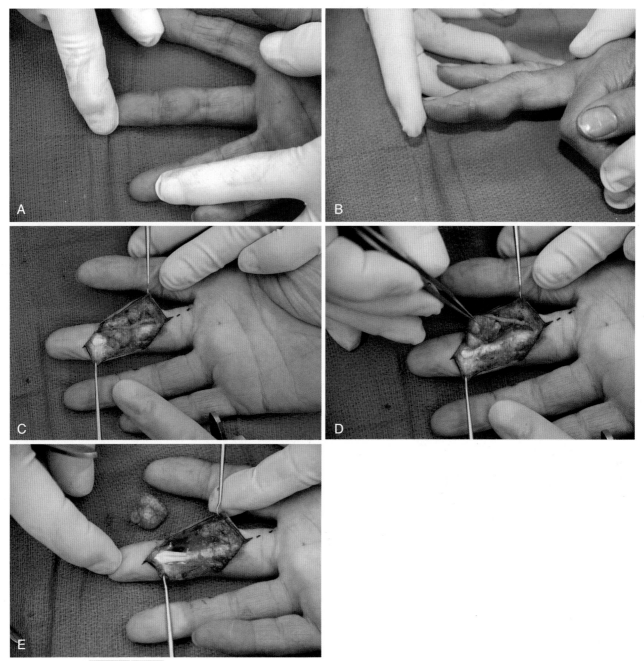

FIGURE 15.5   Giant cell tumor. **A** and **B,** A 77-year-old woman with 6-month history of enlarging nonpainful mass in right middle finger. **C,** Surgical dissection showing well-encapsulated giant cell tumor with typical yellowish brown color. **D,** Marginal tumor resection. **E,** Finger appearance after flexor sheath and distal interphalangeal joint inspection for additional tumor.

recurrence has been associated with tumor beneath the nail bed and those poorly differentiated from the tumor bed. A retrospective, multicenter study of 72 patients (Kim et al.) found a recurrence rate of 6.9%. No significant difference in outcomes were noted between microscopic procedures and loupe procedures, and no risk factors for recurrence were noted.

HEMANGIOMA

The following remarks are limited to the cavernous hemangioma and do not include the capillary superficial infantile hemangioma, which tends to involute by age 7 years. A cavernous hemangioma can be slightly-to-moderately tender and may enlarge a digit with distended venous sinuses. It produces a bluish color when it occurs close to the surface and forms a soft, collapsible mass (Fig. 15.10). Calcifications may be visible on radiographs. Custom-fitted compression garments can be a useful conservative treatment. Radiation therapy is discouraged. Surgery is the treatment of choice for cavernous hemangiomas if symptoms justify it. The tumor can be so extensive that a staged procedure is required for its removal. Sometimes, vessel ligation can assist a second-stage lesion excision. A rare coagulopathy, Kasabach-Merritt syndrome, can occur with lesions larger than 5 cm as a result of secondary platelet sequestration. Early treatment is indicated with this syndrome. With careful tourniquet control, blood partially fills the sinuses and outlines the extent of the tumor at the time of surgical excision. Complete excision is usually curative if the tumor is fairly

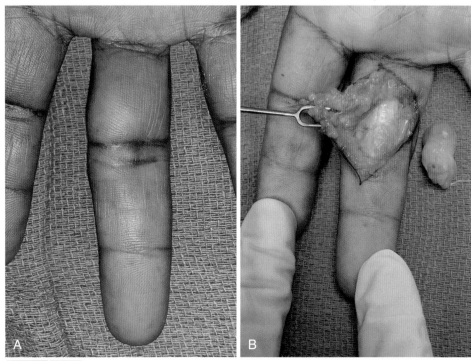

FIGURE 15.6 **A,** Painless fibroma resulting in enlargement of middle finger base. **B,** Well-encapsulated lesion removed en bloc through Bruner incision.

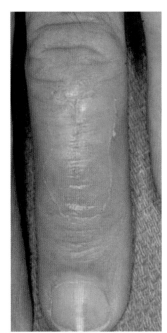

FIGURE 15.7 Desmoid tumor of finger. (From Maher J, Smith D, Parker WL: Desmoid tumor of the hand: a case report, *Ann Plast Surg* 73:390, 2014.)

well localized (Fig. 15.11); however, in diffuse lesions, persistence rather than recurrence is common. If complete excision is impossible, tumor debulking should be the emphasis of the procedure.

LYMPHANGIOMA

Lymphangiomas are benign soft-tissue tumors that consist of an abnormal proliferation of lymph vessels and lymphoid tissue. They rarely occur in the hand. Their tendency to occur

during childhood and to recur after excision, and the pain associated with the condition, make them especially troublesome for the patient, the patient's parents, and the surgeon. They have no malignant potential and overly aggressive surgery should be avoided because hypertrophic scarring may follow. Parents and surgeons should have realistic expectations and goals. Excisional biopsy is recommended for diagnostic confirmation and tumor debulking.

NEURILEMOMA (SCHWANNOMA)

Neurilemomas arise from Schwann cells or sheath cells (Fig. 15.12) and are rarely found in the hand despite being the most common solitary tumor of the peripheral nerves. Proliferation of the Schwann cells begins around one nerve fascicle and results in an eccentric or a centrally located tumor. Two types of Schwann cells are present: hypercellular (Antoni A) cells, which are arranged in palisades and are composed of plump and fusiform nuclei known as Verocay bodies, and hypocellular (Antoni B) cells, which are nonuniform cells dispersed in a myxomatous matrix. These tumors are not extremely tender and are more mobile at right angles to the course of the nerve than in line with the nerve. Neurilemomas are frequently misdiagnosed as ganglions and are rarely multifocal. With careful microsurgical technique, these tumors can usually be dissected from the surrounding nerve. Malignant degeneration is rare and excision is curative. An alternative diagnosis or malignancy should be considered if the mass cannot be dissected free from the nerve trunk or is adherent to adjacent tissue. In such situations, incisional biopsy is indicated.

OSTEOID OSTEOMA

Osteoid osteomas are characterized by pain that gradually increases from mild to severe and is usually worse at night. Although dramatic pain relief can be obtained from salicylates, a small proportion of patients get no or only partial relief with

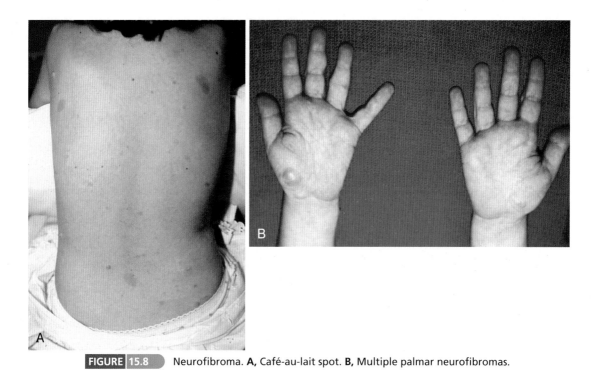

FIGURE 15.8 Neurofibroma. **A,** Café-au-lait spot. **B,** Multiple palmar neurofibromas.

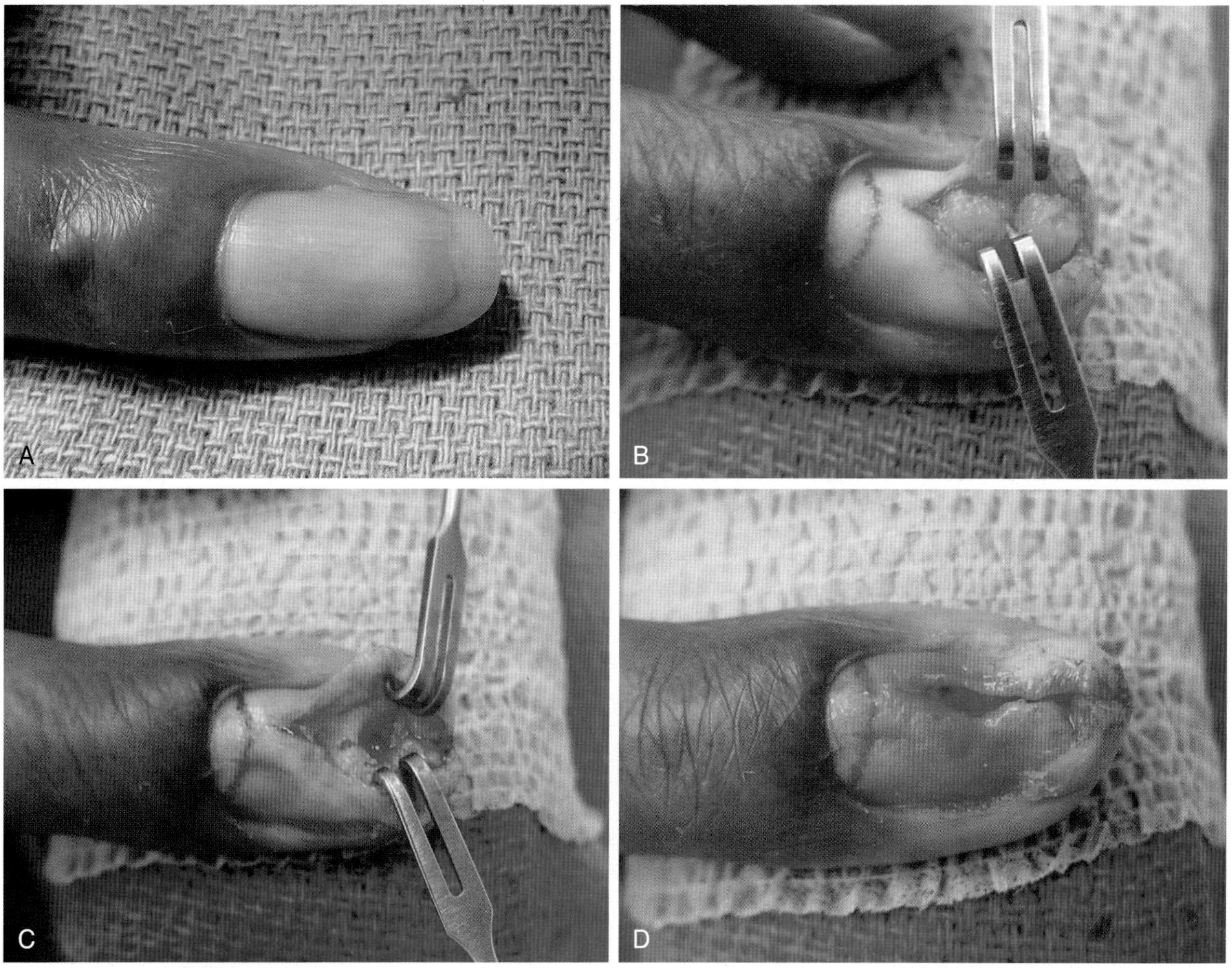

FIGURE 15.9 **A,** Subungual glomus tumor with bluish discoloration. **B,** Nail removed and nail bed incised to expose underlying glomus tumor. **C,** Glomus tumor excised with preservation of nail bed. **D,** Nail bed sutured.

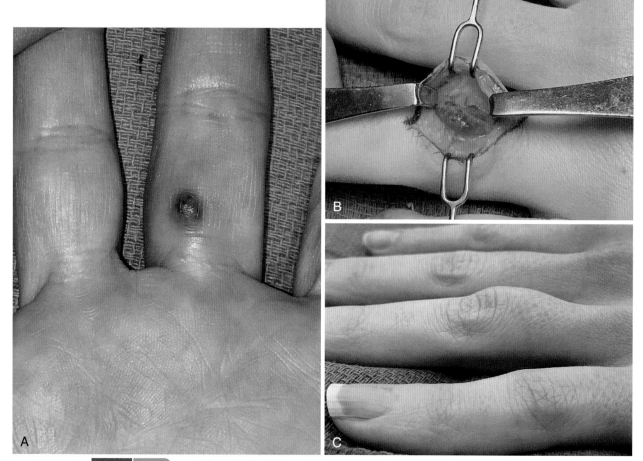

FIGURE 15.10 **A,** Solitary isolated hemangioma in 35-year-old woman with mild tenderness. Treatment was by marginal excision **(B)**.

nonsteroidal antiinflammatory medications. In one study, more than half of upper extremity osteoid osteomas occurred in the wrist and hand; the lesion occurred twice as often in men as in women, and the average age at diagnosis was 19 years (range 4 to 40 years). Some osteoid osteomas of the phalanges are painless, presumably because of the lack of nerve fibers trapped within the tumor. Generalized swelling of the involved part and tenderness to pressure are frequent findings. The carpus, especially the scaphoid, may be the site of involvement. The radiographic appearance depends on the area of bone involved. A small oval or round sclerotic nidus (Fig. 15.13) is surrounded first by an area of less dense bone, similar to a halo, and then by an area of sclerotic bone. Lesions in cortical bone or near the cortex may exhibit extreme sclerosis, requiring special imaging studies to reveal the nidus. A bone scan can be helpful in making the diagnosis. Treatment consists of creating a cortical window for complete removal of the nidus; recurrence may be expected if excision is incomplete. CT-guided radiofrequency ablation may also be used successfully for tumor management.

ENCHONDROMA

Enchondromas are the most common and destructive primary bone tumors of the hand (Fig. 15.14). The most common location is the proximal metaphysis of the proximal phalanx, where the enchondroma is eccentric and expansile (Fig. 15.15). Occasionally, some enlargement of the finger is seen if the loculated medullary tumor has expanded the bony cortex. Pathologic fracture is a common complication

because only minimal trauma is required to fracture the thin shell of bone. The fracture is usually allowed to heal before the tumor is excised. For tumor excision, a window is typically made where the cortical bone is expanded maximally and is the weakest, and the soft, blue, friable cartilaginous material is curetted thoroughly. Although the lesion may be treated successfully by curettage alone, we prefer to fill the cavity with bone graft and verify the filling by intraoperative imaging. Curettage and cementation supplemented with Kirschner wires, calcium phosphate defect packing, high-speed burring, and curettage with alcohol irrigation have also been described. Amputation may be necessary if all useful finger function has been lost. Malignant degeneration of an isolated enchondroma is rare; however, when these tumors are found in multiplicity, as in Ollier disease and Maffucci syndrome, the incidence of sarcomatous degeneration increases. Only multiple enchondromas are associated with Ollier disease, and symmetric hemangiomas visible on the hand and legs are associated with Maffucci syndrome. The diagnosis can usually be made from radiographs and the physical examination, but other destructive lesions, such as inclusion cysts, giant cell tumors, and aneurysmal bone cysts, should be considered.

BENIGN OSTEOBLASTOMA

Benign osteoblastomas are rare, but when they do arise they commonly occur in the small bones of the hands and feet. They are similar in appearance clinically and histologically to osteoid osteomas. In general, osteoblastomas tend to be larger

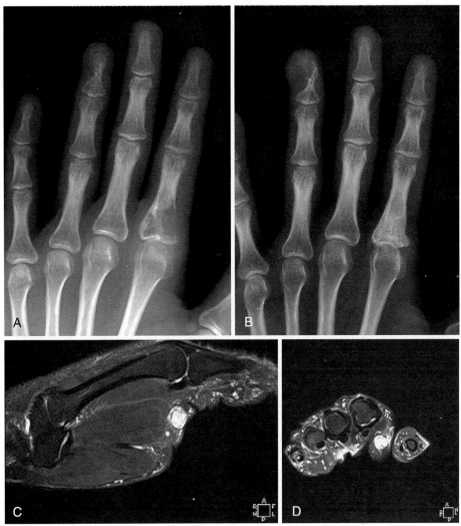

FIGURE 15.11 **A** and **B,** Anteroposterior radiographs showing finger hemangiomas. **C** and **D,** MRI of palmar hemangioma in 59-year-old man before marginal resection.

than osteoid osteomas, cause less pain, and are more expansile radiographically (Fig. 15.16). These tumors have a ground-glass appearance, producing gross metacarpal deformities, although the cortical shells remain intact. Histologically, areas of mature bone, osteoid, and plump osteoblasts are seen. Treatment is with curettage and bone grafting. Locally aggressive or recurrent lesions may require excision and interpositional bone grafting.

ANEURYSMAL BONE CYST

Aneurysmal bone cysts typically begin as eccentric ballooning lesions (metaphyseal, not epiphyseal) that enlarge to become centrally located, causing pain and limitation of motion (Fig. 15.17). Radiographically, they are almost indistinguishable from giant cell tumors or enchondromas. Tremendous cortical expansion and loss of mechanical stability make en bloc resection and autogenous bone grafting the treatment of choice for tubular bone involvement.

GIANT CELL TUMORS OF BONE

Giant cell tumors of bone are uncommon in the hand and have been reported more commonly in the distal radius than the carpal bones (hamate being most common) or phalanges. Despite being

benign, these tumors are aggressive and respond poorly to marginal excision and have a tendency to metastasize. Multicentric tumors have been reported, suggesting that a full bone survey is indicated to discover remote sites of tumor when a giant cell tumor is suspected. This tumor should not be confused with an enchondroma, and a biopsy is indicated to confirm the diagnosis. The Campanacci classification system may help in guiding treatment. Grade I lesions are well marginated, and cortical margins are thinned but not deformed and become grade II lesions when the cortex is expanded. Grade III lesions result when there is soft-tissue invasion and cortical containment has been lost.

Generally, curettage and bone grafting are insufficient treatment for this tumor. Giant cell tumors of the hand are just as aggressive as those found elsewhere. If the cortex is not eroded, resection of the bone and reconstructive surgery are indicated. Cortical invasion and destruction and recurrence may require en bloc excision and allograft reconstruction or ablation of the part (Fig. 15.18). Radiation therapy for giant cell tumors of bone has proved ineffective and has resulted in radiation sarcoma in 20% of patients. Cryosurgery may be useful as adjunctive treatment when simple curettage and bone grafting are performed.

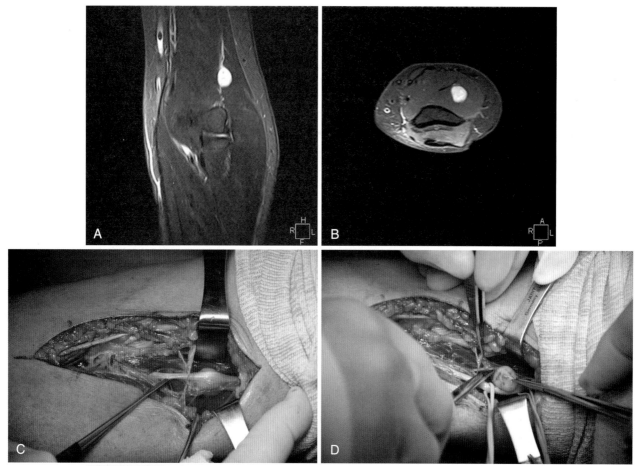

FIGURE 15.12 Schwannoma. **A** and **B**, MRI of elbow demonstrating a 1.3 cm painful mass in 60-year-old woman. **C**, Schwannoma of lateral antebrachial nerve. **D**, Tumor freed from nerve trunk.

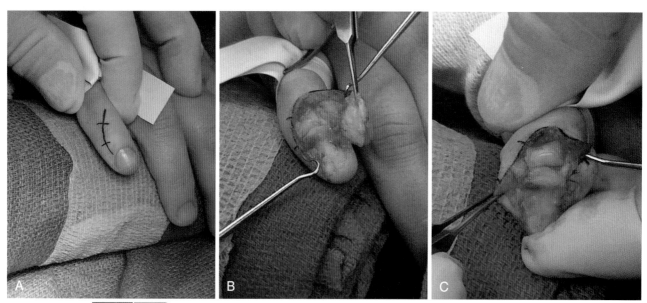

FIGURE 15.13 **A**, Approach to small finger distal phalanx in 30-year-old woman with intractable pain from osteoid osteoma. **B** and **C**, Exposures to lesion in base of distal phalanx successfully treated by curettage.

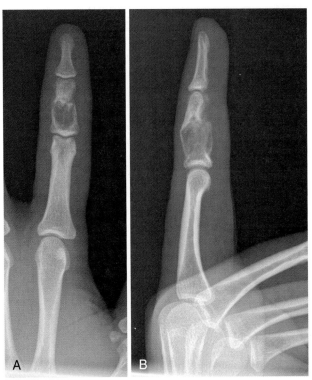

FIGURE 15.14 **A** and **B,** Enchondroma in middle phalanx in a 26-year-old man remained asymptomatic until pathologic fracture.

OSTEOCHONDROMA

Osteochondromas are rare in the hand but are seen occasionally on a phalanx (Fig. 15.19). They are most common in the metaphyseal area and can continue to grow until skeletal maturity. Excisional biopsy may be indicated because of pain, deformity, or mechanical symptoms.

SYNOVIAL CHONDROMATOSIS

Synovial chondromatosis is an unusual monarticular mechanical condition, usually of a large joint such as the knee, hip, elbow, or shoulder, caused by osteocartilaginous loose bodies that vary in size from microscopic to 2 cm in diameter. It most often affects middle-aged men and has been found in the proximal interphalangeal joint and wrist. Cartilaginous metaplasia from joint, tendon, or bursal synovial lining differentiates this entity from loose bodies arising from degenerative arthritis, osteochondritis dissecans, and osteochondral fractures. The plain films are usually characteristic, portraying multiple loose bodies of various sizes. Noncalcified, cartilaginous bodies may be detected by arthrography or MRI with contrast enhancement. Treatment involves removal of the loose bodies and perhaps synovectomy (Fig. 15.20).

MALIGNANT TUMORS

Malignant hand tumors (Table 15.5) are rare, and of the primary bone malignancies of the hand, chondrosarcoma is the most common. A variety of soft-tissue sarcomas occur in the hand and these include, more frequently, malignant fibrous histiocytomas and epithelioid sarcomas; however, liposarcoma,

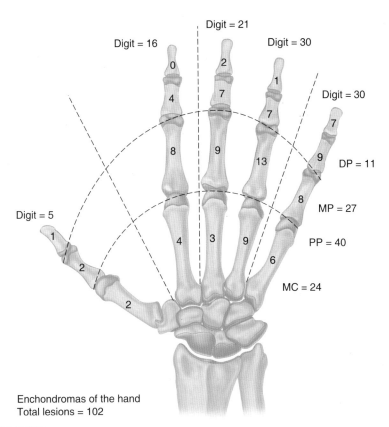

Enchondromas of the hand
Total lesions = 102

FIGURE 15.15   Location of enchondromas. (From Sassoon AA, Fitz-Gibbon PD, Harmsen WS, Moran SL: Enchondromas of the hand: factors affecting recurrence, healing, motion, and malignant transformation, *J Hand Surg* 37A:1229, 2012.)

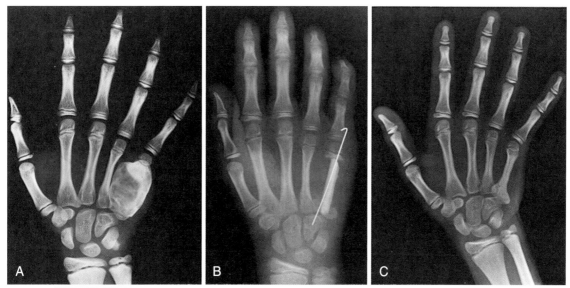

FIGURE 15.16   **A,** Expanding intraosseous tumor of fifth metacarpal with ground-glass appearance. Cortical shell is intact and has caused deformity of fourth metacarpal from pressure. **B,** Partial-thickness fibular graft has been interposed after excision of osteoblastoma. Physis and subchondral cortex of proximal metacarpal have been preserved. **C,** Graft has remodeled 15 months after operation. Evidence of tumor is absent, and physis and carpometacarpal joint have been maintained. (From Mosher JF, Peckham AC: Osteoblastoma of the metacarpal: a case report, *J Hand Surg* 3A:358, 1915.)

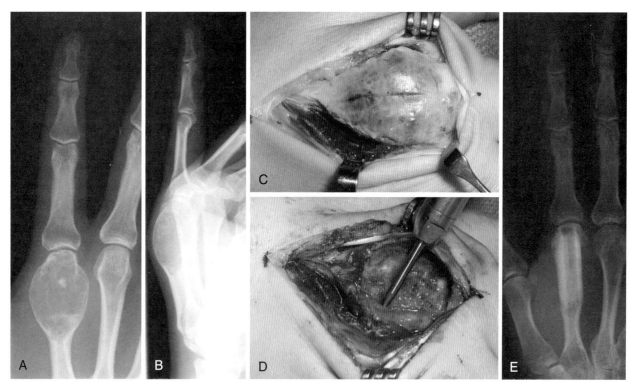

FIGURE 15.17   Aneurysmal bone cyst. **A** and **B,** Anteroposterior and lateral hand radiographs in 19-year-old woman with right hand mass. **C,** Surgical exposure of mass. **D,** Cavity after wide unroofing. **E,** Anteroposterior radiograph showing allograft strut reconstruction and incorporation 5 months after surgery. (From Crowe MM, Houdek MT, Moran SL, Kakar S: Aneurysmal bone cysts of the hand, wrist, and forearm, *J Hand Surg Am* 40:2052, 2015.)

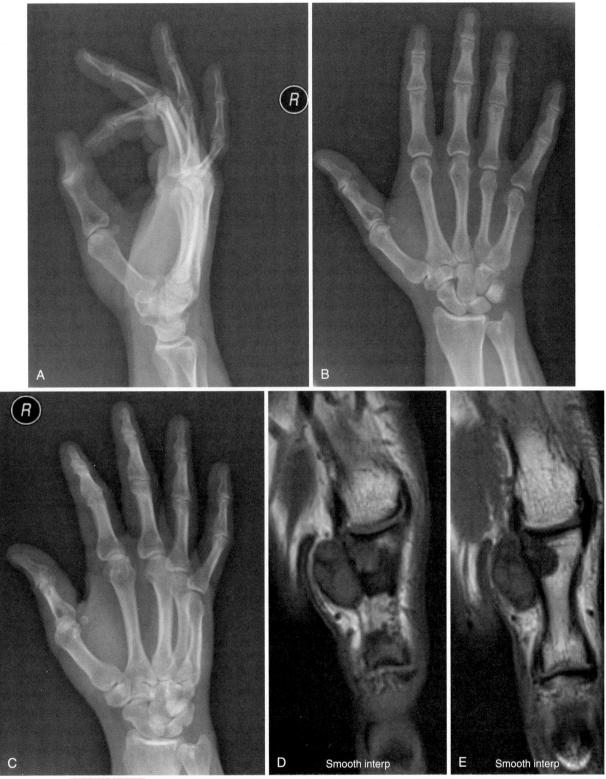

FIGURE 15.18 Giant cell tumor within base of thumb proximal phalanx. **A** through **C**, Plain images showing intraosseous lesion of giant cell tumor in 50-year-old man. **D** and **E**, MRI indicating extraosseous lesion.

leiomyosarcoma, synovial sarcoma, fibrosarcoma, rhabdomyosarcoma, angioleiomyosarcoma, and malignant nerve sheath tumors as well as a mixture of other rarer sarcomas are also reported. Epithelioid sarcoma in some series is reported just as frequently as fibrosarcoma and rhabdomyosarcoma. Metastatic tumors to the hand seldom occur even though bronchogenic

malignancies are associated with distal extremity involvement. Peculiar malignant lesions may initially present as indolent masses simply interfering with hand function (Fig. 15.21).

Proper surgical treatment of malignant hand tumors requires the removal of some normal hand tissue and, occasionally, limb-sparing techniques are not possible. The success

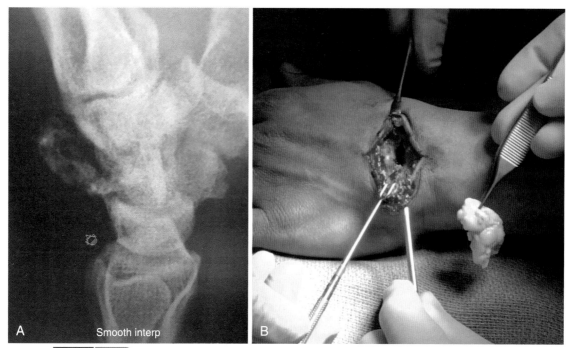

FIGURE 15.19   **A,** Lateral wrist view of osteochondroma of 1-year duration in 40-year-old man. **B,** Gross pathology of dense, white, well-encapsulated mass.

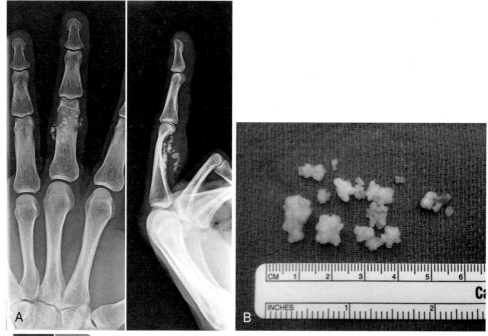

FIGURE 15.20   Synovial chondromatosis. **A,** Anteroposterior and lateral radiographs of 32-year-old man with insidious swelling of left middle finger. **B,** Multiple loose bodies removed from proximal interphalangeal joint and flexor sheath.

of surgery depends on whether residual tumor is left behind. Although some authors have stated that malignant bone tumors of the hand almost never metastasize, this can occur. Local recurrence of the tumor has not been shown to affect survival. Larger tumor size (>5 cm) and advanced tumor stage have been found to have a negative impact on survival, although significant tumor size in the hand is considerably smaller. A review of 198 acral soft-tissue sarcomas from 1998 to 2013 at the Mayo Clinic found that local recurrence after a wide excision was observed infrequently, yet distant disease was relatively common. Tumors 2 cm or more in size were associated with a worse disease-free and overall survival, highlighting the aggressive nature of these tumors.

Although one study reported a 70% survival rate at 5-year follow-up in patients with high-grade soft-tissue sarcomas of the extremity treated with limb-sparing surgery and brachytherapy, others found that amputation was better than other forms of treatment. Sentinel lymph node biopsy and/or dissection are

TABLE 15.5

Malignant Tumors of the Hand

TUMOR	AGE AT ONSET M:F	LOCATION	IMAGING	TREATMENT	SURVIVAL	SPECIAL NOTES
Osteogenic sarcoma	Fourth to sixth decades M=F	Rare in hand	Osteolysis and osteosclerosis	Wide excision Amputation Chemotherapy	Long-term survival after aggressive treatment better for lesions in the hand than elsewhere	Arise from primitive mesenchymal cells
Synovial sarcoma	<Fourth decade M=F	Carpus Rarely in fingers	Radiograph: spotty calcifications	Surgical excision wide margins Multidisciplinary treatment		
Chondrosarcoma	Second to fifth decades 2M:F1	Phalanges Metacarpal Carpus	Radiograph: cortical expansion and calcification	Curettage and bone grafting En bloc excision Chemotherapy	Prognosis good after excision	Second most common primary malignant bone tumor Locally aggressive May metastasize
Epithelioid sarcoma	Second to fourth decades 2M:1F	Hand 3-6 cm Flexor surface	Metastatic workup	Surgery Lymph node resection Chemotherapy	85% 5 and 10 years (F better than M)	Second most common soft-tissue malignancy
Squamous cell carcinoma	Fifth decade M>F	Hand Nail bed Uncommon in palm		Excision ± skin grafting Amputation in recurrent or deep tumors Lymph node dissection in recurrence with symptoms	Prognosis good	Histology: spindle cell, acantholytic, and verrucous Rarely metastasize
Basal cell carcinoma	Middle age M>F	Sun-exposed areas of hand		Excision ± skin grafting	Prognosis good	1% recurrence
Malignant melanoma	Average age 40-50 years M=F (depending on location of lesion)	Sun-exposed areas of hand Subungual thumb		Should be managed by oncologist/cancer surgeon	Survival related to tumor thickness	
Clear cell sarcoma	Wide age distribution M=F	Occurs near tendons and aponeurosis		Wide surgical excision Lymph node biopsy		Can be misdiagnosed as metastatic melanoma
Fibrosarcoma	Most common in third to fourth decades unless congenital M=F	Rare in the hand		Wide excision Amputation Multidisciplinary treatment		
Rhabdomyosarcoma	Alveolar more common in adolescents Slight male predilection	Alveolar more common in hand	Bone erosion seen in hand or foot	Total excision of extremity tumors Multidisciplinary treatment	Most are fatal	Improvement in survival rates observed with total excision and multidisciplinary treatment
Ewing sarcoma	First to second decades M>F	Rare in hand	Permeative pattern of bone destruction and periosteal reaction	Surgical excision combined with irradiation and chemotherapy	50%-75%	Highly aggressive

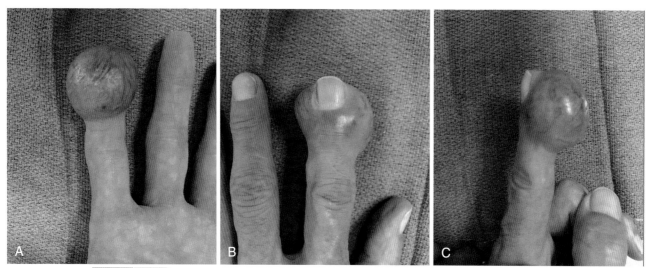

FIGURE 15.21 Aggressive digital papillary adenocarcinoma gradually enlarging over 1-year period in 60-year-old male labor superintendent. Treatment was proximal interphalangeal level disarticulation with clear margins and oncologic referral.

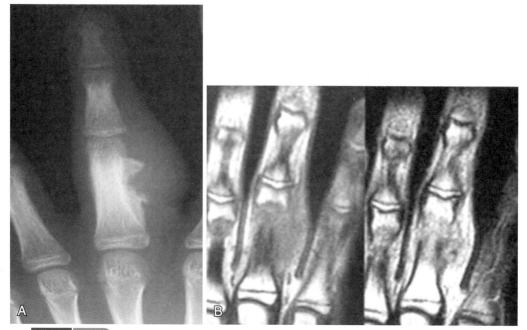

FIGURE 15.22 **A,** Osteogenic sarcoma of proximal phalanx. Note irregular mass of new bone with sunburst appearance. **B,** T1- and T2-weighted MRI reveals extent inside and outside cortex. (From Hanoki K, Miyauchi Y, Yajima H: Primary osteogenic sarcoma of a finger proximal phalanx: a case report and literature review, *J Hand Surg Am* 26:1151, 2001.)

somewhat controversial in the management of these tumors, and the reported benefit for disease-free and survival may not be influenced by such interventions. Although metastatic disease appears to be rare with malignant tumors, our practice is to let our oncology colleagues decide on appropriate metastatic workup and treatment because oncologic treatment continues to evolve and falls outside the scope of our practice.

OSTEOGENIC SARCOMA

Osteogenic sarcoma has rarely been reported to occur in the hand (Fig. 15.22). Irradiation from overexposure to x-rays or ingestion of radium salts has been cited as causative in some patients. The average age at presentation is 49 years. Careful wide excision of the tumor offers a good prognosis. The periosteal variant of osteogenic sarcoma can be treated by digital amputation, whereas ray and below-elbow amputation may be more appropriate for the other forms. The rarity of osteosarcoma in the hand makes treatment decisions based on data limited. The prognosis seems to be better, however, than for the same lesions located elsewhere.

CHONDROSARCOMA

Chondrosarcomas are the most common primary malignant bone tumors of the hand. Radiographically, chondrosarcoma

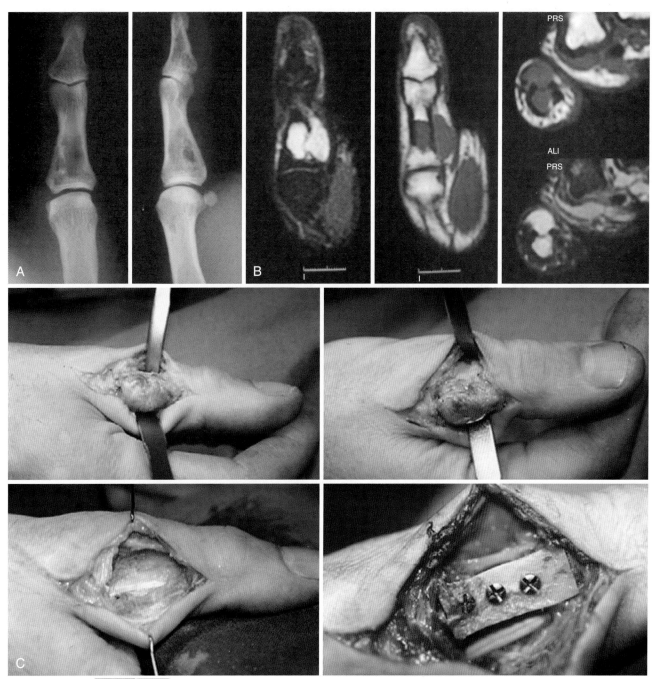

FIGURE 15.23 Patient with low-grade chondrosarcoma of left index finger treated with wide resection of the ray. **A,** Preoperative radiographs. **B,** MRI T1-weighted sequences without *(left)* and with *(right)* contrast. **C,** Excision and curettage and reconstruction with structural allograft.

may mimic osteoarthritis. Some chondrosarcomas have been reported in preexisting enchondromas, but this is rare.

Chondrosarcomas of the bones of the hands and feet are rare and can be difficult to differentiate from enchondromas. Pain is a presenting symptom, whereas it occurs rarely in other chondromas. A fracture may occur as the bone is weakened. A chondrosarcoma should be suspected if a lesion is painful or if it recurs after routine curettage of an enchondroma. When high-grade chondrosarcoma has been diagnosed, anything short of total or en bloc resection, such as ray resection, is usually unsuccessful. If radical surgery is the primary procedure, however, recurrence of the tumor is unlikely and the prognosis is good. Low-grade

chondrosarcomas, however, may be managed by digit sparing techniques rather than wide local excision by intralesional curettage and grafting (Fig. 15.23). Despite the aggressive appearance of the lesions histologically and radiographically, the lesions are less likely to metastasize. According to del Pino et al., only one of six lesions so treated had recurrence, and of those with recurrence treated similarly, there was a one in three chance of recurrence.

EPITHELIOID SARCOMA

Epithelioid sarcomas are commonly misdiagnosed initially because of their benign course. They usually present as unremarkable, subcutaneous, firm masses in young adults.

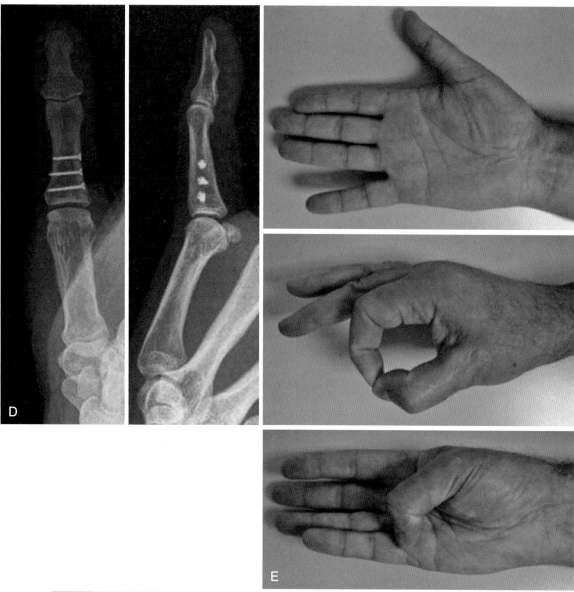

FIGURE 15.23, Cont'd D, Postoperative radiographs. E, Functional outcome at follow-up. (From Del Pino JG, Calderon SAL, Chebib I, Jupiter JB: Intralesional versus wide resection of low-grade chondrosarcoma of the hand, *J Hand Surg Am* 41[4]:541, 2016.)

They have a predilection to grow along fascial or tendinous structures, forming multiple nodules, and may appear to be a simple inflammatory process. At times, the overlying skin ulcerates with necrosis of the underlying lesion. The histologic appearance of these tumors can also be confusing, but there is a basic granulomatous pattern with central necrosis and surrounding inflammatory cells. Under high magnification, tumor cells take on the appearance of epithelial cells. Metastasis to regional lymph nodes is common, and metastasis to the lungs usually follows multiple recurrences. Local recurrence has been noted in 85% of patients, usually within 6 months after excision. An inadequate excision is invariably followed by recurrence. A primary wide excision or an amputation of a digit or entire ray is indicated (Fig. 15.24). Even after a wide excision, the tumor may be present within the margins of the specimen, requiring further excision. A below-elbow amputation may be necessary after any recurrence in the hand proximal to the metacarpophalangeal joints.

Regional node dissection in combination with the primary excision is recommended. The role of adjuvant chemotherapy is currently unclear.

SQUAMOUS CELL CARCINOMA

Squamous cell carcinomas usually occur in individuals in their 50s and are four times more common in men than in women. They account for 58% to 90% of all hand malignancies and exceed malignant melanomas as the most common malignancy of the nail bed. Squamous cell carcinomas have a predilection for the sun-exposed areas of skin and are uncommon on the palm. They vary in appearance from small, desquamating, and erythematous lesions to large, fungating, and ulcerative lesions. Histologic types include conventional (differentiated), spindle cell, acantholytic, and verrucous forms. They grow slowly, rarely metastasize, and are usually superficial and low grade. Recurrence rates vary from 7% to 22%. Recurrence-free survival was 67% and 50% at 5 and 10 years, respectively,

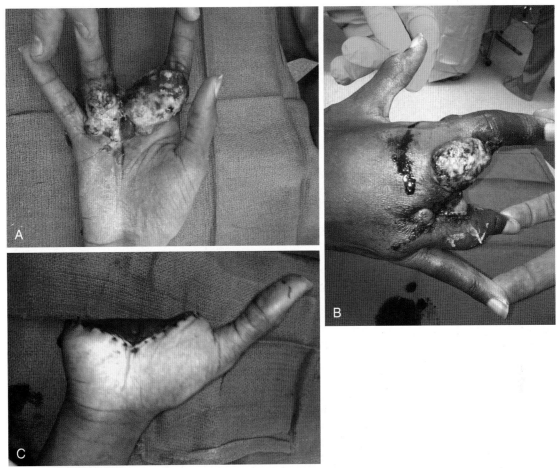

FIGURE 15.24   **A** and **B,** A 17-year-old boy with a rapidly progressing epithelioid sarcoma after middle finger ray amputation. **C,** After hand amputation.

according to Askari et al. in a 20-year review of 86 patients with squamous cell carcinomas. Rate of metastasis was 4%. Survival, free of squamous cell carcinoma in the same upper extremity, was 72% and 54% at 5 and 10 years, respectively. Younger age, history of transplantation, multiple tumors, and use of flap or skin graft for closure were associated with an increased risk of another squamous cell carcinoma developing in the same extremity. Poor risk factors include size greater than 2 cm, poor differentiation, immunosuppression, increased depth of invasion, perineural involvement, and recurrence, which is the only factor that depends on surgery. Tumor-free margins should be at least 0.5 cm for small lesions and 3 cm for recurrent or fixed lesions; however, no benefit was noted with wide, Mohs, or shave resection in terms of overall survival, recurrence-free survival, or squamous cell occurrence in the ipsilateral upper extremity (Fig. 15.25). Skin grafting is commonly is used after excision of larger tumors, and amputation may be required for fixed or recurrent lesions, especially when there is penetration into deeper structures. Lymph node dissection is usually is reserved for patients with fixed or recurrent tumors or for patients presenting with lymph node enlargement.

Squamous cell cancer of the nail unit is most commonly an in-situ form, although 15% may become invasive. Any nail bed lesion not responding to topical treatment should have a biopsy. The thumb is most commonly involved and presentation is usually late. Because the vast majority of the lesions are slow growing and not invasive, metastatic work-up is

usually not required. A literature review suggested that physical examination for regional lymph node involvement is sufficient work-up before surgery unless there is bone involvement or other signs of invasion. Tumor recurrence is unlikely after amputation, and 8.7% recurrence has been reported after wide local excision. Safe margins for excision have not been published; however, higher recurrence rates are reported with Mohs technique.

BASAL CELL CARCINOMA

A raised, pearly-bordered lesion should make basal cell carcinoma a likely diagnosis in a middle-aged, fair-skinned man. Basal cell carcinomas are the most common cancer, yet in the hand they are far less common than the more aggressive squamous cell carcinomas. Despite the dorsum of the hand having the most ultraviolet light exposure, basal cell tumors in this area are rare, presumably because they occur in sebaceous glands. The tumor cells are located at the raised areas of the nodular tumors, which makes the excision boundaries fairly clear. These relatively benign tumors can be excised with a 0.5 cm free margin. Recurrence rates of 1% have been reported.

MALIGNANT MELANOMA

Melanomas are reported to occur in 1 in 70 white men, and the incidence continues to increase 6% per year, faster than any other cancer (Fig. 15.26). The death rate is increasing 2% per year. Exposure to ultraviolet radiation has been proposed

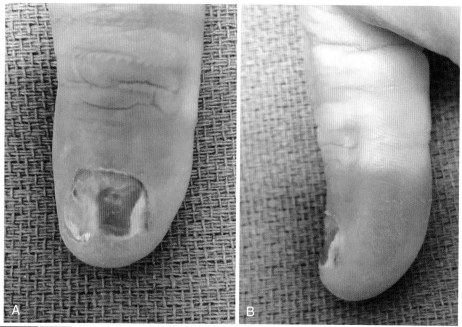

FIGURE **15.25** Moderately differentiated squamous cell carcinoma of nail bed in a 53-year-old man.

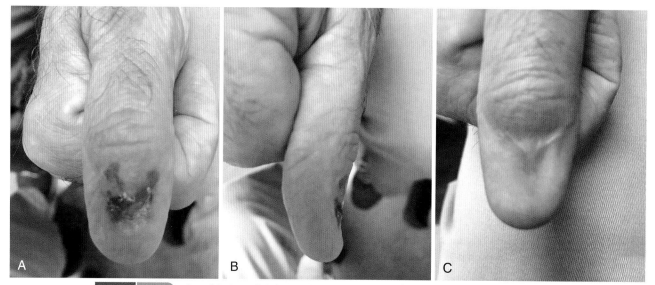

FIGURE **15.26** **A** and **B,** Superficial spreading subungual malignant melanoma of thumb with characteristic eponychial and lateral fold pigmentation (Hutchinson's sign). **C,** Appearance after marginal excision, skin grafting, and secondary healing.

to be the primary risk factor. Survival, which is related to tumor thickness, ranges from 97% for lesions 0.75 mm thick or less, to 50% for lesions 3 mm thick or more. Melanomas are generally asymmetric and have irregular borders, uneven colors, and diameters larger than 6 mm. Awareness of these distinguishing characteristics is essential for early detection. An oncologist and a cancer surgeon should manage lesions that are thicker than 1 mm because chemotherapy and immunotherapy regimens are still evolving, and lymph node biopsy and dissection may be integral to the management.

Melanotic lesions under the nail may not be malignant; however, characteristics such as new onset hyperpigmentation, variable bandwidth of discoloration, irregular lesion border and

pigmentation, ulceration, and nail splitting or bleeding should raise the suspicion for a subungual melanoma. *Acral lentiginous, nodular, desmoplastic, superficial spreading,* and *unclassified* are common subtype classifications of subungual melanomas. Nonetheless, suspicious lesions require a biopsy, ideally performed under local anesthesia after atraumatic nail plate removal. The specimen should be full thickness and longitudinally oriented with excision of the entire lesion if nail bed approximation is possible. Specialized stains aside from hematoxylin and eosin include HMB-45 and MART-1 (melanocytic antigen recognized by cytotoxic T-lymphocytes) immunostains. According to Terushkin et al. the use of MART-1 immunostain allowed better tumor detection and excision using a digit-sparing Mohs technique, resulting in no local disease recurrence. Lesions that do not extend vertically through the entire matrix are considered melanoma in situ, and all others are considered invasive. According to Yang et al., malignant melanoma of the finger is usually diagnosed at a late stage. Nearly 60% of their 22 patients had metastases at the time of presentation; hence, a comprehensive approach is not limited to surgical intervention. Cytokine-induced killer (CIK) cell therapy uses tumor-specific T lymphocytes capable of effectively attacking tumors. At present, CIK cell therapy achieves 60% to 90% cytotoxic activity in the treatment of kidney cancer, malignant melanoma, leukemia, and malignant lymphoma; however, detection of distant disease remains inaccurate, and the use of sentinel lymph node biopsy, although frequently recommended, may not detect metastatic disease, has a high false negative rate, and does not confer a survival benefit.

FIBROSARCOMA

Fibrosarcomas are of mesothelial origin. The enlargement of a mass on the hand or pressure on peripheral nerves may cause the patient to seek help; however, painless masses are more common. Fibrosarcomas can occur years after radiation exposure and in scars from burn injuries. Congenital and infantile fibrosarcomas that occur in the extremity are also rare. Wide excision or amputation is indicated.

METASTATIC TUMORS

Metastatic tumors occurring in the hand have been reported as arising most frequently from bronchogenic carcinomas, but they have also been reported as arising from carcinoma of the kidney, prostate gland, breast, uterus, and colon. They are rare, representing approximately 0.1% of all metastatic lesions, and occur in the distal phalanges most commonly, especially the thumb. They can be confused with infection because usually there is tenderness, swelling, and redness. Radiographs may show osteolytic lesions that are usually destroying the adjacent cortical bone; however, prostate and breast tumors may produce osteoblastic lesions. Hand metastatic lesions are accompanied 66% of the time by metastatic lesions elsewhere. Whole body bone scans are commonly employed in the workup, and local hand imaging should be performed. Other than infection, the differential diagnosis includes gout, giant cell tumor of bone, enchondroma, epidermoid cyst, and aneurysmal bone cyst. A tissue diagnosis is imperative. The patient's general condition may determine the treatment. If a phalangeal lesion is painful, an amputation through the joint proximal to the level of involvement should relieve pain and provide rapid healing. The presence of a metastatic lesion in the hand carries an ominous prognosis for patient survival, with a median survival of 5 to 6 months.

RHABDOMYOSARCOMA

Another rare malignant tumor of the hand is rhabdomyosarcoma. Most reported rhabdomyosarcomas have been fatal, in contrast to other malignant bone tumors in the hand. Any one of the three types can occur (alveolar, embryonal, and pleomorphic). The alveolar form seems to be more common in the limbs. Most limb rhabdomyosarcomas are deeply situated and intimately associated with striated muscle and are painless despite rapid growth. Bone erosion is common with tumors affecting the hands and feet. The location of these tumors in the extremities may account for an unfavorable prognosis. Survival rates in general have increased with a multidisciplinary approach that includes total excision of extremity tumors.

EWING SARCOMA

Ewing sarcoma, similar to other malignant tumors, rarely involves the hand. It occurs more frequently in males and usually manifests during the second decade of life. Clinically, the tumor is often mistaken for a local infection because the patient may report pain, swelling, fever, and general malaise. Leukocytosis and elevation in the erythrocyte sedimentation rate are common. Radiographs of the hand show a permeative pattern of bone destruction with periosteal reaction. Ewing sarcoma is a highly aggressive tumor. In the past, 5-year survival rates were reported to be 10% to 15%; however, with newer chemotherapy and radiation therapies combined with surgical excision, survival rates have improved to 50% to 75%.

TUMOROUS CONDITIONS
GANGLION

Ganglions are the most common cause of focal hand masses and characteristically arise from the synovium of joints or tendon sheaths. They can be intratendinous, causing snapping or triggering. Ganglion cysts may fluctuate in size, distinguishing them from true tumors. The cause of ganglion cysts is unclear; however a history of acute or recurrent stress may suggest an etiology.

The most common upper extremity ganglion cyst is found on the dorsal wrist and is usually visible or palpable between the second and fourth extensor tendon compartments. However, cysts in this region may also be too small to detect on physical examination and require advanced imaging to confirm the diagnosis. Nonetheless, in the absence of trauma, a dorsal ganglion cyst should be suspected when there is focal tenderness directly over the scapholunate region even with nonconfirmatory advanced imaging. Cyst size may not be proportional to the patient's pain symptoms, and even small and imperceptible cysts may cause incapacitating pain in some patients. Dorsal wrist ganglions are usually firm, smooth, fluctuant, and round.

Ganglion-like cysts may extend proximally along the extensor tendons and be confused with true dorsal ganglion cysts. If the cystic masses move with the extensor tendons they may represent a rheumatologic condition. Likewise, dorsal ganglion cysts may be confused with anomalous extensor digitorum brevis manus muscles, which, unlike true dorsal ganglion cysts, become firmer with resisted finger extension. Last, firm and noncompressible dorsal wrist masses located slightly more distal and radial may represent carpal bossing and be confused with dorsal wrist ganglion cysts.

True dorsal ganglion cysts represent intraarticular capsular and ligamentous pathology and almost uniformly arise just distal to or from the dorsal portion of the scapholunate interosseous ligament. Dorsal wrist ganglions can be ruptured by digital pressure (such as being struck by a book), aspiration, or surgical excision. Success rates of 90% can be expected with either open or arthroscopic excision and 65% with a needle after cyst puncture and injection of cortisone. Arthroscopic resection of dorsal wrist ganglion cysts has been reported to have a low complication rate, but this more challenging technique has not substantially lowered the recurrence rate when compared with open techniques, which we prefer. Surgical excision of a ganglion should include removal of a generous capsular margin around the cyst base and ligament debridement, and no attempt should be made to close the joint capsule.

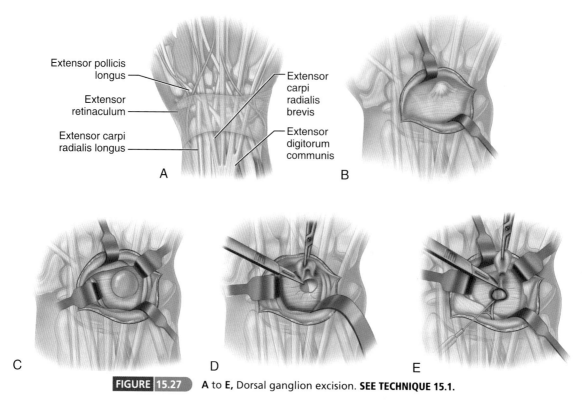

Extensor pollicis longus

Extensor retinaculum

Extensor carpi radialis longus

Extensor carpi radialis brevis

Extensor digitorum communis

A

B

C

D

E

FIGURE 15.27 A to E, Dorsal ganglion excision. **SEE TECHNIQUE 15.1.**

The second most frequent ganglion cyst arises from the volar wrist, often just radial to the flexor carpi radialis tendon. The origination sites for these cysts include the volar scapholunate ligament and/or capsule, radioscaphoid joint, scaphotrapezial joint, trapeziometacarpal joint, and the flexor carpi radialis tendon sheath. Rarely, cysts in this region may be volar expressions of dorsal carpal ganglion cysts. Although aspiration of these cysts may be possible, the proximity of the radial artery and uncertainty of origin may make surgical management in symptomatic cysts more reasonable.

Volar retinacular ganglion cysts arise from the flexor tendon sheath commonly near the metacarpophalangeal joint flexor skin crease. Here the masses are frequently round, usually isolated, not moveable, hard, and often tender to firm pressure. Volar retinacular ganglion cysts may be managed by needle puncture, but we favor open excision.

Ganglion cysts may be associated with various wrist and finger degenerative conditions (discussed elsewhere). However, even in the absence of pisotriquetral degenerative arthritis, cysts on the volar ulnar wrist may be first suspected with manifestations of low ulnar nerve compression, such as atrophy of the ulnar intrinsic muscles.

EXCISION OF A DORSAL WRIST GANGLION

TECHNIQUE 15.1

- Under tourniquet control, make a 2.0 to 3.0 cm transverse incision in one of the dorsal wrist extension creases centered over the scapholunate interval. This incision will often be proximal to the cystic prominence and roughly along a

line connecting the ulnar and radial styloids (Fig. 15.27A). The incision should not be too far radial or ulnar because the radial and ulnar dorsal sensory nerve branches, respectively, may be encountered. Carry the incision through the dermis only and spread the underlying subcutaneous tissues away from underlying extensor retinaculum.
- Protect all cutaneous nerves by carefully elevating the soft tissues off the extensor retinaculum, especially the often-visible superficial sensory branch of the radial nerve (Fig. 15.27B and C).
- Open the ulnar border of extensor pollicis longus from the radiocarpal joint distally for several centimeters and retract this tendon and the underlying radial wrist extensor tendons radialward.
- Enter the fourth dorsal compartment and expose the common extensor tendons by opening the extensor retinaculum longitudinally. Extend the exposure from the radiocarpal joint and far enough distally to allow ulnarward retraction of the extensor digitorum communis tendons.
- Identify the dorsal intercarpal and radiocarpal ligaments and retract them distally and proximally, respectively. At this point, with sharp and blunt dissection, dissect the ganglion cyst in its entirety, including a portion of its capsular origin at the dorsal scapholunate interosseous ligament (Fig. 15.27D). Preserve the scapholunate interosseous ligament, especially the distal dorsal portion, which is where most of the cysts arise and is the most important portion of this ligament. Dissect this portion of the ligament cleanly to expose the remaining normal portions of scapholunate interosseous ligament. Note that sometimes the cyst may originate from the ligament, and the degenerative portions of this ligament can be carefully debrided. Remove redundant capsular synovial tissue from the midcarpal and radiocarpal joints.
- The posterior interosseous nerve terminal branch can be located on the radial floor of the fourth extensor compartment

either at this stage or during entry into and dissection of the fourth extensor compartment tendons. Gently dissect and retract this nerve from the radial floor of the fourth compartment, divide the nerve by electrocautery, and allow its divided end to retract proximal to the radiocarpal joint (Fig. 15.27E).

- After hemostasis is achieved, close the wound. We prefer a 5-0 subcuticular suture reinforced with Steri-Strip over a skin adhesive. The wound is then infiltrated with a regional block if a general anesthetic was used. Apply a soft compressive dressing.

POSTOPERATIVE CARE The patient may remove the dressing at home 2 to 3 days after surgery and initiate a range-of-motion program. The first postoperative appointment is at 2 weeks, at which time the sutures (if required) can be removed, and a more aggressive therapy program is encouraged. Usually 6 weeks is required to achieve full range of motion and return to unrestricted activities.

EXCISION OF A VOLAR WRIST GANGLION

TECHNIQUE 15.2

- Perform an Allen test preoperatively to assess the integrity of the radial and ulnar artery contributions to the hand.
- Under tourniquet control, make a longitudinal incision, centered over the ganglion, which is usually situated just radial to the flexor carpi radialis tendon. Avoid injury to cutaneous sensory branches in this area.
- Carefully dissect the radial artery from the cystic mass. The dissection is simplified by beginning proximal to the lesion where the artery can be clearly delineated from the abnormal tissue.
- Carry the dissection down along the stalk of the ganglion to its origin, which may arise from several regions including the radioscaphoid, scapholunate, scaphotrapezial, and trapeziometacarpal; on rare occasion it may be a projection of a dorsal ganglion cyst coming under the first extensor compartment tendons.
- Excise the origin with a small portion of the surrounding capsule.
- Cauterize the capsular margins and irrigate the wound.
- Deflate the tourniquet to inspect the integrity of the radial artery. Use electrocautery to control any further bleeding.
- After meticulous hemostasis is achieved, irrigate the wound, close with suture, and infiltrate the wound with a local anesthetic.
- Apply a soft, lightly compressive sterile dressing.

POSTOPERATIVE CARE The soft dressing allows for wrist motion early and can usually be removed at 2 to 3 days postoperatively. The sutures are removed at 2 weeks, and active range-of-motion exercises continued; rarely is supervised therapy required.

ARTHROSCOPIC RESECTION OF A DORSAL WRIST GANGLION

TECHNIQUE 15.3

(OSTERMAN AND RAPHAEL; LUCHETTI ET AL.)
- Apply distraction by finger traps attached to the index, long, and ring fingers and countertraction of 3 to 4 kg at the arm.
- Use an axillary block or general anesthesia and a tourniquet to allow good exposure of the joint.
- Make two portals for access to the radiocarpal joint.
- Place a 1.9 or 2.7 mm arthroscope into the 3-4 portal to examine the joint. If this portal does not offer clear exposure, move the arthroscope to the 4-5, 1-2, or 6R portals (see chapter 6).
- Locate the scapholunate ligament and direct the arthroscope dorsally to view the ganglion or its stalk.
- Introduce the probe through the 3-4 portal to palpate the scapholunate ligament and dorsal capsule to determine the consistency of the ligament and the stalk of the ganglion.
- Use a 2.0 or 2.9 mm full-radius shaver or end-cutting resector to excise a 1 cm diameter area of dorsal capsule and the stalk.
- When the extensor tendons are seen, stop the capsular resection. If an intraligamentous ganglion is found, avoid damaging the scapholunate ligament during resection. Occasionally, midcarpal portals are necessary to locate the ganglion and identify its stalk.
- Convert to an open procedure if there is doubt about complete arthroscopic resection.
- Close the portals with a single stitch or Steri-Strip, or leave them open to allow drainage of the fluid. Apply a palmar wrist splint.

POSTOPERATIVE CARE The wrist is mobilized twice a day, and the splint is removed after 1 week. Physiotherapy is continued for 2 weeks. The patient is advised to avoid strenuous work for at least 3 weeks after arthroscopy.

EPIDERMOID CYST (INCLUSION CYST)

Epidermoid cysts can develop from implantation of epithelial cells by trauma. The history usually involves a penetrating wound around the palm or fingertip several months before a hard, rubbery, nontender subcutaneous mass develops. The fingertips are prone to epithelial implantation, and the distal phalanx is the most common site of osseous involvement (Fig. 15.28). The cyst commonly occurs at the base of a fingernail and may resemble an enchondroma on radiographs; the cortex is expanded, and a central lytic lesion the only bony reaction. Surgical removal of the cyst is curative. If the bone is involved, curettage and bone grafting may be recommended.

SEBACEOUS CYST

Sebaceous cysts are rare in the hand because the palmar skin contains no sebaceous glands. They can be confused with

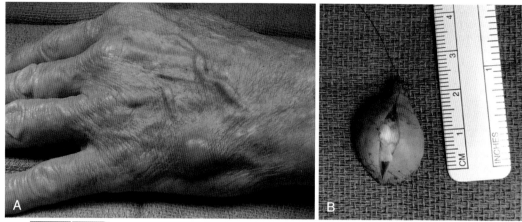

FIGURE 15.28 **A,** Epidermoid inclusion cyst on dorsomedial hand. **B,** Encapsulated gross cystic specimen enclosing characteristic amorphous white paste.

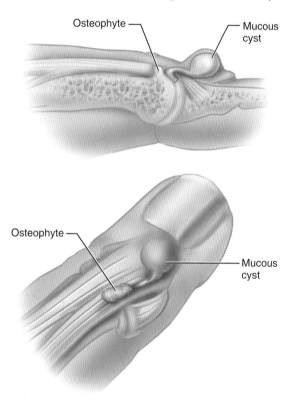

FIGURE 15.29 Relationship between mucous cyst and marginal osteophyte of distal interphalangeal joint. Cyst communicates with joint. This thin communication may become pinched off, but at some stage in development it is in direct communication with joint space. Marginal osteophyte produces attrition of extensor tendon expansion with motion.

epidermoid cysts in the subcutaneous tissues, with mobile overlying skin.

MUCOUS CYST

Mucous cysts occur frequently on the dorsum over the distal interphalangeal joints in women (Fig. 15.29). They are thought to result from myxomatous degeneration of the corneum. The overlying skin is often so thin and translucent that clear mucoid fluid can be seen within. Mucous cysts are frequently associated with Heberden nodes. Anteroposterior,

lateral, and oblique radiographic views usually show an osteophyte near the cyst. This osteophyte should be sought and excised along with the cyst and its stalk, which frequently leads to the joint (Fig. 15.30). A small split skin graft is rarely required. The skin graft is easily removed freehand from a variety of sites from the same arm. Some surgeons prefer to rotate a small local skin flap over the defect.

CONGENITAL ARTERIOVENOUS FISTULA

Congenital arteriovenous fistulas are produced by lack of differentiation of the common embryonic anlage into a true artery and vein. Shunts exist between the arterial and venous circulation. Several may extend over one small area, such as a finger, or over a large area or even involve an entire extremity. Varicose veins of the upper extremity should suggest a congenital arteriovenous fistula, especially if healing is slow or absent after minor trauma. The temperature of the surrounding skin is usually elevated, and the limb may be hypertrophied.

This lesion is not characterized by pain, as is the glomus tumor; however, secondary chronic ulceration can be painful. It is most accurately diagnosed by an arteriogram that reveals dilation of the arteries just proximal to the fistula, abnormal filling of the arteries distal to it, and presence of the contrast medium within the fistula.

All communications between the arterial and venous parts of the fistula should be ligated. This is difficult because they are so small and numerous. Early surgery is indicated in very rare cases to prevent destruction by infection and gangrene. It may be necessary to perform surgery in stages and, at times, skin grafting.

PYOGENIC GRANULOMA

Pyogenic granuloma is a proliferation of granulation tissue frequently overhanging normal skin (Fig. 15.31). Minimal trauma to this unstable tissue typically incites easy bleeding and may be preceded by trauma and infection. Topical silver nitrate application may be curative; however, surgical excision of the lesion, including the vascular base, is almost uniformly successful. Wounds created by such excisions may be difficult to close and secondary intention healing usually leads to a very satisfactory cosmetic result.

FOREIGN BODY GRANULOMA

The granulomatous reaction to centralized foreign material is commonly surrounded by a firm, fibrous capsule. The

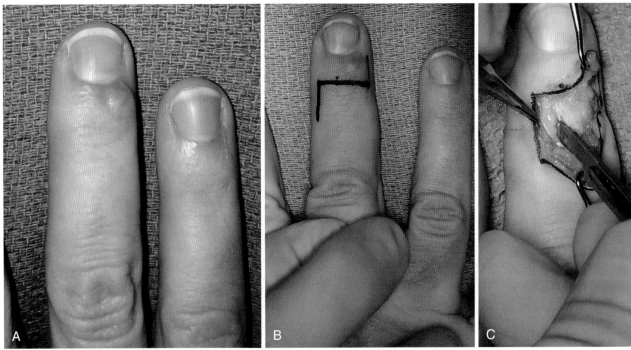

FIGURE 15.30 **A,** Mucous cyst in finger of patient with osteoarthritis. **B,** Surgical excision outlined with marking pen. **C,** Excision of cyst. (From Wu JC, Calandruccio JH, Weller WJ, Henning PR, Swigler CW: Arthritis of the thumb interphalangeal and finger distal interphalangeal joint, *Orthop Clin North Am* 50:489, 2019.)

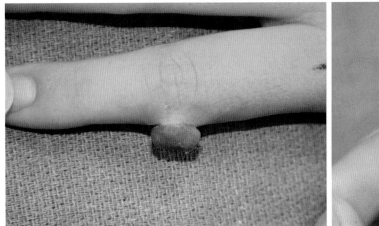
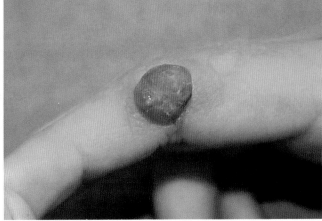

FIGURE 15.31 Pyogenic granuloma of finger.

diagnosis of a foreign body granuloma is easily established with an accurate history. Removal of the foreign body is curative.

GOUT

Some patients with advanced gout have such large deposits of urate crystals within the ligaments, tendons, tendon sheaths, and metaphysis, causing erosion of the diaphysis, that the resultant bone destruction may resemble a lytic tumor on radiographs (Fig. 15.32). Usually, soft-tissue swelling and other findings quickly establish the diagnosis. Clinically, the lesion can be easily confused with an infection because the gouty lesions are also accompanied by increased heat, swelling, and extreme tenderness.

TRAUMATIC NEUROMA

Traumatic neuromas result from an attempt by peripheral nerves to regenerate after their fibers have been interrupted. The neuroma is a bundle of all the nerve elements in one tangled mass at the distal end of the proximal nerve segment. Because this attempted growth occurs to some degree in all individuals, it is not considered a true neoplasm. It can be extremely tender, especially if it involves sensory fibers. This is especially true of an injured digital nerve that adheres to scar and is unprotected by soft tissue. Surgical techniques for painful neuromas usually require neuroma resection more proximally, and placement of the nerve endings in an area less susceptible to trauma.

DÉJÉRINE-SOTTAS DISEASE

Déjérine-Sottas disease, a rare lesion, is a localized enlargement of a peripheral nerve caused by hypertrophic interstitial neuropathy. It is usually present as a tender mass at the wrist and sometimes is quite painful. Surgical exploration reveals enlargement of the median nerve (Fig. 15.33). It cannot be excised without nerve resection, which should be done as a last resort. Dividing the transverse carpal ligament may help to relieve pain and has occasionally decreased the size of the nerve distally. The swelling occasionally subsides spontaneously after surgery. The lesion is sometimes associated with macrodactyly (see chapter 17). The same clinical picture has been caused by infiltration of the nerve by various lipofibromatous neural tumors.

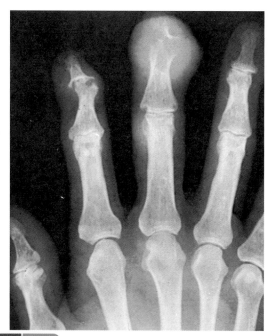

FIGURE 15.32 Destructive lesions around distal interphalangeal joints in gout.

CALCINOSIS

The exact cause of calcium deposits is unknown, but they may result from connective tissue degeneration, with amorphous calcium deposition developing secondarily. Approximately one third of patients give a history of trauma. Calcium deposits occur in the hand much less frequently than around the shoulder and hip, but in the hand the pain, tenderness, and erythema may be more alarming and can easily be confused with an infection because of the inflammatory reaction. Radiographs taken soon after the onset of symptoms may show only a light cloud, suggesting a deposit but, later, the picture is usually diagnostic. Calcium deposits around the hand are more common near the insertion of the flexor carpi ulnaris tendon; the wrist area accounts for approximately two thirds of the cases reported (Fig. 15.34). Deposits do occur, however, in the collateral ligaments of the fingers and thumb, the thumb extensor tendons, and the tendons of the intrinsic muscles. Rarely, multiple deposits are seen.

Treatment usually consists of heat, rest, and injection of a local anesthetic with or without a steroid preparation. Aspiration of the deposit, if possible, may give more immediate relief. The tension may be relieved, however, by spontaneous rupture or by gradual deposit resorption. Only large deposits require surgical treatment.

■ CALCINOSIS CIRCUMSCRIPTA

Calcinosis circumscripta is associated with collagen diseases, such as lupus erythematosus, rheumatoid arthritis, dermatomyositis, and especially scleroderma, with an incidence of 50% in this disease. The pathologic mechanism of deposit of these calcific lobules in the skin and subcutaneous tissues is unknown. Calcinosis circumscripta is rare but is frequently preceded by Raynaud phenomenon for many years. Deposits occur more densely over pressure areas such as fingertips and may sometimes erode through the skin (Fig. 15.35). Partial excision may be indicated when the deposits cause pain or interfere with function, but wound breakdown and skin necrosis are common when dissection is extensive.

TURRET EXOSTOSIS

Turret exostosis is a smooth, dome-shaped extracortical mass of bone lying beneath the extensor apparatus on the middle or proximal phalanx of a finger. It is caused by

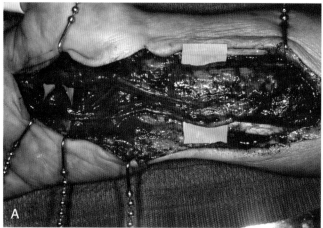
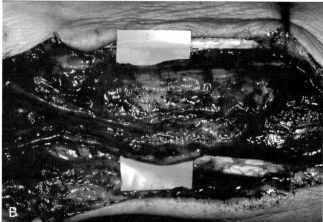

FIGURE 15.33 Déjérine-Sottas disease. **A,** Severe enlargement of median nerve. **B,** Closer view of extensive involvement of median nerve coursing from distal third of forearm into palm.

traumatic subperiosteal hemorrhage that eventually ossifies. Clinically, a firm mass develops on the dorsum of the phalanx and limits excursion of the extensor apparatus (Fig. 15.36), limiting flexion of the interphalangeal joints distal to the lesion. Radiographs that reveal negative results during the first few weeks after injury later reveal subperiosteal new bone located on the dorsum of the phalanx. Conservative treatment has not been beneficial. Any indicated surgery should be delayed until the subperiosteal bone becomes mature, usually 4 to 6 months after injury; at that time, recurrence is less likely.

To excise the exostosis, a midlateral incision (see chapter 1) is made, the extensor apparatus is elevated, and the

periosteum is incised laterally and carefully elevated from the underlying bone; care is taken not to tear the periosteum dorsally, preserving a smooth surface over which the extensor apparatus can glide. The lesion is resected so that the periosteum and the wound can be closed.

CARPOMETACARPAL BOSS

Carpometacarpal bosses are fixed dorsal osteophyte protuberances of mating (commonly the second and third) carpometacarpal joints. These tender osteophytes are normally visible on a tangential radiograph, a feature that distinguishes them from dorsal ganglions.

Most lesions are relatively asymptomatic and constitute only a cosmetic problem; however, extensor tendons occasionally sublux over the dome of the lesions causing pain. Pain can also be caused by local pressure over the lesion or by forced wrist extension.

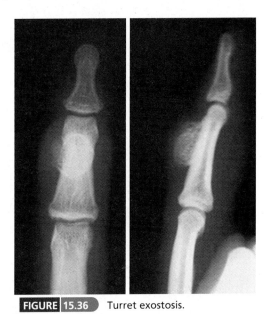

FIGURE 15.36 Turret exostosis.

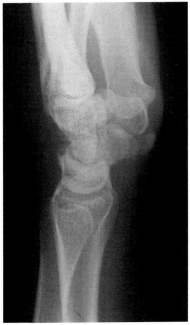

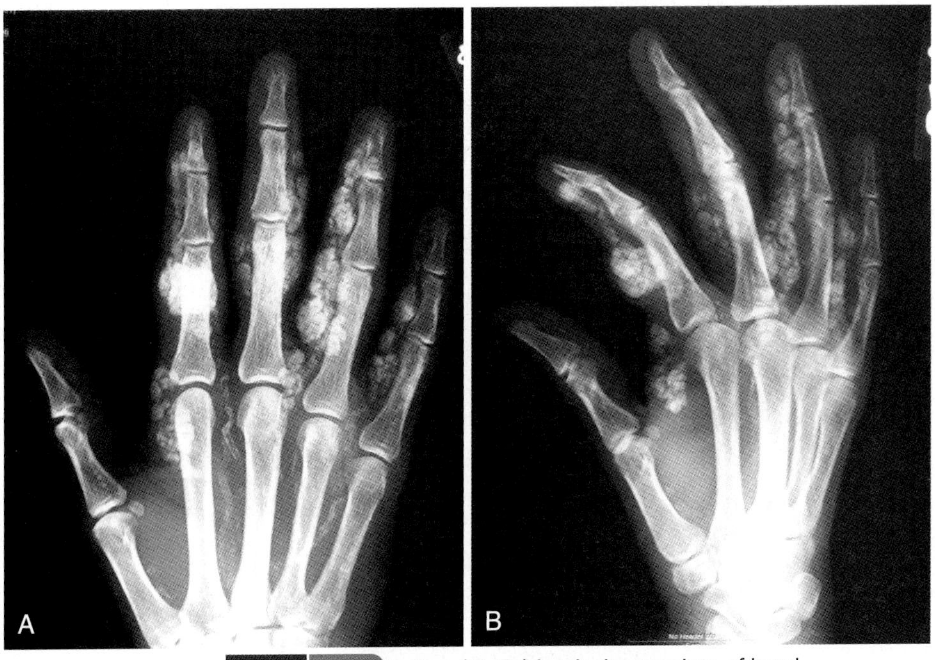

FIGURE 15.34 Calcium deposit near flexor carpi ulnaris insertion into pisiform.

FIGURE 15.35 **A** and **B,** Calcinosis circumscripta of hand.

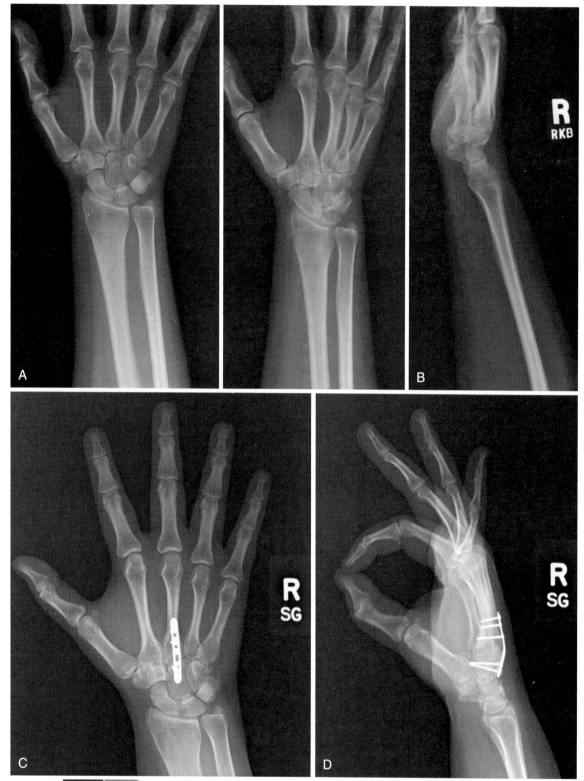

FIGURE 15.37   **A** and **B,** Symptomatic carpometacarpal boss after simple osteophyte excision. **C** and **D,** Appearance after successful re-fusion following failed fusion of middle finger carpometacarpal joint.

Recurrence after excision is a concern, and repeat surgery for recurrence probably warrants carpometacarpal joint fusion. Whatever method is chosen, care must be taken to protect the insertion of the radial wrist extensor tendons, especially that of the extensor carpi radialis brevis (Fig. 15.37).

EPIDERMOLYSIS BULLOSA

The severe form of epidermolysis bullosa is a hereditary disorder that occurs in 1 of every 300,000 births. At birth or soon after, bullae are present over the extremities because the process affects the entire dermis and

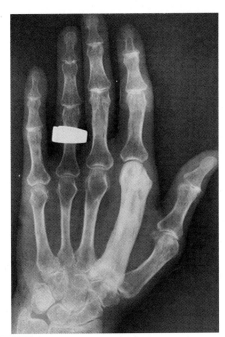

FIGURE 15.38 Paget disease of second metacarpal. (From Haverbush TJ, Wolde AH, Phalen GS: The hand in Paget's disease of bone: report of two cases, *J Bone Joint Surg* 54A:173, 1972.)

sometimes the mucous membranes. Its ultimate course is chronic infection of the bullae and the continuing formation of a cocoon-like epidermis over all the fingers of each hand. Surgical release of these digits is discouraging because recurrence of the webbing and flexion contractures of the fingers is rapid. Free skin grafts and distant flaps have been used to limited advantage; no effective treatment of the disease process is known. These patients are poor surgical risks because of chronic infection. Some authors have reported a death rate of 25% during childhood or adolescence, apparently because of debilitation. Surgical procedures, if any are indicated, are repetitious degloving procedures that give limited hand function over a limited time. The less severe types of the disease may not need surgical treatment.

PAGET DISEASE

Paget disease may occur in the long bones of the hand, although this is rare, especially compared with the incidence of Paget disease of bone in the general population. Radiographs reveal the same sclerotic fusiform enlargement of the long bones as elsewhere in the body. Paget disease should not be confused with fibrous dysplasia (Fig. 15.38).

REFERENCES

GENERAL

Farzan M, Ahangar P, Mazoochy H, et al.: Osseous tumours of the hand: a review of 99 cases in 20 years, *Arch Bone Jt Surg* 1:68, 2013.
Henderson M, Neumeister MW, Bueno RA: Hand tumors: II. Benign and malignant bone tumors of the hand, *Plast Reconstr Surg* 133:814e, 2014.
Simon MJK, Pogoda P, Hövelbom F, et al.: Incidence, histopathologic and distribution of tumours of the hand, *BMC Musculoskelet Disord* 15:182, 2014.

BENIGN TUMORS

Agarwal S, Haase SC: Lipofibromatous hamartoma of the median nerve, *J Hand Surg Am* 38A:392, 2013.
Al-Qattan MM: Biopolar electric cauterization as adjuvant treatment after curettage of aneurysmal bone cysts of the hand, *Ann Plast Surg* 72:348, 2014.
Athanasian EA: Bone and soft tissue tumors. In Wolfe SW, Hotchkiss RN, Pederson WC, et al.: *Operative hand surgery*, Philadelphia, 2011, Elsevier.
Balazs GC, Donohue MA, Drake ML, et al.: Outcomes of open dorsal wrist ganglion excision in active-duty military personnel, *J Hand Surg Am* 40(9):1739, 2015.
Chick G, Hollevoet N, Victor J, Bianchi S: The role of imaging in isolated benign peripheral nerve tumors: a practical review for surgeons, *Hand Surg Rehabil* 35:320, 2016.
Corominas L, Sanpera I, Sanpera-Iglesias J, et al.: Calcifying aponeurotic fibroma in children: our experience and a literature review, *J Pediatr Orthop B* 26:560, 2017.
Giugale JM, Fowler JR: Glomus tumors: a review of preoperative magnetic resonance imaging to detect satellite lesions, *Orthopedics* 38(10):e888, 2015.
Cha SM, Shin HD, Kim KC, et al.: Extensive curettage using a high-speed burr versus dehydrated alcohol instillation for the treatment of enchondroma of the hand, *J Hand Surg Eur* 40E:384, 2015.
Crowe MM, Houdek MT, Moran SL, et al.: Aneurysmal bone cysts of the hand, wrist, and forearm, *J Hand Surg Am* 40:2052, 2015.
Cuesta HE, Villagran JM, Horcajadas AB, et al.: Percutaneous radiofrequency ablation in osteoid osteoma: tips and tricks in special scenarios, *Eur J Radiol* 102:169, 2018.
Georgiannos D, Lampridis V, Bisbinas I: Phenolization and coralline hydroxyapatite grafting following meticulous curettage for the treatment of enchondroma of the hand. A case series of 82 patients with 5-year follow-up, *Hand* 10:111, 2015.
Gosk J, Gutkowska O, Urban M, et al.: Benign nerve tumours of the hand (excluding wrist), *Arch Orthop Trauma Surg* 135:1763, 2015.
Ho YY, Choueka J: Synovial chondromatosis of the upper extremity, *J Hand Surg Am* 38A:804, 2013.
Houdek MT, Rose PS, Cakar S: Desmoid tumors of the upper extremity, *J Hand Surg Am* 39:1761, 2014.
Jafari D, Jamshidi K, Njdmazhar F, et al.: Expansile aneurysmal bone cyst in the tubular bones of the hand treated with en bloc excision and autograft reconstruction: a report of 12 cases, *J Hand Surg Eur* 36E:648, 2011.
Kim YJ, Kim DH, Park JS, et al.: Factors affecting surgical outcomes of digital glomus tumour: a multicentre study, *J Hand Surg Eur* 43(6):652, 2018.
Lancigu R, Rabarin F, Jeudy J, et al.: Giant cell tumors of the tendon sheaths in the hand: review of 96 patients with an average follow-up of 12 years, *Orthop Traumatol Surg Res* 995:5251, 2013.
Lanzinger WD, Bindra R: Giant cell tumor of the tendon sheath, *J Hand Surg Am* 38A:154, 2013.
Lin YC, Hsiao PF, Wu YH, et al.: Recurrent digital glomus tumor: analysis of 75 cases, *Dermatol Surg* 36:1396, 2010.
Lubahn JD, Bachoura A: Enchondroma of the hand: evaluation and management, *J Am Acad Orthop Surg* 24:625, 2016.
Morey VM, Garg B, Kotwal P: Glomus tumours of the hand: review of the literature, *J Clin Orthop Trauma* 7:286, 2016.
Morii T, Mochizuki K, Tajima T, et al.: Treatment outcome of enchondroma by simple curettage without augmentation, *J Orthop Sci* 15:112, 2010.
Nazerani S, Motamedi MHK, Keramati MR: Diagnosis and management of glomus tumors of the hand, *Tech Hand Up Extrem Surg* 14:8, 2010.
Nikci V, Doumas C: Calcium deposits in the hand and wrist, *J Am Acad Orthop Surg* 23:87, 2015.
Payne WT, Merrell G: Benign bony and soft tissue tumors of the hand, *J Hand Surg Am* 35A:1901, 2010.
Sassoon AA, Fitz-Gibbon PD, Harmsen WS, et al.: Enchondromas of the hand: factors affecting recurrence, healing, motion, and malignant transformation, *J Hand Surg Am* 37A:1229, 2012.
Spingardi O, Zoccolan A, Venturino E: Infantile digital fibromatosis: our experience and long-term results, *Chir Main* 30:62, 2011.

Tahiri Y, Xu L, Kanevsky J, Luc M: Lipofibromatous hamartoma of the median nerve: a comprehensive review and systematic approach to evaluation, diagnosis, and treatment, *J Hand Surg Am* 38A:2055, 2013.

Toma R, Ferris S, Coombs CJ, et al.: Lipoblastoma: an important differential diagnosis of tumours of the hand in children, *J Plast Surg Hand Surg* 44:257, 2010.

Trehan SK, Athanasian EA, DiCarlo EF, et al.: Characteristics of glomus tumors in the hand not diagnosed on magnetic resonance imaging, *J Hand Surg Am* 40(30):542, 2015.

Tuncer S, Sezgin B, Kaya B, et al.: An algorithmic approach for the management of hand deformities in dystrophic epidermolysis bullosa, *J Plast Surg Hand Surg* 52:80, 2018.

Williams J, Hodari A, Janevski P, et al.: Recurrence of giant cell tumors in the hand: a prospective study, *J Hand Surg Am* 35A:451, 2010.

Wu JC, Calandruccio JH, Weller WJ, et al.: Arthritis of the thumb interphalangeal and finger distal interphalangeal joint, *Orthop Clin North Am* 50:489, 2019.

MALIGNANT TUMORS

Afshar A, Farhadnia P, Khalchali H: Metastases to the hand and wrist: an analysis of 221 cases, *J Hand Surg Am* 39:923, 2014.

Askari M, Kakar S, Moran SL: Squamous cell carcinoma of the hand: a 20-year review, *J Hand Surg Am* 38A:2124, 2013.

Bowen CM, Landau MJ, Badash I, et al.: Primary tumors of the hand: functional and restorative management, *J Surg Oncol* 118:873, 2018.

Chakera AH, Quinn MJ, Lo S, et al.: Subungual melanoma of the hand, *Ann Surg Oncol* 26(4):1035, 2019.

Chen X, Yu LJ, Peng HM, et al.: Is intralesional resection suitable for central grade 1 chondrosarcoma: a systematic review and updated meta-analysis, *EJSO* 43:1718, 2017.

Cochran AM, Buchanan PJ, Bueno RA, et al.: Subungual melanoma: a reivew of current treatment, *Plast Reconstr Surg* 134:259, 2014.

Dean BJF, Branford-White H, Giele H, et al.: Management and outcome of acral soft-tissue sarcomas, *Bone Joint Lett J* 100-B:1518, 2018.

Del Pino JG, Calderon SAL, Chebib I, et al.: Intralesional versus wide resection of low-grade chondrosarcoma of the hand, *J Hand Surg Am* 41(4):541, 2016.

Dijksterhuis A, Friedeman E, van der Heijden B: Squamous cell carcinoma of the nail unit: review of the literature, *J Hand Surg Am* 43(4):374, 2018.

English C, Hammert WC: Cutaneous malignancies of the upper extremity, *J Hand Surg* 37A:367, 2012.

Houdek MT, Walczak BE, Wilke BK, et al.: What factors influence the outcome of surgically treated soft tissue sarcomas of the hand and wrist? *Hand* 12(5):493, 2017.

Loh TY, Rubin AG, Jiang SIB: Basal cell carcinoma of the dorsal hand: an update and comprehensive review of the literature, *Dermatol Surg* 42:464, 2016.

Martin DE, English JC, Goitz RJ: Squamous cell carcinoma of the hand, *J Hand Surg Am* 36A:1377, 2011.

Martin DE, English JC, Goitz RJ: Subungual malignant melanoma, *J Hand Surg Am* 36A:704, 2011.

Nguyen JT, Bakri K, Nguyen EC, et al.: Surgical management of subungual melanoma. Mayo clinic experience of 124 cases, *Ann Plast Surg* 71:346, 2013.

Parida L, Fernandez-Pineda I, Uffman J, et al.: Clinical management of Ewing sarcoma of the bones of the hands and feet: a retrospective single-institution review, *J Pediatr Surg* 47:1806, 2012.

Puhaindran ME, Athanasian EA: Malignant and metastatic tumors of the hand, *J Hand Surg Am* 35A:2010, 1895.

Reilly DJ, Aksakal G, Gilmour RF, et al.: Subungual melanoma: management in the modern era, *J Plast Reconstr Aesth Surg* 70:1746, 2017.

Sinno S, Wilson S, Billig J, et al.: Primary melanoma of the hand: an algorithmic approach to surgical management, *J Plast Surg Hand Surg* 49(6):339, 2015.

Stubblefield J, Kelly B: Melanoma in non-caucasian populations, *Surg Clin N Am* 94:1115, 2014.

Reilly DJ, Aksakal G, Gilmour RF, et al.: Subungual melanoma: management in the modern era, *J Plast Reconstr Aesthet Surg* 70:1746, 2017.

Terushkin V, Brodland DG, Sharon DJ, et al.: Digit-sparing Mohs surgery for melanoma, *Dermatologic Surg* 42:83, 2016.

Woodward JF, Jones NF: Malignant glomus tumors of the hand, *Hand* 11(3):287, 2016.

Yang Z, Xie L, Huang Y, et al.: Clinical features of malignant melanoma of the finger and therapeutic efficacies of different treatments, *Oncol Lett* 2:811, 2011.

The complete list of references is available online at ExpertConsult.com.

CHAPTER 16

HAND INFECTIONS

Norfleet B. Thompson

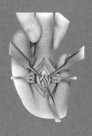

FACTORS INFLUENCING HAND INFECTIONS

The clinical course of most hand infections is affected by anatomic, local, and systemic factors, in addition to bacterial virulence and the size of the inoculum. Anatomic factors that to some extent determine the ease of penetration, localization, and spread of infection include: (1) the thin layer of skin and subcutaneous tissue over the tendons, bones, and joints; (2) the closed space of the distal digital pulp; (3) the proximity of the flexor tendon sheath to bone and joint; (4) the proximal extent of the flexor sheath into the palm, connecting with the radial and ulnar bursae; and (5) the location of the thenar and midpalmar spaces in the hand and the space of Parona proximal to the wrist near the flexor tendon sheaths.

Local factors predisposing to infection include: (1) the extent and nature of soft-tissue damage, (2) the amount and virulence of bacterial contamination, and (3) the type and amount of foreign material present and persistent in the wound. Systemic factors relevant to the course of an infection involve ones that affect the immunocompetence of the patient. Examples include (1) malnutrition, (2) alcoholism, (3) intravenous drug abuse, (4) diabetes mellitus, (5) long-term use of corticosteroids and antitumor necrosis factor-α medicines, (6) immunosuppression following solid organ and bone marrow transplant, and (7) infection with human immunodeficiency virus.

Surgical site infections are uncommon after hand surgery. A database study that included 44,305 patients who had outpatient hand surgery procedures identified infections in fewer than 1%. Predictive factors were government-funded insurance and residence in a rural area; diabetes, obesity, and tobacco use were not associated with an increased risk of infection. The use of preoperative prophylactic antibiotics for small elective soft-tissue procedures, such as carpal tunnel or trigger finger release, remains an area of some debate; however, most agree that prophylactic antibiotics are not necessary for clean, elective procedures lasting less than 2 hours, even in patients with diabetes. A large study of clean, elective hand procedures based on 516,986 patients identified through an insurance claims database found no difference in the risk of postoperative infection in patients who received prophylactic antibiotics and those who did not. The overall 30-day surgical site infection rate was 1.5% in the antibiotic prophylaxis group and 1.4% in the group not receiving antibiotics. This finding applied to all clean soft-tissue hand procedures even after controlling for patient demographics, use of steroids or immunosuppressive agents, and comorbidities such as diabetes, HIV/AIDS, tobacco use, and obesity. With the rising use of wide-awake techniques for certain hand surgery procedures, attention has been given to infection risk in cases done outside the operating room under field sterility instead of full sterility characteristic of an operating room. One systematic review of six studies based on low-level evidence suggested that for some minor hand operations, such as carpal tunnel, trigger finger, or de Quervain release, undertaking the procedure outside the operating room may not alter the baseline infection rate.

Treatment of hand infections depends on the identification of the specific organism, the specific anatomic area involved in the hand and fingers, and the condition of the host whose comorbidities may influence treatment decisions. Identification of organisms with culture and antibiotic sensitivity studies allows proper medical treatment. Surgical procedures, including drainage of abscesses and debridement of necrotic tissues, also may be required.

GENERAL APPROACH TO HAND INFECTIONS

With a careful history and physical examination, the location of the infection, the extent of spread, and the presence of swelling, lymphangitis, lymphadenitis, and joint involvement can be determined. Consideration should be given to other conditions that can be confused with infections, including gout, acute calcium deposition, pseudogout, pyogenic granuloma, insect bites, pyoderma gangrenosum, foreign bodies, factitious lesions, herpetic lesions, metastatic lesions, silicone synovitis, granuloma annulare, rheumatoid arthritis, nonspecific tenosynovitis, reactions to intravenous medications (e.g., chemotherapeutic agents), and Sweet syndrome, an aseptic neutrophilic dermatosis affecting the hand and resembling an infection. If the likelihood of infection is high, an attempt should be made to determine whether an abscess is present that requires drainage. Fluctuance can be difficult to identify in the hand. Radiographs are helpful in revealing bone injury. Radionuclide scanning may show bone infection, and MRI and ultrasound may localize an abscess. A complete blood cell count is obtained, along with determination of the serum C-reactive protein level and erythrocyte sedimentation rate. Strub et al. found significantly higher C-reactive protein levels in patients with infection "mimickers" (gout and pseudogout), and slightly fewer than half of patients with finger infections had elevated C-reactive protein levels. These authors concluded that the specificity of all inflammation markers (WBC, C-reactive protein, ESR) was inadequate for diagnosis. If any fluid or tissue is obtained, it is sent to the laboratory for Gram stain, crystals, culture, and antibiotic sensitivity determinations. Specific requests usually are made of the laboratory to culture for aerobic and anaerobic bacteria and for mycobacteria and fungi. In some cases, viral testing also can be helpful.

Initial antibiotic therapy traditionally has been empirical, depending on the results of the Gram stain and the most likely organism. Consideration should be given to the possibility of mixed flora as the cause of hand infections. Reviews of surgical infections of the hand and upper extremity have shown an increased incidence of gram-negative enteric and anaerobic organisms, even though the most common organisms were gram-positive aerobes (streptococcal species, *Staphylococcus aureus,* and coagulase-negative *Staphylococcus*). Generally, the organism most commonly isolated from community-acquired hand infections is *S. aureus.* Methicillin-resistant *S. aureus* (MRSA) infections have had a rising incidence, especially in many urban medical centers. Typically, 80% or more of wounds cultured from swabs produce multiple organisms, whereas tissue specimens may produce a single causative organism in about 75%. Other organisms that commonly cause hand infections include streptococci, enterobacteria, *Pseudomonas,* enterococci, and *Bacteroides.* Less common causes include the various mycobacteria, gonococcus, *Pasteurella multocida* (in cat or dog bites), *Eikenella corrodens* (in human bites), *Aeromonas hydrophila* from standing fresh water (e.g., ditches, puddles, and ponds), *Haemophilus influenzae* (in children 2 months to 3 years old), a variety of anaerobic organisms (including clostridia), and other rare bacteria, such as those that cause anthrax, erysipeloid, and brucellosis. Postoperative or surgical site infections of the hand usually are caused by gram-positive organisms, including *S. aureus* and *Staphylococcus epidermidis.* Gram-negative organisms also may be isolated from surgical site infections. Overall, community-acquired MRSA has become the most common cause of culture-positive hand infections in the United States.

Antibiotics traditionally recommended for hand infections include a penicillinase-resistant penicillin or cephalosporin.

When selecting antibiotics, it is important to be aware of the prevalence of antibiotic-resistant bacteria, such as MRSA. Vancomycin is effective against gram-positive organisms, whereas ciprofloxacin is mostly effective against gram-negative organisms. The addition of antibiotics effective against gram-negative organisms has been recommended for high-risk situations, such as infections in intravenous drug users and contaminated outdoor or farm injuries (Table 16.1). Antibiotic options for outpatient coverage of community-acquired MRSA include clindamycin (although clindamycin resistance is increasing), trimethoprim-sulfamethoxazole, a tetracycline (doxycycline or minocycline), linezolid, and daptomycin. A recent study of 815 culture-positive hand infections over a 10-year period found clindamycin resistance to MRSA rising from 4% to 31% and levofloxacin resistance rising from 12% to 56% in the same study period (2005–2014). The authors suggested that clinicians should consider alternatives to the use of clindamycin, levofloxacin, penicillin, and other beta-lactam antibiotics, such as cephalosporins for treating common hand infections empirically, especially in urban centers.

Because of the constantly changing inventory of antibiotics and the variations in patient populations and wound flora, antibiotic selection should be based on a variety of considerations, including local antibiotic resistance information and the assistance of an infectious disease specialist when needed.

A protocol of early, aggressive surgical incision and drainage combined with intravenous antibiotic therapy should result in a shorter hospital stay, faster healing, and fewer complications. A randomized trial comparing cefazolin to vancomycin as a first-line agent in patients with community-acquired MRSA found no statistically significant differences in outcomes or cost of treatment. The authors emphasized the importance of early aggressive empiric antibiotic therapy with coverage for MRSA in all hand infections. Current recommendations for outpatient antibiotic treatment include amoxicillin and clavulanate plus trimethoprim and sulfamethoxazole. A comparison of patients who had differing antibiotic regimens after surgical treatment of simple hand infections (systemic cephalosporins and gentamicin bead chain, gentamicin bead chain alone, and no antibiotics) found no difference in outcomes, leading the authors to conclude that the use of antibiotics after surgical treatment of simple hand infection seems to be unnecessary.

Failure to recognize the polymicrobial nature of hand infections and inadequate surgical debridement are frequent causes of poor results. The importance of adequate surgical treatment cannot be overemphasized because antibiotics alone may be insufficient to control the infection.

INCISION AND DRAINAGE OF HAND INFECTION

TECHNIQUE 16.1

- Use a general anesthetic or distant regional block because a local anesthetic may not function in the septic environment, may spread the infection, and add to an already swollen part.

TABLE 16.1

Antibiotic Recommendations for Common Organisms

ORGANISM	ANTIBIOTIC	ADDITIONAL INFORMATION
Methicillin-sensitive *Staphylococcus aureus*	Cephalexin, amoxicillin clavulanate (orally)	
Methicillin-resistant *S. aureus*	Trimethoprim/sulfamethoxazole (orally), linezolid (orally or IV) If sulfa allergy, clindamycin or doxycycline	Linezolid: expensive, avoid in endocarditis or meningitis, weekly complete blood cell monitoring
	Vancomycin (IV), daptomycin (IV) Quinupristin/dalfopristin (IV) Tigecycline (IV) Ceftaroline (IV)	Dapto: weekly creatinine phosphokinase monitoring
Vancomycin-resistant Enterococci	Daptomycin, linezolid (orally or IV), tigecycline (IV), quinupristin/dalfopristin (IV)	
Gram negative	Piperacillin/tazobactam Ceftriaxone Ertapenem Quinolones/ciprofloxacin	
Pseudomonas	Piperacillin/tazobactam Cefepime Meropenem	
Anaerobic infections	Ampicillin/sulbactam, Piperacillin/tazobactam, Ertapenem, meropenem Metronidazole Clindamycin Tigecycline	
Vibrio vulnificus	Ceftriaxone and doxycycline Imipenem and doxycycline	
Nocardia	Trimethoprim/sulfamethoxazole If sulfa allergy: imipenem, ceftriaxone, amikacin	6 mo of treatment in immune-suppressed patients
Sporothrix schenckii	Itraconazole Fluconazole and voriconazole	
Mycobacterium marinum	Clarithromycin/azithromycin Trimethoprim/sulfamethoxazole minocycline Ethambutol	
Aeromonas hydrophilia	Ciprofloxacin Imipenem Trimethoprim/sulfamethoxazole	
Cutaneous anthrax	Ciprofloxacin Doxycycline	Treatment for 60 d to treat any remaining spores
Tularemia	Gentamicin and doxycycline	

From Osterman M, Draeger R, Stern P: Acute hand infections, *J Hand Surg* 39:1628, 2014.

- Use a tourniquet, but before inflating it, elevate the hand for 3 to 6 minutes to avoid limb exsanguination with an elastic wrap and the potential for the proximal spread of the infection.
- After properly preparing and draping the area, make the incision for drainage as described for specific infections.
- After making the skin incision, always spread the deeper structures with blunt dissection to avoid injury to important nerves, vessels, and tendons. These structures may be difficult to see in swollen, infected tissue.
- Although an incision for drainage relieves pain and reduces the spread of infection, it also creates an open infected wound subject to further contamination. Copious irrigation is an effective way to decrease contamination. Although wound closure after abscess drainage has been advocated, it probably is safer to return to the operating room in 3 to 5 days and close the wound secondarily if the condition of the wound permits. If joints or flexor tendons have been exposed by skin necrosis, however, cover them at once to preserve their vital functions. In most instances, leave the wound open. Infections involving the tendon sheaths and joints usually result in some loss of function. Such loss of function is seen less often in superficial infections, unless surgical scars have adhered to adjacent structures, such as nerves or tendons.

POSTOPERATIVE CARE Immediately after surgery, the hand is wrapped with bulky layers of gauze to hold it in the position of function and to pad the wound. A metal, plaster, or fiberglass splint is applied to support the wrist in about 30 degrees of extension, the metacarpophalangeal joints in about 60 to 70 degrees of flexion, the interphalangeal joints in full extension, and the thumb in a palmar abducted-opposed position. The hand is continuously elevated after surgery. Active motion of digits is begun as soon as possible. Therapist-supervised dressing changes in a whirlpool bath are included in the rehabilitation routine. Usually, the dressing is first changed 24 to 48 hours after drainage and then is changed daily or every other day. Moist dressings may help remove infected drainage. Sterile technique should be observed during dressings to prevent further contamination. After several days, further debridement of necrotic material may be necessary if the infection is extensive. As soon as drainage has ceased and healthy granulation tissue appears, the wound is closed secondarily; a free skin graft or flap coverage may be necessary, but usually only when a skin slough has occurred.

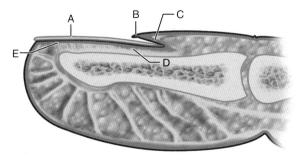

FIGURE 16.1 Diagram of nail and nail bed. *A,* Nail. *B,* Eponychium. *C,* Dorsal roof of nail fold. *D,* Ventral floor of nail fold (germinal matrix). *E,* Nail bed (sterile matrix). (From Bednar MS, Lane LB: Eponychial marsupialization and nail removal for surgical treatment of paronychia, *J Hand Surg* 16A:314, 1991.)

PARONYCHIA

A paronychia ("runaround") infection usually is caused by the introduction of bacteria into the soft-tissue fold around the fingernail (eponychium) associated with a hangnail or poor nail hygiene (Fig. 16.1). In three studies of paronychia, with a total of 61 patients, 25% were caused by anaerobic bacteria, 25% by aerobic bacteria, and 50% by mixed aerobic and anaerobic bacteria. Nonbacterial pathogens such as yeast and viruses also have been identified as causative organisms. The diagnosis is recognized by pain, redness, swelling, and possibly fluctuance at the paronychial and eponychial regions of the nail fold.

Initial treatment may include warm water or chlorhexidine soaks with or without topical or oral antibiotics. When an abscess is present, it should be drained. After drainage, antibiotics should be prescribed judiciously based on patient comorbidities and clinical judgment. A number of case studies have suggested that antibiotics are probably unnecessary in most cases. A prospective study of 46 acute fingertip infections treated with drainage and no antibiotics demonstrated only one recurrence attributed to inadequate resection. When an abscess forms in the eponychial or paronychial fold, it usually begins at one corner of the horny nail and travels under either the eponychium or the nail toward the opposite side. If an abscess is on one side only, it should be incised, angling the knife away from the nail to avoid cutting the nail bed, which would cause a ridge later. If the abscess is under one corner of the nail root, this corner should be removed. If it has already migrated to the opposite side and under the nail, a second incision should be made there, the skin folded back proximally, and the proximal one third of the nail excised. The wound is loosely packed with iodoform gauze for 48 hours for drainage (Fig. 16.2).

Ogunlusi et al. described using the tip of a 21- or 23-gauge needle to lift the nail fold and drain the abscess; drainage was followed by oral antibiotic therapy. Resolution of acute paronychia occurred within 2 days in 8 of 10 patients. No anesthesia or daily dressing changes were required.

Infections caused by herpes simplex virus type 1 or 2 may be confused with bacterial paronychia. The "herpetic whitlow" is seen more often in health care workers and in

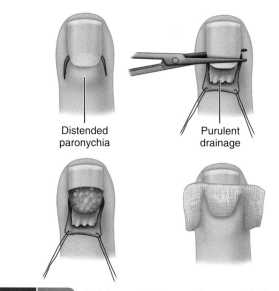

Distended paronychia   Purulent drainage

FIGURE 16.2 Incision and drainage of paronychia (see text).

immunocompromised patients and begins as a localized area of swelling with clear vesicle formation. Lymphangitis and lymphadenopathy may be present. The diagnosis can be confirmed with viral cultures of fluid from the vesicles, a Tzanck smear, and serum antibody titers. The condition is self-limiting, usually resolving over 3 to 4 weeks, and does not require surgical treatment. For immunocompromised patients, a course of an antiviral (acyclovir, valacyclovir, famciclovir, or foscarnet) can be used.

CHRONIC PARONYCHIA

Chronic paronychia typically occurs in patients whose activities require prolonged exposure to water. With chronic inflammation and recurring infection or colonization, the eponychium appears thickened and prominent. Organisms obtained from the cultures of these lesions include *Staphylococcus pyogenes, S. epidermidis, Candida albicans,* colonic gram-negative bacteria, or a mixture of these. Treatment focuses on modifying activity to mitigate the source of inflammation and restore the nail fold. Tosti et al. compared topical methylprednisolone with two oral antifungal medicines in the treatment of chronic paronychia of 45 patients with multiple nail involvement. Methylprednisolone cured or improved 85% of the nails. Of the oral antifungal

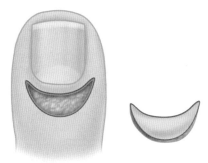

FIGURE 16.3   Eponychial marsupialization for treatment of paronychia. Symmetric, crescent-shaped segment of skin is excised from dorsum of distal phalanx, leaving adequate bridge of skin and cuticle. **SEE TECHNIQUE 16.2.**

medications, terbinafine was effective in 52% and itraconazole in 45%, suggesting the possibility that a chronic paronychia is more likely a dermatitis related to environmental exposure. A more recent study has shown better results using the topical ointment tacrolimus 0.1% (Protopic) compared to betamethasone 17-valerate 0.1%. If avoiding the irritant and topical applications are ineffective, treatment may involve marsupialization of the proximal nail fold.

EPONYCHIAL MARSUPIALIZATION

Bednar and Lane found the eponychial marsupialization technique of Keyser and Eaton to be effective in curing patients of chronic paronychia. They further noted that if nail irregularities are present, removing the nail leads to healing without recurrence.

TECHNIQUE 16.2

(BEDNAR AND LANE; KEYSER AND EATON)
- After administering a digital block anesthetic, cleanse the finger with antiseptic and drape it appropriately.
- Excise a crescent of skin 3 mm wide parallel to the eponychium and extending from the radial to the ulnar borders (Fig. 16.3).
- When using the Keyser and Eaton technique, remove all thickened tissue from the skin. Bednar and Lane leave the subcutaneous fat intact.
- If nail irregularities are present, remove the nail.
- Cover the wound with petroleum/bismuth tribromophenate–impregnated gauze (Xeroform). If the nail is removed, place this gauze beneath the nail fold.

POSTOPERATIVE CARE   Therapy with an oral antibiotic (cephalexin or erythromycin) is begun postoperatively. The patient is instructed to soak the finger in hydrogen peroxide and to wash it with chlorhexidine gluconate skin cleanser (Hibiclens) three times daily, beginning on postoperative day 3. The daily washings are continued until all drainage stops. Antibiotics should be continued for 2 weeks. If the culture results are negative, antibiotics can be discontinued in 3 to 5 days.

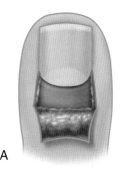

A

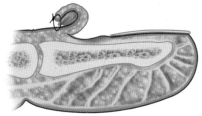

B

FIGURE 16.4   "Swiss roll" technique for treatment of paronychia. **A,** Inflamed germinal matrix is exposed and thoroughly irrigated. **B,** Elevated nail fold is reflected proximally over a nonadherent dressing, rolled like a Swiss roll, and secured to the skin with nonabsorbable suture. (From Pabari A, Iyer S, Khoo CT: Swiss roll technique for treatment of paronychia, *Tech Hand Up Extrem Surg* 15:75, 2011.)

Pabari et al. described a "Swiss roll" technique for the treatment of both acute and chronic paronychia in which the nail fold is elevated and reflected proximally over a nonadherent dressing and secured to the skin with a nonabsorbable suture (Fig. 16.4). For chronic paronychia, the nail bed should be exposed for 7 to 14 days versus 2 to 3 days for acute cases. Cited advantages of this technique are the retention of the nail plate, rapid healing, and avoidance of a skin defect in the finger.

FELON

A felon is an abscess in the subcutaneous tissues of the distal pulp of a finger or thumb. The distal digital pulp is divided into tiny compartments by strong fibrous septa that traverse it from skin to bone. A transverse fibrous curtain also is present at the distal flexor finger crease. Because of these septa, any swelling causes immediate pain that is intensified because of increased pressure within the pulp. Infection can be caused by a penetrating injury from a foreign body or from "finger sticks" for medical reasons (e.g., hematocrit and blood glucose determinations). S. aureus is the organism most commonly isolated from fingertip infections. Swelling, redness, and pain, typical of cellulitis, are present initially. Abscess formation may follow rapidly. The pulp abscess (felon) can extend into the periosteum around the nail bed causing paronychia, or proximally through the fibrous curtain into the flexor sheath, leading to flexor tenosynovitis. Abscesses beginning deep, especially if untreated, penetrate the periosteum and cause osteomyelitis or a septic joint; the more superficial ones cause skin necrosis. Abscesses may form occasionally in the middle and proximal digital pulps.

Treatment generally consists of incision and drainage with antibiotics. Early presentation may be treatable with rest, elevation, warm soaks, and antibiotics. Because MRSA is becoming much more frequent, empiric treatment with antibiotics that cover MRSA is prudent until cultures dictate treatment. The diagnosis of an abscess in this area is sometimes difficult, but one usually is present if severe pain has lasted for 12 hours or longer.

INCISION AND DRAINAGE OF FELONS

TECHNIQUE 16.3

- When the abscess points volarly, causing necrosis of the overlying skin, drain it by excising the necrotic skin.
- When the abscess is in the distal pulp area pointing volarly toward the whorl of the fingerprint, it is best drained by a vertical incision begun distal to the skin crease and placed precisely in the midline to avoid the lateral branches of the digital nerve and allow healing with minimal scarring (Fig. 16.5).
- If the abscess is deep and partitioned by the septa, make a longitudinal incision, usually away from the contact area of the finger, cutting through the partitions (Fig. 16.6).
- This incision must be accurate. Make the incision dorsal to the tactile surface of the finger and not more than 3 mm from the distal free edge of the nail; otherwise, the ends of the digital nerve would be painfully damaged. Blunt dissection with the tip of a small pair of scissors or a mosquito hemostat avoids sharp injury to nerve endings, allowing disruption of the fibrous septa and adequate drainage. A J-shaped incision is sufficient; a fish mouth incision around the whole fingertip is slow to heal and can result in painful scarring, especially if it is placed too far palmarly.
- Irrigate the wound copiously and pack it with iodoform gauze or sterile gauze bandage.

POSTOPERATIVE CARE The finger is splinted, and elevation is maintained. The bandage is changed at about 48 hours. Dressing changes are then begun, soaking the hand in saline solution and allowing secondary healing. Active range-of-motion exercises, edema control, and gradual reincorporation of the finger into activities of daily living are emphasized. Antibiotic treatment with first-generation cephalosporins has usually been sufficient; however, changes in antibiotic therapy should be made on the basis of the results of culture and sensitivity studies. Infections in patients with diabetes or immunosuppression may be difficult to control, and amputation may be the end result.

SUBFASCIAL SPACE INFECTIONS

The potential spaces in the subfascial and deeper layers of the hand are infrequently infected (Table 16.2). A high level of suspicion should lead to their detection and treatment. The recognized deep spaces of the hand include the interdigital web spaces, the midpalmar space, the thenar space, a less

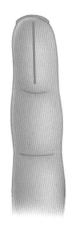

FIGURE 16.5   Midline vertical incision for drainage of abscess pointing volarly in distal pulp of finger. **SEE TECHNIQUE 16.3.**

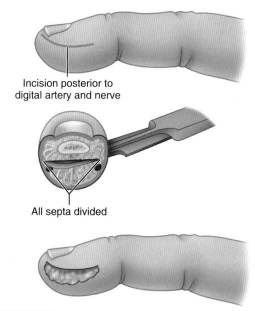

Incision posterior to digital artery and nerve

All septa divided

FIGURE 16.6   Incision and drainage of felon. **SEE TECHNIQUE 16.3.**

well-defined hypothenar space, the Parona space, and the dorsal subaponeurotic space (Fig. 16.7).

WEB SPACE INFECTION (COLLAR BUTTON ABSCESS)

Web space infection usually localizes in one of the three fat-filled interdigital spaces just proximal to the superficial transverse ligament at the level of the metacarpophalangeal joints. The adjacent fingers often are held in an abducted position with the locus of swelling between them. Typically, the infection begins beneath palmar calluses in laborers. It may begin near the palmar surface, but because the skin and fascia here are less yielding, it may localize to drain dorsally. Here the tissue becomes obviously swollen, but the greater part of the abscess remains nearer the palm. This may be the more dangerous part because, unless drained, it may spread through the lumbrical canal into the middle palmar space. Two longitudinal incisions usually are necessary for drainage: one on the dorsal surface between the metacarpal heads and the other

TABLE 16.2

Anatomy, Presentation, and Treatment of Deep Hand Space Infections

DEEP HAND SPACE	BORDERS	PRESENTATION	SURGICAL POINTS
Dorsal subaponeurotic	Dorsal: extensor tendons; volar: metacarpals and interossei	Dorsal hand swelling and fluctuans	Longitudinal incisions over index and ring metacarpals, not directly over extensor tendons
Thenar	Dorsal: adductor pollicis; volar: index flexor tendons; ulnar: septum of Legueu and Juvara; radial: adductor pollicis insertion at P1 of thumb	Thenar and first webspace swelling; thumb abduction with painful adduction or opposition; pantaloons-shaped abscess if involvement of first dorsal webspace through contiguous spread (Burkhalter)	Palmar, dorsal, or two-incision approaches; for pantaloons, abscess may drain through dual incisions or single incision perpendicular to first webspace to minimize webspace contracture
Midpalmar/deep palmar	Dorsal: middle and ring finger metacarpals and second and third interossei; volar: flexor tendons and lumbricales; ulnar: hypothenar muscles; radial: septum of Legueu and Juvara	Loss of normal palmar concavity with marked palm tenderness, painful passive motion of middle and ring fingers; substantial dorsal swelling may be present	Transverse incision in distal palmar crease; curvilinear incision along thenar crease
Webspace	Subfascial palmar space between digits	Abducted posture of adjacent digits with accompanying dorsal swelling and volar tenderness at webspace	Must drain both dorsal and volar aspects of abscess; incisions both dorsally and volarly; avoid webspace incisions to prevent contracture
Parona	Volar: pronator quadratus; dorsal: digital flexor tendons; ulnar: flexor carpi ulnaris; radial: flexor pollicis longus	Pain with passive finger flexion; acute carpal tunnel syndrome may be present	Avoid placing incisions directly over flexor tendons or median nerve to avoid desiccation.

From Osterman M, Draeger R, Stern P: Acute hand infections, *J Hand Surg* 39:1628, 2014.

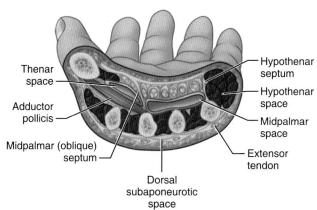

FIGURE 16.7 Cross-sectional anatomy of hand showing thenar, midpalmar, hypothenar, interdigital (web), and dorsal subaponeurotic spaces. (Redrawn from Jebson PJ: Deep subfascial space infections, *Hand Clin* 14:557, 1998.)

on the palm, beginning distal to the distal palmar crease and curving proximally. Crossing the palmar creases at right angles to the crease should be avoided (Fig. 16.8). The web should not be incised.

DEEP FASCIAL SPACE INFECTIONS

The palmar fascial space lies between the fascia covering the metacarpals and their contiguous muscles and the fascia dorsal to the flexor tendons. Its ulnar border is the fascia of the hypothenar muscles, and its radial border is the fascia of the adductor and other thenar muscles. This space is divided into a middle palmar space and a thenar space by a fascial membrane that passes obliquely from the third metacarpal shaft to the fascia of the palmar aponeurosis palmar to the flexor tendons of the index finger (Fig. 16.9). The hypothenar space has as its boundaries: the hypothenar septum laterally, the fifth metacarpal dorsally, and the hypothenar muscle fascia medially and palmarly. The space of Parona is bordered by the pronator quadratus dorsally, the flexor pollicis longus laterally, the flexor carpi ulnaris medially, and the flexor tendons on the palmar aspect; it rarely is the site of abscess formation. Infections in these spaces are now rare because less extensive infections nearby usually are controlled by antibiotics before they spread. Abscesses in these spaces usually result from the spread of infection from other parts of the hand, typically from purulent flexor tenosynovial infections.

A middle palmar abscess can cause a severe systemic reaction, local pain and tenderness, inability to move the long and ring fingers actively because of pain, and generalized swelling of the hand and fingers, which resembles an inflated rubber glove. A thenar abscess causes similar symptoms, but the thumb web is more swollen, the index finger is held flexed, and active motion of the index finger and the thumb is impaired because of pain.

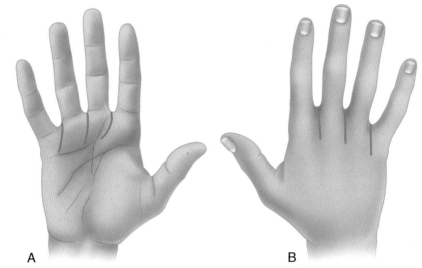

FIGURE 16.8 **A,** Lines show palmar incisions for web abscess drainage. **B,** Dorsal incision.

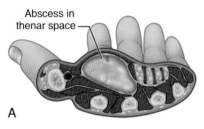

Abscess in thenar space

A

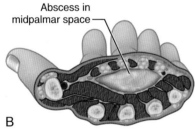

Abscess in midpalmar space

B

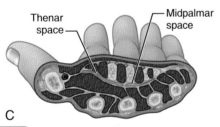

Thenar space — — Midpalmar space

C

FIGURE 16.9 Boundaries of deep palmar space, which is divided into thenar space and middle palmar space (see text). **A,** Abscess in thenar space. **B,** Abscess in middle palmar space. **C,** Relationships of spaces when not distended by pus.

INCISION AND DRAINAGE OF DEEP FASCIAL SPACE INFECTION

TECHNIQUE 16.4

- Drain the middle palmar space through a curved incision beginning at the level of the distal palmar crease, in line with the long finger and extending ulnarly to just inside the hypothenar

eminence (Fig. 16.10). Other options include the longitudinal distal palm incision and the transverse palm incision.

- Enter the space on either side of the long flexor tendon of the ring finger with a blunt instrument, such as a hemostat, to avoid injury to the neurovascular structures. Leave a drain in place if necessary.
- Drain the thenar space through a curved incision in the thumb web parallel to the border of the first dorsal interosseous muscle or along the medial side of the thenar crease (Fig. 16.11). Avoid the recurrent branch of the median nerve at the proximal end of this crease. Avoid sharp, deep dissection, using blunt dissection to delineate the extent of the abscess. Infected, swollen tissue makes identification of small nerves and vessels more difficult.
- Drain Parona space infections through a straight or curved incision on the palmar forearm. Begin the incision just proximal to the wrist flexion crease, slightly medial to the midaxial line. Extend the incision proximally and sufficiently to allow exposure of the flexor tendons and median nerve that lie immediately beneath the fascia. Alternatively, the commonly used approach through the floor of the flexor carpi radialis tendon sheath can be used. In this approach, the flexor tendons and median nerve are retracted ulnarly while the radial artery is retracted radially.
- Retract the flexor tendons and median nerve, protecting them. With use of the midline incision, the flexor tendons and median nerve may be retracted radially while protecting the ulnar neurovascular bundle and flexor carpi ulnaris tendon with ulnar-directed retraction.
- Drain the abscess, and irrigate the wound. If needed, place a Penrose drain or tube for irrigation in the wound.
- Apply a nonadherent gauze and bulky absorbent dressing. Splint the wrist in a position to allow functional motion of the fingers.
- Change the bandage frequently, irrigating as required. Usually, healing by secondary intention is satisfactory. If the infection and drainage can be controlled rapidly, secondary closure or skin grafting may be appropriate.
- If the infection and drainage cannot be controlled rapidly, healing by secondary intention is preferred.

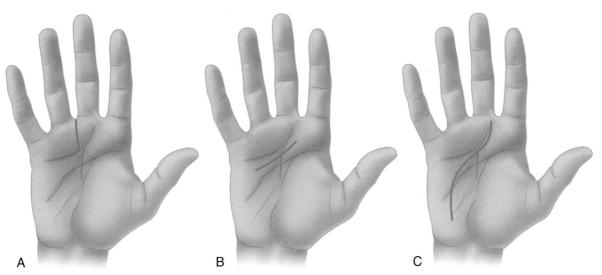

FIGURE 16.10 **A,** Distal longitudinal palmar incision. **B,** Transverse palmar incision. **C,** Extended longitudinal palmar incision. **SEE TECHNIQUE 16.4.**

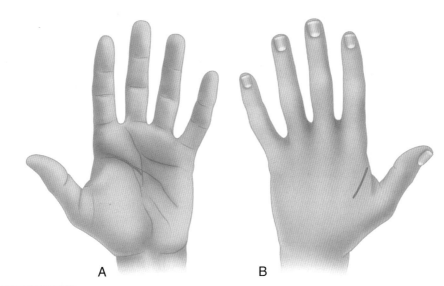

FIGURE 16.11 **A,** Thenar crease incision (palmar). **B,** Dorsal longitudinal incision. **SEE TECHNIQUE 16.4.**

SUBAPONEUROTIC SPACE INFECTIONS

Subaponeurotic space infections on the dorsum of the hand and wrist can be caused by penetrating injury and local spread from other infection in the hand. Dorsal hand swelling, redness, increased heat, tenderness to palpation, painful finger extension, and purulent drainage from areas of penetration may be seen. Although difficult in the presence of cellulitis, it is important to determine the presence of an abscess. If this cannot be done with palpation, needle aspiration can be used to locate a purulent collection. Radionuclide scanning, MRI, and ultrasound may be helpful, but usually are not needed. Most dorsal subaponeurotic abscesses can be drained through one dorsal incision, although the presence of a large dorsal abscess may require two dorsal parallel incisions, usually placed over the second metacarpal and between the fourth and fifth metacarpals. If necessary, these incisions usually are short (2 to 3 cm) and should not compromise the circulation of the skin between them. A single incision is made longitudinally and dorsally, centered over the abscess. Sharp deep dissection is avoided so as not to injure the tendons. The abscess is located and drained with blunt dissection, and the wound is thoroughly irrigated. A drain is placed if the cavity is sufficiently large to create a "dead space." A bulky absorbent bandage with a splint is applied to support the wrist and allow free movement of the fingers.

TENOSYNOVITIS

An infection within the flexor tendon sheath may be the result of local injury or puncture wound to the volar aspect of the finger near a flexor crease. While direct inoculation is the most common cause of infectious tenosynovitis, adjacent spread from a local infection or hematogenous spread also are possible causes. Although the flexor sheath usually is involved, the radial and ulnar bursae may be involved as well. Kanavel considered tenderness over the involved sheath, rigid

TABLE 16.3

Michon Classification for Severity of Flexor Tenosynovitis

INTRAOPERATIVE STAGE	CHARACTERISTIC FINDINGS	TREATMENT RECOMMENDATION
I	Increased fluid in sheath, primarily serous exudate	Minimally invasive drainage and catheter irrigation
II	Cloudy/purulent fluid, granulomatous synovium	Minimally invasive drainage ± indwelling catheter irrigation
III	Septic necrosis of tendon, pulleys, or tendon sheath	Extensile open debridement; possible amputation

From Michon J: Phlegmon of the tendon sheaths, *Ann Chir* 28:277, 1974.

positioning of the finger in flexion, pain on attempts to hyperextend the fingers, and swelling of the involved part to be the four cardinal signs of suppurative tenosynovitis. Of these, tenderness over the flexor sheath is considered the most significant. When early tenosynovitis is suspected, immediate treatment with antibiotics and splinting may abort the spread of infection if the patient's symptoms have been present for less than 48 hours. If nonsurgical treatment is selected, these patients should be followed closely with a low threshold for hospital admission, because the consequences of noncompliance can be devastating to the digit and hand. Good results have been reported in patients with pyogenic flexor tenosynovitis treated with surgical drainage, followed by outpatient management with intravenous antibiotics, wound care, and rehabilitation. Patients with infection after penetrating injuries usually are infected with *S. aureus*. However, *Streptococcus* also may be found. Under ideal circumstances, fluid should be obtained from the sheath for Gram stain, culture, and antibiotic sensitivity testing. If gross pus is obtained from the aspiration of the digital flexor sheath, surgical drainage usually is indicated. Purulent fluid might not be present in the flexor sheath with overlying cellulitis; however, needle aspiration of the sheath through cellulitic tissue creates the risk of inoculating the uninfected sheath with bacteria. An increasing frequency of MRSA hand infections has been documented in clinical studies. Vancomycin is effective for infections caused by gram-positive bacteria, whereas ciprofloxacin is most effective for gram-negative organisms, including *Pseudomonas*. With persistent tenosynovial infection, pressures within the flexor sheath can exceed 30 mm Hg, rendering the tendons ischemic in the presence of infection. Delay in treatment may lead to damage to the flexor tendon and sheath, with resulting adhesion, loss of excursion, finger stiffness, and impaired function. The prognosis for function is poor if an infection here produces pus that must be drained. If drainage is required, an open or closed irrigation technique can be used. If an open technique is used, healing and rehabilitation are prolonged and full motion may not be regained. The use of a continuous postoperative irrigation catheter has not been shown to improve outcomes, but rather increases postoperative pain and adds difficulty to postoperative care. The Michon classification has been proposed as a method to help surgeons make decisions on how aggressively to approach treatment, recommending minimally invasive drainage and catheter irrigation for stage I or II flexor tenosynovitis (Table 16.3). This classification has not been validated, however. In this author's practice, indwelling catheter irrigation is not used. Pang et al. have identified factors

predisposing to poor outcome. Patients presenting with subcutaneous purulence and those with ischemic changes had amputation rates of 8% and 59%, respectively, with increasing loss of total active motion.

POSTOPERATIVE CLOSED IRRIGATION

Closed postoperative irrigation is appropriate and effective for infections that yield serous exudate or purulent fluid on opening the flexor sheath and for infections that are relatively acute. Some have found that closed catheter irrigation is as effective as open drainage of pyogenic flexor tenosynovitis. Chung and Foo modified the closed irrigation technique by introducing an intraluminal 24-gauge wire to stiffen the catheter for easier cannulation and manipulation; they also fenestrated the catheter along its middle portion to increase the turbulence of intrathecal flow. Jing and Iyer described the use of a metal ear suction catheter for irrigation of a flexor tendon sheath infection, citing ease of insertion under direct vision, effectiveness, and low cost among its advantages. If the infection is chronic, or if the flexor tendon is grossly necrotic, open drainage may be necessary.

TECHNIQUE 16.5

(NEVIASER, MODIFIED)

- With the patient under suitable anesthesia and after appropriately preparing and draping the hand and arm, inflate a pneumatic tourniquet. However, to reduce the risk of spreading the infection, do not wrap the limb.
- Expose the proximal end of the flexor sheath in the region of the A1 pulley making a straight transverse incision parallel to the distal palmar crease or a zigzag incision in this area (Fig. 16.12). Expect to see serosanguineous or purulent fluid in the sheath.
- Open the sheath proximal to the A1 pulley, and swab the fluid to send for cultures.
- Make a second incision in the midaxial line on either side of the finger in the distal portion of the middle segment of the digit.
- As an alternative, carefully make a transverse incision over the distal flexion crease.
- Open the flexor sheath distal to the A4 pulley.
- Using smooth forceps or hemostats, pass a 16-gauge or 18-gauge polyethylene catheter beneath the A1 pulley from proximal to distal in the flexor sheath for 1.5 to 2 cm. Distally place a small piece of rubber drain beneath

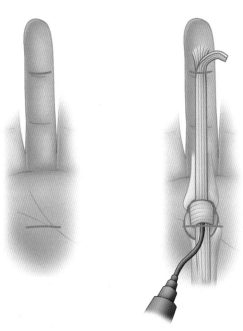

FIGURE 16.12 Closed irrigation for tenosynovitis (modified Neviaser technique). **SEE TECHNIQUE 16.5.**

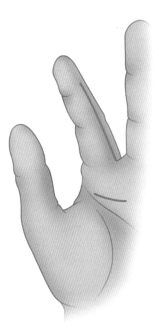

FIGURE 16.13 Open drainage for advanced infection and necrosis of tendon and sheath. **SEE TECHNIQUE 16.6.**

the A4 pulley and bring it out through the skin incision. Irrigate the sheath from proximal to distal with saline. Alternatively, use a 16-gauge angiocatheter attached to a small syringe (20 to 50 mL). The tip can be cut to bevel the end of the angiocatheter. Use the catheter to flush fluid from proximal to distal, watching for outflow of fluid from the distal incision. Irrigate until the outflow fluid is clear.

- Close the wounds around the catheter and the rubber drain, leaving the distal wound sufficiently loose to allow fluid to drain. Suture the catheter to the palmar skin. Test the system for patency by irrigating freely with saline. Alternatively, do not use the postoperative catheter. Monitor the patient and return to the operating room for another drainage procedure if necessary.
- Wrap the hand in a bulky dressing supported with a splint, leaving the tip of the rubber drain exposed to observe the outflow. Bring the inflow catheter out through the dressing, tape it to the dressing, and attach it to a 30-mL syringe.
- When the radial or ulnar bursa is involved, place a second catheter in the palmar wound and pass it proximally in the sheath, securing it to the palmar skin with a suture to prevent dislodgment. Alternatively, a small Penrose drain can be placed.
- Open the respective bursa proximally through a longitudinal incision on the radial or ulnar side of the distal forearm just proximal to the wrist. Place a piece of rubber drain in the bursa, and bring it out through the skin.
- Irrigate in proximal and distal directions for these combined digital and bursal infections.

POSTOPERATIVE CARE If postoperative catheter irrigation has been chosen, the wounds are irrigated with 30 mL of saline every 2 hours, and the wound at the distal end of the finger is checked for catheter patency and flow of irrigant. After 48 hours, the dressing is removed so that the fingers can be examined. If signs of persistent infection are present, irrigation is continued for another 24 hours. The dressings are removed at that time, and the fingers are examined. If no residual signs of infection remain, the catheter and drain are removed, a lighter dressing is applied, and active motion exercises are begun. If pain or drainage persists, irrigation may be necessary for several days. Lille et al. found no significant differences in outcome between patients who received only intraoperative irrigation and patients who received postoperative irrigation for 24 to 48 hours. This author prefers to return to the operating room if symptoms are not improving instead of using continuous catheter irrigation.

OPEN DRAINAGE

Open drainage rarely is used but may be necessary in fingers with advanced infection and necrosis of the tendon and sheath that requires debridement.

TECHNIQUE 16.6

- With the patient under suitable anesthesia, inflate the tourniquet but do not wrap the limb.
- Use two incisions. Make the first incision midaxial on either side of the finger, extending from the distal flexion crease nearly to the web, staying dorsal to the neurovascular bundles (Fig. 16.13). Avoid injury to the annular pulleys, opening the sheath at the cruciform pulleys and debriding the flexor tenosynovium. Make the second incision on the palm, parallel to and near the palmar crease over the A1 pulley.

- Identify the flexor sheath in the distal wound, open the sheath, and obtain swab specimens or fluid to send for culture determination.
- If the thumb or small finger flexor tendons are involved, make an additional longitudinal incision over the respective flexor tendons proximal to the wrist flexion crease.
- Carefully identify the radial or ulnar bursa with blunt dissection, and debride the infected flexor tenosynovium (see next section on infections of the radial and ulnar bursae).
- Irrigate from the proximal wound distally with saline. Leave the wound open, wrap the hand in a bulky dressing, and place it in a splint.

POSTOPERATIVE CARE Active finger motion is encouraged as soon as possible after 36 to 48 hours. The bandages are removed, the wounds inspected, and whirlpool treatments begun daily or twice daily. Active motion exercises are encouraged during and between treatments. Although delayed closure may be considered, usually the resolution of drainage is so prolonged that secondary healing is allowed to occur to minimize the recurrence of infection.

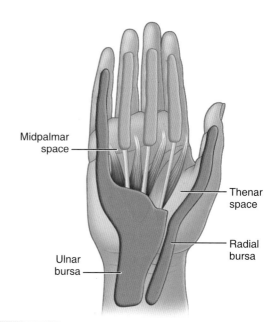

FIGURE 16.14 Flexor tendon sheaths and proximal extensions into radial and ulnar bursae. (Redrawn from Neviaser RJ, Gunther SF: Tenosynovial infections of the hand-diagnosis and management: I. Acute pyogenic tenosynovitis of the hand, *Instr Course Lect* 29:108, 1980.)

INFECTIONS OF RADIAL AND ULNAR BURSAE

The radial and ulnar bursae are the tenosynovial sheaths of the flexor tendons at the wrist (Fig. 16.14). The proximal prolongation of the thumb flexor sheath is the radial bursa (Fig. 16.15). The flexor sheaths communicate from the proximal palmar crease to the level of the pronator quadratus and extend distally as the tendon sheath of the little finger to form the ulnar bursa. Often the two bursae communicate with one another and allow infection to spread from one to the other in a "horseshoe abscess."

INCISION AND DRAINAGE OF RADIAL AND ULNAR BURSAE

TECHNIQUE 16.7

- To drain the radial bursa, first make a lateral incision along the proximal phalanx of the thumb and open the bursa at its distal end.
- Introduce a probe here, advance it proximally to the wrist, and make a second incision over its end.
- Insert small 16- or 18-gauge polyethylene drainage tubes proximally and rubber drains distally for irrigation.
- Make a palmar incision, and pass drainage tubes proximally as described for tenosynovitis.
- Open the ulnar bursa on the ulnar side of the little finger and again proximal to the wrist with the help of a probe. If both bursae are involved, one proximal ulnar incision may be sufficient to drain both because the two bursae communicate proximally in most patients.

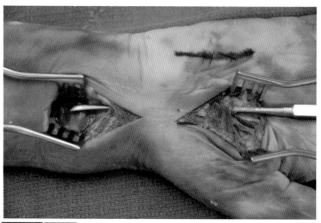

FIGURE 16.15 Passage of instrument from thenar space to radial bursa in cadaver specimen demonstrates how easily infections can propagate proximally. (From McDonald LS, Bavaro MR, Hofmeister EP, Kroonen LT: Current concepts. Hand infections, *J Hand Surg* 36A:1403, 2011.)

SEPTIC ARTHRITIS
FINGER JOINT INFECTIONS

Finger joint infections usually result from the spread of infection in adjacent structures, direct penetration of the joint, and less commonly, hematogenous spread. When hematogenous spread occurs, the primary source should be identified. The involved joints usually are swollen, tender, and warm, and the finger usually is held in slight flexion. Careful inspection and palpation may reveal a fluctuant joint effusion, and active and passive motions usually are quite painful. In addition to the history, physical examination, and radiographic evaluation, diagnosis is accomplished by joint aspiration and synovial fluid analysis, Gram stain, and cultures. Fluid obtained from a septic joint usually is turbid, opaque, or grossly purulent. The joint fluid WBC usually is greater than 50,000/mm³. More recent studies have shown that lowering the cell count threshold to 17,500 increases the sensitivity of the diagnosis to 83%. The polymorphonuclear count usually is greater than 75%, and the synovial fluid glucose is 40 mg or less. *S. aureus* usually is the organism isolated from septic hand and wrist joints.

Because septic arthritis can cause articular cartilage destruction and osteomyelitis in the underlying phalanx, it should be treated as an emergency when pus has been identified in the joint. Cartilage destruction and osteomyelitis can be delayed or avoided if aggressive treatment with incision and drainage and the appropriate antibiotics is pursued. If the joint and adjacent bone have been destroyed and require removal, antibiotic-impregnated polymethyl methacrylate spheres can be a useful adjunct in reconstruction with arthrodesis or bone grafting. Amputation may be required to salvage the hand. Usually little is lost by such an amputation because the chronically infected finger retains little useful function. In children, antibiotics, drainage, and splinting are continued longer than in adults in an attempt to salvage the hand.

OPEN DRAINAGE OF SEPTIC FINGER JOINTS

TECHNIQUE 16.8

- With the patient under appropriate anesthesia, apply and inflate a tourniquet but do not wrap the arm.
- To drain the metacarpophalangeal joint, make an incision on either side of the metacarpal head, retract the extensor expansion distally, and open the joint capsule dorsal to the collateral ligament sufficiently to allow free drainage and irrigation of the joint.
- Leave the capsule and skin incisions open.
- To drain the thumb and finger interphalangeal joints and the thumb metacarpophalangeal joint, use a midaxial incision on either side of the joint. Avoid injury to the neurovascular bundles.
- In the fingers, section the transverse retinacular ligament, retract the extensor lateral band dorsally, and retract the neurovascular bundle toward the palm.
- Identify the collateral ligament and make a longitudinal incision parallel to the ligament and palmar to it, separating the accessory collateral ligament from it.
- Remove a portion of the accessory collateral ligament, drain the joint, and send specimens for aerobic and anaerobic cultures.
- Irrigate the wound with saline and leave it open.
- Apply a bulky dressing and a splint.

POSTOPERATIVE CARE The hand is elevated for about 24 hours. The bandage is changed, and motion exercises begun. The dressing is changed daily or twice daily, and exercise periods in a whirlpool bath begun. When the wound is satisfactorily clean, it can be closed secondarily; otherwise, it should be allowed to heal by secondary intention.

WRIST INFECTIONS

The incidence of septic arthritis of the wrist is unknown, but the wrist is less frequently involved than other large joints. Approximately 25% of cases of septic arthritis in the upper extremity occur in the wrist. As in the finger, septic arthritis of the wrist usually results from the spread of infection in adjacent structures, direct penetration of the joint, and, less commonly, hematogenous spread. In patients older than 60 years, comorbidities such as rheumatoid arthritis, diabetes, and gout or pseudogout, and immunosuppression are known risk factors. Immunosuppressive drugs used for inflammatory arthritis, corticosteroids, and chemotherapy also may predispose patients to septic arthritis. *S. aureus* is the most common organism, with an almost 40% frequency of MRSA reported. Localized warmth, swelling, tenderness, and painful passive motion are typical presenting signs. Prompt irrigation and debridement, along with the appropriate antibiotic therapy, are indicated to prevent articular destruction. Open arthrotomy may include the radiocarpal, ulnocarpal, midcarpal, and distal radioulnar joints and can be accomplished through a standard dorsal approach (see Techniques 6.5 and 6.6). A transverse skin incision also can be used, with better cosmetic results, but may not provide adequate exposure. Arthroscopic irrigation and debridement have been shown to produce outcomes similar to those obtained with open procedures, with fewer operations and shorter hospital stays. Contraindications to arthroscopic irrigation and debridement include postoperative infections, previous wrist surgery, osteomyelitis, purulence that has extended outside of the radiocarpal and midcarpal joints, and an arthroscopically inaccessible joint. Techniques of wrist arthroscopy are described in chapter 6. Regardless of the procedure, open or arthroscopic, 90-day perioperative mortality has been reported to be approximately 20%, likely because of the severity of the disease process and the high rate of comorbidities.

OSTEOMYELITIS

Osteomyelitis of the metacarpals and phalanges can be caused by infection of the neighboring soft tissues; an open fracture; the open treatment of a closed fracture; and the consequences of peripheral vascular disease, diabetes mellitus, and immunodeficiency states. Hematogenous osteomyelitis is rare in the hand and is more likely in immunocompromised patients. *S. aureus* is reported as the most commonly isolated organism. The principles of diagnosis and treatment, including drainage, intravenous antibiotics, and early mobilization, that apply to large bones apply here. If diagnostic measures, including radiographs and radionuclide studies (technetium-labeled, gallium-labeled, and indium-labeled leukocyte scans), suggest bone infection with no sequestrum formation, the process is considered acute or subacute and may resolve without surgical drainage if appropriate antibiotics are instituted for organisms obtained by needle aspiration. If no organisms can be obtained, open drainage of pus and debridement of necrotic material provide adequate material for culture and ensure decompression of the abscesses. If the process has lingered and sequestra have formed, it is considered a chronic infection. Although salvage of the digits is possible with diaphysectomy, sequestrectomy, external fixation, the use of antibiotic-impregnated polymethyl methacrylate, and subsequent bone grafting, frequently it is difficult to

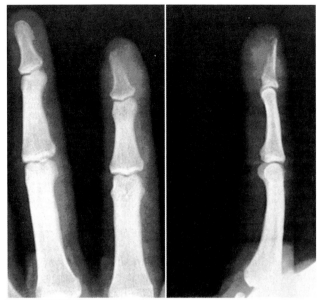

FIGURE 16.16 Osteitis of distal phalanx caused by infection in finger pulp.

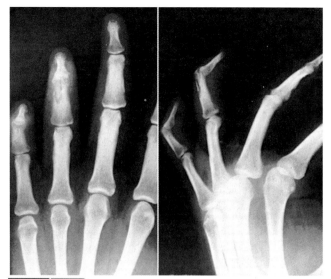

FIGURE 16.17 Sequestrating osteomyelitis of middle phalanx.

preserve a functioning digit and hand because of the severe stiffness that develops in the involved digit and in the remaining digits. Especially in adults, unless the infection can be controlled to preserve satisfactory function in the involved digit and hand, amputation should be considered. The amputation should be at the joint proximal to the involved bone. Although multiple imaging modalities beyond radiographs are available, MRI has been suggested as the initial choice for advanced imaging because it is more readily available and offers assessment for possible sinus tracks, extent of infection, and differentiation of bone and soft-tissue infection. CT may be helpful to identify a sequestrum that may develop in chronic osteomyelitis.

Infection of the distal finger pulp may erode the distal phalanx, as radiographs would show, especially if the abscess is deep and located proximally (Fig. 16.16). This area of osteitis regenerates to some extent after the abscess is drained, especially in children, and should not be confused with sequestrating osteomyelitis (Fig. 16.17).

HUMAN BITE INJURIES

Human bite injuries occur in two ways. The first is inadvertent and relatively innocent, involving nail biting and similar activities. The second, although at times accidental, usually involves intentionally violent attacks and includes the more common full-thickness bites, bite amputations, and injuries related to striking a tooth with the clenched fist. Clenched-fist injuries account for some of the most severe infections related to human tooth wounds. Most often, the third and fourth digits are injured at the metacarpophalangeal joint. Although fractures of the metacarpal neck may occur, chondral and osteochondral fractures are present in 6% to 59% of patients. The chance of inoculating the hand with virulent organisms is great because 42 different bacterial species have been identified in the normal human mouth flora. Although many reports cite *S. aureus* as the most common infecting organism, followed by streptococci, others have found α-streptococcus to be the most common single organism in 24 patients. Other organisms found are *E. corrodens, Micrococcus, Clostridium, Spirochaeta,* and *Neisseria.* An average 2.5-day delay in seeking medical attention has been reported, and patients frequently are noncompliant. Reported complications from the injury include osteomyelitis, fracture, pain, permanent joint stiffness, arthritis, digital amputation, systemic sepsis, and death. The incidence of complications ranges from 25% to 50%.

The mechanism for introducing anaerobic bacteria into the joint is understood best by realizing that the injury occurs when the hand is in a fist. When the finger is next extended, the injured joint is closed because the tendon that was lacerated by the tooth glides proximally (Fig. 16.18). This provides an anaerobic environment for growth of the bacteria introduced.

Generally, all patients with small lacerations over the metacarpophalangeal joint should be assumed to have tooth injuries, regardless of the history given. Radiographs should be obtained to rule out fractures and foreign bodies, and the wound should be explored to rule out intraarticular injury. Several authors have observed that patients who seek treatment less than 24 hours after injury usually do not have signs of sepsis, so joint exploration, swabbing for cultures (aerobic and anaerobic with attention to *E. corrodens*), treatment with antibiotics, and close observation usually are sufficient. Some surgeons advise all patients who have sustained human bites to be admitted to the hospital. Patients who seek treatment 24 hours or more after injury may have definite signs and symptoms of sepsis and may require open joint drainage and irrigation, close observation (usually in the hospital), and intravenous antibiotics. Patients presenting with bite infections more than 8 days after the initial injury have been reported to have an 18% chance of requiring amputation. At this time, the antibiotics usually recommended include penicillin G, ampicillin, carbenicillin, or tetracycline for infection with *E. corrodens* and a cephalosporin for infection with *Staphylococcus* organisms. It is necessary to be aware of the prevalence of penicillin-resistant organisms when antibiotics are selected. Antibiotics can be changed at 36 to 48 hours, depending on the culture and sensitivity results. Tetanus prophylaxis is ensured, and the wound is left open.

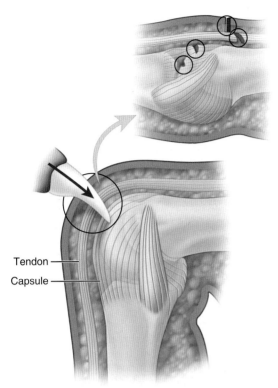

FIGURE 16.18 Tooth penetrates skin, tendon, and joint capsule while metacarpophalangeal joint is flexed. When joint is extended, these tissues shift to occupy different sites; this results in inoculated, closed, intraarticular wound.

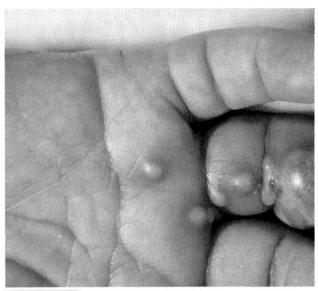

FIGURE 16.19 Vesicle eruption typical of herpetic infection. (From McCarthy JJ, Dormans JP, Kozin SH, Pizzutillo PD. Musculoskeletal infections in children, *J Bone Joint Surg* 86A:850–863, 2004.)

If the healing is progressing satisfactorily, motion exercises can be started at 24 hours after drainage. Daily washing of the wound with soap and water usually provides sufficient cleansing. In some patients with other conditions, such as diabetes, and in patients taking corticosteroids, final resolution and healing may be prolonged, leading to some of the previously mentioned complications. Depending on the clinical course of the infection, antibiotics usually are continued for 7 to 10 days.

ANIMAL BITE INJURIES

Dog bites to the hand may appear as puncture wounds or as superficial or deep lacerations. Canine oral flora include *S. aureus, Streptococcus viridans, Bacteroides,* and *Pasteurella multocida.* Most of these organisms usually are sensitive to penicillin. Tetanus prophylaxis should be accompanied by the use of antibiotics in healing dog bites. Deep wounds should be debrided, cleansed, irrigated, and left open for secondary closure. More superficial lacerations can be loosely closed after the wound has been thoroughly cleansed, the margins debrided, and the wound irrigated thoroughly with copious amounts of normal saline.

Cat bites more often are seen as puncture wounds and can progress to serious infections requiring hospitalization. In a group of 193 patients with cat bites to the hand, 30% were hospitalized for an average of 3 days. *P. multocida* is commonly isolated from cat bites and usually is sensitive to penicillin. If the bites are minor or superficial, treatment includes cleansing and observation. If the cat bites are deep, they can be connected with a scalpel blade to allow thorough wound debridement and irrigation. A severe wound is left open, whereas more superficial wounds can be loosely closed. Amoxicillin clavulanate is a common choice for empiric antibiotic therapy. Systemic signs of toxicity, rapid progression of infection, concern for deep-space infection, inability of the patient to tolerate oral therapy, or ineffective oral therapy are all indicators of the need for intravenous antibiotic therapy.

MISCELLANEOUS AND UNUSUAL INFECTIONS
HERPETIC INFECTIONS

Herpes simplex was first reported by Adamson in 1909. It often resembles a pyogenic infection and frequently involves the paronychial region, but it may involve the palm, usually distal to the metacarpophalangeal joint. It occurs most often on the thumb and index finger. Herpes simplex virus types 1 and 2 are the most common in the hand. The lesions begin as swelling with pain and the development of vesicles. The vesicles progress to ulcers over about 2 weeks. In the next 7 to 10 days, the vesicles begin to dry and heal; however, viral shedding may make the lesions infective for another 12 days or so (Fig. 16.19). The reported recurrence rate is 20%. Laboratory techniques to confirm the diagnosis include viral cultures, Tzanck and other smears and stains, and serologic tests for primary infections. The diagnosis can be confirmed by herpes antibody titers. It is often found in individuals involved in the care of the oral or respiratory system, such as dental hygienists and medical personnel. It may be accompanied by axillary and epitrochlear adenopathy with lymphangitis of the forearm. The lesions should be kept clean to avoid bacterial infection. Current treatment is medical and includes the use of acyclovir in some patients, especially the immunocompromised. Although surgical drainage is not usually indicated for herpetic infections, concomitant pyogenic infection with abscess formation may require incision and drainage. Intravenous antibiotics and acyclovir are added to their treatment.

INFECTIONS IN DRUG ADDICTS

Intravenous drug users are more likely to have MRSA as the organism of infection. The lack of asepsis in cleaning the skin and preparing injectable substances probably accounts for most infections associated with intravenous drug abuse. Although infection may appear as septicemia, usually the sepsis is localized because of subcutaneous extravasation. These hand infections have been categorized into four types, depending on the depth and location of infection. Type I infection is in the skin and subcutaneous tissues, usually on the dorsum of the fingers. Type II infection includes the extensor tendon and possibly the periosteum and bone. Type III involves the flexor tendon sheath of the finger and has the worst prognosis. Type IV includes the sequelae of arterial injection, such as digital necrosis and pain. Dorsal swelling may be caused by chronic lymphedema and fibrosis instead of infection. Treatment includes hospitalization; aggressive incision, drainage, and debridement; culturing for aerobic and anaerobic organisms; copious lavage; open treatment of the wound; splinting; multiple daily dressing changes; appropriate intravenous antibiotics; and progressive rehabilitation of the hand.

INFECTIONS IN PATIENTS WITH ACQUIRED IMMUNODEFICIENCY SYNDROME

Patients with hand infections and acquired immunodeficiency syndrome (AIDS) or AIDS-related complex may have an atypical presentation and course of the infections. Herpetic infections can be more virulent than usual and may not resolve spontaneously; intravenous antiviral therapy may be necessary. Dorsal bacterial abscesses may not respond to early drainage and can progress to osteomyelitis.

NECROTIZING FASCIITIS

During the late 1800s, necrotizing infections were known as "hospital gangrene." Other terms were used until *necrotizing fasciitis* was used by Wilson in 1952. The term *necrotizing fasciitis* generally has been used to describe streptococcal infections of the soft tissues; however, some severe infections are caused by streptococci in combination with anaerobic and other aerobic bacteria. These infections have been placed into four groups, depending on the causative organisms. Type 1 is polymicrobial infection caused by mixture of non–group A streptococci with anaerobic or facultative anaerobic organisms. Type 2 is monomicrobial infection caused by group A streptococci alone or by a species of *Staphylococcus*. Type 3 infection may be caused by gram-negative, marine-related organisms such as *Vibrio* species. Finally, type 4 is a fungal infection, often *Candida* species or *Zygomycetes*, that occurs in patients with severe trauma or those who are immunocompromised.

Although commonly related to traumatic events, such as open fractures, lacerations, contusions, cutaneous abscesses, steroid injections, insect bites, burns, and frostbite, necrotizing infections may occur in the absence of known trauma. Patients who may be susceptible to necrotizing infections include those who are immunosuppressed as a result of AIDS or chemotherapy. Patients with a history of diabetes, peripheral vascular disease, alcoholism, intravenous drug abuse, multiple myeloma, discoid lupus, and porphyria cutanea tarda may also be at increased risk. A systematic review identified a history of intravenous drug use, smoking, and trauma as the most common associated risk factors and diabetes as the most common comorbidity. Although the skin may appear normal early in the course of the illness, the clinical course of a necrotizing infection is one of rapid progressions from a skin abscess with redness around it accompanied by pain and swelling to severe, nonpitting edema. Skin bullae and blue discoloration in the skin may develop over several days; however, lymphangitis and lymphadenopathy may not be present. Similarly, the WBC and body temperature may be normal. A WBC of more than 15,400 cells/mm^3 and serum sodium concentration of less than 135 mmol/L have been reported to have a sensitivity of 90%, specificity of 76%, a negative predictive value of 99%, and a positive predictive value of 26%. Radiographs may reveal subcutaneous gas. Computed tomography scanning has been reported to be 100% sensitive and 81% specific in identifying necrotizing fasciitis, with a positive predictive value of 76% and negative predictive value of 100%. Magnetic resonance imaging has not been found to be helpful and may even confound the diagnosis, because many of the findings with necrotizing fasciitis can overlap with other soft-tissue infections.

Progressing from the skin and subcutaneous tissue, the necrotizing infection spreads along the fascial planes, liquefying the fascia, producing a thin exudate that may be foul smelling with anaerobic infections. Bruising and irregular areas of skin necrosis are apparent, but the extent of fascial involvement extends beyond the area of the apparent skin involvement, and myonecrosis may follow bacterial spread to muscle. Tenderness to palpation often is out of proportion to the examination, and the area of tenderness extends beyond the abnormal soft tissue. When it is well established, necrotizing fasciitis spreads rapidly. In the upper extremity, the proximal spread to the chest wall may have a mortality rate of 75%. Although thrombosis of digital vessels leads to gangrene, necrotizing fasciitis also may be complicated by abscess formation in the liver, spleen, brain, and lungs; disseminated intravascular coagulopathy; septic shock; and death. Mortality rates range from 23% to 76%, with organ failure and sepsis the major causes. Delays in diagnosis and appropriate treatment are significantly associated with increased mortality. The Laboratory Risk Indicator for Necrotizing Fasciitis (LRINEC) score has been utilized to aid clinicians in the diagnosis of a necrotizing soft-tissue infection (Table 16.4). A score ≥6 provides a positive predictive value of 96%. The score has not been shown to correlate with disease severity or outcome but may help in ruling out necrotizing fasciitis. The final diagnosis is still clinical, and aggressive treatment is warranted in equivocal cases.

Successful treatment is aided by the prompt recognition of the spreading soft-tissue involvement. Several studies have determined that the time from diagnosis to first debridement is a primary factor in outcome, with 93% chance of survival when debridement is done within 24 hours, decreasing to 75% at 48 hours. Aggressive debridement of all the necrotic tissue, especially the liquefying fascia, is essential (Fig. 16.20). Cultures for anaerobic organisms should be obtained from the areas of the worst involvement. The use of extensile incisions preserves skin flaps and decreases the risk of injury to viable underlying structures. Wounds are left open, and patients are returned to the operating room for repeat inspection and debridement every 24 to 48 hours, depending on the appearance of the wound. When all the necrotic tissue has been

TABLE 16.4		
LRINEC Score (Laboratory Risk Indicator for the Necrotizing Fasciitis)		
VARIABLE	β	**SCORE**
C-reactive protein level	0	0
<150	3.5	4
>150		
Total white cell count (cells/	0	0
mm³)	0.5	1
<15	2.1	2
15-25		
>25		
Hemoglobin level (g/dL)	0	0
<13.5	0.6	1
11-13.5	1.8	2
<11		
Sodium level (mmol/L)	0	0
>/= 135	1.8	2
<135		
Creatinine level (mcg/L)	0	0
</= 141	1.8	2
>141		
Glucose level (mmol/L)	0	0
</= 10	1.2	1
>10		

From Wong CH, Khin LW, Heng KS, Tan KC, Low CO: The LRINEC (Laboratory Risk Indicator for Necrotizing Fasciitis) score: a tool for distinguishing necrotizing fasciitis from other soft tissue infections, *Crit Care Med* 32:1535, 2004.

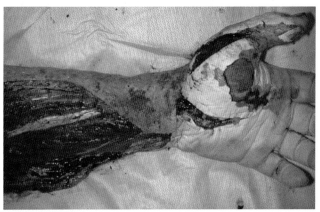

FIGURE 16.20 Necrotizing fasciitis in 78-year-old man. Early and aggressive management with serial wide surgical debridement, negative pressure therapy, and subsequent delayed closure allowed preservation of the limb. (From McDonald LS, Bavaro MR, Hofmeister EP, Kroonen LT: Current concepts. Hand infections, *J Hand Surg Am* 36:1403, 2011.)

removed, and the infection is under control with a healthy, granulating wound, closure with direct suture, skin grafts, or flaps can be done. Amputations may be required to remove necrotic tissue and to control infection; reported amputation rates in patients with necrotizing fasciitis of the extremities range from 18% to 28%.

While bacterial cultures are pending, Gram stains help to determine the initial antibiotic selection. General recommendations include intravenous broad-spectrum antibiotics for *Staphylococcus* and *Streptococcus* (cephalosporin), penicillin for anaerobic organisms, and gentamicin for gram-negative organisms. An awareness of the prevalence of penicillin-resistant organisms and the assistance of an infectious disease consultant help in determining the most appropriate antibiotic therapy.

Hyperalimentation has been beneficial in helping patients heal wounds and combat infection. Hyperbaric oxygen treatments may be helpful with difficult anaerobic infections.

GAS GANGRENE (CLOSTRIDIAL MYONECROSIS)

Gas gangrene, although rarely encountered, when established, threatens life and limb. In a 1947 report, Altmeier and Furste estimated the incidence of gas gangrene to be 0.03% to 5.2%. More recently, the occurrence in the United States has been estimated to be 1000 to 3000 cases per year. *Clostridium perfringens (C. welchii)*, the organism most often associated with gas gangrene, was first isolated in the late 1800s in the United States, Germany, and France. Other clostridial species produce toxins and may be associated with gas gangrene. Nonclostridial organisms are found in an estimated 85% of gas gangrene infections. Readily found in the environment and on human mucous membranes, clostridia are anaerobic, saprophytic gram-positive rods that grow best in necrotic tissue and blood and in conditions of low oxygen concentration, where spores become vegetative and produce a variety of toxins. Toxins produced by clostridia include alpha toxin (myonecrosis and hemolysis), theta toxin (hemolysis and cardiotoxicity), kappa toxin (collagenase), nu toxin (deoxyribonuclease), and mu toxin (hyaluronidase). The production of toxins results in necrosis of muscle, fat, and subcutaneous tissue and in the production of hydrogen sulfide and carbon dioxide. Laboratory isolation of clostridial organisms requires an anaerobic environment and a medium containing a reducing agent (sodium thioglycolate).

Although frequently associated with open fractures, gas gangrene also may be seen with closed fractures. Crushing injuries, soil contamination, and primary closure of contaminated wounds are major factors contributing to the development of gas gangrene. Other predisposing factors include surgery, immunosuppression, penetrating foreign body, chronic edema, shock, and infection with aerobic organisms. Three types of clostridial infections have been described: type 1, clostridial contamination with a positive bacteriologic culture without clinical signs of infection; type 2, clostridial cellulitis, in which the infection of tissue produces foul-smelling gas but there is no systemic infection; and type 3, gas gangrene, clostridial myonecrosis, and systemic signs of severe infection.

The onset and clinical course of gas gangrene is rapid. Rapidly progressing edema, severe and worsening pain in the limb, soft-tissue gas that is visible on radiographs early, and palpable within 24 hours (Fig. 16.21), mild fever, tachycardia, and anxiety may occur early in the course of the infection. Myonecrosis, occurring in the first few days after the initiating lesion, leads to limb edema and the subsequent development of hemorrhagic skin bullae, and blebs, and foul-smelling purulent drainage. Progressive systemic sepsis, leading to hemolysis, renal failure, and septic shock, may lead rapidly to an overall mortality of 19%, with a 5% mortality in patients with posttraumatic clostridial myonecrosis of the extremities.

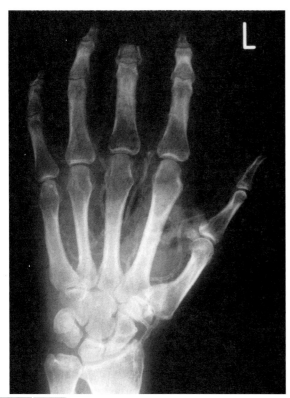

FIGURE 16.21 Radiographic appearance of gas gangrene in left hand. (From Goyal RW, Ng ABY, Bale RS: Case report: bilateral gas gangrene of the hand—a unique case, *Ann R Coll Surg Engl* 85:408, 2003.)

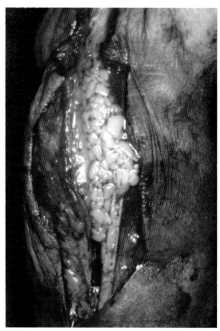

FIGURE 16.22 Tuberculous tenosynovitis presenting as compound palmar ganglion and carpal tunnel syndrome. Note multiple rice bodies. (From Al-Qattan MM, Al-Namla A, Al-Thunayan A, Al-Omawi M: Tuberculosis of the hand, *J Hand Surg Am* 36:1413, 2011.)

Patients with clostridial infections require close monitoring for hemolysis and renal failure. For severe involvement in patients with septic shock, endotracheal intubation and intensive supportive measures may be required. Proper management of wounds susceptible to clostridial infections includes prompt and thorough debridement of all open wounds, especially open fractures, followed by repeat wound debridement every 24 to 48 hours depending on the wound condition. Gram stains, obtained from drainage and from wound debridements, usually are helpful in identifying clostridial infections. All necrotic skin, subcutaneous tissue, muscle, and bone should be debrided initially. Tissue with questionable viability may be left and reinspected at the time of subsequent debridements. Amputation may be required in extreme cases. All wounds suspected to have clostridial infection and questionable tissue, including amputation stumps, should be left open until the infection is controlled.

The assistance of an infectious disease consultant may be helpful in determining appropriate antibiotic therapy. Patients with straightforward, open fractures should receive intravenous cephalosporins. Patients with large dirt-contaminated or grease-contaminated wounds should receive cephalosporin and aminoglycoside. Patients with crushing wounds or farm contamination, especially with a positive Gram stain, should receive penicillin, cephalosporin, and aminoglycoside. Although hyperbaric oxygen is a controversial treatment, several reports suggest that it may be an effective adjunct. Administered at 2 to 2.5 atm, three times daily for acute infections, hyperbaric oxygen has been found to help stabilize limb amputations secondary to clostridial infections.

MYCOBACTERIAL INFECTIONS
■ TUBERCULOSIS

The most common presentation of *Mycobacterium tuberculosis* in the hand is tenosynovitis (Fig. 16.22). Appearing as an extensive palmar "ganglion," it can cause compression of the median nerve in the carpal tunnel. Although uncommon in the hand, tuberculosis infection should be considered when unexplained tenosynovitis is encountered, and tissue cultures and specimens should be examined for *M. tuberculosis*. Rice bodies, or nodules of caseous necrosis that contain live mycobacteria, may be encountered intraoperatively. A combination of antituberculous medication and tenosynovectomy generally is recommended. *M. tuberculosis* also may manifest as osteomyelitis, septic arthritis, and dactylitis in the hand and involve the bones of the wrist. When the hand and wrist bones and joints are involved, treatment frequently includes debridement of bone and joint, and arthrodesis. In some cases of tuberculosis that are refractory to antituberculous medication and radical surgery, amputation may be required.

■ NONTUBERCULOUS MYCOBACTERIAL INFECTIONS

The nontuberculous mycobacteria that most commonly infect the hand are *M. marinum* and *M. kansasii*. Hand infections by *M. fortuitum, M. chelonei,* and other mycobacterial species rarely have been reported. *M. marinum* and *M. kansasii* may cause infections in the skin, tenosynovium, and deeper structures.

Any poorly healing ulcer on the hand should have a culture for *M. marinum* at 30°C and 37°C in Lowenstein-Jensen medium. Many nontuberculous mycobacterial species grow best at 30°C, and Mycobacterium tuberculosis grows at 37°C. Skin testing is not as reliable for this

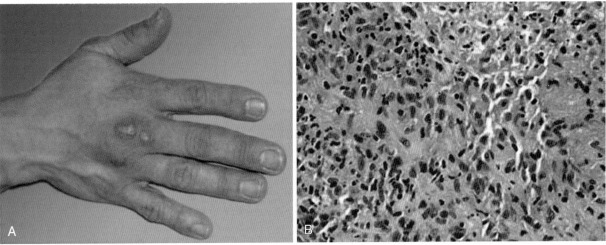

FIGURE 16.23 **A,** Three erythematous, tender, exophytic nodules on dorsum of hand caused by Mycobacterium marinum infection. **B,** Histopathology shows suppurative and granulomatous inflammation with central necrosis. (From Cassetty CT, Sanchez M: Mycobacterium marinum infection, *Dermatol Online J* 10:21, 2004.)

organism as it is for tuberculosis. In the early stages, the infection frequently is confused with gout or rheumatoid arthritis, and nearly all the reported cases have had a cortisone injection. Typically, the organism is found around swimming pools or fish tanks, from whence it derives its name, "swimming pool granuloma," and may infect an open wound or abrasion. It can attack bone, joint, synovium, or skin (Fig. 16.23).

M. kansasii may behave in a similar manner and should be considered when chronic synovitis is not obviously a complication of rheumatoid arthritis, especially if only a single digit or joint is involved. A typical case is one in which a synovectomy of the wrist has been done for compression of the median nerve, only to be followed by the recurrence of swelling and compression of the nerve several weeks later. A slowly healing sinus may also be present. When persistent or recurring synovitis of the wrist or finger is encountered, a mycobacterial infection should be suspected. In a study of 166 patients with *M. marinum* tenosynovitis of the hand, an initial wrong diagnosis resulted in a delay in the appropriate management in 60% of patients, resulting in established stiffness and flexion contractures at presentation of these patients to a hand specialist. When a part is aspirated for routine bacterial cultures, fungus cultures and cultures for tuberculosis also should be ordered. The results of the cultures may not be known for several weeks because these organisms grow slowly. MRI may show changes consistent with tenosynovitis; however, typical rice bodies may be mistaken for synovial chondromatosis.

Treatment is by synovectomy or other excisional surgery for diagnostic and therapeutic reasons. If the diagnosis has not already been established, material is sent for bacteriologic and histologic identification of the organisms. When the diagnosis has been established, the appropriate antimicrobial therapy is started. Infectious disease consultation frequently is helpful.

Mycobacterium leprae, or Hansen disease, also has manifestations in the hand. The condition affects the skin and peripheral nerves. It is most prevalent in developing countries, although the bacterium is carried by armadillos in the Southwestern United States. The diagnosis is established by clinical signs and confirmed by skin biopsy. The three cardinal signs are (1) a hypopigmented skin lesion, (2) an anesthetic skin patch, and (3) enlarged, tender peripheral nerves. Paresthesias and motor paralysis develop as nerve function declines. Patients may also present with painless wounds, sores, or burns on the extremities. Ulnar nerve dysfunction is a common manifestation. There is a spectrum of disease based on the immunocompetence of the host. Medical treatment includes dapsone and rifampin or clofazimine. Tendon transfers or contracture releases may be necessary for those with advanced nerve dysfunction, whereas nerve decompression can be considered in less severe cases.

FUNGAL INFECTIONS

Several types of manifestations of fungal infections in the extremities have been described: (1) cutaneous infections including onychomycosis caused by dermatophytes (Trichophyton/tinea, Microsporum, and Epidermophyton), (2) subcutaneous infections, and (3) deep or systemic infections. Fungal infections of the hand may mimic other conditions, such as neoplasms, and hand surgeons should be aware of the characteristic clinical features of these infections to ensure early diagnosis and treatment (Table 16.5). Diagnosis suspected by clinical findings may be confirmed by potassium hydroxide preparation, fungal culture, or such techniques as histopathology and molecular polymerase chain reaction testing. Treatment of superficial skin infection often consists of topical antifungal agents (imidazoles, Tolnaftate, ciclopirox, and butenafine). Usual causes of deep or systemic infections include sporotrichosis, cryptococcus, mucormycosis, histoplasmosis, coccidioidomycosis, blastomycosis, and aspergillosis; these infections frequently occur in immunocompromised hosts and have a poor prognosis. Table 16.6 summarizes these deep infections. In addition to the appropriate medical treatment, surgical therapy is indicated for flexor or extensor tenosynovitis, fungal arthritis, and osteomyelitis.

TABLE 16.5

Characteristic Clinical Features and Signs of Subcutaneous and Deep Fungal Infections of the Hand

TYPE OF INFECTION	CHARACTERISTIC FEATURE/SIGN
Lymphocutaneous sporotrichosis	Multiple nodules along the lymphatics (lymphatic resider)
Dematiaceous fungal infections	All are subcutaneous tissue residers
Eumycetoma	Chronic inflammatory mass of the skin and subcutaneous tissue with multiple sinuses and granular discharge
Phaeohyphomycosis	Localized multiple subcutaneous masses with dermal microabscesses
Chromoblastomycosis	Localized subcutaneous mass with wart-like epidermis
Deep candidiasis	Chronic arthritis/tenosynovitis (synovial resider)
Invasive aspergillosis	Necrotic ulcer or necrotic muscle (soft-tissue necrotizer)
Mucormycosis	Subdermal plexus invasion resulting in skin necrosis followed by invasion of major blood vessels (blood vessel resider)
Cryptococcosis	Tenosynovitis or osteomyelitis (synovial or bone resider)
Deep sporotrichosis	Variable sites (joint, bursa, bone, muscle, tenosynovium). Rice bodies are common in tenosynovial disease.
Coccidioidomycosis	Osteomyelitis of ends of long bones and bony prominences. Symmetric bilateral involvement may be seen (red marrow resider)
Histoplasmosis	Granulomatous tenosynovitis (sarcoidosis mimic)
Deep blastomycosis	Commonly presents as osteomyelitis that may mimic sarcoma (sarcoma mimic)

From Al-Qattan MM, Helmi AA: Chronic hand infections, *J Hand Surg* 39:1636, 2014.

TABLE 16.6

Epidemiology, Diagnosis, and Treatment of Systemic and Local Fungal Infections

ORGANISM	RISK FACTORS OR EPIDEMIOLOGY	DIAGNOSIS	TREATMENT
Histoplasmosis	Ohio and Mississippi River Valleys	Biopsy: Grocott silver stain, large round single-celled spores Serology: complement fixation test Culture: often negative	Surgical + medical (ketoconazole or itraconazole or IV amphotericin B)
Mucormycosis	Contaminated trauma, diabetes, immunocompromised	Clinical: enlarging black skin eschar, gangrene Biopsy: organisms scattered within areas of necrosis, 90 degrees hyphae on KOH stain Culture: positive in less than half	Early, radical surgical debridement + high-dose IV amphotericin B
Sporotrichosis	Soil, rose thorn	Biopsy: cigar-shaped (narrow-based) budding yeasts Culture: growth can be delayed up to 8 weeks	Cutaneous: itraconazole Deep: surgery + IV amphotericin B
Coccidioidomycosis	US Southwest, San Joaquin Valley	Biopsy: noncaseating granuloma, characteristic spherules, and hyphae Serology: complement fixation	Surgical + medical (Fluconazole or itraconazole or IV amphotericin B)
Blastomycosis	Ohio and Mississippi River Valleys	Biopsy: periodic acid-Schiff stain, silver stain, large broad-based buds	Medical (ketoconazole or itraconazole) ± surgical
Cryptococcus	Pigeon droppings, immunocompromised	Biopsy: encapsulated, ovoid yeasts Serology: cryptococcal antigen titer Culture: growth within 48 hours	Fluconazole or itraconazole or flucytosine or IV amphotericin
Aspergillosis	Immunocompromised (burns, wounds, IV sites)	Clinical: hemorrhagic vesicle or necrotic ulcer Biopsy: numerous fungal hyphae on KOH Culture: growth from tissue specimen (blood cultures often negative)	Early, radical surgical debridement + voriconazole

Modified from Chan E, Bagg M: Atypical hand infections, *Orthop Clin North Am* 48(2):229, 2017.

PYODERMA GANGRENOSUM

Pyoderma gangrenosum is a cutaneous ulcer that develops rapidly and can be mistaken for an infection, leading to unsuccessful surgical treatment. It is a diagnosis of exclusion. There may be associated systemic conditions, such as ulcerative colitis. Surgery should be avoided in this condition. Treatment often involves topical steroid applications or systemic immunosuppressive drugs for more severe disease, but there are no definitive guidelines defining best practice. Dermatologic consultation may help avoid inappropriate surgical treatments.

REFERENCES

Akdemir O, Lineaweaver W: Methicillin-resistant *Staphylococcus aureus* hand infections in a suburban community hospital, *Ann Plast Surg* 66:486, 2011.

Al-Qattan MM, Helmi AA: Chronic hand infections, *J Hand Surg [Am]* 39:1636, 2014.

Babovic N, Cayci C, Carlsen BT: Cat bite infections of the hand: assessment of morbidity and predictors of severe infection, *J Hand Surg [Am]* 39:286, 2014.

Bryant AE, Stevens DL: Clostridial myonecrosis: new insights in pathogenesis and management, *Curr Infect Dis Rep* 12:383, 2010.

Chan E, Bagg M: Atypical hand infections, *Orthop Clin North Am* 48(2):229, 2017.

Chauhan A, Wigton MD, Palmer BA: Necrotizing fasciitis, *J Hand Surg [Am]* 39:1598, 2014.

Cheung JP, Fung BK, Ip WY: Mycobacterium marinum infection of the deep structures of the hand and wrist: 25 years of experience, *Hand Surg* 15:211, 2010.

Cheung JP, Fung B, Wong SS, Ip WY: Review article: *Mycobacterium marinum* infection of the hand and wrist, *J Orthop Surg* 18:98, 2010.

Chong CW, Ormston VE, Tan AB: Epidemiology of hand infection—a comparative study between year 2000 and 2009, *Hand Surg* 18:307, 2013.

Choueka J, De Tolla JE: Necrotizing infections of the hand and wrist: diagnosis and treatment options, *J Am Acad Orthop Surg* 28(2):e55, 2020.

Chung SR, Foo TL: Modifications to simplify intrathecal irrigation for pyogenic flexor tenosynovitis, *Hand (N Y)* 9:258, 2014.

Crosswell S, Vanat Q, Jose R: The anatomy of deep hand space infections: the deep thenar space, *J Hand Surg [Am]* 39:2550, 2014.

Draeger RW, Bynum Jr DK: Flexor tendon sheath infections of the hand, *J Am Acad Orthop Surg* 20:373, 2012.

Eberlin KR: Ring D: infection after hand surgery, *Hand Clin* 31:355, 2015.

Fowler JR, Ilyas AM: Epidemiology of adult acute hand infections at an urban medical center, *J Hand Surg [Am]* 38:1189, 2013.

Franko OI, Abrams RA: Hand infections, *Orthop Clin North Am* 44:625, 2013.

Giuffre JL, Jacobson NA, Rizzo M, et al.: Pyarthrosis of the small joints of the hand resulting in arthrodesis and amputation, *J Hand Surg* 36A:1273, 2011.

Harrison B, Ben-Amotz O, Sammer DM: Methicillin-resistant S*taphylococcus aureus* infection in the hand, *Plast Reconstr Surg* 135:826, 2015.

Henry M: Septic flexor tenosynovitis, *J Hand Surg* 36A:332, 2011.

Imahara SD, Friedrich JB: Community-acquired methicillin-resistant S*taphylococcus aureus* in surgically treated hand infections, *J Hand Surg* 35A:97, 2010.

Jagodzinski NA, Ibish S, Furniss D: Surgical site infection after hand surgery outside the operating theatre: a systematic review, *J Hand Surg Eur* 42(3):289, 2017.

Janis JE, Hatef DA, Reece EM, et al.: Does empiric antibiotic therapy change MRSA hand infection outcomes? Cost analysis of an randomized prospective trial in a county hospital, *Plast Reconstr Surg* 133:511e, 2014.

Jing SS, Iyer S: Simplifying irrigation in flexor tenosynovitis, *J Hand Surg Eur* 40:321, 2015.

Jing SS, Teare L, Iwuagwu F: *Mycobacterium kansasii* flexor tenosynovitis of the finger, *Hand Surg* 19:249, 2014.

Kennedy SA, Stoll LE, Lauder AS: Human and other mammalian bite injuries of the hand: evaluation and management, *J Am Acad Orthop Surg* 23:47, 2015.

Kistler JM, Thoder JJ, Ilyas AM: MRSA incidence and antibiotic trends in urban hand infections: a 10-year longitudinal study, *Hand (NY)* 14(4):449, 2019.

Kowalski TJ, Thompson LW, Gundrum JD: Antimicrobial management of septic arthritis of the hand and wrist, *Infection* 42:379, 2014.

Kwo S, Agarwal JP, Meletiou S: Current treatment of cat bites to the hand and wrist, *J Hand Surg* 36A:152, 2011.

Leggit JC: Acute and chronic paronychia, *Am Fam Physician* 96(1):44, 2017.

Li K, Sambare TD, Jiang SY, et al.: Effectiveness of preoperative antibiotics in preventing surgical site infection after common soft tissue procedures of the hand, *Clin Orthop Relat Res* 476:664, 2018.

Manoli T, Rahmamian-Schwarz A, Konheiser K, et al.: The role of antibiotics after surgical treatment of simple hand infections: a prospective pilot study, *J Invest Surg* 26:229, 2013.

McDonald LS, Bavaro MF, Hofmeister EP, et al.: Hand infections, *J Hand Surg* 36A:1403, 2011.

Menendez ME, Lu N, Unizony S, et al.: Surgical site infection in hand surgery, *Int Orthop*, 2015, [Epub ahead of print].

Nourbakhsh A, Papafragkou S, Dever LL, et al.: Stratification of the risk factors of community-acquired methicillin-resistant *Staphylococcus aureus* hand infection, *J Hand Surg* 35A:1135, 2010.

Osterman M, Dreager R, Stern P: Acute hand infections, *J Hand Surg* 39:1628, 2014.

Pabari A, Iyer S, Khoo CT: Swiss roll technique for treatment of paronychia, *Tech Hand Up Extrem Surg* 15:75, 2011.

Patel DM, Emmanuel NB, Stevanovic MV, et al.: Hand infections: anatomy, types and spread of infection, imaging findings, and treatment options, *Radiographics* 34:1968, 2014.

Pierrart J, Delgrande D, Mamane W, Tordjman D, Masmejean EH: Acute felon and paronychia: antibiotics not necessary after surgical treatment. Prospective study of 46 patients, *Hand Surg Rehabil* 35(1):40, 2016.

Pinder R, Barlow G: Osteomyelitis of the hand, *J Hand Surg Eur* 41(4):431, 2016.

Rigopoulos N, Dailiana ZH, Varmitimidis S, et al.: Closed-space hand infections: diagnostic and treatment considerations, *Orthop Rev* 4:e19, 2012.

Roodsari GS, Zahedi F, Zehtabchi S: The risk of wound infection after simple hand laceration, *World J Emerg Med* 6:44, 2015.

Rubright JH, Shafritz AB: The herpetic whitlow, *J Hand Surg* 36A:340, 2011.

Ryssel H, Germann G, Kloeters O, et al.: Necrotizing fasciitis of the extremities: 34 cases at a single centre over the past 5 years, *Arch Orthop Trauma Surg* 130:1515, 2010.

Sammer DM, Shin AY: Comparison of arthroscopic and open treatment of septic arthritis of the wrist. Surgical technique, *J Bone Joint Surg Am* 92((Suppl 1) Pt 1):107, 2010.

Shafritz AB, Coppage JM: Acute and chronic paronychia of the hand, *J Am Acad Orthop Surg* 22:165, 2014.

Sharma KS, Rao K, Hobson MI: Space of Parona infections: experience in management and outcomes in a regional hand centre, *J Plast Reconstr Aesthet Surg* 66:968, 2013.

Strub B, Von Campe A, Meuli-Simmen C: The value of different inflammatory markers in distinguishing deep closed hand infections from noninfective causes, *J Hand Surg Eur* 40:207, 2015.

Tannan SC, Deal DN: Diagnosis and management of the acute felon: evidence-based review, *J Hand Surg [Am]* 37:2603, 2012.

Tosti R, Ilyas AM: Empiric antibiotics for acute infections of the hand, *J Hand Surg* 35A:125, 2010.

Tosti R, Iorio J, Fowler JR, et al.: Povidone-iodine soaks for hand abscesses: a prospective randomized trial, *J Hand Surg [Am]* 39:962, 2014.

Tosti R, Samuelsen BT, Bender S, et al.: Emerging multidrug resistance of methicillin-resistant *Staphylococcus aureus* in hand infections, *J Bone Joint Surg Am* 96:1535, 2014.

Tosti R, Trionfo A, Gaughan J, et al.: Risk factors associated with clindamycin-resistant, methicillin-resistant *Staphylococcus aureus* in hand abscesses, *J Hand Surg [Am]* 40:673, 2015.

Wegener EE, Johnson WR: Identification of common nail and skin disorders, *J Hand Ther* 23:187, 2010.

The complete list of references is available online at ExpertConsult.com.

CHAPTER 17

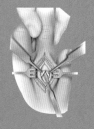

CONGENITAL ANOMALIES OF THE HAND

Benjamin M. Mauck

PRINCIPLES OF MANAGEMENT

The difficulties in treating congenital anomalies of the hand have long been recognized. Milford observed, "a single surgical procedure cannot be standardized to suit even similar anomalies."

Treatment of a congenital hand deformity may be sought at birth or later in the child's development. Involvement may be unilateral or bilateral; the anomaly may be an isolated condition, or it may be a single manifestation of a malformation syndrome or skeletal dysplasia. Early evaluation by a hand surgeon usually is desirable, not because of urgency to begin treatment but to help parents with their concerns. Parents usually have considerable anxiety concerning the appearance of the hand, the future function of the hand, and the possibility of subsequent siblings being similarly affected; they also may feel a sense of guilt. To inform the parents adequately and to dispel as much anxiety as possible, it is helpful for the surgeon to be familiar with the modes of inheritance and the preferred treatment and prognosis of each condition. Although specific considerations and indications for surgical and nonsurgical treatment are discussed for each individual condition, the amazing ability of children to compensate functionally for deformity should be remembered.

INCIDENCE AND CLASSIFICATION

Congenital malformations of the hand encompass myriad deformities, all of which carry different functional and cosmetic implications for the patient and parents. Congenital malformations occur with relative infrequency and have remained unchanged in recent epidemiologic studies. Incidences of 5.25 to 19 per 10,000 live births have been reported. Up to two thirds of patients with congenital hand defects have additional birth defects. The 1-year mortality of live infants with congenital upper limb anomalies has been reported as 14% to 16%. Therefore, early recognition of associated syndromes and appropriate workup is of substantial importance. The most commonly encountered anomalies of the hand are syndactyly, polydactyly, congenital amputations, camptodactyly, clinodactyly, and radial clubhand (Tables 17.1 and 17.2). Approximately 10% of patients with congenital anomalies of the upper extremity have significant cosmetic or functional deficits.

The Oberg-Manske-Tonkin (OMT) classification system proposed in 2010 by Oberg et al. sought to provide an updated classification system. This system incorporates the current molecular knowledge of embryological development and basis for pathogenetic etiology. The OMT classification separates congenital deformities into three groups: malformations, deformations, and dysplasias. Malformations are further subdivided according to the

TABLE 17.1

Distribution of Primary Diagnoses in Descending Order of Incidence

TYPE OF ANOMALY	NO. CASES	%
Syndactyly	443	17.5
Polydactyly—all	361	14.3
Polydactyly, radial	162	6.4
Polydactyly, ulnar	130	5.2
Polydactyly, central	69	2.7
Amputation—all	179	7.1
Amputation, hand/digits	77	3.0
Amputation, arm/forearm	75	3.0
Amputation, wrist	27	1.1
Camptodactyly	173	6.9
Clinodactyly	142	5.6
Brachydactyly	131	5.2
Radial clubhand	119	4.7
Central defects	99	3.9
Thumb, hypoplastic	90	3.6
Acrosyndactyly	83	3.3
Trigger digit	59	2.3
Poland syndrome	56	2.2
Apert syndrome	52	2.1
Constriction bands	51	2.0
Musculotendinous defects	49	1.9
Madelung deformity	43	1.7
Thumb, absent	34	1.4
Ulnar finger/metacarpal absent	31	1.2
Ulnar hypoplasia	31	1.2
Synostosis, radioulnar	29	1.2
Ulnar clubhand	25	1.0
Thumb, triphalangeal	21	0.8
Hypoplasia, whole hand	21	0.8
Macrodactyly	21	0.8
Phocomelia	19	0.8
Thumb, adducted	18	0.7
Radial hypoplasia	17	0.7
Symphalangism	13	0.5
Other	115	4.6
Total	2525	100

From Flatt A: *The care of congenital hand anomalies,* St. Louis, 1977, Mosby.

TABLE 17.2

Diagnoses in Yokohama Patients

TYPE OF ANOMALY	NO. CASES	%
Syndactyly	23	10.1
Polydactyly	65	28.6
Brachydactyly	19	8.4
Brachysyndactyly	10	4.4
Symphalangism	1	0.5
Annular grooves	3	1.3
Ectrodactyly	—	—
Cleft hand	12	5.3
Ectrosyndactyly	17	7.5
Amputation	16	7.0
Microdactyly	5	2.2
Floating thumb	5	2.2
Hypoplasia of the thumb	3	1.3
Five finger	2	0.9
Monodactyly	1	0.5
Floating small finger	1	0.5
Defect of fifth metacarpus	1	0.5
Macrodactyly	3	1.3
Clinodactyly	3	1.3
Clubhand	14	6.1
Phocomelia	2	0.9
Other	21	9.3

Modified from Yamaguchi S, et al: Incidence of various congenital anomalies of the hand from 1961 to 1972. In *Proceedings of the Sixteenth Annual Meeting of the Japanese Society for Surgery of the Hand,* Fukuoka, 1973.

EMBRYOLOGY

The arm arises as a small bud of tissue on the lateral body wall beginning on day 26 of gestation, preceding leg bud formation by only 24 hours. Normal limb bud growth and development occur by a complicated and coordinated collaboration between three distinct signaling centers. Each signaling center is responsible for its own axis of growth but can also interact with the remaining centers to influence genetic expression. This coordinated effort produces a proportionate functional limb. The apical ectodermal ridge (AER) is the primary signaling center of proximal to distal growth. Its location is seated at the very tip, or apex, of the limb bud. A family of fibroblast growth factors (FGFs), most commonly FGF8, mediates AER activity and can influence core-polarizing activity. FGFs also have been shown to influence interdigital necrosis. The zone of polarizing activity (ZPA) located at the ulnarmost portion of the limb bud controls development primarily in the anteroposterior or radioulnar axis (Fig. 17.1). The ZPA produces a family of proteins called "sonic hedgehog (SHH)." Signaling by the ZPA can be divided further into distinct zones that influence specific portions of radial and ulnar limb development. Zone I, the ulnar portion of the limb bud, contains primarily SHH expressing cells and is responsible for development of the small finger, ring finger, and ulnar half of the middle finger. Zone II is responsible for development of the radial half of the middle finger and index finger and is

axis of formation and differentiation and distinguished between anomalies involving the entire limb and the hand. The OMT classification system was adopted by the International Federation of Societies for Surgery of the Hand (IFSSH) in 2014 as the new universal classification system for congenital anomalies. This classification system has demonstrated excellent intraobserver and interobserver reliability among pediatric hand surgeons (Box 17.1).

BOX 17.1

Oberg-Manske-Tonkin Classification of Congenital Differences in the Upper Extremity

I. Malformations
  A. Abnormal axis formation/differentiation-entire upper limb
    1. Proximal-distal axis
      i. Brachymelia with brachydactyly
      ii. Symbrachydactyly
      iii. Transverse deficiency
      iv. Intersegmental deficiency
      v. Whole limb duplication/triplication
    2. Anteroposterior axis
      i. Radial longitudinal deficiency
      ii. Ulnar longitudinal deficiency
      iii. Ulnar dimelia
      iv. Radioulnar synostosis
      v. Congenital dislocation of radial head
      vi. Humeroradial synostosis
      vii. Madelung deformity
  B. Abnormal axis formation/differentiating-hand plate
    1. Proximal-distal axis
      i. Brachydactyly
      ii. Symbrachydactyly
      iii. Transverse deficiency
    2. Anteroposterior axis
      i. Radial (thumb) deficiency
      ii. Ulnar deficiency
      iii. Radial polydactyly
      iv. Triphalangeal thumb
      v. Ulnar dimelia
      vi. Ulnar polydactyly
    3. Dorsal ventral
      i. Dorsal dimelia (palmar nail)
      ii. Hypoplastic/aplastic nail
    4. Unspecified
      i. Soft tissue
        (a) Syndactyly
        (b) Camptodactyly
        (c) Thumb in palm deformity
        (d) Distal arthrogryposis
      ii. Skeletal deficiency
        (a) Clinodactyly
        (b) Kirner deformity
        (c) Metacarpal synostosis
        (d) Carpal synostosis
        (e) Phalangeal synostosis (symphalangism)
      iii. Complex
        (a) Synpolydactyly
        (b) Cleft hand
        (c) Apert hand
II. Deformation
  A. Constriction ring syndrome
  B. Trigger fingers
  C. Not otherwise specified
III. Dysplasias
  A. Hypertrophy
    1. Hypertrophy
      i. Hemihypertrophy
      ii. Aberrant flexor/extensor/intrinsic muscle
    2. Partial limb
      i. Macrodactyly
      ii. Aberrant intrinsic muscles of hand
  B. Tumorous conditions
    1. Vascular
      i. Hemangioma
      ii. Malformation
      iii. Others
    2. Neurological
      i. Neurofibromatosis
      ii. Other
    3. Connective tissue
      i. Juvenile aponeurotic fibroma
      ii. Infantile digital fibroma
      iii. Other
    4. Skeletal
      i. Osteochondromatosis
      ii. Enchondromatosis
      iii. Fibrous dysplasia
      iv. Epiphyseal abnormalities
      v. Other
IV. Syndromes

From Bae DS, Canizares MF, Miller PE, et al: Intraobserver and interobserver reliability of the Oberg-Manske-Tonkin (OMT) classification: establishing a registry on congenital upper limb differences, *J Pediatr Orthop* 38(1):69, 2018.

influenced by long-range diffusion of SHH proteins. Zone III develops only in the absence of SHH proteins and is under the influence of other signaling factors (SALI4, HOXA13, and FGF8). This zone is responsible for the development of the radial column of the carpus, radius, and thumb. The WNT signaling pathway controls the development of the dorsoventral axis. Specifically, the primary signaling protein WNT 7a guides dorsalization. Restricted to the dorsum of the limb bud by FN-1, WNT 7a influences the expression of the HOX gene *LMX1*, which is responsible for dorsal hand development (i.e., dorsal hairy skin, nails, and extensor tendons).

LMX1 also is important in the maintenance of SHH expression. EN1 is expressed in the palmar ectoderm and is essential to the growth of palmar structures, such as glabrous skin and flexor tendons. By day 31 of gestation, the hand paddle is present. Through a process of programmed cellular death, fissuring of the hand paddle is completed by day 36, with central rays forming first, followed by preaxial and postaxial digits. Formation of the chondral elements; endochondral ossification; and joint, muscle, and vascular development follow, with the entire process completed by 8 weeks of gestation (Table 17.3).

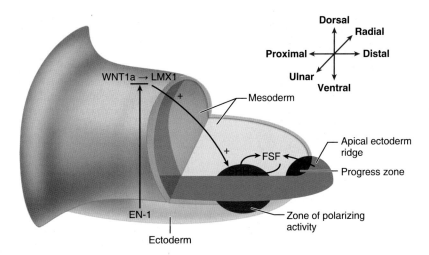

FIGURE 17.1 Limb bud. Apical ectodermal ridge extends from anterior to posterior along dorsal/ventral boundary of growing limb bud. Proximal to apical ectodermal ridge is progress zone (an area of proliferating mesodermal cells). Within posterior mesoderm is zone of polarizing activity, which is important signaling center. These centers are interconnected, so limb patterning and growth partly depend on coordinated function.

TABLE 17.3

Important Steps of Upper Limb Development in the Human Embryo

EMBRYO STAGE	INTRAUTERINE AGE (D)	EVENTS
9	21-22	Notochord expressing SHH
12	26	Limb bud appears
14	31	Limb bud curves, marginal vessel appears
15	33	Hand "paddle" appears; subclavian-axillary-brachial axial arteries appear
16	36	Nerve trunks enter the arm; chondrification of the humerus, radius, and ulna; shoulder joint interzone is apparent
17	41	Digital rays evident within the hand paddle; chondrification of the metacarpals; ulnar artery appears
18	44	Splitting of pectoral muscle mass into a clavicular head and a costal head; chondrification of the proximal phalanges; radial artery appears
19	47	Splitting of the costal head of the pectoral mass into the pectoralis minor and the sternocostal head of the pectoralis major; chondrification of the middle phalanges; initial separation of the fingers; joint interzones are apparent in the hand
20	50	Chondrification of the proximal parts of the distal phalanges; further separation of the fingers
22	54	Ossification of the humerus; fingers are completely separated
23	56	Nutrient vessel penetrates the humerus; the tips of the distal phalanges ossify (intramembranous ossification)

SHH, Sonic hedgehog.

From Al-Qattan M, Kozin SH: Update on embryology of the upper limb, *J Hand Surg* 38A:1835, 2013.

MALFORMATIONS UPPER EXTREMITY
PROXIMAL-DISTAL AXIS
■ TRANSVERSE DEFICIENCIES

Transverse deficiencies include deformities in which there is complete absence of parts distal to some point on the upper extremity, producing amputation-like stumps that allow further classification by naming the level at which the remaining stump terminates. Wynne-Davies and Lamb reported the incidence of transverse deficiencies to be 6.8 per 10,000. Most transverse deficiencies (98%) are unilateral, and the most common level is the upper third of the forearm. There is no particular sex predilection. The cause generally has been believed to be a failure of the AER possibly secondary to infarct. The use of misoprostol to induce abortion has been shown to cause vascular disruption in utero and transverse deficiencies in infants. In the usual unilateral transverse deficiency, there

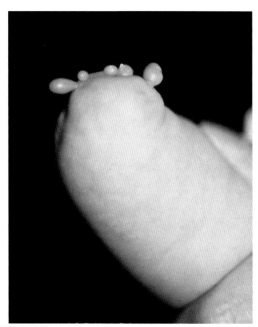

FIGURE 17.2   Transverse deficiency (digital nubbins). Wrist motion allows use as assisting hand.

is no genetic basis, although rare bilateral or multiple transverse deficiencies may be inherited as an autosomal recessive trait. Transverse deficiencies usually do not occur in association with malformation syndromes, but anomalies reported to occur in association with transverse deficiencies include hydrocephalus, spina bifida, myelomeningocele, clubfoot, radial head dislocation, and radioulnar synostosis.

A newborn with a transverse deficiency usually has a slightly bulbous, well-padded stump. In the more distal deficiencies, rudimentary vestigial digital "nubbins" are common (Fig. 17.2). Hypoplasia of the more proximal muscles helps differentiate these deficiencies from deficiencies associated with congenital bands. In the more common upper forearm amputation, the forearm usually is no more than 7 cm long at birth and can be expected to measure no more than 10 cm by skeletal maturity. In midcarpal amputations, the second most frequent level of deficiency, the rudimentary digital remnants usually are nonfunctional. Although the affected forearm may be relatively shorter than the normal side, pronation and supination usually are possible.

PROSTHETIC MANAGEMENT

For patients who do not require surgery, treatment usually consists of early prosthetic fitting of the deficient limb, preferably by the time the child is crawling and certainly by the time of independent ambulation. The child's development of manual and bimanual skills progresses in an orderly and predictable pattern. Until the age of 9 months, prehension is achieved primarily by bilateral palmar grasp. Single-hand grasp develops next, and by age 12 to 18 months, thumb-to-finger pinch is possible. The ability to grasp an object is believed to precede the ability to release. By age 24 months, the child should have developed coordinated shoulder positioning, grasp, and release. The fitting of the upper limb prosthesis should complement and enhance these developmental milestones and improve the chances of myoelectric prosthetic use in the future. The choice of prosthetic design is based on the level of amputation and the age and function of the child.

For the rare case of a child with complete arm amputation, especially if the amputation is bilateral, conventional body-powered prostheses that include an elbow are unlikely to be of functional benefit. For most children with congenital above-elbow amputations, a rigid elbow is used initially. When the passive mitten initially used as a terminal device is exchanged for an actively opened split hook, usually at age 18 months, the rigid elbow is replaced by a friction elbow. At about 3 years of age, dual-terminal devices and elbow controls may be tried. For bilateral above-elbow amputations, only the preferred or dominant side is fitted with a dual-control, articulated prosthesis. For a child with an amputation at the upper third of the forearm, a passive plastic mitten prosthesis is introduced between the ages of 3 and 6 months or when the child has achieved sitting balance (sit to fit). This is followed by the addition of an actively opened, plastisol-covered, split hook at 12 to 18 months of age. A Child Amputee Prosthetic Program (CAPP) terminal device may be substituted if preferred. Training with a functional device begins at 18 months of age. The CAPP device can be used until the child is about 6 years old. The prosthesis also is beneficial in providing stability during sitting and may assist the child in pulling to a standing position. Although standard prosthetic fitting usually is satisfactory, a myoelectrical prosthesis (Fig. 17.3) has been shown to be useful and appropriate for preschool children and may be considered between the ages of 2 and 4 years.

Prosthetic treatment for a child with a midcarpal amputation is more controversial. Although the carpal bones cannot be seen radiographically until about age 6 to 8 months, their presence improves the prognosis because minimal shortening of the forearm can be expected. Delay in carpal bone maturation rarely is encountered. The long, below-elbow stump is so useful for stabilizing objects and assisting in bimanual functions for which sensibility is required that the benefits of a prosthesis are debatable. Options include an open-ended volar plate secured to the forearm that permits simple grip between stump and plate, an open-ended volar plate with a terminal hook, and an artificial hand driven by the radiocarpal motion. Terminal sensibility is sacrificed with the last option, but a good cosmetic effect is achieved. Regardless of the prosthesis chosen, therapist-supervised training sessions are essential. These sessions should be scheduled at regular intervals, particularly when a new prosthesis is introduced, and coordinated follow-up should be maintained among the patient, family members, therapist, orthotist, and physician. Most children do well with prostheses, although it is common for adolescents, particularly boys, to reject the prosthesis for a time before resuming its use.

SURGICAL TREATMENT

There are few indications for surgical intervention in children with transverse deficiencies of the upper extremity. Amputation of nonfunctional digital remnants often is performed for psychologic and cosmetic benefits. Complete amputation of all digits often gives the hand the bizarre appearance of a little paw with small nubbins attached. As stated by Littler and emphasized by Flatt, it often is wise to alter the "stigma of congenitalism" and make the deformity appear acquired. Simple elliptical excision is appropriate.

METACARPAL LENGTHENING

Metacarpal lengthening usually is reserved for transverse deficiencies at the level of the metacarpophalangeal joints in a child with at least one remaining digit. Matev first described in 1967 osteotomy of a digital ray with gradual distraction and subsequent bone grafting for a deficient thumb, and a few reports have advocated this procedure for congenital absence of fingers. The procedure requires judgment and experience and should be performed by surgeons knowledgeable in the special needs and expectations of these patients and in the techniques and realistic results of the procedure. Metacarpal lengthening is best performed in patients between ages 5 and 11 years. An average of 4 to 5 cm of length can be gained, but improved function and cosmesis may not be achieved. Complications include pin track infection, neurovascular compromise, and distal ulcerations. Ilizarov et al. reported gains in length and improved function with his distraction/fixation apparatus.

TECHNIQUE 17.1

(KESSLER ET AL.)
- Under tourniquet control, make longitudinal dorsal incisions over or between the metacarpals to be lengthened.
- Perform an osteotomy of the appropriate metacarpals and insert two wires transversely through the skin and metacarpals, proximal and distal to the osteotomy.
- Close the incisions in a routine manner and apply the distraction apparatus.

POSTOPERATIVE CARE The hand is elevated continuously for 48 hours. Distraction is done at a rate of 1 mm/day and should be painless. Distraction is terminated at any sign of vascular or neurologic impairment. Bone grafting is performed after maximal safe lengthening has been accomplished.

■ INTERSEGMENTAL DEFICIENCY

Intersegmental deficiency includes failure-of-formation not considered as a transverse deficiency. Phocomelia is in this category.

■ PHOCOMELIA

The term *phocomelia* is derived from the Greek words for "seal limb" or "flipper." The term is used to describe a condition in which the hand is suspended from the body near the shoulder; the hand usually is deformed and contains only three or four digits. No definite inheritance pattern has been established; the anomaly was extremely rare (0.8% of congenital hand malformations) until the appearance of thalidomide-related deformities in the 1950s. Sixty percent of infants born to mothers taking thalidomide between days 38 and 54 after conception had this deformity.

Frantz and O'Rahilly described three anatomic types of phocomelia: (1) complete phocomelia with absence of all limb bones proximal to the hand, (2) absence or extreme hypoplasia of proximal limb bones with forearm and hand attached to the trunk, and (3) hand attached directly to the humerus (Fig. 17.4). Associated deformities include radial ray deficiencies in thalidomide-related phocomelia and cleft lip and cleft palate (Robert syndrome). Scoliosis and cardiac, skin, chromosomal, and calcification aberrations also have been reported.

Although children with phocomelia show slight differences in the overall length and appearance of the limb and different degrees of humeral, forearm, and hand deficiencies, the clavicle and scapula always are present. The scapula often is deficient laterally, and active abduction of the extremity is difficult; it is usually achieved by a sudden, jerking type of motion. The abducted position usually can be maintained only by the patient gripping his or her ear. There is no true elbow joint. The hand usually has only three or four digits, and the thumb usually is absent. Active and passive motion at the metacarpophalangeal and proximal interphalangeal joints varies considerably. Marked difficulty in moving the hand to the midline progresses as the patient grows and the chest

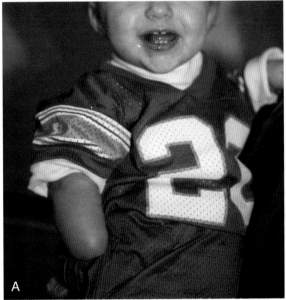
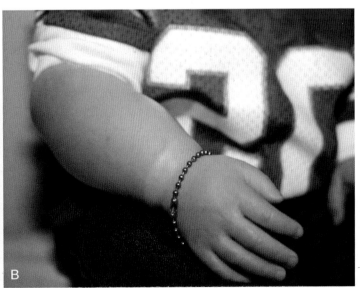

FIGURE 17.3 A and B, Early fitting of passive prosthesis in child with congenital forearm amputation may encourage the use of prosthesis.

widens. By maturity, the patient usually is unable to reach the mouth, face, and genitalia and is unable to clasp the hands together, resulting in considerable functional and psychologic impairment.

TREATMENT

Treatment of these patients generally is conservative. Various ingenious devices have been developed to assist in hygiene, feeding, and dressing, and these play a major role in the child's achieving independence. Conventional prostheses designed to increase length usually are rejected. Surgery plays a minor role in treatment of phocomelia and generally is indicated only for shoulder instability, limb shortening, or inadequate thumb opposition. Rotational osteotomy of one of the digits with web space deepening may improve thumb opposition, but the specific technique for phocomelia has not been well described or tested.

ANTEROPOSTERIOR AXIS
■ RADIAL LONGITUDINAL DEFICIENCY

Radial ray deficiencies include all malformations with longitudinal failure of formation of parts along the preaxial or radial border of the upper extremity: deficient or absent thenar muscles; a shortened, unstable, or absent thumb; and a shortened or absent radius, commonly referred to as radial

clubhand. These conditions may occur as isolated deficiencies, but more commonly they occur to some degree in association with each other. Radial clubhand occurs in an estimated 1 per 50,000 live births. Bilateral deformities occur in approximately 50% of patients; when the deformity is unilateral, the right side is more commonly affected. Both sexes are equally affected. Complete radial absence is more common than partial absence.

In most cases of radial clubhand the cause is unknown and the deformities are believed to occur sporadically outside of the cases caused by thalidomide use, although genetic and environmental factors have been suggested. According to the OMT classification, radial longitudinal deficiency is a malformation caused by disrupted development along the radioulnar axis. Radial longitudinal deficiency commonly occurs in conjunction with other congenital abnormalities. One third is associated with a named syndrome and two thirds have an associated medical or musculoskeletal anomaly. The more severe the radial longitudinal deficiency the greater the association. Some recent studies have suggested an association with the same developmental error or insult as preaxial polydactyly (Table 17.4).

The currently accepted and most useful classification of the congenital radial dysplasias is a modification of that proposed by Heikel, in which four types are described

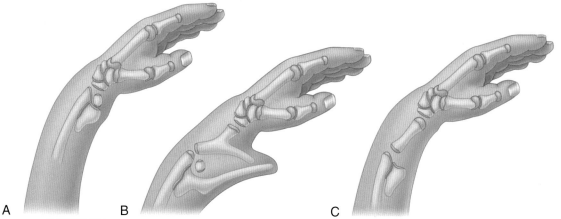

FIGURE 17.4   Three types of phocomelia described by Frantz and O'Rahilly. **A,** Hand attached to shoulder with no intermediate humeral or forearm segment. **B,** Hand attached to shoulder with abnormal humeral, radial, and ulnar segment intervening. **C,** Hand attached to shoulder with intervening humeral segment without forearm segment.

TABLE 17.4

Common Syndromes Associated With Radial Longitudinal Deficiency

ASSOCIATED SYNDROMES	INHERITANCE PATTERN	SYSTEMIC COMORBIDITIES	RECOMMENDED TESTS
Holt-Oram	AD	Congenital heart abnormalities	CBC
Fanconi anemia	AR	Blood dyscrasias	Abdominal ultrasound
Thrombocytopenia absent radius	AR	Renal dysfunction	Scoliosis XR*
VACTERL association	Sporadic	Gastrointestinal dysfunction	Chromosomal breakage test

AD, Autosomal dominant; *AR*, autosomal recessive; *CBC*, complete blood count; *VACTERL*, vertebral defects, anal atresia, cardiac defects, tracheoesophageal fistula, renal anomalies, and limb abnormalities.
*To be performed at an older age.
From Wall LB, Ezaki M, Oishi SN: Management of congenital radial longitudinal deficiency: controversies and current concepts, *Plast Reconstr Surg* 132:122, 2013.

Variable degrees of thumb deficiencies are frequent with all patterns. Manske and Halikis devised a classification system, which has since been modified, that incorporates thumb and carpal deficiencies (Table 17.5). Associated cardiac, hematopoietic, gastrointestinal, and renal abnormalities occur in approximately 25% to 44% of patients with radial clubhand and may pose significant morbidity and mortality risks. The most frequently associated syndromes are Holt-Oram syndrome, Fanconi anemia, thrombocytopenia-absent radius (TAR) syndrome, and the VACTERL syndrome (vertebral defects, anal atresia, cardiac malformation, tracheo esophageal fistula, esophageal atresia, renal abnormalities, and limb anomalies). In Holt-Oram syndrome, the cardiac abnormality (most commonly an atrial septal defect) requires surgical correction before any upper limb reconstruction. The extremity in Holt-Olram syndrome also may have an atypical presentation component to the classic radial longitudinal deficiency. Radioulnar synostosis often is present with syndactyly of the radial two digits. Presence of this combination should prompt workup for Holt-Olram syndrome. Fanconi anemia, which presents at 2 to 3 years after birth, is characterized by pancytopenia of early childhood and has a very poor prognosis. Historically, this condition has been fatal. However, early detection by chromosomal challenge tests and bone marrow transplants have contributed to a longer life expectancy. In TAR syndrome, the thrombocytopenia usually resolves by age 4 to 5 years, and although it may delay reconstruction, it is not a contraindication to surgical treatment. The radii are typically absent bilaterally, but the thumbs are always present, although lacking in extension. Oishi et al. reported the consistent presence of a brachiocarpalis muscle in TAR infants that arises from the humerus and inserts onto the radial carpus, contributing significantly to the deformity of both the wrist and elbow. In a series of 164 patients with radial longitudinal deficiency, 25 were found to have TAR syndrome, 22 VACTERL syndrome, seven Holt-Oram syndrome, and one Fanconi anemia. Radial deficiency also is associated with trisomy 13 and trisomy 18; these children have multiple congenital defects and mental deficiency that may make reconstruction inappropriate despite significant deformity.

The anatomic abnormalities of congenital absence of the radius have been extensively reviewed. The scapula, clavicle, and humerus often are reduced in size, and the ulna is characteristically short, thick, and curved, with an occasional synostosis with any radial remnant. Total absence of the radius is most frequent, but in partial deficiencies the proximal end of the radius is present most often. The scaphoid and trapezium are absent in more than half of these patients; the lunate, trapezoid, and pisiform are deficient in 10%; and the thumb, including the metacarpal and its phalanges, is absent in more than 80%, although a rudimentary thumb is common. The capitate, hamate, triquetrum, and ulnar four metacarpals and phalanges are the only bones of the upper extremity that are present and free from deficiencies in nearly all patients. The muscular anatomy always is deficient, although the deficiencies vary. Muscles that frequently are normal are the triceps, extensor carpi ulnaris, extensor digiti quinti proprius, lumbricals, interossei (except for the first dorsal interosseous), and hypothenar muscles. The long head of the biceps almost always is absent, and the short head is hypoplastic. The brachialis often is deficient or absent as well. The brachioradialis

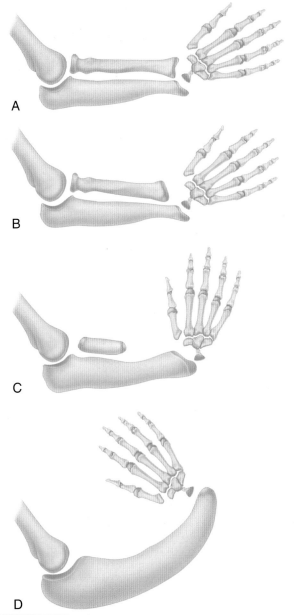

FIGURE 17.5 Heikel's classification of radial dysplasia. **A,** Type I: short distal radius. **B,** Type II: hypoplastic radius. **C,** Type III: partial absence of radius. **D,** Type IV: total absence of radius.

(Fig. 17.5). In type I (short distal radius), the distal radial physis is present but is delayed in appearance, the proximal radial physis is normal, the radius is only slightly shortened, and the ulna is not bowed. In type II (hypoplastic radius), distal and proximal radial physes are present but are delayed in appearance, which results in moderate shortening of the radius and thickening and bowing of the ulna. Type III deformity (partial absence of the radius) may be proximal, middle, or distal, with absence of the distal third being most common; the carpus usually is radially deviated and unsupported, and the ulna is thickened and bowed. The type IV pattern (total absence of the radius) is the most common, with radial deviation of the carpus, palmar and proximal subluxation, frequent pseudoarticulation with the radial border of the distal ulna, and a shortened and bowed ulna.

TABLE 17.5

Modified Classification of Radial Longitudinal Deficiency

TYPE	THUMB	CARPUS	DISTAL RADIUS	PROXIMAL RADIUS	HUMERUS	RELATIVE INCIDENCE (*N* = 245)*
N	Hypoplastic or absent	Normal	Normal	Normal	Normal	16.3%
0	Hypoplastic or absent	Absence, hypoplasia, or coalition	Normal	Normal, radio-ulnar synostosis, congenital radial head dislocation	Normal	
1	Hypoplastic or absent	Absence, hypoplasia, or coalition	>2 mm shorter than ulna	Normal, radio-ulnar synostosis, congenital radial head dislocation	Normal	12.2%
2	Hypoplastic or absent	Absence, hypoplasia or coalition	Hypoplasia	Hypoplasia	Normal	6.9%
3	Hypoplastic or absent	Absence, hypoplasia or coalition	Physis absent	Variable hypoplasia	Normal	7.3%
4	Hypoplastic or absent	Absence, hypoplasia, or coalition	Absent	Absent	Normal	52.2%
5	Hypoplastic or absent	Absence, hypoplasia, or coalition	Absent	Absent	Proximal upper extremity hypoplasia including abnormal glenoid and proximal humerus Distal humerus articulates with ulna	4.9%

*From Tonkin et al: Classification of congenital anomalies of the hand and upper limb: development and assessment of a new system, *J Hand Surg Am* 38(9):1845, 2013.

From Colen DL, et al: Radial longitudinal deficiency: recent developments, controversies, and an evidence-based guide to treatment, *J Hand Surg Am* 42(7):546, 2017.

is absent in nearly 50% of patients. The extensors carpi radialis longus and brevis frequently are absent or may be fused with the extensor digitorum communis. The pronator teres often is absent or rudimentary, inserting into the intermuscular septum, and the palmaris longus often is defective. The flexor digitorum superficialis usually is present and is abnormal more frequently than is the flexor digitorum profundus. The pronator quadratus, extensor pollicis longus (EPL), abductor pollicis longus, and flexor pollicis longus (FPL) muscles usually are absent. The peripheral nerves generally have an anomalous pattern, with the median nerve being the most clinically significant. The nerve is thicker than normal and runs along the preaxial border of the forearm just beneath the fascia. In 25% of patients, it bifurcates distally, with a dorsal branch running a course similar to that of the dorsal cutaneous branch of the superficial radial nerve, which frequently is absent. This nerve is at considerable risk during radial dissections because it is quite superficial and, as stated by Flatt, "represents a strong and unyielding bowstring of the radially bowed forearm and hand." The radial nerve frequently terminates at the level of the lateral epicondyle just after innervating the triceps. The ulnar nerve characteristically is normal according to most authors, and the musculocutaneous nerve usually is absent. The vascular anatomy usually is represented by a normal brachial artery, a normal ulnar artery, a well-developed common interosseous artery, and an absent radial artery.

The obvious deformity of a short forearm and radially deviated hand is almost invariably present at birth. A prominent knob at the wrist usually is caused by the distal end of the ulna. The forearm is between 50% and 75% of the length of the contralateral forearm, a ratio that usually remains the same throughout periods of growth. The thumb characteristically is absent or severely deficient; the contralateral thumb is deficient in unilateral and bilateral cases. Duplication of the thumb also has been reported. The hand often is relatively small. The metacarpophalangeal joints usually have limited flexion and some hyperextensibility. Flexion contractures often occur in the proximal interphalangeal joints. Stiffness of the elbow in extension, probably the result of weak elbow flexors, frequently is associated with a radial clubhand. Most authors emphasize the elbow extension contracture as an extremely important consideration in evaluating these patients for reconstruction. Because of the radial deviation of the hand, the child usually can reach the mouth without elbow flexion. If untreated, the deformity does not seem to worsen over time, but prehension is limited and the hand is used primarily to trap objects between it and the forearm. Lamb found that unilateral involvement did not significantly affect the activities of daily living, but bilateral involvement reduced activities by one third. Associated cardiac or hematologic problems may worsen the overall prognosis.

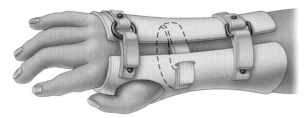

FIGURE 17.6 Plastic splint for congenital absence of radius. Note especially middle strap that is placed over wrist at apex of angulation. Splint is useful for hands that can be properly aligned passively and for maintaining proper position after surgery.

The goals of treatment for radial longitudinal deficiency are to (1) straighten (when necessary) the radial bow of the forearm, (2) correct radial and volar subluxation of the carpus, (3) optimize limb length, and (4) reconstruct the thumb when necessary.

NONOPERATIVE TREATMENT
Immediately after birth, the radial clubhand often can be corrected passively, and early casting and splinting generally are recommended (Fig. 17.6). A light, molded plastic, short arm splint is applied along the radial side of the forearm and is removed only for bathing until the infant begins to use the hands; then the splint is worn only during sleep. Riordan recommended applying a long arm corrective cast as soon after birth as possible. The cast is applied in three stages by means of a technique similar to that used for clubfoot casting. The hand and wrist are corrected first, and the elbow is corrected as much as possible. Although correction usually is achieved in an infant, Milford concluded that casting and splinting in a child younger than 3 months old often is impractical. Lamb reported that elbow extension contracture can be improved by splinting with the hand and wrist in neutral position; 20 of his 27 patients improved to 90 degrees. He cautioned that elbow flexion never improves after centralization procedures. As the child matures and ulnar growth continues, splinting is inadequate to maintain correction. There is no satisfactory conservative therapy for the significant thumb deformities associated with radial clubhand.

OPERATIVE TREATMENT
Although surgery may be postponed for 2 to 3 years with adequate splinting, there is general agreement favoring operative correction at 3 to 6 months of age in children with inadequate radial support of the carpus. Pollicization, when indicated, follows at 9 to 12 months of age if possible. The management of neglected deformities might include external distraction fixation before formal centralization. Specific contraindications to operative treatment include severe associated anomalies not compatible with long life, inadequate elbow flexion, mild deformity with adequate radial support (type I and some type II deformities), and older patients who have accepted the deformities and have adjusted accordingly. Reconstruction of these limbs requires familiarity with the concepts and surgical details of three types of procedures: centralization of the carpus on the forearm, thumb reconstruction, and occasionally transfer of the triceps to restore elbow flexion.

Centralization of the Hand. In 1893, Sayre first reported centralization of the hand over the distal ulna; he suggested sharpening the distal end of the ulna to fit into a surgically created carpal notch. Lidge modified this method by leaving the ulnar epiphysis intact, providing the forerunner of modern centralization techniques.

Incisions and surgical approaches have varied. Manske and McCarroll used transverse ulnar incisions, as described by Riordan, removing an ellipse of skin. Watson, Beebe, and Cruz recommended ulnar and radial Z-plasty incisions to allow removal of the distal radial anlage, which they believe is essential. Evans et al. described a clever bilobed incision that allows the rotation of dorsal skin into the radial incision and excessive ulnar skin into the dorsal defect (Fig. 17.7). Vuillermin et al. evaluated 16 patients 3 years postoperatively after soft-tissue release with a bilobed flap. This procedure did not appear to affect ulnar growth like other centralization procedure; however, recurrence rates were similar to formal centralizations. Van Heest et al. described a simple dorsal rotation flap that allows rotation of the skin in a radial direction while the hand and carpus are rotated in an ulnar direction (Fig. 17.8).

The creation of a carpal notch to stabilize the carpus on the ulna is controversial. Although some authors do not recommend removing the carpus because of the possibility of affecting growth, Lamb believed it to be essential and that the depth of the notch should equal the transverse diameter of the distal ulna, which usually requires removal of all the lunate and most of the capitate. Results have been comparable with or without creation of a notch. Buck-Gramcko promoted overcorrection or radialization.

When a carpal notch is not created, the distal ulna is reported to broaden and take on the radiographic appearance of a normal distal radius. Bora et al. recommended adjunctive tendon transfers in which the flexor digitorum superficialis from the central digits is transferred around the postaxial side of the forearm into the dorsal aspect of the metacarpal shafts, the hypothenar muscles are transferred proximally along the ulnar shaft, and the extensor carpi ulnaris is transferred distally along the shaft of the metacarpal of the little finger; however, according to their report, this procedure failed to prevent 25 to 35 degrees of recurrent radial deviation. Bayne and Klug recommended transfer of the flexor carpi ulnaris into the distally advanced extensor carpi ulnaris to help prevent radiovolar deformity. Most authors agree that it is beneficial to use a Kirschner wire to secure alignment of the long or index metacarpal with the ulna for at least 6 weeks. Ulnar osteotomy is required if the ulna is so bowed that the Kirschner wire cannot be passed along its medullary canal; this usually is when bowing is greater than 30 degrees. When the radius is absent bilaterally, one hand should be surgically fixed in about 45 degrees of pronation and the other in about 45 degrees of supination.

Circumferential and unilateral external fixators can be used to stretch the soft tissues gradually and facilitate centralization (Fig. 17.9). We have found them mostly useful in older children in whom a single-stage centralization procedure would not be possible. Manske et al. evaluated soft-tissue distraction and its effect on recurrence and concluded that, although distraction facilitated correction, recurrence was not prevented and was associated with worse final radial deviation and volar subluxation when compared with centralization alone.

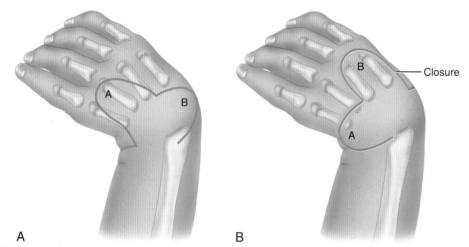

FIGURE 17.7 Evans technique. **A,** The incision should start at point of greatest tension when ulnar force is applied to radial side of wrist. Defect that opens up should be length of proximal flap A and another flap B at 90 degrees on ulnar side. **B,** Flap after transposition. Flap A has been rotated from dorsal to radial on wrist, and flap B rotated from ulnar to dorsal.

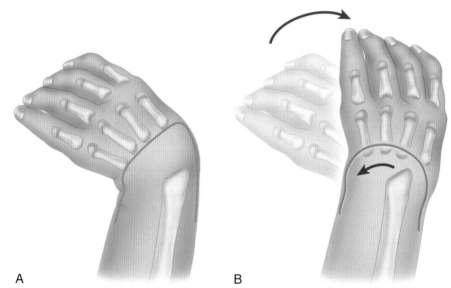

FIGURE 17.8 Van Heest technique. **A,** Incision for dorsal rotation flap, extending from ulnar midlateral border of wrist, transversely across dorsum of wrist in Langer's lines and to radial midlateral border of wrist. **B,** Dorsal rotation flap allowing for rotation of skin in radial direction while hand and carpus are rotated ulnarly. Redundant skin on ulnar side of wrist rotated to compensate for shortage of skin on radial side. Flap naturally falls into place as hand and carpus are rotated ulnarly for centralization.

Centralization has been shown to improve function, particularly in bilateral involvement despite high rates of recurrence. Bora et al. reported total active digital motion of 54% of normal after surgery compared with 27% in untreated patients. Forearm length was functionally doubled, and the metacarpal-ulnar angle averaged 35 degrees after surgery compared with 100 degrees in untreated patients. Kotwal et al. analyzed radiographic and functional outcomes in 446 patients with types 3 and 4 radial longitudinal deficiency over 20 years and compared conservative management with passive stretching followed by surgical management. Significant improvement in hand-forearm angle and digital range of

motion were noted in the surgically treated group. Bayne and Klug reported that 52 of 53 patients believed cosmesis and function had been improved by centralization. Good results had the following factors in common: (1) all had adequate preoperative soft-tissue stretching; (2) surgical goals were obtained; (3) there were no problems with postoperative bracing; (4) most had less severe soft-tissue contractures; and (5) most were younger than 3 years old at the time of centralization. Others have found no correlation between improved wrist alignment or increased forearm length and improved upper extremity function. Despite functional gains, one study found that only half of the patients were satisfied with

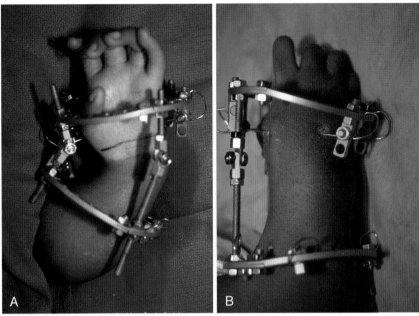

FIGURE 17.9 **A** and **B,** Thin-wire circular external fixator used for gradual distraction and correction of radial clubhand deformity in 9-year-old girl.

the result. In a large retrospective review, surgically treated patients exhibited improved function and appearance when compared with patients treated nonoperatively.

Complications of centralization include growth arrest of the distal ulna, ankylosis of the wrist, recurrent instability of the wrist, damage to neural structures (particularly the anomalous median nerve), vascular insufficiency of the hand, wound infection, necrosis of wound margins, fracture of the ulna, and pin migration and breakage. Major neurovascular complications are rare. Recurrence of the deformity is expected regardless of the procedure and tends to correlate with the severity of the initial deformity. In recent studies evaluating patient function as adulthood is reached, activity and participation were influenced primarily by grip, key pinch, forearm length, and elbow motion as opposed to wrist angulation.

Vilkki described the use of a vascularized second metatarsophalangeal joint as a strut for the radial platform of the ulna as an alternative to centralization. This technique avoids trauma to the ulnar physis, supports the radial carpus, and provides a growing bony support to minimize recurrence. The vascularized metatarsophalangeal joint strut placement is preceded by soft-tissue distraction. Similarly, Yang et al., in a limited study, utilized a vascularized fibular head transfer after soft-tissue distraction with similar results. The surgical results of these techniques are promising and may provide a further alternative to standard centralization techniques.

Abductor digiti minimi opponensplasty, as described by Huber, may be appropriate for rare patients with only isolated thenar aplasia in association with the radial clubhand or for patients with weakness in apposition after pollicization. Manske and McCarroll reported improvement in appearance, dexterity, strength, and usefulness of the thumb in 20 of 21 patients with an average age at operation of 4 years, 9 months.

An elbow stiff in extension is a contraindication to centralization; rarely, a child may have passive elbow flexion but minimal or no active flexion because of complete absence of elbow flexors. Menelaus performed triceps transfer to restore elbow flexion 2 to 3 months after centralization.

CENTRALIZATION OF THE HAND USING TRANSVERSE ULNAR INCISIONS

TECHNIQUE 17.2

(MANSKE, MCCARROLL, AND SWANSON)

- Begin the incision just radial to the midline on the dorsum of the wrist at the level of the distal ulna and proceed ulnarward in a transverse direction to a point radial to the pisiform at the volar wrist crease. Pass the incision through the bulbous soft-tissue mass on the ulnar side of the wrist, incising considerable fat and subcutaneous tissue (Fig. 17.10A).
- Identify and preserve the dorsal sensory branch of the ulnar nerve, which is deep in the subcutaneous tissue and lies near the extensor retinaculum.
- Expose the extensor retinaculum and the base of the hypothenar muscles. It is not necessary to identify the ulnar artery or nerve on the volar aspect of the wrist (Fig. 17.10B).
- Identify and dissect free the extensor carpi ulnaris tendon at its insertion on the base of the fifth metacarpal and detach and retract it proximally.
- Identify and retract radially the extensor digitorum communis tendons. This exposes the dorsal and ulnar aspects of the wrist capsule. Incise the capsule transversely, exposing the distal ulna (Fig. 17.10C).

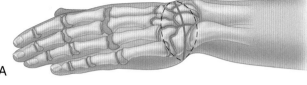

A

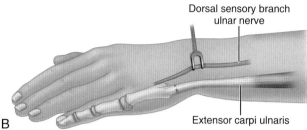

Dorsal sensory branch
ulnar nerve

Extensor carpi ulnaris

B

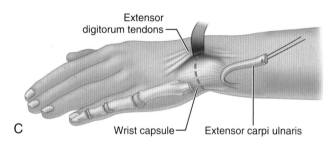

Extensor
digitorum tendons

Wrist capsule   Extensor carpi ulnaris

C

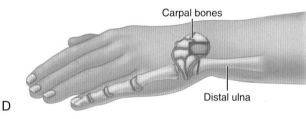

Carpal bones

Distal ulna

D

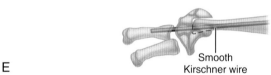

Smooth
Kirschner wire

E

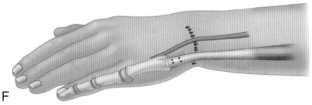

F

FIGURE 17.10 Manske et al. centralization arthroplasty technique, transverse ulnar approach (see text). **A,** Incision. **B,** Exposure of muscle, tendon, and nerve. **C,** Capsular incision. **D,** Exposure of carpoulnar junction and excision of segment of carpal bones. **E,** Insertion of Kirschner wire. **F,** Reattachment of extensor carpi ulnaris tendon. **SEE TECHNIQUE 17.2.**

- The carpal bones are a cartilaginous mass deep in the wound on the radial side of the ulna. The carpoulnar junction is most easily identified by dissecting from proximal to distal along the radial side of the distal ulna. Do not mistake one of the intercarpal articulations for the carpoulnar junction.

- Define the cartilaginous mass of carpal bones and excise a square segment of its midportion (measuring approximately 1 cm) to accommodate the distal ulna.
- Dissect free the distal ulnar epiphysis from the adjacent soft tissue and square it off by shaving perpendicular to the shaft (Fig. 17.10D). Avoid injury of the physis or the attached soft tissue.
- Place the distal ulna in the carpal defect and stabilize it with a smooth Kirschner wire (Fig. 17.10E). In practice, this is usually accomplished by passing the Kirschner wire proximally down the shaft of the distal ulna to emerge at the olecranon (or at the midshaft if the ulna is bowed). Pass the wire distally across the carpal notch into the third metacarpal. Cut off the proximal end of the wire beneath the skin.
- Stabilize the ulnar side of the wrist by imbricating the capsule or by suturing the distal capsule to the periosteum of the shaft of the distal ulna. (If there is insufficient distal capsule, suture the cartilaginous carpal bones to the periosteum.)
- Obtain additional stabilization by advancing the extensor carpi ulnaris tendon distally and reattaching it to the base of the fourth or fifth metacarpal (Fig. 17.10F).
- Advance the origin of the hypothenar musculature proximally and suture it to the ulnar shaft to provide additional stability to the wrist.
- Excise the bulbous excess of the skin and soft tissue and suture the skin. This results in a pleasing cosmetic closure and helps stabilize the hand in the ulnar position (Fig. 17.11).

POSTOPERATIVE CARE The wrist is immobilized in a plaster cast for 6 weeks and then is placed in a removable Orthoplast splint. The Kirschner wire is removed at 6 to 12 weeks. Children are encouraged to wear the splint until they reach skeletal maturity.

CENTRALIZATION OF THE HAND WITH REMOVAL OF THE DISTAL RADIAL ANLAGE

TECHNIQUE 17.3

(WATSON, BEEBE, AND CRUZ)
- Under pneumatic tourniquet control, make two skin incisions (Fig. 17.12A). On the radial aspect, perform a standard 60-degree Z-plasty with a longitudinal central limb to obtain lengthening along the longitudinal axis of the forearm. On the ulnar aspect, perform a similar Z-plasty, but with a transverse central limb to take up skin redundancy in this area, transposing the excess tissue to the deficient radial wrist area (Fig. 17.12B).
- When the skin incisions are completed, carry the dissection along the radial side, identifying the median nerve (Fig. 17.12C). The median nerve is more radially located

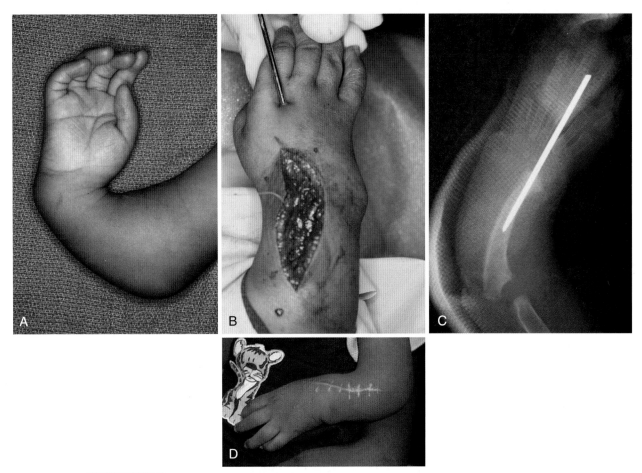

FIGURE 17.11 **A,** Radial clubhand deformity. **B,** Intraoperative photograph during centralization. **C,** Correction of deformity after insertion of smooth pin. **D,** One year after surgery. **SEE TECHNIQUE 17.2.**

than usual and may be the most superficial structure encountered after the radial skin incision is made. Identification and preservation of the "radial-median" nerve are vital to the resulting functional capacity of the hand.

- Continue the dissection ulnarward, resecting the fibrotic distal radial anlage, which may act as a restricting band to maintain the hand in radial deviation (Fig. 17.12D).
- Identify and protect the ulnar nerve and artery through the ulnar incision to allow complete dissection around the distal ulna without damage to crucial structures (Fig. 17.12E).
- Perform a complete capsular release of the ulnocarpal joint, avoiding injury to the ulnar physis. At this point, the hand should be fully movable, attached to the forearm only by the skin, the dorsal and palmar tendons, and the preserved neurovascular structures.
- Remove all the fibrotic material in the "center" of the wrist and forearm area. The ulna and ulnar incision should be clearly visible through the radial incision, and the reverse should be true. It should not be necessary to remove any carpal bones or to remodel the distal ulna to maintain the hand in a centralized position.

- Pass a 0.045-inch Kirschner wire through the lunate, capitate, and long finger metacarpal, exiting through the metacarpophalangeal joint (Fig. 17.12F).
- Centralize the hand in the desired position and pass the Kirschner wire in a retrograde fashion into the ulna to maintain the position of the hand (Fig. 17.12G).
- Deflate the tourniquet and obtain hemostasis before skin closure, or deflate the tourniquet immediately after the application of the dressing and splint.
- Apply a bulky hand dressing with a dorsal plaster splint extending above the elbow.
- Before discontinuing anesthesia, ensure that circulation in the hand is satisfactory.

POSTOPERATIVE CARE The hand is elevated for 24 to 48 hours. The dressing is changed and sutures are removed 2 weeks after surgery. A long arm cast is applied and worn for an additional 4 weeks. The Kirschner wire is removed at 6 weeks, and a short arm cast is worn for an additional 3 weeks. Night splinting is continued until physeal closure to avoid recurrence of radial deviation.

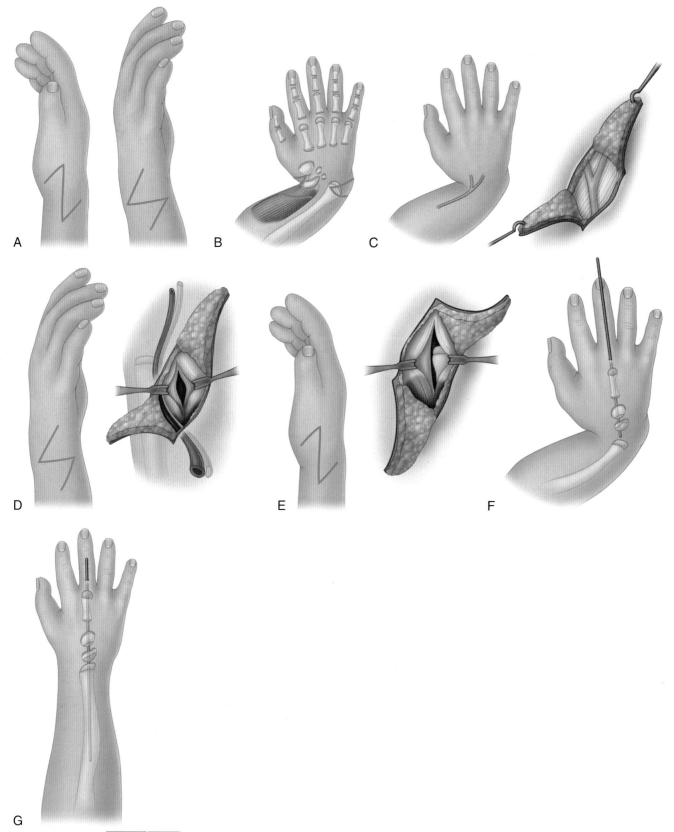

FIGURE **17.12** Watson et al. centralization of radial clubhand (see text). **A,** Z-plasties on radial and ulnar sides of wrist. **B,** Incisions allow lengthening on radial side. Ulnar incision takes up skin redundancy, transposing it to deficient radial side. **C,** Radial incision in wrist for identification of median nerve. **D,** View from ulnar incision across wrist to radial incision after resection of all nonessential central structures. **E,** Distal ulna seen through radial incision at wrist. **F,** Kirschner wire passed through lunate, capitate, and long finger metacarpal. **G,** After centralization, Kirschner wire passed into ulna to maintain position. **SEE TECHNIQUE 17.3.**

CENTRALIZATION OF THE HAND AND TENDON TRANSFERS

Bora et al. suggested that treatment be started immediately after birth with corrective casts to stretch the radial side of the wrist. When the patient is 6 to 12 months old, the hand is centralized surgically over the distal end of the ulna and tendon transfers are done 6 to 12 months later.

TECHNIQUE 17.4　　　*Figure 17.13*

(BORA ET AL.)

STAGE I

- Make a radial S-shaped incision and excise the radiocarpal ligament. Isolate and excise the lunate and capitate.
- Make a longitudinal incision over the distal ulnar epiphysis, free it from the surrounding tissue, and preserve the tendons of the extensor carpi ulnaris and extensor digitorum quinti minimus.
- Transpose the distal end of the ulna through the plane between the flexor and extensor tendons and into a slot formed by the removal of the lunate and capitate.
- With the distal end of the ulna at the base of the long finger metacarpal, transfix it with a smooth Kirschner wire.
- Check the position of the ulna and carpus by radiographs in the operating room to ensure that the ulna is aligned with the long axis of the long finger metacarpal.
- Suture the dorsal radiocarpal ligament over the neck of the ulna, close the skin, and apply a long arm cast with the elbow at 90 degrees.
- If the deformity is unilateral, the wrist and hand should be placed in neutral; and if it is bilateral, they should be placed in 45 degrees of pronation on one side and 45 degrees of supination on the other. The cast is removed at 6 weeks, and a splint is applied at night.

STAGE II

- Three tendon transfers are performed 6 to 12 months after the centralization procedure.
- Before attempting to transfer the flexor digitorum sublimis tendons, test for function because in some instances the sublimis tendon is nonfunctioning in one or more of the three ulnar digits.
- Passively maintain the metacarpophalangeal joints and the wrist joint in hyperextension and the interphalangeal joints in extension, and release one finger at a time. An intact sublimis tendon flexes the proximal interphalangeal joint of the released finger.
- Make a midlateral incision on the ulnar side of the long finger at the level of the proximal interphalangeal joint.
- Divide the sublimis tendon at the level of the middle phalanx and divide the chiasm of the decussating

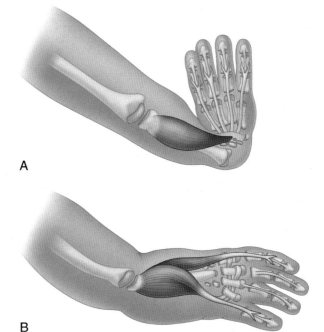

A

B

FIGURE 17.13 Bora et al. centralization of hand and tendon transfer (see text). **A,** Volar aspect of radial clubhand deformity showing right-angle relationship of hand and forearm and acute angulation of extrinsic flexor tendons. **B,** Volar aspect after centralization and transfer of sublimis tendons of ring and long fingers. **SEE TECHNIQUE 17.4.**

fibers. Perform a similar procedure on the ring finger.
- Make a short transverse incision on the volar aspect of the forearm and pull the two tendons into it. At the site of the previous dorsal incision, reenter the wrist and transfer the sublimis tendons subcutaneously around the ulnar side of the ulna to the dorsum of the hand.
- Loop the tendon from the long finger around the shaft of the index finger metacarpal and the tendon from the ring finger around the shaft of the long finger metacarpal (see Fig. 17.13B).
- Transpose the tendons extraperiosteally and suture them back to themselves with the wrist in 15 degrees of dorsiflexion and maximal ulnar deviation.
- Transfer the extensor carpi ulnaris tendon distally along the shaft of the little finger metacarpal and transfer the origin of the hypothenar muscles proximally along the ulnar shaft. An effort is made to maintain balance and prevent recurrence of the deformity.

POSTOPERATIVE CARE A cast is applied after the procedure and is worn for 1 month; after this, a night splint is worn for at least 3 months. Careful follow-up is recommended to observe for possible recurrence of deformity. A night splint can be used for several years.

CENTRALIZATION WITH TRANSFER OF THE FLEXOR CARPI ULNARIS

TECHNIQUE 17.5

(BAYNE AND KLUG)

- Make a transverse wedge incision over the end of the ulna to excise the redundant skin and fibrofatty tissue (Fig. 17.14A). A Z-plasty incision also may be necessary on the radial surface of the distal forearm and wrist to give extra length to the tight skin on the radial side and make the wrist flexors and tight capsular attachments more accessible. If the radial contracture has been corrected before surgery, a Z-plasty incision may not be necessary.
- Through the ulnar incision, identify the dorsal sensory branch of the ulnar nerve, the extensor carpi ulnaris, and the flexor carpi ulnaris.
- Expose the distal ulna, avoiding damage to the epiphyseal blood supply.
- Develop a distally based ulnocarpal flap. Locate the interval between the carpus and the radial aspect of the ulna. Using sharp dissection, free the capsular attachments to the carpal structures, flex the elbow, and reduce the carpus over the end of the ulna. If this cannot be done easily, use the radial incision.
- Elevate the skin flaps and identify and protect the anomalous superficial branch of the median nerve.
- The flexor carpi radialis and frequently the brachioradialis are attached to the radial carpal bones, producing a strong tethering force; release these if necessary.
- If reduction is still difficult, lightly shave the cartilage of the distal ulna to flatten the surface, avoiding exposure of the epiphyseal bone. Because carpal bone excision or excessive shaving often leads to intercarpal fusion and a stiff wrist, Bayne and Klug recommend ulnar osteotomy rather than carpal bone excision if reduction cannot be obtained.
- Select a Kirschner wire slightly smaller than the one to be used for final fixation and use it to make a pilot channel from distal to proximal through the center of the ulna.
- Introduce the larger Kirschner wire into the carpal bones and the third metacarpal, crossing the metacarpophalangeal joint.
- Place the proximal end of the wire in the pilot hole in the central portion of the end of the ulna and drive it retrograde proximally through the ulna (Fig. 17.14B).
- Withdraw the pin so that it does not block motion of the third metacarpophalangeal joint.
- Obtain radiographs to ensure that the carpus is perfectly centralized on the distal ulna; failure to achieve perfect reduction is a common cause of subsequent loss of centralization.
- After fixation of the hand, advance the ulnocarpal flap proximally and suture it in place.
- Advance the extensor carpi ulnaris as far distally as possible on the fifth metacarpal.
- Suture the flexor carpi ulnaris into the extensor carpi ulnaris as far distally and dorsally as possible (Fig. 17.14C). The force of the transfer should be directed dorsally and ulnarward to counteract the palmar- and radial-deviating structures and balance the hand dynamically on the end of the ulna.
- Close the incisions.

- Place the hand in a neutral position, release the tourniquet and evaluate circulation, and apply a bulky dressing and long arm plaster splint.
- If the ulna is severely bowed, a closing wedge osteotomy may be necessary; bowing of more than 30 degrees should be corrected. Make the osteotomy at the apex of angulation of the ulna.

POSTOPERATIVE CARE The dressing is changed in 2 weeks, and sutures are removed. A long arm plaster cast is applied. Mobilization of the fingers is encouraged. The cast and Kirschner wire are removed at 6 to 8 weeks. A short arm Orthoplast splint is applied with the fingers and elbow free. The splint is worn full time until the child is 6 years old, after which time it is used at night until skeletal maturity is reached.

CENTRALIZATION OF THE HAND

TECHNIQUE 17.6

(BUCK-GRAMCKO)

- With the use of general anesthesia and a tourniquet, make an S-shaped incision from the dorsum of the hand to the proximal third of the forearm (Fig. 17.15A), carefully preserving the superficial vessels and nerves, especially the most radial branch of the median nerve and its artery.
- Incise the extensor retinaculum from the radial side in an ulnar direction.
- Identify and preserve the extensor tendons.
- Generally, the radial extensor and flexor muscles have a common muscle mass with almost no tendon and can be detached from the radial carpal bones; occasionally, they have separate masses and a true tendon and should be detached from their metacarpal insertion.
- Incise the dorsal and palmar joint capsule transversely; prepare one or two flaps that can be transposed later in the new joint.
- Save the well-developed ulnar collateral ligament.
- Excise most of the fibrosed and contracted tissue and muscle fasciae because they prevent the necessary extensive mobilization of the hand.
- If a fibrocartilaginous anlage of the distal radius is present, excise it because it would prevent the distal and ulnar movement of the hand.
- Free the distal end of the ulna, carefully preserving the cartilage and all the arteries supplying the epiphysis.
- Position the hand with its radial carpal bones over the head of the ulna. Position the hand in slight ulnar deviation. Insert a Kirschner wire in a retrograde fashion through the full length of the ulna and, under image control, pass it distally through the radial carpal bones and obliquely through the second metacarpal (Fig. 17.15B).
- If marked curvature of the ulna is present, make a wedge osteotomy in its middle third before the Kirschner wire is inserted (Fig. 17.15A).

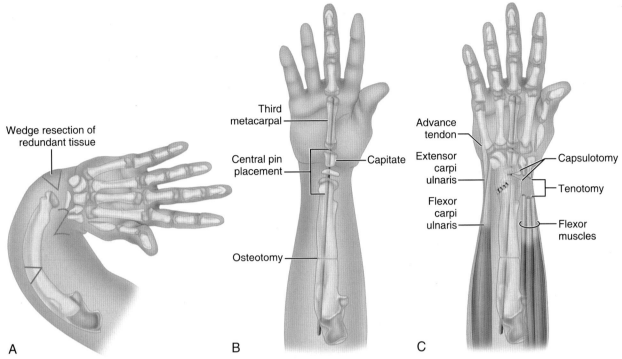

FIGURE 17.14 Bayne and Klug centralization of radial clubhand. **A,** Radial release and resection of redundant soft tissue. **B,** Centralization and pin fixation with ulnar osteotomy. **C,** Radial capsular release and tendon transfer. **SEE TECHNIQUE 17.5.**

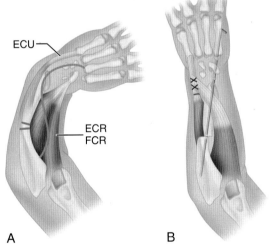

FIGURE 17.15 Buck-Gramcko centralization (radialization) of radial clubhand. **A,** S-shaped incision. **B,** Retrograde insertion of Kirschner wire. *ECR,* Extensor carpi radialis; *ECU,* extensor carpi ulnaris; *FCR,* flexor carpi radialis. **SEE TECHNIQUE 17.6.**

- Suture the ulnar ligaments and capsular flap to the periosteum as a new collateral ligament. Reinforce the muscles on the ulnar side by transposing as many radial muscles as are available, including the extensor carpi radialis and flexor carpi radialis. Pass these muscles between the ulna and the extensor tendons to the ulnar side and suture them end-to-side to the extensor carpi ulnaris tendon that also is shortened by reefing.
- Bring the retinaculum back over the radial carpal bones and place it between joint and tendons to prevent adhesions.

- After careful hemostasis, excise the excess skin on the ulnar side of the wrist; preserve the dorsal branch of the ulnar nerve.
- Apply a long arm plaster splint.

POSTOPERATIVE CARE The cast is worn for 3 weeks. The Kirschner wire usually is removed at the time of pollicization of the second metacarpal (at least 4 weeks after centralization). After wire removal, a night splint is worn for several months.

TRICEPS TRANSFER TO RESTORE ELBOW FLEXION

TECHNIQUE 17.7

(MENELAUS)
- Make a lateral incision to expose the lower end of the triceps muscle and the anterior, lateral, and posterior aspects of the proximal end of the ulna. Identify the triceps insertion and dissect a tongue of periosteum from the proximal end of the ulna in continuity with the triceps tendon.
- Dissect the triceps proximally to the midarm level. Identify and mobilize the ulnar nerve; perform a posterior capsulotomy of the elbow.

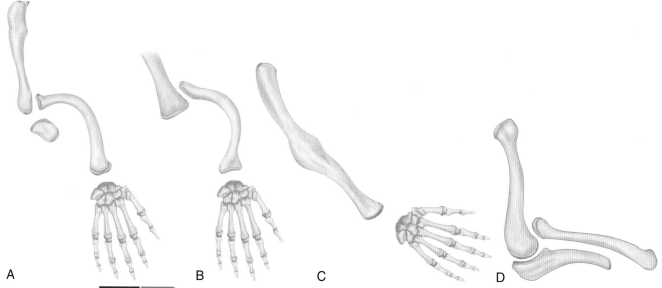

FIGURE 17.16 Swanson classification of ulnar deficiency. **A,** Type 1: hypoplasia or partial defect of ulna. **B,** Type 2: total defect of ulna. **C,** Type 3: total or partial defect of ulna with humeroradial synostosis. **D,** Type 4: total or partial defect of ulna with congenital amputation at wrist.

- Roll the periosteal tongue and the triceps tendon and pass this through a tunnel created in the coronoid process of the ulna.
- Secure the transfer with a nonabsorbable suture.
- Close the wound and apply a splint or cast with the elbow in 120 degrees of flexion.

POSTOPERATIVE CARE The transfer is protected in a long arm cast for 4 to 6 weeks. The sutures are removed at 2 weeks. After cast removal, gentle active exercises are begun, supporting the limb in a 90-degree, long arm, posterior splint that is worn between exercise periods and during sleep.

■ ULNAR LONGITUDINAL DEFICIENCY

Ulnar deficiencies are malformations in which there is longitudinal failure of formation along the postaxial border of the upper extremity. The most common form is a partial deficiency of the ulna and the ulnar two digits, commonly referred to as ulnar clubhand. Other terms for this deformity include ulnar dysmelia, paraxial ulnar hemimelia, and congenital absence of the ulna. Ulnar deficiencies are rare congenital hand anomalies, with a relative incidence one tenth to one third that of radial deficiencies.

The cause of this rare anomaly is unknown, and its occurrence is sporadic. The only report that suggests a familial pattern is that of Roberts in 1886, in which he reported the deformity in three successive generations.

Swanson, Tada, and Yonenobu described four types of ulnar deficiency (Fig. 17.16): type 1, hypoplasia or partial defect of the ulna; type 2, total defect of the ulna; type 3, total or partial defect of the ulna with humeroradial synostosis; and type 4, total or partial defect of the ulna associated with congenital amputation at the wrist. A type 0 has been proposed by Havenhill et al. to describe a subgroup of patients with an ulnar deficient ray and carpus but normal ulna. Partial absence of the ulna is more common than total absence, the reverse of radial deficiencies. Cole and Manske classified ulnar-deficient hands based on the involvement of the thumb and first web (Table 17.6). In their series, 73% of ulnar-deficient limbs had thumb and first web abnormalities.

Anomalies associated with ulnar deficiencies, in contrast to radial deficiencies, are almost solely limited to the musculoskeletal system and include clubfoot, fibular deficiencies, spina bifida, femoral agenesis, mandibular defects, and absence of the patella. Carpal bone deformities are common because of severe deformity and coalition. Digital malformation occurs in 89% of patients, and radial head dislocation is frequent.

Varying degrees of deficiency along the ulnar side of the hand are present at birth. The forearm usually is shortened and frequently bowed. The small and ring fingers usually are absent. Syndactyly of the remaining digits is common. The long and index fingers and the thumb are absent in about two thirds of patients. Forearm bowing with radial convexity is caused by the tethering effect of the ulnar anlage. Ulnar deviation of the hand usually correlates with the degree of radial bowing and increased ulnar slope to the distal radius, as does supination deformity of the forearm. The elbow usually is restricted in motion and may be fused. El Hassan et al. reported 14 patients with associated radiohumeral synostosis and noted that the elbow was fixed on average at 63 degrees of flexion (10 to 90 degrees). Nine of 11 patients with unilateral deformity reported no limitations in their activities of daily living, and five participated in sports. The deformity is more commonly unilateral.

Radiographs usually show a typical pattern (Fig. 17.17) of an absent distal ulna and a bowed radius with an increased ulnar slope along its distal articular surface. The pisiform and hamate usually are absent, and coalitions of the other carpal bones frequently are present. It often is difficult to determine

TABLE 17.6	
Classification of Ulnar Deficiency	
TYPE	**DESCRIPTION**
A	Normal first web space and thumb
B	Mild first web and thumb deficiency
C	Moderate-to-severe first web and thumb deficiency; potential loss of opposition, malrotation of the thumb into the plane of the other digits, thumb-index syndactyly, absent extrinsic tendon function
D	Absent thumb

Modified from Cole RJ, Manske PR: Classification of ulnar deficiency according to the thumb first web, *J Hand Surg* 22A:479, 1997.

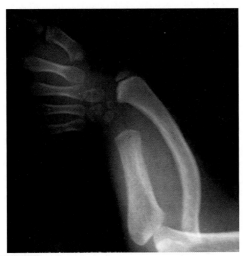

FIGURE 17.17   Radiographic appearance of type I ulnar clubhand.

the presence or absence of the proximal ulna because mineralization may not occur until the child is 1 year old.

NONOPERATIVE TREATMENT

Initial management of ulnar clubhand in infants consists of corrective casting and splinting. A long arm cast is applied in the method of Riordan, applying the hand section first, then joining the hand to the forearm in the corrected position, and finally joining the forearm to the arm in 90 degrees of elbow flexion. Frequent cast changes are necessary and should be continued until correction is achieved. Removable splints can be used to maintain correction. This should be continued until the child is 6 months old, at which time exploration and excision of the ulnar anlage should be considered if significant radial bowing is present.

OPERATIVE TREATMENT

Indications for surgical intervention are syndactyly, radial bowing and presence of an ulnar anlage, dislocation of the radial head with limited elbow extension and forearm pronation and supination, and internal rotation deformity of the humerus. Surgical separation of the syndactyly should be performed in accordance with standard syndactyly protocol:

separation of the thumb and index finger by 6 months of age and of the central syndactyly by 18 months of age. Malrotation and syndactyly of the thumb may require first metacarpal derotational osteotomy to correct the supination deformity. This procedure usually requires a local rotational flap to create the web and should be performed 6 months after syndactyly release.

Most authors agree that an ulnar anlage should be excised to prevent further radial bowing and shortening. Straub first called attention to the fibrocartilage anlage that spans the gap between proximal ulna and distal radius and ulnar carpus. This anlage does not seem to grow and acts as a tether to deform the radius and carpus with subsequent bowing of the radial shaft and dislocation of the radial head. Resection of the distal end of the fibrocartilaginous mass before age 2 to 3 years or as early as 6 months has been recommended, especially if there is progressive or severe ulnar deviation of the hand at the radiocarpal joint, increased radial bowing, or gradual dislocation of the radial head. If bowing is severe, wedge osteotomy of the radius may be necessary at the time of anlage excision.

If radial head dislocation blocks extension of the elbow, creation of a one-bone forearm should be considered. If the block in extension is acceptable and functional pronation and supination are preserved, surgical treatment probably would not improve function. If marked shortening and bowing of the radius with considerable forearm instability and restriction of elbow motion are present, creation of a one-bone forearm probably would improve function. For this procedure to be successful, some proximal ulna must be present. The proximal radius usually is excised several months before the creation of the one-bone forearm because simultaneous performance of the two procedures might be too extensive. Internal rotation deformity of the humerus may be present with humeroradial synostosis and requires correction if it impairs function.

ROTATIONAL OSTEOTOMY OF THE FIRST METACARPAL

TECHNIQUE 17.8

(BROUDY AND SMITH)

- Under tourniquet control, make a transverse, racquet-shaped skin incision on the volar aspect and extend it to a V-shaped tongue at the middorsum of the first metacarpal. The apex of the "V" lies at the level of the first metacarpal base (Fig. 17.18A) to allow adequate exposure for osteotomy.
- Make a proximal longitudinal incision on the radiovolar side of the first metacarpal, 120 degrees from the apex of the "V" (Fig. 17.18B).
- Perform an osteotomy of the base of the first metacarpal and position the metacarpal in the desired amount of pronation.
- Fix the metacarpal in position with Kirschner wires, suture the V flap into the opened linear incision, and close the V defect in a side-to-side manner.
- Apply a long arm cast.

POSTOPERATIVE CARE The cast is removed 6 weeks after surgery, and progressive activity is allowed. Kirschner wires are removed 6 weeks after surgery or when bone healing is complete. A removable, short arm–thumb spica splint is worn during sleep for another 6 weeks.

EXCISION OF AN ULNAR ANLAGE

TECHNIQUE 17.9

(FLATT)
- Under tourniquet control, make a lazy-"S" incision along the postaxial border, carrying it across the wrist crease to the midcarpal level.
- Because of the absence of the extrinsic flexor muscles, the ulnar neurovascular bundle and the anlage lie close together in the subcutaneous tissues. Free and protect the neurovascular bundle before dissecting the anlage off its carpal attachment.
- Remove at least one third of the forearm length. Incise the soft tissues on the ulnar side of the wrist joint sufficiently to allow full correction of the hand on the distal radial articular surface.
- The hand should flop over into neutral or even slight radial deviation; if it must be pushed into neutral, release more soft tissue.
- Close the wound with nonabsorbable sutures and apply a well-molded, long arm cast.

POSTOPERATIVE CARE The sutures are removed at 3 weeks, and the cast is changed. The cast is removed 6 weeks after surgery, and normal activities are resumed gradually during the next 4 to 6 weeks.

CREATION OF A ONE-BONE FOREARM

TECHNIQUE 17.10

(STRAUB)
- Make a curved longitudinal dorsoradial incision beginning just proximal to the elbow and ending at the middle or distal third of the forearm.
- Expose and excise the fibrocartilaginous band that extends distally from the ulnar fragment; in excising this band, free its proximal end by performing an osteotomy on the distal end of the fragment.
- Expose the radial nerve at the elbow and trace it distally to its interosseous branch; this branch and its enclosing

supinator muscle may be grossly displaced by the dislocation of the proximal radius.
- Develop the cleavage between the dorsal and volar muscles of the forearm, while carefully protecting the important neurovascular structures in the antecubital area.
- At the level of the distal end of the ulnar fragment, divide the radial shaft and excise its proximal part, including the radial head (Fig. 17.19A).
- Place the proximal end of the distal radial fragment against the distal end of the ulnar fragment (Fig. 17.19B) and fix them together with a Kirschner wire passed distally through the olecranon (Fig. 17.19C).
- Close the skin with absorbable or nonabsorbable sutures.
- Apply a long arm cast with the elbow flexed about 90 degrees.

POSTOPERATIVE CARE The cast is changed 2 weeks after surgery, and any remaining sutures are removed. A long arm cast is worn for 8 weeks after surgery. The cast and Kirschner wire or Steinmann pin fixation are removed at 8 weeks or when bone healing is complete. Normal activities are resumed after another 6 to 8 weeks.

▣ CONGENITAL PSEUDARTHROSIS OF THE ULNA; RADIOULNAR SYNOSTOSIS; CONGENITAL DISLOCATION OF THE RADIAL HEAD (SEE CHAPTER 31)

▣ MADELUNG DEFORMITY

Madelung deformity is an abnormality of the palmar ulnar part of the distal radial physis in which progressive ulnar and volar tilt develops at the distal radial articular surface, with dorsal subluxation of the distal ulna. The deformity probably was first described by Malgaigne in 1855 and later by Madelung in 1878. It is believed to be a congenital disorder, although it seldom is obvious until late childhood or adolescence. It is a rare anomaly, accounting for only 1.7% of hand anomalies. The cause of Madelung deformity is uncertain; however, it has been transmitted in an autosomal dominant pattern. Vickers described an abnormal ligament that tethers the lunate to the distal radius proximal to the physis. This ligament is believed to impede the growth of the ulnopalmar aspect of the distal radius and is commonly known as the ligament of Vickers. More recently, Hanson et al. described the presence of an anomalous volar radiotriquetral ligament on MRI in a small number of patients. Other Madelung-like deformities have occurred after trauma and also after infection or neoplasm. There is no definitive method of distinguishing these deformities from idiopathic Madelung deformity. Vender and Watson classified Madelung and Madelung-like deformities into four groups: posttraumatic, dysplastic (dyschondrosteosis or diaphyseal aclasis), genetic (e.g., Turner syndrome), and idiopathic. They suggested that acquired deformities usually can be distinguished by a lack of appropriate physical findings, unilaterality, less severe carpal deformities, and the appropriate history of repetitive injury or stress.

A deformity of the wrist similar to Madelung deformity frequently is associated with dyschondrosteosis, the most common form of mesomelic dwarfism. This disorder consists of mild shortness of stature, shortness of the middle segment of the upper and lower extremities, and Madelung deformity. Mutations in the homeobox gene *SHOX*, which is located at the pseudoautosomal region 1 of both the X and Y chromosomes, have been shown to be causative. Other associated conditions include mucopolysaccharidosis, Turner syndrome, achondroplasia, multiple exostoses, multiple epiphyseal dysplasia, and dyschondroplasia (Ollier disease).

Madelung deformity typically consists of increased radial inclination and volar tilt of the distal radius, proximal migration of the lunate with triangulation of the carpus, and dorsal displacement and prominence of the distal ulna. It is more commonly bilateral and affects girls four times more than boys. Bilateral deformities often are more severe at presentation. If bilateral deformities and short stature are present, Leri-Weill dyschondrosteosis should be suspected, especially if atypical deformities are present. A family history of the deformity often is present. The deformity usually manifests in late childhood or early adolescence, with decreased motion and minimal pain. As growth occurs, the deformity worsens in appearance. Radiographic abnormalities are seen in the radius, ulna, and carpal bones (Fig. 17.20). The radius is curved, with its convexity dorsal and radial, and there is a similar angulation of the distal radial articular surface. A "flame-shaped" notch at the ulnar metaphysis of the radius can indicate the presence of a Vickers ligament and can be confirmed by its presence on MRI. The forearm is relatively short. The distal radial epiphysis is triangular because of the failure of growth in the ulnar and volar aspects of the physis; early closure of these aspects of the physis also is frequent. Osteophyte formation may be visible at the volar ulnar border of the radius. The ulna is subluxated dorsally, the ulnar head is

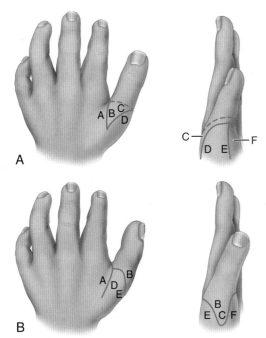

FIGURE 17.18   Broudy and Smith rotational osteotomy of first metacarpal. **A,** Incision. **B,** After osteotomy, dorsal V-flap is rotated volarly. **SEE TECHNIQUE 17.8.**

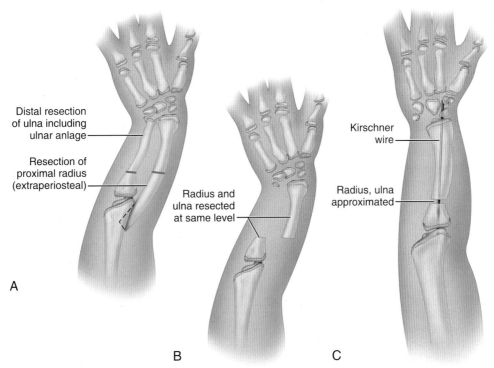

Distal resection of ulna including ulnar anlage

Resection of proximal radius (extraperiosteal)

Radius and ulna resected at same level

Kirschner wire

Radius, ulna approximated

FIGURE 17.19   Creation of one-bone forearm. **A,** Resection of distal ulnar anlage and proximal radius *(shaded areas)*. **B,** Alignment of distal radius and proximal ulna. **C,** Kirschner wire extending into carpals used to stabilize radial and ulnar segments. **SEE TECHNIQUE 17.10.**

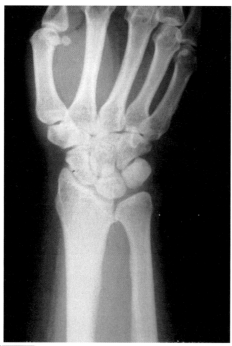

FIGURE 17.20 Radiographic appearance of Madelung deformity. Note abnormalities of radius, ulna, and carpal bones.

enlarged, and the overall length of the ulna is decreased. The carpus appears to have subluxated ulnarward and palmarward into the distal radioulnar joint, which usually is spread apart. The carpus appears wedge shaped, with its apex proximal within the lunate. Advanced imaging rarely is required, although recent literature has supported the use of three-dimensional CT for surgical correction in complex cases.

TREATMENT

Because children with Madelung deformity usually have minimal pain and excellent function, a conservative approach is warranted initially. Surgery should be considered for severe deformity or persistent pain, usually from ulnocarpal impingement of the carpus. Vickers and Nielson reported some success with resection of the abnormal portion of the radial physis and insertion of fat as a form of surgical prophylaxis. In their series, all 17 patients had pain relief and no progression of the deformity after surgery. Historically, the most favored early intervention is a release of Vickers ligament with physiolysis or a Langenskiöld procedure. The abnormal ligament is released from its radial attachment combined with physeal bar resection and fat interposition. The addition of guided growth can be utilized to augment this procedure. Distal radial osteotomy with ulnar shortening (Milch recession) is a preferred treatment in skeletally immature patients. The radial osteotomy may be a closing or opening wedge as needed for alignment. Osteotomy combined with a judicious Darrach excision of the distal ulnar head may be used in skeletally mature patients. Watson, Pitts, and Herber performed balanced radial osteotomies combined with a matched ulnar resection in 10 patients. They reported that radial length was preserved better using this technique; we have had no experience with this technique (Fig. 17.21).

Carter and Ezaki recommended excision of the ligament of Vickers alone in very young patients or in combination

with a dome distal radial osteotomy if considerable deformity already exists. The dome osteotomy tends to provide better volar coverage to the lunate and corrects some of the ulnar positive variance. Long-term radiographic and functional results can be improved when combined with Vickers ligament release and physiolysis. Ulnar shortening may be required at a later date if ulnar wrist pain persists in association with positive ulnar variance. In their series of 23 wrists, they noted a Vickers ligament in 91%, 10 of which required ulnar shortening to relieve persistent ulnar-sided wrist pain. Dome osteotomy was used in 16 wrists and relieved pain in all. Long-term follow-up at an average of 25 years demonstrated maintenance of correction and good-to-excellent functional results. However, in more severe disease, poorer outcomes have been reported. Farr et al. reviewed radiographic criteria for requiring ulnar shortening osteotomy. These criteria included lunate subsidence, ulnar variance, and palmar displacement and were associated with a higher rate of ulnar shortening. An ulnar epiphysiodesis performed at the time of radial osteotomy can prevent the need for ulnar shortening in skeletally immature patients over the age of 10 years.

RESECTION OF A DYSCHONDROSTEOSIS LESION

TECHNIQUE 17.11

(VICKERS AND NIELSEN)

- Under tourniquet control, make a volar transverse incision 1.5 cm proximal to the most proximal wrist crease, passing either on the ulnar side to the flexor carpi radialis and palmaris longus or on the radial side. Protect the median nerve and radial artery.
- Continue the approach radial to the mass of the digital flexor tendons to the distal edge of the pronator quadratus muscle, some of which can be mobilized at the radial end.
- Using an osteotome, make the initial longitudinal osteotomy in the radius, parallel to the long axis of the forearm, about 5 mm from the radioulnar joint. In patients with extreme volar subluxation of the carpus, take care not to mistake the lunate for the underlying radius.
- Reflect the small fragment of the distal radius ulnarward with the osteotome to preserve what exists of the flimsy connections between it and the ulna and to leave some support for the lunate. A sagittal section of the distal radius should be visible. Magnification is recommended.
- If the initial osteotomy is too shallow, a white sheet of fibrous tissue and cartilage is seen.
- Make successive osteotomy cuts 1 mm thick until the physis is clearly identified. When first seen, the physis is thin and wavy and significantly narrowed. When the physeal cartilage is clearly defined, carefully remove bone from the metaphyseal side with a gouge or burr so that the profile of the cartilage is above the bone and is intact from the dorsal periosteum to the volar periosteum to prevent a new bar of bone from forming.

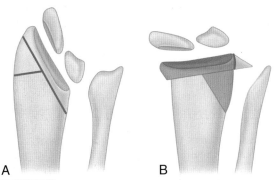

FIGURE 17.21 Watson et al. balanced radial osteotomy. **A,** Osteotomies marked on distal radius with radial-sided bone wedge. **B,** Bone wedge inserted into opening osteotomy on ulnar side. Matched ulnar resection has been performed; radial spike must be excised.

- Identify and excise the abnormal volar ligament tethering the lunate to the radius.
- Deflate the tourniquet and obtain hemostasis, using bone wax if necessary.
- Reinflate the tourniquet and flush with normal saline to remove all bone chips and blood.
- Obtain a generous quantity of fat from the proximal forearm medially and insert to fill the surgical cavity completely. This fat must make intimate contact with the entire length of the physeal cartilage, isolating the bony epiphysis from the bony metaphysis. Soft tissues fall together to hold the fat in place.
- Suture the skin and apply a short arm volar slab or a crepe bandage.

POSTOPERATIVE CARE The bandage should be worn for 2 weeks depending on the degree of the deformity.

CLOSING WEDGE OSTEOTOMY COMBINED WITH DARRACH EXCISION OF THE DISTAL ULNAR HEAD

TECHNIQUE 17.12   *Figure 17.22*

(RANAWAT, DEFIORE, AND STRAUB)
- Make a dorsal longitudinal incision over the distal forearm, detach the extensor retinaculum from the radius over the extensor digitorum communis tendons, and reflect the retinaculum and the tendon of the extensor digiti minimi ulnarward.
- If the patient is skeletally mature, expose the distal radioulnar joint and excise about 1 cm of the distal ulna.

- If the patient is skeletally immature, expose the ulnar shaft and perform an appropriate cuff recession as described by Milch.
- Perform an osteotomy parallel with the distal articular surface of the radius.
- Resect an appropriate wedge of bone based radially and dorsally from the distal end of the proximal fragment of the radius and appose the raw surfaces.
- Stabilize the osteotomy with Kirschner wires so that the distal articular surface of the radius is facing volarward 0 to 15 degrees to the long axis of the radius and ulnarward 60 to 70 degrees.
- Close the incision in routine fashion and apply a long arm cast.

POSTOPERATIVE CARE The cast and pins are removed 4 weeks after surgery, and active exercises of the wrist are begun. The osteotomy incision is protected with a cast or splint until there are sufficient radiographic and clinical signs of bone healing. Normal activities are progressively resumed. After the final cast is removed, protective splinting may be necessary for 8 to 10 weeks after surgery.

DOME OSTEOTOMY AND EXCISION OF VICKERS LIGAMENT

TECHNIQUE 17.13

(CARTER AND EZAKI)
- Under tourniquet control, expose the distal radius through a standard anterior approach in the interval between the flexor carpi radialis and radial artery.
- Incise the pronator quadratus along its radial border and retract ulnarward.
- Identify the Vickers ligament and reflect it off the distal radius beginning proximal to the physis and continue distally until it is released off the physis and the epiphysis (Fig. 17.23A).
- Remove any fibrous tissue or bone noted within the physis.
- Fat can be placed within the physeal defect.
- With curved osteotomes, create a biplanar dome osteotomy in the metaphysis (Fig. 17.23B).
- Rotate the distal radial fragment by pronating it at the osteotomy site and secure it with a Steinmann pin (Fig. 17.23C).
- Remove any palmar step-off of the proximal fragment with a rongeur.
- Repair the pronator quadratus and do a routine closure.
- Apply a long arm splint.

POSTOPERATIVE CARE The long arm splint is worn for 6 weeks. Sutures are removed at 2 weeks, and the pin is removed at 6 weeks, followed by a short arm cast or splint until the osteomy is healed.

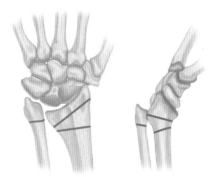

FIGURE 17.22 Ranawat et al. reconstruction of Madelung deformity. Dorsal-based and radial-based closing wedge osteotomy of radius is performed in conjunction with Darrach excision. Correct alignment is obtained, and plate and screws are used for fixation. **SEE TECHNIQUE 17.12.**

UNSPECIFIED
■ SHOULDER (SPRENGEL DEFORMITY, CONGENITAL MUSCULAR TORTICOLLIS, PSEUDARTHROSIS OF THE CLAVICLE)
See *Pediatric Orthopaedics Volume.*

■ ARTHROGRYPOSIS
See *Pediatric Orthopaedics Volume.*

MALFORMATIONS OF HAND PLATE
PROXIMAL DISTAL AXIS
■ BRACHYDACTYLY (HYPOPLASTIC HANDS AND DIGITS)

Hypoplastic hands or digits are those in which development of the part is defective or incomplete. Similar to syndactyly, elements of hypoplasia are seen in almost all hand deformities, and this term is best limited to fingers and hands in which there is relatively symmetric deficiency of the part without associated deformity. Hypoplasia of the entire hand accounted for 0.8% of the deformities in the Iowa series, and brachydactyly ("short fingers") accounted for 5.2%. The most common hypoplastic bony segment is the middle phalanx (brachyphalangia or brachymesophalangia). Brachymetacarpia ("short metacarpal") also is included with the hypoplastic deformities if it is present early, but this is extremely rare; it usually is not noted until after the adolescent growth spurt.

Brachydactyly has played an important role in the genetic literature as the first example of mendelian inheritance shown in humans. Shortening of the fingers usually is considered a dominant trait, but further genetic variations also have been described. If an individual with brachydactyly marries an individual without this anomaly, their offspring have a 50% chance of having brachydactyly. Sporadic cases do occur, but no specific causative factor has been identified.

Brachyphalangia usually occurs alone, but it may occur in association with similar toe deformities. Shortening of the middle phalanges is common in malformation syndromes, such as Treacher Collins, Bloom, Cornelia de Lange, Holt-Oram, Silver, and Poland syndromes. In Poland syndrome, the shortening usually is unilateral. Brachydactyly E, as defined by Bell, consists of brachymetacarpia of the long, ring, and little fingers in association with pseudohypoparathyroidism. Other conditions associated with brachymetacarpia include Turner, Biemond, and Silver syndromes.

There is no useful classification for the hypoplastic hand or digits. Geneticists have devised several detailed groupings of this disorder in an attempt to record patterns of inheritance better, but for the most part these serve no useful purpose in determining management of the deformities.

Hypoplasia of the digits may range from simple shortening (most common) to a small hand with nothing more than nubbins for fingers. In some patients, this may represent an intermediate entity between congenital amputation and hypoplastic digits. There usually is some degree of hypoplasia of all tissues, not just the osseous structures. Except for the nubbin-like fingers, function usually is near-normal. Brachymetacarpia usually is noted during the teenage growth spurt as a depression of one or more metacarpal heads with the fist clenched. The ulnar two fingers are most commonly affected.

■ NONOPERATIVE TREATMENT
Single-digit shortening, particularly of the little finger, requires no surgical correction. Although a single short digit surrounded by digits of normal length may be cosmetically unsatisfactory, functional limitation usually is minimal; also, digital lengthening would not improve function and may result in stiffness.

■ OPERATIVE TREATMENT
Lengthening procedures have been recommended for brachymetacarpia to improve the appearance of the metacarpal row and to increase grip strength. More than 1 cm of shortening can disrupt the metacarpal arch and cause decreased grip strength. Tajima described a single-stage lengthening using a V-shaped metacarpal osteotomy with an interpositional bone graft. Buck-Gramcko detached the interossei and intermetacarpal ligaments at the time of osteotomy (Fig. 17.24). Single-stage procedures usually are limited to about 1 cm of lengthening. Gradual callotasis lengthening has been described, achieving 10 to 19 mm (average 15.2 mm) of additional length. Two-stage procedures can be done with gradual lengthening and bone grafting. Despite success with lengthening procedures, these should be discouraged for adult patients whose only concern is the appearance of the hand.

For a hypoplastic hand with no functioning digits or with preservation of only one digit, more complex and less predictable procedures may be considered, but this is a controversial area of reconstructive hand surgery. It generally is accepted that, with the exception of the soft-tissue nubbin, any digit regardless of size would be of some use to the patient. The musculotendinous structures in these fingers usually are extremely deficient, with little, if any, excursion. Added length created by distraction techniques or web deepening may produce a sense of improved function. Even if the periosteum and physis are preserved, growth of the transferred phalanx is limited. The usual technique of thumb metacarpal lengthening includes division of the

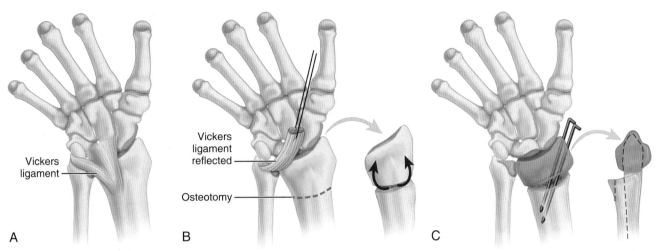

FIGURE 17.23 Carter and Ezaki dome osteotomy for reconstruction of Madelung deformity. **A,** Ligament of Vickers is excised. **B,** Biplanar dome osteotomy is made in metaphysis. Inset, Fat can be placed in physeal defect. **C,** Distal fragment is rotated at osteotomy and secured with Steinmann pins. **SEE TECHNIQUE 17.13.**

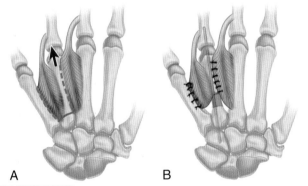

FIGURE 17.24 Buck-Gramcko technique for lengthening brachymetacarpia in hypoplastic hand. **A,** Detachment of interossei and intermetacarpal ligaments and metacarpal osteotomy. **B,** Interposition bone graft fixed with Kirschner wire.

5 to 13 years old. Radiographic growth measurements have shown an average phalangeal growth of 90%, provided that the physis remained open. If a suitable soft-tissue envelope and adequate bony support are available in a child younger than 18 months old, phalangeal transfer can be performed with a reasonable expectation that digital length would be improved. Goldberg and Watson described a dorsal approach for inserting the phalanges, as opposed to Toby et al., who used a volar approach for identification of the flexor tendon, tenolysis and attachment to the phalangeal transfer, and reconstruction of the joint volar plate and collateral ligament complex. Radocha et al. reported mean growth rates of 1 mm per year in 73 children who had toe phalangeal transplantation on or before 1 year of age; tendon and collateral ligament reattachment was beneficial.

metacarpal bone and periosteum, application of external fixation, and gradual distraction of approximately 1 mm per day until the desired length is achieved or neurovascular or cutaneous limits are reached. Cowen and Loftus reported lengthening of the entire palm through the carpometacarpal joints with the use of distal metacarpal and proximal carpal pins. Although the usual length achieved is 25 to 50 mm, Cowen and Loftus reported gaining 7 cm. Lengthening of hand and forearm bones with an Ilizarov distraction apparatus has been reported. Lengthening within a digit should be avoided; the shortest bone to which the device can be applied is about 3 cm.

A one-stage, nonvascularized, extraperiosteal toe-phalanx transplantation as an interpositional or terminal graft may be beneficial for the extremely hypoplastic digit. Physeal patency has been shown in 90% of children operated on between 6 and 18 months of age, in 67% of children 18 months to 5 years old, and in 50% of children

METACARPAL LENGTHENING

TECHNIQUE 17.14   *Figure 17.25*

(TAJIMA)
- Under tourniquet control, make a dorsal longitudinal incision over the shortened metacarpal.
- Retract the extensor tendon to one side and expose the metacarpal shaft subperiosteally.
- Make two V-shaped osteotomies at the junction of the proximal and middle thirds of the bone.
- Expose the deep transverse metacarpal ligament distally and incise it.
- Sharply detach the interosseous muscle on both sides of the metacarpal.

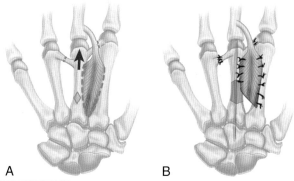

FIGURE **17.25** Tajima technique for metacarpal lengthening in hypoplastic hand. **A,** Chevron osteotomy is made in shortened metacarpal; interosseous muscle and transverse metacarpal ligaments are released. **B,** Bone graft is interposed and secured with axial Kirschner wire; transverse metacarpal ligaments are repaired if possible. **SEE TECHNIQUE 17.14.**

■ Manually distract the metacarpal to ensure that the osteotomy incisions are adequate.
■ Harvest the iliac crest bone graft and fashion it to fill the gap in the lengthened bone.
■ Insert the graft and secure it with a longitudinal Kirschner wire.
■ Reattach the interosseous muscle to the periosteum through separate drill holes into either the bone graft or the metacarpal, depending on where the interosseous muscle falls into place after lengthening.
■ Suture the skin in routine fashion and apply a cast or splint.

POSTOPERATIVE CARE The osteotomy is protected with a cast or splint until union occurs, but motion of the finger is begun 3 weeks after surgery. The Kirschner wire can be removed at 6 weeks.

LENGTHENING WITH DISTRACTION STAGE I

TECHNIQUE 17.15

(COWEN AND LOFTUS)
■ In stage I under tourniquet control, make a Z-type incision on the dorsum of the hand and make an osteotomy of the involved metacarpals.
■ Manually distract the bone to ensure complete release of the soft tissues.
■ Insert a transverse 0.062-inch Kirschner wire through the metacarpal distal to the osteotomy site. Insert this wire into the rectangular blocks of the distraction device.
■ Using the device as a drill guide, place two additional Kirschner wires transversely through the metacarpal if possible.
■ Use the same technique to insert the proximal wires.
■ Release the tourniquet and observe circulation.
■ Make a few turns of the distraction device.
■ Close the incision in routine fashion.
■ If complete closure is impossible after distraction, the open portion of the incision can be allowed to granulate or can be covered with a split-thickness graft.

POSTOPERATIVE CARE The patient is kept in the hospital for a few days after the procedure for careful observation. The patient or parents are instructed to increase the distraction by one third of a turn three times daily or by one-half turn twice daily. This amounts to approximately 1 mm of lengthening per day. This process is continued until the desired length is achieved and may require 3 months. Close observation by the surgeon and the parents during this process is mandatory to recognize any neurovascular compromise. When desired lengthening is obtained or neurovascular or cutaneous limits have been reached, the second stage of the procedure is performed.

LENGTHENING WITH DISTRACTION STAGE II

TECHNIQUE 17.16

(COWEN AND LOFTUS)
■ In stage II, make a dorsal incision over the metacarpals that are to be grafted.
■ Harvest donor bone graft from the iliac crest, ulna, fibula, or toe phalanx, and insert this into the bony defect created by distraction.
■ Stabilize the graft with a longitudinal Kirschner wire, or leave the external fixator in place.
■ Close the incision, deflate the tourniquet, and apply a short arm cast with a protective plaster bow in older children or a long arm cast in infants.

POSTOPERATIVE CARE After 1 to 2 weeks, the cast is replaced by a sling or wrap that covers the entire hand and distraction device. The apparatus and Kirschner wires are removed when sufficient time has passed to allow bone healing (usually ≥8 weeks). The hand is protected with a cast or splint as needed, depending on the radiographic and clinical progress.

CALLOTASIS METACARPAL LENGTHENING

TECHNIQUE 17.17

(KATO ET AL.)
- For lengthening of the long finger, make a straight skin incision on the dorsoradial side; for the little finger, make the incision on the dorsoulnar side.
- Preserve and retract the subcutaneous sensory nerve and the extensor tendons.
- Incise the periosteum longitudinally at the intended osteotomy site and carefully retract it.
- Apply a unilateral external fixation with four half-pins (1.5 or 2.0 mm)
- Under fluoroscopic control, using the external fixator frame as a guide, insert two half-pins into the distal metacarpal and two into the proximal metacarpal. These pins should be placed so as not to impinge on the extensor mechanism of the metacarpophalangeal joint or irritate the extensor or flexor tendon. Insert them from a slight radial-to-ulnar direction in the long finger and from an ulnar-to-radial direction in the little finger.
- After all four pins are inserted, mount the external fixator and adjust all blocks and screws.
- Remove the frame and use an osteotome to make a transverse osteotomy between the center of the distal and proximal pins.
- Adjust the fixator and firmly secure all clamps.
- Close the bone gap caused by the osteotomy, suture the periosteum and close the skin.

POSTOPERATIVE CARE Lengthening is begun 5 days after the operation. Patients are discharged for home recovery and resumption of school activities. Parents conduct lengthening at a rate of 0.25 mm twice a day. For the first 3 weeks, the distance of the distraction gap, the alignment of the metacarpal, and the callus formation are monitored with twice-weekly radiographs. Based on the status of the callus formation, the rate of distraction is increased from 0.25 to 1 mm per day. Four weeks after surgery, radiographs are obtained once a week. Throughout the period of fixator wear, patients are encouraged to move the elongated digits through a full range of motion and to use the hand actively in daily life. When the expected length is achieved and abundant callus formation is present, the fixator and pins are removed.

TOE-PHALANX TRANSPLANTATION

TECHNIQUE 17.18

- Under tourniquet control, make a dorsal longitudinal incision over the second toe, which usually is excessively long

and is the donor of choice; similar grafts can be harvested from the third or fourth toes if desired. Carry the incision through the skin, subcutaneous tissue, and extensor mechanism.
- Harvest the proximal phalanx, including the periosteum, as described by Goldberg and Watson, in an attempt to retain physeal growth.
- Close the donor site with simple sutures.
- The cartilage over each end of the donor phalanx may or may not be retained, depending on whether some pseudojoint function is desirable.
- Make a dorsal longitudinal incision over the hypoplastic digit, which may be represented only by an empty skin tube.
- Place the toe phalanx within the hypoplastic digit in axial alignment with the adjacent bone and secure it with a longitudinal Kirschner wire. This can be used as an interpositional graft or terminal graft.
- Close the skin with interrupted sutures and apply a supportive dressing.
- After the digit viability is certain, apply a cast of appropriate length.

POSTOPERATIVE CARE The cast is maintained for approximately 6 weeks. Kirschner wires are removed, and activities are increased gradually.

TOE-PHALANX TRANSPLANTATION

TECHNIQUE 17.19

(TOBY ET AL.)
- Make a volar zigzag incision over the distal palm and soft-tissue bud of the absent digit. Protect the neurovascular elements.
- Using a small hemostat, gently spread the soft tissue to produce a cavity where the toe phalanx is to be placed.
- Dissect the flexor tendons and their anlagen to the absent digit and preserve the attachments to the soft-tissue pouch.
- Lyse adhesions proximal to the distal insertion to improve excursion of the flexor tendon.
- Select a suitable proximal toe phalanx from the third or fourth toe. Make a dorsal diagonal incision over the proximal phalanx of the toe and harvest the phalanx extraperiosteally.
- Incise the soft-tissue attachments of the proximal interphalangeal joint close to the bone.
- Incise the volar plate and collateral ligaments at the metatarsal origin en bloc.
- Remove the toe phalanx capsule, volar plate, medial and lateral collateral ligaments, and accessory collateral ligament of the metatarsophalangeal joint as a single unit.
- Pass a small Kirschner wire proximally into the harvested toe phalanx.

- After placing the composite phalanx transfer into the soft-tissue pouch, advance the Kirschner wire distally and pass it in a retrograde manner into the recipient metacarpal so that the skin of the pouch is not compromised by the pin.
- Align the volar plate and collateral ligament structures of the toe phalanx in a nearly anatomic position over the metacarpal head.
- Because of their secured position with the Kirschner wire, the volar plate and collateral ligaments can be sutured to adjacent soft tissue or left to heal to the adjacent tissue.
- Center the flexor tendon over the transferred phalanx by suturing it to the periosteum.
- Fix the donor toe with a longitudinal Kirschner wire holding the middle phalanx at a distance from the metatarsal head.

POSTOPERATIVE CARE The pins are removed from the hand and the foot at 6 weeks, and the child is encouraged to actively flex and extend the digits of both.

ANTEROPOSTERIOR AXIS
■ RADIAL (THUMB) DEFICIENCY/HYPOPLASTIC THUMB

The designation "hypoplastic thumb" generally applies to any thumb with some degree of deficiency in any of its anatomic parts—osseous, musculotendinous, or ectodermal. The thumb may be functional but simply shorter than normal or, in the most severe manifestation, totally absent. The hypoplastic thumb constituted 3.6% of anomalies in Flatt's series and 1.3% in the Yokohama series; hypoplasia of the whole hand represented 0.8% in Flatt's series, and absence of the thumb represented 1.4%. Because of the wide variety of deformities produced by hypoplasia of the thumb, etiologic factors also vary. Many of these deformities are sporadic occurrences, but some are transmitted genetically or are associated with specific syndromes. Thumb hypoplasia can occur with radial hypoplasia and is bilateral in 20% to 60% of cases. The six types of hypoplastic thumb are based on the appearance of the deformity and the deficient structures and include short thumb, adducted thumb, abducted thumb, floating thumb, absent thumb, and clasped thumb. An alternative classification system that has become popular is the Blauth system, in which the hypoplastic thumb is classified into five types: type I, minor generalized hypoplasia (short thumb); type II, adduction contracture with deficient intrinsics and an unstable metacarpophalangeal joint (adducted thumb or abducted thumb); type III, deficient extrinsic muscles; type IV, deficient osseous structures, specifically the thumb metacarpal (floating thumb); and type V, absent. Manske suggested dividing the type III thumbs into type IIIA, which has thumb metacarpal hypoplasia with a stable carpometacarpal joint, and type IIIB, which has partial metacarpal aplasia and an unstable carpometacarpal joint. In this classification scheme, the presence of a stable carpometacarpal joint determines whether the thumb should be reconstructed or amputated and pollicization done (Table 17.7). McDonald et al. recommended a staged procedure to reconstruct type IIIA thumbs at 2 years of age, with the first stage including web space deepening, stabilization of the metacarpophalangeal joint, and transfer of the flexor digitorum sublimis to FPL followed later by an extensor indicis proprius to EPL transfer and Huber opponensplasty (see Technique 17.26).

▌TYPE I HYPOPLASIA (SHORTENED THUMB)

The normal thumb extends to about the level of the proximal interphalangeal joint of the index finger; a thumb is considered "short" if its length is less than this. Hypoplasia of any or all osseous components produces a thumb that is significantly shorter than normal. The short thumb frequently is associated with other anomalies and syndromes. When the metacarpal is short and slender, it may be a manifestation of a syndrome such as Fanconi, Holt-Oram, or Juberg-Hayward syndrome; it also may be associated with other malformations of the spine and cardiovascular and gastrointestinal systems. When the metacarpus is short and broad, it may be associated with Cornelia de Lange syndrome, hand-foot-uterus syndrome, diastrophic dwarfism, or myositis ossificans progressiva. Shortening of the proximal phalanx of the thumb may be associated with brachydactyly. The distal phalanx may be broad and short in association with Rubinstein-Taybi, Apert, Carpenter, or hand-foot-uterus syndrome. The thumb may be radially deviated ("hitchhiker's thumb") or very short and stubby ("potter's thumb" or "murderer's thumb"). A slender distal phalanx may be associated with Fanconi or Holt-Oram syndrome.

Treatment. If a hypoplastic thumb is only short, surgical correction rarely is indicated. If prehension is significantly limited, deepening of the web space may be sufficient to create a relative lengthening of the thumb in relation to objects that are grasped. This can be achieved with a two-limb or four-limb Z-plasty.

▌TYPE II HYPOPLASIA (ADDUCTED THUMB)

An adducted thumb usually is caused by absence or partial absence of the thenar muscles, which results in deficient opposition. These thumbs often lack a functional FPL muscle. The radial collateral ligament of the thumb metacarpophalangeal joint also may be deficient. The thumb usually is shortened and tapered, with a flattened thenar eminence and a deficient first web space. The deformity usually is transmitted as an autosomal dominant trait and usually is unilateral.

Treatment. The goals of surgical reconstruction of the adducted thumb are correction of the adduction contracture and restoration of opposition. The adduction contracture can be corrected by a two-limb or four-limb Z-plasty or a sliding dorsal flap raised from the radial side of the index finger. The two-limb Z-plasty rarely attains adequate correction. Less than 50% of web space spread generally is considered inadequate. The two most popular techniques for restoration of opposition are the ring flexor superficialis tendon opponensplasty and the abductor digiti quinti opponensplasty, as described by Huber and popularized by Littler and Cooley. The Huber procedure allows creation of a more nearly normal-appearing thenar eminence. An overlying hypothenar skin paddle can be incorporated with the abductor digiti minimi as described initially by Chase et al. and more recently by Upton and Taghinia. This eliminates routing the muscle through tight palmar tissues and improves thenar bulk

TABLE 17.7

Thumb Deficiency Classification and Treatment Paradigm

TYPE	FINDINGS	TREATMENT
I	Minor generalized hypoplasia	No treatment
II	Intrinsic thenar muscles hypoplasia First web space narrowing UCL insufficiency	Opponensplasty First web release UCL reconstruction
III	Similar findings as type II plus: Extrinsic muscle and tendon abnormalities Bone deficiency A: Stable CMC joint B: Unstable CMC joint	A: Reconstruction B: Pollicization
IV	Pouce flottant or floating thumb	Pollicization
V	Absent thumb	Pollicization

CMC, carpometacarpal; *UCL,* ulnar collateral ligament.
From Soldado F, Zlotolow DA, Kozin SH: Thumb hypoplasia, *J Hand Surg* 38A: 1435, 2013.

and appearance. Littler and Cooley also described the use of an abdominal flap (Fig. 17.26) for reconstruction of the adducted thumb. Upton et al. reported excellent results after the use of pedicled, distally based radial and dorsal interosseous forearm fasciocutaneous island flaps. This technique is described in chapter 2. Often the metacarpophalangeal joint is unstable and the ulnar collateral ligament is in need of reconstruction. This can be accomplished by reefing the ulnar ligamentous tissues, advancing them distally, and augmenting them with the distal portion of the sublimis tendon when performing an opponensplasty, free tendon reconstruction, or metacarpophalangeal chondrodesis (Fig. 17.27).

SIMPLE Z-PLASTY OF THE THUMB WEB

TECHNIQUE 17.20

- Before inflating the tourniquet, diagram the appropriate skin incision, designing the flap with its longitudinal axis along the distal ridge of the first web space and extending from the proximal thumb crease to approximately 1 cm proximal to the proximal digital crease of the index finger at a point that corresponds to the radial confluence of the proximal and middle palmar creases. Draw an oblique proximal palmar limb and a distal dorsal limb at an approximately 60-degree angle, with the lengths of both limbs corresponding to the longitudinal incision (Fig. 17.28A). In designing these flaps, keep in mind the basic principle of all Z-plasty procedures: all flap sides must be of equal lengths.
- Inflate the tourniquet and make the appropriate incisions as outlined.

- Elevate the flaps sharply, carefully undermining to avoid vascular compromise.
- If additional depth is needed, sharply dissect the distal edge of the web space musculature to obtain a partial recession.
- Reverse the flaps and carefully suture them with interrupted 6-0 nylon sutures or absorbable skin sutures (Fig. 17.28B). Mattress sutures can be used to help prevent tip necrosis.
- Deflate the tourniquet, check for adequate blood supply to the flaps, and apply a sterile dressing with the thumb splinted in the abducted, opposed position.

POSTOPERATIVE CARE The splint and sutures are removed 2 weeks after surgery, and free use of the hand is allowed if healing has progressed adequately.

FOUR-FLAP Z-PLASTY

TECHNIQUE 17.21

(BROADBENT AND WOOLF, MODIFIED)
- Before inflating the tourniquet, outline the flaps.
- Make the longitudinal axis of the Z-plasty along the distal edge of the thumb web ridge, extending from the ulnar margin of the proximal thumb crease to an area approximately 1 cm proximal to the proximal digital crease of the index finger.
- Draw proximal palmar and distal dorsal limbs at 90-degree angles to the longitudinal axis; the lengths of these limbs should equal that of the longitudinal incision (Fig. 17.29A). Bisect each angle with an additional oblique

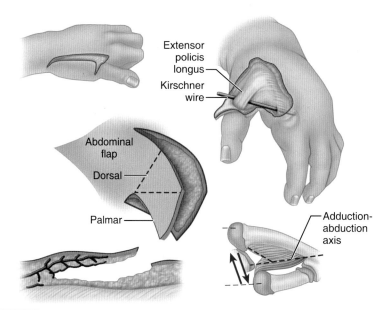

FIGURE 17.26 Littler correction of adduction contracture of thumb using abdominal flap based on thoracoepigastric vessels.

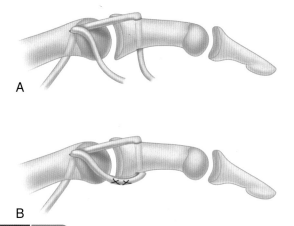

FIGURE 17.27 **A** and **B,** Flexor digitorum sublimis opposition transfer with collateral ligament repair.

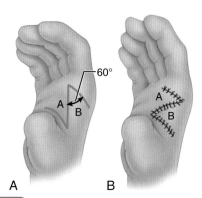

FIGURE 17.28 Simple Z-plasty of thumb web. **A,** Incisions. **B,** Closure after reversal of flaps. **SEE TECHNIQUE 17.20.**

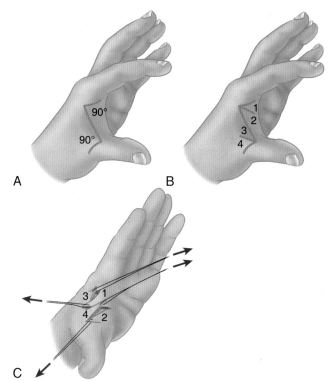

FIGURE 17.29 Broadbent and Woolf four-flap Z-plasty for lengthening first web in adducted thumb. **A,** Ninety-degree dorsal and volar flaps are marked in first web. **B,** These two flaps are bisected to create four flaps. **C,** Flaps are elevated, transposed, and interdigitated to complete lengthening. **SEE TECHNIQUE 17.21.**

limb, again with the length corresponding to the length of the other flap margins (Fig. 17.29B).
- Inflate the tourniquet and make the appropriate incisions.

- Sharply elevate the flaps, elevating the skin and a small amount of subcutaneous tissue.

- For further deepening, perform a small recession of the thumb web musculature in its midsubstance. Do not perform a complete myotomy.
- Interdigitate the appropriate flaps and suture them with 6-0 monofilament nylon. It is helpful to label the flaps before incision; if the flaps are labeled 1, 2, 3, and 4, beginning from the radialmost flap and ending at the ulnarmost flap, the sequence after interdigitation should be 3, 1, 4, 2 (Fig. 17.29C).
- Deflate the tourniquet, inspect the flaps for viability, and apply a bulky dressing with the thumb splinted in the abducted position.

POSTOPERATIVE CARE The sutures and splint are removed 2 weeks after surgery. If desired, a small web-spacer splint can be used for an additional 2 weeks.

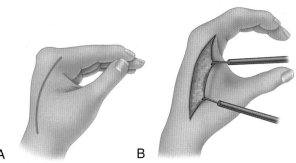

A   B

FIGURE **17.30** Dorsal sliding flap for correction of adduction deformity of first web. **A,** Incision. **B,** Radial flap is undermined, and dorsal defect is covered with split-thickness skin graft. **SEE TECHNIQUE 17.22.**

WEB DEEPENING WITH A SLIDING FLAP

TECHNIQUE 17.22   *Figure 17.30*

(BRAND AND MILFORD)
- Before inflating the tourniquet, design the flaps by drawing a line dorsally from the apex of the first and second metacarpals and extending it distally to the radial side of the proximal phalanx of the index finger. Curve the line back across the web space into the palm proximally to the apex of the first and second metacarpals.
- Exsanguinate the arm, inflate the tourniquet, and make the skin incisions as outlined.
- Sharply elevate the skin flaps with a small amount of subcutaneous tissue.
- Release any thickened dorsal and volar fascia carefully to avoid injury to the neurovascular structures.
- If severe contracture is present, incise the capsule of the carpometacarpal joint of the thumb.
- Pull the thumb away from the palm and hold it with a Kirschner wire.
- Allow the flap to slide with the thumb and use it to cover the thumb and palmar web.
- Cover the dorsal defect with a split-thickness skin graft.
- Suture the flaps in place with interrupted 6-0 nylon sutures and secure and bolster the skin graft.
- Deflate the tourniquet, inspect the flaps for viability, and apply a sterile dressing with the thumb splinted in the abducted position.

POSTOPERATIVE CARE Sutures are removed at 2 weeks, and the Kirschner wire is removed at 4 weeks, after which unrestricted motion of the thumb is allowed.

OPPONENSPLASTY

TECHNIQUE 17.23

(MANSKE AND MCCARROLL)
- Make an incision beginning over the ulnar border of the proximal phalanx of the little finger and palm, curving radialward proximal to the metacarpophalangeal joint and crossing the wrist crease on the radial side of the pisiform (Fig. 17.31A).
- Detach the tendinous insertions into the extensor hood and the proximal phalanx of the little finger, retaining as much tendon length as possible (Fig. 17.31B).
- Starting distally, dissect the abductor digiti minimi muscle out of its fascial sheath to its origin at the pisiform, avoiding dissection on the proximal and radial sides of the muscle where the neurovascular structures enter.
- Make a second incision over the dorsoradial aspect of the metacarpophalangeal joint of the thumb and pass the muscle through a large subcutaneous tunnel between the thumb incision and the proximal ulnar incision (Fig. 17.31C). Ensure that the muscle glides freely in the tunnel and is not restricted by soft tissue.
- The method of insertion of the transferred tendon at the metacarpophalangeal joint (Fig. 17.32A) depends on the patient's deformity. In patients with thenar aplasia with other radial anomalies, suture one of the transferred slips to the soft tissue at the radial aspect of the base of the proximal phalanx and the other to the extensor pollicis longus muscle at the level of the metacarpophalangeal joint as recommended by Riordan, Powers, and Hurd (Fig. 17.32B).
- In patients with isolated thenar aplasia, stabilize the metacarpophalangeal joint by imbricating the ulnar capsule in a pants-over-vest fashion (Fig. 17.32C). Suture one of the tendinous insertions to the radial capsule and the other to the imbricated ulnar capsule and to the extensor pollicis longus tendon (Fig. 17.32D).
- If the opponensplasty is performed after pollicization, suture one slip to the radial lateral band and the other to the central slip at the proximal interphalangeal joint of the pollicized finger (Fig. 17.32E).
- Close the incisions in routine fashion and apply a bulky dressing and splint, holding the thumb in opposition.

POSTOPERATIVE CARE Three weeks after surgery, the bulky dressing is removed and the thumb is taped into opposition for an additional 3 weeks; the child is encouraged to use the hand. Six weeks after surgery, all dressings are discontinued. Formal retraining of the transfer usually is unnecessary.

RING SUBLIMIS OPPONENSPLASTY

TECHNIQUE 17.24

(RIORDAN)

- Expose the sublimis tendon of the ring finger through an ulnar midlateral incision over the proximal interphalan-

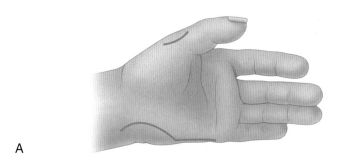

A

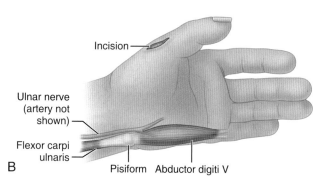

Incision

Ulnar nerve (artery not shown)

Flexor carpi ulnaris

B

Pisiform   Abductor digiti V

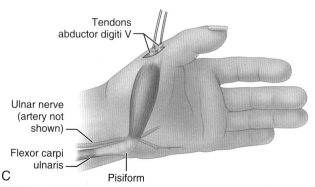

Tendons abductor digiti V

Ulnar nerve (artery not shown)

Flexor carpi ulnaris

C

Pisiform

FIGURE 17.31 Manske and McCarroll abductor digiti minimi opponensplasty (see text). **A,** Incisions. **B,** Detachment of tendinous insertions. **C,** Abductor digiti minimi passed through subcutaneous tunnel. **SEE TECHNIQUE 17.23.**

geal joint and divide the tendon at the level of the joint or just proximal to it.

- Divide the chiasm, separating the two slips of tendon at the level of the joint so that they pass around the profundus and can be easily withdrawn at the wrist.

- Expose the flexor carpi ulnaris tendon through an L-shaped incision that extends proximally along the flexor carpi ulnaris tendon and distally turns radialward, parallel with the flexor creases of the wrist.

- To make a pulley, cut halfway through the flexor carpi ulnaris tendon at a point approximately 6.3 cm proximal to the pisiform (Fig. 17.33).

- Strip the radial half of the tendon distally almost to the pisiform and create a loop large enough for the sublimis tendon to pass through easily; carry the end of the radial segment of the flexor carpi ulnaris through a split in the remaining half of the tendon, loop it back, and suture it to the remaining half.

- Make a wide C-shaped incision on the thumb as follows. Begin on the dorsum of the thumb just proximal to the interphalangeal joint and proceed proximally and volarward around to the radial aspect of the thumb. At a point just proximal to the metacarpophalangeal joint, curve the incision dorsalward in line with the major skin creases of the thenar eminence.

- Preserve on the dorsoradial aspect of the thumb the fine sensory nerve from the superficial branch of the radial nerve.

- Expose and define the extensor pollicis longus tendon over the proximal phalanx, the extensor aponeurosis over the metacarpophalangeal joint, and the tendon of the abductor pollicis brevis.

- At the wrist, identify the sublimis tendon to the ring finger and withdraw it into the forearm incision.

- Pass the tendon through the loop fashioned from the flexor carpi ulnaris.

- With a small hemostat or a tendon carrier, pass the tendon subcutaneously across the thenar eminence in line with the fibers of the abductor pollicis brevis.

- Make a small tunnel for insertion of the transfer by burrowing between two small parallel incisions in the abductor pollicis brevis tendon.

- Split the end of the sublimis tendon for approximately 2.5 cm, or more if necessary, and pass one half of it through the tunnel.

- Separate the extensor aponeurosis from the periosteum of the proximal phalanx of the thumb, make a small incision in it 6 mm distal to the first tunnel, and pass the same strip of sublimis through it.

- Bring the slip out from beneath the aponeurosis through a small longitudinal slit in the long extensor tendon about 3 mm proximal to the interphalangeal joint.

- Determine the proper tension for the transfer. Grasp the two slips of sublimis with small hemostats and cross them. With the thumb in full opposition and the wrist in a straight line, place the two overlapping slips of sublimis under some tension. Releasing the thumb and passively flexing the wrist should completely relax the transfer so that the thumb can be brought into full extension and abduction; extending the wrist 45 degrees should place

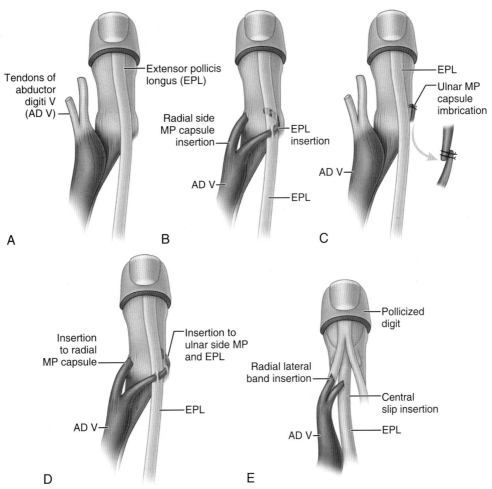

FIGURE 17.32 Manske and McCarroll technique. **A,** Tendon insertion at thumb metacarpophalangeal joint depends on patient's deformity. **B,** Insertion in patients with thenar aplasia and other radial anomalies. **C** and **D,** Insertion in patients with isolated thenar aplasia. **E,** Insertion when opponensplasty follows pollicization. **SEE TECHNIQUE 17.23.**

enough tension on the transfer to bring the thumb into complete opposition and the tip of the thumb into complete extension.

- If the tension is insufficient, increase it and repeat the test.
- When the correct tension has been determined, suture the slips of sublimis together with the cut ends buried (Fig. 17.33, inset).
- Anchor the transfer and the tendon of the abductor pollicis brevis to the joint capsule with a single nylon or wire suture so that the transfer passes over the exact middle of the metacarpal head; this prevents later displacement of the tendon toward the palmar aspect of the joint during opposition.
- Close the wound with nonabsorbable sutures and immobilize the hand in a pressure dressing and a dorsal plaster splint as follows.
- Place the wrist in 30 degrees of flexion, the fingers in the functional position, and the thumb in full opposition with the distal phalanx extended; place a few layers of gauze

between the individual fingers to prevent maceration of the skin.

POSTOPERATIVE CARE At 3 weeks, the dressing and splint are removed and active motion is begun, but the thumb is supported with an opponens splint for an additional 6 weeks. Many patients can oppose the thumb as soon as the splint is removed. When the sublimis of the ring finger has been used for the transfer, as in the Riordan technique, training in its use may be facilitated by asking the patient to place the tip of the thumb against the ring finger; this maneuver produces flexion of the ring finger and an automatic attempt to oppose the thumb with the transferred sublimis. In patients with weak quadriceps muscles who habitually rise from a sitting position by pushing up with the flattened hands or in patients who use crutches, the transfer must be protected for 3 months or longer, or it becomes overstretched and ceases to function.

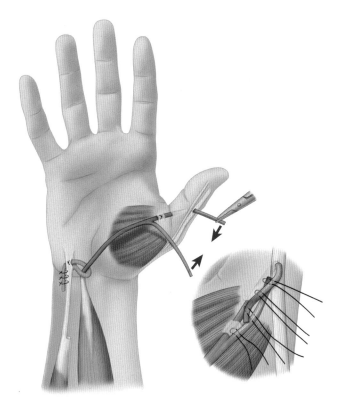

Opponensplasty of ring sublimis for adduction contracture of thumb. **SEE TECHNIQUE 17.24.**

2 to 3 cm of flexor carpi ulnaris tendon and harvest one half of the tendon preserving its distal attachment. Pass the harvested half through the retained flexor carpi ulnaris at the pisiform to create a loop. Suture the tendon weave with nonabsorbable braided suture. Pass the ring finger flexor digitorum superficialis through the flexor carpi ulnaris (Fig. 17.34D,E).

- Create a subcutaneous tunnel between the radial side of the thumb and volar forearm incision for passage of the ring finger flexor digitorum superficialis tendon. Pass the flexor digitorum superficialis tendon under the skin to the radial side of the thumb (Fig. 17.34F).
- Isolate the metacarpal head and drill a 0.45-inch Kirschner wire across the metacarpal head parallel to the joint surface. Using mini-fluoroscopy to ensure proper wire placement, direct the wire from the volar aspect of the radial side of the metacarpal to the ulnar and dorsal aspects. Enlarge the hole with a drill bit to allow passage of the flexor digitorum superficialis tendon (Fig. 17.34G).
- Reduce the metacarpophalangeal joint and stabilize it with a longitudinal 0.45-inch Kirschner wire drilled antegrade from the tip of the thumb. Cut the wire short and apply a Jurgan Pin Ball (RFO Medical, London, UK).
- Pass the flexor digitorum superficialis through the drill hole to the ulnar side of the thumb for ligament reconstruction (Fig. 17.34H). If the tendon is too large in diameter, one flexor digitorum superficialis slip can be removed.
- Place the wrist into slight extension and tension the flexor digitorum superficialis tendon until the thumb moves into opposition. Tenodesis is used to assess tension; once correct tension has been achieved, suture the flexor digitorum superficialis tendon to the surrounding bone and periosteum along the radial side of the thumb. This maneuver sets the tension in the opposition transfer.
- Use the remaining flexor digitorum superficialis tendon along the ulnar side of the thumb to reconstruct the ulnar collateral ligament. Direct the flexor digitorum superficialis tendon to the base of the proximal phalanx and suture it directly onto bone. Usually there is adequate length to pass the extra flexor digitorum superficialis tendon back onto itself to complete a double-stranded repair.
- Close the skin with absorbable suture and immobilize the limb in a long arm–thumb spica cast.

POSTOPERATIVE CARE   The thumb spica cast and Kirschner wire are removed at 3 weeks. A short arm–thumb spica splint is then applied. Active motion and therapy are initiated at this time.

RING SUBLIMIS OPPONENSPLASTY WITH ULNAR COLLATERAL LIGAMENT RECONSTRUCTION

TECHNIQUE 17.25

(KOZIN AND EZAKI)
- To widen the narrow thumb index web space, create a four-flap Z-plasty, extending the radial limb proximally to expose the ulnar collateral ligament and the metacarpophalangeal joint (Fig. 17.34A).
- Isolate the ring finger flexor digitorum superficialis tendon at the base of the finger and in the distal forearm. Make a short oblique incision at the base of the ring finger and a zigzag or oblique incision along the ulnar portion of the volar forearm. Isolate the flexor carpi ulnaris tendon. Make an additional skin incision along the radial side of the thumb metacarpophalangeal joint to expose the site for the flexor digitorum superficialis tendon attachment (Fig. 17.34B).
- Identify the ring finger flexor digitorum superficialis in the base of the finger and within the forearm (Fig. 17.34C). Tag the flexor digitorum superficialis with a suture and cut it at the base of the ring finger while protecting the underlying flexor digitorum profundus tendon.
- Place a forceps around the ring flexor digitorum superficialis tendon in the forearm and use it to roll the tendon through the carpal tunnel and into the forearm.
- Use a loop of flexor carpi ulnaris tendon to construct a pulley for the flexor digitorum superficialis tendon. Isolate the distal

ABDUCTOR DIGITI QUINTI OPPONENSPLASTY

TECHNIQUE 17.26

(HUBER; LITTLER AND COOLEY)
- Make a curved palmar incision along the radial border of the abductor digiti quinti muscle belly, extending from the proximal side of the pisiform proximally to the ulnar border of the little finger distally.

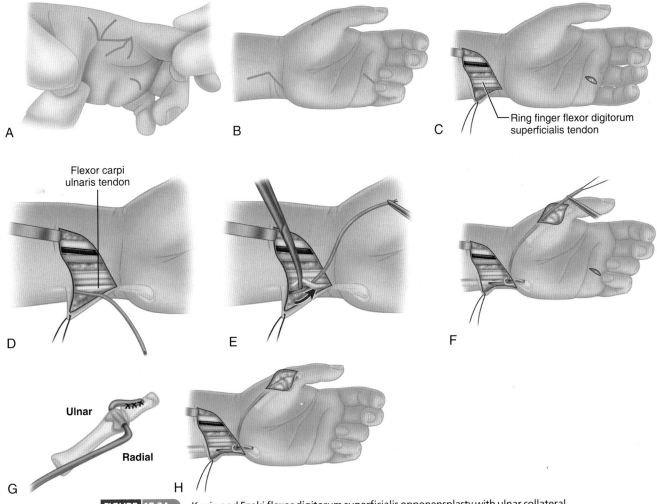

FIGURE 17.34 Kozin and Ezaki flexor digitorum superficialis opponensplasty with ulnar collateral ligament reconstruction. **A,** Four-flap Z-plasty. **B,** Incisions. **C,** Ring finger flexor digitorum superficialis identified at base of finger. **D** and **E,** Pulley construction. **E,** Ring finger flexor digitorum passed through flexor carpi ulnaris loop. **F,** Flexor digitorum superficialis tendon passed through subcutaneous tunnel to radial side of thumb. **G,** Kirschner wire drilled across metacarpal head. **H,** Flexor digitorum superficialis tendon passed through metacarpal head to ulnar side of thumb. **SEE TECHNIQUE 17.25.**

- Free both tendinous insertions of the muscle, one from the extensor expansion and the other from the base of the proximal phalanx.
- Lift the muscle from its fascial compartment and carefully expose its neurovascular bundle. Isolate the bundle, taking care not to damage the veins.
- Free the origin of the muscle from the pisiform but retain the origin on the flexor carpi ulnaris tendon; now the muscle can be mobilized enough for its insertion to reach the thumb.
- Make a curved incision on the radial border of the thenar eminence and create across the palm a subcutaneous pocket to receive the transfer.
- Fold the abductor digiti quinti muscle over about 170 degrees (like a page of a book) and pass it subcutaneously to the thumb.
- Suture its tendons of insertion to the insertion of the abductor pollicis brevis.
- Throughout the procedure, avoid compression of and undue tension on the muscle and its neurovascular pedicle.

- Apply a carefully formed light compression dressing and a volar plaster splint to hold the thumb in abduction and the wrist in slight flexion.

POSTOPERATIVE CARE The plaster splint is removed in 4 weeks, at which time active motion and active-assisted range of motion are begun. A removable thumb splint is worn for 3 months during sleep.

TYPE II AND TYPE III HYPOPLASIA (ABDUCTED THUMB)

The abducted thumb deformity was described in 1969 by Tupper, who reported four patients with mildly hypoplastic thumbs and associated abduction deformities. He called this pollex abductus and believed it resulted from an abnormal insertion of the FPL muscle into an otherwise normal EPL muscle, causing marked abduction of the proximal phalanx of the thumb. This was verified at the time of reconstruction, when he also noted deficiencies in the thenar musculature, adduction contracture of the first metacarpal with web space deficiency, marked laxity of the ulnar collateral ligament, radial and superficial displacement of the FPL, and inability to flex the interphalangeal joint of the thumb. This is an extremely rare deformity, and few cases have been reported. In some cases of type IIIA hypoplasia, extrinsic tendons may be severely hypoplastic or absent. When absent, the FPL can be reconstructed from the sublimis of the long finger, and pulley reconstruction is done with a tendon graft. A Huber opponensplasty can then be performed in a staged manner. In the presence of an EPL deficiency an extensor indicis proprius transfer to the base of the distal phalanx can be performed in staged fashion at the time of opponensplasty. Often, severe limitation of interphalangeal joint motion is present. Appropriate passive range of motion must exist for extrinsic tendon reconstruction. Some authors advocate passive range of motion of at least 35 degrees.

Treatment. There have been almost as many surgical procedures described for an abducted thumb as there have been cases reported: release of the bifurcated tendon insertion and reattachment to the metacarpal neck; release of the tendon distally, withdrawal at the wrist, and reattachment to the distal phalanx; and release of the anomalous slip to the EPL muscle, with an ulnarward shift of the EPL at the metacarpophalangeal joint. All procedures have been combined with release of the radial collateral ligament and reefing of the ulnar collateral ligament of the metacarpophalangeal joint, and some have required a secondary opponensplasty. Blair and Omer described a technique in which the FPL is released from its abnormal tendinous insertion and centralized by being moved ulnarward. To complete the transfer, the abductor pollicis brevis musculotendinous junction is divided, the FPL tendon is transferred under the intrinsic muscle, and the intrinsic muscle is reattached. They did not find it necessary to reconstruct the ulnar collateral ligament. For severe web space contracture, Bayne recommended a staged procedure in which the web space is first released and maintained with a Kirschner wire (Fig. 17.35), followed in 6 weeks by a Riordan opponensplasty that uses the ring sublimis and by reconstruction of the ulnar collateral ligament that uses one slip of the sublimis.

Type IIIB hypoplastic thumbs are best characterized by type IIIA deficiencies with extrinsic tendon abnormalities, partial metacarpal aplasia and, most important, instability of the first carpometacarpal joint. Much like types IV and V hypoplasia, type IIIB hypoplasia is best treated with pollicization attempts at thumb preservation. Reconstructive procedures have afforded inferior functional and cosmetic results when compared with pollicization. The most difficult portion of care is management of parental emotions and expectations. Before proceeding with pollicization, multiple office visits, multiple opinions, postoperative photographs, and referral to reputable websites or support groups may be required before the parents settle on a final surgical plan.

Although reconstruction procedures exist, the procedure of choice is amputation of the hypoplastic thumb and index finger pollicization. Further discussion of pollicization is in the treatment of type IV and type V hypoplastic thumbs.

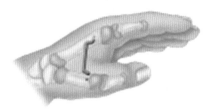

FIGURE 17.35 Staged reconstruction for abducted thumb in which adduction contracture is released and maintained with interposed Kirschner wire; this may be followed in 6 weeks by reconstruction of ulnar collateral ligament and ring sublimis opponensplasty.

REROUTING OF THE FLEXOR POLLICIS LONGUS

TECHNIQUE 17.27

(BLAIR AND OMER)

- Under tourniquet control, make a zigzag palmar incision along the thumb to allow exploration of the flexor pollicis longus, the ulnar collateral ligament, and the extensor pollicis longus.
- Develop the flaps and identify and protect the digital nerves.
- Identify the abnormal tendinous slip of the flexor pollicis longus that passes over the radial border of the thumb and into the extensor pollicis longus, usually between the metacarpophalangeal joint and the interphalangeal joint. Release this abnormal insertion sharply.
- Release the insertion of the abductor pollicis brevis (Fig. 17.36A).
- Transfer the flexor pollicis longus tendon ulnarward under the abductor pollicis brevis tendon (Fig. 17.36B). If the abduction deformity of the thumb metacarpophalangeal joint cannot be corrected, release the radial collateral ligament.
- Suture the abductor pollicis brevis tendon into its normal insertion (Fig. 17.36C). This technique centralizes the flexor pollicis longus and constructs a sling at the metacarpophalangeal joint.
- If there is continued laxity of the ulnar collateral ligament of the thumb metacarpophalangeal joint, use the abnormal tendon slip to reinforce the ligament.
- Suture the skin with simple interrupted sutures and apply a modified thumb spica cast that extends beyond the interphalangeal joint dorsally and stops proximal to the metacarpophalangeal joint on the volar side. This prevents hyperextension and abduction of the thumb but allows metacarpophalangeal flexion and flexor tendon excursion.

POSTOPERATIVE CARE The cast is removed at 6 weeks, and unlimited motion of the hand is allowed.

TYPE IV HYPOPLASIA (POUCE FLOTTANT OR FLOATING THUMB)

"Floating thumb" refers to a small, slender thumb that appears to dangle from the radial border of the hand. Typically, there

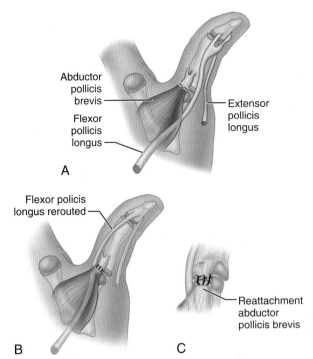

Abductor
pollicis
brevis

Flexor
pollicis
longus

Extensor
pollicis
longus

A

Flexor policis
longus rerouted

Reattachment
abductor
pollicis brevis

B   C

FIGURE 17.36 **A** to **C**, Rerouting of flexor pollicis longus for abducted thumb (Blair and Omer; see text). Flexor pollicis is centralized after tenotomy and reattachment of abductor pollicis brevis. **SEE TECHNIQUE 17.27.**

are two phalanges, a fingernail, no metacarpophalangeal joint, and no first metacarpal (Fig. 17.37). The trapezium and scaphoid also often are absent. The thumb originates more distally than usual, and there is neither extrinsic nor intrinsic muscle function.

Treatment. Amputation is the treatment of choice, followed by index finger pollicization. Despite valiant attempts to restore stability and function to these severely deficient and useless thumbs, the results have not been as rewarding as with pollicization. In bilateral cases, pollicization of one side should be performed early; the parents may decide what to do concerning the other side.

TYPE V HYPOPLASIA (ABSENT THUMB)

Absent thumb is the most severe manifestation of the hypoplastic thumb and may be associated with radial ray deficiencies, ring D chromosome abnormalities, Holt-Oram syndrome, trisomy 18 syndrome, Rothmund-Thomson syndrome, and thalidomide use. Radial clubhand also is associated with an absent thumb except in the TAR syndrome. Absence of the thumb creates an extreme functional impairment, particularly if the anomaly is bilateral. The development of a strong lateral pinch between the index and long fingers compensates for the absence of the thumb, and a fairly strong grip may be developed. Rotational deformity of the fingers allows limited opposition.

Treatment. Function and appearance can be improved with satisfactory pollicization of the index finger. The timing of pollicization is based on the child's natural development of prehensile activities. Because this occurs early,

beginning at age 3 months, the best time for pollicization is between age 6 and 12 months to allow some growth of the hand before surgery. Staines et al. reviewed functional outcomes in children having pollicization for thumb aplasia and found that grip and pinch strengths were about half of the uninvolved hand. Activities that required simultaneous pinch and manipulation of small objects such as buttoning clothes were the most difficult. The choice of procedure usually is between recession and pollicization of the index finger. Recession is preferable in an older child with a strong lateral pinch between the index and long fingers because this pattern may persist despite pollicization. This operation recesses the index finger to make it resemble a thumb more and provides a wider gap between the index and long fingers.

RECESSION OF THE INDEX FINGER

TECHNIQUE 17.28

(FLATT)
- Under tourniquet control, make a dorsal longitudinal 1-cm incision in the first web space.
- Divide the deep transverse metacarpal ligament, palmar and dorsal fascia, and intertendinous connections between the index and middle finger metacarpals. Avoid injury to the neurovascular structures.
- Make a second short, curved dorsoradial incision at the base of the index metacarpal.
- Expose the base of the index metacarpal and perform an osteotomy (Fig. 17.38A). The metacarpal may be easily grasped and maneuvered.
- Reposition the metacarpal into 20 degrees of radial abduction, 35 degrees of palmar abduction, and 100 to 110 degrees of axial rotation (Fig. 17.38B).
- Recess the metacarpal by removing 1.5 to 2.0 cm of the metacarpal shaft.
- When the desired position and recession are achieved, pass a Kirschner wire into adjacent metacarpals to fix the index metacarpal in this position.
- Close the incision routinely (Fig. 17.38C) and apply a well-padded, long arm cast that holds the repositioned index finger in abduction.

POSTOPERATIVE CARE The cast is changed 2 weeks after the operation, and the skin sutures are removed. A long arm cast that supports the pollicized index finger is applied and worn for 4 more weeks. The Kirschner wire is removed when bone healing is complete, usually 4 to 6 weeks after the operation, and progressively increasing activities are allowed. The thumb is splinted in a resting position for another 4 to 6 weeks.

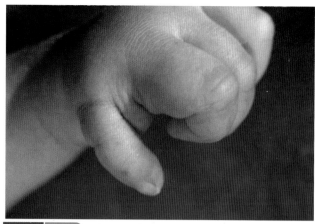

FIGURE 17.37   Floating thumb (pouce flottant) deformity.

POLLICIZATION FOR RECONSTRUCTION OF THE THUMB

Pollicization or transposition of a finger to replace an absent or severely hypoplastic thumb is the procedure of choice for types IIIB, IV, and V thumb hypoplasia. The thumb frequently is absent in patients with radial hypoplasia. Children can adapt to a thumbless hand, with prehension possible using the ulnar side of the index finger and radial side of the long finger. Despite this adaptability, overall function and self-care activities are impaired and can be drastically improved with successful pollicization. Because normal and compensatory prehensile patterns are firmly established within the first year of life, it is desirable that surgical reconstruction be performed early. Pollicization is recommended for unilateral and bilateral cases. If a "floating" thumb deformity is present, with inadequate musculotendinous and bony elements, the remnant should be amputated before pollicization to allow reconstruction of a stable thumb. The parents must be clearly informed that the floating thumb is of no functional use and will be discarded after the operation.

RIORDAN POLLICIZATION

In the Riordan technique, the index ray is shortened by resection of its metacarpal shaft. To simulate the trapezium, the second metacarpal head is positioned palmar to the normal plane of the metacarpal bases, and the metacarpophalangeal joint acts as the carpometacarpal joint of the new thumb. The first dorsal interosseous is converted to an abductor pollicis brevis, and the first volar interosseous is converted to an adductor pollicis. The technique as described is for an immature hand with congenital absence of the thumb, including the greater multangular bone, but it can be modified appropriately for other hands.

TECHNIQUE 17.29

(RIORDAN)

- Beginning on the proximal phalanx of the index finger, make a circumferential oval incision (Fig. 17.39A,B) on the dorsal surface.
- Place the incision level with the middle of the phalanx and on the palmar surface level with the base of the phalanx. From the radiopalmar aspect of this oval, extend the inci-

sion proximally, radially, and dorsally to the radial side of the second metacarpal head, then palmarward and ulnarward to the radial side of the third metacarpal base in the middle of the palm, and finally again radially to end at the radial margin of the base of the palm.

- Dissect the skin from the proximal phalanx of the index finger, leaving the fat attached to the digit and creating a full-thickness skin flap.
- Isolate and free the insertion of the first dorsal interosseous and strip from the radial side of the second metacarpal shaft the origin of the muscle.
- Isolate and free the insertion of the first volar interosseous and strip from the ulnar side of the metacarpal shaft the origin of this muscle. Take care to preserve the nerve and blood supplies to the muscle in each instance.
- Separate the second metacarpal head from the metacarpal shaft by cutting through its epiphysis with a knife; preserve all of its soft-tissue attachments.
- Divide the second metacarpal at its base, leaving intact the insertions of the extensor carpi radialis longus and flexor carpi radialis; discard the metacarpal shaft.
- Carry the index finger proximally and radially and relocate the second metacarpal head palmar to the second metacarpal base so that it simulates a trapezium (Fig. 17.39C); take care to rotate and angulate it so that the new thumb is properly positioned.
- Anchor it in this position with a wire suture (Fig. 17.39D). Anchor the insertion of the first dorsal interosseous to the radial lateral band of the extensor mechanism of the new thumb and its origin to the soft tissues at the base of the digit; this muscle now functions as an abductor pollicis brevis (Fig. 17.39E).
- Anchor the insertion of the first volar interosseous to the opposite lateral band and its origin to the soft tissues; this muscle now functions as an adductor pollicis. Shorten the extensor indicis proprius by resecting a segment of its tendon; this muscle now functions as an extensor pollicis brevis. Also, shorten the extensor digitorum communis by resecting a segment of its tendon.
- Anchor the proximal segment of the tendon to the base of the proximal phalanx; this muscle now functions as an abductor pollicis longus.
- Trim the skin flaps appropriately; fashion the palmar flap so that when sutured it places sufficient tension on the new thumb to hold it in opposition.
- Suture the flaps, but avoid a circumferential closure at the base of the new thumb.
- Apply a pressure dressing of wet cotton and a plaster cast.

POSTOPERATIVE CARE   At 3 weeks, the cast is removed, and motion therapy is begun. The thumb is appropriately splinted.

BUCK-GRAMCKO POLLICIZATION

Buck-Gramcko reported experience with 100 operations for pollicization of the index finger in children with con-

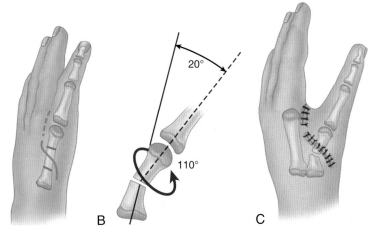

FIGURE 17.38   Flatt recession of index finger. **A,** Two incisions are required: intermetacarpal ligament is cut through distal incision, and osteotomy of index metacarpal is performed through proximal incision. **B,** Distal portion of index is rotated 110 degrees and abducted 20 degrees radialward. **C,** Skin closure. **SEE TECHNIQUE 17.28.**

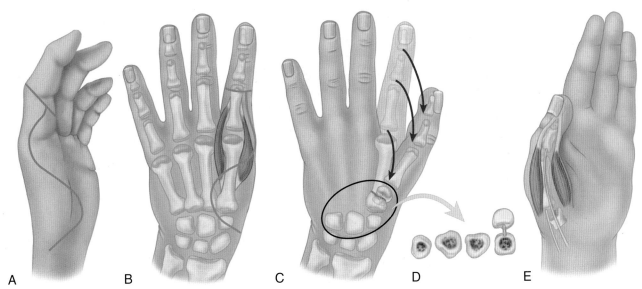

FIGURE 17.39   Riordan pollicization for congenital absence of thumb, including greater trapezium, in an immature hand. **A** and **B,** Incision (see text). Skin of proximal phalanx (blue area in **A**) is elevated as full-thickness skin flap. **C** and **D,** Second metacarpal has been resected by dividing base proximally and by cutting through epiphysis distally, and finger has been relocated proximally and radially. Second metacarpal head has been anchored palmar to second metacarpal base and simulates greater trapezium (see text). **E,** Insertion of first dorsal interosseous has been anchored to radial lateral band of extensor mechanism of new thumb and origin to soft tissues at base of digit; insertion of first volar interosseous has been anchored to opposite lateral band and origin to soft tissues. **SEE TECHNIQUE 17.29.**

genital absence or marked hypoplasia of the thumb. He emphasized a reduction in length of the pollicized digit trapezium. For best results, the index finger has to be rotated initially approximately 160 degrees during the operation so that it is opposite the pulp of the ring finger. This position changes during the suturing of the muscles and the skin so that at the end of the operation there is rotation of approximately 120 degrees. In addition, the pollicized digit is angulated approximately 40 degrees into palmar abduction.

TECHNIQUE 17.30

(BUCK-GRAMCKO)
- Make an S-shaped incision down the radial side of the hand just onto the palmar surface.
- Begin the incision near the base of the index finger on the palmar aspect and end it just proximal to the wrist.
- Make a slightly curved transverse incision across the base of the index finger on the palmar surface, connecting at right angles to the distal end of the first incision. Con-

nect both ends of the incision on the dorsum of the hand (Fig. 17.40A).

- Make a third incision on the dorsum of the proximal phalanx of the index finger from the proximal interphalangeal joint extending proximally to end at the incision around the base of the index finger (Fig. 17.40B).
- Through the palmar incision, free the neurovascular bundle between the index and middle fingers by ligating the artery to the radial side of the middle finger.
- Separate the common digital nerve carefully into its component parts for the two adjacent fingers so that no tension is present after the index finger is rotated.
- Sometimes an anomalous neural ring is found around the artery; split this ring carefully so that angulation of the artery after transposition of the finger does not occur. If the radial digital artery to the index finger is absent, it is possible to perform the pollicization on a vascular pedicle of only one artery. On the dorsal side, preserve at least one of the great veins.
- On the dorsum of the hand, sever the tendon of the extensor digitorum communis at the metacarpophalangeal level.
- Detach the interosseous muscles of the index finger from the proximal phalanx and the lateral bands of the dorsal aponeurosis.
- Partially strip subperiosteally the origins of the interosseous muscles from the second metacarpal, being careful to preserve the neurovascular structures.
- Osteotomize and resect the second metacarpal as follows. If the phalanges of the index finger are of normal length, the whole metacarpal is resected with the exception of its head. When the phalanges are relatively short, the base of the metacarpal must be retained to obtain the proper length of the new thumb.
- When the entire metacarpal is resected except for the head, rotate the head as shown in Fig. 17.40C and attach it by sutures to the joint capsule of the carpus and to the carpal bones, which in young children can be pierced with a sharp needle.
- Rotate the digit 160 degrees to allow opposition (Fig. 17.40D).
- Bony union is not essential, and fibrous fixation of the head is sufficient for good function. When the base of the metacarpal is retained, fix the metacarpal head to its base with one or two Kirschner wires in the previously described position. In attaching the metacarpal head, bring the proximal phalanx into complete hyperextension in relation to the metacarpal head for maximal stability of the joint. Unless this is done, hyperextension is likely at the new "carpometacarpal" joint (Fig. 17.40E).
- Suture the proximal end of the detached extensor digitorum communis tendon to the base of the former proximal phalanx (now acting as the first metacarpal) to become the new "abductor pollicis longus."
- Section the extensor indicis proprius tendon, shorten it appropriately, and suture it by end-to-end anastomosis.
- Suture the tendinous insertions of the two interosseous muscles to the lateral bands of the dorsal aponeurosis by weaving the lateral bands through the distal part of the interosseous muscle and turning them back distally to form a loop that is sutured to itself. In this way, the first palmar interosseous becomes an "adductor pollicis"

and the first dorsal interosseous becomes an "abductor brevis" (Fig. 17.40F).

- Close the wound by fashioning a dorsal skin flap to close the defect over the proximal phalanx and fashion the rest of the flaps as necessary for skin closure as in Fig. 17.40G,H.

POSTOPERATIVE CARE The hand is immobilized for 3 weeks, and then careful active motion is begun.

FOUCHER POLLICIZATION

Despite good sensibility, mobility, growth, and integration of pollicized digits, grip and pinch strength reduction (55% and 42% of the uninvolved side, respectively) have prompted technique modifications. Weakness in abduction and adduction, as well as the slenderness and cleftlike appearance of the pollicized digit, are corrected with the Foucher technique.

TECHNIQUE 17.31

(FOUCHER ET AL.)

- Outline the incisions on the index finger and palm (Fig. 17.41A). Line AB, as depicted in Figure 19.31A, is situated on the midlateral line and crosses the proximal interphalangeal joint. Line DE is on the volar aspect of the index-middle web, and line EF is volar to the midlateral line elongating the web incision. Line F is more distal than line A. Line GHI is a longitudinal incision to the volar wrist crease. Begin the dissection volarly to allow refilling of the dorsal veins and simplify the dorsal dissection. Elevate the arteries and veins, noting absence or hypoplasia of the radial digital artery. Preserve the fat around the digital arteries to protect the small vena comitantes. Divide the radial digital artery to the middle finger and be aware of the Hartmann boutonniere deformity (nerve loop around artery). Divide the intermetacarpal ligament and resect the lumbrical.
- Dissect the first dorsal interosseous muscle from distal to proximal to avoid denervation.
- Begin the dorsal dissection over the proximal interphalangeal joint and preserve the veins and sensory branches. Expose the extensor mechanism. Longitudinally separate the extensor indicis proprius and extensor indicis communis and extensor digitorum communis tendons along the length of the proximal phalanx to form two separate bands that are sectioned at the proximal phalangeal base.
- Separate the metacarpal head from its shaft through the physis, which is destroyed by curettage to prevent overgrowth of the pollicized finger. Dissect the first palmar osseous muscle from the index metacarpal shaft and remove the shaft by sectioning the bone with a palmar slope at its base. Maintain 1 cm of bone at the metacarpal base to preserve the flexor carpi radialis and extensor carpi radialis longus insertions. If present, destroy the pseudoepiphysis at the metacarpal base and open the base like a flower to

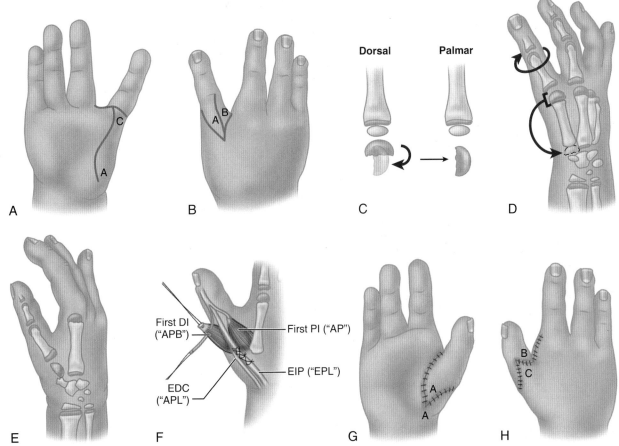

FIGURE 17.40   Buck-Gramcko pollicization of index finger. **A** and **B**, Palmar and dorsal skin incisions. **C**, Rotation of metacarpal head into flexion to prevent postoperative hyperextension. **D**, Index finger rotated about 160 degrees along long axis to place finger pulp into position of apposition. **E**, Final position of skeleton in about 40 degrees of palmar abduction with metacarpal head secured to metacarpal base or carpus. **F**, Reattachment of tendons to provide control of new thumb. First palmar interosseous (PI) functions as adductor pollicis (AP); first dorsal interosseous (DI) as abductor pollicis brevis (APB); extensor digitorum communis (EDC) as abductor pollicis longus (APL); and extensor indicis proprius (EIP) as extensor pollicis longus (EPL). **G** and **H**, Appearance after wound closure. **SEE TECHNIQUE 17.30.**

provide stability for the metacarpal head. Shift the metacarpal head onto the metacarpal base and avoid kinking of the vessels. Rotate the metacarpal head to allow opposition and fix in flexion to prevent hyperextension of the new carpometacarpal joint (Fig. 17.41B). A suture anchor may facilitate this fixation.

- Next, balance the thumb through tendon transfers (Fig. 17.41C). To provide adduction strength, attach the hypoplastic adductor pollicis, which often is present, to the extensor indicis communis and attach the second palmar interosseous muscles to the distal tendon ulnar slip.
- Abduction and pronation are achieved by transfer of the extensor indicis proprius (through a proximoradial fibrous sling of the first dorsal interosseous muscle) and the first dorsal interosseous muscle to the radial half of the distal tendon slip over the proximal phalanx. The thumb should rest in 135 degrees of pronation and 45 degrees of palmar abduction.
- Suture the skin, maintaining some tension on the dorsal web fold from the dorsal flap. To prevent circular scarring, make a Z-plasty on the radial aspect of the thumb (Fig. 17.41D).

POSTOPERATIVE CARE A fluffy dressing is placed in the new web space, and a drop of super glue maintains contact between the new thumb and middle finger. A dorsal plaster shell is applied, incorporating the elbow with two straps of Elastoplast to prevent escape. No therapy is used, and an opposition splint is used nightly for 2 months. Scar compression may be required if the pollicization is performed early because scar hypertrophy is more common in younger children. At 6 weeks if interphalangeal and metacarpophalangeal joint flexion are limited, a splint is worn for 1 hour in the morning and evening until full active flexion is achieved (in 4 to 5 months).

COMPLICATIONS

Pollicization is a complex, demanding, and intricate procedure. Complications, although rarely reported, can occur. Minor complications stem from wound problems, such as contracture or necrosis. Early major complications are related

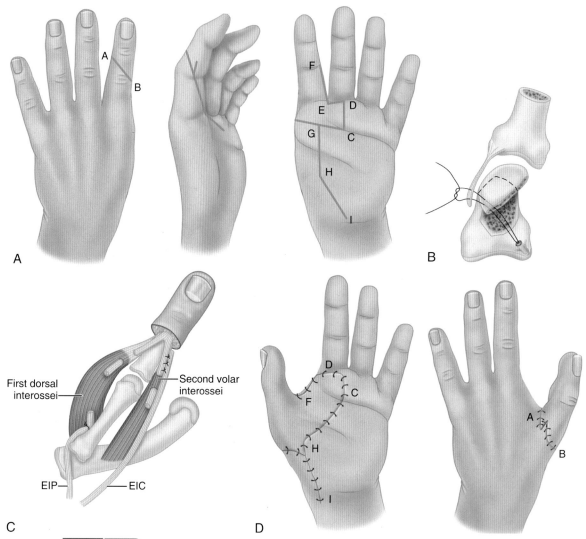

FIGURE 17.41 Foucher index pollicization. **A,** Proposed skin incisions providing a large dorsal flap and a distally based palmar flap, which provide a more weblike fold. **B,** Metacarpal head rotated into flexion and fixed into the metacarpal base with a bone anchor. **C,** New thumb balanced by tendon transfers; adduction is provided by the extensor indicis communis (EIC), second volar interosseous muscle (2nd VI), and adductor pollicis (not shown), and abduction is provided by extensor indicis proprius (EIP) and first dorsal interosseous muscle (1st DI). **D,** Sutured skin flaps showing weblike space between new thumb and middle finger and circular scar prevention by the radially based Z-plasty. **SEE TECHNIQUE 17.31.**

to rare vascular compromise. Long-term complications are more frequent and stem from suboptimal functional results (Table 17.8).

PREAXIAL POLYDACTYLY (DUPLICATE THUMB)

The duplicate thumb represents a complete or partial duplication of the thumb (Fig. 17.42). It is the most common duplication pattern in white and Asian populations, occurring in one per 3000 births. It usually is unilateral. The cause of the bifid thumb is unknown. Some evidence suggests preaxial polydactyly and forearm radial deficiencies share a common embryological pathway involving sonic hedgehog (SHH) signaling. However, most occur sporadically, which suggests environmental factors rather than genetic predisposition. Preaxial polydactyly has been produced in the offspring of rats by the administration of cytarabine during pregnancy.

When the thumb duplication is associated with a triphalangeal thumb, an autosomal dominant pattern and sporadic occurrence have been identified. Bifid thumb typically occurs as an isolated deformity unassociated with other malformation syndromes, but visceral anomalies, although rare, have been reported, particularly hand-heart or Holt-Oram syndrome, Rubinstein-Taybi syndrome, or Fanconi anemia.

Wassel presented a now widely used classification (Fig. 17.43):

Type I: partial duplication of the distal phalanx and a common epiphysis

Type II: complete duplication, including the epiphysis of the distal phalanx

Type III: duplication of the distal phalanx and bifurcation of the proximal phalanx

Type IV: complete duplication of the distal and proximal phalanges

TABLE 17.8		
Pollicization Pitfalls and Complications		
TYPE OF FAILURE	**ETIOLOGY**	**TREATMENT**
First web space contracture	Insufficient web space reconstruction or loss of skin flap	Revision web space deepening via Z-plasty or dorsal rotational flap
Stiffness	May be ascribed to preoperative condition of index finger or secondary to scarring related to surgery	Inherent stiffness not correctable. Surgical adhesions can be treated by tenolysis.
Excessive length	Failure to ablate index metacarpal physis	Epiphysiodesis and ostectomy of metacarpal
Malrotation	Technical error (under or over rotation) or loss of fixation during postoperative care	Rotational osteotomy
Lack of opposition	Primary deficiency in intrinsic muscles or inability to reconstruct interossei	Opposition transfer

From Kozin SH: Pollicization: the concept, technical details, and outcome, *Clin Orthop Surg* 4:18, 2012.

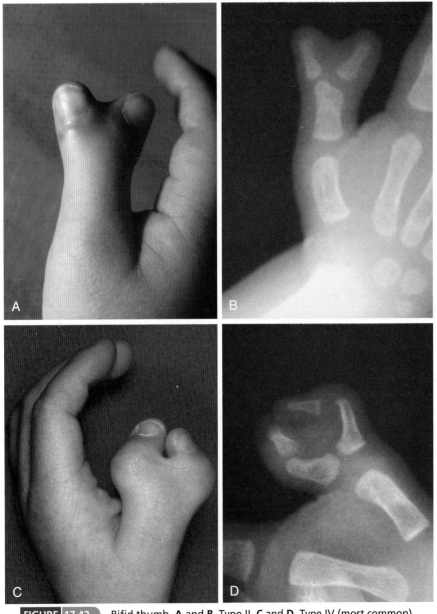

FIGURE 17.42 Bifid thumb. **A** and **B,** Type II. **C** and **D,** Type IV (most common).

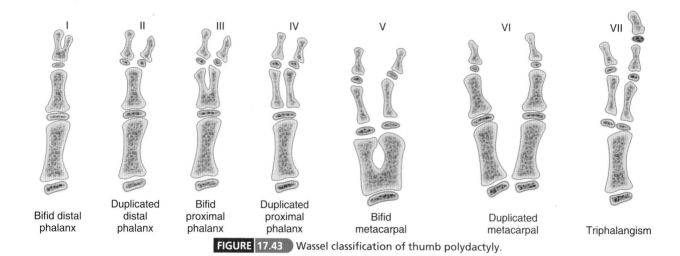

I	II	III	IV	V	VI	VII
Bifid distal phalanx	Duplicated distal phalanx	Bifid proximal phalanx	Duplicated proximal phalanx	Bifid metacarpal	Duplicated metacarpal	Triphalangism

FIGURE 17.43 Wassel classification of thumb polydactyly.

Type V: complete duplication of the distal and proximal phalanges with bifurcation of the metacarpal

Type VI: complete duplication of the distal and proximal phalanges and the metacarpal

Type VII: variable degrees of duplication associated with a triphalangeal thumb

In Wassel's series, type IV was the most common pattern (47%), followed by type VII (20%) and type II (15%). Type IV (Table 17.9) and type VII deformities have been subdivided further, depending on the extent of duplication and triphalangism.

The deformity usually is unilateral, and clinical appearance varies from mild widening of the thumb tip to complete duplication of the entire thumb. Typically, there is some degree of hypoplasia of both duplicates, and, more commonly, the radial duplicate is the more hypoplastic. Duplication of the thumb can occur in both divergent-convergent and parallel forms. In the divergent-convergent or zigzag pattern, the deformity is secondary to abnormal extrinsic insertion and bony alignment. After connection of a zigzag pattern, a higher frequency of recurrent deformity can occur. Special attention is needed to ensure proper extrinsic tendon rebalancing and bony alignment. There may be convergence or divergence of the duplications. Occasionally, the thumb has decreased pronation, placing it in the same plane as the other digits. Anatomic dissections have revealed fibrous interconnections between the two thumbs. The nail may be one large, conjoined nail with a central longitudinal groove, or it may be completely duplicated. The ulnar-innervated intrinsic muscles to the thumb (adductor pollicis and deep head of the flexor pollicis brevis) typically insert on the ulnarmost thumb duplicate, and the median-innervated intrinsic muscles to the thumb (abductor pollicis, superficial head of the flexor pollicis brevis, and opponens pollicis) typically insert on the radialmost thumb duplicate. Extrinsic flexor and extensor tendons may be duplicated and usually are eccentrically placed along each thumb. The phalanges may be angulated, and there may be an associated delta phalanx. The joints usually are stiff, with a widened joint surface. Thumb polydactyly with true symphalangism occurs rarely. The collateral ligaments of the duplicated joints often are shared, with insufficiency in the space along the adjacent sides. Wide variations may occur in the neurovascular anatomy. Radial and ulnar neurovascular bundles to the digits may be completely duplicated or may be shared with small separate branches that supply the individual digits.

■ TREATMENT

Surgical correction of the bifid thumb almost always is indicated, not only for the obvious cosmetic improvement but also for better function. Occasionally, if the thumb appears only slightly broader than expected, with underlying radiographic evidence of duplication, surgery might not improve the condition. Surgical reconstruction generally is performed when the child is between 1 and 2 years old, but no later than 5 years old if possible. Later revisions may be required, and fusions needed for late angular deformities and instability may be performed at 8 to 10 years old. Simple excision of the more hypoplastic digit rarely results in a satisfactory thumb because of progressive angulation and instability. For type I and possibly type II bifid thumbs in which there is only partial duplication of the nail, a combination procedure (Bilhaut-Cloquet) is recommended. This technique is useful when there is a conjoined nail. Baek et al. recommended a modification of this procedure in Wassel type II thumbs in which one epiphysis is preserved with a portion of its diaphysis (Fig. 17.44). More proximal duplication requires excision of the most hypoplastic thumb, narrowing of the widened proximal articular surface, ligament reconstruction, intrinsic transfer, and centralization of the extrinsic flexor and extensor tendons if necessary. In general, the ulnarmost thumb should be preserved. Preoperative splinting, as recommended by Iwasawa et al., may be beneficial; however, we have not attempted this. Long-term results of duplicate thumb reconstruction have shown excellent functional and cosmetic outcomes as the patient matures. However, revision rates tend to rise, with revisions being performed at an average of 8 years after the primary procedure. Parents should also be counseled that the treated thumb will, as a rule, remain weaker than the untreated "normal" thumb in the long term. Diminished interphalangeal joint range of motion is common, and although there is an initial catch-up growth after surgery, most thumbs remain proportionally smaller than the contralateral side. Long-term angular deformity can occur up to 46% of the time, and revision rates have been reported to be from 19% to 40%.

Late angular deformity and instability are the most frequent complications, and these may require further ligament reconstruction, corrective closing wedge osteotomy, or perhaps arthrodesis. Miura has treated this Z-collapse at the thumb interphalangeal joint successfully with a rotation

TABLE 17.9

Type IV Preaxial Polydactyly Subtypes

TYPE	DESCRIPTION	FREQUENCY (%)
IV A	Hypoplastic	12
IV B	Ulnar deviated	64
IV C	Divergent	15
IV D	Convergent	9

From Hung L, Cheng JC, Bundoc R, Leung P: Thumb duplication at the metacarpophalangeal joint. Management and a new classification, *Clin Orthop Relat Res* 323:31, 1996.

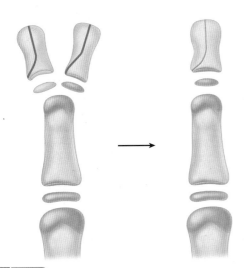

FIGURE 17.44 Baek et al. modified Bilhaut-Cloquet procedure applied to a Wassel type II bifid thumb. Shaded area resected and two distal phalangeal bones combined extraarticularly.

skin flap on the concave side of the deformity, combined with excision of the radial half of the extensor tendon and transfer of the flexor tendon into the ulnar side of the distal phalanx. Other reported complications include infection and deformity, scar contracture, joint stiffness, inadequate tendon excursion, residual prominence at the previous site of duplication, and a narrowed first web space. Loss of sensibility or viability of the digit rarely is encountered if surgical details are carefully observed. Unsatisfactory results are reportedly relatively high in Wassel types III, V, and VI and triphalangeal-type thumbs. Goldfarb et al. attempted to measure the appearance of reconstructed thumbs in 26 children and concluded that the appearance was quite satisfactory despite the narrowed nail. Residual angulation significantly affected the appearance and parental satisfaction. Wassel type VII thumbs had lower ratings using a visual analog scale. When both thumbs in types I and II are notably small without a clear dominant thumb, a modified Bilhaut-Cloquet procedure is recommended. However, when the duplicated thumbs are of normal size, as seen more frequently in type II deformities, reconstruction can be performed through a zigzag incision and standard reconstruction procedures. The soft tissues can be preserved to restore the thumb to a more normal-appearing girth.

CORRECTION OF TYPES I AND II BIFID THUMBS

TECHNIQUE 17.32   *Figure 17.45*

(BILHAUT-CLOQUET)
- Under tourniquet control, make a central wedge-shaped incision from dorsal to palmar over the involved thumb tip, extending proximally to the level of bifurcation. The dorsal component of the incision passes through the nail and nail bed.
- Incise the central component of the underlying tendon and bone of the duplicated structures in line with the skin incision.
- Carefully approximate the articular surface and epiphysis of the remaining parts of the distal phalanx and secure them with a transverse Kirschner wire. This may be difficult because of tightening of the collateral ligaments.
- Carefully suture the nail bed with 6-0 absorbable suture and close the skin with interrupted sutures.
- Apply a short or long arm–thumb spica cast, depending on the patient's age. Younger children require a long arm cast.

POSTOPERATIVE CARE The cast is removed 4 to 6 weeks after surgery, and the Kirschner wire can be removed 6 weeks after surgery. Progressively increased use is allowed after removal of the cast and wire.

CORRECTION OF TYPES III THROUGH VI BIFID THUMBS

TECHNIQUE 17.33

(LAMB, MARKS, AND BAYNE)
- Under tourniquet control, make a racquet-shaped incision over the most hypoplastic thumb (usually the radialmost

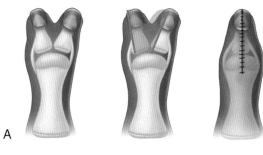

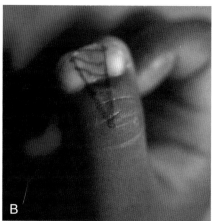
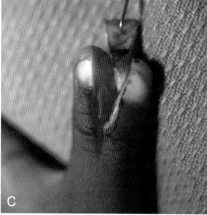
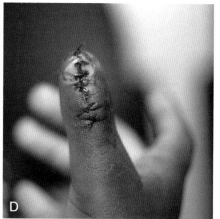

FIGURE 17.45 **A,** Bilhaut-Cloquet technique for symmetric thumb duplication in which duplicate digits are joined at midline after excision of excess central soft and osseous tissue. **B,** Planned resection. **C,** Wedge-shaped portion of central soft and osseous tissue removed. **D,** After closure. **SEE TECHNIQUE 17.32.**

digit). The tail of the incision can be extended in a zigzag or a curvilinear fashion proximally and distally for better exposure.

- If the ulnar thumb is the more affected, it should be removed instead.
- Through the incision, expose the abductor pollicis brevis tendon as it inserts into the proximal phalanx of the radial-almost thumb and carefully preserve this tendon. Identify the neurovascular bundles. The radial bundle is often hypoplastic or may be absent.
- Identify the nerve of the thumb to be excised and sharply incise.
- If the ulnar thumb is to be excised, identify the adductor pollicis and carefully preserve it.
- Detach the collateral ligament distally from the phalanx that is to be excised. Remove with the periosteum to extend the relative length of the collateral ligament if needed.
- Strip the collateral ligament proximally off the metacarpal or phalanx with a strip of periosteum to allow adequate exposure of the joint.
- Excise the supernumerary digit with the part of the metacarpal or phalanx with which it articulates (Fig. 17.46A).
- Examine the metacarpal head and, if widened or bifid, narrow it with a scalpel or osteotome, reserving the proximal attachment of the collateral ligament.
- Assess bony alignment and perform closing or opening wedge osteotomies of the proximal phalanges or metacarpal as necessary. Kirschner wires are used for stabilization.

- Centralize the remaining digit over the remaining articular surface (Fig. 17.46B) and suture the collateral ligament and intrinsic tendon securely to the phalanx (Fig. 17.46C).
- Secure this alignment with a longitudinal Kirschner wire placed across the joint (Fig. 17.46D).
- Check the alignment of the extensor and flexor tendons to ensure that they track centrally along the digit. Partial resection or transfer of the tendons may be required to achieve a central line of pull.
- Close the skin with simple interrupted sutures.
- A Z-plasty also may be required if the skin is inadequate along the ulnar border for a tension-free closure.

POSTOPERATIVE CARE The thumb is immobilized for 4 to 6 weeks, at which time the wire can be removed and the hand mobilized. A protective splint may be required for another 3 to 4 weeks.

■ TRIPHALANGEAL THUMB

As the name implies, the triphalangeal thumb has three phalanges instead of the normal two. This uncommon anomaly, which can be inherited as an autosomal dominant trait, has been associated with the maternal use of thalidomide. Two major types of triphalangeal thumbs are most common: one has a small, wedge-shaped extra ossicle (delta phalanx; see Fig. 17.68) that causes an angular deformity without significantly increasing thumb length; the other has an extra phalanx that is normal or nearly normal and creates the appearance of

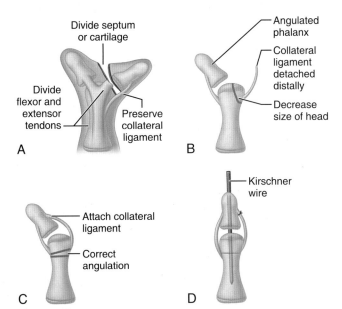

FIGURE 17.46 Lamb, Marks, and Bayne technique for asymmetric duplication (see text). **A,** Removal of less functional component. **B,** Transfer of collateral ligament. **C,** Osteotomy of proximal phalanx. **D,** Kirschner wire fixation. **SEE TECHNIQUE 17.33.**

a five-fingered hand (Fig. 17.47). Buck-Gramcko described a transitional type in which a trapezoidal extra phalanx causes increased length and angular deformity (Fig. 17.48). The triphalangeal thumb also has been classified as opposable or nonopposable. The most common hand anomaly associated with a triphalangeal thumb is a bifid thumb; other associated conditions include cleft foot, tibial defects, congenital heart disease, Fanconi anemia, anomalies of the gastrointestinal tract, and chromosomal anomalies.

In type I deformities (delta phalanx), the thumb is deviated ulnarward in the area of the interphalangeal joint. Radiographs show a delta phalanx or a trapezoidal extra phalanx. In type II deformities (five-fingered hand), the thumb is longer than normal and lies in the same plane as the other fingers. Extra skin creases overlie the additional interphalangeal joint. Patients with type II deformities are unable to oppose the thumb to the other digits and tend to use side-to-side prehension. Hypoplasia of the thenar muscles often is associated with type II deformities and further hinders opposition. Polydactyly usually is present, and 60% of patients have significant web space contractures. Radiographs show a complete extra, rectangular phalanx; the duplicated phalanx typically is the middle phalanx.

▌TREATMENT

Although nonoperative treatment does not correct the condition, operative intervention is not required for all children with triphalangeal thumbs, especially children with type I deformities. The goals of operative treatment are correction of angular deformity, restoration of normal length, correction of web contracture, and improvement of opposition. Removal of the abnormal phalanx along with reconstruction of the collateral ligament allows remodeling of the joint surfaces and usually provides adequate stability, especially if performed during the first year of life; however, late instability and angular deformity have been reported after ligamentous

reconstruction. Reduction osteotomy, as described by Peimer, corrects the angulation deformity with less chance of ligamentous instability. This osteotomy is best performed when the child is 24 to 30 months old and the physis is clearly visible on the radiograph. Late instability can be treated with arthrodesis. Contracture of the first web space may be released with a four-part Z-plasty as described by Woolf and Broadbent (Technique 17.21). Severe contracture may require a dorsal rotation flap as described by Strauch and Spinner. Thenar hypoplasia may require opponensplasty with the use of the abductor digiti minimi (see Technique 17.26) or ring sublimis (see Technique 17.24). For type II deformity (five-fingered hand), pollicization of the radialmost digit, as described by Buck-Gramcko (see Technique 17.30), is recommended.

Surgical correction also may be required for associated anomalies, such as polydactyly. If the duplication is a Wassell type IV, the radialmost digit should be excised when the child is about 6 months old. In a Wassell type VII duplication (complete duplication), the triphalangeal thumb should be removed. The remaining thumb may require web reconstruction and metacarpal osteotomy to complete the pollicization. For a nonopposable triphalangeal thumb, a two-stage procedure has been described by El-Karef. The first stage consists of excision of the extra joint, metacarpal shortening osteotomy in pronation and abduction, and web deepening. The second stage includes an opponensplasty and any necessary revision of the first stage.

REDUCTION OSTEOTOMY

TECHNIQUE 17.34

(PEIMER)
- Mark the preoperative radiographs, or make a sketch of the phalangeal and epiphyseal deformities, to plan the location of the osteotomies and the amount to be resected. Use a skin-marking pen to mark the curved dorsal incision, including the nail and matrix that must be removed (Fig. 17.49A).
- Make a curved incision through the nail, matrix, and skin down to the level of the paratenon.
- Elevate skin flaps and expose the middle and distal phalanges by dividing and reflecting the extensor pollicis longus tendon just proximal to its insertion on the distal phalanx.
- Use a scalpel or fine bone-cutting forceps to narrow the distal phalanx to the desired width; avoid fragmenting the phalanx.
- Expose the distal phalangeal epiphysis with the first longitudinal cut (Fig. 17.49B).
- With a scalpel, make a transverse osteotomy, completely excising the epiphysis (Fig. 17.49C).
- Make a second transverse osteotomy in the middle of the middle phalanx distal to the normal horizontal portion of the epiphysis. Confirm that the second osteotomy is parallel with the proximal interphalangeal joint by inserting a thin hypodermic needle into the joint to determine the joint line (Fig. 17.49D).

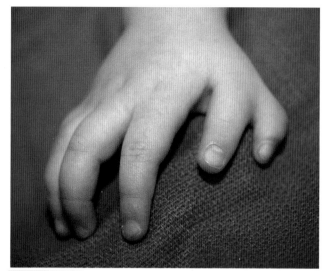

FIGURE 17.47 Clinical appearance of triphalangeal thumb associated with duplication (Wassel type VII).

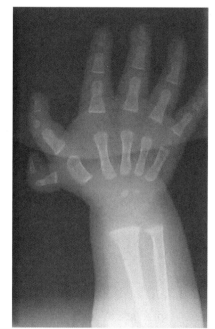

FIGURE 17.48 Radiographic appearance of triphalangeal thumb.

- With the second transverse osteotomy, expose the abnormal longitudinal portion of the C-shaped middle phalangeal epiphysis, and completely excise the distal portion of the middle phalanx and the abnormal epiphysis without cutting the collateral ligament (Fig. 17.49E).
- After removing the bone fragments, place the remaining bone in a closing-wedge position to realign and shorten the thumb (Fig. 17.49F).
- If necessary, use bone-cutting forceps or a small rasp to contour the bony surfaces.
- Align the bone ends and fix them with one or two smooth 0.028-inch or 0.035-inch Kirschner wires (Fig. 17.49G). Transfix the retained interphalangeal joint if additional stability is needed.

- Check the adequacy of resection and realignment and confirm the Kirschner wire placement and phalangeal position with radiographs.
- Shorten and repair the extensor pollicis longus tendon with fine sutures.
- Release the tourniquet, excise redundant skin, and close the wound.
- Cut and bend the Kirschner wires, leaving them protruding through the skin.
- Apply a long, plaster, opponens gauntlet splint that extends above the elbow.

POSTOPERATIVE CARE If necessary, the splint can be removed for wound inspection during the first 2 to 3 weeks after surgery, but the hand is kept well splinted for 6 to 8 weeks. The Kirschner wires are removed after 6 to 8 weeks or when bone healing is evident on radiographs. Splinting usually is not required after pin removal. Physical therapy may be helpful in regaining motion in older patients.

■ ULNAR DIMELIA

Ulnar dimelia, commonly called mirror hand, refers to radial and ulnar clusters of fingers in the same hand that are near-mirror images of each other (Fig. 17.50). It is considered a duplication phenomenon of the ulnar half of the forearm, wrist, and hand, but because there is complete substitution of the radial components as well, this anomaly is not so easily classified as pure duplication. It is an exceedingly rare anomaly, with few reports in the literature. The largest reported series is that of Harrison, Pearson, and Roaf, in which they describe the deformity in three patients. The etiology has been attributed to the replication of the zone of polarizing activity (ZPA), which controls radioulnar development. Transplantation of the ZPA or its signaling protein SHH causes this mirror duplication. When associated with fibular dimelia, it may be explained as a single gene mutation transmitted as an autosomal dominant trait. Ulnar dimelia usually is associated with some degree of hypoplasia of the arm and scapula. The only distant associated anomaly is fibular dimelia with absence of the tibia.

The deformity usually is unilateral, with multiple fingers dangling from a normal palm. The hand usually has six to eight well-formed fingers that all may lie in nearly the same plane or with slight opposition between the two halves. The postaxial digits appear slightly more normal than the preaxial digits; there is no thumb, and syndactyly may be present. The digits may be flexed because of deficient extensors, the hand usually is radially deviated at the wrist, and extension of the wrist may be impossible due to deficiency of unit extensors. The wrist and elbow appear thick, elbow motion is decreased, and the arm is shortened. The ulna and ulnar carpal bones are completely duplicated, the scaphoid and trapezium are replaced, and the distal ulnar epiphysis is broadened. At the elbow, each of the duplicated ulnae articulates with the distal humerus separately and they tend to face each other. There is no capitellum on the distal humerus.

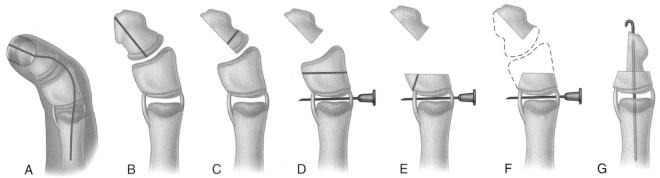

FIGURE 17.49 Peimer reduction osteotomy. A, Dorsal incision. B, Narrowing of distal phalanx. C, Excision of distal epiphysis. D, Needle placed across interphalangeal joint to orient transverse osteotomy. E, Completion of osteotomy. F, Combined osteotomies form closing wedge to shorten and realign thumb. G, Bone ends are fixed with smooth wires. SEE TECHNIQUE 17.34.

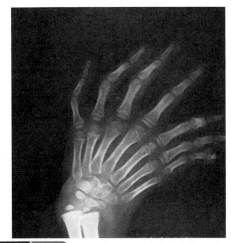

FIGURE 17.50 Duplication of ulna (mirror hand).

▌TREATMENT

The primary goal of treatment is to reduce the number of digits and reconstruct a thumb from the deleted digits. Parents should be encouraged to maintain passive range of motion in the fingers, wrist, elbow, and shoulder by gentle stretching exercises until the child reaches an appropriate age for reconstruction, usually age 2 years. During this period, the child should be carefully observed during play to determine which radial digit may function best as the thumb. Surgical intervention should be performed early to prevent the inevitable psychologic trauma to the parents, which also may be sensed by the child. No single surgeon has accumulated enough experience to delineate clearly the best method of treating the many complex problems involved with this deformity. Problems that require correction include limited movement of the elbow, limited pronation and supination, limited movement of the wrist, excessive number of fingers, inadequate finger extension, absence of the thumb, and inadequate first web space.

To improve elbow flexion, Harrison et al. excised the upper 1-inch portion of the lateral ulna in a 1-year-old patient and achieved 40 degrees of elbow flexion; however, by the time the child was 12 years old the elbow again had stiffened into extension. Most authors recommend this treatment method for limited elbow flexion but emphasize postoperative muscle strengthening. Pronation and supination also may be improved, but rotation osteotomy may be required to place the forearm in a more functional position. Limitation of wrist extension by palmar and radial contractures may require Z-plasty and lengthening of the contracted tendons and capsule. The flexor carpi radialis muscle may be transferred to the dorsum to aid extension. Transferring the flexor digitorum superficialis of the pollicized finger to the dorsum of the index metacarpal also has been recommended. Wrist arthrodesis may be necessary for recurrent wrist instability; this procedure can be performed when the child is about 12 years old. Pollicization can be done in one stage according to the principles of Buck-Gramcko, using the most functional of the radial digits. The excess radial digits are deleted, including the metacarpal and carpal bones. The excess skin is used as a filleted flap to re-create a first web space. Entin recommended deleting the first and third rays, with pollicization of the second digital ray (Fig. 17.51). Tendon transfers, with the use of donor tendons from the amputated digits or the flexor carpi ulnaris if duplicated, may be necessary to improve finger extension. Tendon transfers are used to augment thumb function as described previously.

EXCISION OF THE PROXIMAL ULNA

TECHNIQUE 17.35

- Under tourniquet control if possible, place a longitudinal incision over the proximal aspect of the preaxial ulnar bone.
- Expose the proximal ulna extraperiosteally, preserving a sufficient periosteal and ligamentous strip to reconstruct a collateral ligament.
- Excise a sufficient amount of the ulna, along with its remaining periosteum, to allow adequate extension and flexion, usually approximately 1 inch of bone.
- Check the stability of the elbow, close the incision in layers, and apply a long arm cast with the elbow in 90 degrees of flexion.

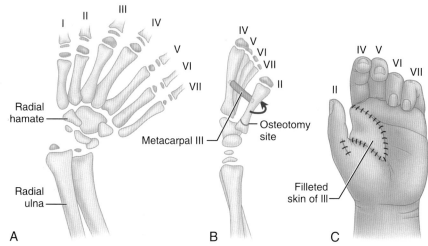

FIGURE 17.51 Entin reconstruction for duplication of ulna (mirror hand). **A,** Appearance of mirror hand with extra digits. Digits I and III were discarded; digit II was retained for pollicization. **B,** Pollicization of digit II. This digit was properly positioned by osteotomy through base of its metacarpal and by intermetacarpal graft cut from metacarpal of discarded digit III. **C,** Filleted skin of digit III was used as flap to cover space created by pollicization.

POSTOPERATIVE CARE The cast is worn for 3 to 6 weeks depending on the stability of the elbow. The neurovascular status must be carefully monitored. After the cast is removed, active assisted flexion and extension exercises are begun. A night splint is recommended to hold the elbow in 90 degrees of flexion until the child can actively flex the elbow against resistance. Emphasis should be placed on strengthening the elbow flexors and extensors to maintain the motion achieved at surgery.

RECONSTRUCTION OF THE HAND AND WRIST

TECHNIQUE 17.36

- Before inflation of the tourniquet, carefully plan the incision to allow pollicization of the most functional digit and fillet-type amputations of the excessive digits and exposure of the neurovascular bundles to the digit chosen for pollicization.
- After the incisions and skin flaps have been designed, exsanguinate the limb and inflate the tourniquet.
- Make the incisions and carefully dissect the common neurovascular bundles to the middle digit in each web space.
- Ligate the bifurcation to each adjacent digit.
- Carefully dissect the common digital nerves to the thenar level before division. Carefully preserve the digital nerves and dorsal veins to the pollicized digit.

- Dissect out the tendons to the pollicized digit; if there are bifurcations of these tendons, divide the abnormal insertions to the neighboring tendons.
- Amputate the extra digits, including the metacarpal and articulating carpal bones. Preserve the extensor tendons to the excised digits, if present, to use later to reinforce finger extension or thumb abduction.
- Shorten the metacarpal of the pollicized digit by performing an osteotomy just proximal to the metacarpal neck and scarring the remaining shaft.
- Rotate the head of the metacarpal into 120 degrees of flexion and 90 degrees of pronation and secure it in this position with two sutures or a Kirschner wire, which allows appropriate shortening and opposition of the pollicized digit.
- Suture the intrinsic muscles to the lateral bands of the extensor mechanism of the pollicized digit to augment adduction and abduction.
- Use the fillet flaps from the deleted digits to reconstruct a first web space.
- Remove any excess skin to allow appropriate closure of the shortened, pollicized digit.
- If increased extension of the wrist is needed, divide the flexor digitorum sublimis muscle at the level of the A1 pulley into the pollicized digit and transfer it to the dorsal base of the second metacarpal.
- Deflate the tourniquet, check the viability of the remaining digits and flaps, and apply a bulky dressing with a long arm posterior splint supporting the elbow at 90 degrees, the wrist at neutral or in slight extension, and the thumb in the abducted position.

POSTOPERATIVE CARE The splint is worn for 3 weeks but can be changed for suture removal and wound inspection. After splint removal, an exercise program is begun, and a removable night splint is used to hold the thumb in the opposed position for an additional 3 months.

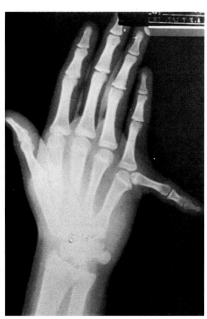

FIGURE 17.52 Type 2 postaxial polydactyly: partial duplication of digit, including osseous structures.

BOX 17.2

Associated Anomalies With Type A Postaxial Polydactyly

Cornelia de Lange
Chondroectodermal dysplasia
Schinzel syndrome
Clubfeet, tracheomalacia, renal reflux
Clubfeet
Tongue malformation, gastroesophageal reflux, aortic insufficiency
Imperforated anus, renal insufficiency, sacral agenesis, vertebral anomalies
Pectus excavatum
Tracheomalacia, gastroesophageal reflux, developmental delay

Modified from Pritsch T, Ezaki M, Mills J, Oishi SN: Type A ulnar polydactyly of the hand: a classification system and clinical series, *J Hand Surg* 38A:453, 2013.

■ POSTAXIAL POLYDACTYLY

Duplication of the small finger is the most common pattern of duplication in the black population. It occurs in approximately one per 300 black births, with a relative frequency of 8:1 compared with duplication of other digits. The true incidence is impossible to determine because many of these children have the extra digit removed in the nursery, although this probably is done less frequently than in the past. Stelling and Turek originally classified postaxial polydactyly into three subtypes based on the degree of duplication: type 1, duplication of soft parts only; type 2, partial duplication of the digit, including osseous structures (Fig. 17.52); and type 3, complete duplication of the ray. Later, Temtamy and McKusick simplified the classification into type A, a fully developed extra digit; or type B, a rudimentary supernumerary digit attached to the small finger in a pedunculated manner. Pritsch et al. further classified type A into five subgroups based on osseous anatomy. Hypoplasia of both subtypes with angular deformity is common.

Duplication of the small finger is believed to be genetically determined. Type B patterns often are multifactorial involving two genes with incomplete penetrance. It is 10 times more common in people of African descent. In isolated nonsyndromic cases of postaxial polydactyly, the inheritance pattern appears to be autosomal. Type A patients typically produce offspring of both types, whereas type B patients produce offspring with type B patterns only. Autosomal recessive inheritance has been identified in association with multiple abnormalities. Type A postaxial polydactyly is rare and has equal incidence in black and white races. In the black population, supernumerary digits are common and usually are not associated with more serious anomalies. However, postaxial polydactyly in the white population is frequently associated with more serious abnormalities, most commonly syndactyly, although multiple deformities and chromosomal abnormalities can be present.

Infants with postaxial polydactyly may have a well-formed extra digit along the ulnar border of the small finger (type 2) or may have only a rudimentary soft-tissue tag (type 1). Both digits usually are hypoplastic to some degree. Angular deformity may be present at birth or may occur later during growth (Box 17.2).

▌TREATMENT

The use of ligatures around the base of type B postaxial duplication is commonly performed in the nursery with sutures or a vascular clip such that blood flow is ceased. The digit becomes necrotic and falls off. Although good to excellent results have been reported with these techniques, complications can occur, including failure of the digit to fall off, infection, traction neuroma, or most commonly residual bumps. Surgical excision also can be performed in the operating room. Katz and Linder reported a prospective series of 11 infants having pedunculated extra digits in which they simply excised the digit at its base, while maintaining digital traction under topical anesthesia with a single swipe of the scalpel. They used pressure to control the bleeding and closed the skin with a sterile adhesive strip. All infants cried for "a few seconds after the excision," but no complications were encountered, and at 1-year follow-up the site of excision was barely seen. Type B duplications should be excised in the operating room under tourniquet control because of the complexity of the duplication when the patient is about 1 year old. A frequent complication is an unsightly bump caused by a retained segment of duplicated metacarpal head.

EXCISION OF EXTRA DIGIT

TECHNIQUE 17.37

- Under tourniquet control, make an elliptical incision around the base of the extra digit. Leave excess skin at the time of initial incision and excise this as appropriate at the time of closure.

- Identify, ligate, and divide the neurovascular bundle to the extra digit.
- For type 1 duplication, complete the excision at this point and close the skin with simple closure.
- For type 2 duplication, identify and preserve the abductor digiti quinti minimi tendon.
- Expose the area of bone bifurcation subperiosteally.
- Identify and preserve the ulnar collateral ligament if the bifurcation is in the area of the joint.
- Amputate the extra digit and trim any excess bone in the area of the bifurcation.
- Reconstruct the collateral ligament and abductor insertion if violated.
- Close the skin with simple interrupted sutures and apply a soft bandage.

POSTOPERATIVE CARE A very young child may require a cast for a short time (10 days), but generally no immobilization is necessary. Sutures are removed at 2 weeks, and unlimited activity is allowed.

MALFORMATIONS UNSPECIFIED
SOFT TISSUE
▓ SYNDACTYLY

Syndactyly, or "webbed fingers," is caused by the failure of the fingers to separate during embryologic development. It is the most common congenital anomaly of the hand, with an occurrence of 1 per 2000 births. The specific cause is unknown, but syndactyly is believed to result from an abnormal slowing of growth and development of the finger buds during weeks 7 and 8 of gestation. Although most are sporadic occurrences, Flatt found a family history of syndactyly in 40% of his patients, which suggests heredity as one factor. Several pedigrees have shown an autosomal dominant trait for long-ring finger syndactyly, but penetrance has been incomplete.

Syndactylies are classified as complete or incomplete and as simple or complex. Complete syndactyly is present when the fingers are joined from the web to the fingertip; incomplete syndactyly indicates that the fingers are joined from the web to a point proximal to the fingertips. Simple syndactyly exists when only skin or other soft-tissue bridges the fingers (see Fig. 17.61); complex syndactyly occurs when there are common bony elements shared by involved fingers (Figs. 17.53 and 17.54). Acrosyndactyly refers to lateral fusion of adjacent digits at their distal ends with proximal fenestrations between the joined digits. Brachysyndactyly denotes associated shortening of the syndactyly digits. Anomalies that may be found in association with syndactyly include webbing of the toes, polydactyly, constriction rings, brachydactyly, cleft feet, hemangioma, absence of muscles, spinal deformities, funnel chest, and heart disorders. In Poland syndrome, the sternocostal portion of the ipsilateral pectoralis major muscle is absent. The hand deformity includes unilateral shortening of the index, long, and ring fingers; multiple simple incomplete syndactylies; and hypoplasia of the hand (Fig. 17.55). Apert syndrome also characteristically includes multiple syndactylies.

Syndactyly occurs between the long and ring fingers in more than 50% of patients (Fig. 17.56); the fourth web, second web, and first web are affected in diminishing frequencies. The syndactyly is bilateral in about half of patients, and boys are more frequently affected than girls. The intervening skin usually is normal, although deficient in surface area compared with the normal hand, a fact that is important in the consideration of surgical correction. The two nails may be completely separate, or the digits may share a common nail without intervening eponychium referred to as *synonychia*. If the fingers are of relatively similar length, flexion and extension usually are normal. Abnormally tight fascial bands usually are present within the web, minimizing any lateral movement between the involved digits. Frequently, there is anomalous sharing of musculotendinous units, nerves, and vessels between joined digits. The phalanges usually are normal in the simple pattern; however, in the complex pattern, various interosseous connections range from duplication patterns, to branching patterns, to shared patterns. Differentiation of the joints also may be incomplete. Rarely is there any angular deformity of the digits at birth, unless a delta phalanx is present. If a central syndactyly involves the long and ring or long and index fingers, angular deformities develop slowly. If the syndactyly involves the ring and little fingers or index finger and thumb, however, a gradual flexion contracture, lateral deviation, and rotation deformity usually develop in the longer of the two digits within the first year of life.

▌TREATMENT

Surgical intervention is not urgent. While waiting for their child to reach the appropriate age for reconstruction, parents should be encouraged to massage the web in an attempt to stretch the intervening skin to facilitate later surgery. Surgical reconstruction is best done before the child is of school age. Results are reportedly better in children older than 18 months at the time of correction, especially in the final appearance of the commissure. There is a tendency for the web to migrate distally and the commissure to contract if surgery is performed at an earlier age. If the syndactyly involves the second or third web space, and there are no other deformities of the involved fingers, surgery should be delayed until the child is at least 18 months old. When digits of different sizes are completely involved, whether the syndactyly is simple or complex, early separation, between age 6 and 12 months, is best because of the likelihood of angular, rotational, and flexion deformities. These deformities are difficult to correct, and preventing them takes precedence over the possibility of distal web migration and commissure contracture. When multiple digits are involved, the border digits should be released early, followed by subsequent releases after a 6-month waiting period. Simultaneous releases of the radial and ulnar sides of a finger are contraindicated and may jeopardize the viability of the finger.

The surgical procedure includes three technical steps: (1) separation of the digits, (2) commissure reconstruction, and (3) resurfacing of the intervening borders of the digits. Early attempts at separation incorporated such techniques as passage of setons, use of ligatures, and straight linear incisions. Pieri, in 1949, condemned the use of straight incisions and favored a zigzag incision to prevent linear contracture along the long axis of the finger; all currently accepted methods

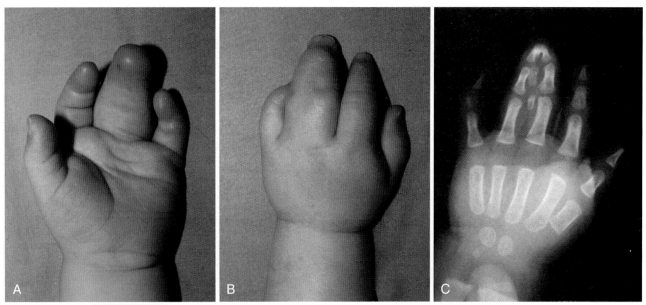

FIGURE 17.53 Complex syndactyly. **A,** Palmar view. **B,** Dorsal view. **C,** Radiograph.

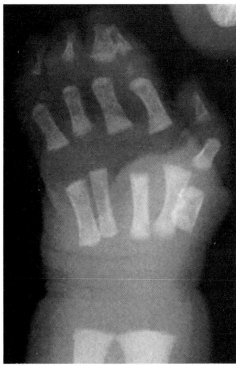

FIGURE 17.54 Note common bony elements shared by involved fingers in complex syndactyly.

incorporate this principle. Shared digital nerves are carefully split longitudinally to preserve innervation to both digits. Common digital arteries may extend into the web and require ligation of one or more branches. Care should be taken to avoid devascularizing the digit. When the nail is shared, an additional longitudinal strip of nail and underlying matrix usually must be removed to match the normal nail width. Osseous structures usually are divided longitudinally with a scalpel if the procedure is performed at an early age.

Special attention must be given to the reconstruction of the web commissure. The normal commissure has a sloping configuration from proximal dorsal to distal palmar. Dorsally, it begins at about the level of the transverse metacarpal ligament and extends distally and palmarward to about the level of the proximal digital flexion crease, usually at about the midpoint of the bony proximal phalanx. Distally, the commissure forms a rectangle between the small, ring, index, and long fingers. In some hands, the commissure between the long and ring fingers forms a "V" or "U" shape. The distal web span must be greater than the proximal web span to allow abduction of the fingers around the axis of the metacarpophalangeal joint. In re-creating a commissure with normal appearance and function, a properly designed local flap generally is preferable to a skin graft to minimize commissure contracture. Numerous local flaps have been designed, but the most commonly used are the dorsal "pantaloon" flap described by Bauer, Tondra, and Trusler; the matching volar and dorsal proximally based V-shaped flaps popularized by Cronin and by Skoog; and the "butterfly" flap devised by Shaw et al. Woolf and Broadbent described the butterfly flap as useful for partial simple syndactyly that ends proximal to the proximal interphalangeal joint (Fig. 17.57). Mericili et al. retrospectively reviewed 30-year outcomes of a tapered M to V flap for commissure reconstruction, reporting 14% web creep without flap loss. Miyamoto et al. performed a finite element analysis using CT reconstruction to assess wound stress or web displacement. A dorsal rectangular flap demonstrated greater stress than a dorsal flap with a palmar rectangular tip or dorsal flap with a V-shaped tip. In a review of 131 web reconstructions, Vekris et al. found that the dorsal rectangular flap required revision less often (3%) than volar and dorsal triangular flaps (63%).

Regardless of flap design, in resurfacing the intervening borders of the digits there usually is not enough skin for primary closure of each digit. This phenomenon can be clearly demonstrated to the patient's parents by comparing the sum

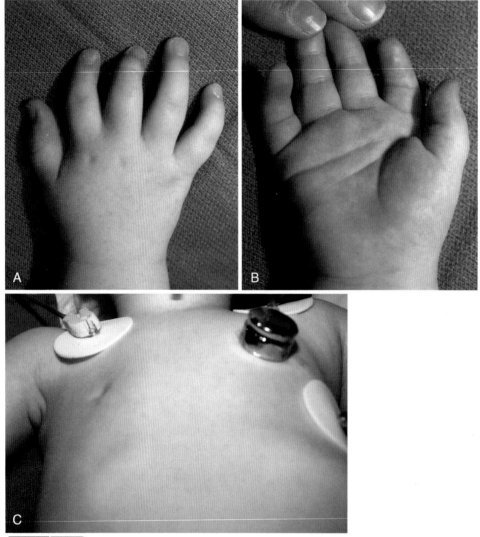

FIGURE 17.55 Poland syndrome in 18-month-old child. **A** and **B,** Brachysyndactyly. **C,** Hypoplasia of pectoralis major muscle.

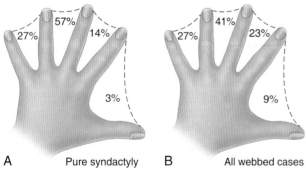

FIGURE 17.56 Site of syndactyly. **A,** Percentage incidence when only true syndactyly of simple or complex type is considered. **B,** Total count incidence in which associated conditions (all webbed digits) are included.

of the circumferences of two individual fingers with that of the circumference of two fingers held together; the latter is always less. Occasionally, there is redundant skin between the syndactylized digits, which may make primary closure possible. Rarely, defatting allows for primary closure without

grafting. The zigzag incision is designed to create interdigitating volar and dorsal flaps for one finger; the other finger requires either full-thickness or split-thickness skin grafting (full-thickness grafting usually is preferred). More contracture has been shown to occur in webs that are split grafted; however, more web creep, hyperpigmentation, and hair have been reported in full-thickness grafts. To minimize ectopic hair growth, the skin from the volar medial wrist or lateral inguinal region should be chosen. Grafts should be avoided at the base of the ring finger where wearing of a ring may be bothersome. Multiple graftless techniques have been reported, with multiple studies comparing graftless with skin grafting. Studies reveal conflicting results as to which technique is superior. However, there does not appear to be a statistically significant difference in patient satisfaction with either technique, although longer operative times are reported in grafting procedures and potentially higher complication rates.

When synonychia is present, eponychial folds are reconstructed. Balic et al. demonstrated improved aesthetic outcomes utilizing Buck-Gramcko flaps (Fig. 17.58) when compared with full-thickness skin grafts.

The patient's parents should be informed that recurrence and angular deformity are possible despite a well-designed and well-executed reconstruction and that future revision may be necessary. Reoperation has been reported to be necessary in 59% of patients with major associated anomalies and in 30% of patients with syndactyly as the primary abnormality. Overall complication rates appear to be approximately 2% with a postoperative infection rate of 1.6% in some studies. However, the most common complication of syndactyly reconstruction is scar deformity of the digit or web. Distal migration of the web may occur, particularly if surgery is performed before the child is 18 months old. Web creep is associated with poor flap design, skin graft loss, use of split-thickness skin grafting, and wound dehiscence. Nail and bony deformities are common in complex syndactyly and are secondary to bony angulation and insufficient paronychial fold reconstruction. The most catastrophic complication is circulatory insufficiency to the finger, resulting in loss of the digit. This rarely has been reported and should not occur if the syndactyly on each side of the finger is released in stages.

OPEN FINGER SYNDACTYLY RELEASE

Withey et al. described an open finger technique. They compared eight patients who had the open technique with

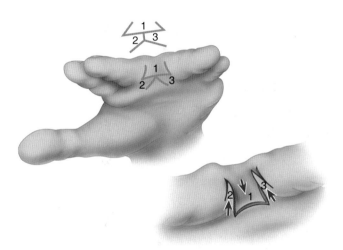

FIGURE 17.57 Woolf and Broadbent butterfly flap technique for release of syndactyly. Flaps are designed in web space to form dorsal rectangle, then flaps are rotated to deepen web.

12 patients who had the standard closed grafting technique. No defatting of the flaps was performed in the open technique, and flap design allowed for more numerous and narrow flaps. The flaps were secured without tension using one stitch, and no grafting was performed. Scar quality and contracture were significantly better with the open-finger technique.

TECHNIQUE 17.38　　*Figure 17. 59*

(WITHEY ET AL. MODIFIED)

- Create a proximally based rectangular flap dorsally for web commissure coverage. The flap should extend approximately two thirds the length of the metacarpophalangeal joint to the proximal interphalangeal joint.
- Dorsally, carry the incision distally in a zigzag pattern until the nail bed is reached. The incision should extend to but not beyond the midsagittal lines of each digit.
- Continue the incision to the volar aspect of the finger, mirroring the zigzag incision of the corresponding dorsal flaps.
- At the proper height make a reciprocating incision to accept the dorsal web commissure flap.
- Raise the dorsal flaps first, preserving the veins when possible. Neurovascular bundles can be identified in a dorsal to ventral manner or through the volar aspect.
- Once the neurovascular bundles are identified raise the volar skin flaps.
- Release the fibrous connections between the digits, distal-to-proximal, protecting the neurovascular bundles.
- Insert the dorsal web commissure flaps.
- Allow the skin flaps to interdigitate and secure into place with simple interrupted suture.
- Harvest full-thickness skin grafts from the inguinal area, antecubital fossa, or hypothenar eminence and use to cover the dorsoradial and dorsoulnar aspects of the ulnar and radial digits, respectively.
- Release the tourniquet and confirm vascularity.
- Place Xeroform gauze on the graft and apply a moistened cotton dressing between the fingers over the grafts.

POSTOPERATIVE CARE The patient is placed in a long arm cast for 4 to 6 weeks. The cast is then discontinued, and the patient is released to unrestricted activity.

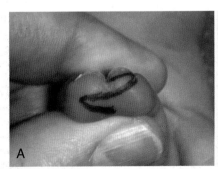
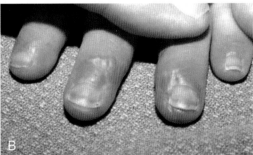

FIGURE 17.58 **A,** Buck-Gramcko nail fold flaps. **B,** Postoperative result. (From Tonkin M: Failure of differentiation part I: syndactyly, *Hand Clin* 25:171, 2009.)

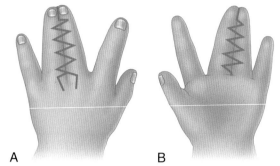

FIGURE 17.59 Withey et al. open technique of syndactyly release (see text). **A,** Dorsal incisions. **B,** Palmar incisions. **SEE TECHNIQUES 17.38 AND 17.39.**

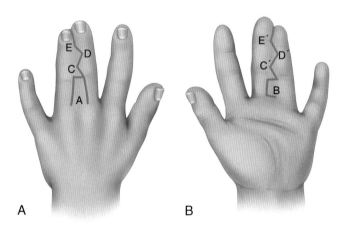

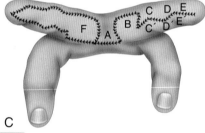

FIGURE 17.60 Bauer et al. syndactyly release. **A,** Dorsal skin incisions. Rectangular dorsal flap (*A*) is designed for web; alternating flaps (*C, D,* and *E*) are arranged to interdigitate with volar flaps. **B,** Palmar skin incisions. Rectangular flap (*B*) is arranged to cover radial side of ring finger; remaining flaps (*C′, D′,* and *E′*) are arranged to interdigitate with dorsal flaps. **C,** Separation is completed; flaps have been sutured into place, covering radial side of ring finger and web. Skin graft is required for ulnar side of long finger. **SEE TECHNIQUE 17.39.**

SYNDACTYLY RELEASE WITH DORSAL FLAP

TECHNIQUE 17.39

(BAUER ET AL.)
▪ Outline all incisions carefully with a skin-marking pen (Fig. 17.60A,B). It also is helpful to draw a dotted line

along the central axis of each involved digit to determine the limits of the triangular flaps. Draw the dorsal flap "A" so that it begins at the level of the metacarpal heads and extends two thirds of the length of the proximal phalanx.
▪ Incise the dorsal flaps and defat the proximal flap, carefully identifying the neurovascular bundles through the dorsal incision.
▪ Incise the palmar flaps, taking care during the midline dissection to spare the neurovascular bundles. The proximal limb of the palmar flap "B" should be just proximal to the adjacent commissures (Fig. 17.60B).
▪ Remove the dorsal fat from the web space and suture the dorsal flap "A" first to restore the commissure; suture the proximal ring finger flap "B" to resurface the radial and proximal border of the ring finger.
▪ Suture the triangular flaps to resurface as much of the intersurface of the digits as possible (Fig. 17.60C).
▪ Release the tourniquet and ensure that perfusion to the triangular flaps is adequate; if perfusion is inadequate after the hand is slightly warmed, resuture the flaps under less tension.
▪ Cover the remaining defects with a full-thickness skin graft taken from the groin or elbow crease.
▪ If the fingernails are confluent, separate them and remove the matrix at their margins so that the grafts can be brought around to the edge of each nail.
▪ When a finger is webbed on both sides, it is safer to separate only one side at a time.
▪ Place Xeroform gauze over the grafts and carefully insert a wet contour dressing between the fingers; begin at the web space and pack distally so that the fingers are held in wide abduction and extension. Apply a dry dressing and a plaster splint to immobilize the fingers and wrist.

POSTOPERATIVE CARE The hand is elevated for 1 week or more before redressing (Fig. 17.61).

SYNDACTYLY RELEASE WITH MATCHING VOLAR AND DORSAL PROXIMALLY BASED V-SHAPED FLAPS

TECHNIQUE 17.40

(SKOOG)
▪ With a skin pencil, outline the incisions to be made on the fingers. Design dorsal and volar flaps so that when mobilized they cover most of the denuded side of one finger without tension (Fig. 17.62A,B). Make the free borders of the flaps irregular by designing small triangular points at the level of the interphalangeal joints.
▪ In planning the flaps so that they fit each other, first outline the incision on one side and then establish the key

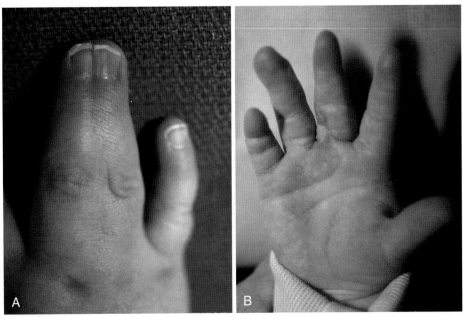

FIGURE 17.61 A, Complete simple syndactyly. B, After syndactyly release. **SEE TECHNIQUE 17.39.**

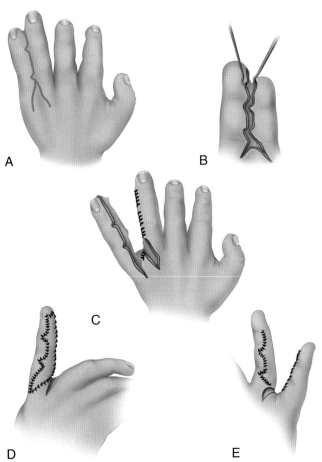

FIGURE 17.62 Skoog technique for syndactyly. **A** and **B,** Dorsal and volar skin incisions. **C,** Web space reconstruction; closure of ring finger. **D** and **E,** Dorsal and volar views: skin graft in place on little finger and graft in web space. **SEE TECHNIQUE 17.40.**

points for the incision on the opposite side by pushing straight needles vertically through the web.

- Inflate the tourniquet and raise the flaps consisting mainly of the skin that forms the abnormal web.
- In raising the flaps, preserve all subcutaneous tissue and take care not to sever digital nerves and arteries.
- Release the tourniquet and control all bleeding.
- Using the triangular flaps, reconstruct the web space (Fig. 17.62C).
- On one finger, close the flaps as planned and cover the small remaining defect at the dorsomedial aspect of the base of this finger (Fig. 17.62D) by a full-thickness skin graft obtained from the inguinal region.
- Make a pattern of the denuded area on the adjacent finger and on the new web and obtain a matching full-thickness graft again from the inguinal region.
- Carefully suture the graft in place (Fig. 17.62E) and close the donor area.
- Apply a pressure dressing: place Xeroform gauze over the grafts and suture lines, spread the fingers widely and place between them wet cotton pressed to fit the contours of the fingers and web, and wrap on dry gauze and Webril. Apply a plaster splint; extend it proximal to the elbow, if necessary, to ensure sufficient immobilization.
- If more than two fingers are involved in the syndactyly, it is safer to separate only one side of a single finger at a time.

POSTOPERATIVE CARE The hand is elevated for at least 3 days after surgery. At 10 to 14 days, the dressing is changed, with the patient under general anesthesia if necessary. Sutures can be removed at this time. Another bandage is maintained for an additional 10 to 14 days, and gradual resumption of normal activities is allowed.

■ CAMPTODACTYLY

Camptodactyly is a flexion deformity of the proximal interphalangeal joint, is often nontraumatic, and often occurs bilaterally (Fig. 17.63). This type of bent finger deformity should be distinguished from clinodactyly, in which the finger is bent either radialward or ulnarward. Camptodactyly occurs in less than 1% of the population and was found in 6.9% of the anomalies in Flatt's series. There is a strong hereditary predisposition in many patients, in whom the deformity is transmitted as an autosomal dominant trait. Sporadic cases also occur. All structures that could possibly cause flexion deformity at the proximal interphalangeal joint have been considered as possible causative factors, including a stout band of tissue in association with the Landsmeer ligament, an abnormal insertion of the lumbrical tendon into the flexor superficialis tendon, the capsule of the metacarpophalangeal joint, or the extensor expansion of the adjacent finger. This finding seems to support that camptodactyly is caused by a relative imbalance between the flexors and extensors. Relative shortening in the flexor superficialis muscle-tendon unit has been suggested as a cause because the deformity usually can be corrected with simultaneous flexion of the wrist (Fig. 17.64). Other theories include contractures of the collateral ligaments or volar plate, insufficient palmar skin, and congenital fibrous substrata in the subcutaneous tissues.

There seem to be three types of camptodactyly, based on the age at which the deformity occurs. The first type occurs in infancy and affects both sexes equally. This is the more common type and occurs in about 80% of patients. The second type occurs during adolescence and affects mostly girls. The third, or syndromic type, is commonly associated with many syndromes, including trisomy 13, oculodentodigital, orofaciodigital, Aarskog, and cerebrohepatorenal syndromes. A subgroup of camptodactyly has been reported in which severe flexion deformities of the proximal interphalangeal joints are present at birth. Often several digits of the same hand are affected, and there is no predilection for the small finger. Pathologic findings in this subtype primarily involve the extensor mechanism (attenuation of the central slip, palmar subluxation of the lateral bands, and hypoplasia of the radial extensor structure). Postoperative impingement has been noted only in patients whose extensor mechanism was realigned and augmented by release or transfer of the flexor digitorum superficialis.

Most patients are seen with a flexion deformity of the proximal interphalangeal joint during the first year of life. About two thirds have bilateral deformities, which are not symmetric in severity. The metacarpophalangeal joint usually is held in hyperextension to compensate for the flexed posture. Rotational deformity can cause mild overlapping of fingers. In young children the deformity disappears when the wrist is flexed, but in older children the flexion deformity usually is fixed. If left untreated, 80% worsen, especially during the period of growth acceleration. The deformity usually does not progress after age 18 to 20 years. Rarely, pain and swelling are present.

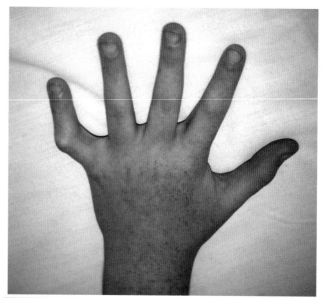

FIGURE 17.63 Camptodactyly (flexion deformity of proximal interphalangeal joint) involving little finger only.

▌TREATMENT

Neither nonoperative nor operative treatment of camptodactyly has been particularly predictable or satisfying. Twenty percent of patients improve with nonoperative treatment and only 35% with operative treatment. Good results have been obtained with dynamic splinting, but some flexion deformity recurred when splinting was discontinued. Baek reported the results of passive stretching in children younger than 3 years of age. A fairly time intense protocol of 5-minute stretches 20 times each daily (i.e., 1 hour and 40 minutes per day) was found to improve mild camptodactyly from 20 degrees to 1 degree, moderate camptodactyly from 39 to 12 degrees, and severe camptodactyly from 75 to 28 degrees. It is reasonable to advise patients with mild deformities to live with their deformities. For young children in whom the deformity disappears with wrist flexion and for whom the parents desire surgical correction, release of the sublimis tendon may correct the deformity and prevent worsening during growth. This usually should be performed by 4 years of age. In older children and young adults in whom the deformity can be corrected with splinting, but who continue to have weak extension at the proximal interphalangeal joint, release of the flexor digitorum sublimis muscle and transfer into the extensor apparatus is advised. A volar release, including local skin flap and volar plate release, has been used before tendon transfer to allow passive correction of the flexion deformity. Smith et al. emphasized the importance of treating all abnormal structures related to camptodactyly. The relative frequency of abnormalities is shown in Table 17.10. With Smith's approach, the postoperative arc of motion was 85 degrees (range 45 to 100 degrees). Recent studies have evaluated the effectiveness of early release, and no improvement was shown between preoperative and postoperative total proximal interphalangeal joint motion. However, the digits did tend to rest in a more extended position.

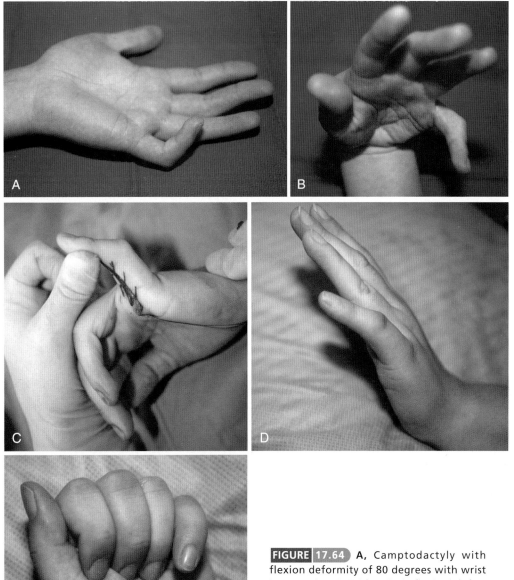

FIGURE 17.64 **A,** Camptodactyly with flexion deformity of 80 degrees with wrist in extension. **B,** With wrist in flexion, deformity measures 40 degrees. **C,** After superficialis tenotomy, flexion deformity measures 40 degrees and is unrelated to wrist position. **D** and **E,** After postoperative rehabilitation, active proximal interphalangeal joint motion from 20 to 90 degrees.

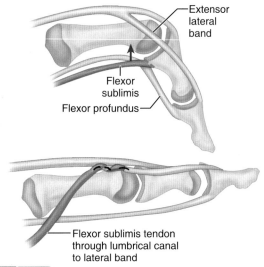

—Extensor
lateral
band

Flexor
sublimis

Flexor profundus—

—Flexor sublimis tendon
through lumbrical canal
to lateral band

FIGURE 17.65 Technique for correction of camptodactyly. Flexor sublimis tendon is transferred to extensor apparatus. **SEE TECHNIQUE 17.42.**

TENDON RELEASE

TECHNIQUE 17.41

(SMITH)
- Make a volar linear incision and convert it to multiple Z-plasties, placing the central limbs over the flexion creases of the joints.
- Reflect the skin and release the tough linear fibrous bands of the digital fascia, including the bony attachment of Grayson ligaments.
- Free the lateral bands of the intrinsic apparatus and the interosseous muscles from their abnormal and widespread attachments to the sides of the proximal phalanx, which may prevent extension of the proximal interphalangeal joint. Proximal pull on the lateral bands confirms that proximal interphalangeal joint extension can occur.
- To determine if there is attenuation of the central slip, flex the wrist and the metacarpophalangeal joints. If attenuation is present, there is an extensor lag at the proximal interphalangeal joint. Do not surgically explore or expose the central slip. Attenuation of the central slip responds to postoperative extension splinting.
- The lumbrical muscle is abnormally inserted and often adherent to the proximal phalanx. It also may have an abnormal origin and occasionally may be inserted into the flexor digitorum superficialis tendon proximal to the A1 pulley.
- Test the flexor digitorum superficialis tendon by a tenodesis test to determine whether it is short. If the proximal interphalangeal joint cannot be fully extended when the wrist is in extension, the flexor digitorum superficialis is short and must be released. Two types of flexor digitorum superficialis abnormalities exist: (1) the flexor digitorum superficialis is shortened; and (2) when there is proximal aplasia, only the distal portion of the flexor digitorum superficialis is present, and this distal part produces a flexion contracture of the proximal interphalangeal joint. If the latter is the case, release completely by division.

- If the flexor digitorum superficialis tendon is normal proximally (no aplasia), perform a lengthening and transposition of the insertions at a chiasma level. Divide both flexor digitorum superficialis insertions eccentrically so that a long proximal and radial insertion can be sutured to the ulnar insertion in such a way that lengthening is achieved.
- In some patients, release of the flexor tendon sheath, volar plate, or accessory collateral ligaments may be necessary. Do not explore any preoperatively detected bony abnormalities at the neck of the proximal phalanx or involving the articular surfaces of the proximal interphalangeal joint because there does not seem to be any benefit.

POSTOPERATIVE CARE The proximal interphalangeal joint is maintained in extension for 4 weeks after surgery in a cast. After that time, a splint is applied that allows active-resisted flexion, unless the flexor digitorum superficialis was lengthened, in which case this should be delayed another 8 weeks. At 6 weeks, daytime motion is allowed with splinting at night. The postoperative regimen corrects any central slip attenuation.

TRANSFER OF THE FLEXOR SUPERFICIALIS TENDON TO THE EXTENSOR APPARATUS

TECHNIQUE 17.42   *Figure 17.65*

(MCFARLANE ET AL.)
- Under tourniquet control, make a straight midline incision over the finger so that a Z-plasty closure can be achieved as necessary.
- Divide the flexor digitorum sublimis tendon just proximal to the vinculum longum and transfer it through the lumbrical canal to the dorsal surface of the finger.
- Suture the sublimis tendon to the extensor apparatus with nonabsorbable sutures. Tension the transferred tendon so that normal stance of the digit is achieved in all wrist positions.
- If correction of the deformity is incomplete, consideration can be given to a proximal release of the volar plate; however, it is best to accept a flexion deformity of approximately 20 degrees.
- Insert a Kirschner wire through the proximal interphalangeal joint to maintain extension.
- Close the skin with single or multiple Z-plasty procedures.
- Apply a short arm cast with the metacarpophalangeal joints in 90 degrees of flexion and the digits fully extended.

POSTOPERATIVE CARE The cast and Kirschner wire are removed 4 weeks after surgery. A dorsal splint with a metacarpal stop to prevent overstretching of the transferred tendon is worn for another 4 weeks.

TABLE 17.10

Structures Involved in Patients With Camptodactyly

NO. DIGITS	STRUCTURES INVOLVED	% OF CASES
18	Skin	100
12	Flexor digitorum superficialis and tendon sheaths	66.6
10	Retinaculum cutis	55.5
4	Lumbricals	22.0
3	Bone (abnormal proximal interphalangeal joint surfaces and neck of proximal phalanx)	16.6
3	Volar plate	16.6
2	Central slip	11.0
2	Adherence of lateral bands to proximal phalanx	11.0
1	Accessory collateral ligaments	5.6

From Smith PJ, Grobbelaar AO: Camptodactyly: a unifying theory and approach to surgical treatment, *J Hand Surg* 23A:14, 1998.

THUMB IN PALM (CLASPED THUMB)

Congenital clasped thumb is an unusual condition in which the thumb is positioned in adduction and extreme flexion at the metacarpophalangeal joint. Underlying hypoplasia or absence of the extensor pollicis brevis muscle is usual, and the extensor pollicis brevis or EPL may be absent. Some degree of total thumb hypoplasia may be present. This may be an isolated deformity or associated with clubfoot deformities and several well-defined syndromes. There is no single cause; the deformity results from an imbalance between the flexors and extensors of the thumb. Weckesser, Reed, and Heiple called this deformity a syndrome and classified it into four distinct types on the basis of etiologic factors: group 1, deficient extension only; group 2, flexion contracture combined with deficient extension; group 3, hypoplasia of the thumb, including tendon and muscle deficiencies; and group 4, deformities that do not fit easily into any of the other three categories. Group 1 syndrome seems to be transmitted as a sex-linked recessive gene because it is more common in boys and frequently is bilateral.

At birth, the thumb usually is flexed into the palm, with the deformity typically located at the metacarpophalangeal joint, in contrast to trigger thumb deformity. During the first few weeks of life, it is typical for an infant to clutch the thumb, but normally the thumb is released intermittently. If no active extension at the metacarpophalangeal joint is shown after prolonged observation and particularly by age 3 months, the diagnosis of congenital clasped thumb is established.

NONOPERATIVE TREATMENT

Most clasped thumb deformities are deficiencies of extension only (group 1) and usually respond to early splinting in extension and abduction. A plaster splint may be applied. It is changed every 6 weeks and continued for 3 to 6 months. The long-term results of this protocol seem satisfactory if the initial response to splinting is good. If at the end of 3 to 6 months of splinting there is no evidence of active extension of the metacarpophalangeal joint, further splinting probably would not be beneficial. This lack of response to splinting usually indicates that the extrinsic extensors are extremely deficient (the usual case) or totally absent and that a tendon transfer is required to restore function.

OPERATIVE TREATMENT

Useful donor tendons for an inadequate EPL muscle are the palmaris longus, brachioradialis, extensor carpi radialis longus, extensor indicis proprius, and flexor superficialis muscles. The extensor indicis proprius is an ideal motor muscle, but it may be absent as well. The brachioradialis with a tendon graft may be used. The extensor pollicis brevis muscle may be replaced with the extensor indicis proprius muscle. Significant web space contracture also may require reconstruction.

For group 3 deformities with significant hypoplasia of the thenar muscles and abductor pollicis longus and instability of the metacarpophalangeal joint, Neviaser recommended a single-stage operation involving chondrodesis of the metacarpophalangeal joint, replacement of the EPL with the extensor indicis proprius, replacement of the abductor pollicis longus with the palmaris longus, and a Huber opponensplasty (see Technique 17.26). Web space reconstruction usually is necessary in these patients. With this protocol, Neviaser obtained useful grasp and pinch in eight patients with no complications, despite the magnitude of the surgery. These procedures should be done after the first year of life and before the child reaches school age.

GROUP 2 CLASPED THUMB DEFORMITY

TECHNIQUE 17.43

- Stage I is release of web space contracture, which is performed as described elsewhere (see Technique 17.20). Stage II is restoration of thumb extension (Fig. 17.66) with the use of the extensor indicis proprius.
- Under tourniquet control, make a short transverse incision at the base of the index metacarpophalangeal joint and locate the extensor indicis proprius tendon.
- Divide the tendon at its confluence with the extensor hood.
- Make a short transverse incision over the dorsum of the wrist in line with the extensor indicis proprius tendon and withdraw the tendon into this wound.

- Make a bayonet-shaped incision over the dorsoulnar aspect of the thumb centered over the metacarpophalangeal joint. Identify the extensor pollicis longus tendon, if present, and retract it to one side.
- Create a tunnel through the base of the proximal phalanx from the ulnar aspect to the radial aspect distal to the epiphysis.
- Reroute the tendon of the extensor indicis proprius subcutaneously from the wrist to the base of the thumb, passing it through the osseous tunnel and suturing it back onto itself.
- If the extensor indicis proprius is absent or severely deficient, choose either the flexor digitorum sublimis to the ring finger or the brachioradialis, with a palmaris longus tendon graft for the donor muscle.
- If the flexor digitorum sublimis is selected, make a transverse incision at the base of the ring finger on the palmar aspect and release the sublimis tendon just proximal to the Camper chiasm.
- Make a short longitudinal incision over the palmar aspect of the wrist proximal to the flexion crease and identify the ring sublimis tendon (see Fig. 17.66A).

- Deliver the sublimis tendon into this wound, reroute it subcutaneously around the radial border of the wrist deep to the abductor pollicis longus tendon, and suture it into the remnants of the extensor pollicis longus at the distal phalanx (see Fig. 17.66B).
- If there is no distal tendon in which to suture the donor, create a periosteal flap to anchor the distal insertion of the tendon.
- Fix the thumb in extension with a Kirschner wire, close the incision in routine fashion, and apply a splint with the thumb in extension and abduction.

POSTOPERATIVE CARE Six weeks after surgery, the Kirschner wire is removed. The hand is held in a plaster splint for an additional 2 months. Some type of thumb support, such as a removable splint, should be continued for about 4 months before unrestricted activity is allowed.

GROUP 3 CLASPED THUMB DEFORMITY

TECHNIQUE 17.44

(NEVIASER, MODIFIED)
- Under tourniquet control, make a dorsal incision over the thumb metacarpophalangeal and interphalangeal joints (Fig. 17.67A).
- If the metacarpophalangeal joints are unstable to radial and ulnar stresses, perform a dorsal capsulotomy and identify the articular surfaces of the metacarpal and proximal phalanx.
- Shave the articular cartilage with a scalpel to expose the epiphyseal bone and pin the joint with a Kirschner wire.
- Make a short transverse dorsal incision at the base of the index finger to expose the extensor indicis proprius tendon.
- Make a transverse dorsal incision over the wrist in line with the tendon, divide the tendon distally, and deliver it into the wound (Fig. 17.67B).

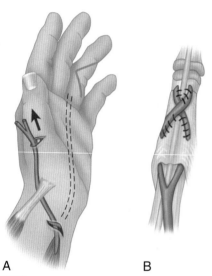

FIGURE 17.66 Littler technique for correction of congenital clasped thumb. **A,** Path of transferred tendon. **B,** Suture of transferred tendon. **SEE TECHNIQUE 17.43.**

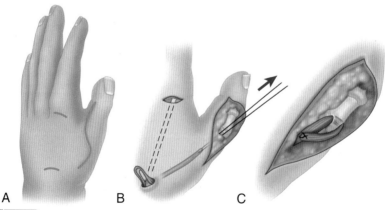

FIGURE 17.67 Neviaser transfer of extensor indicis proprius for absent extensor pollicis brevis. **A,** Incisions. **B** and **C,** Extensor indicis proprius is passed through bony tunnel in proximal phalanx of thumb **(B)** and sutured to itself **(C)**. **SEE TECHNIQUE 17.44.**

- Reroute the tendon subcutaneously and suture it into the soft tissue around the base of the distal phalanx or beneath a periosteal flap.
- Make a short transverse palmar incision at the wrist over the palmaris longus tendon.
- Divide this tendon at its insertion into the palmar fascia and route it subcutaneously, passing it through an osseous tunnel created at the base of the thumb proximal phalanx just distal to the epiphysis; suture the tendon back onto itself (Fig. 17.67C).
- Perform an opponensplasty (see Technique 17.26), perform a Z-plasty reconstruction of the web space contracture (see Technique 17.21), and derotate the thumb metacarpal, if necessary, by sharply incising the capsule of the trapeziometacarpal joint and pronating the thumb 90 degrees.
- Fix this with a Kirschner wire.
- Close the incisions in routine fashion and apply a splint with the thumb in the corrected position.

POSTOPERATIVE CARE The Kirschner wires are removed 6 weeks after surgery, and progressive motion is allowed. The thumb is protected in a night splint for another 3 to 4 weeks.

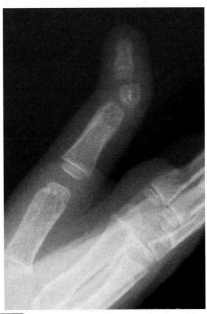

FIGURE 17.68 Radiographic appearance of delta phalanx.

SKELETAL
■ CLINODACTYLY (DELTA PHALANX)

Clinodactyly is the radioulnar deviation of a finger caused by an abnormally shaped phalanx (Fig. 17.68). One or more of the phalanges are either triangular (delta) or trapezoidal in shape owing to an abnormal epiphysis. The abnormal epiphysis is usually C- or J-shaped and tends to bracket the shorter side of the phalanx. The deformity most commonly presents as an isolated radially deviated small finger. When the deformity is in the border digits, the finger tends to deviate toward the hand. In the thumb, this anomaly occurs in the proximal phalanx in association with an abnormal hypertrophic epiphysis or triphalangeal thumb. In the small finger, the middle phalanx is affected and in the ring finger the proximal phalanx. The angulation frequently is mild, but when it is severe it may cause an unacceptable appearance. Progressive angulation is inevitable because this deformity worsens with growth.

The incidence of clinodactyly in the general population has been difficult to establish, ranging from 1% to 19.5%. The specific cause is unknown, but in 44% of patients there is a strong family history with autosomal dominant inheritance. Clinodactyly can be an isolated abnormality or can occur in association with polydactyly, syndactyly, symphalangism, cleft foot, triphalangeal thumb, central hand deficiencies, ulnar longitudinal deficiency, Apert syndrome, Poland syndrome, Rubinstein-Taybi syndrome, diastrophic dwarfism, and Holt-Olram syndrome (Table 17.11)

▌TREATMENT

Moderate angulation of the finger produced by the delta phalanx may be cosmetically unacceptable. With border digits, compensatory abduction prevents functional obstruction to range of motion. However, in the thumb or central digits, angulation can cause functional impairment due to limitation of pinch or interference with flexion, respectively. Nonoperative treatment would not alter progression, and operative intervention (usually indicated with deviation of >20 degrees) should be aimed at narrowing the digit, straightening the phalanx, and destroying the abnormal portion of the epiphysis. If it is associated with central polydactyly, the delta phalanx should be excised along with the extra digit with a syndactyly-type reconstruction. If it is associated with a triphalangeal thumb, the delta phalanx should be excised or reduction osteotomy performed and the joint ligaments reconstructed. The deformity may recur after osteotomy. Reverse wedge osteotomy, as described by Carstam and Theander, is preferable to simple opening wedge osteotomy. Carstam and Theander reported elimination or marked reduction of clinodactyly in all of their patients. Vickers described a procedure in which he resected the isthmus of the continuous epiphysis and inserted an interpositional fat graft. He reported spontaneous angular correction and growth of the phalanx in 11 patients. Caouette-Laberge et al. also reported spontaneous improvement after physiolysis. Strauss and Goldfarb recommended a Vickers type procedure in younger children (<5 years) and an opening wedge osteotomy in older children (Fig. 17.69). Others have described opening or closing wedge osteotomy with or without bone grafting with satisfactory results. Gilles et al. compared outcomes of physiolysis with osteotomy for clinodactyly correction and concluded that physiolysis is more effective in deformities with less than 55 degrees of angulation with higher rates in the osteotomy group. Early intervention (age younger than 6 years) is thought to provide greater correction with physiolysis prior to skeletal maturity.

TABLE 17.11

Clinodactyly Classification

TYPE OF DEFORMITY	AREA OF DEFORMITY	ANGULATION OF DEFORMITY	ASSOCIATED DEFORMITY
Simple	Middle phalanx	<45 degrees	—
Simple complicated	Middle phalanx	>45 degrees	—
Complex	Bone and soft tissue	<45 degrees	Syndactyly
Complex complicated	Bone and soft tissue	>45 degrees	Polydactyly or macrodactyly

From Cooney WP: Camptodactyly and clinodactyly. In Carter P, editor: *Reconstruction of the child's hand*, Philadelphia, 1991, Lea & Febiger.

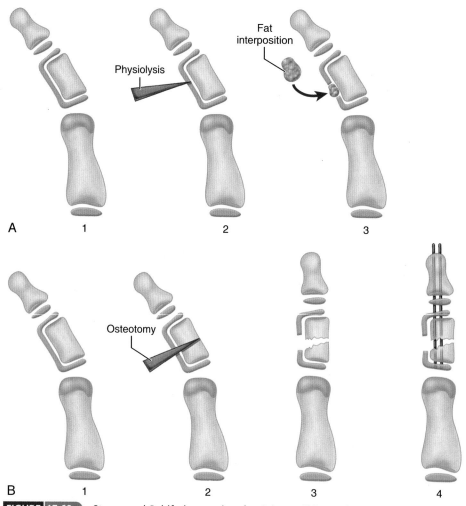

FIGURE 17.69 Strauss and Goldfarb procedure for right small finger clinodactyly. **A,** Physiolysis. **B,** Osteotomy. (Redrawn from Strauss NL, Goldfarb CA: Surgical correction of clinodactyly: two straightforward techniques, *Tech Hand Up Extrem Surg* 14:54, 2010.)

REVERSE WEDGE OSTEOTOMY

TECHNIQUE 17.45   *Figure 17.70*

(CARSTAM AND THEANDER)

- Under tourniquet control, make a curved dorsal incision over the involved phalanx, extending from the distal portion of the proximal phalanx, over the entire length of the middle phalanx, and onto the proximal portion of the distal phalanx.
- Carefully mobilize the edges of the extensor tendon so that both borders of the delta phalanx in the middle phalanx can be seen.
- Identify and protect the insertion of the central extensor slip.
- Remove a wedge-shaped piece of bone from the central portion of the delta phalanx, either by using a scalpel if it is mostly cartilaginous or by carefully picking away at it with sharp bone cutters, as described by Flatt.

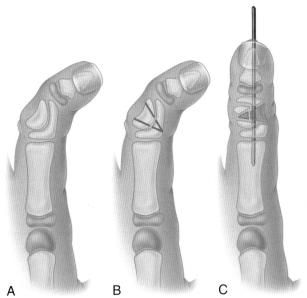

FIGURE 17.70 Carstam and Theander reverse wedge osteotomy for correction of delta phalanx. **A,** Delta phalanx involving middle phalanx. **B,** Wedge-shaped piece of bone is removed from central portion. **C,** Wedge is reversed and reinserted after correction of angular deformity; Kirschner wire is used for fixation. **SEE TECHNIQUE 17.45.**

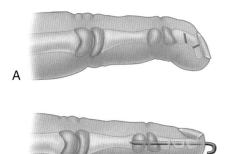

FIGURE 17.71 Carstam and Eiken correction of Kirner deformity. **A,** Deformity. **B,** Multiple opening wedge osteotomy cuts in distal phalanx fixed with Kirschner wire. **SEE TECHNIQUE 17.46.**

- Reverse this wedge-shaped piece of bone and insert it into the defect after correcting the angular deformity.
- Place a longitudinal Kirschner wire through the distal phalanx and into the proximal phalanx to hold the corrected position; leave the wire protruding through the distal end of the finger.
- Close the incision in routine fashion and apply a long or short arm splint.

POSTOPERATIVE CARE The splint and Kirschner wire are removed 4 to 6 weeks after surgery. Gradually increased activity is permitted depending on clinical and radiographic healing.

KIRNER DEFORMITY

The Kirner deformity, originally described in 1927, consists of palmar and radial curving of the distal phalanx of the little finger. It is an unsightly deformity that occurs infrequently (1 per 410 live births). The deformity occurs more frequently in girls and rarely may affect several fingers. Sporadic and familial occurrences have been reported, and there is no known specific causative factor. A similar deformity may result from frostbite, physeal fracture, and infection. Kirner deformity has been associated with Cornelia de Lange, Silver, and Turner syndromes.

The deformity typically is seen when the child is 8 to 10 years old and appears as a beaked little fingertip with increased convexity of the fingernail. The fingertip curves radially and toward the palm. The deformity usually is bilateral and symmetric. Although it can be progressive, usually it is not painful. Radiographs reveal a broadened epiphysis with irregularities of the metaphysis. The typical curvature can be seen within the distal phalanx (Fig. 17.71A).

TREATMENT

For mild deformities, either splinting or no treatment may be appropriate. More severe deformities in skeletally mature patients require one or more osteotomies of the terminal phalanx, as described by Carstam and Eiken. No effective treatment has been described for correction of the nail deformity.

OPENING WEDGE OSTEOTOMY OF THE TERMINAL PHALANX

TECHNIQUE 17.46

(CARSTAM AND EIKEN)
- Under tourniquet control, make a radial midlateral incision over the distal phalanx of the involved finger.
- Expose the distal phalanx subperiosteally and perform two osteotomies through the volar three fourths of the diaphysis.
- Using a periosteal hinge left intact on the dorsum of the phalanx, correct the deformity. This periosteal hinge also helps control rotation of the fragments.
- Complete correction of the deformity may be blocked by a curved nail deformity.
- Place a longitudinal Kirschner wire through the phalanx and the distal interphalangeal joint to hold the correction (Fig. 17.71B).
- If the phalanx is extremely small, insert a Kirschner wire extraperiosteally along the volar aspect of the phalanx to act as an internal splint.
- Close the incisions in routine fashion and apply a long or short arm splint.

POSTOPERATIVE CARE The splint and Kirschner wire are removed 4 to 6 weeks after surgery. Usually no specific postoperative therapy is necessary. Activities are permitted depending on the clinical and radiographic signs of healing.

TABLE 17.12

Classification of Central Synpolydactyly

CLASSIFICATION TYPE	LEVEL OF DUPLICATION	DESCRIPTION
1 A B	Metacarpal Metacarpal	■ 3rd metacarpal bifurcates ■ Affects long and ring fingers ■ 3- or 4-boned digit between long and ring fingers ■ Syndactylized to ring or both ring and long fingers
2 A B	Proximal phalanx Proximal phalanx	■ Duplication of ring finger ■ Syndactyly may involve long finger ■ Delta phalanx of ring P1 ■ Duplication of ring or long fingers ■ Parallel of divergent orientation
3	Middle or distal phalanx	■ Duplication at P2 or P3 level between long and ring fingers

From Wall LB, Bae DS, Oishi SN, Calfee RP, Goldfarb CA: Synpolydactyly of the hand: a radiographic classification, *J Hand Surg Eur* 41(3):301, 2016.

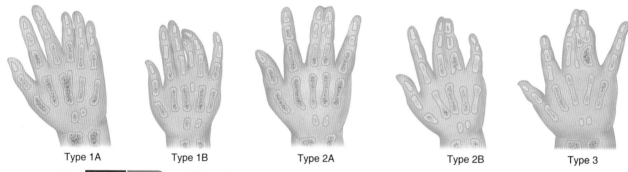

| Type 1A | Type 1B | Type 2A | Type 2B | Type 3 |

FIGURE 17.72 Wall classification system for synpolydactyly. (Redrawn from Wall LB, Bae DS, Oishi SN, Calfee RP, Goldfarb CA: Synpolydactyly of the hand: a radiographic classification, *J Hand Surg Eur* 41(3):301, 2016.)

COMPLEX
■ SYNPOLYDACTYLY (CENTRAL POLYDACTYLY)

Central polydactyly or synpolydactyly is an uncommon congenital anomaly characterized by duplication of the index, long, or ring finger and is usually associated with a complex syndactyly or cleft hand. It is much less common than preaxial or postaxial polydactyly. Synpolydactyly is most commonly inherited in an autosomal dominant fashion with variable expression and incomplete penetrance. Up to 55% of patients had a family history of similar hand differences in some studies. It often is bilateral and can involve the lower extremity. In 2016 Wall et al. proposed a classification system for synpolydactyly (Table 17.12 and Fig. 17.72).

▌TREATMENT

In isolated central polydactyly, excision of the most hypoplastic digit is performed in keeping with surgical principles of polydactyly reconstruction. In the central polysyndactyly pattern, surgical options include syndactyly reconstruction with excision of the extra digit or creation of a three-fingered hand. The complexity of these deformities requires astute surgical judgment and an individualized approach. Surgical reconstruction should be performed by the time the child is 6 months old to prevent further angular deformity. As many normal-appearing fingers as possible should be reconstructed. Amputation of a functionless digit may be performed later.

■ CLEFT HAND

Central deficiencies of the hand include malformations in which there is a longitudinal failure of formation of the second, third, or fourth ray. Also included in this category are deformities in which there is severe suppression of the radial four rays, leaving a one-digit (fifth-ray) hand. Further suppression that results in a digitless hand is considered a transverse deficiency. Common names for this deformity include ectrodactyly, crab claw, lobster claw, and cleft hand. It is exceedingly rare, with an incidence of approximately 1 per 90,000 live births.

Central deficiencies commonly are classified into two main patterns of deformity: typical and atypical. The typical pattern is a central V-shaped cleft with variable degrees of deficiency of the long ray (Fig. 17.73). Syndactyly between the ulnar and radial two digits is common. The deformity typically is bilateral with similar bilateral foot deformities. The atypical pattern, initially described by Lange, is a severe U-shaped deficiency that involves the index, long, and ring ray, leaving only a thumb and little finger attached to the hand (Fig. 17.74). This deformity usually is unilateral without associated foot deformities. According to Ogino, the atypical pattern should be considered a form of symbrachydactyly and is now recognized as such. Flatt's classification of these malformations includes four groups: group 0, all bones present; group 1, one ray involved; group 2, two rays involved; and

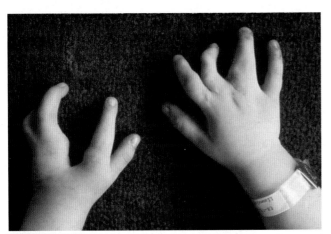

FIGURE 17.73 Typical pattern of central deficiency with central V-shaped cleft.

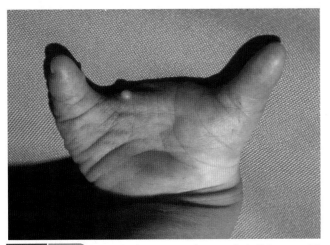

FIGURE 17.74 Atypical pattern of central deficiency with U-shaped deficiency involving index, long, and ring fingers.

group 3, three rays involved. These groups are divided further into three subgroups based on the degree of finger involvement (Fig. 17.75).

The cause of central deficiencies is unknown, and most cases occur sporadically. An autosomal dominant mode of inheritance frequently is seen in the typical pattern, but penetrance often is incomplete. Maisels suggested a centripetal suppression theory according to which milder deformities have only a simple cleft without significant tissue loss, but as the severity of suppression increases, absence of the central ray is seen first, followed by loss of the radial rays and eventually loss of all rays (Fig. 17.76). Müller emphasized the etiologic differences between cleft hand and symbrachydactyly, noting that cleft hand seems to result from primary insufficiency of the central ectodermal ridge, whereas symbrachydactyly may result from primary failure of formation of the underlying bone. This would explain the absence of terminal digital remnants in pure central longitudinal deficiencies. The association of cleft hand and central polydactyly also has been established, emphasizing the complexity of these deformities. A rarer ulnar-sided cleft hand also has been described. These patients have clefting between the small and ring fingers or the small and long fingers with possible absence of the ring ray and hypoplasia of the small finger.

Anomalies that occur most often in association with central hand deficiencies include cleft foot, cleft lip, and cleft palate; congenital heart disease, imperforate anus, anonychia, cataracts, and deafness also have been reported. Reported major musculoskeletal anomalies in addition to hand deformities have included hypoplasia or pseudarthrosis of the clavicle, absent pectoralis major muscle, short humerus, synostosis of the elbow, short forearm, absent ulna, radioulnar synostosis, bilateral absence of the tibia, bilateral dislocation of the hip, short femur, hypoplastic patella, clubfoot, calcaneovalgus foot, cavovarus foot, deviated nasal septum, and congenital ptosis; genitourinary system anomalies also have been reported. The most common associated syndromes are split-hand/split-foot (SHSF) and ectrodactyly ectodermal dysplasia and cleft lip/palate (EEC). SHSF syndrome usually has autosomal dominant inheritance with incomplete penetrance.

The typical cleft hand pattern of a central V-shaped defect in the palm is present at birth. The long finger usually is entirely missing, and frequently the two remaining digits on each side of the cleft have varying degrees of syndactyly and a deficient first web. Similar foot deformities are frequent. Occasionally, the index finger also may be missing, but rarely are the ring and long fingers absent. In the atypical pattern, only two fingers are present, one along the radial border and one along the ulnar border. A shallow U-shaped defect intervenes along the distal palm. The most lateral (radial) ray often lies in the same plane as the most medial (ulnar) ray. The deformity usually is unilateral, without associated foot deformity. In the most severe forms, all digits except for the small finger may be absent.

Radiographic findings vary. Transversely oriented bones and occasionally a delta phalanx may be seen. There may appear to be two metacarpals supporting one digit or a split metacarpal supporting two digits. Goldfarb et al. described and used a metacarpal and phalangeal divergence angle measured between the index and ring finger to assist in preoperative planning and postoperative assessment (Fig. 17.77). Carpal coalition is present in older children.

Children with these deformities develop amazing dexterity but frequently hide their hand in a pocket to avoid drawing attention to its clawlike appearance. This is particularly true in grade school and in new surroundings but seems to diminish as the patient matures.

TREATMENT

No appropriate nonoperative treatment is available for these deformities, and prostheses have been essentially abandoned except on rare occasions when they are requested for cosmesis. The operative management must be individualized according to the deformity and available anatomy. A single cleft can be highly functional. Adaptive function can be significant even in the presence of significant bilateral deformities. General principles of hand surgery are applicable, in that good pinch and grasp are the primary goals, followed by acceptable cosmesis if possible. Surgical reconstruction should maintain or improve hand function and include closure of the cleft, release of syndactyly, correction of thumb adduction contracture, removal of transverse or other deforming bony elements, and correction of delta phalanx. Goldfarb et al. retrospectively reviewed reconstruction

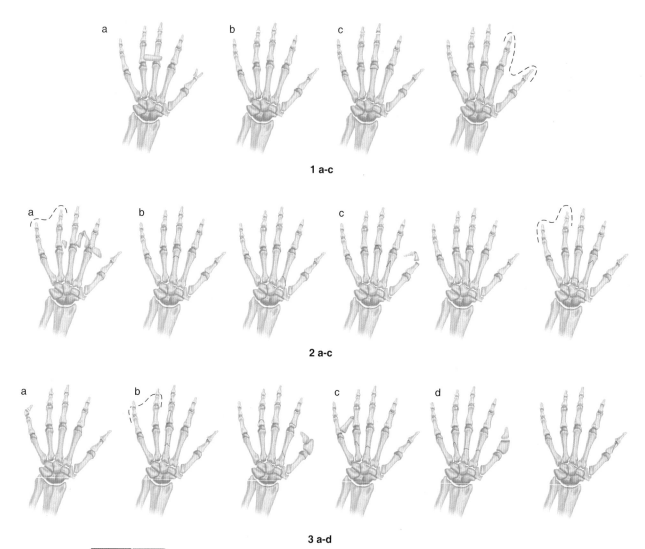

a　b　c

1 a-c

a　b　c

2 a-c

a　b　c　d

3 a-d

FIGURE 17.75 Flatt's classification of central deficiencies. Group 0, all bones present; group 1, one ray involved; group 2, two rays involved; and group 3, three rays involved.

with and without a transverse bone within the cleft, finding similar outcomes between the groups. Worse functional outcomes were associated with preoperative first web space narrowing and postoperative index metacarpophalangeal joint abnormalities. In the atypical pattern, deepening of the palm for grasp, osteotomies of the ulnar or radial metacarpals to allow better opposition, tendon transfers in the hypoplastic hand to restore digital motion, and possibly single-stage toe-to-hand transfer for the one-digit hand occasionally are needed.

In planning the sequence and timing of surgery, the recommendations of Flatt should be carefully reviewed. Syndactyly should be released in the normal time sequence: the border digits by 6 months of age and the central digits by 18 months of age. After a recovery period of 6 months, closure of the cleft alone or closure of the cleft with correction of thumb adduction contracture can be performed. It is often difficult to determine the extent of thumb mobility required by the patient. A minor adduction contracture usually does not require correction. To close the cleft, bony elements that block closure should be removed sparingly

because central metacarpal loss may weaken the palm and lead to cleft recurrence. If cleft closure is performed simultaneously with first web space deepening, the index metacarpal can be transferred to the long metacarpal position by means of the Snow and Littler or Miura and Komada technique. The technique described by Miura and Komada is less demanding technically and produces comparable results with less risk of complications. Recent reports of 20-year outcomes have shown long-term functional success. Ueba also described a technique helpful for palmar cleft with absence of the long finger, especially when the cleft hand is combined with a narrow thumb web. Upton and Taghinia have suggested avoiding all complicated dorsal and volar flaps because of possible flap necrosis and using a simple incision separating the glabrous from the dorsal skin surfaces (Fig. 17.78). All functioning digits with any proximal phalanx should be spared because these usually significantly improve grasp. A delta phalanx should be corrected at about 3 years of age, especially if it is causing radial deviation of the thumb or ulnar deviation of the little finger. Reconstruction of the intermetacarpal ligaments is essential to reinforce the cleft closure and to prevent late

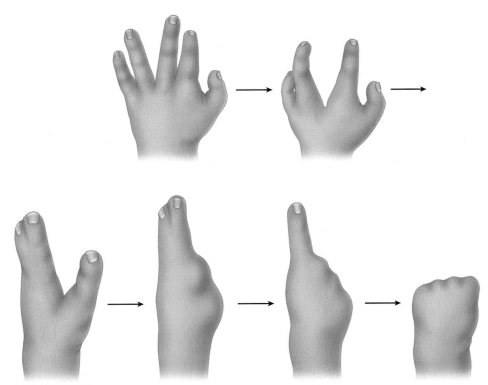

FIGURE 17.76 Maisels' suppression theory. Milder deformities have only simple cleft without significant tissue loss, but as severity of suppression increases, absence first of central ray is followed by loss of radial rays and eventually loss of all rays.

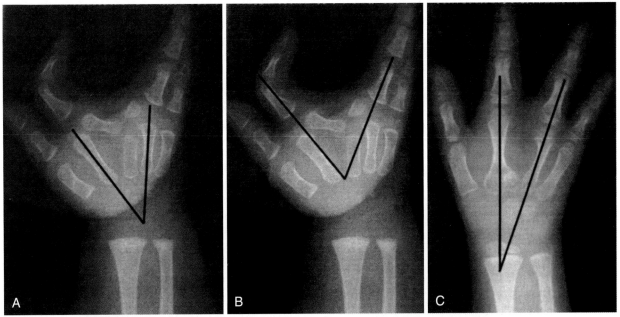

FIGURE 17.77 Radiographic measurement technique for **(A)** metacarpal and **(B)** phalangeal divergence angles. **C,** Radiographic divergence measurement after reconstruction.

diversion of the digits. This can be performed using tendon grafts or using the A1 pulleys from the digits. Described by Saito et al. or Ogino, the A1 pulleys are released and unfolded toward one another, overlapped, then secured using nonabsorbable suture (Fig. 17.79).

In the atypical pattern, the thumb or little finger or both usually are hypoplastic to some extent, making pinch impossible. Deepening of the palm and possibly metacarpal osteotomies performed between age 2 and 3 years should improve grasp. In hands of nearly normal size, tendon transfers usually are unnecessary; however, in severely hypoplastic hands (<50% of normal), tendon transfers may be needed to supplement the available motors. These transfers should be delayed until age 3 years.

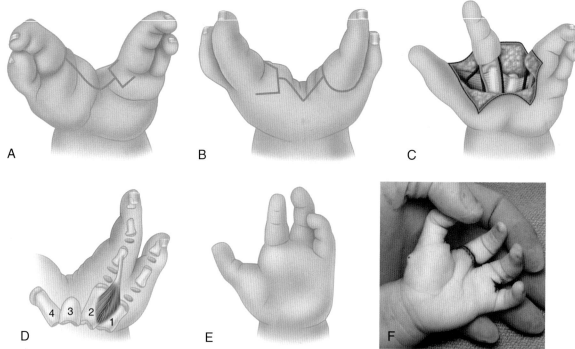

FIGURE 17.78 Upton and Taghinia technique for type II cleft hand. **A,** Incisions within cleft are at juncture of glabrous and dorsal skin. **B,** Small trap door flap is used for commissure lining between ring and transposed index finger. Fibrous band is in contracted first web space. All neurovascular structures isolated on both sides of the index digit. **C,** Flap elevation provides wide exposure to entire palm, including the ring ray. Subperiosteal dissection and removal of long metacarpal. Intrinsic muscles exposed. **D,** Bipennate first dorsal interosseous muscle released from thumb and index ray transposed into long ray position at carpometacarpal level. **E,** Flaps are draped into new first web space and closed. Z-plasties and other local flaps can be used as appropriate. **F,** Final appearance. (From Upton J, Taghinia AH: Correction of the typical cleft hand, *J Hand Surg* 35A:480, 2010.) **SEE TECHNIQUE 17.48.**

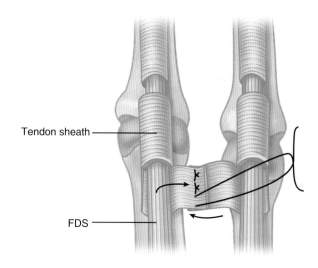

FIGURE 17.79 Cleft closure.

If only one digit exists, a single-stage toe-to-hand transfer may be performed around age 18 months. The strongest indications for this procedure in a child are complete adactyly, complete absence of a thumb, or a nonfunctional thumb with two or fewer fingers on the same hand. Although success has been reported with this technique, numerous problems are associated with the procedure: incorporation of the transferred digit into a functional pattern may be difficult for a child who has never had a thumb, tendon transfers may be required because of deficient donor tendons, anomalous vascular patterns may be present, identification of a recipient branch of the median nerve may be difficult, and a branch of the superficial radial nerve or an adjacent digital nerve may be required to reinnervate the transferred toe.

Manske and Halikis proposed a classification system based on the condition of the thumb-index web that can be used to guide surgical decisions. They identified five progressive narrowings of the thumb web: type 1, normal web (Fig. 17.80); type 2, narrowed web; type 3, syndactylized web; type 4, merged web; and type 5, absent web. Surgical recommendations based on this classification are summarized in Table 17.13.

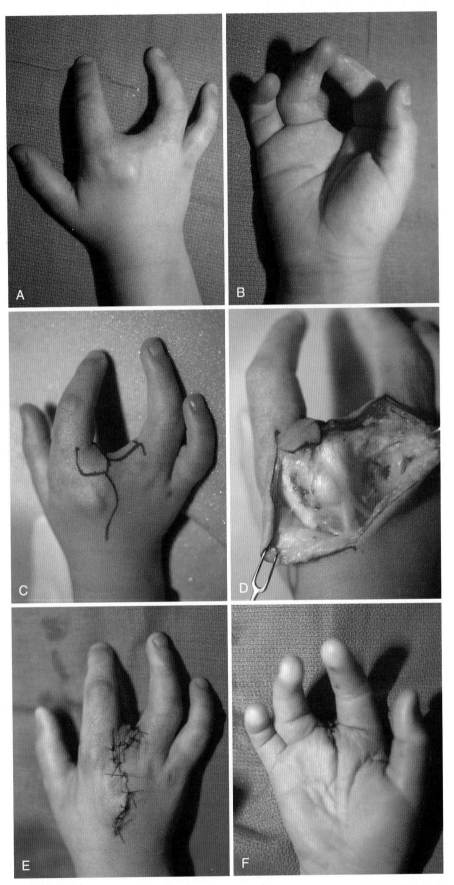

FIGURE 17.80 **A** and **B,** Preoperative appearance of type I central deficiency. **C,** Incision marked for cleft reconstruction. **D,** Exposure for metacarpal excision and index transposition. **E** and **F,** Postoperative appearance.

TABLE 17.13

Surgical Recommendations for Central Deficiency

TYPE	THUMB WEB RECONSTRUCTION	CENTRAL DEFICIENCY CLOSURE
I	None	Cleft closure with local tissue reduction of intermetacarpal space; circumferential tendon graft; local tissue attached to heads (index to middle metacarpal transposition); excise polydactylous bony ossicles when needed
IIA	Local pedicle flaps (Z-plasty)	As noted above
IIB	Dorsal/volar pedicle flaps	As noted above
III	Syndactyly release with skin grafts dorsal/volar pedicle flaps from cleft or excise index bony elements	As noted above or excise index bony elements
IV	None or tissue reduction with metacarpophalangeal stabilization	None (cleft is web space)
V	Consider toe-to-hand transfer or metacarpal lengthening	None

From Manske PR, Halikis MN: Surgical classification of central deficiency according to the thumb web, *J Hand Surg* 20:687, 1995.

CLEFT CLOSURE

TECHNIQUE 17.47

(BARSKY)

- Under tourniquet control, sharply elevate a distally based, diamond-shaped flap from one side of the opposing sides of the involved fingers (Fig. 17.81A). Place the flap slightly dorsally to allow for a gentle slope of the commissure. Make the flap approximately 1 cm at the base and 1.5 times longer than wide. Defat the flap down to the subdermal vascular plexus.
- Make an incision from the free end of the flap along the opposing surfaces of the cleft.
- Expose the metacarpals extraperiosteally.
- Excise excess soft tissue and bony elements that would prevent apposing of the metacarpals.
- Drill two holes in each metacarpal just proximal to the heads and place a heavy suture through the holes (Fig. 17.81B).
- Approximate the metacarpals and tie the suture to secure the correction.
- Close the dorsal and palmar skin incisions from proximal to distal.
- Excise excess skin to create interdigitating flaps along the dorsal and palmar surfaces.
- Place the finger flap into the commissure, and before suturing the flap, excise excess skin from the dorsum of the hand, rather than from the flap (see Fig. 17.81C).
- Apply a well-molded, long arm cast to the level of the metacarpal heads over a minimal amount of bandages.

POSTOPERATIVE CARE   The cast is worn for 3 to 4 weeks. If the thumb tends to separate excessively, another cast is applied for an additional 2 to 3 weeks and then regular use of the hand is allowed. Special therapy usually is not required.

SIMPLE CLOSURE OF TYPE I AND II CLEFT HANDS

TECHNIQUE 17.48

(UPTON AND TAGHINIA)

- Make a simple incision around the index ray and a straight-line incision within the cleft.
- Create a new index-to-ring space by raising a small flap on the radial side of the ring ray with a 45-degree dorsal-to-palmar inclination (see Fig. 17.78A,B).
- Create dorsal and volar skin flaps (see Fig. 17.78C)
- If the first dorsal interosseous muscle is present, release it from the radial origin or ulnar side of the thumb metacarpal. Preserve attachments of the adductor pollicis if present.
- If the metacarpal is hypoplastic, excise the metacarpal subperiosteally and leave the muscle attached to the periosteum.
- Transpose the index metacarpal at the carpometacarpal level and seat it within the long metacarpal periosteal sleeve.
- The index ray should be pronated to allow good thumb-to-pulp contact. Release of flexion contractures, Z-plasty, or skin grafting may be required.
- After skeletal transposition and fixation (see Fig. 17.78D), secure the transposed index finger with nonabsorbable sutures as close as possible to the adjacent digit.
- Use Kirschner wires to maximally abduct the thumb and index rays (see Fig. 17.78D).
- Drape the dorsal and volar flaps without tension into the first web space (see Fig. 17.78E) and close the web commissure between the index and ring fingers.

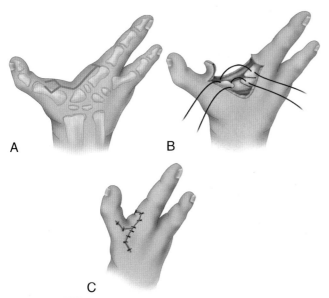

FIGURE 17.81 Barsky technique of cleft closure. **A,** Skin incision. **B,** Approximation of metacarpals with heavy sutures passed through holes drilled in bone. **C,** Flap used to create new web and skin on dorsal and palmar surfaces. **SEE TECHNIQUE 17.47.**

POSTOPERATIVE CARE A dressing and long arm cast are applied. Kirschner wires are removed at 3 to 4 weeks, and a well-contoured spacer or splint is fabricated and worn at night for an additional 6 weeks. Yearly follow-up with radiographs is recommended.

COMBINED CLEFT CLOSURE AND RELEASE OF THUMB ADDUCTION CONTRACTURE

TECHNIQUE 17.49

(SNOW AND LITTLER)
- Make incisions that outline the sides of the cleft on the dorsal surfaces of the index and ring fingers, joining the incisions where the V-shaped apex extends proximal to the level of the metacarpal head.
- Make a small, straight incision on the ulnar side of the index finger to accommodate a small flap that will be used to make a commissure (Fig. 17.82A). Raise this flap on the radial side of the ring finger.
- As the incisions pass the metacarpal heads, curve them back proximally onto the palm, almost parallel with each other and lying to the cleft side of the midline of the two fingers (Fig. 17.82B). Do not extend the incisions any farther into the palm than a point opposite the V-shaped apex of the dorsal incision. This is the palmar flap to create the new thumb web.
- To release the thumb adduction contracture, make another incision beginning on the dorsum of the thumb web at the same level as the V-shaped cleft incision.
- Extend the incision distally, parallel with the index split incision until it reaches the distal edge of the thumb-index web. This creates a strip of dorsal skin that is left connected to the index finger and the dorsum of the hand and that covers the dorsal veins and extensor tendons of the index finger.
- Develop the split flap from the dorsum, carefully tying the dorsal veins in the incision; do not dissect them off the flap. The flap becomes compromised unless venous drainage is good. Also carefully protect and preserve the branches of the median nerve.
- Develop the thumb-index incision and release the fibrous bands between the two metacarpals.
- Detach the origins of the first dorsal interosseous from these bones.
- The adductor muscle and the radial belly of the flexor pollicis brevis muscle may have to be elevated from their origins; the radial artery must be protected during this step. Occasionally, the dissection has to be carried down to the capsule of the carpometacarpal joint, and sometimes the capsule must be incised to permit full thumb abduction.
- Perform an osteotomy of the index ray at its base and transfer it to the third metacarpal (Fig. 17.82C).
- If the third metacarpal is small, shape the index ray into a peg and impale it into the base of the third metacarpal.
- If enough bone is present, fix the index metacarpal to the base of the third metacarpal with a Kirschner wire (Fig. 17.82D). Carefully align the metacarpals so that the transposed ray maintains the transverse and longitudinal arches of the hand and allows the fingers to flex into the palm normally without overlap.
- Suture the skin between the ring and index fingers. Inset the small, longitudinal incision on the ulnar side of the index finger to make a commissure. Use a small drain in the wound as needed.
- Place the large palmar-based cleft flap between the index finger and the newly abducted thumb (Fig. 17.82E). If this flap does not completely cover the area of defect, use a split skin graft for complete coverage. Never place these flaps under tension; if necessary, use a skin graft over the index finger.
- Apply a well-padded long arm cast, maintaining the arches of the hand and leaving the fingers and thumb enough freedom to move.

POSTOPERATIVE CARE The cast is worn for 6 weeks. Sutures are removed at about 2 weeks, and the Kirschner wire is removed at about 6 weeks or after bone healing has occurred. After cast and pin removal, normal activities are permitted on a graduated basis over 6 to 8 weeks.

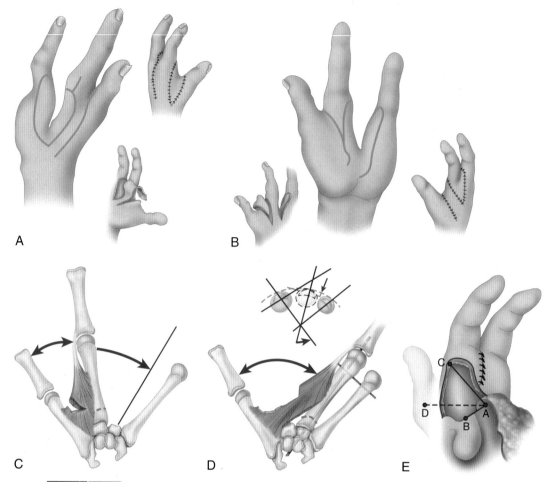

FIGURE 17.82 Snow and Littler technique of combined cleft closure and release of thumb adduction contracture (see text). **A,** Dorsal view. Skin incisions, flap elevation, and wound closure. **B,** Palmar view. Skin incisions, flap elevation, and wound closure. **C,** Index finger is transposed after osteotomy of base of index metacarpal and release of first dorsal interosseous muscle. **D,** Additional release of first dorsal interosseous subperiosteally from base of index allows transposition of index metacarpal to ring metacarpal base. Inset shows rotation necessary (possibly 45 degrees) for transposed digit to prevent overlap. **E,** Relationship of thumb adduction contracture release and palmar flap. Although release allows thumb mobility, area at C may not be covered by palmar flap and may require skin grafting. **SEE TECHNIQUE 17.49.**

CLEFT CLOSURE AND RELEASE OF THUMB ADDUCTION CONTRACTURE

TECHNIQUE 17.50   *Figure 17.83*

(MIURA AND KOMADA)
- Make a linear incision beginning on the radial side of the base of the ring finger and continuing to the ulnar side of the base of the index finger and crossing the cleft space.
- Make a curved incision around the base of the index finger at the level desired for the new thumb web space.
- Detach the index metacarpal at its base, along with the first dorsal interosseous muscle.

- If exposure is inadequate, make another dorsal skin incision to expose just the bases of the index and long metacarpals.
- Release the fascia of the adductor pollicis and the first dorsal interosseous.
- If the base of the third metacarpal is present, impale the index ray on the base of the third metacarpal and fix it with Kirschner wires.
- Reconstruct the transverse metacarpal ligament with two or three soft-tissue sutures between the index and ring fingers.
- Fashion the flap for the thumb web from the skin radial to the curved incision along the original cleft.
- Close the skin. Apply a long arm cast molded over the metacarpals to prevent separation of the cleft.

POSTOPERATIVE CARE The cast and skin sutures are removed at 3 weeks. Additional casting may be required if there is any laxity in the cleft. After final cast removal, gradual resumption of normal activities is permitted over 6 to 8 weeks.

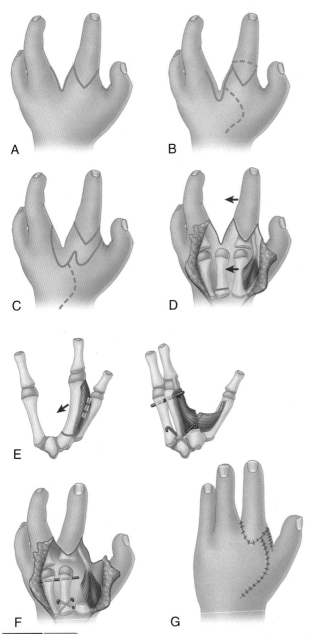

A

B

C

D

E

F

G

FIGURE 17.83 Miura and Komada reconstruction of cleft hand with adducted thumb. **A,** Initial skin incision on dorsum of hand. **B,** Additional incisions *(broken line)* to expose metacarpal dorsally and finger on palmar surface. **C,** Index finger skin flaps. **D,** Scheme for transposing index metacarpal to middle metacarpal position. **E,** Bone transposition: fasciae of first dorsal interosseous and adductor pollicis are released, and muscle may require release. **F,** Transposition of index and release of thumb completed. **G,** Appearance after wound closure. **SEE TECHNIQUE 17.50.**

PALMAR CLEFT CLOSURE

TECHNIQUE 17.51

(UEBA)

- Make a V-shaped skin incision in the form of a triangular skin flap on the radial side of the ring finger (Fig. 17.84A). This flap is used to form the commissure.

- Make a second skin incision beginning from the palmar end of the previous skin incision and extending to the ulnar side of the palm (Fig. 17.84B).
- Make a third skin incision around the base of the index finger; place an incision at the bottom of the cleft to connect the previous incisions (Fig. 17.84C).
- Elevate the interdigital palmar and dorsal skin flaps and sever the fibrous bands between the thumb and index finger to widen the thumb web as much as possible (Fig. 17.84D).
- Elevate the periosteum around the second metacarpal and transfer the metacarpal ulnarward, avoiding injury to the ulnar nerve.
- Shift the second metacarpal slightly ulnarward and supinate it so that the index finger flexes without overlapping the ring finger.
- Fix the second metacarpal to the fourth metacarpal with one or two Kirschner wires and a nonabsorbable suture or long-lasting absorbable suture around the metacarpal necks.
- Connect the common extensor tendons to the index and ring fingers with a free tendon graft taken from the palmaris longus muscle. Pass this tendon graft through the extensor tendons at the level of the metacarpophalangeal joints, reflect its ends, and suture them to the extensor aponeurosis (Fig. 17.84E).
- After rotating the flaps (Fig. 17.84F), make suture lines transversely to conceal the original cleft and deepen the thumb web (Fig. 17.84G).
- Close the skin with absorbable sutures.
- Apply a long arm cast, molded to avoid recurrence of the cleft.

POSTOPERATIVE CARE The cast and any remaining sutures are removed at 3 weeks, when a second cast is applied. The cast and Kirschner wires are removed at about 6 weeks or when bone healing is complete. Resumption of normal activities is allowed during the next 4 to 6 weeks.

DEEPENING OF WEB AND METACARPAL OSTEOTOMY

TECHNIQUE 17.52

- It usually is safer to undertake correction in two stages.
- First, deepen the web by Z-plasty and remove any redundant bone segments or rudimentary digits.
- Later, shorten a metacarpal if needed or rotate one or both to provide oppositional pinch between the digits.
- Apply a long arm cast.

POSTOPERATIVE CARE The sutures are removed at 2 weeks, and the cast is removed at 4 to 6 weeks. Normal activities are resumed during the next 4 to 6 weeks.

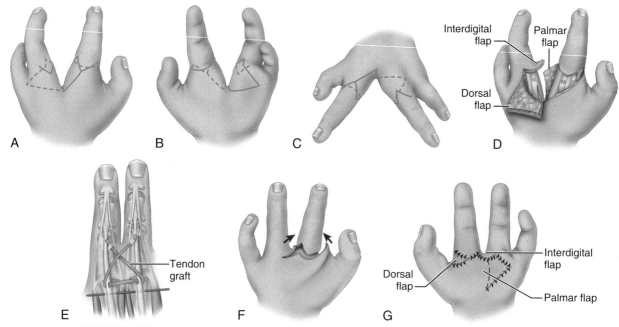

FIGURE 17.84 Ueba technique for cleft hand. **A,** Dorsal view of incisions. Solid line indicates dorsal incisions; broken line indicates palmar incisions. **B,** Palmar view of incisions. Solid line indicates palmar incisions; broken line indicates dorsal incisions. **C,** Incisions from web space. Solid line indicates dorsal incisions; broken line indicates palmar incisions. **D,** Flaps developed and elevated. **E,** Reconstruction of extensor tendon with graft; Kirschner wire stabilizes index to ring metacarpal. **F,** Flaps rotated. **G,** Appearance of palm after wound closure. **SEE TECHNIQUE 17.51.**

TENDON TRANSFER FOR TYPE II DEFORMITIES

TECHNIQUE 17.53

(FLATT)

- This procedure requires good, stable, passive range of motion in the border digits.
- Identify the donor tendons, either wrist flexors or extensors, through appropriate incisions.
- Harvest the palmaris longus tendon to be used as a graft for the transfers.
- Secure the graft to the donor tendons with a Pulvertaft weave and secure the distal ends into the terminal phalanges of the border digits with a pull-out wire.

POSTOPERATIVE CARE The wrist is splinted in mild flexion for 3 weeks, and then the pull-out wire and skin sutures are removed. Normal activities are resumed gradually during the next 4 to 6 weeks.

■ APERT SYNDROME

In 1906, Apert described a patient with a group of deformities that included atypical facies and multiple complex syndactylies of the hand, which he called acrocephalosyndactyly.

Despite its rarity (1 per 200,000 births), much has been written about the management of the complex hand deformities in this syndrome. The condition is believed to result from a single gene mutation in one of the parents and can be passed in dominant and recessive forms; sporadic occurrences also are possible. The abnormal gene is located on chromosome 10q26 and has been identified as *FGFR-2*. Apert syndrome was classified into two main categories by Blank: (1) true, or typical, characterized by multiple complex syndactylies, and (2) atypical, with only partial syndactylies.

At birth, these patients have a high, broad forehead and a flattened occiput. The eyes are widely set, with the outer canthus lower than the inner canthus. The lower jaw is prominent, and the maxilla is shortened (Fig. 17.85A). Mental retardation is common but not universal. There may be associated visceral abnormalities. These patients usually can be expected to live well into adulthood. The hand deformities are typically symmetrical. Upton classified the Apert hand into three types. Type 1 or "spade hand" has a separate thumb with complete syndactyly of the remaining digits. Type 2 or "spoon hand" has syndactyly involving all the digits. The hand is spoon shaped, with a tapering terminal end and complex syndactyly of the index, long, and ring fingers (Fig. 17.85B). The little finger usually shows complete simple syndactyly with the ring finger. Often a nail is shared between the index, long, and ring fingers. The fingers have limited motion because of incomplete joint development, and they usually are shortened. Type 3 or "rosebud hand" has complex syndactyly with distal synostosis between the thumb and the index finger with a broad conjoined nail overlying the thumb, index long,

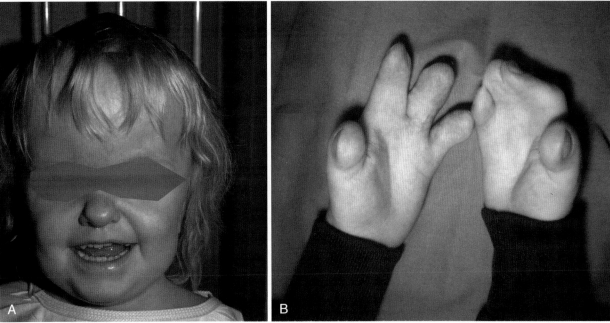

FIGURE 17.85 Apert syndrome. **A,** Characteristic facial features of high forehead and wide-set eyes. **B,** Complex syndactyly involving all fingers of both hands; left hand has had syndactyly release.

and ring fingers. Five digits usually are present, distinguishing Apert syndrome from Carpenter syndrome (acrocephalopolysyndactyly), in which polydactyly also is present. The arm and forearm frequently are shortened with limited elbow motion. The untreated hand functions in a spoonlike fashion with either a two-handed or a thumb-to-side-of-index finger prehensile pattern.

TREATMENT

Reconstructive surgery usually improves hand function in these patients by creating a three-fingered hand with an opposable thumb. Early cranial surgery if recommended should take priority over hand surgery and should not be performed simultaneously. The surgical management should follow the protocol outlined by Flatt. In children younger than 2 years old, bilateral simultaneous reconstructive procedures may be performed because children at this age are not dependent on self-care. In older children, only one hand at a time should be reconstructed. The border digits should be released before 1 year of age. If the thumb is not included in the syndactyly, a simple four-part Z-plasty is used to deepen the first web; 6 to 9 months later, release of the central syndactylies and deletion of the middle finger at the metacarpophalangeal joint are performed. This deletion provides the necessary skin coverage and good sensibility to the remaining digits. Flatt found more deformity in patients with a ray amputation of the long finger and ulnar transposition of the index finger, and this procedure is not recommended.

Split grafts can be used to cover any residual defect. Ring and small metacarpal synostosis release should be done at the time of digital separation. For radially angulated thumbs, Dao et al. recommended a release of the abnormal abductor pollicis brevis tendon insertion into the distal phalanx and reinsertion into the proximal phalanx, excision of the metacarpal

head ulnar prominence, and pinning of the interphalangeal and metacarpophalangeal joints. Oishi and Ezaki proposed that the thumb be reconstructed by releasing the abnormal abductor pollicis brevis insertion, opening or closing wedge osteotomy of the proximal phalanx, and a V-Y advancement flap on the radial side of the thumb.

RECONSTRUCTION OF THE HAND IN APERT SYNDROME

TECHNIQUE 17.54

(FLATT)

STAGE I
- Release of the border digits is performed before 1 year of age.
- Begin with the first web space opening.
- For partial syndactyly, a four-flap Z-plasty can be used.
- For complete syndactyly, a dorsal flap as described by Buck-Gramcko can be useful to restore the first web.
- Perform a simple release of the aberrant distal adductor pollicis brevis insertion on the distal phalanx when necessary and repair it to the base of the proximal phalanx.
- Release the fourth web space as described by Bauer et al. (see Technique 17.39) using zigzag incisions and standard dorsally based flaps for restoration of the web commissure.
- Close the flaps with simple interrupted sutures.

- Use full-thickness skin grafts for coverage of remaining defects.

STAGE II

- This stage is performed 6 to 9 months after the initial operation to allow for scar maturation and revascularization.
- Release the fourth and second web spaces as described by Bauer et al., using all the skin on the middle digit.
- After flap elevation and when necessary, amputate the long digit below the metacarpophalangeal joint.
- Use the remaining skin to reconstruct the remaining web commissure and for coverage of remaining digits.
- Interdigitate the flaps and close in routine fashion. Use a full-thickness skin flap to cover any remaining defect as necessary.
- Dress the wounds with moistened nonstick sterile dressing and apply a long arm cast.

POSTOPERATIVE CARE The splint is worn for 4 weeks. Active motion of the hand is encouraged.

DEFORMATIONS

CONSTRICTION RING SYNDROME (AMNIOTIC BAND SYNDROME)

Congenital ring, or congenital constriction band, syndrome occurs when deep cutaneous creases encircle a limb as if a string were tightly tied around the part (Fig. 17.86). Its frequent association with congenital amputations and acrosyndactyly led to this malformation's designation as a syndrome. Other terms used to describe this condition include Streeter bands or dysplasia, annular grooves or defects, and intrauterine amputation. Patterson reported an incidence of one per 15,000 births. Constriction bands represented 2% of anomalies in Flatt's series. More distal rings are more common, as is involvement of the central digits.

There is no evidence that congenital ring syndrome is an inherited condition. An external effect of amniotic adhesions formed in utero after hemorrhages in the distal rays has been suggested as a cause as has failure of development of subcutaneous tissue in the same manner that normal skin creases are formed. There is general agreement that these malformations occur later than at 5 to 7 weeks of gestation, when most hand anomalies occur; the youngest fetus described with this anomaly was at 10 weeks of gestation.

Patterson included four types of deformity in congenital ring syndrome: (1) a simple ring usually occurring transversely, but occasionally obliquely, around the limb or digit; (2) a deeper ring often associated with abnormality of the part distally, usually lymphedema; (3) fenestrated syndactyly (acrosyndactyly) or lateral fusion of adjacent digits at their distal ends with proximal fenestrations between the intervening skin and soft tissue; and (4) intrauterine amputation, in which the soft tissues are more affected than the bone, which may protrude as in a guillotine amputation—there are no rudimentary parts distally and the proximal limb parts are normally developed. These four types may be present in any combination in a single child, but they do not occur constantly with any other type of anomaly of the limbs.

Syndactyly, hypoplasia, brachydactyly, symphalangism, symbrachydactyly, and camptodactyly have been reported in 80% of patients with congenital ring syndrome, and clubfoot, cleft lip, cleft palate, and cranial defects have been reported in 40% to 50% of patients with this syndrome. Generally, there are no associated visceral malformations, but one of Flatt's patients had a patent ductus arteriosus.

These malformations usually are asymmetric. The grooves, or rings, vary in circumferential extent and depth and at times appear as normal but misplaced skin creases. Lymphedema distal to the crease is frequent. With shallow rings, the skin often is normal, but subcutaneous tissue usually is deficient. With deeper rings, the superficial blood vessels that run across the ring are absent, although deep vessels are intact. Digits distal to the rings may be shortened or completely amputated. Terminal simple syndactyly with small fenestrations through the proximal web is frequent. The rings are not static in their effect. If the ring is deep and unrelenting, there may be progressive necrosis beneath the ring, with increased scarring, constriction, and vascular impairment. Distal lymphedema, cyanosis, and worsening at the site of constriction have been reported before surgical intervention; rarely does the ring progress to cause frank necrosis of the distal part.

■ TREATMENT

For shallow, incomplete creases with no distal lymphedema, surgical intervention usually is unnecessary except to improve appearance. The creases should be observed for gradual improvement in appearance, which may occur as "baby fat" is lost. If creases are deep enough to cause lymphedema or impairment of circulation, they should be excised down to normal tissue, and the defect should be closed with multiple Z-plasty procedures. If the ring completely encircles the part, the safer approach is staged excision of one half of the groove with Z-plasty closure, followed by a second operation 2 to 3 months later. Lymphedema and cyanosis usually improve gradually after release. Simple excision of the groove with simple everting closure generally is inadequate because circumferential scar contracture may occur. In refute of this principle, several investigators have been pleased with excision of the scar and simple advancement of the normal proximal and distal fasciocutaneous tissue. The approach described includes simple excision with direct closure combined with limited Z-plasty. Ulnar nerve palsy was associated with congenital ring syndrome in one study.

Acrosyndactyly is a frequent component of this syndrome. Because all fingertips frequently are bound together, permanent deformity results, unless early syndactyly reconstruction is performed. Release of the border digits should be done within the first 6 months of life, followed by release of the central digits when the child is about 18 months old. Finger stiffness at the proximal interphalangeal joints is common after syndactyly release. Short digits may require lengthening by osteotomy and distraction. The shortened thumb may require deepening of the web space or lengthening by the method of Søiland, in which an extremely shortened index finger is added to the top of the thumb. Amputations in this syndrome usually have adequate or abundant soft-tissue coverage and rarely require surgical reconstruction.

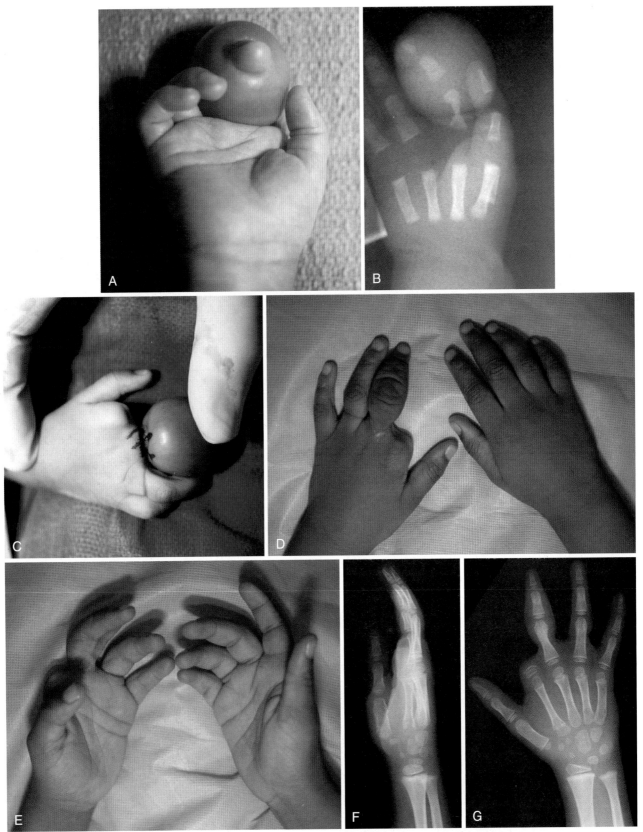

FIGURE 17.86 **A,** Congenital ring syndrome with amputation of index finger and severe lymphedema of long finger. Good capillary refill was present at birth despite severe lymphedema; surgery was postponed for 1 month to lessen surgical risk. **B,** Radiograph showing hourglass deformity of proximal phalanx. **C,** Staged multiple Z-plasties performed. **D,** Lymphedema gradually diminished after Z-plasties. Active flexion and extension of digit were present. **E to G,** At 2 years' follow-up.

MULTIPLE Z-PLASTY RELEASE OF A CONGENITAL RING

TECHNIQUE 17.55

- If the congenital ring is deep and completely encircles the limb or finger, plan to correct only half of the ring in the initial procedure.
- Before inflating the tourniquet, mark out the multiple Z-plasty sites along the constricting ring (Fig. 17.87A).
- Exsanguinate the limb and inflate the tourniquet.
- Excise half the constricting ring and sharply incise the Z-plasty sites to elevate the flaps.

- Suture the flaps in an appropriate interdigitating fashion to allow for lengthening of the constricting ring (Fig. 17.87B).
- Deflate the tourniquet and apply a bulky dressing with a short arm or long arm splint.

POSTOPERATIVE CARE The splinting is maintained for 2 to 3 weeks. Sutures are removed after 10 to 14 days. The other half of the constricting ring can be similarly reconstructed after 2 to 3 months.

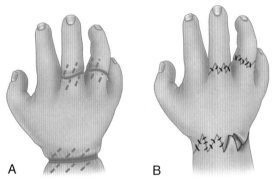

FIGURE 17.87 Multiple Z-plasties for severe congenital ring syndrome. **A,** Band is completely excised after it is ascertained that no deep fascial constriction remains. Only volar half of ring should be corrected at initial procedure. **B,** Z-plasty closure. **SEE TECHNIQUE 17.55.**

TRIGGER FINGERS

Congenital trigger digit occurs when the normal gliding movement of the flexor tendon is impeded within the digital flexor sheath. In contrast to the situation in adults with stenosing tendovaginitis, the congenitally involved finger usually shows a persistent flexion deformity, rather than actual "triggering" (Fig. 17.88A). This is a relatively rare condition (2.3%). It occurs far more commonly in the thumb and is bilateral in about 25% of patients. The condition occurs sporadically and is not believed to be an inherited trait. Trigger digits typically occur without other anomalies, but an association with trisomy 13 has been reported. Its association with mucopolysaccharidosis also has been described.

Trigger digits in children are more commonly acquired; 25% are noted at birth. A prospective study of 5765 newborns did not reveal a single case of congenital trigger thumb. Frequently, the condition is not noted until age 1 or 2 years, at which time the child has a relatively fixed flexion posture of the interphalangeal joint of the thumb. Even with some force, it may be impossible to extend the interphalangeal joint of the thumb fully, although an occasional extension posture of the thumb and involvement of multiple digits have been reported. The abnormal clicking or snapping usually is not the presenting complaint as seen in adults. This condition

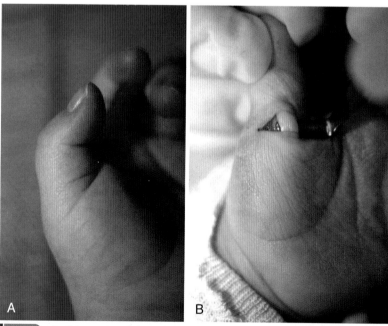

FIGURE 17.88 **A,** Trigger thumb in 2-year-old child. **B,** After release. **SEE TECHNIQUE 17.56.**

must be differentiated from the clasped thumb deformity, in which there is primarily metacarpophalangeal flexion.

The pathologic anatomy responsible for trigger digits includes narrowing and thickening of the sheath, with occasional formation of a ganglion cyst. An intratendinous nodule may be present proximal to the first annular pulley often referred to as Notta's nodule. Chronic inflammation also is frequent. Fixed contractures are unlikely if the condition resolves or is corrected before the child is 3 years old. Spontaneous resolution occurs in about 30% of children in whom the condition appears within the first year of life and in about 12% of children in whom it appears between 6 months and 2 years of age. Baek et al. noted spontaneous resolution in 63% over a median of 48 months. Timing of surgical intervention has been called into question. Han et al. reported excellent results in surgical A1 pulley release in children with an average age of 7.5 years. He noted return of motion to near normal by an average of 2.7 weeks postoperatively. Several articles have emphasized the differences between the congenital trigger finger and trigger thumb. Trigger finger is not often associated with a fixed flexion deformity, and, more importantly, it may not respond to a simple A-pulley release. When surgical intervention for trigger finger is undertaken, the surgeon should be prepared for a more extensive exploration of the flexor mechanism, which may include excision of one or both slips of the flexor digitorum superficialis tendon and release of the A3 pulley.

■ TREATMENT

Because spontaneous resolution can be expected in about 30% of children whose condition becomes apparent within the first year of life, observation and gentle manipulation are appropriate. Splinting can be attempted; a success rate of 92% has been reported. If the thumb is locked or painful, then surgical release is recommended. Intermittent nonpainful triggering can be followed safely in hopes of resolution if this is preferred by the parents; the timing of surgery probably has no effect on the ultimate outcome. Shiozawa et al. showed improvement in 20 of 24 patients with splinting. Only seven patients required surgery. However, there is little justification in subjecting a child to years of triggering, especially because surgical release has been found safe and effective. Early surgical intervention should be considered in patients with bilateral locked trigger thumb because conservative treatment frequently fails. Ignoring the problem in hopes of resolution is not appealing. Surgical release of the first annular pulley should be performed at about age 2 years if spontaneous resolution has not occurred. In the rare instance in which multiple trigger digits fixed in extension prevent the child from making a fist, surgical intervention should be earlier (around 1 year of age). In recent low-powered studies, open A1 pulley release has shown more reliable and rapid recovery when compared with nonoperative treatment. Accidental nerve injury may be avoided by first making a shallow incision and identifying the digital nerves. Lacerated digital nerves and tendons should be repaired. Percutaneous trigger thumb release in children has been reported without complications, although we cannot recommend this currently. Recurrence is unlikely if release is adequate.

RELEASE OF A CONGENITAL TRIGGER THUMB

TECHNIQUE 17.56

- Under tourniquet control, make a transverse incision at the volar crease of the metacarpophalangeal joint of the thumb.
- Carefully protect the two digital nerves.
- The flexor sheath usually is quite prominent just beneath the subcutaneous fat.
- Identify the proximal edge of the first annular pulley and completely incise it longitudinally under direct vision.
- Shaving the nodule and excising a segment of the A1 pulley usually are unnecessary.
- Close the wound (Fig. 17.88B) and apply a soft dressing. No particular immobilization is required.
- This procedure can be done in a similar fashion in other involved digits.

RELEASE OF A TRIGGER FINGER

TECHNIQUE 17.57

- Make a Bruner incision centered over the A1 pulley to allow for proximal and distal exposure of the flexor tendon sheath and its contents.
- Identify and protect the digital nerves.
- Incise the A1 pulley completely and assess the finger for further triggering.
- Inspect the flexor tendons for nodules.
- Passively flex and extend the digit and inspect the motion of the flexor tendons.
- If there is no triggering and normal gliding of flexor digitorum superficialis and profundus is present, routine closure is carried out.
- If further triggering or abnormal motion is observed, inspect the superficialis tendon for a more proximal than normal decussation or an abnormal insertion into the flexor digitorum profundus tendon.
- Excise a slip of the flexor digitorum superficialis tendon if necessary.
- Inspect the A3 pulley area and release the A3 pulley if there is triggering at this level. Place the finger through a passive range of motion to ensure that the triggering has resolved.
- Apply proximal traction to both flexor tendons together and individually, and passively extend the finger to verify that there is no further triggering.
- Close the skin and apply a soft hand dressing.

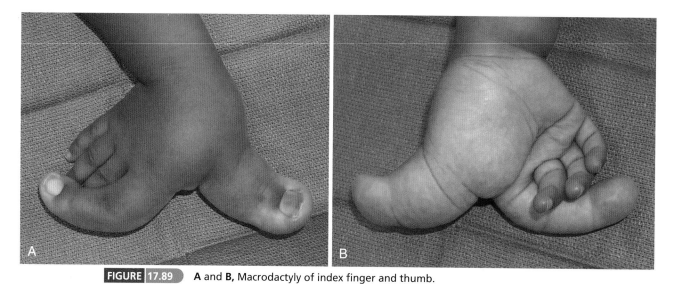

FIGURE 17.89 A and B, Macrodactyly of index finger and thumb.

TABLE 17.14

Flatt Classification of Macrodactyly

TYPE	DESCRIPTION
Type I: Gigantism and lipofibromatosis	Macrodactyly associated with enlarged nerves infiltrated with fat within the digit and extending proximally through carpal tunnel; most common form of macrodactyly deformity
Type II: Gigantism and neurofibromatosis	Macrodactyly usually occurs in conjunction with plexiform form of neurofibromatosis and is often bilateral; may be osteochondral masses associated with the enlarged skeleton
Type III: Gigantism and digital hyperostosis	Hyperostotic form of macrodactyly with osteochondral periarticular masses developing in infancy; no significant nerve enlargement; very rare and not hereditary; the digits are nodular and stiff, and there may be other skeletal anomalies
Type IV: Gigantism and hemihypertrophy	Rare anomaly without know inheritance pattern or etiologic pattern; macrodactyly part of hemihypertrophy; all digits involved, but less severe than type I or II; deformity marked by intrinsic muscle hypertrophy or abnormal intrinsic anatomy; deformities present with flexion contracture, ulnar deviation, and an adducted thumb deformity

From Kay SP, McCombe DB, Kozin SH: Deformities of the hand and fingers. In Wolfe SW, Hotchkiss RN, Pederson WC, Kozin SH, Cohen MS, editors: *Green's Operative Hand Surgery*, ed 3, Philadelphia, 2017, Elsevier, pp. 1276.

DYSPLASIAS
HYPERTROPHY
■ MACRODACTYLY

Macrodactyly is a rare congenital anomaly (0.9%) in which there is fibrofatty enlargement of the finger. The index finger is involved most frequently (Fig. 17.89). Macrodactyly does not seem to be an inherited condition. However, recent discoveries have shown mutations of the PIK3CA pathway associated with many overgrowth disorders, including isolated macrodactyly. Although its cause is uncertain, three possible factors are strongly suspected: abnormal nerve supply, abnormal blood supply, and abnormal humoral mechanism. Vascular malformations, lymphedema, or tumors can cause overgrowth but are not considered true macrodactyly. Barsky described two types of true macrodactyly: static enlargement of the digit without progression as the child grows and progressive enlargement out of proportion to normal growth. The latter form may not enlarge during infancy but begins to enlarge rapidly during early childhood; this form frequently is associated with angular deformity

(Table 17.14). Macrodactyly most commonly exists without other conditions, but syndactyly is associated with macrodactyly in about 10% of patients. Macrodactyly involving the hands and the feet has been reported by Keret, Ger, and Marks. Some patients with neurofibromatosis develop macrodactyly.

In static macrodactyly, the deformity is present in infancy. There usually is diffuse enlargement of the digit; however, the distal and palmar tissues usually appear more enlarged than the dorsal and proximal tissues. The finger grows, but in proportion to normal digital growth. Progressive macrodactyly occurs in early childhood as a rapidly enlarging digit, frequently with an angular deformity that makes the finger banana shaped (Fig. 17.90). The skin may be thickened, and the nails may be hypertrophied. The phalanges always are involved, and the metacarpals may be enlarged. With maturity, the enlarged digit begins to lose motion. Later in life, symptoms of carpal tunnel syndrome may develop, with complaints of paresthesias and hypesthesias. Trophic ulcers also may develop over the involved digit. Involvement usually is unilateral, and multiple digits are affected two to three times as often as single digits. If the thumb is involved, a characteristic

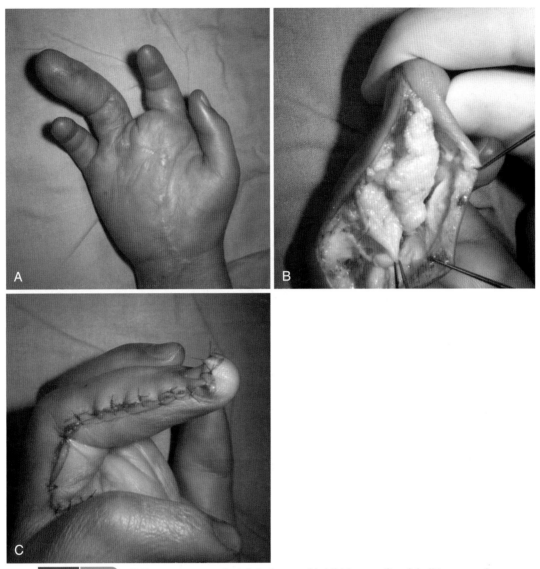

FIGURE 17.90 **A,** Recurrent macrodactyly in 6-year-old child 2 years after debulking procedure of ring finger and amputation of long finger. **B,** Intraoperative photograph shows enlargement of digital nerve. **C,** Wound closure after debulking.

abduction and hyperextension deformity results. It generally is believed that all the tissues of the involved finger are enlarged; however, some authors have noted sparing of the tendons and vessels. The nerves that innervate the involved territory are characteristically enlarged. In a rare type of macrodactyly (hyperostotic), there may be osteocartilaginous deposits around the joints; a traumatic cause for this condition has been reported.

TREATMENT

There are no satisfactory nonsurgical methods of controlling macrodactyly. Attempts to compress the digit with elastic wrapping have been unsuccessful. Indications for surgery include enlargement, angulation, carpal tunnel syndrome, and causalgia. For a progressively enlarging digit, a debulking procedure usually is needed. With this procedure, as much excess tissue as possible is excised from one half of the digit; 3 months later, the other half is debulked. This procedure may be required several times during the growth period.

Tsuge proposed that the disproportionate growth is a result of excessive neural input and recommended that the digital nerves be stripped of one half of their fascicles at the time of debulking. He also recommended complete excision of the enlarged digital nerves during debulking as the most effective way to control progressive macrodactyly, believing that this causes only minimal neural impairment in children. Kelikian recommended segmental resection of the tortuous digital nerves with end-to-end repair.

Physeal arrest by drilling holes through the physes, resection of the physes, or epiphysiodesis of all phalanges frequently is recommended after the digit has reached the estimated length of same-sex parent's. Various methods of digital shortening also have been described, including simple amputation of the distal phalanx and filleting of the distal phalanx, with transfer of the nail and matrix onto the end of the middle phalanx, with or without some of the underlying distal phalanx. In the angulated finger, closing wedge osteotomies through the proximal or middle phalanx are necessary for correction. Tan et al. performed middle phalangectomy in one patient with macrodactyly as their preferred surgical option. Millesi described a complicated technique for shortening the enlarged thumb, in which parts of the distal and middle phalanges are removed and the distal interphalangeal joint is preserved. However, shortening procedures are prone to stiffness and development of contractures. Amputation is used to provide relief only as a last resort in an adult with a severe and bothersome deformity. Although not routinely performed, long finger pollicization has been reported for severe, nonreconstructable macrodactyly of the index finger and thumb.

The most common complication is recurrence, which is expected after debulking. Flap necrosis is a major surgical complication, and some authors have recommended excision of the overlying skin and replacement with a full-thickness skin graft to avoid this problem. Careful attention to flap design may help prevent skin necrosis. Operating on only one side of the finger at a time minimizes the risk of circulatory disturbance.

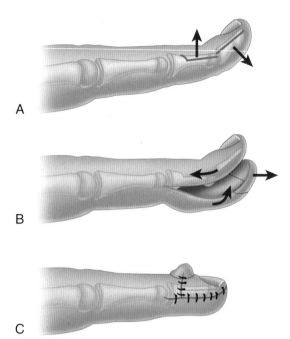

FIGURE 17.91 Digital shortening for macrodactyly (Tsuge). **A,** Matching sections *(shaded areas)* of volar half of distal phalanx and dorsal half of middle phalanx are removed. **B,** Distal phalanx is reduced on middle phalanx, with preservation of dorsal skin bridge, but removal of excess soft tissue. **C,** Soft-tissue closure is completed, accepting some excess dorsal soft tissue. **SEE TECHNIQUE 17.58.**

DEBULKING

TECHNIQUE 17.58

(TSUGE)
- Under tourniquet control, make a midlateral incision the length of the involved digit.
- Identify and dissect out the digital nerve.
- Excise all excessive adipose tissue.
- If the digital nerve is grossly enlarged, half the fascicles may be stripped and excised as recommended by Tsuge. If the digital nerve is excessively tortuous, a section can be resected and an end-to-end repair performed as described by Kelikian.
- Resect matching sections of the volar half of the distal phalanx and the dorsal half of the middle phalanx (Fig. 17.91A) and reduce the fragments (Fig. 17.91B).
- Remove excessive skin, close the incision (Fig. 17.91C), and apply a bulky hand dressing.
- No particular postoperative protection is required.
- Debulking of the opposite side of the digit can be done 3 months after the first procedure.

EPIPHYSIODESIS

TECHNIQUE 17.59

- Under tourniquet control, make a midlateral incision the length of the entire finger.

- Identify the physes of the proximal, middle, and distal phalanges, and perform epiphysiodesis of these with a high-speed burr or curet and cautery.
- Close the incision and apply a finger splint, which is worn for 3 weeks.

DIGITAL SHORTENING

TECHNIQUE 17.60

(BARSKY)
- Under tourniquet control, make an L-shaped incision beginning at the midlateral aspect of the proximal interphalangeal joint and extending distally to a level just proximal to the germinal matrix (Fig. 17.92A).
- Carry the incision transversely across the dorsum of the finger.
- Remove the distal half of the middle phalanx and the proximal part of the distal phalanx.
- Using a rongeur, sharpen the distal end of the remaining middle phalanx to a point to fit into the medullary canal of the distal phalanx (Fig. 17.92B).
- Place the distal phalanx onto the middle phalanx and fix it with a Kirschner wire to recess the finger (Fig. 17.92C).
- Excess volar soft tissue can be removed at a later stage.
- Close the incision and apply a finger splint to be worn for 3 weeks.

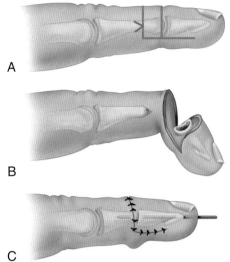

FIGURE 17.92 Digital shortening for macrodactyly (Barsky). **A,** L-shaped midlateral and dorsal incisions allow removal of excess dorsal tissue, distal half of middle phalanx, and proximal portion of distal phalanx *(shaded area).* **B,** Bone ends are prepared for pencil-cone reduction. **C,** Distal phalanx is reduced on middle phalanx and secured with Kirschner wire. **SEE TECHNIQUE 17.60.**

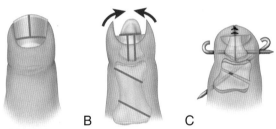

FIGURE 17.93 Thumb reduction for macrodactyly (Millesi). **A,** Removal of distal half of nail and distal phalanx, preserving eponychial tissue. **B,** Reduction osteotomies performed through dorsal incision. **C,** Remaining bone reduced and pinned. **SEE TECHNIQUE 17.61.**

THUMB SHORTENING

TECHNIQUE 17.61

(MILLESI)
- Under tourniquet control, excise the distal half of the nail and nail matrix and the underlying distal phalangeal tuft (Fig. 17.93A).
- Through a dorsal longitudinal incision overlying the proximal and distal phalanx, remove the middle third of the distal phalanx and the middle third of the overlying nail and matrix.
- Remove the middle third of the proximal phalanx by making parallel oblique osteotomies (Fig. 17.93B).

- Reduce the two remaining longitudinal components of the distal phalanx and pin them with a transverse Kirschner wire.
- Reduce the distal and proximal fragments of the proximal phalanx in a shortened fashion and pin them with an oblique Kirschner wire (Fig. 17.93C).
- Close the wound by carefully approximating the skin edges and the nail matrix, leaving the Kirschner wires protruding through the skin.
- Apply a thumb splint.

POSTOPERATIVE CARE The splint is worn for 3 weeks. The Kirschner wires are removed when the osteotomy incisions are healed, usually by 4 to 6 weeks.

REFERENCES

GENERAL
Al-Qattan M, Kozin SH: Update on embryology of the upper limb, *J Hand Surg Am* 38A:1835, 2013.
Bae DS, Canizares MF, Miller PE, et al.: Intraobserver and interobserver reliability of the Oberg-Manske-Tonkin (OMT) classification: establishing a registry on congenital upper limb differences, *J Pediatr Orthop* 38(1):69, 2018.
Gold NB, Westgate M-N, Holmes LB: Anatomic and etiological classification of congenital limb deficiencies, *Am J Med Genet* 155:1225, 2011.
Koskimies E, Lindfors N, Gissler M, et al.: Congenital upper limb deficiencies and associated malformations in Finland: a population based study, *J Hand Surg Am* 36A:1058, 2011.
Oberg KC, Feenstra JM, Manske PR, Tonkin MA: Developmental biology and classification of congenital anomalies of the hand and upper extremity, *J Hand Surg Am* 35A:2066, 2010.

RADIAL LONGITUDINAL DEFICIENCIES
Colen DL, Lin IC, Levin LS, Chang B: Radial longitudinal deficiency: recent developments, controversies, and an evidence-based guide to treatment, *J Hand Surg Am* 42(7):546, 2017.
Kotwal PP, Varshney MK, Soral A: Comparison of surgical treatment and nonoperative management for radial longitudinal deficiency, *J Hand Surg Eur* 37(2):161, 2012.
Manske MC, Wall LB, Steffen JA, Goldfarb CA: The effect of soft tissue distraction on deformity recurrence after centralization for radial longitudinal deficiency, *J Hand Surg Am* 39:895, 2014.
Oishi SN, Carter P, Bidwell T, et al.: Thrombocytopenia absent radius syndrome: presence of brachiocarpalis muscle and its importance, *J Hand Surg Am* 34A:1696, 2009.
Tonkin MA: Classification of congenital anomalies of the hand and upper limb, *J Hand Surg Eur* 42(5):448, 2017.
Vuillermin C, Wall L, Mills J, et al.: Soft tissue release and bilobed flap for severe radial longitudinal deficiency, *J Hand Surg Am* 40(5):894, 2015.
Wall LB, Ezaki M, Oishi SN: Management of congenital radial longitudinal deficiency: controversies and current concepts, *Plast Reconstr Surg* 132:122, 2013.
Yang J, Qin B, Li P, et al.: Vascularized proximal fibular epiphyseal transfer for Bayne and Klug type III radial longitudinal deficiency in children, *Plast Reconstr Surg* 135(1):157e, 2015.

MADELUNG DEFORMITY
Farr S, Kalish LA, Bae DS, Waters PM: Radiographic criteria for undergoing an ulnar shortening osteotomy in Madelung deformity: a long-term experience from a single institution, *J Pediatr Orthop* 36:310, 2016.

Hanson TJ, Murthy NS, Shin AY, et al.: MRI appearance of the anomalous volar radiotriquetral ligament in true Madelung deformity, *Skel Radiol* 48(6):915, 2019.

Steinman S, Oishi S, Mills J, et al.: Volar ligament release and distal radial dome osteotomy for the correction of Madelung deformity: long-term follow-up, *J Bone Joint Surg Am* 95(13):1198, 2013.

HYPOPLASTIC THUMB

De Roode CP, James MA, McCarroll Jr HR: Abductor digit minimi opponensplasty: technique, modifications, and measurement of opposition, *Tech Hand Up Extrem Surg* 14:51, 2010.

Kozin SH: Pollicization: the concept, technical details, and outcome, *Clin Orthop Surg* 4:18, 2012.

Kozin SH, Ezaki M: Flexor digitorum superficialis opponensplasty with ulnar collateral ligament reconstruction for thumb deficiency, *Tech Hand Up Extrem Surg* 14:46, 2010.

Light TR, Gaffey JL: Reconstruction of the hypoplastic thumb, *J Hand Surg Am* 35A:474, 2010.

Soldado F, Zlotolow DA, Kozin SH: Thumb hypoplasia, *J Hand Surg Am* 38A:1435, 2013.

Vekris MD, Beris AE, Lykissas MG, Soucacos PN: Index finger pollicization in the treatment of congenitally deficient thumb, *Ann Plast Surg* 66:137, 2011.

TRIPHALANGEAL THUMB

Wang AA, Hutchinson DT: Results of treatment of delta triphalangeal thumbs by excision of the extra phalanx, *J Pediatr Orthop* 35(5):474, 2015.

ULNAR DIMELIA

Al-Qattan MM, Al-Kahtani AR, Al-Sharif EM, Al-Otaibi NJ: Thumb reconstruction without formal pollicization in mirror hand deformity: a series of four cases, *J Hand Surg Eur* 38:940, 2013.

Takagi T, Seki A, Takayama S: Elbow and forearm reconstruction in patients with ulnar dimelia can improve activities of daily living, *J Shoulder Elbow Surg* 323:e68, 2014.

POSTAXIAL POLYDACTYLY

Abzug JM, Kozin SH: Treatment of postaxial polydactyly type B, *J Hand Surg Am* 38:1223, 2013.

Katz K, Linder N: Postaxial type B polydactyly treated by excision in the neonatal nursery, *J Pediatr Orthop* 31:448, 2011.

Mills JK, Ezaki M, Oishi SN: Ulnar polydactyly: long-term outcomes and cost-effectiveness of surgical clip application in the newborn, *Clin Pediatr (Phila)* 53:470, 2014.

Pritsch T, Ezaki M, Mills J, Oishi SN: Type A ulnar polydactyly of the hand: a classification system and clinical series, *J Hand Surg Am* 38A:453, 2013.

SYNDACTYLY

Hutchinson DT, Frenzen SW: Digital syndactyly release, *Tech Hand Up Extrem Surg* 14:33, 2010.

Jose RM, Timoney N, Vidyadharan R, Lester R: Syndactyly correction: an aesthetic reconstruction, *J Hand Surg Am* 35E:446, 2010.

Lumenta DB, Kitzinger HB, Beck H, Frey M: Long-term outcomes of web creep, scar quality, and function after simple syndactyly surgical treatment, *J Hand Surg Am* 35A:1323, 2010.

Mericli AF, Black JS, Morgan RF: Syndactyly web space reconstruction using the tapered M-to-V flap: a single-surgeon, 30-year experience, *J Hand Surg Am* 40:1755, 2015.

Miyamoto J, Nagasao T, Miyamoto S: Biomechanical analysis of surgical correction of syndactyly, *Plast Reconstr Surg* 125:963, 2010.

Tolerton SK, Tonkin MA: Keloid formation after syndactyly release in patients with associated macrodactyly: management with methotrexate therapy, *J Hand Surg Am* 36E:490, 2011.

Vekris MD, Lykissas MG, Soucacos PN, et al.: Congenital syndactyly: outcome of surgical treatment in 131 webs, *Tech Hand Up Extrem Surg* 14:2, 2010.

CAMPTODACTYLY

Hamilton KL, Netscher DT: Evaluation of a stepwise surgical approach to camptodactyly, *Plast Reconstr Surg* 135:568, 2015.

Rhee SH, Oh WS, Lee HJ, et al.: Effect of passive stretching on simple camptodactyly in children younger than three years of age, *J Hand Surg Am* 35A:1768, 2010.

CLINODACTYLY (DELTA PHALANX)

Bednar MS, Bindra RR, Light TR: Epiphyseal bar resection and fat interposition for clinodactyly, *J Hand Surg Am* 35A:834, 2010.

Gillis JA, Nicoson M, Floccari L, et al.: *Comparison of Vickers' physiolysis with osteotomy for primary correction of clinodactyly*, Hand (N Y), 2019, Epub ahead of print.

Strauss NL, Goldfarb CA: Surgical correction of clinodactyly: two straightforward techniques, *Tech Hand Up Extrem Surg* 14:54, 2010.

SYNPOLYDACTYLY

Aleem AW, Wall LB, Manske MC, et al.: The transverse bone in cleft hand: a case cohort analysis of outcome after surgical reconstruction, *J Hand Surg Am* 39:226, 2014.

Upton J, Taghinia AH: Correction of the typical cleft hand, *J Hand Surg Am* 35A:480, 2010.

Wall LB, Bae DS, Oishi SN, et al.: Synpolydactyly of the hand: a radiographic classification, *J Hand Surg Eur* 41(3):301, 2016.

APERT SYNDROME

Oishi SN, Ezaki M: Reconstruction of the thumb in Apert syndrome, *Tech Hand Up Extrem Surg* 14:100, 2010.

CONGENITAL TRIGGER DIGITS

Han SH, Yoon HK, Shin DE, Song DG: Trigger thumb in children: results of surgical treatment in children above 5 years of age, *J Pediatr Orthop* 30:710, 2010.

Marek DJ, Fitoussi F, Bohn DC, Van Heest AE: Surgical release of the pediatric trigger thumb, *J Hand Surg Am* 36A:647, 2011.

Shiozawa R, Uchiyama S, Sugimoto Y, et al.: Comparison of splinting versus nonsplinting in the treatment of pediatric trigger finger, *J Hand Surg Am* 37:1211, 2012.

MACRODACTYLY

Cerrato F, Eberlin KR, Waters P, et al.: Presentation and treatment of macrodactyly in children, *J Hand Surg Am* 38:2112, 2013.

Donohue KW, Zlotolow DA, Kozin SH: Long-finger pollicization for macrodactyly of the thumb and index finger, *J Pediatr Orthop* 34:e50, 2014.

Gluck JS, Ezaki M: Surgical treatment of macrodactyly, *J Hand Surg Am* 40:1461, 2015.

Hardwicke J, Khan MA, Richards H, et al.: Macrodactyly—options and outcomes, *J Hand Surg Eur* 38:297, 2013.

Kay SP, McCombe DB, Kozin SH: Deformities of the hand and fingers. In Wolfe SW, Hotchkiss RN, Pederson WC, Kozin SH, Cohen MS, editors: Green's Operative Hand Surgery, ed 3, Philadelphia, 2017, Elsevier, pp. 1276.

The complete list of references is available online at ExpertConsult.com.